THE OXFORD HANDBOOK OF

THE AUDITORY BRAINSTEM

THE OXFORD HANDBOOK OF

THE AUDITORY BRAINSTEM

Edited by

KARL KANDLER

OXFORD
UNIVERSITY PRESS

OXFORD
UNIVERSITY PRESS

Oxford University Press is a department of the University of Oxford. It furthers the University's objective of excellence in research, scholarship, and education by publishing worldwide. Oxford is a registered trade mark of Oxford University Press in the UK and certain other countries.

Published in the United States of America by Oxford University Press
198 Madison Avenue, New York, NY 10016, United States of America.

Library of Congress Cataloging-in-Publication Data
Names: Kandler, Karl, editor.
Title: The Oxford handbook of the auditory brainstem / edited by Karl Kandler.
Description: New York, NY : Oxford University Press, [2019] | Includes index.
Identifiers: LCCN 2019005704 | ISBN 9780190849061 (hardcover)
Subjects: LCSH: Auditory pathways—Physiology. | Auditory pathways—Diseases. | Brain stem.
Classification: LCC QP461 .O94 2019 | DDC 612.8/51—dc23
LC record available at https://lccn.loc.gov/2019005704

Oxford Handbooks in Neuroscience

The *Oxford Handbooks in Neuroscience* series features authoritative, critical, and original perspectives on the state of the science, research trends, and future research needs in neuroscience, as well as on the relationship of research to applications in health and disease. Written by noted experts, these published review articles provide a critical survey of the current state of research on a topic, and insightful discussions on the future directions of that research in this fast-moving field. *Oxford Handbooks in Neuroscience* is thus a premier source for sophisticated reviews on cutting-edge topics for experienced and new researchers, educators, leaders, technicians, and students. This series provides the kind of critical and original perspectives that readers need to advance the total scope of issues integral to, and associated with, neuroscience and its many related fields.

Gordon M. Shepherd
Editor in Chief
Oxford Handbooks in Neuroscience

Contents

About the Editor xi
Contributors xiii
Introduction and Overview xvii

1. Wiring the Cochlea for Sound Perception 1
   Brikha R. Shrestha and Lisa V. Goodrich

2. The Diversified Form and Function of Cochlear Afferents 37
   Paul Albert Fuchs

3. Efferent Innervation to the Cochlea 59
   Ana Belén Elgoyhen, Carolina Wedemeyer, and Mariano N. Di Guilmi

4. The Cochlear Nuclei: Synaptic Plasticity in Circuits and Synapses in the Ventral Cochlear Nuclei 95
   Donata Oertel, Xiao-Jie Cao, and Alberto Recio-Spinoso

5. In Vitro Studies of Neuromodulation and Plasticity in the Dorsal Cochlear Nucleus 123
   Laurence O. Trussell

6. Molecular and Structural Changes in the Cochlear Nucleus in Response to Hearing Loss 143
   Maria E. Rubio

7. Age-Related and Noise-Induced Hearing Loss: Central Consequences in the Ventral Cochlear Nucleus 163
   Ruili Xie, Tessa-Jonne F. Ropp, Michael R. Kasten, and Paul B. Manis

8. The Cochlear Nucleus as a Generator of Tinnitus-Related Signals 189
   James A. Kaltenbach and Donald A. Godfrey

9. Multimodal Inputs to the Cochlear Nucleus and Their Role in the Generation of Tinnitus 223
Susan E. Shore and David T. Martel

10. Perinatal Development of the Medial Nucleus of the Trapezoid Body 245
Shobhana Sivaramakrishnan, Ashley Brandebura, Paul Holcomb, Daniel Heller, Douglas Kolson, Dakota Jackson, Peter H. Mathers, and George A. Spirou

11. Extraction of Auditory Information by Modulation of Neuronal Ion Channels 273
Leonard K. Kaczmarek

12. The Medial Superior Olivary Nucleus: Meeting the Need for Speed 301
Benedikt Grothe, Christian Leibold, and Michael Pecka

13. Lateral Superior Olive: Organization, Development, and Plasticity 329
Eckhard Friauf, Elisa G. Krächan, and Nicolas I. C. Müller

14. The Superior Paraolivary Nucleus 395
Anna K. Magnusson and Marcelo Gómez-Álvarez

15. Perineuronal Nets in the Superior Olivary Complex: Development, Function, and Plasticity 421
Markus Morawski and Mandy Sonntag

16. The Nuclei of the Lateral Lemniscus 445
Felix Felmy

17. Axon Trajectories in the Auditory Brainstem 473
Nell Beatty Cant

18. Neuron Types, Intrinsic Circuits, and Plasticity in the Inferior Colliculus 503
Tetsufumi Ito, Munenori Ono, and Douglas L. Oliver

19. Changes in the Inferior Colliculus Associated with Hearing Loss: Noise-Induced Hearing Loss, Age-Related Hearing Loss, Tinnitus and Hyperacusis 527
Alan R. Palmer and Joel I. Berger

20. Unifying the Midbrain: The Commissure of the Inferior Colliculus 549
Adrian Rees and Llwyd D. Orton

21. Neuromodulatory Feedback to the Inferior Colliculus 577
LAURA HURLEY

22. Descending Auditory Pathways and Plasticity 611
BRETT R. SCHOFIELD AND NICHOLE L. BEEBE

23. Aging Processes in the Subcortical Auditory System 639
DONALD M. CASPARY AND DANIEL A. LLANO

24. Glial Cells in the Auditory Brainstem 681
GIEDRE MILINKEVICIUTE AND KARINA S. CRAMER

25. Deviance Detection and Encoding Acoustic Regularity in the Auditory Midbrain 707
MANUEL S. MALMIERCA, GUILLERMO V. CARBAJAL, AND CARLES ESCERA

26. Brainstem Encoding of Speech and Music Sounds in Humans 741
NINA KRAUS AND TRENT NICOL

27. The Auditory Brainstem Implant: Restoration of Speech Understanding from Electric Stimulation of the Human Cochlear Nucleus 759
ROBERT V. SHANNON

Index 771

About the Editor

Karl Kandler is Professor in the Department of Neurobiology at the University of Pittsburgh, with secondary appointments in the departments of Otolaryngology and Bioengineering. He was born in Germany, where he studied Biology at the University of Regensburg and the Eberhard Karls University of Tübingen, from which he graduated in 1993 with a PhD. As a Feodor Lynen Research Fellow of the Alexander von Humboldt-Stiftung he then performed postdoctoral research with Lawrence C. Katz at the Howard Hughes Medical Institute and Duke University studying synaptic circuits and plasticity in the visual cortex and hippocampus. Since 1998, Dr. Kandler has been a faculty member in the School of Medicine at the University of Pittsburgh, investigating the development and plasticity of auditory circuits in the mammalian brain, for which he received a number of prestigious awards, including the Presidential Early Career Award in Science and Engineering (2000). From 2007 to 2017, he established and directed the Auditory Research Group in the Department of Otolaryngology. Dr. Kandler is also a faculty member in the Center for the Neural Basis of Cognition and an adjunct professor in the Department of Biological Sciences at Carnegie Mellon University.

Contributors

Nichole L. Beebe, Northeast Ohio Medical University, USA

Joel I. Berger, University of Nottingham, UK

Ashley Brandebura, West Virginia University, USA

Nell Beatty Cant, Duke University Medical Center, USA

Xiao-Jie Cao, University of Wisconsin-Madison, USA

Guillermo V. Carbajal, University of Salamanca & Salamanca Institute for Biomedical Research, Spain

Donald M. Caspary, Southern Illinois University, USA

Karina S. Cramer, University of California, Irvine, USA

Mariano N. Di Guilmi, National Council of Scientific and Technical Research, Argentina

Ana Belén Elgoyhen, National Council of Scientific and Technical Research & University of Buenos Aires, Argentina

Carles Escera, University of Barcelona, Spain

Felix Felmy, University of Veterinary Medicine Hannover, Germany

Eckhard Friauf, University of Kaiserslautern, Germany

Paul Albert Fuchs, Johns Hopkins University, USA

Donald A. Godfrey, University of Toledo, USA

Marcelo Gómez-Álvarez, Karolinska Institute, Sweden

Lisa V. Goodrich, Harvard Medical School, USA

Benedikt Grothe, Ludwig Maximilian University of Munich, Germany

Daniel Heller, West Virginia University, USA

Paul Holcomb, West Virginia University, USA

Laura Hurley, Indiana University, USA

Tetsufumi Ito, Kanazawa Medical University, Japan

Dakota Jackson, West Virginia University, USA

Leonard K. Kaczmarek, Yale University, USA

James A. Kaltenbach, Cleveland Clinic, USA

Michael R. Kasten, University of North Carolina, USA

Douglas Kolson, West Virginia University, USA

Elisa G. Krächan, University of Kaiserslautern, Germany

Nina Kraus, Northwestern University, USA

Christian Leibold, Ludwig Maximilian University of Munich, Germany

Daniel A. Llano, University of Illinois at Urbana-Champaign, USA

Anna K. Magnusson, Karolinska Institute, Sweden

Manuel S. Malmierca, University of Salamanca, Spain

Paul B. Manis, University of North Carolina, USA

David T. Martel, University of Michigan, USA

Peter H. Mathers, West Virginia University, USA

Giedre Milinkeviciute, University of California, Irvine, USA

Markus Morawski, University of Leipzig, Germany

Nicolas I. C. Müller, University of Kaiserslautern, Germany

Trent Nicol, Northwestern University, USA

Donata Oertel, University of Wisconsin-Madison, USA

Douglas L. Oliver, University of Connecticut, USA

Munenori Ono, Kanazawa Medical University, Japan

Llwyd D. Orton, Manchester Metropolitan University, UK

Alan R. Palmer, University of Nottingham, UK

Michael Pecka, Ludwig Maximilian University of Munich, Germany

Alberto Recio-Spinoso, University of Castilla–La Mancha, Spain

Adrian Rees, Newcastle University, UK

Tessa-Jonne F. Ropp, University of North Carolina, USA

Maria E. Rubio, University of Pittsburgh, USA

Brett R. Schofield, Northeast Ohio Medical University, USA

Robert V. Shannon, University of Southern California, USA

Susan E. Shore, University of Michigan, USA

Brikha R. Shrestha, Harvard Medical School, USA

Shobhana Sivaramakrishnan, West Virginia University, USA

Mandy Sonntag, University of Leipzig, Germany

George A. Spirou, West Virginia University, USA

Laurence O. Trussell, Oregon Health and Science University, USA

Carolina Wedemeyer, National Council of Scientific and Technical Research, Argentina

Ruili Xie, University of Toledo, USA

Introduction and Overview

KARL KANDLER

Overview

Sound is created by vibrations that propagate as pressure waves through a medium. The sense of hearing begins with these small pressure changes being detected as tiny, rapid vibrations of the eardrums. Yet when we think about our sense of hearing, our vibrating eardrums are not what come to mind. We assign sounds to specific objects, animals, or people, and are able to place them at specific locations in space. Hearing plays an important role in creating an internal representation of our environment, which is crucial for guiding our movements and actions. For many animals, including humans, another important function of hearing is to share reproductive or emotional states through vocal communication. Humans in particular use speech, language, and music to communicate abstract ideas and emotions. Transforming the vibrations of two eardrums into a detailed representation of the acoustic environment is a challenging task, even for the brain. This task is made even more challenging by the fact that this transformation has to occur very rapidly and accurately, because the fleeting nature of sound excludes the possibility to 'take a second look' at a sound stimulus.

This book is a collection of chapters, written by leading experts in the field, summarizing our current knowledge of how neuronal circuits in the auditory brainstem extract and encode the fundamental acoustic features of sound. As briefly outlined in this "Introduction and Overview" and in more detail in the respective chapters, the challenges of processing even basic sound features led to the evolution of some extreme neuronal and synaptic specializations and very precisely organized neuronal circuits in the auditory brainstem. These specializations and the need to process sound rapidly and reliably led the long-held assumption that auditory brainstem circuits have to be very stable, showing little, if any of the plasticity that is typically encountered in higher brain areas. However, over the past 10 to 15 years an increasing number of studies have revealed unexpected levels of plasticity in almost all auditory brainstem circuits. The highest level of plasticity has been observed during development, when young circuits exhibit use- and activity-dependent plasticity to increase the precision of synaptic connectivity and to fine-tune the intrinsic membrane properties of neurons. Another significant degree of plasticity occurs after cochlear trauma and partial or complete deafness. Peripheral hearing loss can also trigger maladaptive plasticity, which is thought to generate some forms of central hearing impairments such as tinnitus or hyperacusis. A major goal of this book is to illustrate the many forms of plasticity that have been observed in the healthy and pathological auditory brainstem.

The *Handbook* is aimed at readers who already have a basic background in neuroscience, such as more advanced neuroscience students or postdoctoral fellows, who wish to get an introduction and thorough overview of the current state and challenges of the auditory field, including existing areas of controversy. It also can be a valuable resource for basic and clinical neuroscientists not working in the auditory brainstem who would like to get an update as to the current state of research in the auditory brainstem and on the plasticity mechanisms in lower brain areas. Each chapter is designed to stand on its own, but readers without a strong background in auditory neuroscience or readers who want to gain a more comprehensive picture of the current state of the field will benefit greatly from reading the chapters in sequence. This book does not cover all aspects of research on the auditory brainstem. Rather, the chapters will cover areas that have seen significant progress in the past decade and in which significant advancements have been made in revealing new forms of plasticity and their underlying mechanism.

Before I proceed with providing a brief overview of the auditory brainstem and outlining the sequence and content of chapters, I first want to express my sincere gratitude to all the authors who contributed to make this book happen. This book was only possible thanks to the great effort and time each author dedicated to his or her chapter, along with the generosity, patience, and positive attitude they all showed throughout all stages of editing.

A Brief Introduction to the Auditory Brainstem

Sound-evoked vibrations of the tympanic membrane are conducted to the cochlea by the middle ear bones, which elicit traveling waves that propagate along the cochlear spiral from its base to the apex. These waves deflect the stereocilia bundles of cochlear hair cells, the primary sensory cells in the auditory system, leading to their depolarization. Hair cells are arranged linearly along the cochlear spiral. Each hair cell responds best to a specific sound frequency, which gradually shifts along the length of the cochlea. Hair cells close to the base of the cochlea respond to high sound frequencies while hair cells at the apex of the cochlea respond to low frequencies. Thus, sound frequency is represented systematically along the cochlea, giving rise to a tonotopic organization, which is maintained throughout all auditory areas and represents one of the fundamental organization principles of the auditory system.

Upon depolarization, hair cells release the neurotransmitter glutamate, which excites the postsynaptic dendrites of spiral ganglion neurons and leads to the propagation of action potentials down their axons, which form the auditory nerve, through which all cochlear activity is transmitted on its way to the brain. Most of the spiral ganglion neurons form thick, myelinated axons (type 1 category), which make up 95% of the fibers of the auditory nerve. Type 1 spiral ganglion neurons contact a single hair cell, but each hair cell in turn is contacted by 5 to 10 spiral ganglion neurons, which differ in their physiological properties (see *chapter* 2). The information that is encoded by the activity of the auditory nerve is quite limited. Each auditory nerve fiber essentially only encodes three aspects of a sound stimulus: (1) the start and end (encoded by the rise and fall of firing activity); (2) the loudness (encoded by the firing rate); and (3) the frequency (defined by the location of the presynaptic hair cell along the cochlea). The brain is now challenged to make wise use of this limited information in order to create the rich perception of the acoustic environment that most of us take for granted.

One of the basic strategy by which the mammalian brain successfully solves this problem is the extensive use of parallel processing pathways. Parallel processing of different aspects of sound allows for increased processing speed, ensuring that the auditory system can keep up with the rapid arrival of different acoustic stimuli, and for the optimal extraction and encoding of sound features. Parallel pathways allow the auditory system to take advantage of highly specialized synaptic, neuronal, and circuit properties to optimize the extraction and encoding of one sound feature while ignoring most others, which are processed by another specialized pathway. For example, so-called octopus cells in the cochlear nucleus are morphologically and biophysically optimized to faithfully preserve the onset of a sound stimulus down to the level of microseconds, but the specialization that allow them to do this makes them largely insensitive to the frequency of the sound (chapter 4). Other pathways are specialized for sound localization. Unlike other sensory systems in which the location of a stimulus is reflected by the location of the receptors being activated in the sensory epithelium, in the auditory system the receptor location in the cochlea encodes the frequency of sound, not the location of a sound source in space. Thus, the location of a sound source has to be computed *de novo* in the brain by using specialized circuits. Binaural neurons in these circuits faithfully encode very small interaural sound intensity or time differences, which vary according to the incoming direction of sound (see chapters 13 and 14) but provide a relatively poorly representation of the absolute loudness of the sound. As a consequence of this parallel processing strategy, the brainstem contains a vast network of interconnected auditory nuclei and numerous specialized cell types. In fact, the complexity of brainstem pathways in the auditory system exceeds that found in any other sensor system.

The first part of this book (chapters 1–22) is organized such that it follows the ascending auditory pathway, from the cochlea to the inferior colliculus (Figure I.1). Each of the chapters in this part focuses on the anatomy, connectivity, physiology, function,

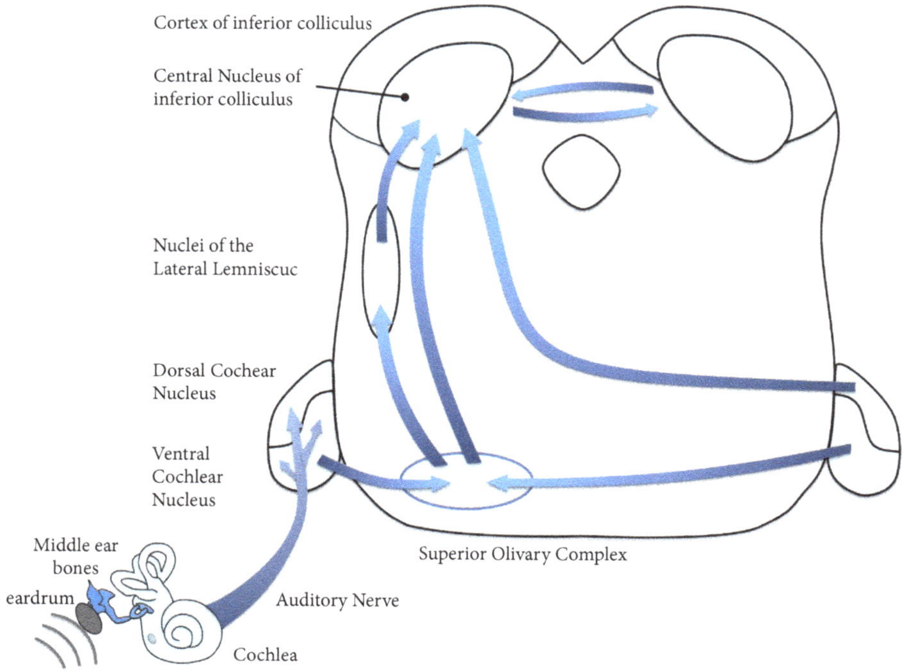

FIGURE I.1. Highly simplified schematic illustration of the mammalian ascending auditory brainstem of mammals, emphasizing the major areas and pathways that are covered in this book. For simplicity, descending and neuromodulatory pathways are not shown here but are described in several chapters of this volume.

and plasticity (normal and pathological) of one particular nucleus. The remaining chapters (chapters 23–27) review aspects of auditory brainstem function or plasticity that are not restricted to a specific area, such as the descending auditory pathways, the role of glial cells, central changes associated with aging, and higher processing functions carried out by the brainstem.

Afferent and Efferent Innervation of the Cochlea

The first three chapters review the afferent and efferent innervation of the cochlea and its development. Chapter 1 by Brikha R. Shrestha and Lisa V. Goodrich summarizes our current understanding of how the cochlea is wired up during development. This chapter begins by illustrating the underlying cellular and molecular mechanisms of the key events involved in the generation and maturation of spiral ganglion neurons. This is followed by a summary of how the peripheral processes from SGNs initially connect to their hair cell partners and how these early connections are subsequently reorganized to correct for any initial errors. Finally, the authors provide an overview of the steps and mechanisms by which the centrally directed axons from SGN connect to the three subdivisions of the cochlear nucleus, the first auditory nucleus in the brainstem.

Parallel ascending auditory pathways begin in the cochlea, where each inner hair cell is innervated by many Type 1 afferent fibers. Type 1 afferent fibers fall into functionally diverse groups, which differ in their spontaneous discharge rates and their sensitivity to sound. In chapter 2, Paul Albert Fuchs summarizes the distinguishing properties of Type 1 afferents and reviews the (still controversial) pre- and postsynaptic mechanisms that give rise to different groups of Type 1 afferents. In addition, he discusses new emerging hypotheses about the function of type 2 afferents, a class of sound-insensitive fibers that contact outer hair cells and whose physiological properties and functional role in hearing has remained enigmatic. Based on recent results, the author proposes a role of Type 2 afferents in signaling the presence of harmful acoustic conditions or in the generation of abnormal gain control after cochlear trauma.

The cochlea not only sends information to the brain but is also directly modulated by the brain via efferent fibers that originate from neurons located in the superior olivary complex in the brainstem. These efferent fibers are part of the lateral or the medial olivocochlear system, depending on their targets in the cochlea and the neuron type from which they originate in the brainstem. In chapter 3, Ana Belén Elgoyhen, Carolina Wedemeyer, and Mariano N. Di Guilmi summarize the differences between these two systems before they go on to review the organization, physiology, and function of the medial olivocochlear system and explain the mechanisms by which cholinergic synapses are used by the medial system to hyperpolarize hair cells. They also summarize the reorganization events that occur during development and the wide-reaching consequences of cholinergic modulation of immature hair cells during the maturation and organization of central pathways.

The Cochlear Nucleus Complex

Upon entering the brain, auditory nerve fibers bifurcate to send collaterals to each of the three subnuclei of the cochlear nucleus complex, the anteroventral cochlear nucleus, the posteroventral cochlear nucleus, and the dorsal cochlear nucleus (Figure I.1). The cochlear nucleus has been investigated extensively and its principle cell types and their responses to sound and biophysical and synaptic properties have been summarized in many excellent reviews and books (listed in chapters 4 and 5). Therefore, the chapters in this book do not focus on these aspects but rather emphasize synaptic and neuronal plasticity in the cochlear nucleus, which is receiving increased attention. This section summarizes how synapses, neurons, and circuits in the cochlear nucleus change with acoustic stimulation, cochlear damage, and aging and will describe how synaptic transmission is influenced by neuromodulatory systems, whose activity levels correlate with different behavioral states.

In chapter 4, Donata Oertel, Xiao-Jie Cao, and Alberto Recio-Spinoso review the forms of short-term plasticity that have been observed at synapses between auditory nerve fibers and neurons in the ventral cochlear nucleus. Although the classic forms of activity-dependent plasticity such as long-term potentiation or long-term depression have never been observed in ventral cochlear nucleus (VCN) neurons, synapses in the VCN exhibit short-term depression when challenged in acute *in vitro* slice preparations. The chapter summarizes current knowledge of this short-term depression and discusses its relationship to sound responses *in vivo* and possible contributions to auditory processing. In contrast to the VCN, where the level of synaptic plasticity is generally weak, perhaps to ensure a stable and reliable processing of acoustic stimuli in this pathway, synapses in the DCN are highly plastic, exhibiting multiple forms of short-term as well as long-term plasticity. In addition, synaptic transmission in the DCN is modulated by a host of neuromodulators, suggesting that processing of auditory information in the DCN is influenced not only by previous acoustic stimulation but also by the animal's internal state.

In chapter 5, Laurence O. Trussell provides a comprehensive summary of the various types of activity-dependent synaptic plasticity in the DCN and their underlying mechanisms, as have been revealed in *in vitro* brain slices preparation. The author also reviews the complex influence of the neuromodulators noradrenalin, dopamine, serotonin, endocanninoids, and zinc on synaptic transmission at DCN synapses and it explores the mutual interactions between neuromodulation and activity-dependent plasticity.

Cochlear hair cells and afferent synapses are sensitive to damage by loud noise, pharmacological drugs, and aging. Cochlear damage not only makes it more difficult to detect sound, but it also frequently triggers the emergence of more complex hearing problems such as understanding speech in noisy environments, the perception of phantom sounds (tinnitus), or even an increased sensitivity to certain sounds (hyperacusis). These secondary hearing impairments arise from changes in central auditory areas, including structural and physiological changes in in the cochlear nucleus, which are summarized and discussed in chapters 6–9. In chapter 6, Maria E. Rubio summarizes the anatomical, structural, and molecular changes that are caused by genetic or acute hearing loss. These changes include both presynaptic and postsynaptic modifications and are influenced by the severity (total or partial), the time course (sudden or slow), and the type (sensorineural or conductive) of hearing loss. These synaptic changes are highly variable, with some occurring surprisingly fast, within hours of hearing loss, while others develop slowly; some changes are temporary, reversing with the restoration of normal hearing, while others are permeant.

These structural changes are accompanied by changes in synaptic transmission and intrinsic neuronal properties, which are summarized in chapter 7 by Ruili Xie, Tessa-Jonne F. Ropp, Michael R. Kasten, and Paul B. Manis. In addition, they discuss how these changes may compensate for decreased auditory nerve activity. As is the case with structural changes, physiologic adaptations vary with the type of hearing loss. While a complete picture has yet to emerge, detailed understanding of how cochlear nucleus circuits change with specific forms of hearing loss will provide important information for predicting how the central auditory system will react when auditory nerve activity is reintroduced, for example by correcting conductive hearing loss or with cochlear implants.

Paradoxically, one of the most consistent changes observed in *in vivo* recordings in the cochlear nucleus after peripheral trauma is an increase in spontaneous spiking activity. This increase in sound-independent activity may be misinterpreted by higher auditory centers as being sound-generated, leading to the hypothesis that this increase in spontaneous spiking activity is, in part, responsible for the perception of phantom sounds (tinnitus). In chapter 8, James A. Kaltenbach and Donald A. Godfrey summarize three decades of research aimed at identifying the changes in the cochlear nucleus circuitry and excitability that may lead to the generation of tinnitus and discuss the major controversies and challenges of this type of research.

Although the auditory nerve provides the majority of synaptic inputs to the cochlear nucleus, the activity of cochlear nucleus neurons is also influenced by other sensory modalities, such as the somatosensory system. In chapter 9, Susan E. Shore and David T. Martel describe how somatosensory inputs to the dorsal cochlear nucleus modulate auditory processing. They discuss how somatosensory inputs engage spike timing-dependent plasticity and how this may contribute to the generation of tinnitus. This chapter also summarizes results from recent studies in animal models showing that bimodal auditory-somatosensory stimulation can induce long-term depression in DCN neurons and that application of similar bimodal sensory stimulation in human tinnitus patients successfully reduces subjective tinnitus loudness and discomfort. These studies provide encouraging examples of how the fundamental biological mechanisms of neuronal plasticity can be harnessed to correct central pathologies in humans that may arise from maladaptive plasticity.

The Nuclei of the Superior Olivary Complex

The major projection target of the VCN is the superior olivary complex (SOC), located ventrally in the brainstem (Figure I.1). The SOC is a collection of nuclei whose size and relative arrangement show considerable variations between species, reflecting adaptations to their particular hearing range and auditory specializations. Approximately 6 to 12 distinct nuclei or cell groups have been identified, depending on the species investigated. SOC neurons are involved in a diverse set of tasks. Cell groups involved in sound localization encode the time or intensity differences of sound signals from the two ears. Other cell groups provide descending inputs to the cochlear nucleus and the cochlea via the olivocochlear fibers (see chapter 3). This book contains six chapters on the SOC. Four chapters focus on the SOC nuclei involved in sound localization: the medial nucleus of the trapezoid body (MNTB), the medial superior olive (MSO), and the lateral superior olive (LSO). One chapter is dedicated to the superior paraolivary nucleus (SPON), a prominent nucleus present in all mammals, including humans, which is hypothesized to be involved in the detection of silent gaps or periodic patterns of sound. The final chapter focuses on the role of the perineuronal nets, a form of extracellular matrix, in SOC function and plasticity. The nuclei in the SOC that contain olivocochlear neurons are discussed in the chapter about the descending auditory system (chapter 22).

Chapters 10 and 11 describe the function, development, and plasticity of the medial nucleus of the trapezoid body (MNTB), a prominent glycinergic nucleus that provides stimulus-locked inhibition to several nuclei in the SOC and beyond. MNTB neurons are unique in that they receive excitatory input from a single giant terminal, the Calyx of Held, which is the largest and fastest synapse in the mammalian brain. The sheer size of the Calyx of Held has allowed researchers to simultaneously record from both the presynaptic Calyx and the postsynaptic MNTB neuron, thus providing detailed insight into the function of individual synapses and making the Calyx of Held one of the best understood synapses in the mammalian brain. In chapter 10, Shobhana Sivaramakrishnan, Ashley Brandebura, Paul Holcomb, Daniel Heller, Douglas Kolson, Dakota Jackson, Peter H. Mathers, and George A. Spirou summarize the development of the MNTB, including the major steps by which the pre- and postsynaptic elements within the MNTB are assembled and the molecular signaling events involved in these processes. They also describe how competition between immature calyces innervating the same postsynaptic MNTB neuron ultimately results in the characteristic single-calyx innervation of mature MNTB neurons.

Despite often being considered a simple relay nucleus, the MNTB continues to exhibit activity-dependent plasticity after development is completed. As described in detail in chapter 11 by Leonard K. Kaczmarek, mature MNTB neurons express experience-dependent plasticity by ways of modulating the expression and function of their voltage-gated potassium channels. MNTB neurons express a large variety of potassium channel subunits whose relative expression levels vary between individual neurons. As a result, different MNTB neurons respond to sound with slightly different delays and temporal accuracy. This cellular diversity is modulated by sound-driven activity and the production of nitro oxide and cyclic GMP, thus creating a means to dynamically adapt the firing patterns of MNTB neurons according to the ongoing acoustic environment.

The MNTB provides synaptic inhibition to two nuclei whose function is to compare the differences in the arrival times and intensity of sound between the ears (interaural time and sound level differences, respectively). These differences vary systematically with the azimuthal direction of the incoming sound and provide highly reliable cues used to compute the location of the sound source in space. Interaural time differences are most useful for lower sound frequencies, which neurons in the sound localization pathway can still phase-lock to. In contrast, interaural sound level differences comprise the major cue for high-frequency sounds, which are more strongly attenuated by the head than low frequency sounds. Thus, animals with low-frequency hearing primarily rely on time difference cues for sound localization, while animals with high-frequency hearing primarily rely on sound level differences, a fact that is also reflected by the size of the respective nuclei.

In chapter 12, Benedikt Grothe, Christian Leibold, and Michael Pecka summarize what is currently known about how MSO neurons encode interaural time differences. The authors illustrate the structural and cellular optimizations that enable these neurons to accomplish the astonishing feat of encoding interaural time differences on a microsecond timescale. Several controversial models have been proposed to describe how these minuscule time differences are represented in the MSO. These models are still highly debated, and chapter 12 will discuss the pros and cons of these models considering recent results from both animal models and human psychophysical studies.

While the MSO encodes interaural time differences, neurons the lateral superior olive (LSO), are specialized for encoding interaural intensity differences. In chapter 13, Eckhard Friauf, Elisa G. Krächan, and Nicolas I. C. Müller take a deep look at both *in vivo* and *in vitro* data from a host of mammalian species to provide a detailed review of our current knowledge of the organization of the LSO across mammalian species, as well as the development of its synaptic inputs and physiological response properties. Studies in the LSO have revealed a number of novel mechanisms involved in the developmental organization of inhibitory circuits and their activity-dependent short-term plasticity, even at later ages. The chapter discusses these phenomena and their mechanisms, and contemplates their implications on the neuronal encoding of interaural intensity differences.

The third major SOC nucleus that derives its inhibition from the MNTB is the SPON. In contrast to the MSO and LSO, which integrate information from both ears, the SPON is a monaural nucleus, receiving excitatory and inhibitory drive only from the contralateral ear. In chapter 14 Anna K. Magnusson and Marcelo Gómez-Álvarez, explain that SPON neurons preferentially fire action potentials after a sound stimulus ends (OFF-response). As described in more detail in the chapter, this OFF-response is made possible by an exquisite combination of strong MNTB-derived inhibition, present during sound presentation, and rapid depolarization when the sound stops, caused by the activation of low-voltage-activated membrane ion channels. The SPON is a prominent nucleus in all mammalian species, including humans, suggesting an important role in hearing; however, this role is still a matter of debate. Magnusson and Gómez-Álvarez discuss some intriguing hypotheses, such as the participation of SPON neurons in the initial processing of prosodic information, that are based on the tuning of SPON neurons to periodic sound stimuli, or rhythm sensitivity, as well as their interesting projection patterns to auditory and non-auditory areas.

The final chapter in the series on the SOC focuses on the role of the extracellular matrix in SOC function and plasticity, an area that has recently received increased attention. In chapter 15, Markus Morawski and Mandy Sonntag describe the distribution of perineuronal nets, a specialized component of the extracellular matrix, in the superior olivary complex. The chapter summarizes the formation and development of perineuronal nets and discusses current ideas on how perineuronal nets regulate synaptic transmission and neuronal excitability, and thus could be closely linked to their plasticity.

The Nuclei of the Lateral Lemniscus

The lateral lemniscus is a thick fiber bundle running dorsoventally on the lateral edge of the brainstem. It contains axons that relay auditory information from the cochlear nucleus and superior olivary complex to the auditory midbrain, the inferior colliculus. Embedded in this fiber bundle are the three nuclei of the lateral lemniscus: ventral, intermediate, and dorsal. Compared to the other areas of the auditory brainstem, many aspects of the nuclei of the lateral lemniscus remain poorly understood. In chapter 16, Felix Felmy summarizes what is currently known about the anatomical connectivity, neuron types, and physiological properties of the neurons in these nuclei and summarizes several recent in vivo studies, which have contributed to current hypotheses on the possible function of these neurons in sound processing.

The Inferior Colliculus

The inferior colliculus (IC), often called the 'auditory hub' of the brainstem, is where the auditory information that has already been processed by lower auditory brainstem nuclei converges for further integration and processing (Figure I.1). Subsequently, this information is transmitted to the auditory thalamus and several non-auditory areas, which include neuromodulator centers, limbic areas, and areas involved in behavioral control. In addition, the IC gives rise to descending projections that modulate the activity of lower brainstem nuclei and it receives descending projections from the auditory cortex (see chapter 23). This book includes five chapters (17–21) that focus on the IC. Certain aspects of IC function are also a major component of subsequent chapters on the descending auditory pathway (chapter 22), aging (chapter 23), and higher-level auditory processing in the brainstem (chapters 25 and 26).

In chapter 17 Nell Beatty Cant describes the trajectories different groups of axons take through the brainstem on their way to the IC and discusses the intrinsic organization of the three main fiber bundles that connect the IC to the rest of the brainstem. This chapter also summarizes the course of fibers that directly connect major auditory nuclei in the brainstem, including the commissural pathways. The chapter provides a comprehensive and unprecedented summary of the organization of the white matter in the auditory brainstem, information that will undoubtedly be valuable for interpreting present and especially future high-resolution imaging studies of the normal and pathological auditory system.

Neurons in the IC are tuned to a large variety of sound stimuli and show a diversity of response patterns, reflecting their different their synaptic inputs, membrane properties, and the influence of the vast intrinsic network in the IC. In chapter 18, Tetsufumi Ito, Munenori Ono, and Douglas L. Oliver give a detailed review on the different neuron classes in the IC based on morphology, neurotransmitter types, synaptic organization, membrane properties, and responses to sound. The authors then cover recent progress in understanding the organization and function of the intrinsic synaptic network in the IC, which has remained enigmatic for a long time. Reflecting its integrative function and performance of higher auditory processing, which often requires adjustments to changing acoustic environments, the IC shows a high degree of plasticity, some forms of which are discussed in this chapter as well. This plasticity is especially pronounced when auditory nerve activity is severely decreased by noise-induced cochlear trauma or by age-related hearing loss. In chapter 19, Alan R. Palmer and Joel I. Berger review and synthesize the large literature describing the many ways in which the IC reacts to hearing loss, including changes in neurotransmitter systems, spontaneous activity, and sound-evoked responses. The authors also summarize previous attempts, using pharmacological approaches as well as acoustic or electrical stimulation, to modulate or reverse pathologic, hearing-loss induced IC activity in animal models.

As described in chapter 20 by Adrian Rees and Llwyd D. Orton, a unique feature of the auditory system is the presence of subcortical commissural connections connecting homologous nuclei on both sides of the brain (see also chapter 17). The most prominent of these commissural connections is the fiber tract that connects the two inferior colliculi. In their chapter, these authors review what type of neurons contribute to this commissure, what targets they project to, and how commissural connections influence sound-evoked responses in the IC. Based on this information, the authors propose a model of how commissural connections in the IC contribute to sound localization by reducing the ambiguities in the encoding of the azimuthal component of incoming sound that are present in the firing rate of neurons in a single IC.

In addition to receiving inputs from ascending and descending auditory pathways, the IC is also the target of several neuromodulatory systems that influence how the IC processes auditory information. As summarized by Laura Hurley in chapter 21, the IC is under the influence of neuromodulatory centers that release acetylcholine, dopamine, noradrenaline, or serotonin. Although these centers are not considered part of the ascending auditory system, neurons in these areas nevertheless can respond to sound and thus can establish auditory-modulatory feedback loops that change the responses of IC neurons according to internal or reproductive state or the saliency of a sound stimulus. This chapter reviews these modulatory influences and their underlying mechanisms, and provides examples as to how and under what conditions modulatory inputs to the IC can change auditory-evoked behaviors.

Descending Auditory Pathways

A characteristic feature of the auditory system is the presence of an extensive top-down modulatory system that arises from multiple stages along the ascending pathway. These descending projections, in turn, influence auditory processing at almost every stage, including the cochlea (see chapter 3). Descending projections are activated under various acoustic stimulation conditions and have been associated with a variety of hearing impairments. In chapter 22, Brett R. Schofield and Nichole L. Beebe summarize the organization and discuss possible functions of the descending auditory system, focusing on pathways that release the neurotransmitters glutamate, GABA, glycine, dopamine, and acetylcholine. Following an overview of the anatomical organization of these systems, the authors highlight research areas that have progressed significantly in recent years, including the influence of corticofugal projections on sound processing and plasticity in the IC as well as the close interactions between modulatory systems and descending pathways. They conclude with a discussion of circuit loops and chains in the descending system, speculate as to whether the ventral nucleus of the trapezoid body (an area in the superior olivary complex) serves as a central hub of the descending system, and identify key questions in the field that remain open.

Age-Related Changes in the Auditory Brainstem and Thalamus

Age-related hearing loss, or presbycusis, is the most common type of sensorineural hearing loss. It is usually a progressive hearing loss that begins with the inability to hear high-frequency sounds and, as aging continues, progresses to include lower frequencies. Although many consider presbycusis a normal part of the aging process, we now know that its progress is greatly accelerated by frequent exposure to even modest noise levels. Presbycusis has become more prevalent and its onset shifted to younger ages in industrialized societies, where ambient or recreational noise levels are on the rise and life expectancy continues to increase. In addition to peripheral hearing loss due to deterioration of the cochlea, age-related hearing loss is accompanied by changes in the central auditory system that arise independently from peripheral damage with age. These central changes are thought to contribute to subtler hearing impairments, for example difficulty understanding speech in noisy environments. In chapter 23, Donald M. Caspary and Daniel A. Llano review age-related changes in neurotransmission that have been observed in the auditory brainstem and thalamus and try to untangle what aspects of these changes are a consequence of decreased peripheral input and what aspects are due to the aging. They also discuss how these synaptic changes contribute to decreased precision in the temporal processing of sound, one of the hallmarks of central presbycusis.

Glial Cells in the Auditory Brainstem

Most neuroscience research, including that on the auditory brainstem, has largely ignored the contribution of glial cells, which make up about 90% of brain cells. In recent years, however, there has been increasing interest in how glial cells participate in the development and function of auditory brainstem neurons and their synaptic connections. In chapter 24, Giedre Milinkeviciute and Karina S. Cramer provide a comprehensive review of the role the three major types of glial cells in the brain (astrocytes, micoglia, and oligodendrocytes) have in auditory brainstem development, function, and injury. Our current understanding of the developmental role of glial cells stems primarily from experiments in the chick brainstem. Studies in this system revealed a critical role of astrocyte-secreted factors in the maturation of inhibitory inputs. In addition, astrocytes seem to play a role in regulating dendritic arborization and axonal targeting. In the primary sound localization nuclei of both chicks and mammals, oligodendrocytes contribute to the fine-adjustment of the conduction velocity of axons, which is critical for regulating the exact arrival time of synaptic inputs to binaural coincidence detector neurons. Finally, the chapter reviews how microglial cells react to cochlear trauma or ablation and act as phagocytic scavengers to remove inactive inputs and play a supportive role in the formation of new, compensatory synaptic connections.

Higher Auditory Functions in the Brainstem

While the faithful encoding of fundamental sound features is undoubtedly the major task of the auditory brainstem, research over the past two decades has provided increasing evidence that subcortical auditory areas also perform surprisingly complex functions that were previously attributed to cortical circuits. Two chapters in this book provide examples of such higher functions performed in the IC. In chapter 25, Manuel S. Malmierca, Guillermo V. Carbajal, and Carles Escera summarize experimental results that link stimulus-specific adaptation (SSA) exhibited by neurons in the non-lemniscal divisions of the IC (cortical regions) to true deviance detection. More than simply adapting to a repeated (predictable) stimulus, these neurons enhance their responses when a novel (unexpected) stimulus occurs, thus acting as deviance detectors. The authors discuss the circuit and neuronal mechanisms by which SSA emerges in the IC, taking into consideration and evaluating results from anatomical, cortical reversible inactivation, and pharmacological studies *in vivo*. They propose that SSA is a neuronal correlate of mismatch negativity, a component of the auditory event-related potential recorded in humans that appears when subjects perceive a change in stimulation. They also discuss SSA in the conceptual framework of predictive coding theory.

In humans, activity in the IC can be recorded non-invasively using scalp electrodes that record the synchronous, sound-evoked activity of populations of auditory neurons. One component of these auditory brainstem responses is the frequency following response (FFR), which reflects the highly temporally precise, phase-locked response of the IC to periodic stimuli. In chapter 26, Nina Kraus and Trent Nicol review studies that use the FFR to investigate representations of speech and music processing in the human IC. The authors give a short tutorial of FFR by describing the general characteristic of FFR and what components of speech are reflected by it. They describe evidence that the encoding of various components of speech is altered by traumatic brain injury and in poor readers, such as those with dyslexia, and is conversely enhanced in subjects who have undergone auditory enrichment or training. Because the FFR to speech and other complex stimuli is closely connected to the listener's level of literacy and ability to listen in noise, the authors argue for increased clinical use of brainstem FFR to objectively assess a listener's ability to encode fast speech signals.

Auditory Brainstem Prosthesis

The cochlear implant is the most successful neuronal prosthesis, providing hearing to hundreds of thousands of otherwise deaf people. Cochlear implants bypass a dysfunctional cochlea by electrically stimulating the spiral ganglion neurons, or their axons, directly; thus their success depends on the presence of a functional auditory nerve. Because patients without an auditory nerve cannot benefit from a cochlear implant, scientists and surgeons have attempted to reestablish hearing in these patients through electrical stimulation of other central auditory structures, such as the cochlear nucleus and inferior colliculus. In chapter 27, Robert V. Shannon reviews the current state of the auditory brainstem implant, which stimulates the cochlear nucleus. After giving an overview of the surgical approach and of the type of hearing experienced by implant users, he discusses possible reasons for the variability in performance observed between patients. Based on data obtained from human and animal studies, he proposes the intriguing hypothesis that the degree of speech perception attained after an auditory brainstem implant critically depends on the surgical preservation of the small cell cap region. This region is especially well developed in humans, compared to other mammals, and is likely to play a critical role in encoding amplitude modulations of sound, a critical cue for speech recognition.

Acknowledgments

My foremost gratitude goes to the authors who contributed to this book by generously sharing their scholarly insight and valuable time. I also want to thank my colleges and laboratory members for many insightful and stimulating discussions, and their patience while my mind was occupied by this book. A special thanks is extended to Ada Brunstein from Oxford University Press for her skillful guidance and encouraging humor throughout the process.

CHAPTER 1

WIRING THE COCHLEA FOR SOUND PERCEPTION

BRIKHA R. SHRESTHA AND LISA V. GOODRICH

Abstract

Sound information enters the auditory brainstem via spiral ganglion neurons (SGNs), which reliably encode and transmit information received from sensory hair cells in the cochlea. SGNs form both a structural and a functional bridge between the cochlea and the auditory brainstem beginning early in development, with long-term consequences for the maturation of central auditory circuits. This chapter summarizes the key events in SGN development, from their origin in the early otic vesicle and the emergence of the basic wiring pattern of the cochlea to the elaboration of specialized synapses and the acquisition of diverse firing properties that enable sound perception even within noisy environments. Key cellular events and molecular players are introduced, with emphasis on the impact of reciprocal interactions between the cochlea and the auditory brainstem throughout development.

Keywords: spiral ganglion neuron, otic vesicle, ribbon synapse, endbulb of Held, tonotopy, spontaneous activity, inner ear development

Spiral ganglion neurons (SGNs) provide the primary conduit for sound information to enter the brainstem from the cochlea, allowing the brain to calculate what was heard and where it is located based on the spatiotemporal pattern of SGN activation. To fulfill this role, SGNs must develop several specialized properties that distinguish them from other primary sensory neurons. This includes formation of tonotopically organized connections in the cochlea and in the cochlear nucleus complex, elaboration of synapses that transmit with high fidelity, and acquisition of distinct firing properties that enable signaling across a wide dynamic range. Given their crucial position as the gateway between the periphery and the central nervous system (CNS), changes in the number, organization, or function of SGNs can have permanent consequences for how auditory information is subsequently represented in the brainstem and along the neuraxis.

Efforts to understand how SGNs develop have established the basic sequence of events and begun to unravel the genetic networks that guide their specification and wiring.

Overview of SGN Development

SGNs develop from a pool of neurosensory progenitors that is progressively subdivided to generate all of the hair cells and neurons in the auditory and vestibular systems (Goodrich, 2016). In birds and rodents, neurosensory progenitors arise in the anteroventral quadrant of the otic cup (Adam et al., 1998; Cole et al., 2000; Morsli, Choo, Ryan, Johnson, & Wu, 1998), which is the embryonic anlage of the inner ear. As development proceeds, the otic cup invaginates and detaches from the hindbrain to form the otic vesicle (Anniko & Wikström, 1984; Hemond & Morest, 1991). Around the same time, neuroblasts begin to delaminate from the pro-neurosensory domain (PNSD) into the mesenchyme, where they aggregate to form a common cochlear-vestibular ganglion (CVG). The CVG is initially attached to the geniculate ganglion, which forms the seventh cranial nerve. In mice, the auditory and vestibular divisions gradually separate from each other (Carney & Silver, 1983; Sher, 1971), and the spiral ganglion grows and extends, due both to ongoing proliferation among the delaminated neuroblasts (Matei et al., 2005; Ruben, 1967) and convergent movements that lengthen the cochlea (J. Wang et al., 2005). Vestibular ganglion neuron (VGN) precursors exit the cell cycle first, followed shortly by an overlapping production of SGN precursors that differentiate along a gradient starting in the base of the cochlea and spiraling toward the apex (Ruben, 1967).

The earliest indication of SGN differentiation is the extension of peripheral and central processes, which eventually form topographically organized synapses in the cochlea and cochlear nucleus complex (CNC), respectively. Activity initiates in the embryonic cochlea and is propagated all the way along the auditory axis during postnatal stages, thus probably influencing the final maturation of auditory circuitry both in the cochlea and in the brainstem (H. C. Wang & Bergles, 2015). Indeed, removal of the cochlea during development has severe consequences for development of the CNC (Harris & Rubel, 2006). SGN development follows a similar progression across species, including humans (Bibas et al., 2006; Streeter, 1906), although the timing can differ. Much of our understanding derives from analysis of mice and other rodents, with additional important insights from chickens, which are more amenable to embryological manipulations.

Development of SGNs in the periphery overlaps temporally with development of olivocochlear neurons (OCNs) in the CNS. OCNs are a specialized population of efferent neurons that reside in the brainstem and provide reciprocal input to the cochlea (Bruce, Kingsley, Nichols, & Fritzsch, 1997; Fritzsch & Elliott, 2017). They comprise two broad subtypes: the lateral and medial olivocochlear neurons (LOCs and MOCs, respectively). LOCs are situated in the lateral superior olive (LSO) and extend largely ipsilateral projections that terminate close to the endings of Type I SGNs underneath the inner hair cells (IHCs). MOCs are located in the ventral nucleus of the trapezoid body (VNTB) and extend both ipsilateral and contralateral projections that directly innervate the outer hair cells (OHCs). Collectively, the olivocochlear efferent system may contribute to binaural processing and also protects the inner ear from noise damage (Darrow, Maison, & Liberman, 2006, 2007; Kujawa & Liberman, 1997). OCN axons arrive in the cochlea during embryonic stages and are closely associated with SGN axons as they innervate their peripheral targets. Hence, SGN development is temporally and spatially coordinated with similar developmental events in the brainstem.

Production of SGNs

As in other regions of the nervous system, SGNs are specified by the sequential action of familiar signaling pathways and networks of transcription factors. In mice, these events start around embryonic day 9 (E9), with an obvious CVG present rostral to the otocyst by E10.5 (Anniko & Wikström, 1984; Carney & Silver, 1983; Sher, 1971). VGNs are born around E8, followed by the SGNs from E9.5 until E13.5 (Matei et al., 2005; Ruben, 1967); staging in rats is similar but shifted by a day. Analogous events occur in fish (Haddon & Lewis, 1996; Riley, 2003) and chickens (Hemond & Morest, 1991). In all species examined, the first step is to set aside the PNSD, which occurs as part of the basic patterning of the early otic cup by signals from surrounding tissues, including the brainstem, notochord, mesenchyme, and overlying ectoderm (Bok, 2005; Bok et al., 2007; A. S. Brown & Epstein, 2011; Liang, Bok, & Wu, 2010; Riccomagno, Takada, & Epstein, 2005).

Within the PNSD, neuronal precursors are selected among a mixed pool that contains progenitors for both neurons and sensory cells, namely the hair cells (HCs) and support cells of the organ of Corti (Raft et al., 2007; Sapède, Dyballa, & Pujades, 2012; Satoh & Fekete, 2005). The decision to follow the neuronal fate depends on Notch pathway activity, which probably biases the outcome of cross-repressive interactions between the pro-neural Neurog1 transcription factor and the pro-sensory Atoh1 transcription factor (Bermingham et al., 1999; Kiernan, 2013; Ma, Anderson, & Fritzsch, 2000; Ma, Chen, del Barco Barrantes, de la Pompa, & Anderson, 1998). A complex and dynamic network of transcription factors, including Neurog1, Six1, Eya1, and Sox2, cooperate to induce neuronal fate and usher inner ear neuroblasts toward maturity (Evsen, Sugahara, Uchikawa, Kondoh, & Wu, 2013; Jahan, Pan, Elliott, & Fritzsch, 2015; E. Y. M. Wong, Ahmed, & Xu, 2013). Layered on top of this generic neurogenic network are additional transcription factors that determine which neuroblasts will populate the spiral versus the vestibular ganglion. This decision occurs early, prior to delamination (Bell et al., 2008; Koundakjian, Appler, & Goodrich, 2007; Sher, 1971). A major determinant of the auditory-vestibular fate decision is the transcription factor Lmx1a, which divides the PNSD into an $Lmx1^-$ vestibular division and an $Lmx1a^+$ auditory division, where it inhibits the vestibular fate in nascent auditory neuroblasts (Koo et al., 2009; Nichols et al., 2008). SGNs are further subdivided into Type I and Type II subtypes, but no transcription factors have been directly implicated in this fate decision.

One of the key regulators of SGN development is the transcription factor Gata3. *Gata3* is expressed from the earliest stages of inner ear development, initially throughout the otic placode (Lawoko-Kerali, Rivolta, & Holley, 2002; Lilleväli et al., 2006). Over time, expression becomes more limited to SGNs (Karis et al., 2001; Lawoko-Kerali et al., 2002; Lilleväli, Matilainen, Karis, & Salminen, 2004; Rivolta & Holley, 1998), although a few VGNs retain expression of *Gata3* as well (Lu, Appler, Houseman, & Goodrich, 2011). Expression is maintained postnatally and into adulthood (Appler et al., 2013; Lu et al., 2011; Nishimura, Noda, & Dabdoub, 2017), raising the possibility that *Gata3* influences multiple stages of SGN development and function. In support of this idea, different phenotypes were observed when *Gata3* was removed from the entire otic vesicle or only from post-delaminated neuroblasts in mice. In *Gata3* null mutants or after early conditional deletion, SGNs were absent altogether, but the VGN persisted (Duncan & Fritzsch, 2013; Duncan, Lim, Engel, & Fritzsch, 2011; Karis et al., 2001). After slightly later conditional deletions, SGNs were specified and delaminated, but were fewer in number (Duncan & Fritzsch, 2013). The mutant SGNs did not differentiate properly and underwent massive cell death beginning around E12.5 (Duncan & Fritzsch, 2013; Luo et al., 2013). Deletion using a neuronal-specific Cre driver circumvented these early phenotypes and revealed further roles for *Gata3* in SGN differentiation (Appler et al., 2013), probably acting upstream of additional transcriptional effectors (Appler et al., 2013; Yu et al., 2013). For instance, upon later deletion, *Gata3* mutant SGNs were present but differentiated prematurely and failed to form orderly radial bundles, although the peripheral axons still reached the organ of Corti. Subsequently, the mutant SGNs were lost, echoing the survival phenotypes observed after early deletion of *Gata3*. Thus, *Gata3* is not only an early indicator of the SGN fate but also a major player in both the execution of this fate and subsequent survival.

Outgrowth and Targeting of SGN Peripheral Processes

In the cochlea, SGN peripheral processes are organized in a stereotypic manner that reflects the basic map of auditory information. Fibers are arranged within radial bundles that project like spokes of a wheel from the "modiolus" of the cochlea out toward the organ of Corti, responding to low sound frequencies in the apex and to high frequencies in the base. Type I SGN processes densely innervate the IHC region, with one neuron contacting one IHC (Figure 1.1). Type II SGNs instead turn toward the base and grow along rows of OHCs, forming synaptic contacts with multiple OHCs. In mice, the emergence of this striking pattern begins around E11.5, when SGNs first extend peripheral processes through the periotic mesenchyme and back toward the developing cochlear

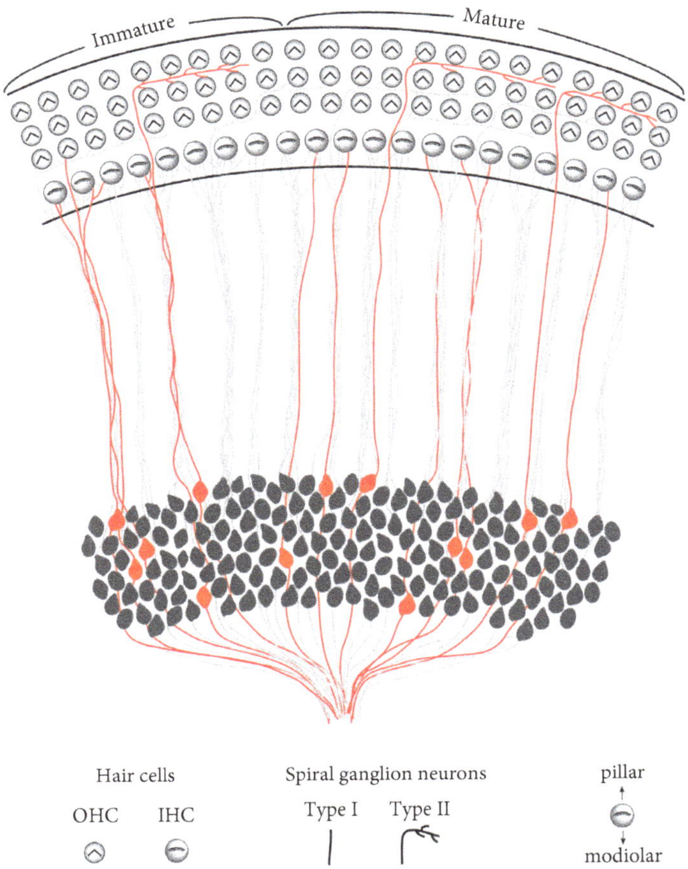

FIGURE 1.1. **Innervation of hair cells by spiral ganglion neurons during development and in maturity.** In the immature cochlea, Type I spiral ganglion neurons (SGNs) project radially toward the cochlear epithelium. Most contact inner hair cells (IHCs), but some branches overshoot and enter the outer hair cell (OHC) region. During development, each Type I SGN terminal may contact multiple IHCs and/or form many contacts with a single IHC. At mature stages, all Type I SGNs exclusively innervate IHCs, with each neuron connected to one IHC. Type II SGNs grow past the IHCs and spiral toward the base, forming *en passant* synapses with OHCs along the way.

duct, arriving in the prosensory domain in the base of the cochlea around E14.5 (Carney & Silver, 1983; Koundakjian et al., 2007; Sandell, Butler Tjaden, Barlow, & Trainor, 2014). Differentiation progresses from the base to the apex, following the gradient of cell cycle exit. By E15.5, SGN peripheral processes lie in nascent radial bundles that line up beneath the IHCs along the length of the cochlea (Coate et al., 2012; Koundakjian et al., 2007).

Little is known about the cues that elicit peripheral process outgrowth during the early stages of cochlear wiring. Outgrowth does not require the presence of HCs (Elliott, Kersigo, Pan, Jahan, & Fritzsch, 2017; Fritzsch et al., 2005), indicating that a classic target-derived mechanism is unlikely to be at work. Instead, SGN peripheral processes may be steered locally by surrounding non-neuronal cells. During the earliest stages of axon outgrowth, young SGNs are surrounded by a "funnel" of mesoderm and glia (Carney & Silver, 1983). Moreover, the SGN peripheral processes are systematically interdigitated with neural crest-derived glia that could form a permissive corridor for outgrowth (Sandell et al., 2014), as occurs in other regions of the nervous system (Freter, Fleenor, Freter, Liu, & Begbie, 2013). Indeed, SGN neurites grow robustly along Schwann cells in vitro (Jeon, Xu, Xu, & Hansen, 2011; Whitlon, Tieu, Grover, Reilly, & Coulson, 2009). More strikingly, SGNs are misplaced and fail to form orderly radial bundles in mice with abnormal glial invasion (Mao, Reiprich, Wegner, & Fritzsch, 2014; Morris et al., 2006). Bundle formation also depends on Ephrin/Eph dependent interactions between SGNs and the surrounding mesenchymal cells (Coate et al., 2012). Neurotrophins are likely to contribute to these early stages (Yang, Kersigo, Jahan, Pan, & Fritzsch, 2011), but it can be difficult to distinguish effects on outgrowth from those on survival, since the final phenotype is reduced innervation in both cases. Overall, although many guidance cues are expressed in the developing inner ear and able to influence neurite outgrowth in vitro, specific roles remain to be defined in vivo (Bank et al., 2013; Battisti, Fantetti, Moyers, & Fekete, 2014; Battisti & Fekete, 2008; Bianchi & Gale, 1998; Bianchi & Gray, 2002; Fantetti & Fekete, 2012; Fekete & Campero, 2007).

During the next stage of cochlear wiring, SGN peripheral processes target appropriate synaptic partners: the IHCs for Type I SGNs and the OHCs for Type II SGNs. In both cases, synaptic communication occurs through glutamate-induced activation of AMPA receptors (AMPARs) in SGNs. In the absence of early molecular markers, studies have relied on morphological distinctions, namely radial versus spiraling fibers, to identify these two subtypes. Based on this criterion, the gross afferent innervation pattern at E16.5 already bears strong resemblance to that seen at maturity in mice, with most SGN processes innervating IHCs and a minority projecting to OHCs (Coate, Spita, Zhang, Isgrig, & Kelley, 2015; Koundakjian et al., 2007). That these patterns are seen before HCs are fully differentiated suggests that the Type I and II identities are established independent of interactions with their peripheral synaptic targets. Acquisition of SGN identities might be under the control of familiar transcriptional networks, as mature Type II SGNs express higher levels of nuclear-localized Gata3 and Mafb, complementing Prox1 expression in mature Type I SGNs (Nishimura et al., 2017). Enrichment of *Gata3* in a subset of SGNs was detected as early as E17.5 in mice, suggesting that the Type I/II decision must occur then or earlier. Type I and Type II SGNs can eventually be identified by differential expression of *EphA4* in Type I SGNs (Defourny et al., 2013) and Peripherin and Tyrosine hydroxylase in Type II SGNs (Hafidi, 1998; Hafidi, Després, & Romand, 1993; Vyas, Wu, Zimmerman, Fuchs, & Glowatzki, 2017), thus underscoring the likelihood that transcription factors such as Gata3, Mafb, and Prox1 may directly control aspects of Type I/II identity.

Segregation of Type I and II afferents to distinct domains of the sensory epithelium is mediated by repulsive interactions that keep Type I fibers away from the OHC zone while permitting entry of Type II fibers (Druckenbrod & Goodrich, 2015). Such interactions are mediated in part by two molecular pathways. On the one hand, Ephrin A5 in the OHC zone repels Type I fibers, all of which express the receptor Epha4 (Defourny et al., 2013). On the other, the secreted chemorepellant Sema3a is expressed in the OHC zone and repels Type I SGNs, which express the cognate Neuropilin receptor Nrp2. How Type II SGNs, which also express *Nrp2*, manage to grow into the Sema3a zone remains unclear, but it may involve a co-receptor (Coate et al., 2015). Disruption of either cue results in increased invasion of the OHC area by Type I fibers. However, most Type I SGNs are still confined to the IHC zone in single mutants, suggesting that multiple mechanisms underlie selective targeting of SGN afferents. Indeed, EphB receptor signaling is required to keep SGN processes from growing even further, past the OHC region, probably via an EphrinB1 ligand (Zhou, Lee, Henkemeyer, & Lee, 2011). Studies so far have not identified the attractive guidance cues that may direct Type II axons to turn toward the base.

Like other nascent neural circuits, target innervation by SGN afferents is initially imprecise, with a fraction of Type I afferents invading the OHC area during late embryonic and early postnatal stages (Figure 1.1). Why ectopic branches are present and how this relates to synapse formation is not fully understood. Classic studies of Golgi-stained processes in the apex of the cochlea suggested that individual fibers branch exuberantly and contact both IHCs and OHCs, followed by a period of refinement (Echteler, 1992; D. D. Simmons, 1994). Likewise, putative Type I fibers, identified based on selective dye uptake, were observed among rows of OHCs (L.-C. Huang, Thorne, Housley, & Montgomery, 2007). Consistent with this interpretation, the putative Type I fibers found near OHCs during early postnatal stages exhibit synaptic AMPAR profiles that match those found at Type I-IHC synapses in mature animals (L.-C. Huang et al., 2012). However, live-imaging of SGNs ex vivo revealed that excess branches from Type I fibers are not positioned to form synapses with the OHCs, arguing against the notion that the IHC-like synapses on OHCs are made by Type I fibers that overextend into the OHC zone (Druckenbrod & Goodrich, 2015). In addition, both AMPAR-mediated current (by pharmacology) and the GluA2 AMPAR subunit (by immunohistochemistry) can be detected at OHC-Type II synapses (Martinez-Monedero et al., 2016), raising questions as to whether GluA2-containing OHC synapses observed at early postnatal stages (P0-P6) are formed by Type II or Type I fibers.

Nevertheless, there is broad agreement that Type I fibers that invade the OHC area undergo retraction, resulting ultimately in subtype-specific confinement to distinct spatial domains of the sensory epithelium. Reconstruction of individual radial and spiral fibers during postnatal stages confirmed a period of extensive branching followed by pruning, but these events appear to be confined to putative Type I SGNs (Druckenbrod & Goodrich, 2015). Among Type I fibers that terminate in the IHC zone, most are branched and innervate multiple IHCs or establish multiple contacts with the same IHC at neonatal stages, as well as extending rare branches to contact pillar cells and the first row of OHCs. All but one of these processes are pruned, resulting in strict mono-innervation of IHC by each SGN. Factors regulating this pruning process are currently unknown. Importantly, Type I SGNs seem to be able to form synapses with OHCs if given the opportunity, as occurs in *EphA4* mutant mice (Defourny et al., 2013). Thus, cochlear wiring specificity may arise through guidance mechanisms rather than being dictated by a molecular recognition code, as occurs in other sensory systems such as the retina (Sanes & Yamagata, 2009).

Formation of Peripheral Synapses

Faithful encoding of acoustic information necessitates high fidelity of synaptic transfer at the IHC-SGN synapse. Reliable signal transmission is achieved in part via specializations such as the presynaptic ribbon, an electron-dense structure consisting of glutamate-filled vesicles arranged in a ring-like pattern and anchored at the active zone. Each ribbon is apposed by an SGN terminal ending, which forms a large post-synaptic density rich with AMPARs (Yu & Goodrich, 2014). The formation and maturation of synaptic connections in the cochlea occur over a prolonged period, starting at neonatal stages and lasting until about the fourth postnatal week in mice (Figure 1.2). The earliest events seem to initiate independently in HCs and SGNs. Subsequently, interactions between pre- and post-synaptic partners promote localization and maturation of the synapses, as well as the final synapse count. In the mature cochlea, the sizes of individual synapses on the modiolar and pillar sides of the IHC differ such that SGNs with different physiological properties receive acoustic information through morphologically distinct synaptic connections.

The onset of synapse development begins with the production of necessary presynaptic components in the IHCs, which produce immature ribbons even in the absence of SGN innervation (Sobkowicz, Rose, Scott, & Levenick, 1986). These events happen quite early, probably during late embryogenesis in rodents (Lenoir, Shnerson, & Pujol, 1980; Shnerson, Devigne, & Pujol, 1981). Synapse development is similar in OHCs, but slightly delayed (Sobkowicz et al., 1986). The ribbons are initially dispersed in the cytoplasm and become gradually localized to the basal pole of the IHC (Sendin, Bulankina, Riedel, & Moser, 2007; Shnerson et al., 1981; Sobkowicz et al., 1986), where they are anchored to the membrane by the scaffolding protein Bassoon (Jing et al., 2013), probably via interactions with the ribbon protein RIBEYE (Dieck et al., 2005). IHCs are capable of evoked exocytosis by late embryogenesis (Beutner & Moser, 2001; Johnson, Marcotti, & Kros, 2005). On the post-synaptic side, AMPARs are detectable in SGN endings at birth and then increase in expression during the first postnatal week (L.-C. Huang et al., 2012). Postsynaptic differentiation also lags behind morphologically, as a well-defined electron-dense PSD appears after the ribbons have already begun to be anchored to the active zone (Sobkowicz et al., 1986). Development of the PSD depends on the transcription factor Mafb, which is expressed in SGNs (but not in VGNs) beginning around E16.5 in mice (Yu et al., 2013). In *Mafb* mouse mutants, SGN peripheral processes reach the IHCs, but do not develop normal PSDs, evidenced by morphological changes and loss of glutamate receptor (GluR) immunoreactivity. Formation of contacts between IHCs

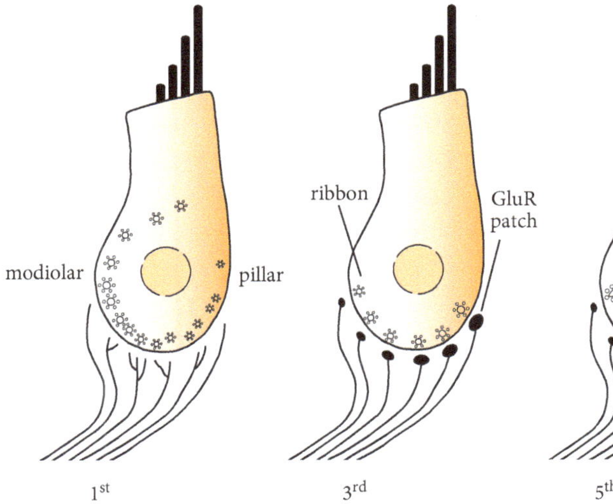

FIGURE 1.2. **Development of IHC-SGN synapses.** During early postnatal life in rodents, immature synaptic ribbons are scattered in the IHC cytoplasm, localizing gradually to the basal pole. A modiolar-pillar gradient of ribbon size is already apparent during the first week of life. This gradient is lost during the third postnatal week, and then reappears at the beginning of the fifth postnatal week. The inverse pillar-to-modiolar gradient of glutamate receptor (GluR) patch is visible by P10 and maintained into adulthood. Although Type I SGN terminals form contacts with IHCs as early as birth, one-to-one pairing of presynaptic ribbons and postsynaptic boutons is not fully established until the third postnatal week.

and SGNs may also involve the Ig superfamily protein Neuroplastin, which is localized to the base of maturing IHCs and is required for cochlear synaptogenesis and hearing in mice (Carrott et al., 2016).

Over the first postnatal week, the pattern of synaptic connectivity changes significantly, both in terms of the morphology and number of IHC-SGN contacts. Immature synapses feature multiple ribbons and diffuse GluR patches, whereas each mature synapse contains a single elongated ribbon at the active zone apposed to an electron-dense PSD with a well-defined GluR patch (Figure 1.2; Sendin et al., 2007; Sobkowicz et al., 1986; A. B. Wong et al., 2013). Even at these early stages, HCs can signal to the SGNs (Beutner and Moser, 2001; Johnson et al., 2005; Tritsch et al., 2010), indicating that these synapses are functional. However, exocytosis is inefficient initially, probably reflecting the relative immaturity of the Ca^{2+} signaling system in the IHCs (Beutner & Moser, 2001; Johnson et al., 2005). During maturation, the number of ribbons per hair cell decreases (L.-C. Huang et al., 2012; Nemzou, Bulankina, Khimich, Giese, & Moser, 2006; Sendin et al., 2007; Sobkowicz, Rose, Scott, & Slapnick, 1982; Sobkowicz et al., 1986), with a corresponding increase in association between presynaptic ribbons and postsynaptic GluR patches, which is seen robustly starting around P10 in mice (L. D. Liberman & Liberman, 2016). At the same time, the ribbons fuse with each other and assume a more elongated morphology (Sendin et al., 2007; Sobkowicz et al., 1982). In addition, the overall number of synapses (i.e., ribbons co-localized with GluR patches) decreases by about 50% through development (L.-C. Huang et al., 2012; Nemzou et al., 2006; Sendin et al., 2007; Sobkowicz et al., 1982, 1986). These changes are particularly evident in the OHC region, with most mature OHCs retaining only one to three ribbons. Thus, the overall ribbon number can be influenced by differences in the initial formation of synapses, pruning of excess synapses, or loss of Type II SGNs during a wave of cell death postnatally (Barclay, Ryan, & Housley, 2011).

Not surprisingly, the formation of properly aligned and functional synaptic contacts involves coordination between HCs and SGNs (Sheets et al., 2011; Sobkowicz et al., 1986). For instance, disruption of post-synaptic differentiation upon loss of *MafB* from SGNs also results in dysmorphic presynaptic ribbons in mouse HCs (Yu et al., 2013). More broadly, the overall number of synapses decreases and the number of orphan ribbons is increased at P12. Conversely, premature overexpression of *Mafb* accelerated the localization of presynaptic ribbons to the basal pole of the IHCs. This *Mafb*-dependent coordination of IHC-SGN synapse development appears to proceed as part of a broader SGN-specific differentiation program orchestrated by the master regulator Gata3.

Following the formation of functional synaptic contacts, the cochlea undergoes an additional phase of maturation during which pre- and postsynaptic structures exhibit dynamic changes before acquiring heterogeneous morphologies that reflect Type I SGN identities. Type I SGNs in mammals are classified as low-SR, medium-SR, and high-SR subtypes based on their spontaneous firing rates (discussed further in the section on "Reciprocal interactions between the cochlea and the brainstem" and covered in the chapter by Fuchs, this volume). In the mature cochlea, these subtypes exhibit spatially ordered heterogeneity in synapse morphology along the basal surface of the IHCs (Figure 1.2). Because the cochlea spirals, the IHC axis is generally described based on the order of cells within the duct, with the "modiolar" side closer to the SGN cell bodies and the "pillar" side closer to the pillar cells (Figures 1.1 and 1.2). At each IHC, the SGN processes that terminate on the modiolar face (low- and medium-SR) have larger presynaptic ribbons and small postsynaptic GluR patches, while those on the pillar face (high-SR) have small ribbons and large GluR patches (L. D. Liberman, Wang, & Liberman, 2011). How these morphological features affect synaptic function, particularly in the context of known afferent physiological diversity, remains unknown. In stark contrast to the prolonged period over which SGN ion channel profiles mature postnatally, heterogeneity in ribbon size is already apparent by P3 in rats (Kalluri & Monges-Hernandez, 2017). However, ribbon morphologies appear to be dynamic throughout the first few weeks of development: the adult-like size gradient that is visible shortly after birth is lost by hearing onset, spatially reversed in the third postnatal week, and then reestablished sometime in the fourth week (Kalluri & Monges-Hernandez, 2017; L. D. Liberman & Liberman, 2016).

SGNs also undergo developmental changes in glutamate receptor composition that alter how they respond to glutamate released from HCs. Although all four AMPAR subunits are detected in SGNs, their expression patterns vary during development (Eybalin, Caicedo, Renard, Ruel, & Puel, 2004). GluA1 is expressed soon after birth but downregulates throughout the first week and is lost after hearing onset. On the other hand, GluA2 is undetectable early on but upregulates toward the end of the first postnatal week, with clear apposition of GluA2 puncta against presynaptic ribbons apparent before hearing onset (Eybalin et al., 2004; L. D. Liberman & Liberman, 2016). Both GluA3 and GluA4 are expressed at all stages, but GluA3 levels progressively decrease beyond the fourth postnatal week. The developmental switch from GluA1- to GluA2-mediated synaptic transmission around hearing onset may hold significance for Ca^{2+} permeability of AMPARs and plasticity (Cull-Candy, Kelly, & Farrant, 2006). Furthermore, it is unknown whether GluA subunits in SGNs exhibit a developmental switch in regulation at the mRNA and protein levels, for instance, via RNA editing, splicing, and phosphorylation, as occurs elsewhere in the CNS (Isaac, Ashby, & McBain, 2007). NMDARs, which shape glutamate-mediated SGN excitation in the neonatal cochlea and influence their spontaneous firing behavior (Zhang-Hooks, Agarwal, Mishina, & Bergles, 2016), also exhibit a developmental switch: GluN1 and GluN2A are expressed in the prehearing cochlea, but GluN1 is downregulated and GluN2A is lost while GluN2B, GluN2C, and GluN2D are upregulated with maturation (Knipper et al., 1997; Sanchez, Ghelani, & Otto-Meyer, 2015). Notably, this transition from a predominantly GluN2A- to GluN2B-containing NMDA receptor profile among SGNs is opposite of the developmental switch that occurs in the CNS (Yashiro & Philpot, 2008), including the auditory brainstem (Sanchez, Wang, Rubel, & Barria, 2010).

In summary, SGNs begin to receive synaptic signals from HCs perinatally while both the cochlea and brainstem are still maturing. The nature of synaptic transmission between the IHCs and SGNs changes as the system develops and matures. Since SGNs can evoke action potentials in post-synaptic targets in the brainstem as early as E15 in mice (Marrs & Spirou, 2012), developmental changes in the pattern of activity in the cochlea could influence the development of circuits in the brainstem.

Development of Central Axons

Acoustic information encoded by SGNs is relayed to a diverse array of neurons in the auditory brainstem that subserve circuits underlying detection of distinct sound features. All SGNs exit the cochlea via the eighth cranial nerve and then bifurcate after they enter the CNC, sending an ascending projection to the anterior ventral cochlear nucleus (aVCN) and a descending projection to the posterior VCN (pVCN) that ultimately terminates in the dorsal cochlear nucleus (DCN; Figure 1.3A). In mice, SGN axons reach the brainstem by E11.5 and bifurcations are obvious one day later (Lu et al., 2011). Thus, the cochlea is connected to the developing brainstem even before all of the SGNs have become post-mitotic. Likewise, neurons in the CNC are produced between E10.5 and E15.5 in mice (Martin & Rickets, 1981), overlapping with eighth nerve development. This

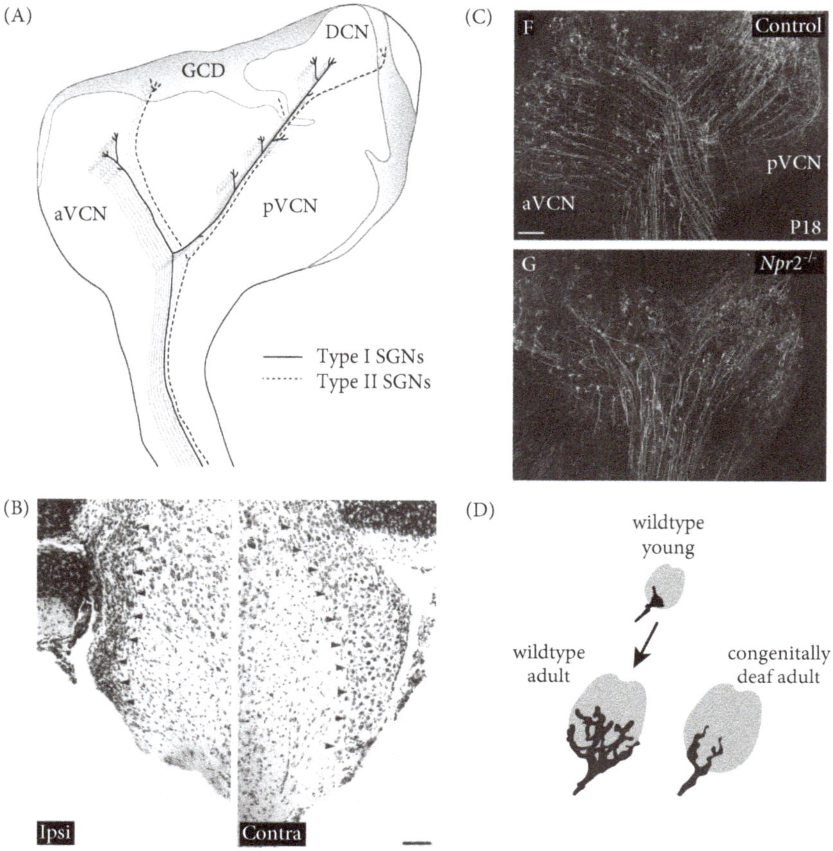

FIGURE 1.3. SGN projections in the cochlear nucleus complex. (A) Axons of Type I SGNs bifurcate in the cochlear nucleus complex (CNC), with one branch innervating the anterior ventral cochlear nucleus (aVCN) and the other branch innervating the posterior ventral nucleus (pVCN) and the dorsal cochlear nucleus (DCN). Each Type I branch gives rise to many collaterals, but they remain restricted to the magnocellular core of the CNC. On the other hand, Type II SGNs, which also bifurcate and exhibit the same basic innervation pattern, target the granule cell domain (GCD). (B) Proper development of the CNC requires cochlear innervation during a postnatal "critical period." Unilateral cochlear ablation at P5 in mice resulted in a gross decrease in the size of the ipsilateral nucleus (Ipsi) relative to the contralateral side (Contra), as shown in coronal sections of the aVCN. Scale bar = 100 μm. Reproduced with permission from (Mostafapour et al., 2000), Copyright © 2000 Wiley-Liss, Inc. (C) Bifurcation of SGNs is regulated by the natriuretic peptide receptor 2 (Npr2). In *Npr2*$^{-/--}$ animals, SGN axons fail to bifurcate, show a bias to turn caudally, and eventually form a blurred tonotopic organization relative to control. Scale bar = 100 μm. Taken from Lu et al. (2014) under the terms of the Creative Commons License. (D) In the aVCN, Type I SGNs envelop principal cells via calyceal synapses called the endbulbs of Held. Maturation of the endbulb of Held involves a striking change in the shape and size of the presynaptic terminal. This process requires activity, as revealed by observations of significantly smaller and less complex endbulbs of Held in congenitally deaf adult cats. Adapted and modified with permission from (Limb & Ryugo, 2000).

has important implications for circuit assembly, since the arrival of SGN axons marks the first time that tonotopic order in the cochlea is communicated to the CNS.

The nascent CNC spans rhombomeres 2 to 5 (R2 to R5) in the brainstem (Cramer, Fraser, & Rubel, 2000; Di Bonito & Studer, 2017; Farago, Awatramani, & Dymecki, 2006), so the first step for SGN axons is to target the correct rostro-caudal position. This might be aided by the presence of a stream of neural crest cells emanating from R4 (Sandell et al., 2014). In support of this idea, the eighth nerve is malformed after ablation of neural crest cells in chick embryos. There is also a band of GFAP-positive cells that is well-positioned to demarcate where 8th nerve fibers should enter (Siddiqui & Cramer, 2005). As expected based on their birth dates, the vestibular axons arrive slightly before the auditory axons, by E10.5 in mice, at about the same time that facial motor neurons have extended axons out through the 7th nerve, which develops in close proximity (Fritzsch & Nichols, 1993). Transplant studies in *Xenopus* suggest that cranial nerve development might be somewhat promiscuous. For instance, motor neurons are able to innervate an ectopic inner ear in the trunk. Conversely, VGNs send projections back to the spinal cord, apparently growing along whichever nerves are available (Elliott & Fritzsch, 2010; Elliott, Houston, & Fritzsch, 2013). Similarly, in mice, SGNs still send central axons into the vicinity of the CNC even when most CNC neurons are missing (Maricich et al., 2009). Thus, it is possible that SGN central axons simply follow the path available to them rather than responding to specific cues, with some contributions from permissive cues at the nerve entry site.

The eighth nerve contains a variety of fibers that are organized in a systematic fashion. For instance, the auditory and vestibular branches of the nerve are segregated from each other, and auditory fibers are further organized tonotopically (Sando, 1965). Axon-axon interactions within and across these different branches may contribute both to the guidance of central axons to the brainstem and the organization of the axons within the nerve. In other regions of the nervous system, such orderly arrangement within nerves and tracts is mediated by selective fasciculation (Sitko and Mason, 2015). Chicken auditory and vestibular axons express different complements of Eph receptors and ligands, but no role in segregation has been confirmed (Siddiqui & Cramer, 2005). However, a disorganized nerve forms when *Pax2-cre* is used to abolish *Neurod1* expression, with intermingling of auditory and vestibular axons that project to inappropriate targets in the hindbrain (Jahan, Kersigo, Pan, & Fritzsch, 2010). Whether this is a primary effect on the guidance behavior of the neurons remains to be determined.

In the auditory system, sound frequency is represented as a place code in the cochlea and relayed via topographically organized projections to higher auditory centers. Tonotopy starts in the cochlea, with HCs and SGNs that respond to high sound frequencies located in the base and those for low frequencies in the apex. The same order is preserved in the 8th nerve, with SGN axons from high frequency regions segregated from those for low frequency regions (Muniak et al., 2013; Sando, 1965). The axons go on to terminate in a cochleotopic manner in all three divisions of the CNC, a pattern that is reiterated along the auditory axis (Kandler, Clause, & Noh, 2009). Topographic maps exist throughout the nervous system and form through a combination of hard-wired and activity-dependent mechanisms, with crucial roles for Ephrin/Eph signaling during the first phase and acetylcholine-driven waves of spontaneous activity in the second (Cang & Feldheim, 2013). In the auditory system, SGN axons are topographically organized before they form synaptic connections either in the periphery or in the CNS (Koundakjian et al., 2007; Molea & Rubel, 2003). For instance, as early as E15 in mice, SGN axons from the apex innervate a restricted region of the developing CNC, with no signs of overshooting that are typical in other sensory systems (Koundakjian et al., 2007). Likewise, SGN axons show a coarse topographic organization in the CNC of newborn kittens (Leake, Hradek, Chair, & Snyder, 2006). It is unclear whether Eph receptors influence topography within the auditory nerve as they do in other regions of the nervous system, but some family members are expressed in gradients within the nerve (Siddiqui & Cramer, 2005) and seem to play a role in the distribution of 8th nerve fibers that enter the hindbrain in chickens (Allen-Sharpley, Tjia, & Cramer, 2013). In addition, reduction of EphrinB2, which is expressed uniformly among SGN axons and in the CNC, leads to slightly blurred tonotopy in DCN (Miko, Nakamura, Henkemeyer, & Cramer, 2007).

Although initial development of SGN-CNC connections may be hard-wired, the maps become more precise with age, possibly due to activity-dependent mechanisms. For instance, the broad maps seen in the newborn kitten are more adult-like by P6 (Snyder & Leake, 1997), but remain coarse if the animals are deafened at birth (Leake et al., 2006). This period of refinement corresponds to a phase during which rhythmic bursts of spontaneous activity occur among SGNs in neonatal cats (Jones, Leake, Snyder, Stakhovskaya, & Bonham, 2007). However, it is unclear whether spontaneous activity was actually disrupted by deafening, which was achieved by neomycin-induced HC death. Additionally, complete removal of the cochlea during early postnatal life reduces the number of neurons in the CNC (Harris & Rubel, 2006): many neurons die in the aVCN, causing reduction in size of the nucleus (Figure 1.3B; Mostafapour, Cochran, Del Puerto, & Rubel, 2000), and there is a loss of Wnt-sensitive progenitors that would otherwise produce neurons during this time frame (Volkenstein et al., 2013). Mass ablation of HCs from neonatal (but not mature) mice had the same effect (Tong et al., 2015). Thus, it is unclear which changes drive the observed degradation of tonotopic organization seen in deafened cats.

Analysis of a mouse mutant with an unusually specific effect on sensory axon development (Lu et al., 2014) hints that SGNs can in fact influence the formation of tonotopically ordered circuits within the CNC. SGN axons exhibit a stereotyped bifurcation that enables distribution of auditory information to all three divisions of the CNC. Bifurcation differs from axon branching in that the primary axon gives rise to two equal axons that go on to navigate independently (Schmidt & Rathjen, 2010). SGN bifurcation (Lu et al., 2014) relies on the same pathway used by sensory neurons in the dorsal root ganglion (DRG), which bifurcate in a similar fashion upon reaching the spinal cord (Schmidt et al., 2002, 2007). Like DRG neurons, SGNs express the natriuretic peptide receptor 2 (Npr2) during the time of bifurcation, which fails to occur in *Npr2* mutant mice (Lu et al., 2014). The Npr2 ligand, c-type natriuretic peptide (CNP), is detectable in mice by E9.5 exactly where the SGN axons enter (Ter-Avetisyan, Rathjen, & Schmidt, 2014), pointing to a model where the localized bifurcation of SGN axons is controlled by CNP-Npr2 interactions. In *Npr2* mutants, peripheral wiring and myelination appear normal, as is the tonotopic organization of SGN axons within the eighth nerve (Lu et al., 2014). However, the unbifurcated axons preferentially turn caudally and tonotopic organization within the CNC becomes blurred (Figure 1.3C). Whether these guidance defects are mediated by Npr2 or are instead secondary to the failure of bifurcation is unclear, as *Npr2* mutant axons also elaborate collateral branches that can innervate multiple divisions of the CNC and hence further degrade tonotopy. Notably, the dramatic change in the pattern of SGN innervation is accompanied by changes in the organization of circuitry within the CNC. Tuberculoventral (TV) cells normally form tonotopically organized connections that link DCN to VCN, and in *Npr2* mutants, this organization is less precise, mirroring effects on the SGN afferents (Lu et al., 2014). Although it remains to be proven that Npr2 acts solely in SGNs, this phenotype underscores the influential role that SGN afferents may play in the organization of central auditory circuits, starting at the very first site of processing.

Targeting and Synaptogenesis in the Cochlear Nucleus Complex

When SGN axons reach each target region within the CNC, they face the challenge of forming a variety of synapses with multiple post-synaptic partners. A particularly important step is the formation of unusually large calyceal synapses, which are crucial for the sound localization pathway. At a broad level, proper targeting and synaptogenesis of SGN afferents in the CNC are critical events that enable parcellation of neural signal onto distinct sub-circuits and extraction of diverse acoustic features.

A fundamental difference in the central innervation patterns of Type I and Type II neurons is that they primarily innervate cells in the magnocellular core and the granule cell domain (GCD), respectively (Figure 1.3A; Berglund & Brown, 1994; M. C. Brown, Berglund, Kiang, & Ryugo, 1988). Within the GCD, Type II fibers establish synaptic contacts mainly with small cells, and to some extent with other principal cell types, particularly the multipolar cells. Notably, the GCD also receives descending input from the auditory cortex (Weedman & Ryugo, 1996), inferior colliculus (Caicedo & Herbert, 1993), and superior olivary nucleus (Ryan, Schwartz, Helfert, Keithley, & Wang, 1987), as well as non-auditory sources (Burian & Gstoettner, 1988; Kevetter & Perachio, 1989; Ohlrogge, Doucet, & Ryugo, 2001; Zhan, Pongstaporn, & Ryugo, 2006; Zhan & Ryugo, 2007) such as the vestibular and somatosensory pathways (Haenggeli, Pongstaporn, Doucet, & Ryugo, 2005; Itoh et al., 1987; Weinberg & Rustioni, 1987; D. D. Wright & Ryugo, 1996). Thus, there is likely multimodal and top-down influence on the neurons targeted by Type II fibers.

Type I fibers exhibit systematic heterogeneity in their central innervation at multiple levels. Most Type I fibers terminate in the magnocellular core of the aVCN and pVCN, and the deep layer of the DCN (Fekete, Rouiller, Liberman, & Ryugo, 1984; M. C. Liberman, 1991, 1993; Ryugo & May, 1993). However, the pattern of innervation differs among the three physiologically defined SR groups, both in terms of the CN subdivisions they innervate and the cell types they contact. Low- and medium-SR fibers provide the sole source of input to the small cell cap (SCC), a thin sheet of small cells at the peripheral margin of the VCN (Ryugo, 2008). Within the SCC, low-SR collaterals ramify extensively, mostly within the neuropil, and likely contact multiple cells. Since cells in the SCC project to MOCs (Ye, Machado, & Kim, 2000), the selective innervation of SCC by low-SR SGNs, which have high thresholds, is thought to be part of a feedback circuit triggered by high sound intensities (Ryugo, 2008). On the other hand, all three SR subtypes project to the aVCN and pVCN, where they synapse with both common and distinct postsynaptic cell types (M. C. Liberman, 1991, 1993). Stellate cells in the aVCN receive input from all SR groups, but multipolar cells are contacted by only low- and medium-SR fibers (M. C. Liberman, 1993). In the pVCN, granule cells are innervated predominantly by high-SR fibers and multipolar cells are innervated by all SR groups. In the DCN, high-SR inputs generally form somatic contacts onto small cells in the deep layer, whereas medium-/low-SR inputs are non-somatic and occur closer to the fusiform cell layer (M. C. Liberman, 1993). That SR subtypes form connections that vary both by the identity of the postsynaptic cell and the subcellular location of the synapse suggests that the Type I SGNs collectively relay acoustic information to distinct circuit motifs within the lower auditory pathway. Although the number and nature of the synapses that link SGNs to the CNS determine how acoustic information is initially encoded in the brain, nothing is known about how the correct pattern is established in development.

Across all SR groups, Type I SGNs are tasked with faithfully conveying the complex temporal properties of sound up the auditory pathway. Fidelity is achieved in part via huge and complex synaptic structures, called the endbulbs of Held (Figure 1.3D), which are found at Type I SGN terminal endings on to globular and spherical bushy cells (SBCs) in the aVCN and are critical for sound localization. They occur as both axodendritic and axosomatic synapses, feature hundreds of presynaptic active zones (Ryugo, Wu, & Pongstaporn, 1996), and are powerful drivers of postsynaptic firing, especially considering that up to three endbulbs contact a single SBC (Brawer & Morest, 1975; Cant & Morest, 1979; Ryugo & Sento, 1991). The endbulbs release glutamate that is detected by the SBCs via both AMPA and NMDA-type receptors (Pliss, Yang, & Xu-Friedman, 2009; Y. X. Wang, Wenthold, Ottersen, & Petralia, 1998). Endbulb morphologies vary extensively between low- and high-SR SGNs with systematic differences in the complexity of the presynaptic terminal, which are accompanied by variations in PSD size and shape (Ryugo & Sento, 1991; Ryugo et al., 1996).

Synapse formation begins during the first postnatal week, when SGN axons contact SBCs and form relatively simple terminals. Over the next few days, these terminals grow much larger and begin to extend thin branches locally. Growth continues for many more weeks, as the terminal gradually envelops most of the SBC cell body and becomes ever more elaborate (Ryugo, Montey, Wright, Bennett, & Pongstaporn, 2006). Why SGN axons form endbulbs only upon contacting SBCs is not known. SGN axons are able to form functionally normal synaptic connections in *Npr2* mutant mice despite the lack of tonotopic order, indicating that synaptic maturation may be controlled by local cell-cell interactions (Lu et al., 2014). The characteristic growth of the endbulbs, on the other hand, is influenced by activity. The role of activity is evident both in the natural variation in endbulb complexity that occurs among SGNs with different spontaneous firing rates (Ryugo & May, 1993), and in the loss of this complexity in congenitally deaf animals (Figure 1.3D; Baker, Montey, Pongstaporn, & Ryugo, 2010). Instead of well-defined and dome-shaped PSDs, deaf cats have significantly enlarged and flattened PSDs. Some aspects of this phenotype, such as enlargement of PSDs and increase in presynaptic vesicle density, may indicate homeostatic plasticity compensating for reduced activity. Consistent with this idea, transmitter release probability is elevated at the endbulb of Held-SBC synapse in *deafness* (*dn/dn*) mutant mice (Oleskevich & Walmsley, 2002), and reintroduction of activity via cochlear implants at three months of age corrects the synaptic morphology defect (O'Neil, Limb, Baker, & Ryugo, 2010). However, rescue does not occur when activity is restored at six months of age, which suggests a critical period during which synaptic morphology remains plastic with respect to activity in the auditory pathway. Little is known about how SGNs select the correct complement of post-synaptic partners and develop the morphologically appropriate type of synapse.

Reciprocal Interactions between the Cochlea and the Brainstem

SGNs provide a direct link between the periphery and the central auditory system that serves as both a physical and an electrical substrate for communication. Physically, the SGN axons offer a roadway for OCN axons into the cochlea. The OCNs, in turn, have important effects on the maturation of HCs and connectivity within the cochlea. Electrically, SGNs convey patterns of activity from the cochlea to the central nervous system, likely further refining tonotopic maps.

OCNs develop together with more canonical motor neurons in the ventral hindbrain (Fritzsch & Elliott, 2017). Like other motor neurons, they are primarily cholinergic, although a subset produce other transmitters and peptides such as GABA and CGRP (Eybalin, 1993; Sewell, 2011). OCNs share a particularly close relationship with the facial branchial motor neurons (FMBNs), which send axons into the 7th nerve. Both populations arise mostly in the fourth rhombomere and then undergo extensive migrations, leaving their axons behind them (Fritzsch & Elliott, 2017; Han, Gupta, & Novitch, 2018). As a result, OCN efferent axons follow along the genu of the 7th nerve. Upon exiting the brainstem, the OCN efferent axons diverge from the FBMN axons and reach the developing otocyst by E11.5 in mice (Bruce et al., 1997). At this stage, the earliest inner ear neuron axons, mostly vestibular, have already reached the brainstem, raising the possibility that the OCN efferents grow along the pre-existing inner ear afferents to reach the ear. There is broad agreement that SGN peripheral processes provide a scaffold for OC efferent growth inside the cochlea, but the idea has not been directly tested experimentally, nor is the molecular mechanism known (Fritzsch, 1996; Simmons, 2002). Nonetheless, in a wide variety of mouse mutants with disorganized SGN peripheral processes, OCN efferents are likewise disorganized (Duncan and Fritzsch, 2013; Duncan et al., 2011; Huang et al., 2001; Ma et al., 2000). Thus, the early extension of SGN peripheral and central processes may enable the subsequent guidance of OCN efferents into the inner ear.

The arrival of OCN efferents initiates reciprocal interactions that influence cochlear maturation and function. The most obvious effect comes from the MOC population. Upon first arriving in the cochlea, the MOC efferents elaborate transient branches that innervate the IHCs, despite the fact that in the mature cochlea, MOC efferents only innervate the OHCs (Glowatzki & Fuchs, 2000; Goutman, Fuchs, & Glowatzki, 2005). This contact may influence IHC maturation (Johnson et al., 2013). Less is known about the impact of LOC efferents, which are harder to study because the axons are thinner and unmyelinated. However, there are indications that input from the LOC neurons is poised to contribute to the different spontaneous firing rates among Type I SGNs (M. C. Liberman, 1980a, 1980b). In support of this idea, severing of the olivocochlear bundle prevents the maintenance of the mature pattern of synaptic heterogeneity associated with SR subtypes (Yin, Liberman, Maison, & Liberman, 2014). With no way to access LOC neurons selectively prior to birth, it is unclear whether they also affect the initial establishment of this pattern (M. C. Liberman, O'Grady, Dodds, Mcgee, & Walsh, 2000). However, analysis of a mouse mutant with early disruption of the efferent system prevented normal emergence of the synaptic gradient during early postnatal life (Hickman, Liberman, & Jacob, 2015). Overall, the olivocochlear system is well-positioned to influence the pattern of activity that emanates from the cochlea during development, either through effects on the HCs or on the SGNs (Johnson et al., 2011, 2013). Indeed, when cholinergic signaling is disrupted during development, the temporal pattern of activity is altered, with long-term consequences for the refinement of tonotopic projections in the lateral superior olive (Clause et al., 2014).

As well as providing a structural bridge between the PNS and CNS, SGNs directly inform the hindbrain about levels of activity in the cochlea, information that could influence assembly of circuits all the way up to the cortex. This activity begins quite early in auditory circuit development, as SGNs are spontaneously active by E14 in mice (Marrs & Spirou, 2012). By E15, stimulation of the auditory nerve can generate responses in the developing VCN, although these responses are slow and small. Thus, activity in the SGNs could influence the CNC even before synapses have formed in the periphery. In the mouse cochlea, IHCs first generate action potentials around E17 (Johnson et al., 2005; Marcotti, Johnson, Holley, & Kros, 2003), about the same time that mechanosensitivity can first be detected (Géléoc & Holt, 2003). The IHCs are functionally connected to the SGNs by birth, although the synapses are still immature (Shnerson et al., 1981; Tritsch et al., 2010). During these early stages, IHCs are activated by waves of ATP and potassium ions released from inner supporting cells (ISC) in Kolliker's organ, a transient structure adjacent to the developing organ of Corti (Tritsch, Yi, Gale, Glowatzki, & Bergles, 2007; H. C. Wang et al., 2015). Bursts of action potentials in IHCs induce similar bursts of activity in SGNs and indeed along the auditory pathway (Tritsch et al., 2010). Spontaneous activity peaks during a time of significant change and maturation in auditory circuits, from the pruning of Type I SGN peripheral contacts with IHCs to the emergence of precise tonotopy and the remarkable growth of endbulbs in the CNC (Tritsch & Bergles, 2010; H. C. Wang & Bergles, 2015). Although cochlear ablation studies confirm that this spontaneous activity originates in the cochlea (Tritsch et al., 2010), it has been challenging to pinpoint the in vivo consequences for cochlear wiring and function.

Electrophysiological Maturation of SGNs

Long after their central and peripheral connections are established, SGNs continue to undergo molecular changes that produce adult electrophysiological signatures. These changes occur in concert with maturation of presynaptic inputs from the HCs and the olivocochlear efferent system, which further sculpt SGN firing behaviors. Intrinsically, developing SGNs must fine-tune the elements that generate and propagate action potentials, including expression and proper localization of a large cohort of voltage- and ligand-gated ion channels (Reijntjes & Pyott, 2016). Although the precise onset or dynamics of expression is unknown for most ion channels, adult profiles likely emerge after gene-specific variation in expression through development. For example, Kv1.1 protein level ramps up between P3 and P8 in mice and may contribute to a change in SGN excitability (Crozier & Davis, 2014). Proper localization of ion channels must go hand-in-hand with such expression changes. Indeed, in rats, the potassium channel Kv3.1b is initially diffuse but co-localizes with the scaffold protein AnkG in nascent nodes by P17 and stabilizes thereafter. Confinement of the sodium channel Nav1.6 to the AnkG domain, however, progresses until P30 (Kim & Rutherford, 2016). Hence, assembly of nodal components, which begins with the onset of myelination toward the end of the first postnatal week (Kim & Rutherford, 2016; Romand & Romand, 1985), continues at least until P30. Although nodes are almost fully assembled around hearing onset, the heminode, which is thought to be the axon initial segment, approaches mature configuration only after hearing begins.

Spatiotemporal changes in SGN ion channel profiles are contemporaneous with multifaceted changes in SGN physiology in the first few postnatal weeks. SGNs exhibit IHC-driven spontaneous activity at birth but undergo a switch from random to burst firing a few days later (Tritsch & Bergles, 2010). Burst firing disappears by the end of the second postnatal week and spontaneous SGN firing patterns instead exhibit temporal features suggestive of a Poisson process (A. B. Wong et al., 2013). It is unknown if such early changes in the temporal structure of SGN firing behavior are influenced by fluxes in SGN molecular profiles. However, cell-intrinsic changes likely occur, since spontaneous action potentials in immature SGNs occur both in response to input from IHCs and via IHC-independent mechanisms. With maturation, intrinsically generated spikes contribute less to SGN spontaneous activity, disappearing sometime in the third postnatal week (Wu, Young, & Glowatzki, 2016). Overall, the increase in the average rate and total range of spontaneous firing with the emergence of progressively higher SR is one key aspect of post-hearing electrophysiological maturation of SGNs (Kim & Rutherford, 2016; Wu et al., 2016). These changes in spontaneous activity are accompanied by maturation of responses to sound-evoked responses, including a decrease in threshold and latency, and an increase in the synchrony of auditory nerve fiber discharge (Geal-Dor, Freeman, Li, & Sohmer, 1993; Uziel, Romand, & Marot, 1981; A. B. Wong et al., 2013).

Whole-cell recordings of cultured SGNs have offered additional insights into intrinsic differences in SGN electrical properties. For example, Type I SGNs from neonatal mice exhibit tonotopic differences in membrane kinetics and degrees of accommodation (Crozier & Davis, 2014), which may be driven by differences in expression of voltage-gated potassium and calcium channels (Chen et al., 2011; Q. Liu, Lee, & Davis, 2014). Furthermore, a decrease in excitability occurs together with an alteration of accommodation properties within the first two postnatal weeks (Crozier & Davis, 2014), thus indicating that SGN maturation includes changes in cell-intrinsic electrical properties. However, the extent to which this accounts for changes observed in vivo is unknown. Likewise, although SGN firing behavior is subject to modulation by neurotrophins in vitro (Crozier & Davis, 2014; T. Wright, Gillespie, O'Leary, & Needham, 2016), the relevance for functional maturation of SGNs in vivo is unclear.

Several presynaptic changes that occur over the same period may further contribute to the emergence of mature SGN firing behaviors. These include transition of IHCs from producing action potentials to graded receptor potentials, maturation of presynaptic ribbon structures, and stronger coupling of Cav1.3 channels and vesicle release sites in IHCs (A. B. Wong et al., 2014), as well as establishment of synaptic contacts by LOC efferent terminals on Type I afferent endings. Indeed, heterogeneities in LOC innervation of SGNs (Yin et al., 2014) and functional diversity across IHC active zones (Meyer et al., 2009) are thought to contribute to the wide spontaneous firing rate diversity among SGNs in the mature cochlea.

How SGN physiological diversity is linked to observed molecular differences is not well understood. It is unclear, for example, which of the many genes that are differentially expressed among Type I SGNs underlie their in vivo physiological properties. For instance, in cultured neonatal SGNs, relative levels of two calcium-binding proteins, calbindin and calretinin, are variable and correlate with a temporal parameter of SGN firing (W. Liu & Davis, 2014). This observation suggests that SGN functional signatures may be shaped by calcium-binding proteins, in addition to the expected variation in ion channel components. More work is needed to establish a causal relation between such candidate molecules and distinct physiological features.

In summary, emerging evidence indicates that SGN molecular profiles undergo spatiotemporal refinement that may underlie the striking shifts in electrophysiological features observed across development. Although the biggest changes coincide with hearing onset around P11, subtler changes continue to shape SGN activity in subsequent weeks, driven both by shifts in the intrinsic properties of SGNs and the extrinsic influence of their presynaptic inputs, which mature over the same time frame.

Conclusion

SGNs are the main conduits through which auditory signals captured by the inner ear reach the brain. During development, SGNs make precise, specialized synaptic connections and acquire unique electrophysiological properties that involve both cell-intrinsic and activity-dependent mechanisms, starting well before animals are able to respond to airborne sounds. SGN processes are in place long before their target cells have matured and therefore play a significant role in auditory circuit assembly and maturation. Indeed, the arrival of SGN processes in the cochlear nucleus anlage marks the first time that cochlear tonotopy coordinates are relayed to the developing auditory brainstem, thus suggesting a crucial role for SGNs in setting up topographic order centrally. Indeed, the cochlea has a strong influence on the development of auditory circuits at multiple levels, from regulating cell survival locally to tonotopic order deeper in the brainstem. Given that SGNs connect the PNS and the CNS both developmentally and functionally, it will be important for the field as a whole to gain a better understanding of the primary effects of congenital mutations on SGNs and their impact on the organization of central auditory circuits.

Acknowledgments

We thank Lorna Wu for figure illustrations, and Michelle Frank, Dr. Austen Sitko, Dr. Kirupa Suthakar, Dr. Paul Fuchs, and Dr. David Ryugo for feedback. Our work is supported by funding from the NIH, the Lefler Family Foundation, and the Harvard Brain Initiative. BRS is a recipient of a F32 Postdoctoral Individual National Research Service Award and a Goldenson Postdoctoral Fellowship.

References

Adam, J., Myat, A., Le Roux, I., Eddison, M., Henrique, D., Ish-Horowicz, D., & Lewis, J. (1998). Cell fate choices and the expression of Notch, Delta and Serrate homologues in the chick inner ear: parallels with Drosophila sense-organ development. *Development*, *125*(23), 4645–4654.

Allen-Sharpley, M. R., Tjia, M., & Cramer, K. S. (2013). Differential roles for EphA and EphB signaling in segregation and patterning of central vestibulocochlear nerve projections. *PLoS ONE*, *8*(10), e78658. https://doi.org/10.1371/journal.pone.0078658

Anniko, M., & Wikström, S.-O. (1984). Pattern formation of the otic placode and morphogenesis of the otocyst. *American Journal of Otolaryngology*, *5*(6), 373–381. https://doi.org/10.1016/S0196-0709(84)80051-4

Appler, J. M., Lu, C. C., Druckenbrod, N. R., Yu, W.-M., Koundakjian, E. J., & Goodrich, L. V. (2013). Gata3 Is a Critical Regulator of Cochlear Wiring. *Journal of Neuroscience*, *33*(8), 3679–3691. https://doi.org/10.1523/JNEUROSCI.4703-12.2013

Baker, C. A., Montey, K. L., Pongstaporn, T., & Ryugo, D. K. (2010). Postnatal development of the endbulb of Held in congenitally deaf cats. *Frontiers in Neuroanatomy*, *4*, 19. https://doi.org/10.3389/fnana.2010.00019

Bank, L. M., Bianchi, L. M., Ebisu, F., Lerman-Sinkoff, D., Smiley, E. C., Shen, Y.-C., . . . Barald, K. F. (2013). Macrophage migration inhibitory factor acts as a neurotrophin in the developing inner ear. *Development*, *140*(139), 4666–4674. https://doi.org/10.1242/dev.066647

Barclay, M., Ryan, A. F., & Housley, G. D. (2011). Type I vs type II spiral ganglion neurons exhibit differential survival and neuritogenesis during cochlear development. *Neural Development*, *6*, 33. https://doi.org/10.1186/1749-8104-6-33

Battisti, A. C., Fantetti, K. N., Moyers, B. A., & Fekete, D. M. (2014). A subset of chicken statoacoustic ganglion neurites are repelled by Slit1 and Slit2. *Hearing Research*, *310*, 1–12. https://doi.org/10.1016/J.HEARES.2014.01.003

Battisti, A. C., & Fekete, D. M. (2008). Slits and robos in the developing chicken inner ear. *Developmental Dynamics*, *237*(2), 476–484. https://doi.org/10.1002/dvdy.21429

Bell, D., Streit, A., Gorospe, I., Varela-Nieto, I., Alsina, B., & Giraldez, F. (2008). Spatial and temporal segregation of auditory and vestibular neurons in the otic placode. *Developmental Biology*, *322*(1), 109–120. https://doi.org/10.1016/J.YDBIO.2008.07.011

Berglund, A. M., & Brown, M. C. (1994). Central trajectories of type II spiral ganglion cells from various cochlear regions in mice. *Hearing Research*, *75*(1–2), 121–130. https://doi.org/10.1016/0378-5955(94)90063-9

Bermingham, N. A., Hassan, B. A., Price, S. D., Vollrath, M. A., Ben-Arie, N., Eatock, R. A., . . . Zoghbi, H. Y. (1999). Math1: an essential gene for the generation of inner ear hair cells. *Science*, *284*(5421), 1837–1841. https://doi.org/10.1126/SCIENCE.284.5421.1837

Beutner, D., & Moser, T. (2001). The presynaptic function of mouse cochlear inner hair cells during development of hearing. *Journal of Neuroscience*, *21*(13), 4593–4599. https://doi.org/10.1523/JNEUROSCI.21-13-04593.2001

Bianchi, L. M., & Gale, N. W. (1998). Distribution of Eph-related molecules in the developing and mature cochlea. *Hearing Research*, *117*(1–2), 161–172. https://doi.org/10.1016/S0378-5955(98)00010-0

Bianchi, L. M., & Gray, N. A. (2002). EphB receptors influence growth of ephrin-B1-positive statoacoustic nerve fibers. *European Journal of Neuroscience*, *16*(8), 1499–1506. https://doi.org/10.1046/j.1460-9568.2002.02248.x

Bibas, A., Hornigold, R., Liang, J., Michaels, L., Anagnostopoulou, S., & Wright, A. (2006). The development of the spiral ganglion in the human foetus. *Folia Morphologica*, *65*(2), 140–144.

Bok, J. (2005). Role of the hindbrain in dorsoventral but not anteroposterior axial specification of the inner ear. *Development*, *132*(9), 2115–2124. https://doi.org/10.1242/dev.01796

Bok, J., Dolson, D. K., Hill, P., Ruther, U., Epstein, D. J., & Wu, D. K. (2007). Opposing gradients of Gli repressor and activators mediate Shh signaling along the dorsoventral axis of the inner ear. *Development*, *134*(9), 1713–1722. https://doi.org/10.1242/dev.000760

Brawer, J. R., & Morest, D. K. (1975). Relations between auditory nerve endings and cell types in the cat's anteroventral cochlear nucleus seen with the Golgi method and nomarski optics. *Journal of Comparative Neurology*, *160*(4), 491–506. https://doi.org/10.1002/cne.901600406

Brown, A. S., & Epstein, D. J. (2011). Otic ablation of smoothened reveals direct and indirect requirements for Hedgehog signaling in inner ear development. *Development*, *138*(18), 3967–3976. https://doi.org/10.1242/dev.066126

Brown, M. C., Berglund, A. M., Kiang, N. Y. S., & Ryugo, D. K. (1988). Central trajectories of type II spiral ganglion neurons. *Journal of Comparative Neurology*, *278*(4), 581–590. https://doi.org/10.1002/cne.902780409

Bruce, L. L., Kingsley, J., Nichols, D. H., & Fritzsch, B. (1997). The development of vestibulocochlear efferents and cochlear afferents in mice. *International Journal of Neuroscience*, *15*(45), 671–692. https://doi.org/10.1016/S0736-5748(96)00120-7

Burian, M., & Gstoettner, W. (1988). Projection of primary vestibular afferent fibres to the cochlear nucleus in the guinea pig. *Neuroscience Letters*, *84*(1), 13–17. https://doi.org/10.1016/0304-3940(88)90329-1

Caicedo, A., & Herbert, H. (1993). Topography of descending projections from the inferior colliculus to auditory brainstem nuclei in the rat. *Journal of Comparative Neurology*, *328*(3), 377–392. https://doi.org/10.1002/cne.903280305

Cang, J., & Feldheim, D. A. (2013). Developmental mechanisms of topographic map formation and alignment. *Annual Review of Neuroscience*, *36*(1), 51–77. https://doi.org/10.1146/annurev-neuro-062012-170341

Cant, N. B., & Morest, D. K. (1979). The bushy cells in the anteroventral cochlear nucleus of the cat. A study with the electron microscope. *Neuroscience*, *4*(12), 1925–1945. https://doi.org/10.1016/0306-4522(79)90066-6

Carney, P. R., & Silver, J. (1983). Studies on cell migration and axon guidance in the developing distal auditory system of the mouse. *Journal of Comparative Neurology*, *215*(4), 359–369. https://doi.org/10.1002/cne.902150402

Carrott, L., Bowl, M. R., Aguilar, C., Johnson, S. L., Chessum, L., West, M., . . . Brown, S. D. M. (2016). Absence of neuroplastin-65 affects synaptogenesis in mouse inner hair cells and causes profound hearing loss. *Journal of Neuroscience*, *36*(1), 222–234. https://doi.org/10.1523/JNEUROSCI.1808-15.2016

Chen, W. C., Xue, H. Z., Hsu, Y. (Lucy), Liu, Q., Patel, S., & Davis, R. L. (2011). Complex distribution patterns of voltage-gated calcium channel α-subunits in the spiral ganglion. *Hearing Research*, *278*(1–2), 52–68. https://doi.org/10.1016/j.heares.2011.01.016

Clause, A., Kim, G., Sonntag, M., Weisz, C. J. C., Vetter, D. E., Ubsamen, R., & Kandler, K. (2014). The precise temporal pattern of prehearing spontaneous activity is necessary for tonotopic map refinement. *Neuron*, *82*(4), 822–835. https://doi.org/10.1016/j.neuron.2014.04.001

Coate, T. M., Raft, S., Zhao, X., Ryan, A. K., Crenshaw, E. III, & Kelley, M. W. (2012). Otic mesenchyme cells regulate spiral ganglion axon fasciculation through a Pou3f4/EphA4 signaling pathway. *Neuron*, *73*(1), 49–63. https://doi.org/10.1016/j.neuron.2011.10.029

Coate, T. M., Spita, N. A., Zhang, K. D., Isgrig, K. T., & Kelley, M. W. (2015). Neuropilin-2/semaphorin-3F-mediated repulsion promotes inner hair cell innervation by spiral ganglion neurons. *eLife*, *4*, 1–24. https://doi.org/10.7554/eLife.07830

Cole, L. K., Le Roux, I., Nunes, F., Laufer, E., Lewis, J., & Wu, D. K. (2000). Sensory organ generation in the chicken inner ear: Contributions of bone morphogenetic protein 4, Serrate1, and lunatic fringe. *Journal of Comparative Neurology*, *424*(3), 509–520. https://doi.org/10.1002/1096-9861(20000828)424:3<509::AID-CNE8>3.0.CO;2-Q

Cramer, K. S., Fraser, S. E., & Rubel, E. W. (2000). Embryonic origins of auditory brain-stem nuclei in the chick hindbrain. *Developmental Biology*, *224*(2), 138–151. https://doi.org/10.1006/dbio.2000.9779

Crozier, R. A., & Davis, R. L. (2014). Unmasking of spiral ganglion neuron firing dynamics by membrane potential and neurotrophin-3. *Journal of Neuroscience*, *34*(29), 9688–9702. https://doi.org/10.1523/JNEUROSCI.4552-13.2014

Cull-Candy, S., Kelly, L., & Farrant, M. (2006). Regulation of Ca^{2+}-permeable AMPA receptors: Synaptic plasticity and beyond. *Current Opinion in Neurobiology*, *16*(3), 288–297. https://doi.org/10.1016/j.conb.2006.05.012

Darrow, K. N., Maison, S. F., & Liberman, M. C. (2006). Cochlear efferent feedback balances interaural sensitivity. *Nature Neuroscience*, *9*(12), 1474–1476. https://doi.org/10.1038/nn1807

Darrow, K. N., Maison, S. F., & Liberman, M. C. (2007). Selective removal of lateral olivocochlear efferents increases vulnerability to acute acoustic injury. *Journal of Neurophysiology*, *97*(2), 1775–1785. https://doi.org/10.1152/jn.00955.2006

Defourny, J., Poirrier, A. L., Lallemend, F., Sánchez, S. M., Neef, J., Vanderhaeghen, P., . . . Malgrange, B. (2013). Ephrin-A5/EphA4 signalling controls specific afferent targeting to cochlear hair cells. *Nature Communications*, *4*, 1438. https://doi.org/10.1038/ncomms2445

Di Bonito, M., & Studer, M. (2017). Cellular and Molecular Underpinnings of Neuronal Assembly in the Central Auditory System during Mouse Development. *Frontiers in Neural Circuits*, *11*, 18. https://doi.org/10.3389/fncir.2017.00018

Dieck, S. T., Altrock, W. D., Kessels, M. M., Qualmann, B., Regus, H., Brauner, D., . . . Brandstätter, J. H. (2005). Molecular dissection of the photoreceptor ribbon synapse: Physical interaction of Bassoon and RIBEYE is essential for the assembly of the ribbon complex. *Journal of Cell Biology*, *168*(5), 825–836. https://doi.org/10.1083/jcb.200408157

Druckenbrod, N. R., & Goodrich, L. V. (2015). Sequential retraction segregates SGN processes during target selection in the cochlea. *Journal of Neuroscience*, *35*(49), 16221–16235. https://doi.org/10.1523/JNEUROSCI.2236-15.2015

Duncan, J. S., & Fritzsch, B. (2013). Continued expression of GATA3 is necessary for cochlear neurosensory development. *PLoS ONE*, *8*(4), e62046. https://doi.org/10.1371/journal.pone.0062046

Duncan, J. S., Lim, K. C., Engel, J. D., & Fritzsch, B. (2011). Limited inner ear morphogenesis and neurosensory development are possible in the absence of GATA3. *International Journal of Developmental Biology*, *55*(3), 297–303. https://doi.org/10.1387/ijdb.103178jd

Echteler, S. M. (1992). Developmental segregation in the afferent projections to mammalian auditory hair cells. *Proceedings of the National Academy of Sciences of the United States of* America, 89(14), 6324–6327. https://doi.org/10.1073/pnas.89.14.6324

Elliott, K. L., & Fritzsch, B. (2010). Transplantation of Xenopus laevis ears reveals the ability to form afferent and efferent connections with the spinal cord. *International Journal of Developmental Biology*, *54*(10), 1443–1451. https://doi.org/10.1387/ijdb.103061ke

Elliott, K. L., Houston, D. W., & Fritzsch, B. (2013). Transplantation of *Xenopus laevis* tissues to determine the ability of motor neurons to acquire a novel target. *PLoS ONE*, *8*(2), e55541. https://doi.org/10.1371/journal.pone.0055541

Elliott, K. L., Kersigo, J., Pan, N., Jahan, I., & Fritzsch, B. (2017). Spiral Ganglion Neuron Projection Development to the Hindbrain in Mice Lacking Peripheral and/or Central Target Differentiation. *Frontiers in Neural Circuits*, *11*, 25. https://doi.org/10.3389/fncir.2017.00025

Evsen, L., Sugahara, S., Uchikawa, M., Kondoh, H., & Wu, D. K. (2013). Cellular/molecular progression of neurogenesis in the inner ear requires inhibition of Sox2 transcription by neurogenin1 and neurod1. *Journal of Neurophysiology*, *33*(9), 3879–3890. https://doi.org/10.1523/JNEUROSCI.4030-12.2013

Eybalin, M. (1993). Neurotransmitters and neuromodulators of the mammalian cochlea. *Physiological Reviews*, *73*(2), 309–373. https://doi.org/10.1152/physrev.1993.73.2.309

Eybalin, M., Caicedo, A., Renard, N., Ruel, J., & Puel, J. L. (2004). Transient Ca^{2+}-permeable AMPA receptors in postnatal rat primary auditory neurons. *European Journal of Neuroscience*, *20*(11), 2981–2989. https://doi.org/10.1111/j.1460-9568.2004.03772.x

Fantetti, K. N., & Fekete, D. M. (2012). Members of the BMP, Shh, and FGF morphogen families promote chicken statoacoustic ganglion neurite outgrowth and neuron survival in vitro. *Developmental Neurobiology*, *72*(9), 1213–1228. https://doi.org/10.1002/dneu.20988

Farago, A. F., Awatramani, R. B., & Dymecki, S. M. (2006). Assembly of the brainstem cochlear nuclear complex is revealed by intersectional and subtractive genetic fate maps. *Neuron*, *50*(2), 205–18. https://doi.org/10.1016/j.neuron.2006.03.014

Fekete, D. M., & Campero, A. M. (2007). Axon guidance in the inner ear. *International Journal of Developmental Biology*, *51*(6–7), 549–556. https://doi.org/10.1387/ijdb.072341df

Fekete, D. M., Rouiller, E. M., Liberman, M. C., & Ryugo, D. K. (1984). The central projections of intracellularly labeled auditory nerve fibers in cats. *Journal of Comparative Neurology*, *229*(3), 432–450. https://doi.org/10.1002/cne.902290311

Freter, S., Fleenor, S. J., Freter, R., Liu, K. J., & Begbie, J. (2013). Cranial neural crest cells form corridors prefiguring sensory neuroblast migration. *Development*, *140*(17), 3595–3600. https://doi.org/10.1242/dev.091033

Fritzsch, B. (1996). Development of the labyrinthine efferent system. *Annals of the New York Academy of Sciences*, *781*, 21–33. https://doi.org/10.1111/j.1749-6632.1996.tb15690.x

Fritzsch, B., & Elliott, K. L. (2017). Evolution and development of the inner ear efferent system: Transforming a motor neuron population to connect to the most unusual motor protein via ancient nicotinic receptors. *Frontiers in Cellular Neuroscience*, *11*, 114. https://doi.org/10.3389/fncel.2017.00114

Fritzsch, B., Matei, V. A., Nichols, D. H., Bermingham, N., Jones, K., Beisel, K. W., & Wang, V. Y. (2005). Atoh1 null mice show directed afferent fiber growth to undifferentiated ear sensory epithelia followed by incomplete fiber retention. *Developmental Dynamics*, *233*, 570–583. https://doi.org/10.1002/dvdy.20370

Fritzsch, B., & Nichols, D. H. (1993). DiI reveals a prenatal arrival of efferents at the differentiating otocyst of mice. *Hearing Research*, *65*(1–2), 51–60. https://doi.org/10.1016/0378-5955(93)90200-K

Geal-Dor, M., Freeman, S., Li, G., & Sohmer, H. (1993). Development of hearing in neonatal rats: Air and bone conducted ABR thresholds. *Hearing Research*, *69*(1–2), 236–242. https://doi.org/10.1016/0378-5955(93)90113-F

Géléoc, G. S. G., & Holt, J. R. (2003). Developmental acquisition of sensory transduction in hair cells of the mouse inner ear. *Nature Neuroscience*, *6*(10), 1019–1020. https://doi.org/10.1038/nn1120

Glowatzki, E., & Fuchs, P. A. (2000). Cholinergic synaptic inhibition of inner hair cells in the neonatal mammalian cochlea. *Science*, *288*(5475), 2366–2368. https://doi.org/10.1126/SCIENCE.288.5475.2366

Goodrich, L. V. (2016). Early development of the spiral ganglion. In A. Dabdoub, B. Fritzsch, R. R. Fay, and A. N. Popper (Eds.), *The primary auditory neurons of the mammalian cochlea* (pp. 11–48). New York, NY: Springer. https://doi.org/10.1007/978-1-4939-3031-9_2

Goutman, J. D., Fuchs, P. A., & Glowatzki, E. (2005). Facilitating efferent inhibition of inner hair cells in the cochlea of the neonatal rat. *Journal of Physiology*, *566*(1), 49–59. https://doi.org/10.1113/jphysiol.2005.087460

Haddon, C., & Lewis, J. (1996). Early ear development in the embryo of the Zebrafish, Danio rerio. *Journal of Comparative Neurology*, *365*(1), 113–128. https://doi.org/10.1002/(SICI)1096-9861(19960129)365:1<113::AID-CNE9>3.0.CO;2-6

Haenggeli, C.-A., Pongstaporn, T., Doucet, J. R., & Ryugo, D. K. (2005). Projections from the spinal trigeminal nucleus to the cochlear nucleus in the rat. *Journal of Comparative Neurology*, *484*(2), 191–205. https://doi.org/10.1002/cne.20466

Hafidi, A. (1998). Peripherin-like immunoreactivity in type II spiral ganglion cell body and projections. *Brain Research*, *805*(1–2), 181–190. https://doi.org/10.1016/S0006-8993(98)00448-X

Hafidi, A., Després, G., & Romand, R. (1993). Ontogenesis of type II spiral ganglion neurons during development: Peripherin immunohistochemistry. *International Journal of Developmental Neuroscience*, *11*(4), 507–512. https://doi.org/10.1016/0736-5748(93)90024-8

Han, A. Y., Gupta, S., & Novitch, B. G. (2018). Molecular specification of facial branchial motor neurons in vertebrates. *Developmental Biology*, *436*(1), 5–13. https://doi.org/10.1016/J.YDBIO.2018.01.019

Harris, J. A., & Rubel, E. W. (2006). Afferent regulation of neuron number in the cochlear nucleus: Cellular and molecular analyses of a critical period. *Hearing Research*, *216–217*(1–2), 127–137. https://doi.org/10.1016/j.heares.2006.03.016

Hemond, S. G., & Morest, D. K. (1991). Ganglion formation from the otic placode and the otic crest in the chick embryo: Mitosis, migration, and the basal lamina. *Anatomy and Embryology*, *184*(1), 1–13. https://doi-org.ezp-prod1.hul.harvard.edu/10.1007/BF01744256

Hickman, T. T., Liberman, M. C., & Jacob, M. H. (2015). Adenomatous polyposis coli protein deletion in efferent olivocochlear neurons perturbs afferent synaptic maturation and reduces the dynamic range of hearing. *Journal of Neuroscience*, *35*(24), 9236–45. https://doi.org/10.1523/JNEUROSCI.4384-14.2015

Huang, E. J., Liu, W., Fritzsch, B., Bianchi, L. M., Reichardt, L. F., & Xiang, M. (2001). Brn3a is a transcriptional regulator of soma size, target field innervation and axon pathfinding of inner ear sensory neurons. *Development*, *128*(13), 2421–2432.

Huang, L.-C., Barclay, M., Lee, K., Peter, S., Housley, G. D., Thorne, P. R., & Montgomery, J. M. (2012). Synaptic profiles during neurite extension, refinement and retraction in the developing cochlea. *Neural Development*, *7*, 38. https://doi.org/10.1186/1749-8104-7-38

Huang, L.-C., Thorne, P. R., Housley, G. D., & Montgomery, J. M. (2007). Spatiotemporal definition of neurite outgrowth, refinement and retraction in the developing mouse cochlea. *Development*, *134*(16), 2925–2933. https://doi.org/10.1242/dev.001925

Isaac, J. T. R., Ashby, M., & McBain, C. J. (2007). The Role of the GluR2 Subunit in AMPA receptor function and synaptic plasticity. *Neuron*, *54*(6), 859–871. https://doi.org/10.1016/j.neuron.2007.06.001

Itoh, K., Kamiya, H., Mitani, A., Yasui, Y., Takada, M., & Mizuno, N. (1987). Direct projections from the dorsal column nuclei and the spinal trigeminal nuclei to the cochlear nuclei in the cat. *Brain Research*, *400*(1), 145–150. https://doi.org/10.1016/0006-8993(87)90662-7

Jahan, I., Kersigo, J., Pan, N., & Fritzsch, B. (2010). Neurod1 regulates survival and formation of connections in mouse ear and brain. *Cell and Tissue Research*, *341*(1), 95–110. https://doi.org/10.1007/s00441-010-0984-6

Jahan, I., Pan, N., Elliott, K. L., & Fritzsch, B. (2015). The quest for restoring hearing: Understanding ear development more completely. *BioEssays*, *37*(9), 1016–1027. https://doi.org/10.1002/bies.201500044

Jeon, E.-J., Xu, N., Xu, L., & Hansen, A. M. R. (2011). Influence of central glia on spiral ganglion neurite outgrowth. *Neuroscience*, *177*, 321–334. https://doi.org/10.1016/j.neuroscience.2011.01.014

Jing, Z., Rutherford, M. A., Takago, H., Frank, T., Fejtova, A., Khimich, D., . . . Strenzke, N. (2013). Disruption of the presynaptic cytomatrix protein bassoon degrades ribbon anchorage, multiquantal release, and sound encoding at the hair cell afferent synapse. *Journal of Neuroscience*, *33*(10), 4456–4467. https://doi.org/10.1523/JNEUROSCI.3491-12.2013

Johnson, S. L., Eckrich, T., Kuhn, S., Zampini, V., Franz, C., Ranatunga, K. M., . . . Marcotti, W. (2011). Position-dependent patterning of spontaneous action potentials in immature cochlear inner hair cells. *Nature Neuroscience*, *14*(6), 711–717. https://doi.org/10.1038/nn.2803

Johnson, S. L., Marcotti, W., & Kros, C. J. (2005). Increase in efficiency and reduction in Ca $^{2+}$ dependence of exocytosis during development of mouse inner hair cells. *Journal of Physiology*, *563*(1), 177–191. https://doi.org/10.1113/jphysiol.2004.074740

Johnson, S. L., Wedemeyer, C., Vetter, D. E., Adachi, R., Holley, M. C., Elgoyhen, A. B., & Marcotti, W. (2013). Cholinergic efferent synaptic transmission regulates the maturation of auditory hair cell ribbon synapses. *Open Biology*, *3*(11), 130–163. https://doi.org/10.1098/RSOB.130163

Jones, T. A., Leake, P. A., Snyder, R. L., Stakhovskaya, O., & Bonham, B. (2007). Spontaneous discharge patterns in cochlear spiral ganglion cells before the onset of hearing in cats. *Journal of Neurophysiology*, *98*(4), 1898–1908. https://doi.org/10.1152/jn.00472.2007

Kalluri, R., & Monges-Hernandez, M. (2017). Spatial gradients in the size of inner hair cell ribbons emerge before the onset of hearing in rats. *Journal of the Association for Research in Otolaryngology*, *18*(3), 399–413. https://doi.org/10.1007/s10162-017-0620-1

Kandler, K., Clause, A., & Noh, J. (2009). Tonotopic reorganization of developing auditory brainstem circuits. *Nature Neuroscience*. https://doi.org/10.1038/nn.2332

Karis, A., Pata, I., Van Doorninck, J. H., Grosveld, F., De Zeeuw, C. I., De Caprona, D., & Fritzsch, B. (2001). Transcription factor GATA-3 alters pathway selection of olivocochlear neurons and affects morphogenesis of the ear. *Journal of Comparative Neurology*, *429*(4), 615–630. https://doi.org/10.1002/1096-9861(20010122)429:4<615::AID-CNE8>3.0.CO;2-F

Kevetter, G. A., & Perachio, A. A. (1989). Projections from the sacculus to the cochlear nuclei in the mongolian gerbil. *Brain, Behavior and Evolution*, *34*(4), 193–200. https://doi.org/10.1159/000116505

Kiernan, A. E. (2013). Notch signaling during cell fate determination in the inner ear. *Seminars in Cell & Developmental Biology*, *24*(5), 470–479. https://doi.org/10.1016/j.semcdb.2013.04.002

Kim, K. X., & Rutherford, M. A. (2016). Maturation of NaV and KV channel topographies in the auditory nerve spike initiator before and after developmental onset of hearing function. *Journal of Neuroscience*, *36*(7), 2111–2118. https://doi.org/10.1523/JNEUROSCI.3437-15.2016

Knipper, M., Kopschall, I., Rohbock, K., Kopke, A. K. E., Bonk, I., Zimmermann, U., & Zenner, H. P. (1997). Transient expression of NMDA receptors during rearrangement of AMPA-receptor-expressing fibers in the developing inner ear. *Cell and Tissue Research*, *287*(1), 23–41. https://doi.org/10.1007/s004410050729

Koo, S. K., Hill, J. K., Hwang, C. H., Lin, Z. S., Millen, K. J., & Wu, D. K. (2009). Lmx1a maintains proper neurogenic, sensory, and non-sensory domains in the mammalian inner ear. *Developmental Biology*, *333*(1), 14–25. https://doi.org/10.1016/j.ydbio.2009.06.016

Koundakjian, E. J., Appler, J. L., & Goodrich, L. V. (2007). Auditory Neurons Make Stereotyped Wiring Decisions before Maturation of Their Targets. *Journal of Neuroscience*, *27*(51), 14078–14088. https://doi.org/10.1523/JNEUROSCI.3765-07.2007

Kujawa, S. G., & Liberman, M. C. (1997). Conditioning-related protection from acoustic injury: Effects of Chronic Deefferentation and Sham Surgery. *Journal of Neurophysiology*, *78*(6), 3095–3106. https://doi.org/10.1152/jn.1997.78.6.3095

Lawoko-Kerali, G., Rivolta, M. N., & Holley, M. (2002). Expression of the transcription factors GATA3 and Pax2 during development of the mammalian inner ear. *Journal of Comparative Neurology*, *442*(4), 378–391. https://doi.org/10.1002/cne.10088

Leake, P. A., Hradek, G. T., Chair, L., & Snyder, R. L. (2006). Neonatal deafness results in degraded topographic specificity of auditory nerve projections to the cochlear nucleus in cats. *Journal of Comparative Neurology*, *497*(1), 13–31. https://doi.org/10.1002/cne.20968

Lenoir, M., Shnerson, A., & Pujol, R. (1980). Cochlear receptor development in the rat with emphasis on synaptogenesis. *Anatomy and Embryology*, *160*(3), 253–262. https://doi.org/10.1007/BF00305106

Liang, J. K., Bok, J., & Wu, D. K. (2010). Distinct contributions from the hindbrain and mesenchyme to inner ear morphogenesis. *Developmental Biology*, *337*(2), 324–334. https://doi.org/10.1016/j.ydbio.2009.11.001

Liberman, L. D., & Liberman, M. C. (2016). Postnatal maturation of auditory-nerve heterogeneity, as seen in spatial gradients of synapse morphology in the inner hair cell area. *Hearing Research*, *339*, 12–22. https://doi.org/10.1016/J.HEARES.2016.06.002

Liberman, L. D., Wang, H., & Liberman, M. C. (2011). Opposing gradients of ribbon size and AMPA receptor expression underlie sensitivity differences among cochlear-nerve/hair-cell synapses. *Journal of Neuroscience*, *31*(3), 801–808. https://doi.org/10.1523/JNEUROSCI.3389-10.2011

Liberman, M. C. (1980a). Efferent synapses in the inner hair cell area of the cat cochlea: An electron microscopic study of serial sections. *Hearing Research*, *3*(3), 189–204.

Liberman, M. C. (1980b). Morphological differences among radial afferent fibers in the cat cochlea: An electron-microscopic study of serial sections. *Hearing Research*, *3*(1), 45–63.

Liberman, M. C. (1991). Central projections of auditory-nerve fibers of differing spontaneous rate. I. Anteroventral cochlear nucleus. *Journal of Comparative Neurology*, *313*(2), 240–258. https://doi.org/10.1002/cne.903130205

Liberman, M. C. (1993). Central projections of auditory nerve fibers of differing spontaneous rate, II: Posteroventral and dorsal cochlear nuclei. *Journal of Comparative Neurology*, *327*(1), 17–36. https://doi.org/10.1002/cne.903270103

Liberman, M. C., O'Grady, D. F., Dodds, L. W., Mcgee, J., & Walsh, E. J. (2000). Afferent innervation of outer and inner hair cells is normal in neonatally de-efferented cats. *Journal of Comparative Neurology*, *423*(1), 132–139. https://doi.org/10.1002/1096-9861(20000717)423:1<132::AID-CNE11>3.0.CO;2-7

Lilleväli, K., Haugas, M., Matilainen, T., Pussinen, C., Karis, A., & Salminen, M. (2006). Gata3 is required for early morphogenesis and Fgf10 expression during otic development. *Mechanisms of Development, 123*(6), 415–429. https://doi.org/10.1016/j.mod.2006.04.007

Lilleväli, K., Matilainen, T., Karis, A., & Salminen, M. (2004). Partially overlapping expression of Gata2 and Gata3 during inner ear development. *Developmental Dynamics, 231*(4), 775–781. https://doi.org/10.1002/dvdy.20185

Limb, C. J., & Ryugo, D. K. (2000). Development of primary axosomatic endings in the anteroventral cochlear nucleus of mice. *Journal of the Association for Research Otolaryngology, 1*(2), 103–119. https://doi.org/10.1007/s101620010032

Liu, Q., Lee, E., & Davis, R. L. (2014). Heterogeneous intrinsic excitability of murine spiral ganglion neurons is determined by Kv1 and HCN channels. *Neuroscience, 257*, 96–110. https://doi.org/10.1016/j.neuroscience.2013.10.065

Liu, W., & Davis, R. L. (2014). Calretinin and calbindin distribution patterns specify subpopulations of type I and type II spiral ganglion neurons in postnatal murine cochlea. *Journal of Comparative Neurology, 522*(10), 2299–2318. https://doi.org/10.1002/cne.23535

Lu, C. C., Appler, J. M., Houseman, E. A., & Goodrich, L. V. (2011). Developmental Profiling of Spiral Ganglion Neurons Reveals Insights into Auditory Circuit Assembly. *Journal of Neuroscience, 31*(30), 10903–10918. https://doi.org/10.1523/JNEUROSCI.2358-11.2011

Lu, C. C., Cao, X. J., Wright, S., Ma, L., Oertel, D., & Goodrich, L. V. (2014). Mutation of Npr2 Leads to Blurred Tonotopic Organization of Central Auditory Circuits in Mice. *PLoS Genetics, 10*(12). https://doi.org/10.1371/journal.pgen.1004823

Luo, X. J., Deng, M., Xie, X., Huang, L., Wang, H., Jiang, L., . . . Gan, L. (2013). GATA3 controls the specification of prosensory domain and neuronal survival in the mouse cochlea. *Human Molecular Genetics, 22*(18), 3609–3623. https://doi.org/10.1093/hmg/ddt212

Ma, Q., Anderson, D. J., & Fritzsch, B. (2000). Neurogenin 1 null mutant ears develop fewer, morphologically normal hair cells in smaller sensory epithelia devoid of innervation. *Journal of the Association for Research in Otolaryngology, 1*(2), 129–43. https://doi-org.ezp-prod1.hul.harvard.edu/10.1007/s101620010017

Ma, Q., Chen, Z., del Barco Barrantes, I., de la Pompa, J. L., & Anderson, D. J. (1998). neurogenin1 is essential for the determination of neuronal precursors for proximal cranial sensory ganglia. *Neuron, 20*(3), 469–482. https://doi.org/10.1016/S0896-6273(00)80988-5

Mao, Y., Reiprich, S., Wegner, M., & Fritzsch, B. (2014). Targeted deletion of Sox10 by Wnt1-cre defects neuronal migration and projection in the mouse inner ear. *PLoS ONE, 9*(4), e94580. https://doi.org/10.1371/journal.pone.0094580

Marcotti, W., Johnson, S. L., Holley, M. C., & Kros, C. J. (2003). Developmental changes in the expression of potassium currents of embryonic, neonatal and mature mouse inner hair cells. *Journal of Physiology, 548*(2), 383–400. https://doi.org/10.1113/jphysiol.2002.034801

Maricich, S. M., Xia, A., Mathes, E. L., Wang, V. Y., Oghalai, J. S., Fritzsch, B., & Zoghbi, H. Y. (2009). Atoh1-lineal neurons are required for hearing and for the survival of neurons in the spiral ganglion and brainstem accessory auditory nuclei. *Journal of Neuroscience, 29*(36), 11123–11133. https://doi.org/10.1523/JNEUROSCI.2232-09.2009

Marrs, G. S., & Spirou, G. A. (2012). Embryonic assembly of auditory circuits: Spiral ganglion and brainstem. *Journal of Physiology, 590*(10), 2391–2408. https://doi.org/10.1113/jphysiol.2011.226886

Martin, M. R., & Rickets, C. (1981). Histogenesis of the cochlear nucleus of the mouse. *Journal of Comparative Neurology, 197*(1), 169–184. https://doi.org/10.1002/cne.901970113

Martinez-Monedero, R., Liu, C., Weisz, C., Vyas, P., Fuchs, P. A., & Glowatzki, E. (2016). GluA2-containing AMPA receptors distinguish ribbon-associated from ribbonless afferent contacts on rat cochlear hair cells. *eNeuro*, *3*(2). https://doi.org/10.1523/ENEURO.0078-16.2016

Matei, V., Pauley, S., Kaing, S., Rowitch, D., Beisel, K. W., Morris, K., . . . Fritzsch, B. (2005). Smaller inner ear sensory epithelia in Neurog1 null mice are related to earlier hair cell cycle exit. *Developmental Dynamics*, *234*(3), 633–650. https://doi.org/10.1002/dvdy.20551

Meyer, A. C., Frank, T., Khimich, D., Hoch, G., Riedel, D., Chapochnikov, N. M., . . . Moser, T. (2009). Tuning of synapse number, structure and function in the cochlea. *Nature Neuroscience*, *12*(4), 444–453. https://doi.org/10.1038/nn.2293

Miko, I. J., Nakamura, P. A., Henkemeyer, M., & Cramer, K. S. (2007). Auditory brainstem neural activation patterns are altered in EphA4- and ephrin-B2-deficient mice. *Journal of Comparative Neurology*, *505*(6), 669–681. https://doi.org/10.1002/cne.21530

Molea, D., & Rubel, E. W. (2003). Timing and topography of nucleus magnocellularis innervation by the cochlear ganglion. *The Journal of Comparative Neurology*, *466*(4), 577–591. https://doi.org/10.1002/cne.10896

Morris, J. K., Maklad, A., Hansen, L. A., Feng, F., Sorensen, C., Lee, K. F., . . . Fritzsch, B. (2006). A disorganized innervation of the inner ear persists in the absence of ErbB2. *Brain Research*, *1091*(1), 186–199. https://doi.org/10.1016/j.brainres.2006.02.090

Morsli, H., Choo, D., Ryan, A., Johnson, R., & Wu, D. K. (1998). Development of the mouse inner ear and origin of its sensory organs. *Journal of Neuroscience*, *18*(9), 3327–3335. https://doi.org/10.1523/JNEUROSCI.18-09-03327.1998

Mostafapour, S. P., Cochran, S. L., Del Puerto, N. M., & Rubel, E. W. (2000). Patterns of cell death in mouse anteroventral cochlear nucleus neurons after unilateral cochlea removal. *Journal of Comparative Neurology*, *426*(4), 561–571. https://doi.org/10.1002/1096-9861(20001030)426:4<561::AID-CNE5>3.0.CO;2-G

Muniak, M. A., Rivas, A., Montey, K. L., May, B. J., Francis, H. W., & Ryugo, D. K. (2013). 3D model of frequency representation in the cochlear nucleus of the CBA/J mouse. *Journal of Comparative Neurology*, *521*(7), 1510–1532. https://doi.org/10.1002/cne.23238

Nemzou, R. M., Bulankina, A. V., Khimich, D., Giese, A., & Moser, T. (2006). Synaptic organization in cochlear inner hair cells deficient for the CaV1.3 (α1D) subunit of L-type Ca^{2+} channels. *Neuroscience*, *141*(4), 1849–1860. https://doi.org/10.1016/J.NEUROSCIENCE.2006.05.057

Nichols, D. H., Pauley, S., Jahan, I., Beisel, K. W., Millen, K. J., & Fritzsch, B. (2008). Lmx1a is required for segregation of sensory epithelia and normal ear histogenesis and morphogenesis. *Cell and Tissue Research*, *334*(3), 339–358. https://doi.org/10.1007/s00441-008-0709-2

Nishimura, K., Noda, T., & Dabdoub, A. (2017). Dynamic expression of Sox2, Gata3, and Prox1 during primary auditory neuron development in the mammalian cochlea. *PLoS ONE*, *12*(1), e0170568. https://doi.org/10.1371/journal.pone.0170568

Ohlrogge, M., Doucet, J. R., & Ryugo, D. K. (2001). Projections of the pontine nuclei to the cochlear nucleus in rats. *Journal of Comparative Neurology*, *436*(3), 290–303. https://doi.org/10.1002/cne.1068

Oleskevich, S., & Walmsley, B. (2002). Synaptic transmission in the auditory brainstem of normal and congenitally deaf mice. *Journal of Physiology*, *540*(2), 447–455. https://doi.org/10.1113/jphysiol.2001.013821

O'Neil, J. N., Limb, C. J., Baker, C. A., & Ryugo, D. K. (2010). Bilateral effects of unilateral cochlear implantation in congenitally deaf cats. *Journal of Comparative Neurology*, *518*(12), 2382–2404. https://doi.org/10.1002/cne.22339

Pliss, L., Yang, H., & Xu-Friedman, M. a. (2009). Context-dependent effects of NMDA receptors on precise timing information at the endbulb of Held in the cochlear nucleus. *Journal of Neurophysiology, 102*(5), 2627–2637. https://doi.org/10.1152/jn.00111.2009

Raft, S., Koundakjian, E. J., Quinones, H., Jayasena, C. S., Goodrich, L. V., Johnson, J. E., . . . Groves, A. K. (2007). Cross-regulation of Ngn1 and Math1 coordinates the production of neurons and sensory hair cells during inner ear development. *Development, 134*(24), 4405–15. https://doi.org/10.1242/dev.009118

Reijntjes, D. O. J., & Pyott, S. J. (2016). The afferent signaling complex: Regulation of type I spiral ganglion neuron responses in the auditory periphery. *Hearing Research, 336*, 1–16. https://doi.org/10.1016/j.heares.2016.03.011

Riccomagno, M. M., Takada, S., & Epstein, D. J. (2005). Wnt-dependent regulation of inner ear morphogenesis is balanced by the opposing and supporting roles of Shh. *Genes and Development, 19*(13), 1612–1623. https://doi.org/10.1101/gad.1303905

Riley, B. B. (2003). Genes controlling the development of the zebrafish inner ear and hair cells. *Current Topics in Developmental Biology, 57*, 357–388. https://doi.org/10.1016/S0070-2153(03)57012-0

Rivolta, M. N., & Holley, M. C. (1998). GATA3 is downregulated during hair cell differentiation in the mouse cochlea. *Journal of Neurocytology, 27*(9), 637–647. https://doi.org/10.1023/A:1006951813063

Romand, R., & Romand, M. R. (1985). Qualitative and quantitative observations of spiral ganglion development in the rat. *Hearing Research, 18*(2), 111–120. https://doi.org/10.1016/0378-5955(85)90002-4

Ruben, R. J. (1967). Development of the inner ear of the mouse: a radioautographic study of terminal mitoses. *Acta Oto-Laryngologica*, Suppl. 220,1–44.

Ryan, A. F., Schwartz, I. R., Helfert, R. H., Keithley, E., & Wang, Z.-X. (1987). Selective retrograde labeling of lateral olivocochlear neurons in the brainstem based on preferential uptake of3H-D-aspartic acid in the cochlea. *Journal of Comparative Neurology, 255*(4), 606–616. https://doi.org/10.1002/cne.902550411

Ryugo, D. K. (2008). Projections of low spontaneous rate, high threshold auditory nerve fibers to the small cell cap of the cochlear nucleus in cats. *Neuroscience, 154*(1), 114–126. https://doi.org/10.1016/j.neuroscience.2007.10.052

Ryugo, D. K., & May, S. K. (1993). The projections of intracellularly labeled auditory nerve fibers to the dorsal cochlear nucleus of cats. *Journal of Comparative Neurology, 329*(1), 20–35. https://doi.org/10.1002/cne.903290103

Ryugo, D. K., Montey, K. L., Wright, A. L., Bennett, M. L., & Pongstaporn, T. (2006). Postnatal development of a large auditory nerve terminal: The endbulb of Held in cats. *Hearing Research, 216–217*, 100–115. https://doi.org/10.1016/j.heares.2006.01.007

Ryugo, D. K., & Sento, S. (1991). Synaptic connections of the auditory nerve in cats: Relationship between endbulbs of held and spherical bushy cells. *Journal of Comparative Neurology, 305*(1), 35–48. https://doi.org/10.1002/cne.903050105

Ryugo, D. K., Wu, M. M., & Pongstaporn, T. (1996). Activity-related features of synapse morphology: A study of endbulbs of Held. *Journal of Comparative Neurology, 365*(1), 141–158. https://doi.org/10.1002/(SICI)1096-9861(19960129)365:1<141::AID-CNE11>3.0.CO;2-T

Sanchez, J. T., Ghelani, S., & Otto-Meyer, S. (2015). From development to disease: Diverse functions of NMDA-type glutamate receptors in the lower auditory pathway. *Neuroscience, 285*, 248–259. https://doi.org/10.1016/j.neuroscience.2014.11.027

Sanchez, J. T., Wang, Y., Rubel, E. W., & Barria, A. (2010). Development of Glutamatergic Synaptic Transmission in Binaural Auditory Neurons. *Journal of Neurophysiology, 104*(3), 1774–1789. https://doi.org/10.1152/jn.00468.2010

Sandell, L. L., Butler Tjaden, N. E., Barlow, A. J., & Trainor, P. A. (2014). Cochleovestibular nerve development is integrated with migratory neural crest cells. *Developmental Biology, 385*, 200–210. https://doi.org/10.1016/j.ydbio.2013.11.009

Sando, I. (1965). The anatomical interrelationships of the cochlear nerve fibers. *Acta Oto-Laryngologica, 59*(2–6), 417–436.

Sanes, J. R., & Yamagata, M. (2009). Many Paths to Synaptic Specificity. *Annual Review of Cell and Developmental Biology, 25*(1), 161–195. https://doi.org/10.1146/annurev.cellbio.24.110707.175402

Sapède, D., Dyballa, S., & Pujades, C. (2012). Cell lineage analysis reveals three different progenitor pools for neurosensory elements in the otic vesicle. *Journal of Neuroscience, 32*(46), 16424–16434. https://doi.org/10.1523/JNEUROSCI.3686-12.2012

Satoh, T., & Fekete, D. M. (2005). Clonal analysis of the relationships between mechanosensory cells and the neurons that innervate them in the chicken ear. *Development, 132*(7), 1687–1697. https://doi.org/10.1242/dev.01730

Schmidt, H., & Rathjen, F. G. (2010). Signalling mechanisms regulating axonal branching in vivo. *BioEssays, 32*(11), 977–985. https://doi.org/10.1002/bies.201000054

Schmidt, H., Stonkute, A., Jüttner, R., Schäffer, S., Buttgereit, J., Feil, R., . . . Rathjen, F. G. (2007). The receptor guanylyl cyclase Npr2 is essential for sensory axon bifurcation within the spinal cord. *Journal of Cell Biology, 179*(2), 331–340. https://doi.org/10.1083/jcb.200707176

Schmidt, H., Werner, M., Heppenstall, P. A., Henning, M., Moré, M. I., Kühbandner, S., . . . Rathjen, F. G. (2002). cGMP-mediated signaling via cGKIalpha is required for the guidance and connectivity of sensory axons. *Journal of Cell Biology, 159*(3), 489–498. https://doi.org/10.1083/jcb.200207058

Sendin, G., Bulankina, A. V., Riedel, D., & Moser, T. (2007). Maturation of ribbon synapses in hair cells is driven by thyroid hormone. *Journal of Neuroscience, 27*(12), 3163–3173. https://doi.org/10.1523/JNEUROSCI.3974-06.2007

Sewell, W. F. (2011). Pharmacology and neurochemistry of olivocochlear efferents. In *Auditory and Vestibular Efferents* (pp. 83–101). https://doi.org/10.1007/978-1-59745-523-7

Sheets, L., Trapai, J. G., Mo, W., Obholzer, N., & Nicolson, T. (2011). Ribeye is required for presynaptic CaV1.3a channel localization and afferent innervation of sensory hair cells. *Development, 138*, 1309–1319. https://doi.org/10.1242/dev.059451

Sher, A. E. (1971). The embryonic and postnatal development of the inner ear of the mouse. *Acta Oto-Laryngologica, 285*, 1–77.

Shnerson, A., Devigne, C., & Pujol, R. (1981). Age-related changes in the C57BL/6J mouse cochlea. II. Ultrastructural findings. *Developmental Brain Research, 2*(1), 77–88. https://doi.org/10.1016/0165-3806(81)90060-2

Siddiqui, S. A., & Cramer, K. S. (2005). Differential expression of Eph receptors and ephrins in the cochlear ganglion and eighth cranial nerve of the chick embryo. *Journal of Comparative Neurology, 482*(4), 309–319. https://doi.org/10.1002/cne.20396

Simmons, D. D. (1994). A transient afferent innervation of outer hair cells in the postnatal cochlea. *Neuroreport, 5*(11), 1309–1312. https://doi.org/10.1097/00001756-199406270-00003

Simmons, D. D. (2002). Development of the inner ear efferent system across vertebrate species. *Journal of Neurobiology, 53*(2), 228–250. https://doi.org/10.1002/neu.10130

Sitko, A., & Mason C. (2015). Organization of axons in their tracts. In K. Rockland (Ed.), *Axons and Brain Architecture* (1st ed., pp. 267–288). Amsterdam: Academic Press.

Snyder, R. L., & Leake, P. A. (1997). Topography of spiral ganglion projections to cochlear nucleus during postnatal development in cats. *Journal of Comparative Neurology*, *384*(2), 293–311. https://doi.org/10.1002/(SICI)1096-9861(19970728)384:2<293::AID-CNE9>3.0.CO;2-X

Sobkowicz, H. M., Rose, J. E., Scott, G. L., & Levenick, C. V. (1986). Distribution of synaptic ribbons in the developing organ of Corti. *Journal of Neurocytology*, *15*(6), 693–714. https://doi.org/10.1007/bf01625188

Sobkowicz, H. M., Rose, J. E., Scott, G. E., & Slapnick, S. M. (1982). Ribbon synapses in the developing intact and cultured organ of Corti in the mouse. *Journal of Neuroscience*, *2*(7), 942–957. https://doi.org/10.1523/JNEUROSCI.02-07-00942.1982

Streeter, G. L. (1906). On the development of the membranous labyrinth and the acoustic and facial nerves in the human embryo. *American Journal of Anatomy*, *6*(1), 139–165. https://doi.org/10.1002/aja.1000060103

Ter-Avetisyan, G., Rathjen, F. G., & Schmidt, H. (2014). Bifurcation of axons from cranial sensory neurons is disabled in the absence of Npr2-induced cGMP signaling. *Journal of Neuroscience*, *34*(3), 737–747. https://doi.org/10.1523/JNEUROSCI.4183-13.2014

Tong, L., Strong, M. K., Kaur, T., Juiz, J. M., Oesterle, E. C., Hume, C., . . . Rubel, E. W. (2015). Selective Deletion of Cochlear Hair Cells Causes Rapid Age-Dependent Changes in Spiral Ganglion and Cochlear Nucleus Neurons. *Journal of Neuroscience*, *35*(20), 7878–7891. https://doi.org/10.1523/JNEUROSCI.2179-14.2015

Tritsch, N. X., & Bergles, D. E. (2010). Developmental Regulation of Spontaneous Activity in the Mammalian Cochlea. *Journal of Neuroscience*, *30*(4), 1539–1550. https://doi.org/10.1523/JNEUROSCI.3875-09.2010

Tritsch, N. X., Rodríguez-Contreras, A., Crins, T. T. H., Wang, H. C., Borst, J. G. G., & Bergles, D. E. (2010). Calcium action potentials in hair cells pattern auditory neuron activity before hearing onset. *Nature Neuroscience*, *13*(9), 1050–1052. https://doi.org/10.1038/nn.2604

Tritsch, N. X., Yi, E., Gale, J. E., Glowatzki, E., & Bergles, D. E. (2007). The origin of spontaneous activity in the developing auditory system. *Nature*, *450*(7166), 50–55. https://doi.org/10.1038/nature06233

Uziel, A., Romand, R., & Marot, M. (1981). Development of cochlear potentials in rats. *International Journal of Audiology*, *20*(2), 89–100. https://doi.org/10.3109/00206098109072687

Volkenstein, S., Oshima, K., Sinkkonen, S. T., Corrales, C. E., Most, S. P., Chai, R., . . . Heller, S. (2013). Transient, afferent input-dependent, postnatal niche for neural progenitor cells in the cochlear nucleus. *Proceedings of the National Academy of Sciences of the United States of America*, *110*(35), 14456–14461. https://doi.org/10.1073/pnas.1307376110

Vyas, P., Wu, J. S., Zimmerman, A., Fuchs, P., & Glowatzki, E. (2017). Tyrosine hydroxylase expression in type ii cochlear afferents in mice. *Journal of the Association for Research in Otolaryngology*, *18*(1), 139–151. https://doi.org/10.1007/s10162-016-0591-7

Wang, H. C., & Bergles, D. E. (2015). Spontaneous activity in the developing auditory system. *Cell and Tissue Research*. https://doi.org/10.1007/s00441-014-2007-5

Wang, H. C., Lin, C.-C., Cheung, R., Ellis-Davies, G., Rock, J., Bergles, D. E., . . . Agarwal, A. (2015). Spontaneous activity of cochlear hair cells triggered by fluid secretion mechanism in adjacent support cells. *Cell*, *163*, 1348–1359. https://doi.org/10.1016/j.cell.2015.10.070

Wang, J., Mark, S., Zhang, X., Qian, D., Yoo, S.-J., Radde-Gallwitz, K., . . . Chen, P. (2005). Regulation of polarized extension and planar cell polarity in the cochlea by the vertebrate PCP pathway. *Nature Genetics*, *37*(9), 980–985. https://doi.org/10.1038/ng1622

Wang, Y. X., Wenthold, R. J., Ottersen, O. P., & Petralia, R. S. (1998). Endbulb synapses in the anteroventral cochlear nucleus express a specific subset of AMPA-type glutamate receptor subunits. *Journal of Neuroscience*, *18*(3), 1148–1160. https://doi.org/10.1523/JNEUROSCI.18-03-01148.1998

Weedman, D. L., & Ryugo, D. K. (1996). Projections from auditory-cortex to the cochlear nucleus in rats - synapses on granule cell dendrites. *Journal of Comparative Neurology*, *371*(2), 311–324. https://doi.org/10.1002/(SICI)1096-9861(19960722)371:2<311::AID-CNE10>3.0.CO;2-V

Weinberg, R. J., & Rustioni, A. (1987). A cuneocochlear pathway in the rat. *Neuroscience*, *20*(1), 209–219. https://doi.org/10.1016/0306-4522(87)90013-3

Whitlon, D. S., Tieu, D., Grover, M., Reilly, B., & Coulson, A. M. T. (2009). Spontaneous association of glial cells with regrowing neurites in mixed cultures of dissociated spiral ganglia. *Neuroscience*, *161*, 227–235. https://doi.org/10.1016/j.neuroscience.2009.03.044

Wong, A. B., Jing, Z., Rutherford, M. A., Frank, T., Strenzke, N., & Moser, T. (2013). Concurrent maturation of inner hair cell synaptic Ca^{2+} influx and auditory nerve spontaneous activity around hearing onset in mice. *Journal of Neuroscience*, *33*(26), 10661–10666. https://doi.org/10.1523/JNEUROSCI.1215-13.2013

Wong, A. B., Rutherford, M. A., Gabrielaitis, M., Pangršič, T., Göttfert, F., Frank, T., . . . Moser, T. (2014). Developmental refinement of hair cell synapses tightens the coupling of Ca2+ influx to exocytosis. *EMBO Journal*, *33*(3), 247–264. https://doi.org/10.1002/embj.201387110

Wong, E. Y. M., Ahmed, M., & Xu, P.-X. (2013). EYA1-SIX1 complex in neurosensory cell fate induction in the mammalian inner ear. *Hearing Research*, *297*, 13–19. https://doi.org/10.1016/j.heares.2012.09.009

Wright, D. D., & Ryugo, D. K. (1996). Mossy fiber projections from the cuneate nucleus to the cochlear nucleus in the rat. *Journal of Comparative Neurology*, *365*(1), 159–172. https://doi.org/10.1002/(SICI)1096-9861(19960129)365:1<159::AID-CNE12>3.0.CO;2-L

Wright, T., Gillespie, L. N., O'Leary, S. J., & Needham, K. (2016). Firing frequency and entrainment maintained in primary auditory neurons in the presence of combined BDNF and NT3. *Scientific Reports*, *6*. https://doi.org/10.1038/srep28584

Wu, J. S., Young, E. D., & Glowatzki, E. (2016). Maturation of spontaneous firing properties after hearing onset in rat auditory nerve fibers: Spontaneous rates, refractoriness, and interfiber correlations. *Journal of Neuroscience*, *36*(41), 10584–10597. https://doi.org/10.1523/JNEUROSCI.1187-16.2016

Yang, T., Kersigo, J., Jahan, I., Pan, N., & Fritzsch, B. (2011). The molecular basis of making spiral ganglion neurons and connecting them to hair cells of the organ of Corti. *Hearing Research*, *278*(1–2), 21–33. https://doi.org/10.1016/J.HEARES.2011.03.002

Yashiro, K., & Philpot, B. D. (2008). Regulation of NMDA receptor subunit expression and its implications for LTD, LTP, and metaplasticity. *Neuropharmacology*, *55*(7), 1081–1094. https://doi.org/S0028-3908(08)00312-2 [pii]\r10.1016/j.neuropharm.2008.07.046

Ye, Y., Machado, D. G., & Kim, D. O. (2000). Projection of the marginal shell of the anteroventral cochlear nucleus to olivocochlear neurons in the cat. *Journal of Comparative Neurology*, *420*(1), 127–138. https://doi.org/10.1002/(SICI)1096-9861(20000424)420:1<127::AID-CNE9>3.0.CO;2-7

Yin, Y., Liberman, L. D., Maison, S. F., & Liberman, M. C. (2014). Olivocochlear innervation maintains the normal modiolar-pillar and habenular-cuticular gradients in cochlear synaptic morphology. *Journal of the Association for Research in Otolaryngology*, *15*(4), 571–583. https://doi.org/10.1007/s10162-014-0462-z

Yu, W.-M., Appler, J. M., Kim, Y.-H., Nishitani, A. M., Holt, J. R., & Goodrich, L. V. (2013). A Gata3–Mafb transcriptional network directs post-synaptic differentiation in synapses specialized for hearing. *eLife*, *2*, e01341. https://doi.org/10.7554/eLife.01341

Yu, W.-M., & Goodrich, L. V. (2014). Morphological and physiological development of auditory synapses. *Hearing Research*. https://doi.org/10.1016/j.heares.2014.01.007

Zhan, X., Pongstaporn, T., & Ryugo, D. K. (2006). Projections of the second cervical dorsal root ganglion to the cochlear nucleus in rats. *Journal of Comparative Neurology*, *496*(3), 335–48. https://doi.org/10.1002/cne.20917

Zhan, X., & Ryugo, D. K. (2007). Projections of the lateral reticular nucleus to the cochlear nucleus in rats. *Journal of Comparative Neurology*, *504*(5), 583–598. https://doi.org/10.1002/cne.21463

Zhang-Hooks, Y., Agarwal, A., Mishina, M., & Bergles, D. E. (2016). NMDA receptors enhance spontaneous activity and promote neuronal survival in the developing cochlea. *Neuron*, *89*(2), 337–350. https://doi.org/10.1016/j.neuron.2015.12.016

Zhou, C. Q., Lee, J., Henkemeyer, M. J., & Lee, K. H. (2011). Disruption of ephrin B/Eph B interaction results in abnormal cochlear innervation patterns. Laryngoscope, *121*(7), 1541–1547. https://doi.org/10.1002/lary.21861

CHAPTER 2

THE DIVERSIFIED FORM AND FUNCTION OF COCHLEAR AFFERENTS

PAUL ALBERT FUCHS

Abstract

Cochlear afferents differ in form and function. The great majority are type I, large diameter, myelinated neurons that contact a single inner hair cell to transmit acoustic information. Each inner hair cell is presynaptic to a pool of 10–30 type I afferents, among which spontaneous activity and acoustic threshold vary widely. Variation in the number, voltage-gating, and density of L-type calcium channels at each presynaptic active zone (ribbon) may dictate this functional diversity. Despite contacting large numbers of outer hair cells, the scarce, unmyelinated type II afferents are acoustically *in*sensitive, and only weakly depolarized by outer hair cell transmitter release. However, type II afferents respond strongly to adenosine triphosphate released by cochlear tissue damage, providing a biological basis for painful hearing (noxacusis).

Keywords: cochlea, type I afferent, type II afferent, ribbon synapse, inner hair cell, outer hair cell, acoustic threshold, adenosine triphosphate (ATP), noxacusis, hyperacusis

EARLY neuroanatomists captured the exquisitely patterned innervation of the cochlea (Figure 2.1) and discussed the implications for functional diversity (Lorente de No, 1937). Certainly this innervation pattern determines the frequency selectivity of each type I cochlear afferent as it matures to contact a single inner hair cell (IHC) along the tonotopic gradient of the cochlea. Additional diversification in activity patterns and acoustic sensitivity correlates with the form and function of each synaptic contact on the IHC. Beyond these quantitative differences among type I afferents, the type II afferents are qualitatively distinct, with extensive arbors that spread hundreds of microns toward the cochlear base, giving off branches to dozens of outer hair cells. These smaller caliber, unmyelinated afferents are poorly, if at all, sensitive to sound, but can be activated

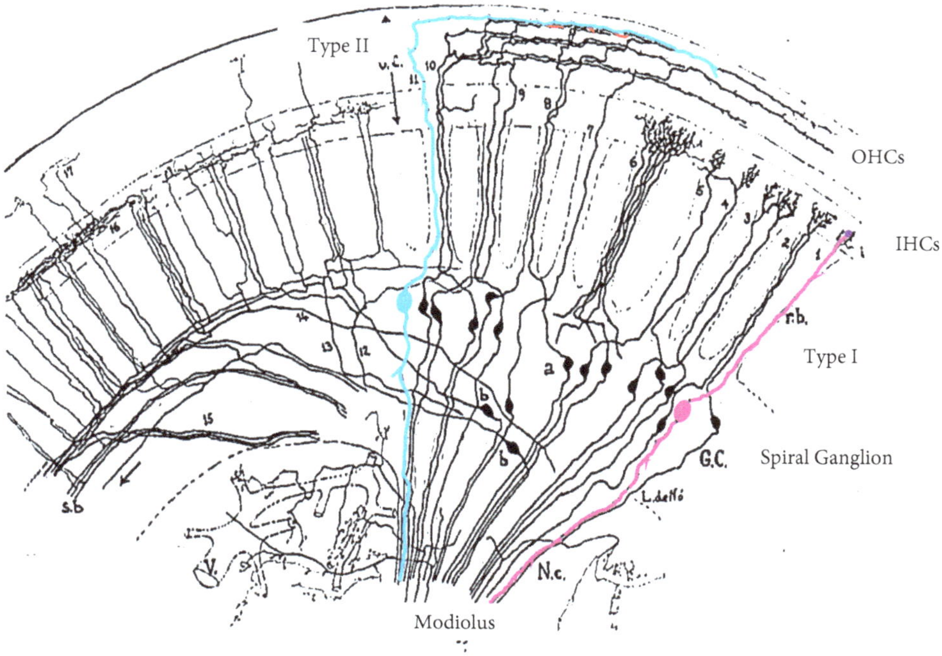

FIGURE 2.1. Drawing of cochlear innervation based on Golgi impregnation in young rat (6–7 days) cochlea. Modified from (Lorente de No, 1937). Type II afferents highlighted in light blue. Type I afferent highlighted in magenta. Type I afferents reduce to a single terminal contact in adult.

strongly by tissue damage. The synaptic determinants of functional diversity among type I afferents and the much greater differences between type I and type II afferents will serve as the focus for this chapter. Details of type I afferent acoustic responses and guidance to the original literature can be found in previous reviews and chapters (e.g., Ruggero, 1992; Young, 2008).

Type I Cochlear Afferents

Myelinated, large caliber type I spiral ganglion neurons (SGNs) constitute 95% of cochlear afferents (Spoendlin, 1972). These bipolar neurons have a cell body in the spiral ganglion within Rosenthal's Canal, with a peripheral process that contacts a single IHC, and a central axon that projects through the modiolus to the cochlear nuclei of the brainstem (Ryugo & Parks, 2003). Decades of research has thoroughly documented the acoustic response properties of type I neurons, and have shown that these can account for the sensitive frequency selectivity of the organism (Young, 2008). Additional features like phase-locking of afferent firing are essential for higher order computations involved in sound localization (Middlebrooks, 2015). Frequency selectivity can be determined by a tuning curve whereby pure tones of different intensity and frequency are used to establish the best (lowest intensity) or characteristic frequency for an individual type I SGN during single unit recording in the VIIIth nerve (Figure 2.2).

Each individual inner hair cell is the sole presynaptic partner of 10 to 30 type I afferents. Thus, this group of afferents will have identical frequency tuning. However, type I afferents differ widely in their acoustic sensitivity and dynamic range (the difference between threshold and saturated sound levels). These differences in acoustic response correlate with their rate of spontaneous activity in the absence of sound (M.C. Liberman, 1978; Sachs & Abbas, 1974; Schmiedt, 1989). Acoustically

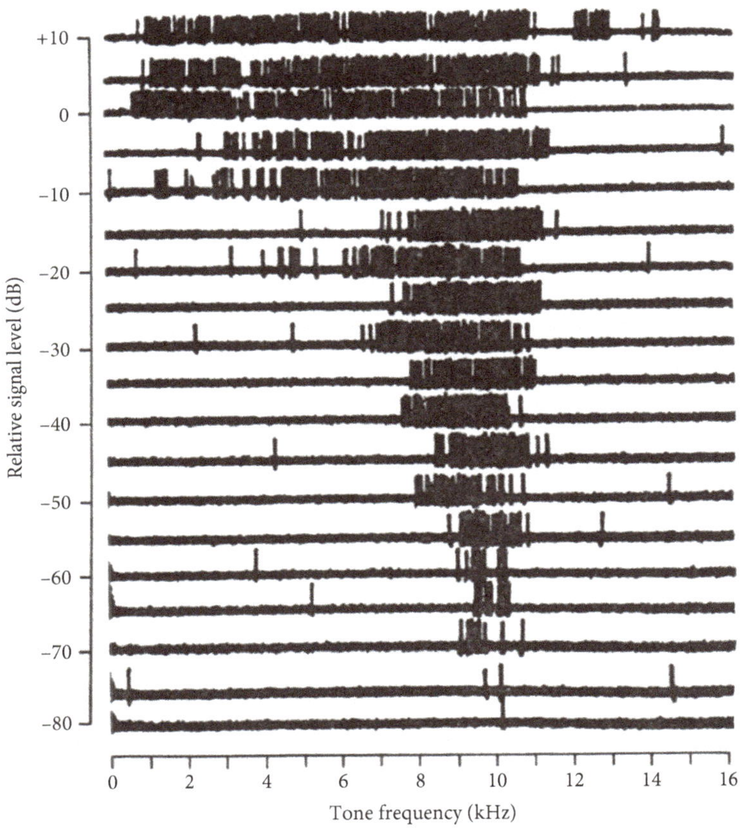

FIGURE 2.2. Constant intensity frequency sweep stimuli were used to determine the selectivity and sensitivity of a single auditory nerve fiber in the guinea pig. Action potentials (vertical ticks) occur at a particular time point, corresponding to a particular frequency during the sweep (on the x-axis). The characteristic frequency (cf) is that which elicits action potentials at the lowest intensity—10 kHz in this example. As intensity rises, action potentials are driven by a wider band of frequencies.

Modified from (Evans, 1972).

sensitive type I afferents with a narrow dynamic range have high rates of spontaneous activity—"high-spont" fibers. "Low-spont" type I afferents are less sensitive to sound (i.e., a high threshold) and have a wider, sloping dynamic range (M.C. Liberman, 1978; Sachs & Abbas, 1974; Schmiedt, 1989). Since low- and high-spont afferents are thought to innervate the same inner hair cell (M. C. Liberman, 1982), these differences can be attributed at least in part to properties of the synaptic contacts. These synaptic properties can be probed by studies of spontaneous activity both in vivo and *ex vivo*.

An important clue is provided by the observation that low frequency tones modulate the spontaneous firing rate both up *and* down (Johnson, 1980). Firing rate increases during the positive (rarefaction) phase, as expected for hair cell depolarization that increases the open probability of voltage-gated calcium channels driving transmitter release. More revealing is the fact that afferent activity *decreases* during the negative (compression) phase. This decrease implies that reduced transduction current hyperpolarized the hair cell from a resting potential that permits ongoing calcium channel gating and transmitter release in the absence of sound. This implication was secured by the fundamental discovery that spontaneous activity is dependent on influx through dihydropyridine-sensitive calcium channels (CaV1.3) that drives transmitter release from the presynaptic inner hair cell (Robertson & Paki, 2002; Sueta, Zhang, Sellick, Patuzzi, & Robertson, 2004; S. Y. Zhang, Robertson, Yates, & Everett, 1999). It seems intuitive that higher rates of spontaneous transmitter release might be related to lower thresholds for acoustic stimulation. What synaptic features might underlie differences in spontaneous release rates?

Several studies have described possible structural correlates of these functional differences, reviewed in (M.A. Rutherford, 2016). In pioneering studies of the cat cochlea, it was proposed that larger caliber, mitochrondion-rich afferents contacting the abneural, or pillar side, of inner hair cells corresponded to high-spont, low-threshold afferents. Smaller, mitochondrion-poor afferents terminating on the neural or modiolar surface of the inner hair cell would be low-spont, high-threshold afferents in this scheme (M.C. Liberman, 1980, 1982). Serial section electron microscopy of inner hair cells showed that modiolar ribbons (i.e., low-spont afferents) were two-fold longer in their principal axis (420 nm), than pillar ribbons—200 nm (i.e., high-spont afferents) that tended to be spherical. Antibody labeling to the ribeye protein that constitutes much of the synaptic ribbon dense body was consistent with this pattern, showing that neural (modiolar) immunolabeled ribbons produced a larger diffraction-limited image (presumably reflecting their greater length) than did abneural (pillar) ribbons (L. D. Liberman, Wang, & Liberman, 2011). In contrast, postsynaptic immunolabeling for an AMPA (α-amino-3-hydroxy-5-methyl-4-isoxazolepropionic acid) receptor subunit showed the opposite pattern, with larger AMPA receptor immunopuncta found on the abneural (pillar—"hi-spont") side, and smaller receptor immunopuncta on the neural (modiolar—"low-spont") side. These innervation patterns may vary somewhat between species and during development (L. D. Liberman & Liberman, 2016). Rather than a strictly neural/abneural organization, afferent synapses were found preferentially on the flattened, rather than rounded side of inner hair cells in the mouse cochlea (Bullen et al., 2015).

Functional studies of afferent synapses on inner hair cells have confirmed some of these features. Thus, direct recording from pairs of afferents contacting individual inner hair cells showed that spontaneous firing could be similar, or different, but there was zero correlation in spike timing for any afferent pair (Wu, Young, & Glowatzki, 2016). Further, this study showed that the detailed statistics of transmitter release (postsynaptic currents) accounted for the pattern of spontaneous action potentials in the afferent neurons. These findings, together with the tight coupling of synaptic input to the nearby spike initiation zone (M. A. Rutherford, Chapochnikov, & Moser, 2012), cement the hypothesis that the responses of individual type I afferents result directly from the properties of their presynaptic ribbon synapse. It remains to be determined whether postsynaptic heterogeneity or modulation by lateral olivocochlear efferents further affect the diversity of afferent response properties.

The number, size and location of ribbons, calcium channel immunopuncta and calcium microdomains (as observed with low affinity indicator dyes) were thoroughly analyzed in mouse inner hair cells (Frank, Khimich, Neef, & Moser, 2009; Meyer et al., 2009; Ohn et al., 2016). These studies showed that the size of calcium hotspots varied widely within individual inner hair cells. That variability reflected differences both in the voltage-dependence of gating (determined from calcium influx revealed with a fluorescent indicator dye), and in the number of channels (from the size of immunopuncta). The number of calcium channels also correlated with the size of the synaptic ribbon. Neural (modiolar—low- spont synapses) had larger ribbons and stronger calcium signals than those of abneural (pillar—high-spont synapses) signals. These correlations run counter to expectation for determination of spontaneous rate. Rather, these workers suggest that the voltage of half activation is positively shifted for modiolar calcium hotspots (low-spont afferents), requiring stronger depolarization to achieve a given level of calcium influx (as measured by low affinity calcium indicator dyes). A molecular mechanism for differences in voltage gating remains to be determined. Another possible factor is the density of channels at each ribbon. If the interchannel distance is greater on average, this would have an effect like that of stronger calcium buffering that reduces the regional calcium signal (Graydon, Cho, Li, Kachar, & von Gersdorff, 2011; Roberts, 1994). In zebrafish hair cells ribbon size and calcium current magnitude co-vary but correlate negatively with the spontaneous activity of afferents (Sheets et al., 2017)—i.e., larger ribbons with larger calcium currents had lower rates of transmitter release. This study also found that calcium channel density (clustering) was lower at larger ribbons—i.e., greater average interchannel distance. A greater interchannel distance would reduce the probability that flux through stochastically opening calcium channels sums to trigger vesicle fusion, thus lowering the rate of spontaneous activity in the postsynaptic afferent.

Other synaptic parameters have been described that could influence transmission efficacy at hair cell synapses. The large range of synaptic current amplitudes led to the suggestion that the ribbon synapse supported coordinate multivesicular release (Glowatzki

& Fuchs, 2002). Spontaneous postsynaptic currents in type I boutons are more or less temporally concise, referred to as monophasic or multiphasic events, with monophasic transmission becoming more prevalent with maturation (Glowatzki & Fuchs, 2002; Grant, Yi, Goutman, & Glowatzki, 2011). The peak postsynaptic depolarization is greater for monophasic transmission, potentially contributing to high-spont, low-acoustic threshold afferent activity and precise temporal coding (M. A. Rutherford et al., 2012). The smaller fraction of synapses that maintain multiphasic transmission in maturity could represent low-spont, high-threshold afferents. An alternative mechanism is that the amplitude and waveform of postsynaptic currents reflects the open time of a fusion pore, so that single vesicles release variable amounts of glutamate over varying time courses (Chapochnikov et al., 2014). Immediate and complete vesicular fusion would produce large, monophasic postsynaptic currents while stuttering opening of the fusion pore would result in multiphasic responses, a variant on the "kiss and run" hypothesis for vesicle cycling (Ceccarelli, Hurlbut, & Mauro, 1972, 1973), reviewed in (J. R. Morgan, Augustine, & Lafer, 2002).

Timing of transmitter release is central to the low frequency phase locking of afferent action potentials. Strikingly, these responses are phase-invariant across a range of stimulus intensities at the characteristic or best frequency of an afferent (Rose, Brugge, Anderson, & Hind, 1967). Phase-constancy also occurs in the timing of postsynaptic events in the type I afferent bouton evoked by cyclical depolarization of the hair cell (Goutman, 2012). Phase constancy results from the opposing effects of increased calcium channel gating to advance transmitter release, with depletion of the readily releasable pool that reduces the probability of release. Together these opposing effects result in constant average timing of release for a range of presynaptic depolarizations. Multivesicular release from ribbons helps to ensure stability in the timing of the afferent response (Wittig & Parsons, 2008). Similar conclusions were reached in a study of phase-locking in afferents of the frog inner ear (G. L. Li, Cho, & von Gersdorff, 2014).

What is clear from the fore-going discussion is that acoustic signaling depends critically on the properties of ribbon synapses between inner hair cells and type I cochlear afferents. Each type I afferent is driven by transmitter release from its private active zone (ribbon), and the release capacities of that ribbon are major determinants of the rate of spontaneous activity, the acoustic sensitivity, the dynamic range and the detailed timing of action potentials. Such synaptic competence is in marked distinction to that found in the cochlea's other afferents, the type II spiral ganglion neurons that innervate the outer hair cells.

Type II Cochlear Afferents

For more than 50 years, the role of type II afferents in the mammalian cochlea has been a matter of some speculation, but little resolution. Despite beautiful and informative anatomical studies defining their arborization and innervation patterns (Berglund,

Benson, & Brown, 1996; Berglund & Brown, 1994; Berglund & Ryugo, 1987; Brown, Berglund, Kiang, & Ryugo, 1988; Perkins & Morest, 1975; Simmons & Liberman, 1988a, 1988b; Smith & Haglan, 1973; Spoendlin, 1972), immunolabeling efforts (e.g., Hafidi, 1998; Hossain, Antic, Yang, Rasband, & Morest, 2005; Huang, Thorne, Housley, & Montgomery, 2007) and intracellular recordings from somata *ex vivo* (Jagger & Housley, 2003; Reid, Flores-Otero, & Davis, 2004), type II function remains somewhat enigmatic. This is due in large part to their scarcity, small caliber and lack of myelination that make single unit recording in vivo exceedingly difficult. Only three studies have attempted to determine their acoustic sensitivity in guinea pigs (Brown, 1994; Robertson, 1984; Robertson, Sellick, & Patuzzi, 1999), reporting on a total of 28 putative type II neurons (only one confirmed anatomically by fill of the distinctive peripheral arbor), the others based on their conduction velocity and waveform during antidromic stimulation). Of these 28, only one had spontaneous activity and only one responded to intense broadband noise, although type I afferents in these preparations could be driven by sound. Although scarce, these data show that type II afferents are acoustically insensitive, despite being postsynaptic to large numbers of OHCs. This poor acoustic sensitivity had led to suggestions that type II afferents may function as a type of peripheral interneuron, possibly to modulate outer hair cells through putative reciprocal synapses (Thiers, Nadol, & Liberman, 2008). Nonetheless type II afferents do project to the brain.

Tonotopically organized type I afferents project through the VIIIth nerve to the magnocellular regions of the cochlear nucleus (Benson, Berglund, & Brown, 1996; Brown, Berglund, et al., 1988; Fekete, Rouiller, Liberman, & Ryugo, 1984; Y. V. Morgan, Ryugo, & Brown, 1994). Type II afferents from the same region of the spiral ganglion, but innervating outer hair cells about ¼ octave higher in frequency (Brown, 1987), project alongside the type I axons. Type II's branch through both the ventral and dorsal cochlear nuclei, but morphological synapses have been described primarily in granule cell lamina that border the nuclear cores (Benson & Brown, 1990; Berglund et al., 1996; Berglund & Brown, 1994; Brown, Berglund, et al., 1988). The granule cell regions are thought to serve as integration zones, also receiving projections from polymodal somatosensory areas (Paloff & Usunoff, 1992; Shore & Zhou, 2006; Wright & Ryugo, 1996; Zhan & Ryugo, 2007) and collaterals from the medial olivocochlear (MOC) efferents to the OHCs (Benson & Brown, 1990; Brown, Liberman, Benson, & Ryugo, 1988). Granule cells project at least to the pyramidal neurons of the dorsal cochlear nucleus (Mugnaini, Osen, Dahl, Friedrich, & Korte, 1980) perhaps to integrate information from type II and type I neurons. While type I and II afferents branch in parallel and tonotopically to the dorsal and ventral cochlear nuclei, type II collaterals uniquely innervate small cells in the granule cell lamina that lie between the core nuclei (Benson & Brown, 2004). The similarity of this arrangement to C-fiber innervation of superficial layers of the dorsal horn has been noted (Brown & Ledwith, 1990; Hurd, Hutson, & Morest, 1999). However, while suggesting some differentiation from type I signaling, these central projections do not designate any particular role for type II afferents.

An alternative strategy has been to make intracellular recordings from type II afferents in excised cochlear tissue from young rats or mice. Somatic recordings in cochlear

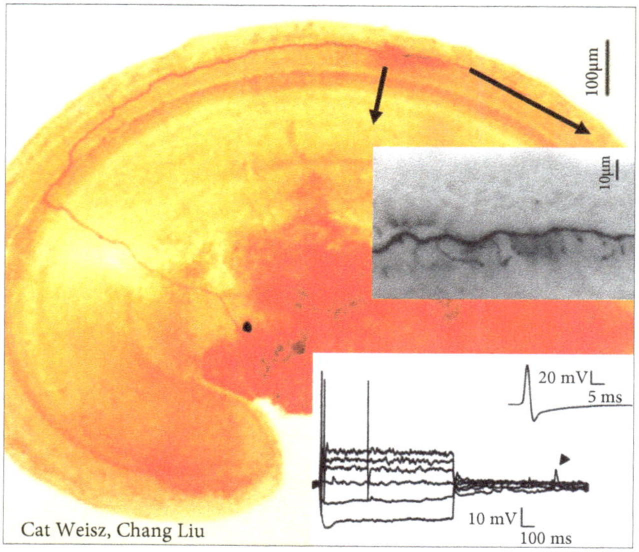

FIGURE 2.3. The intracellular label Biocytin diffused into a type II afferent during intracellular recording, revealing the characteristic dendritic process that spirals toward the cochlear base (to the right). Each type II afferent has one or two terminal arbors from which short branches contact outer hair cells (magnified inset). Intracellular voltage recording shows voltage responses to current steps, including overshooting action potentials. Spontaneous excitatory synaptic potentials are also present (arrowhead).

Modified from (Liu et al., 2015, Weisz et al., 2009).

slices from young rats (postnatal days 7–9) revealed that anatomically-confirmed type II neurons expressed a rapidly-inactivating A-type potassium current and could be depolarized by glutamate or ATP applied to the soma (Jagger & Housley, 2003). Spiral ganglion explants from 6–7 day old mice provided evidence that type II SGNs (identified by peripherin immunolabel) tended to sustained, tonic firing patterns while type I SGNs were phasic (Reid et al., 2004). These differences were more pronounced for SGNs in basal turns of the cochlea.

Tight-seal intracellular recording from the spiral process beneath outer hair cells in apical turns of cochleas excised from young (P5-9) rats (C. Weisz, Glowatzki, & Fuchs, 2009) provided additional information about the excitability and postsynaptic activity of type II afferents. Intracellular labeling revealed the characteristic type II dendritic morphology (Figure 2.3). Action potentials and small (~4 mV) synaptic potentials were observed in these recordings. At least 10 outer hair cells were synaptically connected to an individual type II afferent (C. J. Weisz, Lehar, Hiel, Glowatzki, & Fuchs, 2012). Maximal stimulation of individual outer hair cells (water jet bundle deflection that caused calcium spikes in these immature cells) released single synaptic vesicles with a 25% probability on average. Dual intracellular recordings from single fibers revealed length constants (the distance that a passive voltage change spreads along a fiber) that ranged from 0.6 to 1.2 mm, encompassing the entire spiral process (C. J. Weisz, Glowatzki, & Fuchs, 2014). These dual recordings also showed that action potentials were initiated near the spiral ganglion, and spread decrementally along the spiral process, consistent with the gradient of sodium channel immunolabeling reported previously (Hossain et al., 2005). Data from the dual recordings were used in compartmental modeling to conclude that maximal stimulation of the entire pool of presynaptic outer hair cells would be required to drive a type II afferent to threshold, consistent with their poor acoustic sensitivity in vivo (Brown, 1994; Robertson, 1984; Robertson et al., 1999).

What determines the efficacy of outer hair cell to type II afferent transmission? It is known that outer hair cells have few ribbons and small voltage-gated calcium currents (Knirsch et al., 2007; Michna et al., 2003) that drive limited vesicular fusion (Beurg et al., 2008). The connectivity of outer hair cells with type II afferents has been examined in the light and electron microscopes (Dunn & Morest, 1975; Simmons & Liberman, 1988b; Siegel & Brownell, 1981; Sobkowicz, Rose, Scott, & Slapnick, 1982; Sobkowicz, Rose, Scott, & Levenick, 1986). The spiral process extends several hundred microns toward the cochlear base, giving off numerous short branches to outer hair cells, predominantly in a single row (Berglund & Ryugo, 1987; Brown, 1987; Echteler, 1992; Fechner, Nadol, Burgess, & Brown, 2001; Ginzberg & Morest, 1983). Type II afferents in the apex of young rat cochleas gave off 6-16 short branches, as revealed with intracellular fills after recording in cochlear explants (Jagger & Housley, 2003). Dendritic contacts with outer hair cells can occur with or without associated presynaptic ribbons (Dunn & Morest, 1975; Gulley & Reese, 1977). This issue was given further attention using a combination of intracellular fiber fills, immunolabeling light microscopy and electron microscopy in the rat cochlea (Martinez-Monedero et al., 2016). Fifteen filled type II afferents had on average 16 (± 1.4 SEM) short branches averaging 10.9 μm (± 1.7 SEM) in length. Each such branch contacted one to three outer hair cells for 23.7 (± 1.5 SEM) outer hair cells per type II fiber. Immunolabeled postsynaptic densities that aligned with immunolabeled presynaptic ribbons (half the total) also were positive for the GluA2 AMPA receptor subunit. "Ribbonless" postsynaptic densities lacked GluA2 immunopuncta. Similar findings were obtained from a "reporter" mouse where only some type II afferents contacts were associated with immunolabeled presynaptic ribbons (Vyas, Wu, Zimmerman, Fuchs, & Glowatzki, 2016). Serial section electron microscopy likewise found that only half the afferent boutons on outer hair cells were associated with presynaptic ribbons. Intracellular recording was used to confirm that postsynaptic currents in type II fibers had biophysical properties and pharmacology consistent with AMPA receptor mediation. Others have reported that only ionotropic kainate receptors (related to but distinct from GluA AMPA receptors) were found at OHC to type II synapses in the adult mice (Fujikawa et al., 2014). Intriguingly, the GluK2 subunit was observed only at those synapses associated with hair cell ribbons.

Outer hair cells release glutamate to activate receptor-gated ion channels with rapid kinetics. These responses are quite similar (allowing for the effect of cable loss on waveform shape) to those occurring in type I afferents below inner hair cells that are mediated by GluA2-containing AMPARs. Ribbon-associated synapses in type II afferents included either the GluA2 (rats) or GluK2 subunit (mice). Taken together the literature drives the conclusion that only some type II afferent boutons are classically postsynaptic. The "ribbonless" contacts may correspond to "silent synapses" as found in the CNS (Faber, Lin, & Korn, 1991), and could provide a substrate for plastic changes.

Molecular Specification of Type II Afferents

Given the marked morphological and functional differences between type I and type II cochlear afferents, one can expect differences in gene expression as well, despite their common origin (Koundakjian, Appler, & Goodrich, 2007). Once validated, the responsible gene promoters then could provide selective expression of reporter proteins, or serve to alter type II afferent activity. So for example, it has been noted that the high expression of neurofilaments in the somata of type II neurons enabled them to be distinguished and quantified using a monoclonal antibody (Berglund & Ryugo, 1986). An early and promising genetic candidate was the protein peripherin, antibodies for which labeled type II, but not type I neurons (Hafidi, 1998). Peripherin immunolabel has been used in several studies as a marker for type II afferents (e.g., Reid et al., 2004), however, the suitability of peripherin as a genetic tool remains uncertain. Not all type II afferents are peripherin-positive (to be discussed), and peripherin may be expressed more widely, especially during development (Hafidi, Despres, & Romand, 1993). Nonetheless, co-labeling with peripherin can be a positive identifier of type II neurons. For example, double-immunolabeling for peripherin showed that the transcription factor Gata3 and a downstream effector Mafb, are maintained in mature type II spiral ganglion neurons (Nishimura, Noda, & Dabdoub, 2017).

Considerable progress has been made in the search for molecular markers of differentiation among dorsal root ganglion afferents of the somatic nervous system (Le Pichon & Chesler, 2014; L. Li et al., 2011; Sun & Dong, 2016). These mouse lines include at least two that show selective expression of reporter proteins in type II, but not type I cochlear afferents. Tyrosine hydroxylase is an enzyme that converts the amino acid L-tyrosine to L-3,4-dihydroxyphenylalanine (L-DOPA), leading to synthesis of dopamine, norepinephrine, and epinephrine and so is a marker of catecholaminergic neurons. Unexpectedly, since there is no evidence to date of catecholaminergic function, a TH-CreER mouse line showed expression of reporter protein (green fluorescent protein or TD-tomato) in type II cochlear afferents (Vyas et al., 2016). There was no overlap with immunolabel for Na/K ATPase, a validated marker of type I afferents and medial olivocochlear efferents (McLean, Smith, Glowatzki, & Pyott, 2009). TH-Cre driven reporter expression and immunolabel of the TH protein itself overlapped throughout the characteristic spiral processes of type II afferents. TH-driven expression also was found in sympathetic nerve fibers within the cochlea and in lateral efferents in 3-4 week old cochleas. Some, but not every, TH-CreER positive type II afferent co-labeled with antibody to peripherin, consistent with the heterogeneous expression of peripherin in type II afferents noted elsewhere (Nishimura et al., 2017).

Type II afferents in the cochlear apex express tyrosine hydroxylase more strongly than do those in the cochlear base. This observation was quantified in a study comparing the expression patterns of TH and calcitonin gene related protein (CGRP; Wu, Vyas, Glowatzki, & Fuchs, 2018). CGRP is expressed by a variety of cell types, including small afferents of the dorsal root ganglia where its release increases vasodilation and inflammation to exacerbate pain (Russell, King, Smillie, Kodji, & Brain, 2014). EGFP under control of CGRPα regulatory sequences in a bacterial artificial chromosome was expressed in cochlear efferents, as shown previously by CGRP immunolabel (Kitajiri et al., 1985), and also in a subset of spiral ganglion neurons (Wu et al., 2018). CGRP-positive SGNs had type II-like peripheral arbors, spiraling basally and connecting to outer hair cells. CGRP-dependent reporter expression was completely separate from type I SGNs immunolabeled for Na/K ATPase. As for TH (Vyas et al., 2016), CGRP-positive SGNs overlapped only partially with peripherin immunolabel. Expression patterns of TH and CGRP-positive neurons was quantified by counting labeled somata in 10 equal segments along the entire cochlear spiral. TH expression was consistently higher in apical type II afferents, while CGRP was higher in basal type II afferents (Figure 2.4). Individual SGNs in middle cochlear regions could be positive for both biomarkers. Thus, as suggested by differences in dendritic arborization (Nayagam,

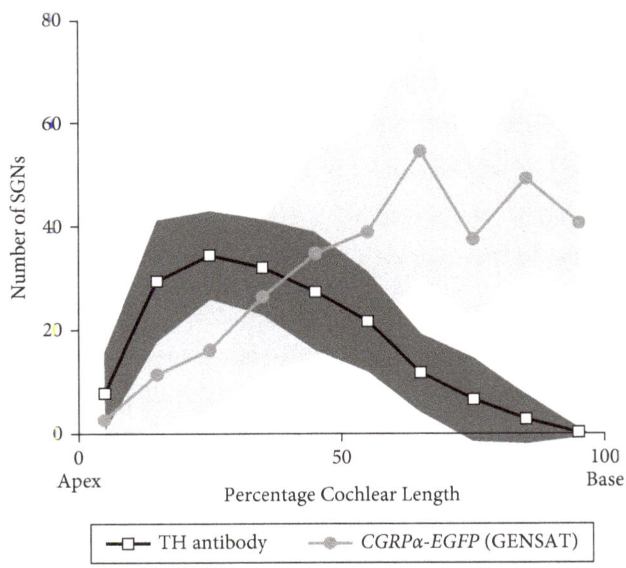

FIGURE 2.4. Tyrosine hydroxylase and calcitonin gene related peptide alpha drive antiparallel expression gradients in type II spiral ganglion neurons. Spiral ganglion neurons ($n = 6$) labeled with an antibody to tyrosine hydroxylase (TH) predominated in the cochlear apex. Antibodies to GFP under control of the CGRPα promoter labeled spiral ganglion neurons ($n = 8$) more heavily in the cochlear base.

Modified from (Wu et al., 2018).

Muniak, & Ryugo, 2011), type II cochlear afferents may be "tonotopically" differentiated, potentially reflecting even further functional sub-specialization.

A Functional Role for Type II Afferents

Since type I cochlear afferents provide acoustic input, what remains for type II afferents to do? Apparently they have something to do with OHCs. In the earliest studies it was suggested that type II afferents might be sensitive to very faint sounds by spatial summation from their numerous presynaptic OHCs (C. Fernandez quoting H. Davis) (Fernandez, 1951; Spoendlin, 1969) a logical but now incorrect assumption. Another idea is that type II afferents are analogous to muscle spindle afferents, providing updates on the mechanical "setpoint" of the cochlea by signaling the activity of OHCs (Berglund & Brown, 1994; Kim, 1984). A peripherin knockout mouse was found to lack sound-evoked suppression of otoacoustic emissions. Type II afferents appeared to be absent from the cochleas of these mice, leading to the suggestion that type II afferents activate the medial olivocochlear efferents that mediate suppression by inhibiting OHCs (Froud et al., 2015). That conclusion was called into question by a subsequent study showing that electrical stimulation of medial olivocochlear efferents also failed to suppress distortion products in these knockout mice, suggesting that peripherin knockout disrupted efferent neurons directly (Maison, Liberman, & Liberman, 2016). More generally, type II afferents are unlikely to be the sole activators of olivocochlear efferents whose acoustic sensitivity is essentially equivalent to that of type I afferents (M. C. Liberman & Brown, 1986; Robertson & Gummer, 1985). Another notion is that type II fibers are a kind of peripheral interneuron, based on a suggestion of reciprocal contacts with OHCs (Nadol, 1983; Thiers et al., 2008) and presynaptic specializations with supporting cells (Fechner et al., 2001). However, even if these peripheral connections are functional (which has not been determined), type II neurons also do project to the cochlear nuclei of the brainstem, distributing branches that largely parallel those of neighboring type I afferents (Berglund & Brown, 1994; Brown, Berglund, et al., 1988) and so they must have central functions as well. More consistent with existing data is the suggestion that type II afferents exist specifically to encode "loudness" (Knirsch et al., 2007).

Type II afferents may serve a still more distinct function, to signal the presence of traumatic, or noxious, levels of sound, as summarized recently (Francis, 2012; K. D. Zhang & Coate, 2017). This hypothesis derives from their morphological similarity to unmyelinated somatic C-fibers, poor acoustic sensitivity (Brown, 1994; Robertson, 1984; Robertson et al., 1999) and weak drive by outer hair cell glutamate release (C. J. Weisz et al., 2012). In support of this hypothesis, when mice with dysfunctional inner hair cell synapses were exposed to traumatizing sound, activity-dependent c-FOS labeling was enhanced in the granule cell domain of the cochlear nucleus (Flores et al.,

2015), the specific brainstem destination of type II afferents (Brown, Berglund, et al., 1988). Still more directly, recordings from type II afferents in excised cochlear segments from young rats showed that type II afferents were strongly excited when outer hair cells were ruptured by a mechanical probe (Liu, Glowatzki, & Fuchs, 2015). This response was due in large part to activation of ionotropic (P2X) and metabotropic (P2Y) purinergic receptors in type II afferents. P2Y receptor activation depolarized the type II neuron by the closure of KCNQ-type potassium channels, making the afferent more excitable and lowering the apparent spike threshold (C. Weisz, J.C., 2011). The minutes-long damage response in type II afferents was similar to that of ATP-dependent calcium waves seen in surrounding support cells upon outer hair cell ablation (Gale, Piazza, Ciubotaru, & Mammano, 2004; Lahne & Gale, 2010). Thus, ATP release from supporting cells may drive type II afferent activation, akin to the transient role of Kolliker's organ cells in spontaneous activity of type I afferents during cochlear maturation (Tritsch, Yi, Gale, Glowatzki, & Bergles, 2007).

The gain of function pathologies tinnitus and hyperacusis arise subsequent to loss of type I afferent input. It is thought that the loss of peripheral input leads to increases in gain at synaptic connections in the central auditory pathway (Auerbach, Rodrigues, & Salvi, 2014). It is not known what, if any contribution type II afferents might make, although their peripheral arbors can persist in damaged cochleas (Ryan, Woolf, & Bone, 1980; Spoendlin, 1971). A guiding analogy can be drawn from the somatic nervous system where the loss of large diameter myelinated afferents (e.g., touch, vibration sensors), but survival of unmyelinated C-fibers, can lead to persistent pain. This was proposed as the "gate theory" (Wall, 1978) whereby rapidly-conducting, large diameter, myelinated somatic afferents normally inhibit the pain pathway. Uncompensated C-fiber input results in chronic pain syndromes. These include hyper-excitability of the peripheral C-fibers as well as changes in central synaptic efficacy (Perl, 1996). In combination with the loss of type I afferent contacts onto inner hair cells (Kujawa & Liberman, 2009; Ruel et al., 2007; Stamataki, Francis, Lehar, May, & Ryugo, 2006), the hyperexcitability of type II afferents could be particularly germane to mechanisms of hyperacusis. Synaptic inputs may increase in number and strength, intrinsic excitability may increase (for example, by down-regulation of KCNQ channels), and sensitivity to ATP may increase. The cellular and synaptic physiology of damaged cochleas (e.g. Zachary & Fuchs, 2015) will receive increased attention as efforts mount to explore both the loss and gain of function after cochlear trauma.

Acknowledgments

Work in the author's laboratory is supported by NIDCD R01DC001508, R01DC016559, R01DC015309, the John E. Bordley Professorship and the David M. Rubenstein Fund for Hearing Research to Johns Hopkins Otolaryngology-HNS. T. Coate and M. Rutherford are thanked for their careful reading of an earlier draft.

References

Auerbach, B. D., Rodrigues, P. V., & Salvi, R. J. (2014). Central gain control in tinnitus and hyperacusis. *Frontiers in Neurology*, 5, 206. doi:10.3389/fneur.2014.00206

Benson, T. E., Berglund, A. M., & Brown, M. C. (1996). Synaptic input to cochlear nucleus dendrites that receive medial olivocochlear synapses. *Journal of Comparative Neurology*, 365(1), 27–41. doi:10.1002/(SICI)1096-9861(19960129)365:1<27::AID-CNE3>3.0.CO;2-L

Benson, T. E., & Brown, M. C. (1990). Synapses formed by olivocochlear axon branches in the mouse cochlear nucleus. *Journal of Comparative Neurology*, 295(1), 52–70. Retrieved from http://www.ncbi.nlm.nih.gov/entrez/query.fcgi?cmd=Retrieve&db=PubMed&dopt=Citation&list_uids=2341636

Benson, T. E., & Brown, M. C. (2004). Postsynaptic targets of type II auditory nerve fibers in the cochlear nucleus. *Journal of the Association for Research in Otolaryngology*, 5(2), 111–125. Retrieved from http://www.ncbi.nlm.nih.gov/entrez/query.fcgi?cmd=Retrieve&db=PubMed&dopt=Citation&list_uids=15357415

Berglund, A. M., Benson, T. E., & Brown, M. C. (1996). Synapses from labeled type II axons in the mouse cochlear nucleus. *Hearing Research*, 94(1–2), 31–46. Retrieved from http://www.ncbi.nlm.nih.gov/entrez/query.fcgi?cmd=Retrieve&db=PubMed&dopt=Citation&list_uids=8789809

Berglund, A. M., & Brown, M. C. (1994). Central trajectories of type II spiral ganglion cells from various cochlear regions in mice. *Hearing Research*, 75(1–2), 121–130. Retrieved from http://www.ncbi.nlm.nih.gov/pubmed/8071139

Berglund, A. M., & Ryugo, D. K. (1986). A monoclonal antibody labels type II neurons of the spiral ganglion. *Brain Research*, 383(1–2), 327–332. Retrieved from http://www.ncbi.nlm.nih.gov/entrez/query.fcgi?cmd=Retrieve&db=PubMed&dopt=Citation&list_uids=3533212

Berglund, A. M., & Ryugo, D. K. (1987). Hair cell innervation by spiral ganglion neurons in the mouse. *Journal of Comparative Neurology*, 255(4), 560–570. doi:10.1002/cne.902550408

Beurg, M., Safieddine, S., Roux, I., Bouleau, Y., Petit, C., & Dulon, D. (2008). Calcium- and otoferlin-dependent exocytosis by immature outer hair cells. *Journal of Neuroscience*, 28(8), 1798–1803. Retrieved from http://www.ncbi.nlm.nih.gov/entrez/query.fcgi?cmd=Retrieve&db=PubMed&dopt=Citation&list_uids=18287496

Brown, M. C. (1987). Morphology of labeled afferent fibers in the guinea pig cochlea. *Journal of Comparative Neurology*, 260(4), 591–604. Retrieved from http://www.ncbi.nlm.nih.gov/entrez/query.fcgi?cmd=Retrieve&db=PubMed&dopt=Citation&list_uids=3611412

Brown, M. C. (1994). Antidromic responses of single units from the spiral ganglion. *Journal of Neurophysiology*, 71(5), 1835–1847. Retrieved from http://www.ncbi.nlm.nih.gov/entrez/query.fcgi?cmd=Retrieve&db=PubMed&dopt=Citation&list_uids=8064351

Brown, M. C., Berglund, A. M., Kiang, N. Y., & Ryugo, D. K. (1988). Central trajectories of type II spiral ganglion neurons. *Journal of Comparative Neurology*, 278(4), 581–590. Retrieved from http://www.ncbi.nlm.nih.gov/entrez/query.fcgi?cmd=Retrieve&db=PubMed&dopt=Citation&list_uids=3230171

Brown, M. C., & Ledwith, J. V., 3rd. (1990). Projections of thin (type-II) and thick (type-I) auditory-nerve fibers into the cochlear nucleus of the mouse. *Hearing Research*, 49(1–3), 105–118. Retrieved from http://www.ncbi.nlm.nih.gov/entrez/query.fcgi?cmd=Retrieve&db=PubMed&dopt=Citation&list_uids=1963423

Brown, M. C., Liberman, M. C., Benson, T. E., & Ryugo, D. K. (1988). Brainstem branches from olivocochlear axons in cats and rodents. *Journal of Comparative Neurology*, 278(4), 591–603.

Retrieved from http://www.ncbi.nlm.nih.gov/entrez/query.fcgi?cmd=Retrieve&db=PubMed&dopt=Citation&list_uids=3230172

Bullen, A., West, T., Moores, C., Ashmore, J., Fleck, R. A., MacLellan-Gibson, K., & Forge, A. (2015). Association of intracellular and synaptic organization in cochlear inner hair cells revealed by 3D electron microscopy. *Journal of Cell Science, 128*(14), 2529–2540. doi:10.1242/jcs.170761

Ceccarelli, B., Hurlbut, W. P., & Mauro, A. (1972). Depletion of vesicles from frog neuromuscular junctions by prolonged tetanic stimulation. *Journal of Cell Biology, 54*(1), 30–38. Retrieved from http://www.ncbi.nlm.nih.gov/pubmed/4338962

Ceccarelli, B., Hurlbut, W. P., & Mauro, A. (1973). Turnover of transmitter and synaptic vesicles at the frog neuromuscular junction. *Journal of Cell Biology, 57*(2), 499–524. Retrieved from http://www.ncbi.nlm.nih.gov/entrez/query.fcgi?cmd=Retrieve&db=PubMed&dopt=Citation&list_uids=4348791

Chapochnikov, N. M., Takago, H., Huang, C. H., Pangrsic, T., Khimich, D., Neef, J., . . . Moser, T. (2014). Uniquantal release through a dynamic fusion pore is a candidate mechanism of hair cell exocytosis. *Neuron, 83*(6), 1389–1403. doi:10.1016/j.neuron.2014.08.003

Dunn, R. A., & Morest, D. K. (1975). Receptor synapses without synaptic ribbons in the cochlea of the cat. *Proceedings of the National Academy of Sciences USA, 72*(9), 3599–3603. Retrieved from http://www.ncbi.nlm.nih.gov/entrez/query.fcgi?cmd=Retrieve&db=PubMed&dopt=Citation&list_uids=1059148

Echteler, S. M. (1992). Developmental segregation in the afferent projections to mammalian auditory hair cells. *Proceedings of the National Academy of Sciences USA, 89*, 6324–6327.

Evans, E. F. (1972). The frequency response and other properties of single fibres in the guinea-pig cochlear nerve. *Journal of Physiolology, 226*, 263–87.

Faber, D. S., Lin, J. W., & Korn, H. (1991). Silent synaptic connections and their modifiability. *Annals of the New York Academy of Science, 627*, 151–164. Retrieved from http://www.ncbi.nlm.nih.gov/pubmed/1883136

Fechner, F. P., Nadol, J. J., Burgess, B. J., & Brown, M. C. (2001). Innervation of supporting cells in the apical turns of the guinea pig cochlea is from type II afferent fibers. *Journal of Comparative Neurology, 429*(2), 289–298.

Fekete, D. M., Rouiller, E. M., Liberman, M. C., & Ryugo, D. K. (1984). The central projections of intracellularly labeled auditory nerve fibers in cats. *Journal of Comparative Neurology, 229*(3), 432–450. Retrieved from http://www.ncbi.nlm.nih.gov/entrez/query.fcgi?cmd=Retrieve&db=PubMed&dopt=Citation&list_uids=6209306

Fernandez, C. (1951). The innervation of the cochlea (guinea pig). *Laryngoscope, 61*(12), 1152–1172. Retrieved from http://www.ncbi.nlm.nih.gov/entrez/query.fcgi?cmd=Retrieve&db=PubMed&dopt=Citation&list_uids=14889888

Flores, E. N., Duggan, A., Madathany, T., Hogan, A. K., Marquez, F. G., Kumar, G., . . . Garcia-Anoveros, J. (2015). A non-canonical pathway from cochlea to brain signals tissue-damaging noise. *Current Biology, 25*(5), 606–612. doi:10.1016/j.cub.2015.01.009

Francis, H. W. (2012). Synaptic transfer from outer hair cells to type II afferent fibers in the rat cochlea. *Neurobiology of Aging, 32*(28), 9528–9536. doi:10.1016/j.neurobiolaging.2012.02.007 10.1523/jneurosci.6194-11.2012

Frank, T., Khimich, D., Neef, A., & Moser, T. (2009). Mechanisms contributing to synaptic Ca2+ signals and their heterogeneity in hair cells. *Proceedings of the National Academy of Sciences USA, 106*(11), 4483–4488. doi:10.1073/pnas.0813213106

Froud, K. E., Wong, A. C., Cederholm, J. M., Klugmann, M., Sandow, S. L., Julien, J. P., . . . Housley, G. D. (2015). Type II spiral ganglion afferent neurons drive medial olivocochlear reflex suppression of the cochlear amplifier. *Nature Communications*, *6*, 7115. doi:10.1038/ncomms8115

Fujikawa, T., Petralia, R. S., Fitzgerald, T. S., Wang, Y. X., Millis, B., Morgado-Diaz, J. A., . . . Kachar, B. (2014). Localization of kainate receptors in inner and outer hair cell synapses. *Hearing Research*, *314*, 20–32. doi:10.1016/j.heares.2014.05.001

Gale, J. E., Piazza, V., Ciubotaru, C. D., & Mammano, F. (2004). A mechanism for sensing noise damage in the inner ear. *Current Biology*, *14*(6), 526–529. Retrieved from http://www.ncbi.nlm.nih.gov/entrez/query.fcgi?cmd=Retrieve&db=PubMed&dopt=Citation&list_uids=15043820

Ginzberg, R. D., & Morest, D. K. (1983). A study of cochlear innervation in the young cat with the Golgi method. *Hearing Research*, *10*(2), 227–246. Retrieved from http://www.ncbi.nlm.nih.gov/pubmed/6863156

Glowatzki, E., & Fuchs, P. A. (2002). Transmitter release at the hair cell ribbon synapse. *Nature Neuroscience*, *5*(2), 147–154. doi:10.1038/nn796

Goutman, J. D. (2012). Transmitter release from cochlear hair cells is phase locked to cyclic stimuli of different intensities and frequencies. *Journal of Neuroscience*, *32*(47), 17025–17035a. doi:10.1523/JNEUROSCI.0457-12.2012

Grant, L., Yi, E., Goutman, J. D., & Glowatzki, E. (2011). Postsynaptic recordings at afferent dendrites contacting cochlear inner hair cells: monitoring multivesicular release at a ribbon synapse. *Journal of Visualized Experiments* (48). doi:10.3791/2442

Graydon, C. W., Cho, S., Li, G. L., Kachar, B., & von Gersdorff, H. (2011). Sharp Ca(2)(+) nanodomains beneath the ribbon promote highly synchronous multivesicular release at hair cell synapses. *Journal of Neuroscience*, *31*(46), 16637–16650. doi:10.1523/JNEUROSCI.1866-11.2011

Gulley, R. L., & Reese, T. S. (1977). Freeze-fracture studies on the synapses in the organ of Corti. *Journal of Comparative Neurology*, *171*(4), 517–543. doi:10.1002/cne.901710407

Hafidi, A. (1998). Peripherin-like immunoreactivity in type II spiral ganglion cell body and projections. *Brain Research*, *805*(1–2), 181–190. Retrieved from http://www.ncbi.nlm.nih.gov/entrez/query.fcgi?cmd=Retrieve&db=PubMed&dopt=Citation&list_uids=9733963

Hafidi, A., Despres, G., & Romand, R. (1993). Ontogenesis of type II spiral ganglion neurons during development: peripherin immunohistochemistry. *International Journal of Developmental Neuroscience*, *11*(4), 507–512. Retrieved from http://www.ncbi.nlm.nih.gov/pubmed/8237466

Hossain, W. A., Antic, S. D., Yang, Y., Rasband, M. N., & Morest, D. K. (2005). Where is the spike generator of the cochlear nerve? Voltage-gated sodium channels in the mouse cochlea. *Journal of Neuroscience*, *25*(29), 6857–6868. Retrieved from http://www.ncbi.nlm.nih.gov/entrez/query.fcgi?cmd=Retrieve&db=PubMed&dopt=Citation&list_uids=16033895

Huang, L. C., Thorne, P. R., Housley, G. D., & Montgomery, J. M. (2007). Spatiotemporal definition of neurite outgrowth, refinement and retraction in the developing mouse cochlea. *Development*, *134*(16), 2925–2933. Retrieved from http://www.ncbi.nlm.nih.gov/entrez/query.fcgi?cmd=Retrieve&db=PubMed&dopt=Citation&list_uids=17626062

Hurd, L. B., Hutson, K. A., & Morest, D. K. (1999). Cochlear nerve projections to the small cell shell of the cochlear nucleus: the neuroanatomy of extremely thin sensory axons. *Synapse*, *33*(2), 83–117. Retrieved from http://www.ncbi.nlm.nih.gov/entrez/query.fcgi?cmd=Retrieve&db=PubMed&dopt=Citation&list_uids=10400889

Jagger, D. J., & Housley, G. D. (2003). Membrane properties of type II spiral ganglion neurones identified in a neonatal rat cochlear slice. *Journal of Physiology*, *552*(Pt 2), 525–533. doi:10.1113/jphysiol.2003.052589

Johnson, D. H. (1980). The relationship between spike rate and synchrony in responses of auditory nerve-fibers to single tones. *Journal of the American Statistical Association*, *68*(4), 1115–1122.

Kim, D. (1984). Functional roles of inner- and outer-hair-cell subsystems in the cochlea and brainstem. In C. I. Berlin (Ed.), *Hearing science: Recent advances* (pp. 241–262). San Diego CA: College Press.

Kitajiri, M., Yamashita, T., Tohyama, Y., Kumazawa, T., Takeda, N., Kawasaki, Y., . . . et al. (1985). Localization of calcitonin gene-related peptide in the organ of Corti of the rat: An immunohistochemical study. *Brain Research*, *358*(1–2), 394–397. Retrieved from http://www.ncbi.nlm.nih.gov/pubmed/3907750

Knirsch, M., Brandt, N., Braig, C., Kuhn, S., Hirt, B., Munkner, S., . . . Engel, J. (2007). Persistence of Ca(v)1.3 Ca2+ channels in mature outer hair cells supports outer hair cell afferent signaling. *Journal of Neuroscience*, *27*(24), 6442–6451. Retrieved from http://www.ncbi.nlm.nih.gov/entrez/query.fcgi?cmd=Retrieve&db=PubMed&dopt=Citation&list_uids=17567805

Koundakjian, E. J., Appler, J. L., & Goodrich, L. V. (2007). Auditory neurons make stereotyped wiring decisions before maturation of their targets. *Journal of Neuroscience*, *27*(51), 14078–14088. doi:10.1523/JNEUROSCI.3765-07.2007

Kujawa, S. G., & Liberman, M. C. (2009). Adding insult to injury: Cochlear nerve degeneration after "temporary" noise-induced hearing loss. *Journal of Neuroscience*, *29*(45), 14077–14085. Retrieved from http://www.ncbi.nlm.nih.gov/entrez/query.fcgi?cmd=Retrieve&db=PubMed&dopt=Citation&list_uids=19906956

Lahne, M., & Gale, J. E. (2010). Damage-induced cell-cell communication in different cochlear cell types via two distinct ATP-dependent Ca waves. *Purinergic Signal*, *6*(2), 189–200. doi:10.1007/s11302-010-9193-8

Le Pichon, C. E., & Chesler, A. T. (2014). The functional and anatomical dissection of somatosensory subpopulations using mouse genetics. *Frontiers in Neuroanatomy*, *8*, 21. doi:10.3389/fnana.2014.00021

Li, G. L., Cho, S., & von Gersdorff, H. (2014). Phase-locking precision is enhanced by multiquantal release at an auditory hair cell ribbon synapse. *Neuron*, *83*(6), 1404–1417. doi:10.1016/j.neuron.2014.08.027

Li, L., Rutlin, M., Abraira, V. E., Cassidy, C., Kus, L., Gong, S., . . . Ginty, D. D. (2011). The functional organization of cutaneous low-threshold mechanosensory neurons. *Cell*, *147*(7), 1615–1627. doi:10.1016/j.cell.2011.11.027

Liberman, L. D., & Liberman, M. C. (2016). Postnatal maturation of auditory-nerve heterogeneity, as seen in spatial gradients of synapse morphology in the inner hair cell area. *Hearing Research*, *339*, 12–22. doi:10.1016/j.heares.2016.06.002

Liberman, L. D., Wang, H., & Liberman, M. C. (2011). Opposing gradients of ribbon size and AMPA receptor expression underlie sensitivity differences among cochlear-nerve/hair-cell synapses. *Journal of Neuroscience*, *31*(3), 801–808. doi:10.1523/JNEUROSCI.3389-10.2011

Liberman, M. C. (1978). Auditory-nerve response from cats raised in a low-noise chamber. *Journal of the Acoustical Society of America*, *63*, 442–455.

Liberman, M. C. (1980). Morphological differences among radial afferent fibers in the cat cochlea: an electron-microcopic study of serial sections. *Hearing Research*, *3*, 45–63.

Liberman, M. C. (1982). Single-neuron labeling in the cat auditory nerve. *Science, 216*, 1239–1241.

Liberman, M. C., & Brown, M. C. (1986). Physiology and anatomy of single olivocochlear neurons in the cat. *Hearing Research, 24*(1), 17–36. Retrieved from http://www.ncbi.nlm.nih.gov/entrez/query.fcgi?cmd=Retrieve&db=PubMed&dopt=Citation&list_uids=3759672

Liu, C., Glowatzki, E., & Fuchs, P. A. (2015). Unmyelinated type II afferent neurons report cochlear damage. *Proceedings of the National Academy of Sciences USA*. doi:10.1073/pnas.1515228112

Lorente de No, R. (1937). The sensory endings in the cochlea. *Laryngoscope, 47*, 373–377.

Maison, S., Liberman, L. D., & Liberman, M. C. (2016). Type II cochlear ganglion neurons do not drive the olivocochlear reflex: Re-examination of the cochlear phenotype in peripherin knock-out mice. *eNeuro, 3*(4). doi:10.1523/ENEURO.0207-16.2016

Martinez-Monedero, R., Liu, C., Weisz, C., Vyas, P., Fuchs, P. A., & Glowatzki, E. (2016). GluA2-containing AMPA receptors distinguish ribbon-associated from ribbonless afferent contacts on rat cochlear hair cells. *eNeuro, 3*(2). doi:10.1523/ENEURO.0078-16.2016

McLean, W. J., Smith, K. A., Glowatzki, E., & Pyott, S. J. (2009). Distribution of the Na, K-ATPase alpha subunit in the rat spiral ganglion and organ of corti. *Journal of the Association for Research in Otolaryngology, 10*(1), 37–49. Retrieved from http://www.ncbi.nlm.nih.gov/entrez/query.fcgi?cmd=Retrieve&db=PubMed&dopt=Citation&list_uids=19082858

Meyer, A. C., Frank, T., Khimich, D., Hoch, G., Riedel, D., Chapochnikov, N. M., . . . Moser, T. (2009). Tuning of synapse number, structure and function in the cochlea. *Nature Neuroscience, 12*(4), 444–453. doi:10.1038/nn.2293

Michna, M., Knirsch, M., Hoda, J. C., Muenkner, S., Langer, P., Platzer, J., . . . Engel, J. (2003). Cav1.3 (alpha1D) Ca2+ currents in neonatal outer hair cells of mice. *Journal of Physiology, 553*(Pt 3), 747–758. Retrieved from http://www.ncbi.nlm.nih.gov/entrez/query.fcgi?cmd=Retrieve&db=PubMed&dopt=Citation&list_uids=14514878

Middlebrooks, J. C. (2015). Sound localization. *Handbook of Clinical Neurology, 129*, 99–116. doi:10.1016/B978-0-444-62630-1.00006-8

Morgan, J. R., Augustine, G. J., & Lafer, E. M. (2002). Synaptic vesicle endocytosis: The races, places, and molecular faces. *Neuromolecular Medicine, 2*(2), 101–114. doi:10.1385/NMM:2:2:101

Morgan, Y. V., Ryugo, D. K., & Brown, M. C. (1994). Central trajectories of type II (thin) fibers of the auditory nerve in cats. *Hearing Research, 79*(1–2), 74–82. Retrieved from http://www.ncbi.nlm.nih.gov/entrez/query.fcgi?cmd=Retrieve&db=PubMed&dopt=Citation&list_uids=7806486

Mugnaini, E., Osen, K. K., Dahl, A. L., Friedrich, V. L., Jr., & Korte, G. (1980). Fine structure of granule cells and related interneurons (termed Golgi cells) in the cochlear nuclear complex of cat, rat and mouse. *Journal of Neurocytology, 9*(4), 537–570. Retrieved from http://www.ncbi.nlm.nih.gov/entrez/query.fcgi?cmd=Retrieve&db=PubMed&dopt=Citation&list_uids=7441303

Nadol, J. B., Jr. (1983). Serial section reconstruction of the neural poles of hair cells in the human organ of Corti. II. Outer hair cells. *Laryngoscope, 93*(6), 780–791. Retrieved from http://www.ncbi.nlm.nih.gov/entrez/query.fcgi?cmd=Retrieve&db=PubMed&dopt=Citation&list_uids=6855401

Nayagam, B. A., Muniak, M. A., & Ryugo, D. K. (2011). The spiral ganglion: Connecting the peripheral and central auditory systems. *Hearing Research, 278*(1–2), 2–20. doi:10.1016/j.heares.2011.04.003

Nishimura, K., Noda, T., & Dabdoub, A. (2017). Dynamic Expression of Sox2, Gata3, and Prox1 during Primary Auditory Neuron Development in the Mammalian Cochlea. *PLoS One, 12*(1), e0170568. doi:10.1371/journal.pone.0170568

Ohn, T. L., Rutherford, M. A., Jing, Z., Jung, S., Duque-Afonso, C. J., Hoch, G., . . . Moser, T. (2016). Hair cells use active zones with different voltage dependence of Ca2+ influx to decompose sounds into complementary neural codes. *Proceedings of the National Academy of Sciences USA, 113*(32), E4716–4725. doi:10.1073/pnas.1605737113

Paloff, A. M., & Usunoff, K. G. (1992). Projections to the inferior colliculus from the dorsal column nuclei. An experimental electron microscopic study in the cat. *Journal fur Hirnforschung, 33*(6), 597–610. Retrieved from http://www.ncbi.nlm.nih.gov/entrez/query.fcgi?cmd=Retrieve&db=PubMed&dopt=Citation&list_uids=1283610

Perkins, R. E., & Morest, D. K. (1975). A study of cochlear innervation patterns in cats and rats with the Golgi method and Nomarkski Optics. *Journal of Comparative Neurology, 163*(2), 129–158. Retrieved from http://www.ncbi.nlm.nih.gov/entrez/query.fcgi?cmd=Retrieve&db=PubMed&dopt=Citation&list_uids=1100684

Perl, E. R. (1996). Cutaneous polymodal receptors: characteristics and plasticity. *Progress in Brain Research, 113*, 21–37. Retrieved from http://www.ncbi.nlm.nih.gov/pubmed/9009726

Reid, M. A., Flores-Otero, J., & Davis, R. L. (2004). Firing patterns of type II spiral ganglion neurons in vitro. *Journal of Neuroscience, 24*(3), 733–742. Retrieved from http://www.ncbi.nlm.nih.gov/entrez/query.fcgi?cmd=Retrieve&db=PubMed&dopt=Citation&list_uids=14736859

Roberts, W. M. (1994). Localization of calcium signals by a mobile calcium buffer in frog saccular hair cells. *Journal of Neuroscience, 14*(5 Pt 2), 3246–3262. Retrieved from http://www.ncbi.nlm.nih.gov/pubmed/8182469

Robertson, D. (1984). Horseradish peroxidase injection of physiologically characterized afferent and efferent neurones in the guinea pig spiral ganglion. *Hearing Research, 15*(2), 113–121. Retrieved from http://www.ncbi.nlm.nih.gov/entrez/query.fcgi?cmd=Retrieve&db=PubMed&dopt=Citation&list_uids=6490538

Robertson, D., & Gummer, M. (1985). Physiological and morphological characterization of efferent neurones in the guinea pig cochlea. *Hearing Research, 20*(1), 63–77. Retrieved from http://www.ncbi.nlm.nih.gov/pubmed/2416730

Robertson, D., & Paki, B. (2002). Role of L-type Ca2+ channels in transmitter release from mammalian inner hair cells. II. Single-neuron activity. *Journal of Neurophysiology, 87*(6), 2734–2740. Retrieved from http://www.ncbi.nlm.nih.gov/entrez/query.fcgi?cmd=Retrieve&db=PubMed&dopt=Citation&list_uids=12037175

Robertson, D., Sellick, P. M., & Patuzzi, R. (1999). The continuing search for outer hair cell afferents in the guinea pig spiral ganglion. *Hearing Research, 136*(1–2), 151–158. Retrieved from http://www.ncbi.nlm.nih.gov/entrez/query.fcgi?cmd=Retrieve&db=PubMed&dopt=Citation&list_uids=10511634

Rose, J. E., Brugge, J. F., Anderson, D. J., & Hind, J. E. (1967). Phase-locked response to low-frequency tones in single auditory nerve fibers of the squirrel monkey. *Journal of Neurophysiology, 30*(4), 769–793. Retrieved from http://www.ncbi.nlm.nih.gov/entrez/query.fcgi?cmd=Retrieve&db=PubMed&dopt=Citation&list_uids=4962851

Ruel, J., Wang, J., Rebillard, G., Eybalin, M., Lloyd, R., Pujol, R., & Puel, J. L. (2007). Physiology, pharmacology and plasticity at the inner hair cell synaptic complex. *Hearing Research, 227*(1–2), 19–27. doi:10.1016/j.heares.2006.08.017

Ruggero, M. A. (1992). Physiology and coding of sound in the auditory nerve. In R. R. Fay & A. N. Popper (Eds.), *The mammalian auditory pathway: Neurophysiology* (vol. 2, pp. 34–93). New York, NY: Springer.

Russell, F. A., King, R., Smillie, S. J., Kodji, X., & Brain, S. D. (2014). Calcitonin gene-related peptide: physiology and pathophysiology. *Physiology Review, 94*(4), 1099–1142. doi:10.1152/physrev.00034.2013

Rutherford, M. A., Chapochnikov, N. M., & Moser, T. (2012). Spike encoding of neurotransmitter release timing by spiral ganglion neurons of the cochlea. *Journal of Neuroscience, 32*(14), 4773–4789. doi:10.1523/JNEUROSCI.4511-11.2012

Rutherford, M. A., & Moser, T. (2016). The ribbon synapse between type I spiral ganglion neurons and inner hair cells. In A. Dabdoub & B. Fritzsch (Eds.), *Springer Handbook of Auditory Research* (vol. 52, pp. 117–156). New York, NY: Springer. doi: 10.1007/978-1-4939-3031-9_5

Ryan, A. F., Woolf, N. K., & Bone, R. C. (1980). Ultrastructural correlates of selective outer hair cell destruction following kanamycin intoxication in the chinchilla. *Hearing Research, 3*(4), 335–351. Retrieved from http://www.ncbi.nlm.nih.gov/entrez/query.fcgi?cmd=Retrieve&db=PubMed&dopt=Citation&list_uids=7451380

Ryugo, D. K., & Parks, T. N. (2003). Primary innervation of the avian and mammalian cochlear nucleus. *Brain Research Bulletin, 60*(5–6), 435–456. Retrieved from http://www.ncbi.nlm.nih.gov/pubmed/12787866

Sachs, M. B., & Abbas, P. J. (1974). Rate versus level functions for auditory-nerve fibers in cats: Tone-burst stimuli. *Journal of the Acoustical Society of America, 56*(6), 1835–1847. Retrieved from http://www.ncbi.nlm.nih.gov/entrez/query.fcgi?cmd=Retrieve&db=PubMed&dopt=Citation&list_uids=4443483

Schmiedt, R. A. (1989). Spontaneous rates, thresholds and tuning of auditory-nerve fibers in the gerbil: Comparisons to cat data. *Hearing Research, 42*(1), 23–35. Retrieved from http://www.ncbi.nlm.nih.gov/pubmed/2584157

Sheets, L., He, X. J., Olt, J., Schreck, M., Petralia, R. S., Wang, Y. X., . . . Kindt, K. S. (2017). Enlargement of ribbons in zebrafish hair cells increases calcium currents but disrupts afferent spontaneous activity and timing of stimulus onset. *Journal of Neuroscience, 37*(26), 6299–6313. doi:10.1523/JNEUROSCI.2878-16.2017

Shore, S. E., & Zhou, J. (2006). Somatosensory influence on the cochlear nucleus and beyond. *Hearing Research, 216–217*, 90–99. Retrieved from http://www.ncbi.nlm.nih.gov/entrez/query.fcgi?cmd=Retrieve&db=PubMed&dopt=Citation&list_uids=16513306

Siegel, J. H., & Brownell, W. E. (1981). Presynaptic bodies in outer hair cells of the chinchilla organ of Corti. *Brain Research, 220*(1), 188–193. Retrieved from http://www.ncbi.nlm.nih.gov/entrez/query.fcgi?cmd=Retrieve&db=PubMed&dopt=Citation&list_uids=7272751

Simmons, D. D., & Liberman, M. C. (1988a). Afferent innervation of outer hair cells in adult cats: I. Light microscopic analysis of fibers labeled with horseradish peroxidase. *Journal of Comparative Neurology, 270*(1), 132–144. doi:10.1002/cne.902700111

Simmons, D. D., & Liberman, M. C. (1988b). Afferent innervation of outer hair cells in adult cats: II. Electron microscopic analysis of fibers labeled with horseradish peroxidase. *Journal of Comparative Neurology, 270*(1), 145–154. doi:10.1002/cne.902700112

Smith, C. A., & Haglan, B. J. (1973). Golgi stains on the guinea pig organ of Corti. *Acta Otolaryngology, 75*(2), 203–210. Retrieved from http://www.ncbi.nlm.nih.gov/pubmed/4120814

Sobkowicz, H. M., Rose, J. E., Scott, G. L., & Levenick, C. V. (1986). Distribution of synaptic ribbons in the developing organ of Corti. *Journal of Neurocytology, 15*(6), 693–714. Retrieved from http://www.ncbi.nlm.nih.gov/entrez/query.fcgi?cmd=Retrieve&db=PubMed&dopt=Citation&list_uids=3819777

Sobkowicz, H. M., Rose, J. E., Scott, G. E., & Slapnick, S. M. (1982). Ribbon synapses in the developing intact and cultured organ of Corti in the mouse. *Journal of Neuroscience*, *2*(7), 942–957. Retrieved from http://www.ncbi.nlm.nih.gov/pubmed/7097321

Spoendlin, H. (1969). Innervation patterns in the organ of corti of the cat. *Acta Otolaryngologica*, *67*(2), 239–254. Retrieved from http://www.ncbi.nlm.nih.gov/pubmed/5374642

Spoendlin, H. (1971). Primary structural changes in the organ of Corti after acoustic overstimulation. *Acta Otolaryngologica*, *71*(2), 166–176. Retrieved from http://www.ncbi.nlm.nih.gov/entrez/query.fcgi?cmd=Retrieve&db=PubMed&dopt=Citation&list_uids=5577011

Spoendlin, H. (1972). Innervation densities of the cochlea. *Acta Otolaryngologica*, *73*(2), 235–248. Retrieved from http://www.ncbi.nlm.nih.gov/entrez/query.fcgi?cmd=Retrieve&db=PubMed&dopt=Citation&list_uids=5015157

Stamataki, S., Francis, H. W., Lehar, M., May, B. J., & Ryugo, D. K. (2006). Synaptic alterations at inner hair cells precede spiral ganglion cell loss in aging C57BL/6J mice. *Hearing Research*, *221*(1–2), 104–118. Retrieved from http://www.ncbi.nlm.nih.gov/entrez/query.fcgi?cmd=Retrieve&db=PubMed&dopt=Citation&list_uids=17005343

Sueta, T., Zhang, S. Y., Sellick, P. M., Patuzzi, R., & Robertson, D. (2004). Effects of a calcium channel blocker on spontaneous neural noise and gross action potential waveforms in the guinea pig cochlea. *Hearing Research*, *188*(1–2), 117–125. Retrieved from http://www.ncbi.nlm.nih.gov/entrez/query.fcgi?cmd=Retrieve&db=PubMed&dopt=Citation&list_uids=14759575

Sun, S., & Dong, X. (2016). Trp channels and itch. *Seminars in Immunopathology*, *38*(3), 293–307. doi:10.1007/s00281-015-0530-4

Thiers, F. A., Nadol, J. B., Jr., & Liberman, M. C. (2008). Reciprocal synapses between outer hair cells and their afferent terminals: Evidence for a local neural network in the mammalian cochlea. *Journal of the Association for Research in Otolaryngology*, *9*(4), 477–489. Retrieved from http://www.ncbi.nlm.nih.gov/entrez/query.fcgi?cmd=Retrieve&db=PubMed&dopt=Citation&list_uids=18688678

Tritsch, N. X., Yi, E., Gale, J. E., Glowatzki, E., & Bergles, D. E. (2007). The origin of spontaneous activity in the developing auditory system. *Nature*, *450*(7166), 50–55. Retrieved from http://www.ncbi.nlm.nih.gov/entrez/query.fcgi?cmd=Retrieve&db=PubMed&dopt=Citation&list_uids=17972875

Vyas, P., Wu, J. S., Zimmerman, A., Fuchs, P., & Glowatzki, E. (2016). Tyrosine hydroxylase expression in type ii cochlear afferents in mice. *Journal of the Association for Research in Otolaryngology*. doi:10.1007/s10162-016-0591-7

Wall, P. D. (1978). The gate control theory of pain mechanisms: A re-examination and restatement. *Brain*, *101*(1), 1–18. Retrieved from http://www.ncbi.nlm.nih.gov/entrez/query.fcgi?cmd=Retrieve&db=PubMed&dopt=Citation&list_uids=205314

Weisz, C., Glowatzki, E., & Fuchs, P. (2009). The postsynaptic function of type II cochlear afferents. *Nature*, *461*(7267), 1126–1129. doi:10.1038/nature08487

Weisz, C. J. C. (2011). *Synaptic inputs and excitability in type II cochlear afferents* (Ph.D. dissertation), Johns Hopkins, ProQuest Dissertations Publishing, Baltimore, MD. (3497142)

Weisz, C. J., Glowatzki, E., & Fuchs, P. A. (2014). Excitability of type II cochlear afferents. *Journal of Neuroscience*, *34*(6), 2365–2373. doi:10.1523/JNEUROSCI.3428-13.2014

Weisz, C. J., Lehar, M., Hiel, H., Glowatzki, E., & Fuchs, P. A. (2012). Synaptic transfer from outer hair cells to type II afferent fibers in the rat cochlea. *Journal of Neuroscience*, *32*(28), 9528–9536. doi:10.1523/JNEUROSCI.6194-11.2012

Wittig, J. H., Jr., & Parsons, T. D. (2008). Synaptic ribbon enables temporal precision of hair cell afferent synapse by increasing the number of readily releasable vesicles: a modeling study. *Journal of Neurophysiology*, *100*(4), 1724–1739. Retrieved from http://www.ncbi.nlm.nih.gov/entrez/query.fcgi?cmd=Retrieve&db=PubMed&dopt=Citation&list_uids=18667546

Wright, D. D., & Ryugo, D. K. (1996). Mossy fiber projections from the cuneate nucleus to the cochlear nucleus in the rat. *Journal of Comparative Neurology*, *365*(1), 159–172. Retrieved from http://www.ncbi.nlm.nih.gov/entrez/query.fcgi?cmd=Retrieve&db=PubMed&dopt=Citation&list_uids=8821448

Wu, J. S., Vyas, P., Glowatzki, E., & Fuchs, P. A. (2018). Opposing expression gradients of calcitonin-related polypeptide alpha (Calca/Cgrpalpha) and tyrosine hydroxylase (Th) in type II afferent neurons of the mouse cochlea. *Journal of Comparative Neurology*. doi:10.1002/cne.24341

Wu, J. S., Young, E. D., & Glowatzki, E. (2016). Maturation of spontaneous firing properties after hearing onset in rat auditory nerve fibers: Spontaneous rates, refractoriness, and interfiber correlations. *Journal of Neuroscience*, *36*(41), 10584–10597. doi:10.1523/JNEUROSCI.1187-16.2016

Young, E. D. (2008). Neural representation of spectral and temporal information in speech. *Philosophical Transactions of the Royal Society of London Ser. B Biological Science*, *363*(1493), 923–945. doi:10.1098/rstb.2007.2151

Zachary, S. P., & Fuchs, P. A. (2015). Re-Emergent inhibition of cochlear inner hair cells in a mouse model of hearing loss. *Journal of Neuroscience*, *35*(26), 9701–9706. doi:10.1523/JNEUROSCI.0879-15.2015

Zhan, X., & Ryugo, D. K. (2007). Projections of the lateral reticular nucleus to the cochlear nucleus in rats. *Journal of Comparative Neurology*, *504*(5), 583–598. Retrieved from http://www.ncbi.nlm.nih.gov/entrez/query.fcgi?cmd=Retrieve&db=PubMed&dopt=Citation&list_uids=17701985

Zhang, K. D., & Coate, T. M. (2017). Recent advances in the development and function of type II spiral ganglion neurons in the mammalian inner ear. *Seminars in Cell & Developmental Biology*, *65*, 80–87. doi:10.1016/j.semcdb.2016.09.017

Zhang, S. Y., Robertson, D., Yates, G., & Everett, A. (1999). Role of L-type Ca(2+) channels in transmitter release from mammalian inner hair cells I. Gross sound-evoked potentials. *Journal of Neurophysiology*, *82*(6), 3307–3315. Retrieved from http://www.ncbi.nlm.nih.gov/entrez/query.fcgi?cmd=Retrieve&db=PubMed&dopt=Citation&list_uids=10601462

CHAPTER 3

EFFERENT INNERVATION TO THE COCHLEA

ANA BELÉN ELGOYHEN, CAROLINA WEDEMEYER, AND MARIANO N. DI GUILMI

Abstract

The auditory system consists of ascending and descending neuronal pathways. The best studied is the ascending pathway, whereby sounds that are transduced in the cochlea into electrical signals are sent to the brain via the auditory nerve. Before reaching the auditory cortex, auditory ascending information has several central relays: the cochlear nucleus and superior olivary complex in the brainstem, the lateral lemniscal nuclei and inferior colliculus in the midbrain, and the medial geniculate body in the thalamus. The function(s) of the descending corticofugal pathway is less well understood. It plays important roles in shaping or even creating the response properties of central auditory neurons and in the plasticity of the auditory system, such as reorganizing cochleotopic and computational maps. Corticofugal projections are present at different relays of the auditory system. This review focuses on the physiology and plasticity of the medial efferent olivocochlear system.

Keywords: olivocochlear, nicotinic receptors, ligand-gated channels, cochlea, critical period

Anatomy of the Olivocochlear Efferent Innervation

Rasmussen (1946) was the first one to provide a subdivision of the efferent pathway into uncrossed and crossed olivocochlear bundles, the latter crossing the midline near the floor of the fourth ventricle. Nowadays, olivocochlear efferents are subdivided into medial (MOC) and lateral (LOC), based on tract-tracing experiments (Brown, 1987; Warr, 1992; Warr, 1975); (Figure 3.1). Thin, unmyelinated lateral LOC efferents originate from

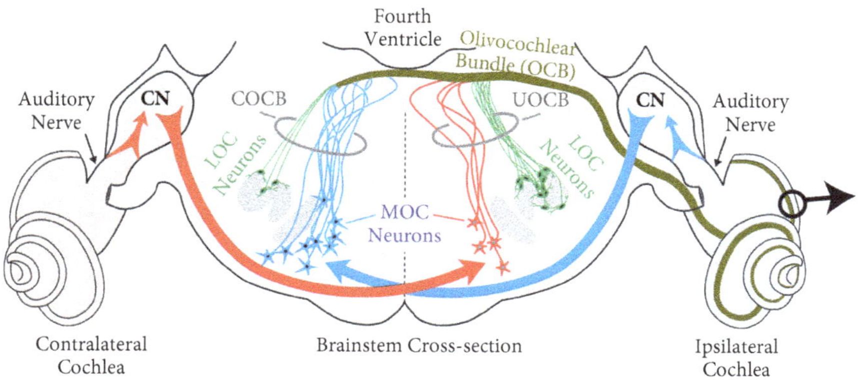

FIGURE 3.1. The olivocochlear reflex. Illustration of a transverse section of the brainstem; lateral olivocochlear (LOC, green) and medial olivocochlear (MOC, blue or red) neurons. The pathways for the ipsilateral and contralateral MOC reflexes to the right ear are shown in blue and red, respectively, and in gold when they join the olivocochlear bundle (OCB). Crossed (COCB) and uncrossed OCB (UOCB) components, are formed by LOC and MOC axons. CN, cochlear nucleus. The S-shaped gray structure is the lateral superior olivary nucleus, and the gray structure medial to it, is the medial superior olivary nucleus.

Reproduced from Guinan, 2006.

small neurons in or around the lateral superior olivary nucleus and project through the vestibular nerve mainly to the region near inner hair cells (IHCs) in the ipsilateral cochlea. They form synaptic contacts on the radial dendrites of Type I auditory afferent fibers postsynaptic to the IHCs. Thick, myelinated MOC efferents originate from larger neurons located in the medial part of the superior olivary nucleus and project through the vestibular nerve mostly contralaterally to make synaptic contacts directly onto outer hair cells (OHCs; Figure 3.2). Both MOC and LOC efferent fibers also send collaterals to brainstem vestibular nuclei and the cochlear nucleus. Lateral and medial efferent innervation patterns differ along the length of the cochlea. LOC inputs spread widely throughout the cochlea (Maison, Adams, & Liberman, 2003; Vetter, Adams, & Mugnani, 1991). In contrast, MOC fibers peaks near the middle of the cochlear spiral with significantly lower innervation densities toward the basal and apical extremes (Maison et al., 2003). Most efferent effects studied to date are mainly attributed to the MOC system (Guinan, 1996). This derives from the fact that experimental approaches involve the electrical stimulation of efferent fibers at the floor of the fourth ventricle where MOC fibers are more exposed. In addition, medial efferents are myelinated and thus have a lower threshold for extracellular current stimulation than do the smaller unmyelinated LOC fibers. MOC and LOC neurons receive auditory innervation and are the final arms of acoustic reflexes. The MOC acoustic reflex is the best understood and has both an ipsilateral and contralateral arm with a relay in reflex interneurons in the posteroventral cochlear nuclei (de Venecia, Liberman, Guinan, & Brown, 2005; Figure 3.1).

Efferent innervation to the cochlea undergoes extensive developmental remodeling. These descending fibers can be detected in the peripheral sensory epithelium around

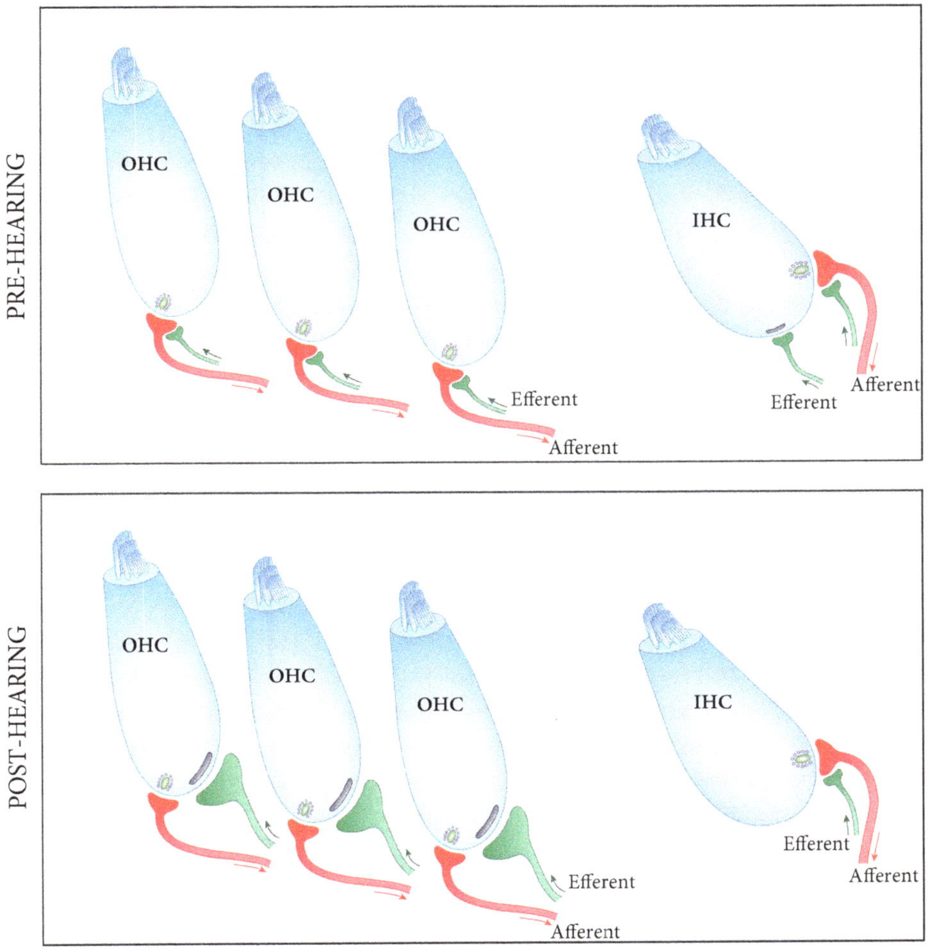

FIGURE 3.2. Innervation of hair cells during development. Before the onset of hearing, the basal pole of cochlear inner hair cells (IHCs) is surrounded by immature afferent axosomatic, transient efferent axosomatic, and efferent axodendritic terminals. At least part of the efferent endings under IHCs in the immature cochlea is represented by medial olivocochlear neurons making direct synaptic contacts with the cell. Pre-hearing OHCs are devoid of direct efferent contacts. In the mature mouse cochlea, afferent synapses typically have a single ellipsoid ribbon per active zone in both inner and outer hair cells. IHCs form afferent synapses only. Lateral olivocochlear neurons synapse onto type I SGNs boutons in close proximity to IHCs, whereas medial olivocochlear neurons contact OHCs directly.

Scheme drawn by Marcelo J. Moglie.

embryonic day 13 in rodents (Bruce, Kingsley, Nichols, & Fritzsch, 1997). MOC efferents transiently project to the IHC area during development, where they make direct axo-somatic contacts (Simmons, 2002). No direct contacts are seen over IHCs around the onset of hearing (P12 in altricial rodents), and only the LOC fibers make axo-dendritic synapses with afferent fibers in the IHC area in adults (Simmons, 2002). Efferents start to appear beneath the OHCs by P2 and to establish the adult-like axo-somatic synaptic contacts by P12 in altricial rodents (Bruce, Christensen, & Warr, 2000; Bruce et al., 1997; Bulankina & Moser, 2012; Rontal & Echteler, 2003; Simmons, 2002) (See Figure 3.2.). This developmental period where efferent fibers make direct contacts with IHCs is known as the "critical period" and appears to be important for the development of the auditory pathway (Clause et al., 2014; Clause, Lauer, & Kandler, 2017).

Physiology of the MOC Efferents to "Mature" OHC

Two alternative mechanisms for sound amplification have been described in the peripheral auditory system. An old one, shared by non-mammalian and mammalian vertebrates, where amplification results from the nonlinearity in the transduction mechanism itself (Chan & Hudspeth, 2005; Jia & He, 2005; Kennedy et al., 2005) and a more recent one, in which the hair cell receptor potential drives a novel motile process within the lateral membrane of the OHC (Brownell, Bader, Bertrand, & de Ribaupierre, 1985; Dallos, 1992, 2008; Dallos & Evans, 1995). In mammals, OHCs are the principal players underlying cochlear amplification, where hyperpolarization causes the cell to expand along its longitudinal axis and depolarization causes it to contract. This process, known as somatic electromotility, is based on the motor-protein prestin (Zheng et al., 2000), a member of the solute carrier anion-transport family 26 (SLC26) (Elgoyhen & Franchini, 2011; Franchini & Elgoyhen, 2006; Mount & Romero, 2004). Thus, at each place along the cochlear partition, OHCs amplify basilar membrane motion. MOC efferents that contact OHCs are in place to modify the action of the OHCs and, through this, to control the gain of the "cochlear amplifier" (Guinan, 1996; Guinan, 2006). Efferent inhibition can be activated by sound presented to the contralateral ear (Chambers, Hancock, Maison, Liberman, & Polley, 2012; Kujawa, Glattke, Fallon, & Bobbin, 1994; Maison et al., 2012; Muller, Janssen, Heppelmann, & Wagner, 2005). However, most studies of efferent inhibition in animals have been performed by electrical stimulation of efferent axons at the floor of the fourth ventricle and measurement of effects in the cochlea (Guinan, 1996). Thus, MOC stimulation reduces the response at the best frequency measured either at the compound (Galambos, 1956) or single unit response of afferent fibers (Gifford & Guinan, 1987; Wiederhold & Kiang, 1970), IHC receptor potential (Brown & Nuttal, 1984) or basilar membrane motion (Murugasu & Russell, 1996; Russell & Murugasu, 1997). Efferent inhibition also affects cochlear tuning, resulting in a broader tuning curve and a diminished selectivity of afferent neurons (Guinan, 1996; Guinan, 2006). The functional roles of MOC activity are still a matter of intense research, including the control of the dynamic range of hearing (Guinan, 1996), enhance selective attention (Delano, Elgueda, Hamame, & Robles, 2007; Oatman, 1976; Terreros, Jorratt, Aedo, Elgoyhen, & Delano, 2016), the improvement of signal detection in background noise

(Dolan & Nuttall, 1988; Kawase, Delgutte, & Liberman, 1993; Winslow & Sachs, 1988), and the protection from acoustic injury (Maison & Liberman, 2000; Maison, Luebke, Liberman, & Zuo, 2002; Patuzzi & Thompson, 1991; Taranda, Maison, et al., 2009).

Synaptic Responses at the MOC-Hair Cell Synapse

Although several neurotransmitters have been described in the efferent system—such as γ-aminobutyric acid (GABA), calcitonin-gene-related peptide, dopamine, and neuropeptides—acetylcholine (ACh) is the main neurotransmitter that mediates fast synaptic transmission between MOC efferents and OHCs (for review see Eybalin, 1993; Sewell, 1996). Schuknecht et al. (1959) provided the first hints of a cholinergic innervation. They reported acetylcholinesterase-labeled processes in the intact cochlea that disappeared after surgical de-efferentation. Further biochemical and immunohistochemical studies supported the hypothesis of a cholinergic innervation in the following years, including choline acetyltransferase immuno-labeled patches in large axosomatic synapses onto OHCs observed by electron microscopy (Eybalin & Pujol, 1987).

The first reports of direct efferent effects onto hair cells came from recordings on fish lateral line, known to have cellular mechanisms similar to those of auditory hair cells (Flock & Russell, 1976; Flock & Russell, 1973). Efferent effects on hair cells were inhibitory, caused hyperpolarizing inhibitory post-synaptic potentials (IPSPs) that were blocked by cholinergic antagonists, and produced a reduction of afferent fiber activity. These results were then extended to auditory hair cells of different vertebrate species, such as frogs (Ashmore & Russell, 1983; Sugai, Yano, Sugitani, & Ooyama, 1992), reptiles (Art, Fettiplace, & Fuchs, 1984; Art, Crawford, Fettiplace, & Fuchs, 1982), birds (Fuchs & Murrow, 1992; Shigemoto & Ohmori, 1991), and guinea pigs (Erostegui, Norris, & Bobbin, 1994; Housley & Ashmore, 1991; Kakehata, Nakagawa, Takasaka, & Akaike, 1993; Nenov, Norris, & Bobbin, 1996; Nenov, Norris, & Bobbin, 1996), indicating that efferent effects are conserved across vertebrate species (Manley & Koppl, 1998). The development of an ex vivo rodent cochlear explant preparation for intracellular recordings from hair cells (Glowatzki & Fuchs, 2000) has accelerated the discovery of the synaptic mechanisms involved in both efferent (Ballestero et al., 2011; Gomez-Casati, Fuchs, Elgoyhen, & Katz, 2005; Goutman, Fuchs, & Glowatzki, 2005; Katz et al., 2004; Lioudyno et al., 2004; Oliver et al., 2000; Wedemeyer et al., 2013) and afferent (Glowatzki & Fuchs, 2002; Goutman, 2012; Goutman & Glowatzki, 2007) synapses of mammalian hair cells. Most experiments in cochlear explants were initially performed in developing IHCs, since they are more tractable for sustained stable recordings. Recently, they have been extended to OHCs and this will be indicated when necessary.

Patch-clamp recordings from hair cells shows that spontaneous or evoked IPSPs and responses to ACh are biphasic and consist of a small inward current followed within milliseconds by a much larger and longer lasting outward K^+ current (Figure 3.3). As described below, the inward current corresponds to the opening of a high-calcium permeable non-selective cationic cholinergic nicotinic receptor (Elgoyhen, Johnson, Boulter, Vetter, & Heinemann, 1994; Elgoyhen et al., 2001; Fuchs & Murrow, 1992; Housley, Batcher, Kraft, & Ryan, 1994) and the outward current which leads to hyperpolarization, to the activation of small-conductance Ca^{2+}-activated SK2 K^+ channels (Dulon, Luo, Zhang, & Ryan, 1998; Matthews, Duncan, Zidanic, Michael, & Fuchs, 2005; Nenov et al., 1996; Yuhas & Fuchs, 1999). Unitary inhibitory postsynaptic currents (IPSCs) occur rapidly, with rise and decay time constants of approximately 6 ms and 30 ms, respectively. Since this time course corresponds to the Ca^{2+} gating of SK channels, it implies a fast coupling between the ionotropic neurotransmitter receptor and the SK channel, which leads to the hyperpolarization of the sensory cell. Moreover, it suggests that rapid, localized changes in subsynaptic Ca^{2+} levels rather than major changes in intracellular Ca^{2+} levels are sufficient for correct coupling (Oliver et al., 2000). Nevertheless, other lines of evidence have led to the proposal that release of calcium from an internal store, contributes to activation of the SK channels (Kakehata et al., 1993; Lioudyno et al., 2004; Shigemoto & Ohmori, 1991; Yoshida, Shigemoto, Sugai, & Ohmori, 1994). This includes the existence of an endoplasmic reticulum membrane that is co-extensive to the efferent synaptic contact in OHCs (Fuchs, Lehar, & Hiel, 2014; Gulley & Reese, 1977; Hirokawa, 1978; Saito, 1983), which resembles the sarcoplasmic reticulum of the skeletal muscle and pharmacological evidence suggesting ryanodine-sensitive calcium stores (Evans, Lagostena, Darbon, & Mammano, 2000; Lioudyno et al., 2004). More recent experiments in chicken hair cells have suggested that synaptic cisterns serve primarily as a calcium barrier and sink during low-level synaptic activity (Im, Moskowitz, Lehar, Hiel, & Fuchs, 2014). Whether Ca^{2+}-induced Ca^{2+}-release from internal stores might explain the slow effects reported for the MOC efferents (Sridhar, Brown, & Sewell, 1997; Sridhar, Liberman, Brown, & Sewell, 1995) is still a matter of debate.

Most recordings from OHCs have been performed in apical regions of the cochlea, since they are less challenging than those from the basal region. Recent findings have shown that large conductance, Ca^{2+}- and voltage-gated (BK) potassium channels also contribute to efferent inhibition in basal, high-frequency rodent OHCs after the onset of hearing (Wersinger, McLean, Fuchs, & Pyott, 2010). BK channels underlie faster synaptic IPSCs waveforms than SK channels. Thus, IPSCs recorded from basal high-frequency OHCs expressing BK channels are briefer than IPSCs recorded from apical low-frequency OHCs that do not express BK channels (Rohmann, Wersinger, Braude, Pyott, & Fuchs, 2015). Moreover, immature high-frequency OHCs before the developmental onset of BK channel expression also have longer IPSCs, as do OHCs of BK $\alpha^{(-/-)}$ mice lacking the pore-forming α-subunit of BK channels compared to $BK\alpha^{(+/+)}$ littermates (Rohmann et al., 2015). In vivo efferent-mediated inhibition of distortion product otoacoustic emissions has been analyzed in BK knockout mice, indicating that both BK and SK channels contribute to the effect (Maison, Pyott, Meredith, & Liberman, 2013). In addition, immunostaining has shown BK- and SK2-positive puncta at the basal pole of OHCs, colabeling with anti-synaptophysin, suggesting that each of these puncta

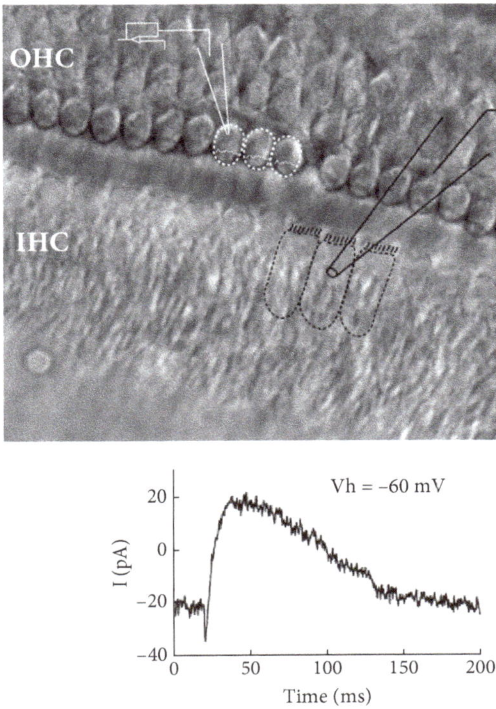

FIGURE 3.3. Efferent synaptic responses. Snapshot of a cochlear explant. IHCs are depicted with a dashed black line, and some OHCs in the first row are shown with a dashed white line. Representative spontaneous synaptic current recorded in a P10 OHC from a mouse apical cochlear coil, voltage-clamped at −60 mV (recording performed by Jimena Ballestero). As can be observed, a rapid inward current (mediated by the α9α10 nAChR) is curtailed by a larger and longer-lasting outward current (mediated by the SK2 potassium channel).

Adapted from Elgoyhen & Katz, 2012.

is located directly opposite to an efferent terminal. A gradient of expression is observed along the cochlea, since BK expression in the OHC area is stronger in the basal half, whereas SK2 expression is stronger in the apical half. The consequence of this BK/SK2 gradient to efferent function is still unknown (but see below).

The Cholinergic Nicotinic Hair Cell Receptor

Although the existence of a cochlear efferent cholinergic innervation was known since the 1960s, an experimental conundrum existed derived from the baroque pharmacological profile of the receptor, which is not activated neither by nicotine nor muscarine and blocked by atropine, nicotine, strychnine, α-bungarotoxin, *d*-tubocurarine, and bicuculline (Blanchet, Erostegui, Sugasawa, & Dulon, 1996; Doi & Ohmori, 1993; Fuchs & Murrow, 1992; Housley & Ashmore, 1991; Kakehata et al., 1993; Shigemori & Ohmori, 1990, 1991; Yoshida et al., 1994). This profile remained at odds with the classical pharmacological classification of cholinergic receptors into either metabotropic muscarinic or ionotropic nicotinic. Indeed, the receptor was in fact proposed to be a muscarinic one, coupled to a guanine nucleotide binding protein (G-protein) which triggers metabolic cascades of InsP3 and Ca^{2+} (Kakehata et al., 1993; Shigemoto & Ohmori, 1990, 1991; Yoshida et al., 1994). It was not until the cloning of the α9 cholinergic nicotinic receptor subunit that the molecular nature of the receptor present at the MOC-hair cell synapse, both in developing IHCs and adult OHCs was deciphered (Elgoyhen et al., 1994). The additional cloning of the α10 subunit (Elgoyhen et al., 2001; Lustig, Peng, Hiel, Yamamoto, & Fuchs, 2001; Sgard et al., 2002) completed the subunit composition of the cholinergic nicotinic receptor present at the MOC-hair cell synapse. Mutant mice lacking either the α9 (Vetter et al., 1999) or the α10 (Vetter et al., 2007) and a α9 knockin mouse model bearing a point mutation in the pore region of the channel (Taranda, Maison, et al., 2009), have unequivocally demonstrated that both nAChR subunits are needed for ACh-mediated MOC efferent effects. By comparison of the properties of recombinant α9α10 nAChRs expressed in *Xenopus* oocytes (Ballestero et al., 2005; Elgoyhen et al., 1994; Elgoyhen et al., 2001; Ellison et al., 2006; Johnson, Martinez, Elgoyhen, Heinemann, & McIntosh, 1995; McIntosh et al., 2005; Rothlin, Verbitsky, Katz, & Elgoyhen, 1999; Rothlin et al., 2003; Verbitsky, Rothlin, Katz, & Elgoyhen, 2000) with those of native receptors present in hair cells (Ballestero et al., 2011; Elgoyhen et al., 2001; Gomez-Casati et al., 2005), it is now well established that the receptor is a pentameric assembly of α9 and α10 subunits (Elgoyhen & Katz, 2012) with a likely $\alpha 9_2 \alpha 10_3$ stoichiometry (Plazas, Katz, Gomez-Casati, Bouzat, & Elgoyhen, 2005). Thus, it belongs to the family of pentameric ligand-gated ion channels which in mammals comprises nicotinic acetylcholine receptors (nAChRs), serotonin type 3 (5-HT_3) receptors, γ-aminobutyric acid type A ($GABA_A$) receptors, glycine receptors, and zinc-activated ion channels (Nemecz, Prevost, Menny, & Corringer, 2016). In this regard, it is worth noting that it retains pharmacological properties of other members of the family, since it is blocked with high potency by the glycinergic antagonist strychnine, the 5-HT_3 receptor antagonists ICS 205-930, ondansetron and granisetron and the $GABA_A$ receptor antagonist bicuculline (Elgoyhen et al., 2001; Rothlin et al., 2003).

An additional peculiarity of the α9α10 nAChR is its evolutionary history. It was originally proposed to be the most primitive of all nAChR subunits, with the closest similarity with the hypothetical ancestor that gave rise to the family (Elgoyhen & Katz, 2012; Fritzsch & Elliott, 2017; Rothlin et al., 1999), based on its pharmacological properties and on the fact that α9 can form functional homomeric receptors. However, this might not be the case since the last common ancestor of chordates and invertebrates had an α7 subunit (possibly several), an α9 subunit and the muscle/neuronal-type subunits (Dent, 2006). Although both α9 and α10 subunits belong to the nAChR family, they are distant members based upon amino acid sequence homology (Elgoyhen et al., 1994; Elgoyhen et al., 2001). Moreover, a phylogenetic and molecular evolutionary analysis has shown that the gene encoding the α10 subunit (*CHRNA10*) has been under positive selection pressure only in the mammalian lineage (Elgoyhen & Franchini, 2011; Franchini & Elgoyhen, 2006). This suggests that *CHRNA9* and *CHRNA10* genes appeared after a gene duplication event from a common ancestor and co-existed without much functional diversion, until at some point during the course of evolution of the mammalian lineage changes started to accumulate in *CHRNA10*. Since during evolution, purifying (or negative) selection, i.e., the removal of functionally deleterious mutations, prevails in most protein-coding DNA sequences, the acquisition of amino acid changes in the coding region of the α10 nAChR subunit might indicate that mammalian α9α10 nAChR increased its fitness by acquiring novel functional properties which might have evolved with the specialization of mammalian hearing (Elgoyhen & Franchini, 2011). It is worth noting that prestin, the protein responsible for somatic electromotility and active mechanism for amplification in mammalian OHCs as well as the giant spectrin βV, a major component of the OHC's cortical cytoskeleton, have also been under positive selection pressure only in mammals (Cortese et al., 2017; Franchini & Elgoyhen, 2006). Cholinergic efferent feedback is found in all vertebrate species (Manley & Koppl, 1998; Simmons, 2002) and α9 and α10 nAChRs have been found expressed in auditory and vestibular hair cells of all vertebrate species analyzed (Elgoyhen et al., 1994; Elgoyhen et al., 2001; Glowatzki et al., 1995; Hiel, Elgoyhen, Drescher, & Morley, 1996; Lustig, Hiel, & Fuchs, 1999; Morley, Li, Hiel, Drescher, & Elgoyhen, 1998; Morley & Simmons, 2002; Simmons & Morley, 1998). Thus, one could speculate that the evolution of *CHRNA10* has endowed the mammalian auditory system feedback an α9α10 nAChR fit to control prestin-driven somatic electromotility, a capacity that is not required in non-mammalian species. One clear feature that differs between mammalian and non-mammalian α9α10 is their Ca^{2+} permeability (Lipovsek et al., 2014; Lipovsek et al., 2012).Whereas rat receptors have a high (pCa^{2+}/pMonovalents ~10) Ca^{2+}, chicken α9α10 receptors have a much lower permeability (~2) to this cation, comparable to that of neuronal α4β2 receptors. It has been speculated that the selection pressure might have derived from the fact that large conductance, calcium and voltage-gated (BK) potassium channels are expressed at efferent contacts and responsible for ACh-mediated hyperpolarization of OHCs in high frequency regions of the rat cochlea (Wersinger et al., 2010). Calcium affinity of BK channels is 2 orders of magnitude lower than that of SK channels (Fakler & Adelman, 2008), thus requiring higher calcium influx for activation compared to SK channels present in cochlear low-frequency regions or the chicken basilar papilla. Taken together these functional adaptations in cochlear proteins might have occurred to accommodate the higher frequency hearing capacities of mammals (Manley, 2017).

All nicotinic receptors serve fast excitatory synaptic transmission in the nervous system (Karlin, 2002). In contrast, neuronal fast inhibition is brought about by the activation of either $GABA_A$ or glycine receptors which are ligand-gated Cl^- channels (Burgos, Yevenes, & Aguayo, 2016; Moss & Smart, 2001). Given the presence of efferent GABAergic innervation to hair cells, the existence of a fast inhibitory neurotransmission brought about by the activation of a nicotinic cholinergic Ca^{2+}- permeable α9α10 receptor coupled to SK and/or BK channels, is a self-standing feature. One could argue that K^+-versus Cl^--driven hyperpolarization needed to modulate electromotility is more pronounced at the -60 mV resting potential of OHCs (O'Beirne & Patuzzi, 2007). In addition, fast K^+ instead of Cl^--mediated hyperpolarization might be required to avoid a direct perturbation of prestin extrinsic voltage sensors which are brought about by the intracellular anions chloride and bicarbonate (Oliver et al., 2001). However, α9α10 nAChR-mediated activation of SK channels is also present in non-mammalian and vestibular hair cells, which lack-prestin-driven electromotility. Thus, the evolutionary pressures leading to the appearance of a Cl^- independent fast synaptic inhibition mechanism are still an enigma.

Molecular Actors at the MOC-Hair Cell Synapse

Neurotransmitter release at central and peripheral synapses is triggered by presynaptic Ca^{2+} entry (Katz & Miledi, 1969) through multiple voltage-gated Ca^{2+} channels (VGCC) including N-type, P/Q- type and R-type (Catterall, 2000; Catterall & Few, 2008). Electrophysiological and pharmacological experiments have shown that at P9-11 release at efferent-IHC synapses derives from the activation of both N ($Ca_v2.2$) and P/Q-type ($Ca_v2.1$) VGCC closely associated with the release machinery (Zorrilla de San Martin, Pyott, Ballestero, & Katz, 2010) (Figure 3.4). In addition, Ca^{2+} influx via L-type VGCCs together with membrane depolarization activates efferent terminal BK channels (Zorrilla de San Martin et al., 2010). As reported in other neurons this would accelerate the repolarization of the terminal membrane (Berkefeld & Fakler, 2008; Berkefeld, Fakler, & Schulte, 2010; Berkefeld et al., 2006) and tight regulate transmitter release by exerting a negative feedback (Raffaelli, Saviane, Mohajerani, Pedarzani, & Cherubini, 2004; Robitaille, Garcia, Kaczorowski, & Charlton, 1993). The Ca^{2+} channels involved in transmitter release at MOC-OHCs are still to be determined. Electron microscopy experiments with immunogold labeling have shown OHC pre and post-synaptic expression of BK channels (Sakai, Harvey, & Sokolowski, 2011), suggesting the presence of a similar negative feedback of transmitter release.

In addition to Ca^{2+}-triggered exocytosis, neuronal transmitter release is regulated by the activation of presynaptic receptors present in the synaptic terminal. Depending on the ligand that activates the presynaptic receptor, they are distinguished into auto- and heteroreceptors, the former controlling the release of their endogenous agonist, the latter controlling the release of transmitters other than their endogenous ligand. The presence of cholinergic presynaptic autoreceptors on MOC efferent terminals has not been investigated. However, presynaptic $GABA_B$ (Wedemeyer et al., 2013) and group I metabotropic glutamate mGluR1 (Ye, Goutman, Pyott, & Glowatzki, 2017) heteroreceptors are present at these cholinergic terminals and provide negative and positive feedback for transmitter release, respectively (Figure 3.4).

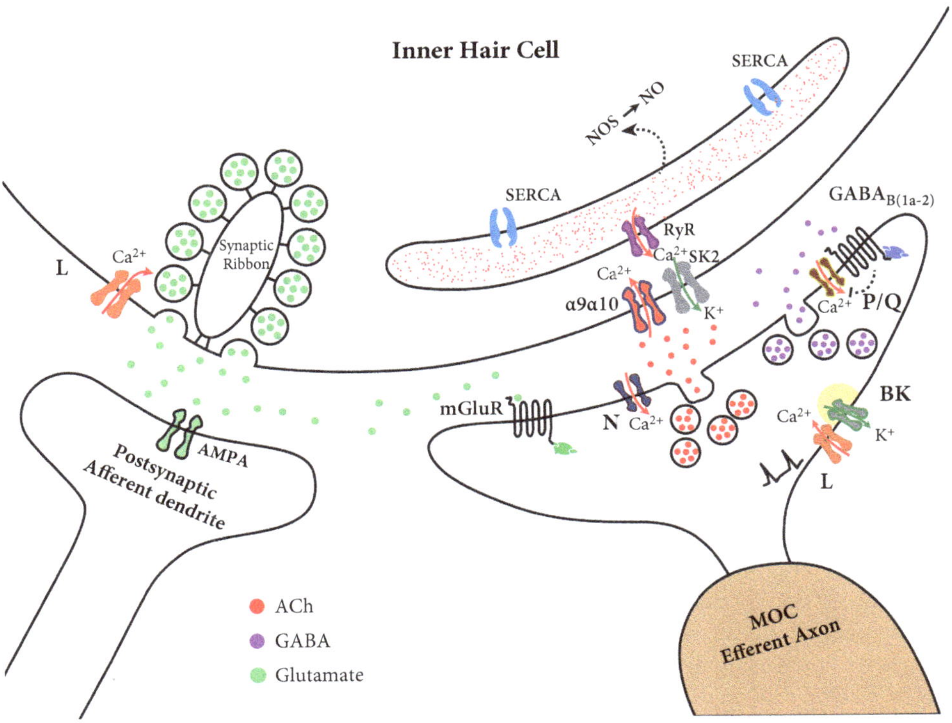

FIGURE 3.4. Representation of the molecules at the efferent synapse. Schematic representation of the molecules and mechanisms involved in synaptic transmission at MOC-hair cell synapses (right side). ACh release is supported by both P/Q and N-type VGCC. BK channels activated by Ca^{2+} entering through L-type VGCC accelerate action potential repolarization and thus diminish the amount of ACh being released. GABA probably co-released with ACh, activates presynaptic $GABA_{B(1a,2)}$ receptors, which inhibit ACh release by altering the activity of P/Q-type VGCC. The inhibitory postsynaptic response is mediated by α9α10 nAChR coupled to the activation of SK2 potassium channels. Ca^{2+}-induced Ca^{2+} release from the postsynaptic cisterns closely apposed to the IHC synaptic region probably also contributes to SK2 activation. Nitric oxide synthetized by the IHC enhances transmitter release by the MOC synaptic terminals acting as a retrograde messenger. Glutamate released from the efferent synapses (left side) activates group I mGluRs on presynaptic efferent terminals and enhances ACh release and efferent synaptic inhibition to the IHC. (SERCA: sarcoendoplasmic reticulum calcium ATPase; RyR: ryanodine receptor; NOS: nitric oxide synthase; NO: nitric oxide).

During the developmental critical period immature IHCs fire action potentials and release glutamate into the synaptic cleft. This activates ionotropic glutamate receptors on afferent dendrites of the spiral ganglion neurons (Grant, Yi, & Glowatzki, 2010). Each IHC action potential can release hundreds of glutamate-filled vesicles (Glowatzki & Fuchs, 2002) and therefore, glutamate spillover is likely to occur under physiological conditions (Ye et al., 2017). In fact, activation of group I metabotropic glutamate receptors (mGluR1s) enhances ACh release, most likely through the activation of presynaptic mGluR1s present in efferent terminals (Ye et al., 2017). It has been reported that in the central nervous system mGluRs reduce currents through L-type Ca^{2+} channels (Pin & Duvoisin, 1995; Sahara & Westbrook, 1993). Thus, group I mGluRs activation in the developing cochlea might provide a positive feedback to enhance efferent inhibition by suppressing L-type Ca^{2+} channels known to be present in efferent terminals (Zorrilla de San Martin et al., 2010), prevent the activation of BK channels, and prolong terminal depolarization and neurotransmitter release (Ye et al., 2017). Whether the same mechanism operates in MOC-OHC synapses has not been evaluated.

Antibodies against either GABA or its synthesizing enzyme, glutamate decarboxylase (GAD), have shown immunoreactivity in cell bodies of the superior olivary complex and in efferent terminals located below IHCs and OHCs. Moreover, cochlear efferent terminals demonstrate GABA uptake, suggesting GABA as a second neurotransmitter of the efferent system (for review see (Eybalin, 1993)). Studies in mice have provided evidence that virtually all olivocochlear endings in OHCs, including cholinergic and GABAergic projections, arise from the MOC system; whereas those in the IHC area arise almost exclusively from the LOC system (Maison et al., 2003). The longitudinal distribution of GABAergic terminals beneath OHCs varies from species to species: apical half in guinea pigs and throughout the cochlea in mouse. Immunoelectron microscopy studies have provided strong evidence for ChAT and GAD colocalization in efferent terminals on OHCs throughout the rat cochlea (Dannhof, Roth, & Bruns, 1991). A study in mice has further suggested the complete congruence of GABAergic and cholinergic markers in the IHC and OHC areas (Maison et al., 2003), suggesting that ACh and GABA are released from the same terminal. In this regard, since the advent of optogenetics, corelease of fast neurotransmitter is emerging as a common theme of central neuromodulatory systems (Granger, Mulder, Saunders, & Sabatini, 2016; Hnasko & Edwards, 2012). For example, corelease of ACh and GABA from cholinergic forebrain neurons has been recently reported (Saunders, Granger, & Sabatini, 2015).The function of the GABAergic innervation to hair cells and the exact molecular targets are poorly understood. Mouse lines with targeted deletions of $GABA_A$ receptor subunits have suggested that the GABAergic component of the OC system is needed for the long-term maintenance of hair cells and neurons in the inner ear (Maison, Rosahl, Homanics, & Liberman, 2006). Furthermore, the analysis of $GABA_{B1}$ knock-out mice has indicated that GABAergic signaling is required for normal OHC amplifier function at low sound levels and OHC responses to high-level sound, since they show increased resistance to permanent acoustic injury (Maison, Casanova, Holstein, Bettler, & Liberman, 2009). GABA-mediated changes in the stiffness and motility of OHCs have been also reported (Batta, Panyi, Szucs, & Sziklai, 2004; Zenner, Gitter, Rudert, & Ernst, 1992). Although one early study reported that guinea pig OHCs hyperpolarize in the presence of GABA (Gitter & Zenner, 1992), recent studies in mouse P9-11 IHCs and P12-14 OHCs show no evidence of currents when GABA is applied, suggesting the lack of postsynaptic $GABA_A$ receptors (Wedemeyer et al., 2013). Lack of $GABA_A$-mediated fast postsynaptic responses is further demonstrated by the fact that no postsynaptic currents in response to either high K^+ or electrical stimulation of MOC efferent axons are seen in

OHCs (Ballestero et al., 2011; Oliver et al., 2000) and IHCs (Glowatzki & Fuchs, 2000; Gomez-Casati et al., 2005) when the α9α10 nAChR is pharmacologically blocked or in α9 knockout mice (Vetter et al., 2007). Moreover, $GABA_B$ receptors are not expressed either in postnatal (Wedemeyer et al., 2013) or adult hair cells (Maison et al., 2009), further indicating a lack of postsynaptic $GABA_B$-mediated action. Therefore, a presynaptic site of action for GABA is expected. This is indeed the case, since GABA downregulates the amount of ACh released both at developing efferent IHC and OHCs. At least in IHCs this is mediated by presynaptic $GABA_{B(1a,2)}$ receptors coupled to the inhibition of P/Q-type VGCCs (Wedemeyer et al., 2013).

In summary, tight control of ACh release from efferent terminals is exerted through the presence of presynaptic neurotransmitter receptors, namely $GABA_B$ (Wedemeyer et al., 2013) and group I metabotropic glutamate receptor mGluR1 (Ye et al., 2017). In brief, whereas GABA inhibits, glutamate enhances ACh release, providing a negative and positive feedback to efferent inhibition, respectively. GABA most likely has a neuronal efferent origin, whereas glutamate is a spillover from the nearby IHC endogenous release of glutamate. This tight regulation of ACh release at MOC terminals might act in concert with the short-term synaptic plasticity phenomena known to shape the strength of cochlear inhibition.

Short-Term Synaptic Plasticity

A common property of most synapses is that they can keep track of their previous activity by means of synaptic plasticity. Each synapse can integrate several forms of plasticity leading to changes in synaptic strength and this plays a critical role in information transfer and neural processing. Thus, synaptic strength can be reduced for hundreds of milliseconds to seconds leading to depression, or it can be enhanced during hundreds of milliseconds to seconds resulting in facilitation. In addition, enhancement can last tens of seconds, a phenomenon known as post-tetanic potentiation (Fioravante & Regehr, 2011; Zucker & Regehr, 2002).

MOC efferents respond to sound with sensitivity and tuning like that of type I cochlear afferents (Liberman & Brown, 1986; Robertson & Gummer, 1985) and provide a feedback loop for cochlear gain control. The correct operation of this feedback requires a careful match between the acoustic stimulus and the strength of cochlear inhibition. This is mainly brought about by efferent synaptic plasticity both at the developing efferent-IHC and MOC-OHC synapses. A low probability of release at rest, and facilitation of responses at high frequency stimulation, is a common feature of efferent synapses (Art et al., 1984; Ballestero et al., 2011; Goutman et al., 2005).

The first reports of short-term synaptic plasticity in efferent terminals were described in turtle hair cells, where the resting probability of release at the hair cell efferent synapse was low, ranging from 0.08 to 0.3, but facilitated markedly during repetitive stimulation of the efferent axons (Art et al., 1984). Thus, single shocks to the efferents generated hair cell membrane hyperpolarization with an average amplitude of less than 1 mV. The size of the post-synaptic potential grew markedly to a maximum of 20–30 mV when trains of shocks were applied. Similar results have been found in rat P7–11 IHCs. Single shocks at frequencies less than 2 Hz evoked small IPSCs with a mean probability of 0.35. With repeated stimulation, IPSCs are both larger and more prolonged, likely due to facilitation and summation. For trains of 10 shocks IPSCs reliably reached more than 100 pA in amplitude (Goutman et al., 2005). Nitric oxide retrograde signaling from the hair cell to the efferent terminal has been proposed to contribute to this facilitation (Kong, Zachary, Rohmann, & Fuchs, 2013).

Similar mechanisms have been reported for the MOC-OHC synapse with a low resting probability of release. Facilitation combined with postsynaptic summation significantly increase the reliability and strength of synaptic transmission during repetitive efferent activity (Ballestero et al., 2011). The poor efficacy of synaptic transmission at the MOC–OHC at low frequency of stimulation is reflected by the low quantum content of transmitter release (m = 0.3). The overlap between spontaneous and evoked IPSCs amplitude histograms has led to the proposal that, on average, one vesicle is released upon arrival of an action potential to the MOC–OHC efferent terminal. The observation that in mice, OHCs from the apical region (where recordings were performed) are usually innervated by one efferent fiber (Maison et al., 2003) and that one efferent axon only rarely makes more than one contact with each OHC (Warr & Boche, 2003; Wilson, Henson, & Henson, 1991) is consistent with the idea that only one bouton will be activated each time an electrical shock is applied (Ballestero et al., 2011). However, shortage of synaptic vesicles cannot account for the low resting probability of release since efferent terminals have large numbers of vesicles (Fuchs et al., 2014; Lenoir, Schnerson, & Pujol, 1980). The implication of this result is that the efferent terminal is prepared to recruit synaptic vesicles when stimulation is repetitive and at sufficiently high frequencies so that facilitation of transmitter release can occur. The unreliability of transmitter release at the MOC–OHC synapse at low frequency stimulation has been attributed to the stochastic nature of release, rather than to axonal threshold variations or conduction failures (Ballestero et al., 2011). The negative feedback loop provided by the coupling between L-type voltage-gated calcium channels and BK channels (Zorrilla de San Martin et al., 2010) may operate to decrease synaptic output. Thus, as reported by Ballestero et al (2011) synaptic events occur sparsely at 10 Hz but increase in frequency and amplitude of individual responses as stimulation frequency increases (Figure 3.5). As expected, a sustained and enhanced hyperpolarization of the OHCs is observed in response to high-frequency MOC stimulation (Figure 3.6). The strengthening of synaptic transmission at high frequency stimulation of MOC terminals is accounted for by both facilitation and summation of OHCs synaptic responses. Ballestero et al. (2011) have evaluated the relative contribution of summation and facilitation by simulating the postsynaptic responses at different stimulation frequencies and concluded that the combined effect of both phenomena are needed to produce a simulated response most closely resembling the experimental data (Figure 3.7). Since the increase in the postsynaptic response during repetitive stimulation correlates with an increase in the probability of release and not with an increase in the mean amplitude of IPSCs, facilitation is due to a presynaptic

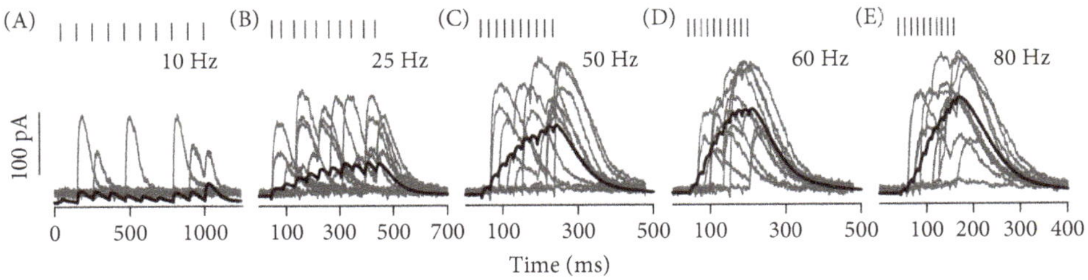

FIGURE 3.5. Facilitation of efferent transmitter release. Facilitation of transmitter release contributes to the increase in the postsynaptic response during high-frequency stimulation. Responses to 10 shock trains (gray traces) were applied at different frequencies (A–E). The black trace is the average response of 100 repetitions at each frequency.

Reproduced from Ballestero et al., 2011.

mechanism. In addition, the relatively slow decay of combined nAChR and SK2 eIPSCs result in temporal summation.

Synapses with low initial probability of release and strong facilitation have been postulated to work as high-pass filters, since they fail to transmit during low frequency action potentials but facilitate during sustained firing in a frequency-dependent manner (Atluri & Regehr, 1996; Jackman & Regehr, 2017). This would allow the MOC efferent feedback to operate in a kind of failsafe mode. Thus, OHCs would ignore spontaneous or inadvertent activity and only respond when efferents are strongly stimulated. Short-term plasticity of the MOC–OHC synapse allows this scaling of inhibition to MOC activity encoding graded levels of efferent feedback. This is important to provide a fine tuning of cochlear amplification, since efferent firing frequency increases linearly with sound intensity (Brown, Kujawa, & Liberman, 1998; Liberman & Brown, 1986; Robertson & Gummer, 1985). In vivo studies of the MOC effect on auditory function highly resemble the properties of the MOC–OHC synapse: brainstem electrical stimulation of MOC neurons

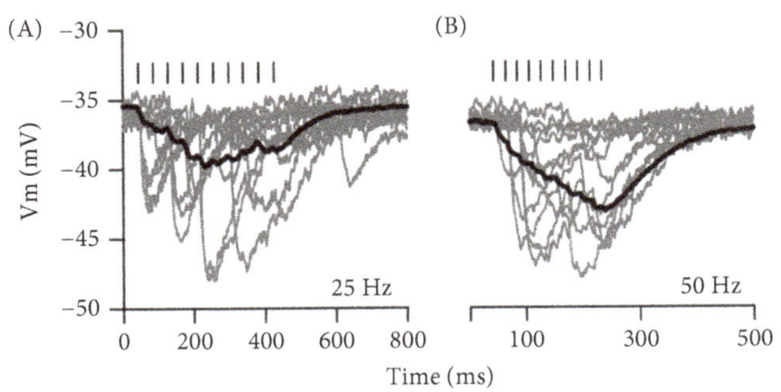

FIGURE 3.6. Hyperpolarization in response to efferent stimulation. IPSPs obtained in OHCs in response to 25 and 50 Hz stimulation trains in the current-clamp mode (gray traces). The black trace is the average response obtained upon 100 repetitions of the train.

Reproduced from Ballestero et al., 2011.

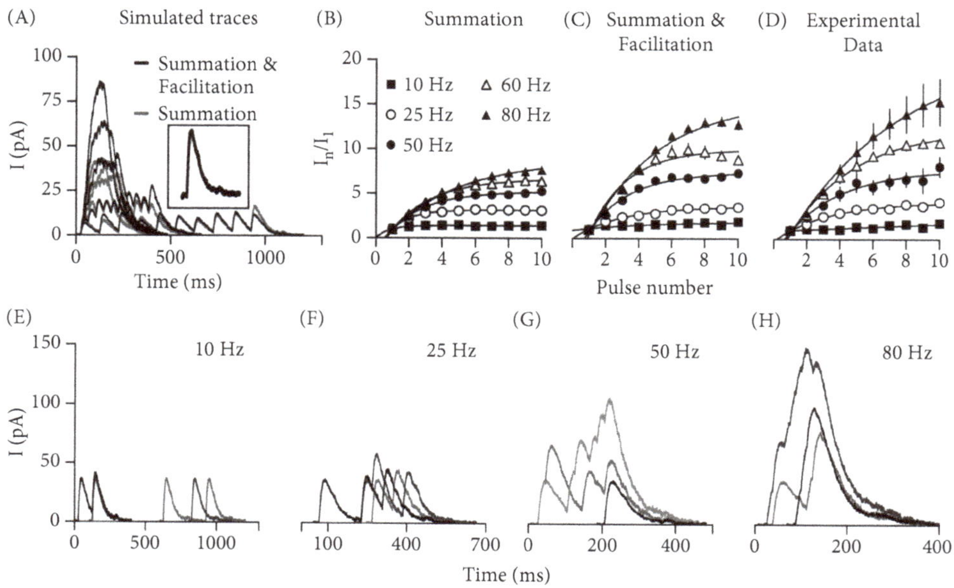

FIGURE 3.7. Summation of efferent responses. Summation contributes to the increment of the postsynaptic response during high-frequency stimulation. Simulated responses were derived from a response (A, inset) considering only temporal summation (gray traces) or facilitation by taking into account the change in the probability of release (black traces) for every shock. Simulation plots of normalized current versus pulse number were constructed considering only summation (B) or summation and facilitation (C). D: Experimental plot of normalized current versus pulse number. Summation and facilitation best fit the experimental data. E–H: Representative traces of the simulated single sweep responses.

Reproduced from Ballestero et al., 2011.

relies on high-frequency trains rather than single shocks to inhibit auditory function (Galambos, 1956; Gifford & Guinan, 1987; Mountain, 1980; Wiederhold & Kiang, 1970) and the strength of the efferent effect increases as the frequency of stimulation increases, (Art et al., 1984; Brown & Nuttal, 1984; Flock & Russell, 1973; Galambos, 1956; Gifford & Guinan, 1987; Wiederhold & Kiang, 1970) (See Figure 3.8.). The increase of MOC firing rate with sound intensity is consistent with the proposal that the efferent system protects the inner ear from noise-induced trauma (Kujawa & Liberman, 1997; Patuzzi & Thompson, 1991; Rajan, 1988; Rajan, 2000; Taranda, Maison, et al., 2009).

MOC Efferent Synaptogenesis

Nearly all vertebrate hair-cell sense organs have an efferent innervation. Efferent innervation of hair cells is as old as hair cells themselves and co-evolved with the vertebrate inner ear (Manley, 2000, 2017; Manley & Koppl, 1998). The most ancient efferents synapsed on a

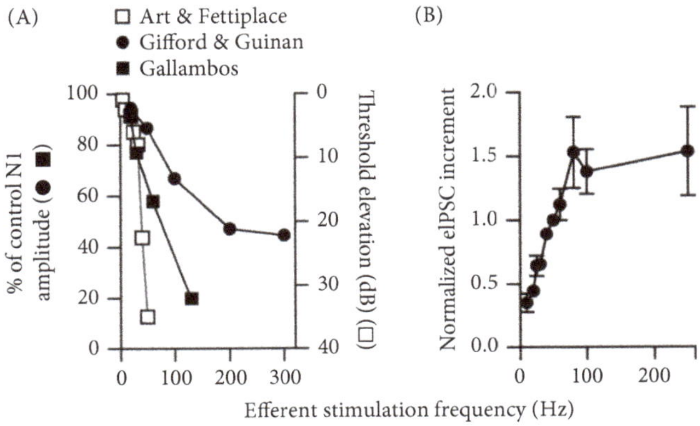

FIGURE 3.8. In vivo studies of the MOC effect on auditory function highly resemble the properties of the MOC–OHC synapse. MOC neurons rely on high-frequency trains rather than single shocks to inhibit auditory function, and the strength of the efferent effect increases as the frequency of stimulation increases. A: Relationship between the frequency of MOC activation and inhibition of afferent activity in the cat (Galambos, 1956; and Gifford & Guinan, 1987) and in the turtle [Art & Fettiplace (1984)]. Left-axis: Efferent effect quantified as the ratio between the amplitude of the N1 component of the compound action potential. Right-axis: Increase in sound intensity (threshold shift in decibels) necessary to evoke an afferent discharge as a function of the efferent stimulation frequency. B: Increment in eIPSC amplitudes in response to efferent stimulation at different frequencies.

Reproduced from Ballestero et al., 2011.

range of vestibular end organs and lateral line providing a gross control of hair cells. It has been suggested that efferents evolutionarily derived from facial branchial motor neurons, based upon their spatial and developmental associations, as well as their cholinergic nature (Fritzsch & Elliott, 2017; Roberts & Meredith, 1992). This hypothesis is further based on the fact that after ear ablation developing efferents join the facial motor neurons, most likely reverting to their ancestral condition (Fritzsch, 1999). Moreover, inner ear efferent neurons and motor neurons share a common embryological origin (Fritzsch, 1999). For an extended review of the development of the efferent system see (Simmons, 2002).

Efferent axons innervate the mouse cochlea as early as embryonic day 13 (Bruce et al., 1997; Fritzsch, 1999). The molecular cues that guide efferent axons to the inner ear are not well understood. Moreover, inner ear afferent fibers may serve as a substrate to direct efferent fibers to their sensory targets (Fritzsch, Pirvola, & Ylikoski, 1999). During cochlear development, there are numerous efferent axosomatic synapses on IHCs that disappear in the adult cochlea (Simmons, Bertolotto, Kim, Raji-Kubba, & Mansdorf, 1998; Simmons, Mansdorf, & Kim, 1996; Simmons, Manson-Gieseke, Hendrix, & McCarter, 1990; Simmons, Moulding, & Zee, 1996). Reconstructions of the efferent innervation in hamsters has shown that anterograde biocytin and horseradish peroxidase labeled efferent axons terminate on or below IHCs prior to P5. After P5, labeled axons terminate on both IHCs and OHCs and after P10, the majority of labeled axons terminate on the OHCs. At the electron microscopy level, small labeled terminals containing densely packed synaptic vesicles are observed both adjacent to IHCs (axosomatic) as well as apposed to afferent and efferent fibers below IHCs prior to P5. By P10, large labeled terminals are found only in direct contact with OHCs and no longer on IHCs (Simmons et al., 1990). Similar results have been obtained in rats and cats (Bruce et al., 2000; Perkins & Morest, 1975). The developmental changes in axosomatic synaptic contacts in IHCs are matched by changes in ultrastructural features such as the synaptic cisterns, which are present at early postnatal ages and disappear from IHCs after the onset of hearing (Ginzberg & Morest, 1984). These transient axosomatic efferent contacts to IHCs are of MOC origin (Simmons et al., 1990) and suggest that MOC axons first innervate IHCs prior to the onset of hearing (second postnatal week in altricial rodents) before terminating on OHCs. This is reminiscent of a waiting period below an intermediate target, similar to that described in the development of thalamocortical projections (Ghosg & Shatz, 1993). The mechanisms involved in this period of MOC synaptic transition from inner to OHCs are not known. Competition of afferent and efferent terminals for synaptic space below OHCs might explain the coincidence of efferent arrival and the decrease of afferent terminals on OHC (Pujol, 1985).

The transient direct efferent innervation of IHCs is mirrored by developmental regulation of expression of the *CHRNA9* and *CHRNA10* genes, suggesting the presence of cholinergic synapses. In situ hybridization studies have shown that α9 nAChR subunit mRNA is expressed as early as E18, reaching its maximum near birth in IHCs and P10 in OHCs. A transgenic mouse with a GFP reporter in the *CHRNA9* locus resolves a similar expression pattern (Zuo, Treadaway, Buckner, & Fritzsch, 1999). Moreover, *CHRNA9* expression is still observed in adult IHCs even after retraction of axosomatic MOC contacts (Elgoyhen et al., 1994; Luo, Bennett, Jung, & Ryan, 1998; Simmons & Morley, 1998; Zuo et al., 1999). On the other hand, α10 nAChR subunit mRNA expression is observed as from E21, peaks around P1 in IHCs and P10 in OHCs (Morley & Simmons, 2002). Contrary to that described for α9, α10 expression is not present in adult IHCs and disappears by P21 (Elgoyhen et al., 2001; Morley & Simmons, 2002). Homomeric α9 receptors expressed in *Xenopus* oocytes are functional, albeit rendering current amplitudes which are ~ 100 times smaller than those of α9α10 heteromeric receptors (Elgoyhen et al., 1994; Elgoyhen et al., 2001). However, although small ACh-gated currents are observed in OHCs of α10 knock-out mice, IHCs lack ACh responses before the onset of hearing in these mice (Vetter et al., 2007). Moreover, IHCs of wild-type mice lack responses after the onset of hearing (Katz et al., 2004). Therefore, the expression of α9 in the absence of α10 subunits in IHCs with no direct efferent contacts after the onset of hearing is intriguing. One could speculate, although it is not tested, that the high permeable α9 nAChR has an alternative, not purely "ionotropic," function in mature IHCs to modulate the release of glutamate through ribbon synapses.

Acetylcholine responses and synaptic currents in developing IHCs were first reported in an acute ex vivo rat cochlear explant by Glowatzki & Fuchs (2000).

Acetylcholine responses, but no synaptic currents, are detected by P0 in rat apical cochlear IHCs and are mediated by α9α10 nAChRs, since they are blocked by strychnine, curare, and RgIA but are not coupled to SK channels (Roux, Wersinger, McIntosh, Fuchs, & Glowatzki, 2011). From P1 onward, punctate α-Btx labeling and the first clusters of SK2-immunoreactivity are detected in a fraction of IHCs, thus indicating histological signs of synapse formation. This is accompanied by SK-coupled ACh responses and the first evidence of synaptic currents. Moreover, IHC with efferent synaptic activity are only seen when the SK current is present, suggesting that SK2 expression is correlated with functional synapses (Roux et al., 2011). This might indicate that the expression of SK2 channels is causally related to the onset of efferent synaptic function and required for the assembly, trafficking, and/or anchorage of the nAChR macromolecular synaptic complex. Although not tested, proteins known to form a macromolecular complex with SK2 channels, such as calmodulin, protein kinase CK2, and protein phosphatase 2A (Bildl et al., 2004), might also be developmentally regulated and be the linking molecules of the SK2 channel with the nAChR macromolecular complex. Given the sign reversal when nAChRs are coupled to SK channels, one could speculate that SK-mediated hyperpolarization compared to ACh-mediated depolarization might be essential for synaptic maturation. In addition, SK channels are also important for the maintenance of the synapse, since synaptic currents disappear with the loss of functional SK currents after the onset of hearing (Katz et al., 2004). A fundamental role for SK2 channel in synapse formation and stability is supported by the lack of ACh response and efferent synaptic activity in P6–P12 IHCs of SK2 knockout mice, despite normal levels of α9 and α10 nAChR mRNAs (Kong, Adelman, & Fuchs, 2008). In addition, efferent innervation progressively degenerates in SK2 (Kong et al., 2008; Murthy, Maison, et al., 2009), but not in either α9 (Murthy, Taranda, Elgoyhen, & Vetter, 2009; Vetter et al., 1999) or α10 (Vetter et al., 2007) deficient mice. Moreover, the finding that in a transgenic mouse with constitutive expression of the α10 subunit, IHCs still lack ACh responses after the onset of hearing (Taranda, Ballestero, et al., 2009), indicates that the expression of the *CHRNA9* and *CHRNA10* genes does not suffice for the assembly of functional α9α10 nAChRs and probably requires chaperon proteins which are not expressed as from ~ P12.

Experiments in isolated OHCs from gerbils and rats suggest that the onset of acetylcholine-induced responses begins on or after P6. At this stage currents are inward and reverse near 0 mV suggesting that the nAChR is not coupled to the SK channel (Dulon & Lenoir, 1996; He & Dallos, 1999). This response becomes functionally mature by P12 when coupling to the SK potassium current is always observed. The developmet of acetylcholine-induced responses in isolated OHCs coincides with the time period when OHCs develop motility before the onset of auditory function (He & Dallos, 1999). Moreover, it mirrors prestin OHCs lateral membrane labeling which is very low at P0, has a prominent increase between P6 and P9 and reaches adult levels at P9 in the basal turn of the cochlea, at P10–P11 in the middle turn, and at P12 in the apical turn (Belyantseva, Adler, Curi, Frolenkov, & Kachar, 2000).

The Critical Period

The precise organization and physiological properties of neuronal circuits and topographic maps in the mature brain are often established by developmental processes that involve reorganization and fine tuning of immature synaptic networks (Goodman & Shatz, 1993). Therefore, establishing correctly organized and appropriately adjusted synaptic circuits is a crucial event during "critical periods" of brain development, an early postnatal epoch of plasticity during which large-scale changes take place. One key issue discussed in developmental neuroscience is the question of how the specificity of synaptic connections in these networks are established in such a precise manner. Several major factors are thought to play a crucial role. In general, internal factors (i.e., genetically determined) must be distinguished from external factors (i.e., environmental). On the other hand, activity-dependent developmental processes play a key role and are subdivided into those associated with spontaneous activity and those depending on sensory-evoked activity.

The auditory system in many mammals is very immature at birth but precisely organized in adults. Hearing onset, defined as the ability of neurons to reliably respond to normal intensities of airborne sound, occurs after the second postnatal week in altricial rodents (Blatchley, Cooper, & Coleman, 1987; Puel & Uziel, 1987). Consequently, the early steps in the generation of the basic auditory brainstem circuitry are not influenced by acoustically driven activity. However, it is not established in an activity-independent manner, because spontaneous activity, giving rise to glutamate release from IHCs and to the subsequent activation of auditory nerve fibers that discharge bursts of Ca^{2+} action potentials, comes into play to guide this process (Glowatzki & Fuchs, 2000; Johnson, Kuhn, et al., 2013; Jones, Jones, & Paggett, 2001; Lippe, 1994). With maturation, a number of changes reduce IHC spiking. These include a reduction in the number of voltage-gated calcium channels, and the onset of a large, voltage-gated potassium conductance (Marcotti, Johnson, Holley, & Kros, 2003). These changes trigger the transformation of a developing epithelium with active synaptogenesis to a sensing epithelium, where synaptic contacts have stabilized and mechanical input is transduced into receptor potentials in IHCs in a graded manner.

The spontaneous activity in auditory nerve fibers before the onset of hearing is propagated to central auditory nuclei (Tritsch et al., 2010) and is essential for the survival of target neurons in the cochlear nucleus, accurate wiring of auditory pathways, and the refinement of tonotopic maps in auditory nuclei (Friauf & Lohmann, 1999; Kandler, 2004; Leake, Hradek, Chair, & Snyder, 2006). Synchronous activity among groups of hair cells along the length of the cochlea could help establish and maintain tonotopic segregation of neuronal projections in auditory pathways through hebbian like plasticity (Kandler, 2004; Kotak & Sanes, 1995) and help further refine and maintain synaptic connections (Erazo-Fischer, Striessnig, & Taschenberger, 2007; Leake et al., 2006). Thus, changes in afferent activity are known to lead to changes in synaptic properties in higher brainstem nuclei (Erazo-Fischer et al., 2007; Lippe, 1994; Sonntag, Englitz, Kopp-Scheinpflug, & Rubsamen, 2009). This could derive from changes in the pattern of action potential activity in IHCs which alter the developmental changes that occur in the Ca^{2+} dependence of neurotransmitter release at the cell's ribbon synapses before the onset of hearing (Johnson, Kuhn, et al., 2013; Johnson, Wedemeyer, et al., 2013).

The origin of this pre-hearing spontaneous activity is still a matter of debate. It has been proposed that supporting cells within Kölliker's organ initiate bursts of electrical activity in spiral ganglion neurons through ATP-dependent excitation of hair cells (Tritsch, Yi, Gale, Glowatzki, & Bergles, 2007). Moreover, it has been shown that ATP stimulates purinergic autoreceptors in inner spiral bundle cells, triggering Cl^- efflux by opening TMEM16A Ca^{2+}-activated Cl^- channels (Wang et al., 2015). However, Johnson Johnson et al. (2011) have further provided evidence that spontaneous action potentials are intrinsically generated by IHCs and only regulated by ATP. Although efferent input is not required to initiate this bursting activity (Tritsch et al., 2010), it modulates the bursting pattern (Johnson et al., 2011; Sendin, Bourien, Rassendren, Puel, & Nouvian, 2014), and this could be directly related to the maturation of the auditory system. High IHC intracellular Ca^{2+} buffering and "subsynaptic" cisterns provide efficient compartmentalization and tight control of cholinergic Ca^{2+} signals to prevent synaptic efferent Ca^{2+} spillover and cross-talk to afferent ribbon synapses (Moglie, Fuchs, Elgoyhen & Goutman, 2018). This preserves the inhibitory signature of the efferent system to ensure normal development of the auditory system. Earlier work showed that surgical lesion of the efferent nerve supply causes kittens to fail to develop normal hearing (Walsh, McGee, McFadden, & Liberman, 1998). Recent in vivo recordings in MNTB neurons from α9 knockout mice have shown no changes on average spontaneous spike rates or overall bursting activity but a modification in the temporal pattern of spontaneous spikes (Clause et al., 2014). This is translated into an impaired refinement of functional MNTB-LSO maps before the onset of hearing (Clause et al., 2014) and deficits in frequency difference limens and sound localization (Clause et al., 2017). This indicates that the precise temporal pattern of spontaneous prehearing activity is important for the formation of tonotopy in the central auditory pathway and that the transient efferent cholinergic innervation to IHCs is crucial to maintain this temporal pattern.

It is interesting to note that during AMPA-mediated excitotoxicity in the adult guinea pig cochleas, which results in swelling and disappearance of radial afferents below IHCs, vesiculated efferents (sometimes with postsynaptic cisterns) make transient direct contacts with IHCs (Ruel et al., 2007). These direct efferent contacts resemble those seen during the critical period of early stages of IHCs synaptogenesis and disappear as efferents make normal axo-dendritic synapses with the regenerated auditory neurites. Moreover, cochlear injury triggers the release of ATP and induces Ca^{2+} waves in supporting cells, as observed during development (Gale, Piazza, Ciubotaru, & Mammano, 2004). In addition, in aged C57BL/6 efferent terminals re-innervate IHCs, making direct synaptic contacts, containing focal presynaptic accumulations of small vesicles and occasional postsynaptic cisterns (Lauer, Fuchs, Ryugo, & Francis, 2012). Surprisingly, electrophysiological recordings from these C57BL/6J mouse IHCs reveal that functional cholinergic synaptic inputs re-emerge during aging. These efferents are inhibitory and recapitulate the same ionic mechanisms (α9 mediated-SK activation) as the transient efferent contacts present during the developmental critical period (Zachary & Fuchs, 2015). The re-appearance of efferent contacts below IHCs during damage and aging is intriguing. Since similar histological changes are seen at the level of radial dendrites between acute exposure to kainate or AMPA and those observed in various pathophysiological conditions such as ischemic events or acoustic trauma, excitotoxicity might be involved in a variety of cochlear diseases such as sudden deafness (or other ischemia-related pathologies), noise-induced hearing loss, and noise-induced tinnitus (Puel, Ruel, Gervais d'Aldin, & Pujol, 1998; Pujol & Puel, 1999; Spoendlin, 1971). If re-appearance of direct efferent contacts in IHCs were to be reported in all these conditions, a re-emergence of a developmental-like critical period could be suggested. This could be important for early therapeutic intervention in these pathological conditions, since critical periods are known to be an epoch of increased plasticity of the central nervous system (de Villers-Sidani, Simpson, Lu, Lin, & Merzenich, 2008; Levelt & Hubener, 2012; Zhou, Panizzutti, de Villers-Sidani, Madeira, & Merzenich, 2011).

Conclusions and Forward

Much progress has been made concerning the anatomy, physiology, and molecules involved in the MOC innervation to the inner ear hair cells. Plasticity features of the MOC-hair cell synapse ensure low probability of release at rest and facilitation of responses at high frequency stimulation. These are important to provide a fine tuning of cochlear amplification, since efferent firing frequency increases linearly with sound intensity. Moreover, the increase of MOC firing rate with sound intensity is consistent with the proposal that the efferent system protects the inner ear from noise-induced trauma. Future studies should provide a deeper insight on the functional roles of MOC activity in audition. The participation of the efferent innervation during the critical period and the "re-opening" of a critical period-like epoch during cochlear damage should be investigated further as a window for intervention during trauma.

References

Art, J. J., Crawford, A. C., Fettiplace, R., & Fuchs, P. A. (1982). Efferent regulation of hair cells in the turtle cochlea. *Proceedings of the Royal Society of London B 216*(1204), 377–384.

Art, J. J., Fettiplace, R., & Fuchs, P. A. (1984). Synaptic hyperpolarization and inhibition of turtle cochlear hair cells. *Journal of Physiology 365*(1), 525–550.

Ashmore, J. F., & Russell, I. J. (1983). Sensory and effector functions of vertebrate hair cells. *Journal of Submicroscopic Cytology 15*(1), 163–166.

Atluri, P. P., & Regehr, W. G. (1996). Determinants of the time course of facilitation at the granule cell to Purkinje cell synapse. *Journal of Neuroscience 16*(18), 5661–5671.

Ballestero, J. A., Plazas, P. V., Kracun, S., Gómez-Casati, M. E., Taranda, J., Rothlin, C. V., . . . Elgoyhen, A. B. (2005). Effects of quinine, quinidine, and chloroquine on alpha9alpha10 nicotinic cholinergic receptors. *Molecular Pharmacology 68*(3), 822–829.

Ballestero, J., Zorrilla de San Martín, J., Goutman, J., Elgoyhen, A., Fuchs, P., & Katz, E. (2011). Short term synaptic plasticity regulates the level of olivocochlear inhibition to auditory hair cells. *Journal of Neuroscience 31*(41), 14763–14774.

Batta, T. J., Panyi, G., Szucs, A., & Sziklai, I. (2004). Regulation of the lateral wall stiffness by acetylcholine and GABA in the outer hair cells of the guinea pig. *European Journal of Neuroscience 20*(12), 3364–3370.

Belyantseva, I. A., Adler, H. J., Curi, R., Frolenkov, G. I., & Kachar, B. (2000). Expression and localization of prestin and the sugar transporter GLUT-5 during development of electromotility in cochlear outer hair cells. *Journal of Neuroscience 20*(24), Rc116.

Berkefeld, H., & Fakler, B. (2008). Repolarizing responses of BKCa-Cav complexes are distinctly shaped by their Cav subunits. *Journal of Neuroscience 28*(33), 8238–8245.

Berkefeld, H., Fakler, B., & Schulte, U. (2010). Ca2+-activated K+ channels: From protein complexes to function. *Physiological Reviews 90*(4), 1437–1459.

Berkefeld, H., Sailer, C. A., Bildl, W., Rohde, V., Thumfart, J. O., Eble, . . . Fakler, B. (2006). BKCa-Cav channel complexes mediate rapid and localized Ca2+-activated K+ signaling. *Science 314*(5799), 615–620.

Bildl, W., Strassmaier, T., Thurm, H., Andersen, J., Eble, S., Oliver, D., . . . Fakler, B. (2004). Protein kinase CK2 is coassembled with small conductance Ca(2+)-activated K+ channels and regulates channel gating. *Neuron 43*(6), 847–858.

Blanchet, C., Erostegui, C., Sugasawa, M., & Dulon, D. (1996). Acetylcholine-induced potassium current of guinea pig outer hair cells: Its dependence on a calcium influx through nicotinic-like receptors. *Journal of Neuroscience 16*(8), 2574–2584.

Blatchley, B. J., Cooper, W. A., & Coleman, J. R. (1987). Development of auditory brainstem response to tone pip stimuli in the rat. *Brain Research 429*(1), 75–84.

Brown, M. C. (1987). Morphology of labeled efferent fibers in the guinea pig cochlea. *Journal of Comparative Neurology 260*(4), 605–618.

Brown, M. C., Kujawa, S. G., & Liberman, M. C. (1998). Single olivocochlear neurons in the guinea pig. II. Response plasticity due to noise conditioning. *Journal of Neurophysiology 79*(6), 3088–3097.

Brown, M. C., & Nuttal, A. L. (1984). Efferent control of cochlear inner hair cell responses in guinea-pig. *Journal of Physiology 354*(1), 625–646.

Brownell, W., Bader, C., Bertrand, D., & de Ribaupierre, Y. (1985). Evoked mechanical responses of isolated cochlear hair cells. *Science 227*(4683), 194–196.

Bruce, L. L., Christensen, M. A., & Warr, W. B. (2000). Postnatal development of efferent synapses in the rat cochlea. *Journal of Comparative Neurology 423*(3), 532–548.

Bruce, L. L., Kingsley, J., Nichols, D. H., & Fritzsch, B. (1997). The development of vestibulocochlear efferents and cochlear afferents in mice. *International Journal of Developmental Neuroscience 15*(4–5), 671–692.

Bulankina, A. V., & Moser, T. (2012). Neural circuit development in the mammalian cochlea. *Physiology 27*(2), 100–112.

Burgos, C. F., Yevenes, G. E., & Aguayo, L. G. (2016). Structure and pharmacologic modulation of inhibitory glycine receptors. *Molecular Pharmacology 90*(3), 318–325.

Catterall, W. A. (2000). Structure and regulation of voltage-gated Ca2+ channels. *Annual Review of Cell and Developmental Biology 16*, 521–555.

Catterall, W. A., & Few, A. P. (2008). Calcium channel regulation and presynaptic plasticity. *Neuron 59*(6), 882–901.

Clause, A., Kim, G., Sonntag, M., Weisz, C. J., Vetter, D. E., Rubsamen, R., & Kandler, K. (2014). The precise temporal pattern of prehearing spontaneous activity is necessary for tonotopic map refinement. *Neuron 82*(4), 822–835.

Clause, A., Lauer, A. M., & Kandler, K. (2017). Mice lacking the alpha9 subunit of the nicotinic acetylcholine receptor exhibit deficits in frequency difference limens and sound localization. *Frontiers in Cellular Neuroscience 11*, 167.

Cortese, M., Papal, S., Pisciottano, F., Elgoyhen, A. B., Hardelin, J. P., Petit, C., . . . El-Amraoui, A. (2017). Spectrin betaV adaptive mutations and changes in subcellular location correlate with emergence of hair cell electromotility in mammalians. *Proceedings of the National Academy of Sciences USA 114*(8), 2054–2059.

Chambers, A. R., Hancock, K. E., Maison, S. F., Liberman, M. C., & Polley, D. B. (2012). Sound-evoked olivocochlear activation in unanesthetized mice. *Journal of the Association for Research in Otolaryngology 13*(2), 209–217.

Chan, D. K., & Hudspeth, A. J. (2005). Ca^{2+} current-driven nonlinear amplification by the mammalian cochlea in vitro. *Nature Neuroscience 8*(2), 149–155.

Dallos, P. (1992). The active cochlea. *Journal of Neuroscience 12*(12), 4575–4585.

Dallos, P. (2008). Cochlear amplification, outer hair cells and prestin. *Current Opinion in Neurobiology 18*(4), 370–376.

Dallos, P., & Evans, B. N. (1995). High-frequency motility of outer hair cells and the cochlear amplifier. *Science 267*(5206), 2006–2009.

Dannhof, B. J., Roth, B., & Bruns, V. (1991). Anatomical mapping of choline acetyltransferase (ChAT)-like and glutamate decarboxylase (GAD)-like immunoreactivity in outer hair cell efferents in adult rats. *Cell and Tissue Research 266*(1), 89–95.

de Venecia, R. K., Liberman, M. C., Guinan, J. J., Jr., & Brown, M. C. (2005). Medial olivocochlear reflex interneurons are located in the posteroventral cochlear nucleus: A kainic acid lesion study in guinea pigs. *Journal of Comparative Neurology 487*(4), 345–360.

de Villers-Sidani, E., Simpson, K. L., Lu, Y. F., Lin, R. C., & Merzenich, M. M. (2008). Manipulating critical period closure across different sectors of the primary auditory cortex. *Nature Neuroscience 11*(8), 957–965.

Delano, P. H., Elgueda, D., Hamame, C. M., & Robles, L. (2007). Selective attention to visual stimuli reduces cochlear sensitivity in chinchillas. *Journal of Neuroscience 27*(15), 4146–4153.

Dent, J. A. (2006). Evidence for a diverse Cys-loop ligand-gated ion channel superfamily in early bilateria. *Journal of Molecular Evolution 62*(5), 523–535.

Doi, T., & Ohmori, H. (1993). Acetylcholine increases intracellular Ca2+ concentration and hyperpolarizes the guinea-pig outer hair cell. *Hearing Research 67*(1–2), 179–188.

Dolan, D. F., & Nuttall, A. L. (1988). Masked cochlear whole-nerve response intensity functions altered by electrical stimulation of the crossed olivocochlear bundle. *Journal of the Acoustical Society of America 83*(3), 1081–1086.

Dulon, D., & Lenoir, M. (1996). Cholinergic responses in developing outer hair cells of the rat cochlea. *European Journal of Neuroscience 8*(9), 1945–1952.

Dulon, D., Luo, L., Zhang, C., & Ryan, A. F. (1998). Expression of small-conductance calcium-activated potassium channels (SK) in outer hair cells of the rat cochlea. *European Journal of Neuroscience 10*(3), 907–915.

Elgoyhen, A. B., & Franchini, L. F. (2011). Prestin and the cholinergic receptor of hair cells: Positively-selected proteins in mammals. *Hearing Research 273*(1–2), 100–108.

Elgoyhen, A. B., Johnson, D. S., Boulter, J., Vetter, D. E., & Heinemann, S. (1994). Alpha 9: An acetylcholine receptor with novel pharmacological properties expressed in rat cochlear hair cells. *Cell* 79(4), 705–715.

Elgoyhen, A. B., & Katz, E. (2012). The efferent medial olivocochlear-hair cell synapse. *Journal of Physiology Paris* 106(1–2), 47–56.

Elgoyhen, A. B., Vetter, D., Katz, E., Rothlin, C., Heinemann, S., & Boulter, J. (2001). Alpha 10: A determinant of nicotinic cholinergic receptor function in mammalian vestibular and cochlear mechanosensory hair cells. *Proceedings of the National Academy of Sciences USA* 98(6), 3501–3506.

Ellison, M., Haberlandt, C., Gomez-Casati, M. E., Watkins, M., Elgoyhen, A. B., McIntosh, J. M., & Olivera, B. M. (2006). Alpha-RgIA: a novel conotoxin that specifically and potently blocks the alpha9alpha10 nAChR. *Biochemistry* 45(5), 1511–1517.

Erazo-Fischer, E., Striessnig, J., & Taschenberger, H. (2007). The role of physiological afferent nerve activity during in vivo maturation of the calyx of Held synapse. *Journal of Neuroscience* 27(7), 1725–1737.

Erostegui, C., Norris, C. H., & Bobbin, R. P. (1994). In vitro characterization of a cholinergic receptor on outer hair cells. *Hearing Research* 74(1–2), 135–147.

Evans, M. G., Lagostena, L., Darbon, P., & Mammano, F. (2000). Cholinergic control of membrane conductance and intracellular free Ca2+ in outer hair cells of the guinea pig cochlea. *Cell Calcium* 28(3), 195–203.

Eybalin, M. (1993). Neurotransmitters and neuromodulators of the mammalian cochlea. *Physiological Reviews* 73(2), 309–373.

Eybalin, M., & Pujol, R. (1987). Choline acetyltransferase (ChAT) immunoelectron microscopy distinguishes at least three types of efferent synapses in the organ of Corti. *Experimental Brain Research* 65(2), 261–270.

Fakler, B., & Adelman, J. P. (2008). Control of K(Ca) channels by calcium nano/microdomains. *Neuron* 59(6), 873–881.

Fioravante, D., & Regehr, W. G. (2011). Short-term forms of presynaptic plasticity. *Current Opinion in Neurobiology* 21(2), 269–274.

Flock, A., & Russell, I. J. (1973). The post-synaptic action of efferent fibres in the lateral line organ of the burbot Lota lota. *Journal of Physiology* 235(3), 591–605.

Flock, A., & Russell, I. (1976). Inhibition by efferent nerve fibres: Action on hair cells and afferent synaptic transmission in the lateral line canal organ of the burbot Lota lota. *Journal of Physiology* 257(1), 45–62.

Franchini, L. F., & Elgoyhen, A. B. (2006). Adaptive evolution in mammalian proteins involved in cochlear outer hair cell electromotility. *Molecular Phylogenetics and Evolution* 41(3), 622–635.

Friauf, E., & Lohmann, C. (1999). Development of auditory brainstem circuitry. Activity-dependent and activity-independent processes. *Cell Tissue Research* 297(2), 187–195.

Fritzsch, B. (1999). Ontogenetic and evolutionary evidence for the motoneuron nature of vestibular and cochlear efferents. In C. Berlin (Ed.), *The efferent auditory system: basic science and clinical applications* (pp. 31–59). New York, NY: Singular Publishing Group, Inc.

Fritzsch, B., & Elliott, K. L. (2017). Evolution and development of the inner ear efferent system: Transforming a motor neuron population to connect to the most unusual motor protein via ancient nicotinic receptors. *Frontiers in Cellular Neuroscience* 11, 114.

Fritzsch, B., Pirvola, U., & Ylikoski, J. (1999). Making and breaking the innervation of the ear: neurotrophic support during ear development and its clinical implications. *Cell Tissue Research* 295(3), 369–382.

Fuchs, P. A., Lehar, M., & Hiel, H. (2014). Ultrastructure of cisternal synapses on outer hair cells of the mouse cochlea. *Journal of Comparative Neurology 522*(3), 717–729.

Fuchs, P. A., & Murrow, B. W. (1992). A novel cholinergic receptor mediates inhibition of chick cochlear hair cells. *Proceedings of the Royal Society of London B 248*(1321), 35–40.

Galambos, R. (1956). Suppression of auditory nerve activity by stimulation of efferent fibers to the cochlea. *Journal of Neurophysiology 19*(5), 424–437.

Gale, J. E., Piazza, V., Ciubotaru, C. D., & Mammano, F. (2004). A mechanism for sensing noise damage in the inner ear. *Current Biology 14*(6), 526–529.

Ghosg, A., & Shatz, C. J. (1993). A role for subplate neurons in the patterning of connections from thalamus to neocortex. *Development 117*(3), 1031–1047.

Gifford, M. L., & Guinan, J. J., Jr. (1987). Effects of electrical stimulation of medial olivocochlear neurons on ipsilateral and contralateral cochlear responses. *Hearing Research 29*(2–3), 179–194.

Ginzberg, R. D., & Morest, D. K. (1984). Fine structure of cochlear innervation in the cat. *Hearing Research 14*(2), 109–127.

Gitter, A. H., & Zenner, H. P. (1992). gamma-Aminobutyric acid receptor activation of outer hair cells in the guinea pig cochlea. *European Archives of Oto-Rhino-Laryngology 249*(1), 62–65.

Glowatzki, E., & Fuchs, P. (2000). Cholinergic synaptic inhibition of inner hair cells in the neonatal mammalian cochlea. *Science 288*(5475), 2366–2368.

Glowatzki, E., & Fuchs, P. (2002). Transmitter release at the hair cell ribbon synapse. *Nature Neuroscience 5*(2), 147–154.

Glowatzki, E., Wild, K., Brandle, U., Fakler, G., Fakler, B., Zenner, H. P., & Ruppersberg, J. P. (1995). Cell-specific expression of the alpha 9 n-ACh receptor subunit in auditory hair cells revealed by single-cell RT- PCR. *Proceedings of the Royal Society of London B 262*(1364), 141–147.

Gomez-Casati, M. E., Fuchs, P. A., Elgoyhen, A. B., & Katz, E. (2005). Biophysical and pharmacological characterization of nicotinic cholinergic receptors in cochlear inner hair cells. *Journal of Physiology 566*(1), 103–118.

Goodman, C. S., & Shatz, C. J. (1993). Developmental mechanisms that generate precise patterns of neuronal connectivity. *Cell 72* Suppl., 77–98.

Goutman, J. D. (2012). Transmitter release from cochlear hair cells is phase locked to cyclic stimuli of different intensities and frequencies. *Journal of Neuroscience 32*(47), 17025–17035a.

Goutman, J. D., Fuchs, P. A., & Glowatzki, E. (2005). Facilitating efferent inhibition of inner hair cells in the cochlea of the neonatal rat. *Journal of Physiology 566*(Pt 1), 49–59.

Goutman, J. D., & Glowatzki, E. (2007). Time course and calcium dependence of transmitter release at a single ribbon synapse. *Proceedings of the National Academy of Sciences USA 104*(41), 16341–16346.

Granger, A. J., Mulder, N., Saunders, A., & Sabatini, B. L. (2016). Cotransmission of acetylcholine and GABA. *Neuropharmacology 100*, 40–46.

Grant, L., Yi, E., & Glowatzki, E. (2010). Two modes of release shape the postsynaptic response at the inner hair cell ribbon synapse. *Journal of Neuroscience 30*(12), 4210–4220.

Guinan, J. J. (1996). Physiology of olivocochlear efferents. In P. J. Dallos, A. N. Popper, & R. R. Fay (Eds.), *The Cochlea* (pp. 435–502). New York, NY: Springer-Verlag.

Guinan, J. J., Jr. (2006). Olivocochlear efferents: anatomy, physiology, function, and the measurement of efferent effects in humans. *Ear and Hearing 27*(6), 589–607.

Gulley, R. L., & Reese, T. S. (1977). Freeze-fracture studies on the synapses in the organ of Corti. *Journal of Comparative Neurology 171*(4), 517–543.

He, D. Z., & Dallos, P. J. (1999). Development of acetylcholine-induced responses in neonatal gerbil outer hair cells. *Journal of Neurophysiology 81*(3), 1162–1170.

Hiel, H., Elgoyhen, A., Drescher, D., & Morley, B. (1996). Expression of nicotinic acetylcholine receptor mRNA in the adult rat peripheral vestibular system. *Brain Research 738*(2), 347–352.

Hirokawa, N. (1978). The ultrastructure of the basilar papilla of the chick. *Journal of Comparative Neurology 181*(2), 361–374.

Hnasko, T. S., & Edwards, R. H. (2012). Neurotransmitter corelease: Mechanism and physiological role. *Annual Review of Physiology 74*, 225–243.

Housley, G. D., & Ashmore, J. F. (1991). Direct measurement of the action of acetylcholine on isolated outer hair cells of the guinea pig cochlea. *Proceedings of the Royal Society of London B 244*, 161–167.

Housley, G. D., Batcher, S., Kraft, M., & Ryan, A. F. (1994). Nicotinic acetylcholine receptor subunits expressed in rat cochlea detected by the polymerase chain reaction. *Hearing Research 75*(1–2), 47–53.

Im, G. J., Moskowitz, H. S., Lehar, M., Hiel, H., & Fuchs, P. A. (2014). Synaptic calcium regulation in hair cells of the chicken basilar papilla. *Journal of Neuroscience 34*(50), 16688–16697.

Jackman, S. L., & Regehr, W. G. (2017). The mechanisms and functions of synaptic facilitation. *Neuron 94*(3), 447–464.

Jia, S., & He, D. Z. (2005). Motility-associated hair-bundle motion in mammalian outer hair cells. *Nature Neuroscience 8*(8), 1028–1034.

Johnson, D. S., Martinez, J., Elgoyhen, A. B., Heinemann, S. F., & McIntosh, J. M. (1995). Alpha-conotoxin ImI exhibits subtype-specific nicotinic acetylcholine receptor blockade: Preferential inhibition of homomeric alpha 7 and alpha 9 receptors. *Molecular Pharmacology 48*(2), 194–199.

Johnson, S. L., Eckrich, T., Kuhn, S., Zampini, V., Franz, C., Ranatunga, K. M., . . . Marcotti, W. (2011). Position-dependent patterning of spontaneous action potentials in immature cochlear inner hair cells. *Nature Neuroscience 14*(6), 711–717.

Johnson, S. L., Kuhn, S., Franz, C., Ingham, N., Furness, D. N., Knipper, M., . . . Marcotti, W. (2013). Presynaptic maturation in auditory hair cells requires a critical period of sensory-independent spiking activity. *Proceedings of the National Academy of Sciences USA 110*(21), 8720–8725.

Johnson, S. L., Wedemeyer, C., Vetter, D. E., Adachi, R., Holley, M. C., Elgoyhen, A. B., & Marcotti, W. (2013). Cholinergic efferent synaptic transmission regulates the maturation of auditory hair cell ribbon synapses. *Open Biology 3*(11), 130–163.

Jones, T. A., Jones, S. M., & Paggett, K. C. (2001). Primordial rhythmic bursting in embryonic cochlear ganglion cells. *Journal of Neuroscience 21*(20), 8129–8135.

Kakehata, S., Nakagawa, T., Takasaka, T., & Akaike, N. (1993). Cellular mechanism of acetylcholine-induced response in dissociated outer hair cells of guinea-pig cochlea. *Journal of Physiology 463*(1), 227–244.

Kandler, K. (2004). Activity-dependent organization of inhibitory circuits: Lessons from the auditory system. *Current Opinion in Neurobiology 14*(1), 96–104.

Karlin, A. (2002). Ion channel structure: emerging structure of the nicotinic acetylcholine receptors. *Nature Reviews Neuroscience 3*(2), 102–114.

Katz, E., Elgoyhen, A. B., Gomez-Casati, M. E., Knipper, M., Vetter, D. E., Fuchs, P. A., & Glowatzki, E. (2004). Developmental regulation of nicotinic synapses on cochlear inner hair cells. *Journal of Neuroscience 24*(36), 7814–7820.

Katz, B., & Miledi, R. (1969). Spontaneous and evoked activity of motor nerve endings in calcium Ringer. *Journal of Physiology 203*(3), 689–706.

Kawase, T., Delgutte, B., & Liberman, M. C. (1993). Antimasking effects of the olivocochlear reflex. II. Enhancement of auditory-nerve response to masked tones. *Journal of Neurophysiology 70*(6), 2533–2549.

Kennedy, H. J., Crawford, A. C., & Fettiplace, R. (2005). Force generation by mammalian hair bundles supports a role in cochlear amplification. *Nature 433*(7028), 880–883.

Kong, J. H., Adelman, J. P., & Fuchs, P. A. (2008). Expression of the SK2 calcium-activated potassium channel is required for cholinergic function in mouse cochlear hair cells. *Journal of Physiology 586*(22), 5471–5485.

Kong, J. H., Zachary, S., Rohmann, K. N., & Fuchs, P. A. (2013). Retrograde facilitation of efferent synapses on cochlear hair cells. *Journal of the Association for Research in Otolaryngology 14*(1), 17–27.

Kotak, V. C., & Sanes, D. H. (1995). Synaptically evoked prolonged depolarizations in the developing auditory system. *Journal of Neurophysiology 74*(4), 1611–1620.

Kujawa, S. G., Glattke, T. J., Fallon, M., & Bobbin, R. (1994). A nicotinic-like receptor mediates suppression of distortion product otoacoustic emissions by contralateral sound. *Hearing Research 74*(1–2), 122–134.

Kujawa, S. G., & Liberman, M. C. (1997). Conditioning-related protection from acoustic injury: Effects of chronic deefferentation and sham surgery. *Journal of Neurophysiology 78*(6), 3095–3106.

Lauer, A. M., Fuchs, P. A., Ryugo, D. K., & Francis, H. W. (2012). Efferent synapses return to inner hair cells in the aging cochlea. *Neurobiology of Aging 33*(12), 2892–2902.

Leake, P. A., Hradek, G. T., Chair, L., & Snyder, R. L. (2006). Neonatal deafness results in degraded topographic specificity of auditory nerve projections to the cochlear nucleus in cats. *Journal of Comparative Neurology 497*(1), 13–31.

Lenoir, M., Schnerson, A., & Pujol, R. (1980). Cochlear receptor development in the rat with emphasis on synaptogenesis. *Anatomy and Embryology 160*(3), 253–262.

Levelt, C. N., & Hubener, M. (2012). Critical-period plasticity in the visual cortex. *Annual Review of Neuroscience 35*, 309–330.

Liberman, M. C., & Brown, M. C. (1986). Physiology and anatomy of single olivocochlear neurons in the cat. *Hearing Research 24*(1), 17–36.

Lioudyno, M., Hiel, H., Kong, J. H., Katz, E., Waldman, E., Parameshwaran-Iyer, S., . . . Fuchs, P. A. (2004). A "synaptoplasmic cistern" mediates rapid inhibition of cochlear hair cells. *Journal of Neuroscience 24*(49), 11160–11164.

Lipovsek, M., Fierro, A., Perez, E. G., Boffi, J. C., Millar, N. S., Fuchs, P. A., . . . Elgoyhen, A. B. (2014). Tracking the molecular evolution of calcium permeability in a nicotinic acetylcholine receptor. *Molecular Biology and Evolution 31*(12), 3250–3265.

Lipovsek, M., Im, G. J., Franchini, L. F., Pisciottano, F., Katz, E., Fuchs, P. A., & Elgoyhen, A. B. (2012). Phylogenetic differences in calcium permeability of the auditory hair cell cholinergic nicotinic receptor. *Proceedings of the National Academy of Sciences USA 109*(11), 4308–4313.

Lippe, W. R. (1994). Rhythmic spontaneous activity in the developing avian auditory system. *Journal of Neuroscience 14*(3 Pt 2), 1486–1495.

Luo, L., Bennett, T., Jung, H. H., & Ryan, A. (1998). Developmental expression of alpha 9 acetylcholine receptor mRNA in the rat cochlea and vestibular inner ear. *Journal of Comparative Neurology 393*(3), 320–331.

Lustig, L., Hiel, H., & Fuchs, P. (1999). Vestibular hair cells of the chick express the nicotinic acetylcholine receptor subunit alpha 9. *Journal of Vestibular Research* 9(5), 359–367.

Lustig, L. R., Peng, H., Hiel, H., Yamamoto, T., & Fuchs, P. (2001). Molecular cloning and mapping of the human nicotinic acetylcholine receptor a10 (CHRNA10). *Genomics* 73(3), 272–283.

Maison, S. F., Adams, J. C., & Liberman, M. C. (2003). Olivocochlear innervation in the mouse: Immunocytochemical maps, crossed versus uncrossed contributions, and transmitter colocalization. *Journal of Comparative Neurology* 455(3), 406–416.

Maison, S. F., Casanova, E., Holstein, G. R., Bettler, B., & Liberman, M. C. (2009). Loss of GABAB receptors in cochlear neurons: threshold elevation suggests modulation of outer hair cell function by type II afferent fibers. *Journal of the Association for Research in Otolaryngology* 10(1), 50–63.

Maison, S. F., & Liberman, M. C. (2000). Predicting vulnerability to acoustic injury with a noninvasive assay of olivocochlear reflex strength. *Journal of Neuroscience* 20(12), 4701–4707.

Maison, S. F., Luebke, A. E., Liberman, M. C., & Zuo, J. (2002). Efferent protection from acoustic injury is mediated via alpha9 nicotinic acetylcholine receptors on outer hair cells. *Journal of Neuroscience* 22(24), 10838–10846.

Maison, S. F., Pyott, S. J., Meredith, A. L., & Liberman, M. C. (2013). Olivocochlear suppression of outer hair cells in vivo: Evidence for combined action of BK and SK2 channels throughout the cochlea. *Journal of Neurophysiology* 109(6), 1525–1534.

Maison, S. F., Rosahl, T. W., Homanics, G. E., & Liberman, M. C. (2006). Functional role of GABAergic innervation of the cochlea: Phenotypic analysis of mice lacking GABA(A) receptor subunits alpha 1, alpha 2, alpha 5, alpha 6, beta 2, beta 3, or delta. *Journal of Neuroscience* 26(40), 10315–10326.

Maison, S. F., Usubuchi, H., Vetter, D. E., Elgoyhen, A. B., Thomas, S. A., & Liberman, M. C. (2012). Contralateral-noise effects on cochlear responses in anesthetized mice are dominated by feedback from an unknown pathway. *Journal of Neurophysiology* 108(2), 491–500.

Manley, G. A. (2000). Cochlear mechanisms from a phylogenetic viewpoint. *Proceedings of the National Academy of Sciences USA* 97(22), 11736–11743.

Manley, G. A. (2017). The mammalian Cretaceous cochlear revolution. *Hearing Research* 352, 23–29.

Manley, G. A., & Koppl, C. (1998). Phylogenetic development of the cochlea and its innervation. *Current Opinion in Neurobiology* 8(4), 468–474.

Marcotti, W., Johnson, S. L., Holley, M. C., & Kros, C. J. (2003). Developmental changes in the expression of potassium currents of embryonic, neonatal and mature mouse inner hair cells. *Journal of Physiology* 548(Pt 2), 383–400.

Matthews, T. M., Duncan, R. K., Zidanic, M., Michael, T. H., & Fuchs, P. A. (2005). Cloning and characterization of SK2 channel from chicken short hair cells. *Journal of Comparative Physiology A* 191(6), 491–503.

McIntosh, J. M., Plazas, P. V., Watkins, M., Gomez-Casati, M. E., Olivera, B. M., & Elgoyhen, A. B. (2005). A novel alpha-conotoxin, PeIA, cloned from Conus pergrandis, discriminates between rat alpha9alpha10 and alpha7 nicotinic cholinergic receptors. *Journal of Biological Chemistry* 280(34), 30107–30112.

Moglie, M. J., Fuchs, P. A., Elgoyhen, A. B., Goutman, J. D. (2018) Compartmentalization of antagonistic Ca^{2+} signals in developing cochlear hair cells. *Proceedings of the National Academy of Sciences USA*. doi/10.1073/pnas.1719077115

Morley, B., Li, H., Hiel, H., Drescher, D., & Elgoyhen, A. B. (1998). Identification of the subunits of the nicotinic cholinergic receptors in the rat cochlea using RT-PCR and in situ hybridization. *Molecular Brain Research 53*(1–2), 78–87.

Morley, B. J., & Simmons, D. D. (2002). Developmental mRNA expression of the alpha10 nicotinic acetylcholine receptor subunit in the rat cochlea. *Developmental Brain Research 139*(1), 87–96.

Moss, S. J., & Smart, T. G. (2001). Constructing inhibitory synapses. *Nature Reviews Neuroscience 2*(4), 240–250.

Mount, D. B., & Romero, M. F. (2004). The SLC26 gene family of multifunctional anion exchangers. *Pflügers Archiv 447*(5), 710–721.

Mountain, D. C. (1980). Changes in endolymphatic potential and crossed olivocochlear bundle stimulation alter cochlear mechanics. *Science 210*(4465), 71–72.

Muller, J., Janssen, T., Heppelmann, G., & Wagner, W. (2005). Evidence for a bipolar change in distortion product otoacoustic emissions during contralateral acoustic stimulation in humans. *Journal of the Acoustical Society of America 118*(6), 3747–3756.

Murthy, V., Maison, S. F., Taranda, J., Haque, N., Bond, C. T., Elgoyhen, A. B., . . . Vetter, D. E. (2009). SK2 channels are required for function and long-term survival of efferent synapses on mammalian outer hair cells. *Molecular and Cellular Neuroscience 40*(1), 39–49.

Murthy, V., Taranda, J., Elgoyhen, A. B., & Vetter, D. E. (2009). Activity of nAChRs containing alpha9 subunits modulates synapse stabilization via bidirectional signaling programs. *Developmental Neurobiology 69*(14), 931–949.

Murugasu, E., & Russell, I. J. (1996). The effect of efferent stimulation on basilar membrane displacement in the basal turn of the guinea pig cochlea. *Journal of Neuroscience 16*(1), 325–332.

Nemecz, A., Prevost, M. S., Menny, A., & Corringer, P. J. (2016). Emerging molecular mechanisms of signal transduction in pentameric ligand-gated ion channels. *Neuron 90*(3), 452–470.

Nenov, A. P., Norris, C., & Bobbin, R. P. (1996). Acetylcholine response in guinea pig outer hair cells. I. Properties of the response. *Hearing Research 101*(1–2), 132–148.

Nenov, A. P., Norris, C., & Bobbin, R. P. (1996). Acetylcholine responses in guinea pig outer hair cells. II Activation of a small conductance Ca^{2+}-activated K^{+} channel. *Hearing Research 101*(1–2), 149–172.

Oatman, L. C. (1976). Effects of visual attention on the intensity of auditory evoked potentials. *Experimental Neurology 51*(1), 41–53.

O'Beirne, G. A., & Patuzzi, R. B. (2007). Mathematical model of outer hair cell regulation including ion transport and cell motility. *Hearing Research 234*(1–2), 29–51.

Oliver, D., He, D. Z., Klocker, N., Ludwig, J., Schulte, U., Waldegger, S., . . . Fakler, B. (2001). Intracellular anions as the voltage sensor of prestin, the outer hair cell motor protein. *Science 292*(5525), 2340–2343.

Oliver, D., Klocker, N., Schuck, J., Baukrowitz, T., Ruppersberg, J. P., & Fakler, B. (2000). Gating of Ca^{2+}-activated K^{+} channels controls fast inhibitory synaptic transmission at auditory outer hair cells. *Neuron 26*(3), 595–601.

Patuzzi, R. B., & Thompson, M. L. (1991). Cochlear efferent neurones and protection against acoustic trauma: Protection of outer hair cell receptor current and interanimal variability. *Hearing Research* 54(1), 45–58.

Perkins, R. E., & Morest, D. K. (1975). A study of cochlear innervation patterns in cats and rats with the Golgi method and Nomarkski optics. *Journal of Comparative Neurology* 163(2), 129–158.

Pin, J. P., & Duvoisin, R. (1995). The metabotropic glutamate receptors: Structure and functions. *Neuropharmacology* 34(1), 1–26.

Plazas, P. V., Katz, E., Gomez-Casati, M. E., Bouzat, C., & Elgoyhen, A. B. (2005). Stoichiometry of the {alpha}9{alpha}10 nicotinic cholinergic receptor. *Journal of Neuroscience* 25(47), 10905–10912.

Puel, J. L., Ruel, J., Gervais d'Aldin, C., & Pujol, R. (1998). Excitotoxicity and repair of cochlear synapses after noise-trauma induced hearing loss. *Neuroreport* 9(9), 2109–2114.

Puel, J. L., & Uziel, A. (1987). Correlative development of cochlear action potential sensitivity, latency, and frequency selectivity. *Brain Research* 465(1–2), 179–188.

Pujol, R. (1985). Morphology, synaptology and electrophysiology of the developing cochlea. *Acta Oto-Laryngologica* 99(421), 5–9.

Pujol, R., & Puel, J. L. (1999). Excitotoxicity, synaptic repair, and functional recovery in the mammalian cochlea: A review of recent findings. *Annals of the New York Academy of Sciences* 884, 249–254.

Raffaelli, G., Saviane, C., Mohajerani, M. H., Pedarzani, P., & Cherubini, E. (2004). BK potassium channels control transmitter release at CA3-CA3 synapses in the rat hippocampus. *Journal of Physiology* 557(Pt 1), 147–157.

Rajan, R. (1988). Effect of electrical stimulation of the crossed olivocochlear bundle on temporary threshold shifts in auditory sensitivity. I. Dependence on electrical stimulation parameters. *Journal of Neurophysiology* 60(2), 549–568.

Rajan, R. (2000). Centrifugal pathways protect hearing sensitivity at the cochlea in noisy environments that exacerbate the damage induced by loud sound. *Journal of Neuroscience* 20(17), 6684–6693.

Rasmussen, G. L. (1946). The olivary peduncle and other fiber projections of the superior olivary complex. *Journal of Comparative Neurology* 84(2), 141–219.

Roberts, B., & Meredith, G. (1992). The efferent innervation of the ear: Variations on an enigma. In D. Webster, R. Fay, & A. Popper (Eds.), *The evolutionary biology of hearing* (pp. 185–210). New York, NY: Springer-Verlag.

Robertson, D., & Gummer, M. (1985). Physiological and morphological characterization of efferent neurones in the guinea pig cochlea. *Hearing Research* 20(1), 63–77.

Robitaille, R., Garcia, M. L., Kaczorowski, G. J., & Charlton, M. P. (1993). Functional colocalization of calcium and calcium-gated potassium channels in control of transmitter release. *Neuron* 11(4), 645–655.

Rohmann, K. N., Wersinger, E., Braude, J. P., Pyott, S. J., & Fuchs, P. A. (2015). Activation of BK and SK channels by efferent synapses on outer hair cells in high-frequency regions of the rodent cochlea. *Journal of Neuroscience* 35(5), 1821–1830.

Rontal, D. A., & Echteler, S. M. (2003). Developmental segregation in the efferent projections to auditory hair cells in the gerbil. *Journal of Comparative Neurology* 467(4), 509–520.

Rothlin, C. V., Lioudyno, M. I., Silbering, A. F., Plazas, P. V., Casati, M. E., Katz, E., . . . Elgoyhen, A. B. (2003). Direct interaction of serotonin type 3 receptor ligands with recombinant and native alpha 9 alpha 10-containing nicotinic cholinergic receptors. *Molecular Pharmacology 63*(5), 1067–1074.

Rothlin, C., Verbitsky, M., Katz, E., & Elgoyhen, A. (1999). The a9 nicotinic acetylcholine receptor shares pharmacological properties with type A g-aminobutyric acid, glycine and type 3 serotonin receptors. *Molecular Pharmacology 55*(2), 248–254.

Roux, I., Wersinger, E., McIntosh, J. M., Fuchs, P. A., & Glowatzki, E. (2011). Onset of cholinergic efferent synaptic function in sensory hair cells of the rat cochlea. *Journal of Neuroscience 31*(42), 15092–15101.

Ruel, J., Wang, J., Rebillard, G., Eybalin, M., Lloyd, R., Pujol, R., & Puel, J. L. (2007). Physiology, pharmacology and plasticity at the inner hair cell synaptic complex. *Hearing Research 227*(1–2), 19–27.

Russell, I. J., & Murugasu, E. (1997). Medial efferent inhibition suppresses basilar membrane responses to near characteristic frequency tones of moderate to high intensities. *Journal of the Acoustical Society of America 102*(3), 1734–1738.

Sahara, Y., & Westbrook, G. L. (1993). Modulation of calcium currents by a metabotropic glutamate receptor involves fast and slow kinetic components in cultured hippocampal neurons. *Journal of Neuroscience 13*(7), 3041–3050.

Saito, K. (1983). Fine structure of the sensory epithelium of guinea-pig organ of Corti: Subsurface cisternae and lamellar bodies in the outer hair cells. *Cell Tissue Research 229*(3), 467–481.

Sakai, Y., Harvey, M., & Sokolowski, B. (2011). Identification and quantification of full-length BK channel variants in the developing mouse cochlea. *Journal of Neuroscience Research 89*(11), 1747–1760.

Saunders, A., Granger, A. J., & Sabatini, B. L. (2015). Corelease of acetylcholine and GABA from cholinergic forebrain neurons. *eLife 4*, e06412. doi: 10.7554/eLife.06412

Schuknecht, H. F., Churchill, J. A., & Doran, R. (1959). The localization of acetylcholinesterase in the cochlea. *A.M.A. Archives of Otolaryngology 69*(5), 549–559.

Sendin, G., Bourien, J., Rassendren, F., Puel, J. L., & Nouvian, R. (2014). Spatiotemporal pattern of action potential firing in developing inner hair cells of the mouse cochlea. *Proceedings of the National Academy of Sciences USA 111*(5), 1999–2004.

Sewell, W. (1996). Neurotransmitters and synaptic transmission. In P. J. Dallos, A. N. Popper, & R. R. Fay (Eds.), *The cochlea* (pp. 503–533). New York, NY: Springer-Verlag.

Sgard, F., Charpentier, E., Bertrand, S., Walker, N., Caput, D., Graham, D., . . . Besnard, F. (2002). A novel human nicotinic receptor subunit, a 10, that confers functionality to the a9-subunit. *Molecular Pharmacology 61*(1), 150–159.

Shigemoto, T., & Ohmori, H. (1990). Muscarinic agonists and ATP increase the intracellular Ca2+ concentration in chick cochlear hair cells. *Journal of Physiology 420*(1), 127–148.

Shigemoto, T., & Ohmori, H. (1991). Muscarinic receptor hyperpolarizes cochlear hair cells of chick by activating Ca($^{2+}$)-activated K^+ channels. *Journal of Physiology 442*(1), 669–690.

Simmons, D. D. (2002). Development of the inner ear efferent system across vertebrate species. *Journal of Neurobiology 53*(2), 228–250.

Simmons, D. D., Bertolotto, C., Kim, J., Raji-Kubba, J., & Mansdorf, N. (1998). Choline acetyltransferase expression during a putative developmental waiting period. *Journal of Comparative Neurology 397*(2), 281–295.

Simmons, D. D., Mansdorf, N. B., & Kim, J. H. (1996). Olivocochlear innervation of inner and outer hair cells during postnatal maturation: Evidence for a waiting period. *Journal of Comparative Neurology* 370(4), 551–562.

Simmons, D. D., Manson-Gieseke, L., Hendrix, T. W., & McCarter, S. (1990). Reconstructions of efferent fibers in the postnatal hamster cochlea. *Hearing Research* 49(1–3), 127–139.

Simmons, D. D., & Morley, B. J. (1998). Differential expression of the alpha 9 nicotinic acetylcholine receptor subunit in neonatal and adult cochlear hair cells. *Brain Research* 56(1–2), 287–292.

Simmons, D. D., Moulding, H. D., & Zee, D. (1996). Olivocochlear innervation of inner and outer hair cells during postnatal maturation: an immunocytochemical study. *Brain Research* 95(2), 213–226.

Sonntag, M., Englitz, B., Kopp-Scheinpflug, C., & Rubsamen, R. (2009). Early postnatal development of spontaneous and acoustically evoked discharge activity of principal cells of the medial nucleus of the trapezoid body: an in vivo study in mice. *Journal of Neuroscience* 29(30), 9510–9520.

Spoendlin, H. (1971). Primary structural changes in the organ of Corti after acoustic overstimulation. *Acta Oto-Laryngologica* 71(2), 166–176.

Sridhar, T. S., Brown, M. C., & Sewell, W. F. (1997). Unique postsynaptic signaling at the hair cell efferent synapse permits calcium to evoke changes on two time scales. *Journal of Neuroscience* 17(1), 428–437.

Sridhar, T. S., Liberman, M. C., Brown, M. C., & Sewell, W. F. (1995). A novel cholinergic "slow effect" of efferent stimulation on cochlear potentials in the guinea pig. *Journal of Neuroscience* 15(5 Pt 1), 3667–3678.

Sugai, T., Yano, J., Sugitani, M., & Ooyama, H. (1992). Actions of cholinergic agonists and antagonists on the efferent synapse in the frog sacculus. *Hearing Research* 61(1–2), 56–64.

Taranda, J., Ballestero, J. A., Hiel, H., de Souza, F. S., Wedemeyer, C., Gomez-Casati, M. E., . . . Elgoyhen, A. B. (2009). Constitutive expression of the alpha10 nicotinic acetylcholine receptor subunit fails to maintain cholinergic responses in inner hair cells after the onset of hearing. *Journal of the Association for Research in Otolaryngology* 10(3), 397–406.

Taranda, J., Maison, S. F., Ballestero, J. A., Katz, E., Savino, J., Vetter, D. E., . . . Elgoyhen, A. B. (2009). A point mutation in the hair cell nicotinic cholinergic receptor prolongs cochlear inhibition and enhances noise protection. *PLOS Biology* 7(1), e18.

Terreros, G., Jorratt, P., Aedo, C., Elgoyhen, A. B., & Delano, P. H. (2016). Selective attention to visual stimuli using auditory distractors is altered in alpha-9 nicotinic receptor subunit knock-out mice. *Journal of Neuroscience* 36(27), 7198–7209.

Tritsch, N. X., Rodriguez-Contreras, A., Crins, T. T., Wang, H. C., Borst, J. G., & Bergles, D. E. (2010). Calcium action potentials in hair cells pattern auditory neuron activity before hearing onset. *Nature Neuroscience* 13(9), 1050–1052.

Tritsch, N. X., Yi, E., Gale, J. E., Glowatzki, E., & Bergles, D. E. (2007). The origin of spontaneous activity in the developing auditory system. *Nature* 450(7166), 50–55.

Verbitsky, M., Rothlin, C., Katz, E., & Elgoyhen, A. B. (2000). Mixed nicotinic-muscarinic properties of the α9 nicotinic cholinergic receptor. *Neuropharmacology* 39(13), 2515–2524.

Vetter, D. E., Adams, J. C., & Mugnani, E. (1991). Chemically distinct rat olivocochlear neurons. *Synapse* 7(1), 21–43.

Vetter, D. E., Katz, E., Maison, S. F., Taranda, J., Turcan, S., Ballestero, J., . . . Boulter, J. (2007). The alpha10 nicotinic acetylcholine receptor subunit is required for normal synaptic function and integrity of the olivocochlear system. *Proceedings of the National Academy of Sciences USA 104*(51), 20594–20599.

Vetter, D., Lieberman, M., Mann, J., Barhanin, J., Boulter, J., Brown, M., . . . Elgoyhen, A. (1999). Role of a9 nicotinic ACh receptor subunits in the development and function of cochlear efferent innervation. *Neuron 23*(1), 93–103.

Walsh, E., McGee, J., McFadden, S., & Liberman, M. (1998). Long-term effects of sectioning the olivocochlear bundle in neonatal cats. *Journal of Neuroscience 18*(10), 3859–3869.

Wang, H. C., Lin, C. C., Cheung, R., Zhang-Hooks, Y., Agarwal, A., Ellis-Davies, G., . . . Bergles, D. E. (2015). Spontaneous activity of cochlear hair cells triggered by fluid secretion mechanism in adjacent support cells. *Cell 163*(6), 1348–1359.

Warr, W. B. (1975). Olivocochlear and vestibular efferent neurons of the feline brain stem: Their location, morphology and number determined by retrograde axonal transport and acetylcholinesterase histochemistry. *Journal of Comparative Neurology 161*(2), 159–181.

Warr, W. (1992). Organization of olivocochlear efferent system in mammals. In W. Douglas, A. Popper, & R. Fay (Eds.), *The mammalian auditory pathway: Neuroanatomy* (pp. 410–448). New York, NY: Springer-Verlag.

Warr, W. B., & Boche, J. E. (2003). Diversity of axonal ramifications belonging to single lateral and medial olivocochlear neurons. *Experimental Brain Research 153*(4), 499–513.

Wedemeyer, C., Zorrilla de San Martin, J., Ballestero, J., Gomez-Casati, M. E., Torbidoni, A. V., Fuchs, P. A., . . . Katz, E. (2013). Activation of presynaptic GABA(B(1a,2)) receptors inhibits synaptic transmission at mammalian inhibitory cholinergic olivocochlear-hair cell synapses. *Journal of Neuroscience 33*(39), 15477–15487.

Wersinger, E., McLean, W. J., Fuchs, P. A., & Pyott, S. J. (2010). BK channels mediate cholinergic inhibition of high frequency cochlear hair cells. *PLOS One 5*(11), e13836.

Wiederhold, M. L., & Kiang, N. Y. S. (1970). Effects of electrical stimulation of the crossed olivocochlear bundle on cat single auditory nerve fibers. *Journal of the Acoustical Society of America 48*(4), 950–965.

Wilson, J. L., Henson, M. M., & Henson, O. W., Jr. (1991). Course and distribution of efferent fibers in the cochlea of the mouse. *Hearing Research 55*(1), 98–108.

Winslow, R. L., & Sachs, M. B. (1988). Single-tone intensity discrimination based on auditory-nerve rate responses in backgrounds of quiet, noise, and with stimulation of the crossed olivocochlear bundle. *Hearing Research 35*(2–3), 165–189.

Ye, Z., Goutman, J. D., Pyott, S. J., & Glowatzki, E. (2017). mGluR1 enhances efferent inhibition of inner hair cells in the developing rat cochlea. *Journal of Physiology 595*(11), 3483–3495.

Yoshida, N., Shigemoto, T., Sugai, T., & Ohmori, H. (1994). The role of inositol triphosphate on ACh-induced outward currents in bullfrog saccular hair cells. *Brain Research 644*, 90–100.

Yuhas, W. A., & Fuchs, P. A. (1999). Apamin-sensitive, small-conductance, calcium-activated potassium channels mediate cholinergic inhibition of chick auditory hair cells. *Journal of Comparative Physiology A 185*(5), 455–462.

Zachary, S. P., & Fuchs, P. A. (2015). Re-emergent inhibition of cochlear inner hair cells in a mouse model of hearing loss. *Journal of Neuroscience 35*(26), 9701–9706.

Zenner, H. P., Gitter, A. H., Rudert, M., & Ernst, A. (1992). Stiffness, compliance, elasticity and force generation of outer hair cells. *Acta Oto-Laryngologica 112*(2), 248–253.

Zheng, J., Shen, W., He, D. Z., Long, K. B., Madison, L. D., & Dallos, P. (2000). Prestin is the motor protein of cochlear outer hair cells. *Nature 405*(6783), 149–155.

Zhou, X., Panizzutti, R., de Villers-Sidani, E., Madeira, C., & Merzenich, M. M. (2011). Natural restoration of critical period plasticity in the juvenile and adult primary auditory cortex. *Journal of Neuroscience 31*(15), 5625–5634.

Zorrilla de San Martin, J., Pyott, S., Ballestero, J., & Katz, E. (2010). Ca($^{2+}$) and Ca($^{2+}$)-activated K($^{+}$) channels that support and modulate transmitter release at the olivocochlear efferent-inner hair cell synapse. *Journal of Neuroscience 30*(36), 12157–12167.

Zucker, R. S., & Regehr, W. G. (2002). Short-term synaptic plasticity. *Annual Review of Physiology 64*, 355–405.

Zuo, J., Treadaway, J., Buckner, T. W., & Fritzsch, B. (1999). Visualization of alpha9 acetylcholine receptor expression in hair cells of transgenic mice containing a modified bacterial artificial chromosome. *Proceedings of the National Academy of Sciences USA 96*(24), 14100–14105.

CHAPTER 4

THE COCHLEAR NUCLEI

Synaptic Plasticity in Circuits and Synapses in the Ventral Cochlear Nuclei

DONATA OERTEL, XIAO-JIE CAO, AND ALBERTO RECIO-SPINOSO

Abstract

Plasticity in neuronal circuits is essential for optimizing connections as animals develop and for adapting to injuries and aging, but it can also distort the processing, as well as compromise the conveyance of ongoing sensory information. This chapter summarizes evidence from electrophysiological studies in slices and in vivo that shows how remarkably robust signaling is in principal cells of the ventral cochlear nucleus. Even in the face of short-term plasticity, these neurons signal rapidly and with temporal precision. They can relay ongoing acoustic information from the cochlea to the brain largely independently of sounds to which they were exposed previously.

Keywords: ventral cochlear nucleus, short-term plasticity, synapse, electrophysiology, sound, slice, temporal precision, signaling

The ventral cochlear nucleus (VCN) serves as the brain's port of entry for acoustic information. The VCN performs two tasks. First, individual neurons extract biologically useful features of sounds from signals in auditory nerve fibers. Some neurons sharpen the encoding of the fine structure of sounds, others detect the onset of spectrally complex sounds that arise from a single source, and a third group tracks spectral peaks and valleys. Second, the VCN distributes acoustic information along parallel ascending pathways to brainstem nuclei, the inferior colliculi and the thalamus. In this chapter we review what is known about responses to sound in view of what has been learned about synaptic plasticity from slices in vitro.

Plasticity is crucial in the functioning of the brain for it allows neuronal circuits to be optimized as animals develop and to adapt to changes as animals suffer injuries. On the other hand, adjustment of the strength of synapses influences the way synapses convey information. Synapses in the VCN balance the need for adjustment with the need to convey ongoing acoustic information robustly. For the purposes of this chapter we will distinguish several distinct types of plasticity that differ in how they are driven, how long they last, and by what mechanisms they are regulated.

1. Over development some neurons die apoptotic deaths while others make or withdraw synaptic connections that can increase or decrease in size and strength. *Developmental plasticity* takes place as animals develop at all stages of the auditory pathway and the consequences last over the lifetime of the animals, months and years. That plasticity will be reviewed in (see Friauf, this volume). Such plasticity is usually rapid early in life and then slows. In development, plastic changes are accompanied by maturation in the morphology of dendritic and axonal arbors of neurons.
2. Plasticity in the adult brain is particularly evident when the brain responds to injury. In the auditory system it is evident when animals suffer hearing loss. *Responses to hearing loss* are evident over days, months or years and are considered in many other chapters of this book and will thus not be reviewed here (see chapters by Caspary & Llano, Manis, and Rubio, this volume).
3. In many parts of the brain, famously in the hippocampus and cerebral cortex where it is thought to underlie the ability to learn and remember, synapses undergo *long-term plasticity,* long-term potentiation and long-term depression. Long-term plasticity adjusts the strength of synapses upward or downward as a function of synaptic traffic they convey and can last for hours and days. This type of plasticity takes place at synapses on spines that form separate biochemical compartments for synapses. It is largely synapse specific but also shows cooperativity and associativity with nearby synapses. Such long-term plasticity occurs in the molecular layer of the dorsal cochlear nucleus (DCN; see Trussell, this volume) but not in the ventral cochlear nucleus (VCN). Neurons in the VCN lack spines and neither long-term potentiation or long-term depression have been observed in electrophysiological recordings from the VCN.
4. Synaptic plasticity can also occur over short periods. *Short-term plasticity* affects the strength of synapses temporarily over tens of milliseconds to seconds. This kind of plasticity will be discussed here.

This chapter summarizes evidence that the synapses that convey acoustic information from auditory nerve fibers to targets in the VCN are striking for how faithfully they convey signals even when signaling is rapid. Neurons differ in manifestation of short-term plasticity of their auditory nerve inputs in their responses to sound. In some neurons plasticity is not evident whereas in others the subtle effects of short-term depression are evident. It also discusses what little is known about plasticity of interconnections between neurons in the VCN.

Spiral Ganglion Cells Impose a Tonotopic Organization on the VCN

Myelinated spiral ganglion cells receive sensory inputs through a peripheral process from a tiny segment of the tonotopic array of inner hair cells, in mice about ~1/3000. Auditory nerve fibers, the axons of spiral ganglion cells, enter the brainstem and bifurcate to innervate the anteroventral cochlear nucleus (aVCN) with the ascending branch and the posteroventral cochlear nucleus (pVCN) and the dorsal cochlear nucleus (DCN) with the descending branch. Like other sensory neurons that innervate the hind brain and spinal cord, auditory nerve fibers grow into the brain from the periphery and bifurcate upon reaching the brain (Lu et al., 2014; Schmidt et al., 2007; Ter-Avetisyan, Rathjen, & Schmidt, 2014). The sturdy ascending branch contacts neurons in the aVCN through collateral branches that end in clusters of boutons, the end bulbs of Held, or with individual terminals while the thinner descending branch innervates neurons in the pVCN and DCN through boutons on collateral branches. In mice that lack *npr2*, neither auditory nerve fibers nor sensory neurons in the spinal cord bifurcate while still generating collateral branches, indicating that the bifurcation of auditory nerve fibers in the nerve root is regulated by mechanisms distinct from collateral branching (Lu et al., 2014).

A fundamental feature of the growth of spiral ganglion cells into the cochlear nuclei is the tonotopic organization. Spiral ganglion cells that receive input from the apical part of the cochlea and encode the lowest frequencies, innervate the most ventral region of the ventral and dorsal cochlear nuclei (Bourk, Mielcarz, & Norris, 1981). Those that receive input from the base of the cochlea and that encode the highest frequencies innervate the most dorsal regions of VCN and DCN. The orderly topographic organization of connections between the cochlea and cochlear nuclear targets develops before animals hear and exists even in animals in which hair cells never function (X. J. Cao, McGinley, & Oertel, 2008) and in which synapses between hair cells and spiral ganglion cells function only weakly over a short period (Beurg et al., 2008; Wright, Hwang, & Oertel, 2014). The tonotopic organization of connections between auditory nerve fibers and their cochlear nuclear targets is thus not dependent on auditory experience but rather on molecular cues (Lu, Appler, Houseman, & Goodrich, 2011). Mutant mice that lack *npr2*, whose auditory nerve fibers fail to bifurcate normally (Lu et al., 2014), mutant mice in which neurons in the VCN are deprived of *Hox2* genes (Karmakar et al., 2017), or where netrin signaling is disrupted (Kim et al., 2016) have a blurred tonotopic organization.

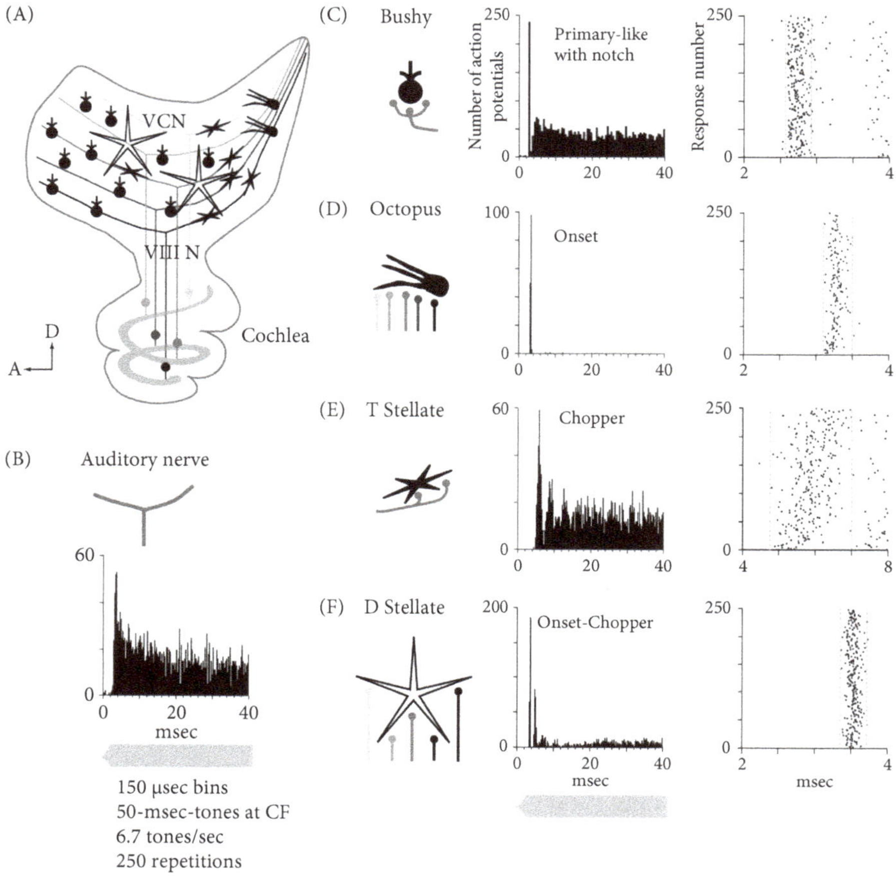

FIGURE 4.1. Principal cells of the VCN respond robustly and characteristically even when driven by 250 tones of 50 msec duration at the cells' characteristic frequency (CF) every 150 msec in vivo. **A.** Schematic representation of the innervation of the VCN by spiral ganglion cells. The axons of spiral ganglion cells, the auditory nerve fibers, bifurcate in the nerve root and innervate target cells of the VCN tonotopically through collateral branches. Those fibers that encode the lowest frequencies (black) innervate targets ventrally in the VCN, whereas those that encode the highest frequencies (light gray) innervate neurons that lie most dorsally, imposing a tonotopic organization on the VCN. Each fiber innervates several types of target neurons—bushy, octopus cells, T stellate, and D stellate—but the patterns differ. Bushy and T stellate cells receive input from only a few similarly tuned neurons that give them narrow tuning, whereas octopus and D stellate cells receive input from many fibers that give them broad tuning. **B.** Peristimulus time histogram of responses of an auditory nerve fiber. As is characteristic of primary-like responses, the fiber fired rapidly after the onset of the tone and then its firing slowed. **C.** (PSTH) Globular bushy cell responds to tones with a sharply timed onset (almost all first spikes fall into a single 250 μsec bin) that also synchronizes the refractory period to give the PSTH its characteristic notch. (Dot raster) The first action potential generally falls into a 500 μsec window and does not change from first to last, indicating that there is no sign of synaptic plasticity. Dashed line is for reference. **D.** (PSTH) Octopus cell responds to tones at the onset but responses fall into several bins. (Dot raster) Responses are sharply timed, in that they fall into a 400 μsec window. The gradual lengthening

Through collateral branches auditory nerve fibers innervate four types of principal neurons, three excitatory and one inhibitory. The three major groups of excitatory principal cells that transmit acoustic information along separate ascending pathways are bushy cells, T stellate cells, and octopus cells (J. R. Brawer, Morest, & Kane, 1974; Cant & Morest, 1979; Lorente de No, 1933; Osen, 1969). D Stellate cells also project out of the VCN to the ipsilateral DCN and to the contralateral cochlear nuclei but these cells are inhibitory (Needham & Paolini, 2003; Wenthold, 1987). The organization is illustrated schematically in Figure 4.1A.

Differences in the way target cells process acoustic information is evident in the transformation of responses to tones at the frequency to which they are tuned, the characteristic frequency (CF; Figure 4.1C–F). In mature mammals auditory nerve fibers have characteristic "primary-like" firing patterns in that they fire rapidly at the onset of a sound and then the firing slows (Figure 4.1B; Liberman, 1978; Rhode & Smith, 1985). Globular bushy cells convert primary-like patterns of auditory nerve fibers to "primary-like with notch" patterns that have a sharply timed first spike followed by a refractory period (Figure 4.1C; P. H. Smith & Rhode, 1987). Octopus cells respond only at the onsets of tones with "onset" patterns when those tones are > 1 kHz (Figure 4.1D; Rhode, Oertel, & Smith, 1983; P. H. Smith, Massie, & Joris, 2005). T Stellate cells fire steadily throughout the tone without conveying information about the fine structure of sounds with "chopper" patterns except at low frequencies (Figure 4.1E; Blackburn & Sachs, 1989; P. H. Smith & Rhode, 1989). D Stellate cells also fire tonically but with a more sharply timed initial spike to produce an "Onset chopper" response (Figure 4.1F; P. H. Smith & Rhode, 1989).

The patterns of convergence of auditory nerve inputs differ as shown schematically in Figure 4.1. Bushy and T stellate cells receive input from a small number of similarly tuned inputs making them sharply tuned whereas octopus and D stellate cells receive input from large numbers of inputs and are broadly tuned. The dynamics of the synaptic currents differs (Figure 4.2). Repeated stimulation of auditory nerve inputs in bushy and octopus cells evokes strong synaptic depression whereas in T and D stellate cells synaptic currents show weak synaptic depression. Neurons also differ in the contribution

of the latency of action potentials is consistent with the build-up of synaptic depression. **E.** (PSTH) T Stellate cell fires regularly at a roughly constant rate. The consistent timing of the first three action potentials appears as modes in the histogram, unrelated to the fine structure of sounds. (Dot raster) Not only does the latency of the first action potential fall over a longer time window, about 2 msec, but the latency of the first action potential is also longer than for other VCN neurons. The latency shifts between first and last responses but it is unclear whether the shift results from synaptic depression or from the accumulation of inhibition. Note that the time scale differs from other dot raster plots. **F.** (PSTH) D Stellate cells respond to tones with sharply timed, regular firing. (Dot raster) The timing of the first action potential is sharply timed, falling into a time window of about 300 μsec. The latency of responses does not change between the first and last responses. Responses to tones were recorded by William S. Rhode and Alberto Recio from cats. Details of methods are described by Rhode & Smith (1986).

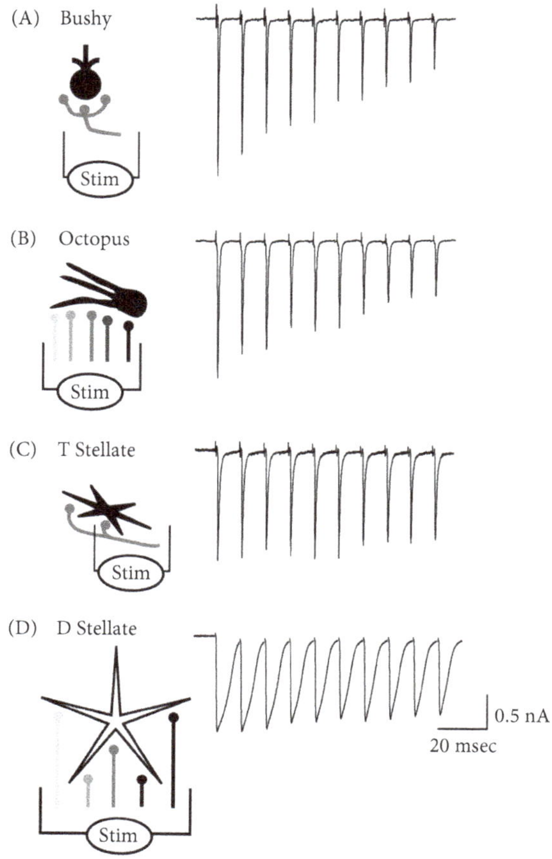

FIGURE 4.2. In slices from mice, synapses between auditory nerve fibers and their targets show varying degrees of synaptic depression. **A–C.** Synaptic depression is strong in bushy and octopus cells and less strong in T stellate cells. Extracellular Ca^{2+} concentration was 2.4 mM. (Traces are from fig. 8, X. J. Cao & Oertel, 2010, used with permission of the American Physiological Society.) **D.** Synaptic responses are broader in D stellate cells than in the other types of neurons. They show relatively little synaptic depression. Recording was made in the presence of 2.5 mM Ca^{2+}. (Trace was kindly provided by Dr. Ruili Xie.)

of inhibitory inputs and in the way the electrical properties of target neurons shape the voltage responses to synaptic currents determine the firing patterns in responses to sounds of the principal cells of the VCN.

It is now possible to assign general functions to the various VCN neurons at least tentatively, as we shall discussed. Bushy cells preserve or sharpen information in the firing patterns of auditory nerve fibers that conveys the fine structure of sounds, including phase locking at low frequencies. Octopus cells detect the coincident firing of large groups of auditory nerve fibers, signaling the presence of onsets and broadband transients. Individual T stellate cells detect the amplitude of sounds over a narrow frequency range and as a population they detect the ongoing spectrum of sounds impinging on the ear. D Stellate cells detect coincident firing from many auditory nerve fibers but the temporal and spatial summation of inputs obscures temporal fine structure.

Connections between Auditory Nerve Fibers and Bushy Cells

Bushy cells sharpen the representation of the fine structure of sounds. The sharpened representations serve as the basis for the comparison of interaural time and intensity in the superior olivary complex that underlie our ability to localize sounds in the horizontal plane (Yin, 2002).

The characteristic "bush" of dendrites gives bushy cells their name (J. R. Brawer et al., 1974; Lorente de No, 1933). Bushy cells are most common in the aVCN. They are of three subtypes that differ in their targets within the brainstem. Large spherical bushy cells, most common ventrally and anteriorly in the aVCN, terminate bilaterally in the medial superior olivary nuclei (MSO). Small spherical bushy cells terminate ipsilaterally in the vicinity of the ipsilateral lateral superior olive (LSO; Cant & Casseday, 1986). Globular bushy cells terminate in the contralateral medial nucleus of the trapezoid body (Tolbert, Morest, & Yurgelun-Todd, 1982). Consistent with their lying ventrally, the tuning of large spherical bushy cells is biased toward the low frequencies, as are their targets in the MSO. Animals that have little low-frequency hearing, as for example mice and bats, have relatively few large spherical bushy cells. Lying more dorsally, small spherical bushy cells are biased toward tuning to the higher frequencies and are numerous in the aVCN of mice and bats.

The number of converging inputs differs between subtypes of bushy cells. Large and small spherical bushy cells that lie anteriorly in the anterior VCN receive input from about 2-4 fibers (J. R. Brawer & Morest, 1975; X. J. Cao & Oertel, 2010; Sento & Ryugo, 1989). They respond to tones resemble those in auditory nerve fibers and are thus termed "primary-like" (P. H. Smith, Joris, & Yin, 1993). Globular bushy cells that lie more caudally near the nerve root receive more inputs, ≥ 5 in mice (X. J. Cao & Oertel, 2010) and about 25 in cats (Ostapoff & Morest, 1991; Spirou, Rager, & Manis, 2005). They respond to tones with an initial well-timed action potential that is followed by a "notch" that reflects the refractory period of auditory nerve inputs (Figure 4.1C; P. H. Smith, Joris, Carney, & Yin, 1991).

Auditory nerve fibers innervate bushy cells through large clusters of terminals, the end bulbs of Held (Held, 1893), that engulf the cell body. End bulbs are capable of releasing large amounts of neurotransmitter that evoke large postsynaptic currents, up to 6 nA in wild type mice and up to 12 nA in deaf mice, through numerous release sites (Cant & Morest, 1979; X. J. Cao & Oertel, 2010; Spirou et al., 2005; Wright et al., 2014). In animals that never hear, end bulbs are smaller and less branched (Lee, Cahill, & Ryugo,

2003; Ryugo, Pongstaporn, Huchton, & Niparko, 1997; Wright et al., 2014). At these synapses, synaptic currents are larger and synaptic depression is greater than in hearing mice reflecting a higher probability of release (Oleskevich & Walmsley, 2002; Wright et al., 2014; Zhuang, Sun, & Xu-Friedman, 2017).

Bushy cells sharpen the encoding of the fine structure of sounds. The presence of a low-voltage-activated K^+ conductance gives bushy cells low input resistances that cause EPSPs to rise and fall rapidly, to minimize temporal summation (X. J. Cao, Shatadal, & Oertel, 2007; Manis & Marx, 1991). Bushy cells are differentiators of excitatory postsynaptic potentials (EPSPs); large, summed synchronous EPSPs rise most rapidly and evoke action potentials most reliably (McGinley & Oertel, 2006). Extracellular recordings often indicate that the firing of bushy cells often follows the firing of auditory nerve fibers, accounting for the similarity of auditory nerve fibers and bushy cells in their responses to tones (Bourk, 1976; Kopp-Scheinpflug, Dehmel, Dorrscheidt, & Rubsamen, 2002). The relatively small number of inputs is consistent with their narrow tuning (Rhode et al., 1983; Rhode & Smith, 1986). However, the responses are subtly altered by convergence. The standard deviation in the first spike latency in the population of globular bushy cells is 0.58 msec compared to 0.73 msec for auditory nerve fibers (Rhode & Smith, 1986). Phase-locked responses to low-frequency sounds, presumably from large spherical bushy cells, are also sharpened (P.X. Joris, Carney, Smith, & Yin, 1994; P. X. Joris, Smith, & Yin, 1994). Tuning is sharpened by inhibitory sidebands, probably from D stellate cells (Caspary, Backoff, Finlayson, & Palombi, 1994; Kopp-Scheinpflug et al., 2002; Oertel, 1983; Oertel, Wu, Garb, & Dizack, 1990).

Responses of bushy cells to sound have long been explored by presenting tones many times in rapid succession and constructing a peristimulus time histogram (PSTH), which plots the probability of the cell's firing with respect to the presentation of the tone. The observation that responses to tones are not perceptibly affected by the rate at which tones are presented shows how subtle the role of plasticity is. The peristimulus time histograms illustrated in Figure 4.1 were generated by summing firing in responses to 250 repetitions of a 50-msec tone at the frequency to which they are tuned. They were generated from responses to tones that were repeated at 150 ms intervals (6.7/sec). These are not substantially different from those generated by others from responses at higher rates (9.5/sec; Rhode & Smith, 1985, 1986), or slower rates (5/sec; Blackburn & Sachs, 1989; Winter & Palmer, 1990). The response of a globular bushy cell (Figure 4.1C) shows that the timing of the first action potential is sharp, sharper than that of auditory nerve fibers, most falling into one 250 μsec bin of the PSTH. The dot raster on the right shows that the first spikes occur over a window that does not change even as the cell responds to a rapid succession of tones. The fact that responses are stable even during stimulation at high rates is an indication that synaptic transmission shows little sign of long-term synaptic plasticity. Large spherical bushy cells also signal with sharp timing (P. X. Joris, Smith, & Yin, 1998).

The question whether short-term plasticity plays a role in vivo has been examined with elegant experiments in large spherical bushy cells. A series of studies has shown that in extracellular recordings three events, the presynaptic action potential, the postsynaptic current, and the postsynaptic action potential, can be separately and reliably monitored, as illustrated in Figure 4.3A (Kuenzel, Borst, & van der Heijden, 2011). The relationship between them can thus also be measured. Short-term synaptic depression or facilitation would be expected to cause correlation of the slope of the EPSP with the interval between responses. Figures 4.3C and 3D show that there is little correlation (Keine, Rubsamen, & Englitz, 2016; Kuenzel et al., 2011).

The relationship between the slopes of EPSPs and the threshold of action potentials did change with activity, however. When auditory nerve fibers were driven slowly by soft tones (20 dB SPL; Figure 4.3C) the threshold slope of EPSPs required to evoke action potentials was lower than when auditory nerve fibers were driven rapidly by loud tones (70 dB SPL; Figure 4.3D; Kuenzel et al., 2011). Findings like these led to the conclusion that while short-term synaptic plasticity does not play a major role, inhibition influences the dynamics of responses to sound in vivo (Englitz, Tolnai, Typlt, Jost, & Rubsamen, 2009; Keine et al., 2016; Keine, Rubsamen, & Englitz, 2017; Kopp-Scheinpflug et al., 2002; Kuenzel et al., 2011; Kuenzel, Nerlich, Wagner, Rubsamen, & Milenkovic, 2015; Winter & Palmer, 1990). Such detailed analyses have not been performed on small spherical or on globular bushy cells.

In contrast with the subtlety or absence of synaptic plasticity in vivo, synaptic transmission between auditory nerve fibers and bushy cells in slices in vitro consistently reveals short-term synaptic depression (Figure 4.2A; Bellingham & Walmsley, 1999; X. J. Cao & Oertel, 2010; Chanda & Xu-Friedman, 2010; Klug et al., 2012; Oleskevich, Clements, & Walmsley, 2000; Y. Wang & Manis, 2008; Y. Wang, Ren, & Manis, 2010; Yang & Xu-Friedman, 2008, 2009). While most recordings from bushy cells in slices are from mice that have few large spherical bushy cells and are thus likely to be from small spherical or globular bushy cells, there is no reason to think the difference in synaptic plasticity reflects a difference in the type of bushy cell. Synaptic depression is a feature of synapses that have a high probability of neurotransmitter release (Oleskevich & Walmsley, 2002; Schneggenburger, Meyer, & Neher, 1999; Silver, Momiyama, & Cull-Candy, 1998). The high probability of release implies that when a resting synapse is stimulated with a train of shocks, a relatively large proportion of the readily releasable pool of vesicles is released in response to the first shock, leaving the pool depleted for subsequent stimuli (Taschenberger, Scheuss, & Neher, 2005). Much has been learned about short-term synaptic depression as investigators have grappled with the question why synaptic plasticity looks so different in large spherical bushy cells in vivo and in vitro.

Synaptic depression is variable. It differs between bushy cells but is matched at inputs that converge on one cell (H. Yang & Xu-Friedman, 2009). It is greater at younger than at more mature synapses (Wu & Oertel, 1987); in vivo studies are generally done on mature animals whereas measurements in slices are generally done on immature rodents.

Desensitization of the AMPA receptors that mediate transmission causes synaptic depression. Especially at immature end bulbs, EPSCs are reduced as a result of progressive desensitization of AMPA receptors (Chanda & Xu-Friedman, 2010; Trussell, Zhang, & Raman, 1993; H. Yang & Xu-Friedman, 2008). It has been demonstrated that

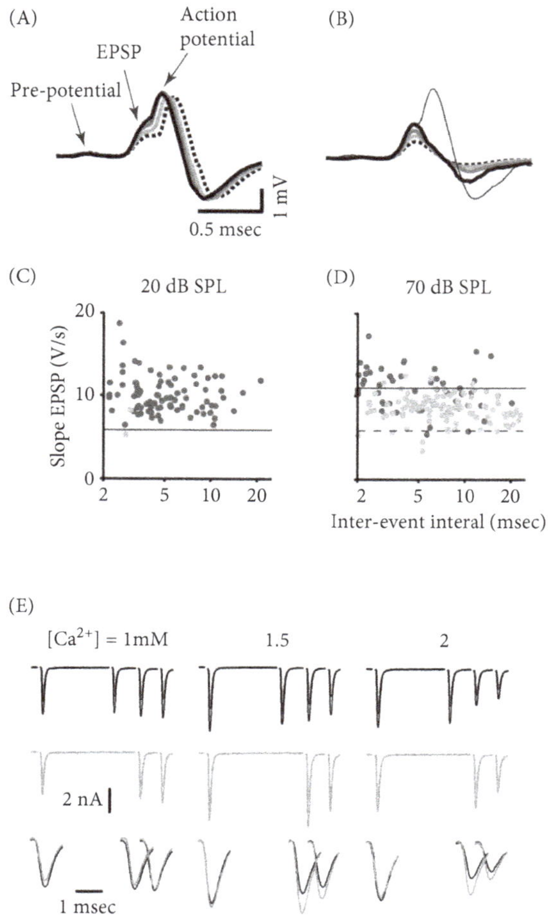

FIGURE 4.3. Short-term depression in bushy cells is evident in vitro but not in vivo. **A.** Juxtacellular recordings in vivo from large spherical bushy cells in gerbils in responses to tones at CF at 20 dB SPL were categorized as a function of the slopes of EPSPs (7.5, 10, and 12.5 V/s) and averaged. In these recordings the prepotential reflects the firing of the auditory nerve fiber. After a synaptic delay, the EPSP rises from the baseline with varying slopes. The EPSPs evoked action potentials but those that were evoked by slowly rising EPSPs (dashed line) were delayed relative to those evoked by rapidly rising EPSPs (solid line). **B.** Responses to tones at 70 dB SPL were analyzed as in A. Many responses were subthreshold. **C.** Inter-event intervals in responses to 20 dB SPL tone plotted against the slope of the EPSP show that the slope of the EPSP is unaffected by the duration of the preceding interval. Most responses are suprathreshold (black dots), with very few being subthreshold (gray dots). Solid horizontal line marks the threshold slope. **D.** In response to 70 dB SPL tones, slopes of EPSPs were not very different but a smaller proportion of responses were suprathreshold (black dots). The threshold slope, marked by the solid horizontal line, increased. The slopes of EPSPs did not generally vary systematically as a function of inter-event intervals, suggesting that EPSPs showed little synaptic depression. Black dots show suprathreshold responses; gray dots show subthreshold responses. The solid line, marking the threshold slope of action potentials, is increased relative to C. (Panels A–D are adapted with

the presence of NMDA receptors at these synapses can counteract synaptic depression in that while AMPA receptors become depressed, currents through NMDA receptors sum and strengthen (Pliss, Yang, & Xu-Friedman, 2009).

Spontaneous firing of auditory nerve fibers could put synapses into a depressed state in vivo but not in slices in vitro. In vivo many auditory nerve fibers fire spontaneously even in the absence of sound stimuli. Spontaneous firing rates vary from 0 to > 100 Hz, with the proportions of fibers firing at low and high rates varying between species and also between strains of mice (Liberman, 1978; Taberner & Liberman, 2005; Tsuji & Liberman, 1997). In mice 30%–50% of fibers fire >20/sec (Taberner & Liberman, 2005) suggesting that in vivo many end bulb synapses are probably in a constantly depressed state so that depression is less evident. Stimulation of synapses at rates similar to those in vivo resulted in reduced synaptic depression (Y. Wang et al., 2010).

Differences in short-term plasticity in vivo and in vitro are exacerbated by differences in the extracellular calcium concentrations in the extracellular fluids. Recordings in slices are often done at > 2 mM Ca^{2+} while in vivo physiological extracellular Ca^{2+} concentrations are lower, between 1.2 and 1.7 mM. High extracellular Ca^{2+} concentrations result in artificially high release probability and artificially high synaptic depression (Borst, 2010; H. Yang & Xu-Friedman, 2015).

In slices, even at physiological extracellular Ca^{2+} concentrations, EPSCs suffer from presynaptically mediated synaptic depression. In an elegant experiment in which investigators presented naturalistic stimulus trains and compared responses when a single stimulus about midway through the train was skipped, it was possible to relate the size of synaptic currents to the length of the previous interstimulus interval (Figure 4.3E; H. Yang & Xu-Friedman, 2015). Figure 4.3E illustrates how lengthening the preceding interval increased the size of EPSPs even when the extracellular Ca^{2+} concentration was near physiological at 1.5 mM. While synaptic depression was evident, recovery from depression was rapid, occurring over about 60 msec, because activity accelerates recovery from inactivation (H. Yang & Xu-Friedman, 2008, 2015).

Sodium channel inactivation also contributes to failure of EPSPs to evoke action potentials (H. Yang & Xu-Friedman, 2015). During the refractory period of an action potential, larger and faster depolarizations are required reach threshold.

It is possible that synapses in vivo are tonically inhibited by GABA or glycine. Bushy cells are contacted by synaptic terminals that contain glycine and GABA (Juiz, Helfert, Bonneau, Wenthold, & Altschuler, 1996). Sound evoked inhibition increased the threshold of action potentials, so that only the largest and most sharply timed EPSPs

permission from Figure 4.5; Kuenzel et al., 2011.) **E.** Synaptic depression is stronger in the presence of elevated extracellular Ca^{2+}. Bushy cells of mice in vitro were stimulated with long trains of shocks whose intervals had a Poisson distribution. Responses are compared in similar trains in which a single shock was skipped when the extracellular Ca^{2+} concentration was varied. Upper traces (black) show control responses. Middle traces (gray) show responses when one shock was skipped. Lower traces show overlapped responses in upper and middle panels. (Traces are adapted with permission from Figure. 4.5; H. Yang & Xu-Friedman, 2015.)

evoked postsynaptic action potentials (Kuenzel et al., 2011). Such inhibition produces a depression in firing.

In summary, no long-term plasticity has been detected at synapses between auditory nerve fibers and bushy cells. Short-term depression is consistently observed in slices but is subtle or absent in vivo. Short-term plasticity at inputs to bushy cells in vivo appears to be regulated by many factors including release probability, desensitization of AMPA receptors, activation of NMDA receptors, accumulation of inhibition, and also Na^+ channel inactivation. When these mechanisms act together at synapses between auditory nerve fibers and bushy cells in vivo, short-term plasticity is not obvious. The properties of auditory nerve inputs to globular bushy cells have not been studied in detail in vivo and may differ somewhat. Published studies indicate that synapses between auditory nerve fibers and bushy cells are remarkably robust, conveying ongoing, precisely timed information both when their inputs fire slowly and also when they fire rapidly.

Connections between Auditory Nerve Fibers and Octopus Cells

While their integrative role is not fully understood, it is likely that octopus cells contribute to the detection of gaps, a feature that is important in the understanding of speech (Oertel, Cao, Ison, & Allen, 2017; F. G. Zeng, Kong, Michalewski, & Starr, 2005; F.G. Zeng, Oba, Garde, Sininger, & Starr, 1999). Octopus cells occupy the most caudal and dorsal part of the VCN where auditory nerve fibers become closely bundled on their way to the DCN. They were named for the unidirectional spread of their dendrites across the tonotopically organized bundle of auditory nerve fibers (Osen, 1969). They project to the contralateral superior paraolivary nucleus (Schofield, 1995) and ventral nucleus of the lateral lemniscus where they terminate in calyceal endings (Adams, 1997).

Octopus cells splay their dendrites across the bundle of auditory nerve fibers from caudal to rostral, enabling them to detect synchronous firing among the many fibers (>60 in mice; Figure 4.1; Golding, Robertson, & Oertel, 1995; McGinley, Liberman, Bal, & Oertel, 2012). Inputs from fibers tuned to a wide range of frequencies generates broad tuning in octopus cells (Godfrey, Kiang, & Norris, 1975; Rhode et al., 1983; P. H. Smith et al., 2005). Each auditory nerve fiber delivers only a small current so that coincident inputs from many fibers are required for octopus cells to reach threshold. They respond to sounds that activate many auditory nerve fibers synchronously: clicks, the onsets of tones, and loud phase-locked sounds at every cycle at frequencies below 800 Hz (Oertel, Bal, Gardner, Smith, & Joris, 2000; Rhode & Smith, 1986; P. H. Smith et al., 2005). In responding at every cycle up to 800 Hz, octopus cells fire at extraordinary rates. They respond only at the onset of tones of higher frequency (Figure 4.1D; Godfrey et al., 1975; Rhode et al., 1983;

P. H. Smith et al., 2005). That single action potential occurs with little temporal jitter, having a standard deviation of only 0.12 msec (Figure 4.1D; Rhode & Smith, 1986).

Short-term depression is evident in responses to sound of octopus cells. In responses to tones (Figure 4.1D) and clicks (Figure 4.4A) octopus cells fire over a time window that gradually shifts while cells are responding rapidly. Responses to tones presented at 6.7/sec shifted by about 100 μsec (Figure 4.1D, right panel); responses to 100 clicks at 500 Hz increased by about 200 μsec in latency between the first and the 100th click (Figure 4.4A; Oertel et al., 2000). While the greatest differences occurred between the first and subsequent responses, the latency continued to change with later responses. These systematic shifts parallel synaptic depression in slices.

In vitro rapid stimulation of auditory nerve fibers evokes responses in octopus cells that show synaptic depression. Synaptic currents evoked by stimulation of auditory nerve fibers diminish in size when they are evoked in rapid succession in the presence of high (2.4 mM) extracellular Ca^{2+} concentrations (Figure 4.2B; X. J. Cao & Oertel, 2010). The voltage changes produced by synaptic currents are determined by the biophysical properties of target cells. Octopus cells have exceptionally low input resistances and short time constants (Golding, Ferragamo, & Oertel, 1999; Golding et al., 1995).

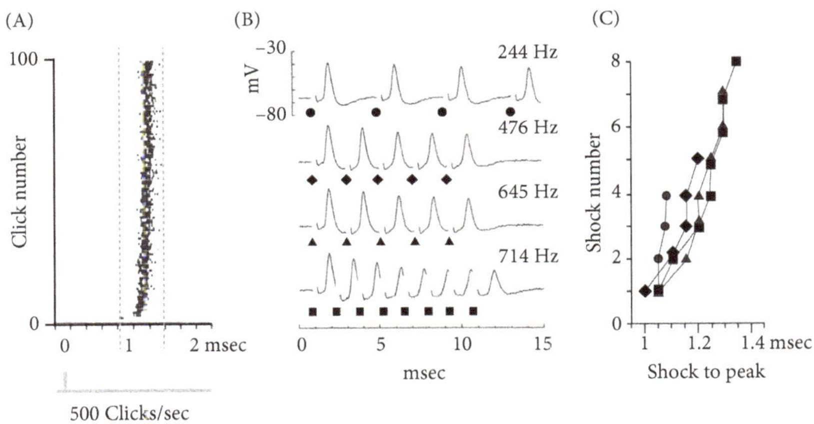

FIGURE 4.4. Short-term depression of auditory nerve inputs to octopus cells is evident when auditory nerve fibers are stimulated roughly synchronously in vivo with clicks and in vitro with shocks to the auditory nerve. **A.** Timing of firing of an octopus cell in vivo to 100 clicks relative to the 2 msec period of clicks presented at 500/sec shows that the intervals lengthen by about 200 μsec as the cell is driven to fire at 500/sec (from Figure 9; Oertel et al., 2000). **B.** Responses to shocks of the nerve root in slices show that as octopus cells are driven at increasing rates, the peaks of responses in which EPSPs and action potentials cannot be distinguished become progressively smaller. (Adapted with permission from Figure 8; Golding et al., 1995.) **C.** Plot of delays from data in B shows that the latency between the beginning of the shock and the peak of action potentials occurs progressively later when synapses are driven rapidly. The symbols correspond to the symbols under the traces in B.

The short time constants are a consequence of the activation of two opposing voltage-sensitive conductances, a slow hyperpolarization-activated, mixed cation conductance and a fast depolarization-activated K^+ conductance (Bal & Oertel, 2000, 2001). In octopus cells, EPSPs are faster than the currents that drive them, only about 1 msec in duration, because EPSPs are actively repolarized by the fast, low-voltage-activated K^+ conductance (X. J. Cao & Oertel, 2010; Golding et al., 1995). The fast K^+ conductance also gives every octopus cell a threshold rate of depolarization (M. J. Ferragamo & Oertel, 2002). To generate action potentials, small unitary EPSPs must sum on their rising phases to generate a depolarization that exceeds the threshold rate of depolarization. Action potentials are generated on the rising phase of EPSPs. This mechanism makes octopus cells excellent coincidence detectors. The need for coincidence in the submillisecond range raised the question how summing occurs for inputs that are subject to traveling wave delays of multiple milliseconds. Dendritic filtering compensates for differences in the cochlear traveling wave delay (McGinley et al., 2012).

In responses to rapid trains of shocks to the auditory nerve, diminishing synaptic currents depolarize octopus cells more and more slowly, generating progressively smaller, albeit suprathreshold, responses (Figure 4.4B). The peaks of suprathreshold postsynaptic responses become smaller (Figure 4.4B). The peaks of responses also become increasingly delayed (Figure 4.4C), much as responses to clicks are delayed when they are presented in rapid succession (Figure 4.4A). How a reduction of extracellular Ca^{2+} to physiological levels affects the degree of depression in slices and whether synaptic depression reflects only depletion of neurotransmitter or also involves other factors is not known. Inhibition may or may not play a role. In guinea pigs glycinergic, but not GABAergic, terminals have been detected (Juiz et al., 1996) but in mice there is a conspicuous absence of inhibition in the octopus cell area (R. E. Wickesberg, Whitlon, & Oertel, 1994). It is also not known whether sodium channel inactivation elevates the thresholds of action potentials.

In summary, responses to tones and clicks in vivo show evidence of short-term depression, but not of long-term synaptic plasticity. Detailed comparisons of short-term plasticity in octopus cells in vivo and in vitro have not been made.

Connections between Auditory Nerve Fibers and T Stellate Cells

T Stellate cells encode features that are critical for understanding speech in humans and for understanding the significance of environmental sounds in all mammals, spectral peaks and valleys and amplitude modulation (Frisina, Smith, & Chamberlain, 1990; Rosen, 1992; Shannon, Zeng, Kamath, Wygonski, & Ekelid, 1995; X. Wang & Sachs, 1992). As a population they encode spectrum (Blackburn & Sachs, 1990; May, Prell, & Sachs, 1998; Recio & Rhode, 2000). The fact that they encode those features known to be conveyed by cochlear implants and that they fail to encode the temporal fine structure of sounds that is not conveyed by cochlear implants, suggests that T stellate cells play a particularly important role in cochlear implant users and that they are important for understanding speech in all listeners.

T Stellate cells are concentrated just caudal to the nerve root in the multipolar cell area. Their dendrites lie parallel to the path of auditory nerve fibers and their axons project out of the VCN through the trapezoid body (hence T stellate (Oertel et al., 1990)). They are known by a confusing array of names. They are referred to as multipolar cells (Osen, 1969), stellate cells (J. R. Brawer et al., 1974), type I cells (Cant, 1981), and planar multipolar cells (Doucet & Ryugo, 1997). T Stellate cells are not only numerous but they project more widely than the other principal cells. T Stellate cells excite targets in the ipsilateral DCN (Doucet & Ryugo, 1997; Oertel et al., 1990; P.H. Smith, Joris, Banks, & Yin, 1993), the contralateral ventral nucleus of the trapezoid body (P.H. Smith et al., 1993; Thompson & Thompson, 1991), the contralateral ventral nucleus of the lateral lemniscus (Schofield & Cant, 1997; P.H. Smith et al., 1993), the inferior colliculi (Adams, 1979; Oliver, 1987; Schofield, Mellott, & Motts, 2014), and the thalamus (Schofield et al., 2014).

T Stellate cells respond tonically to sound stimuli in vivo. That is, they fire at a roughly constant rate in the presence of sounds to which they are tuned (Figure 4.1E). The "chopping" pattern reflects the consistency of the regular firing (Blackburn & Sachs, 1989; Rhode et al., 1983; P. H. Smith & Rhode, 1989; Young, Robert, & Shofner, 1988). The first spike has a narrow range of latencies and produces the first mode in the chopping pattern; the jitter in timing of the second spike sums with the jitter in the timing of the first, producing a broader, smaller mode and so on until the modes are not resolvable. These cells respond to tones as if they are steadily depolarized by sound and fire at a rate monotonically related to the size of the depolarization. The firing pattern thus does not reflect the fine structure of sounds except at low frequencies (Blackburn & Sachs, 1989).

It was noted long ago that the responses of T stellate cells to tones in vivo occur almost 2 msec later than responses of other VCN neurons (Figure 4.1E; Young et al., 1988). Furthermore, the variability of the latency of the first spike is greater than that of other targets of auditory nerve fibers. The firing of T stellate cells at roughly constant rates for the duration of a tone, also stands in contrast with responses of their auditory nerve inputs, which fire most rapidly at the onset of sound stimuli and then slow. How T stellate cells convert the phasic responses of auditory nerve fibers to tonic responses is not understood (Oertel, Wright, Cao, Ferragamo, & Bal, 2011). The consistency of the firing pattern over many repetitions even when those stimuli are presented at high rates is an indication that long-term plasticity does not play a role in shaping responses to tones in T stellate cells. Dot rasters of responses to tones do show that the latency of responses shifts gradually when the cell is driven at high rates. The finding that at physiological Ca^{2+} concentrations, T stellate cells show facilitation rather than depression makes it unlikely that the shift is a consequence of synaptic depression (Chanda & Xu-Friedman, 2010). It could arise from accumulating inhibition.

T Stellate cells/choppers are strongly influenced by inhibition. The tuning of choppers is sharpened by inhibitory sidebands (Palombi & Caspary, 1992; Paolini, Clarey, Needham, & Clark, 2005; Rhode & Greenberg, 1994b). In responses to complex sounds, inhibition would be expected to enhance the encoding of spectral peaks, consistent with the observation that choppers convey information about the spectrum of sounds (Blackburn & Sachs, 1990; May et al., 1998; Recio & Rhode, 2000). Possibly inhibition balances excitation, counteracting strong excitation at the onset of a sound and obscuring the fine structure of excitation (Paolini et al., 2005). The presence of early inhibition could also account for the longer latency of responses of choppers than responses of other VCN neurons (Figure 4.1E, right panel). As T stellate cells receive input directly from auditory nerve fibers and inhibition requires an extra synaptic delay, it is unclear how inhibition can affect the onset of responses to sounds. However, inhibition so rapid that it can reduce responses to single clicks has been observed in vivo (R.E. Wickesberg, 1996).

Studies in slices reveal that shocks to auditory nerve fibers evoke rapid excitation and delayed, long-lasting inhibition in T stellate cells Recordings in slices show that T stellate cells receive input from a relatively small number of auditory nerve fibers, in mice about 5.5, consistent with their sharp tuning (M. J. Ferragamo, Golding, & Oertel, 1998). The latency between shocks to auditory nerve fibers and responses are similar to those in bushy and octopus cells (Wu & Oertel, 1984). T Stellate cells fire steadily and regularly as long as they are depolarized, the firing rate being monotonically related to the injected depolarizing current (Oertel et al., 1990). In contrast with bushy and octopus cells, whose thresholds are a function of the slope of EPSPs, thresholds of action potentials in T stellate cells are more nearly a function of the peak amplitude of EPSPs as result of having somatic voltage-sensitive Na^+ channels (Y. Yang, Ramamurthy, Neef, & Xu-Friedman, 2016).

In slices bathed in extracellular fluid with elevated Ca^{2+} concentrations, synaptic responses to stimulation of the auditory nerve show synaptic depression in T stellate cells. Under voltage-clamp at -65 mV, AMPA-receptor mediated responses can be isolated. These show some synaptic depression, but less than bushy or octopus cells (Figure 4.2C; X. J. Cao & Oertel, 2010). Under lower, more physiological Ca^{2+} concentrations, inputs to T stellate cells show facilitation rather than depression (Chanda & Xu-Friedman, 2010). Synaptic responses in T stellate cells involve not only AMPA but also NMDA receptors that can last for hundreds of milliseconds (X. J. Cao & Oertel, 2010; M. J. Ferragamo et al., 1998).

Slices confirm that inhibition affects the dynamics of signaling (M. Ferragamo, Golding, Gardner, & Oertel, 1998; Paolini et al., 2005). Glycinergic inputs are regularly activated by stimulation of the auditory nerve and can sometimes provide repeated IPSPs for long periods (Figure 4.5A; M. Ferragamo et al., 1998). The observation that inhibition can last for 500 msec, albeit in slices (Figure 4.5A), suggests that responses to tones repeated every 150 msec could be affected by inhibition evoked by previous tones (Figure 4.1E). While GABAergic IPSPs have not been detected in slices, bicuculline, a blocker of $GABA_A$ receptors affects choppers, suggesting that

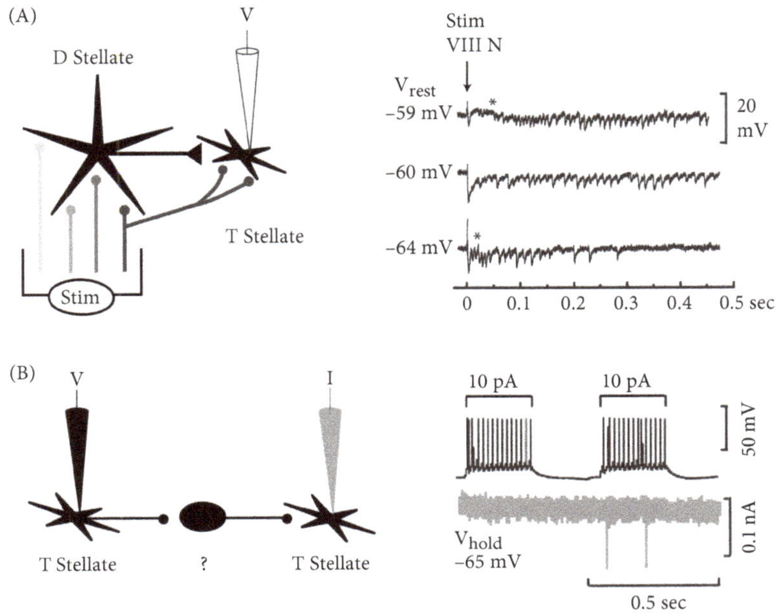

FIGURE 4.5. Properties of interconnections between neurons. **A.** Separate intracellular recordings from three different T stellate cells show that responses to single shocks of the auditory nerve evoke excitation (not well resolved at slow time scale) that can be followed by trains of IPSPs. Because such IPSPs were recorded in slices that lacked any DCN, the source of IPSPs is within the VCN and is likely to be D stellate cells; the amplitudes of IPSPs suggest that they arose from one or two cells that fired repetitively. The complexity of early responses that involve both excitation and inhibition (*) limits resolution of early IPSPs but later IPSPs were uniform in size and shape, showing no evidence of synaptic plasticity. (Traces are from Figure 5; M. J. Ferragamo et al., 1998; used with permission of the American Physiological Society.) **B.** Dual patch-clamp recording from a pair of T stellate cells shows that depolarization of one cell (black, current clamp) resulted in synaptic responses (gray, voltage-clamp) in the other. The connection between these cells was weak, in that 29 presynaptic action potentials only evoked 2 postsynaptic responses. Because synaptic responses did not follow action potentials with a consistent latency, the connection was probably mediated by an unknown interneuron.

$GABA_A$ receptors affect responses to sound in vivo (Caspary et al., 1994). The presence of GABA suggests that release from auditory nerve terminals could be modulated through $GABA_B$ receptors.

In summary, T stellate cells respond robustly to sounds showing no evidence of long-term plasticity. If short-term plasticity plays a role, it is subtle. While responses to tones of T stellate cells become slightly delayed when they are presented in rapid succession, those shifts could arise from shifts in the balance between excitation and inhibition. Like the other principal cells of the VCN, T stellate cells respond robustly to ongoing sounds, largely independently of what happened previously.

Connections between Auditory Nerve Fibers and D Stellate Cells

In contrast with bushy, octopus and T stellate cells, which are excitatory and form the major ascending auditory pathways, D Stellate cells are glycinergic, inhibitory neurons that project within the ipsilateral cochlear nuclei and to the contralateral cochlear nuclei (Needham & Paolini, 2003; Paolini & Clark, 1999; Wenthold, 1987). Being inhibitory, these neurons shape the output of their targets. These neurons are thought to generate inhibitory sidebands that sharpen tuning in their targets, in T stellate cells and also in targets in pyramidal cells of the DCN (Nelken & Young, 1994).

The reach of D stellate cell dendrites across the tonotopic axis gives D stellate cells access to input from numerous auditory nerve fibers and accounts for their broad tuning (Oertel et al., 1990; Xie & Manis, 2017). D Stellate cells fire with "onset-chopper" response patterns (Figure 4.1F; Palmer, Jiang, & Marshall, 1996; Paolini & Clark, 1999; P. H. Smith & Rhode, 1989). In these neurons the regularity of the early spikes in responses to tones generates sharply timed modes at the onset of peristimulus time histograms. The sharpness in timing likely reflects a reduction in temporal jitter by coincidence detection (Rhode & Greenberg, 1994a; Xie & Manis, 2017). As in other VCN neurons, the firing patterns are stable even when they are stimulated rapidly, suggesting that synaptic inputs from auditory nerve fibers are not subject to long-term synaptic plasticity (Figure 4.1F). The dot rasters confirm the consistency in the timing of firing of responses to tones, with first spike latencies largely falling within a 300 μsec window and there being no detectable difference between the early and late responses.

In slices EPSCs activated by stimulation of auditory nerve fibers in slices are slower in D stellate cells than in the other principal cells of the VCN (Xie & Manis, 2017). In the presence of high extracellular Ca^{2+} some synaptic depression is evident (Figure 4.2D). Synaptic depression is, however, even weaker than in T stellate cells (Xie & Manis, 2017). Presumably there would be little synaptic depression or perhaps facilitation in the presence of physiological extracellular Ca^{2+} concentrations but that has not been measured.

In summary, neither responses to sound in vivo nor responses to trains of shocks in slices show signs of synaptic plasticity. Like excitatory neurons of the VCN, D stellate cells fire independently of previous signaling. They are thus able to provide ongoing representations of the acoustic environment.

Interconnections between T and D Stellate Cells

Less is known about the properties of synaptic connections between principal cells than between auditory nerve fibers and principal cells. In vivo two sources of inhibition were identified, with one arising from the DCN (R.E. Wickesberg, 1996). Intracellular recordings from bushy and T stellate cells show that these cells are disynaptically inhibited by shocks to the auditory nerve in slices that contain VCN and DCN (M. J. Ferragamo et al., 1998; Oertel, 1983). That inhibition is glycinergic (Wu & Oertel, 1986). Two groups of inhibitory neurons can be the source of that inhibition, tuberculoventral cells in the deep layer of the DCN (R. E. Wickesberg & Oertel, 1990; R. E. Wickesberg et al., 1994) and D stellate cells in the VCN (M. J. Ferragamo et al., 1998; Wenthold, 1987). In slices that lack the DCN, disynaptic inhibition arising from shocks to the auditory nerve is likely to arise from D stellate cells, the only known group of glycinergic neurons in the VCN (Figure 4.5A). Strong shocks to the root of the auditory nerve evoked brief excitation and then long trains of IPSPs in many T stellate cells. Their regularity and uniformity in amplitude suggest that these come from only a few inhibitory interneurons. Over hundreds of milliseconds, synaptic responses neither grow nor shrink systematically, showing a lack of long-term depression or potentiation. While the early inhibitory responses are obscured by excitation (Figure 4.5A*), the later ones are clear and seem unaffected by the previous interval. There is no indication of short-term depression or facilitation.

The finding that T stellate cells have local axonal collaterals within the same isofrequency as the dendrites within the multipolar cell area suggests that T stellate cells are interconnected within an isofrequency lamina (Oertel et al., 2011; Oertel et al., 1990). To study those connections, paired recordings were made from T stellate cells within an isofrequency lamina. To date only weak indirect connections have been found (Figure 4.5B). Preliminary experiments suggest that these connections are potentiated when firing of one cell is paired with depolarization of another and that this potentiation is mediated by nitric oxide signaling (X.-J. Cao, Oertel, D., 2016, 2017). What role this plasticity plays in responses to sounds in vivo is not known but an interesting possibility is that it enhances the signaling of spectral peaks.

Concluding Remarks

Synaptic connections between auditory nerve fibers and their targets in the VCN show no signs of long-term potentiation or depression. Short-term plasticity varies in different targets of auditory nerve fibers in the VCN. Measurements in slices in the presence of unphysiologically high (>2 mM) Ca^{2+} suggest that synaptic depression between auditory nerve fibers and their targets is greatest in bushy and octopus cells and less in T stellate cells and D stellate cells (Figure 4.2). The story is more interesting than that, however. Not only is synaptic depression weaker in vivo because the probability of release is lower in the presence of lower, more physiological levels of extracellular Ca^{2+}, but other mechanisms including desensitization of AMPA receptors, the presence of NMDA receptors, the presence of inhibition, and perhaps also Na^{+} channel inactivation make signaling dynamic. Synaptic depression in bushy cells that is strong in vitro is only subtly evident in vivo, likely because inhibition reduces the probability of release when firing is rapid. On the other hand, the threshold of action potentials is dynamic. In octopus cells that are not observed to be subject to much inhibition, short-term synaptic depression is evident in vivo as it is in vitro. In T and D stellate cells synaptic depression of auditory nerve inputs is weak in slices and would be expected to be even weaker or facilitatory in vivo in the presence of lower concentrations of Ca^{2+}. Nevertheless, the latency of first spikes shifts in repeated responses to tones.

The usefulness of hearing depends on the faithful transmission of information about what is happening in the acoustic environment no matter what happened previously. Because VCN neurons respond so robustly, the early studies that characterized responses to sound ignored long-term and short-term plasticity. If synapses were to be strengthened or weakened as a function of the synaptic traffic, then the information they convey would be affected by what the animal heard previously. It is perhaps not surprising, therefore, that synapses in the VCN have only short-term plasticity, plasticity that recovers over milliseconds. Cells differ in the way short term plasticity is manifest in vivo. It is subtly present in the latencies of responses of octopus cells and perhaps in T stellate cells. In bushy cells, where synaptic depression is as great as in octopus cells in slices, synaptic depression is difficult to detect in vivo and inhibition seems to govern the dynamics. D Stellate cells have been less intensively studied but show no sign of long-term or short-term plasticity. Nitric oxide-mediated plasticity has been observed only at interconnections between T stellate cells, cells that do not carry information in the precise timing of firing.

While synaptic plasticity is subtle in the VCN, it is not absent. In the two cells that convey information in the timing of firing, bushy and octopus cells, plasticity is subtle or regulated by inhibition. These circuits change dramatically as they mature and when acoustic input is removed. That type of plasticity is covered in other chapters in this book, however.

References

Adams, J. C. (1979). Ascending projections to the inferior colliculus. *Journal of Comparative Neurology*, *183*(3), 519–538. doi:10.1002/cne.901830305

Adams, J. C. (1997). Projections from octopus cells of the posteroventral cochlear nucleus to the ventral nucleus of the lateral lemniscus in cat and human. *Auditory Neuroscience*, *3*(4), 335–350.

Bal, R., & Oertel, D. (2000). Hyperpolarization-activated, mixed-cation current (Ih) in octopus cells of the mammalian cochlear nucleus. *Journal of Neurophysiology*, *84*, 806–817.

Bal, R., & Oertel, D. (2001). Potassium currents in octopus cells of the mammalian cochlear nucleus. *Journal of Neurophysiology*, *86*(5), 2299–2311.

Bellingham, M. C., & Walmsley, B. (1999). A novel presynaptic inhibitory mechanism underlies paired pulse depression at a fast central synapse. *Neuron*, *23*(1), 159–170.

Beurg, M., Safieddine, S., Roux, I., Bouleau, Y., Petit, C., & Dulon, D. (2008). Calcium- and otoferlin-dependent exocytosis by immature outer hair cells. *Journal of Neuroscience*, *28*(8), 1798–1803. doi:10.1523/JNEUROSCI.4653-07.2008

Blackburn, C. C., & Sachs, M. B. (1989). Classification of unit types in the anteroventral cochlear nucleus: PST histograms and regularity analysis. *Journal of Neurophysiology, 62*(6), 1303–1329.

Blackburn, C. C., & Sachs, M. B. (1990). The representations of the steady-state vowel sound phoneme-e in the discharge patterns of cat anteroventral cochlear nucleus neurons. *Journal of Neurophysiology, 63*(5), 1191–1212.

Borst, J. G. (2010). The low synaptic release probability in vivo. *Trends in Neuroscience, 33*(6), 259–266. doi:10.1016/j.tins.2010.03.003

Bourk, T. R. (1976). *Electrical responses of neural units in the anteroventral cochlear nucleus of the cat* (1 ed.). Boston, MA: MIT Press.

Bourk, T. R., Mielcarz, J. P., & Norris, B. E. (1981). Tonotopic organization of the anteroventral cochlear nucleus of the cat. *Hearing Research, 4*, 215–241.

Brawer, J. R., & Morest, D. K. (1975). Relations between auditory nerve endings and cell types in the cat's anteroventral cochlear nucleus seen with the Golgi method and Nomarski optics. *Journal of Comparative Neurology, 160*, 491–506.

Brawer, J. R., Morest, D. K., & Kane, E. C. (1974). The neuronal architecture of the cochlear nucleus of the cat. *Journal of Comparative Neurology, 155*(3), 251–300. doi:10.1002/cne.901550302

Cant, N. B. (1981). The fine structure of two types of stellate cells in the anterior division of the anteroventral cochlear nucleus of the cat. *Neuroscience, 6*(12), 2643–2655.

Cant, N. B., & Casseday, J. H. (1986). Projections from the anteroventral cochlear nucleus to the lateral and medial superior olivary nuclei. *Journal of Comparative Neurology, 247*(4), 457–476. doi:10.1002/cne.902470406

Cant, N. B., & Morest, D. K. (1979). The bushy cells in the anteroventral cochlear nucleus of the cat. A study with the electron microscope. *Neuroscience, 4*(12), 1925–1945.

Cao, X. J., McGinley, M. J., & Oertel, D. (2008). Connections and synaptic function in the posteroventral cochlear nucleus of deaf jerker mice. *Journal of Comparative Neurology, 510*(3), 297–308. doi:10.1002/cne.21788

Cao, X. J., & Oertel, D. (2010). Auditory nerve fibers excite targets through synapses that vary in convergence, strength, and short-term plasticity. *Journal of Neurophysiology, 104*(5), 2308–2320. doi:10.1152/jn.00451.2010

Cao, X.-J., & Oertel, D. (2016). Synaptic plasticity at connections between T stellate cells in the ventral cochlear nucleus. *Association for Research* in *Otolaryngology Abstracts, 2016*.

Cao, X.-J., & Oertel, D. (2017). Nitric oxide donor evokes excitation in the ventral cochlear nucleus. *Association for Research* in *Otolaryngology Abstracts,2017*.

Cao, X. J., Shatadal, S., & Oertel, D. (2007). Voltage-sensitive conductances of bushy cells of the mammalian ventral cochlear nucleus. *Journal of Neurophysiology, 97*(6), 3961–3975. doi:10.1152/jn.00052.2007

Caspary, D. M., Backoff, P. M., Finlayson, P. G., & Palombi, P. S. (1994). Inhibitory inputs modulate discharge rate within frequency receptive-fields of anteroventral cochlear nucleus neurons. *Journal of Neurophysiology, 72*(5), 2124–2133.

Chanda, S., & Xu-Friedman, M. A. (2010). A low-affinity antagonist reveals saturation and desensitization in mature synapses in the auditory brainstem. *Journal of Neurophysiology, 103*(4), 1915–1926.

Doucet, J. R., & Ryugo, D. K. (1997). Projections from the ventral cochlear nucleus to the dorsal cochlear nucleus in rats. *Journal of Comparative Neurology, 385*(2), 245–264.

Englitz, B., Tolnai, S., Typlt, M., Jost, J., & Rubsamen, R. (2009). Reliability of synaptic transmission at the synapses of Held in vivo under acoustic stimulation. *PLoS One*, *4*(10), e7014. doi:10.1371/journal.pone.0007014

Ferragamo, M., Golding, N. L., Gardner, S. M., & Oertel, D. (1998). Golgi cells in the superficial granule cell domain overlying the ventral cochlear nucleus: Morphology and eletrophysiology in slices. *Journal of Comparative Neurology*, *400*, 519–528.

Ferragamo, M. J., Golding, N. L., & Oertel, D. (1998). Synaptic inputs to stellate cells in the ventral cochlear nucleus. *Journal of Neurophysiology*, *79*(1), 51–63.

Ferragamo, M. J., & Oertel, D. (2002). Octopus cells of the mammalian ventral cochlear nucleus sense the rate of depolarization. *Journal of Neurophysiology*, *87*(5), 2262–2270. doi:10.1152/jn.00587.2001

Frisina, R. D., Smith, R. L., & Chamberlain, S. C. (1990). Encoding of amplitude modulation in the gerbil cochlear nucleus: I. A hierarchy of enhancement. *Hearing Research*, *44*(2–3), 99–122.

Godfrey, D. A., Kiang, N. Y., & Norris, B. E. (1975). Single unit activity in the posteroventral cochlear nucleus of the cat. *Journal of Comparative Neurology*, *162*(2), 247–268. doi:10.1002/cne.901620206

Golding, N. L., Ferragamo, M. J., & Oertel, D. (1999). Role of intrinsic conductances underlying responses to transients in octopus cells of the cochlear nucleus. *Journal of Neuroscience*, *19*(8), 2897–2905.

Golding, N. L., Robertson, D., & Oertel, D. (1995). Recordings from slices indicate that octopus cells of the cochlear nucleus detect coincident firing of auditory-nerve fibers with temporal precision. *Journal of Neuroscience*, *15*(4), 3138–3153.

Held, H. (1893). Die zentrale Gehoerleitung. *Archives of Anatomy and Physiology*, 201–248.

Joris, P. X., Carney, L. H., Smith, P. H., & Yin, T. C. (1994). Enhancement of neural synchronization in the anteroventral cochlear nucleus. I. Responses to tones at the characteristic frequency. *Journal of Neurophysiology*, *71*(3),1022–1036.

Joris, P. X., Smith, P. H., & Yin, T. C. (1994). Enhancement of neural synchronization in the anteroventral cochlear nucleus. II. Responses in the tuning curve tail. *Journal of Neurophysiology*, *71*(3), 1037–1051.

Joris, P. X., Smith, P. H., & Yin, T. C. (1998). Coincidence detection in the auditory system: 50 years after Jeffress. [Review] [20 refs]. *Neuron*, *21*(6), 1235–1238.

Juiz, J. M., Helfert, R. H., Bonneau, J. M., Wenthold, R. J., & Altschuler, R. A. (1996). Three classes of inhibitory amino acid terminals in the cochlear nucleus of the guinea pig. *Journal of Comparative Neurology*, *373*(1), 11–26. doi:10.1002/(SICI)1096-9861(19960909)373:1<11::AID-CNE2>3.0.CO;2-G

Karmakar, K., Narita, Y., Fadok, J., Ducret, S., Loche, A., Kitazawa, T., . . . Rijli, F. M. (2017). Hox2 genes are required for tonotopic map precision and sound discrimination in the mouse auditory brainstem. *Cell Rep*, *18*(1), 185–197. doi:10.1016/j.celrep.2016.12.021

Keine, C., Rubsamen, R., & Englitz, B. (2016). Inhibition in the auditory brainstem enhances signal representation and regulates gain in complex acoustic environments. *Elife*, *5*, e19295. doi:10.7554/eLife.19295

Keine, C., Rubsamen, R., & Englitz, B. (2017). Signal integration at spherical bushy cells enhances representation of temporal structure but limits its range. *Elife*, *6*, e29639. doi:10.7554/eLife.29639

Kim, Y. J., Wang, S. Z., Tymanskyj, S., Ma, L., Tao, H. W., & Zhang, L. I. (2016). DCC mediates functional assembly of peripheral auditory circuits. *Science Reports, 6*, 23799. doi:10.1038/srep23799

Klug, A., Borst, J. G., Carlson, B. A., Kopp-Scheinpflug, C., Klyachko, V. A., & Xu-Friedman, M. A. (2012). How do short-term changes at synapses fine-tune information processing? *Journal of Neuroscience, 32*(41), 14058–14063. doi:10.1523/JNEUROSCI.3348-12.2012

Kopp-Scheinpflug, C., Dehmel, S., Dorrscheidt, G. J., & Rubsamen, R. (2002). Interaction of excitation and inhibition in anteroventral cochlear nucleus neurons that receive large endbulb synaptic endings. *Journal of Neuroscience, 22*(24), 11004–11018.

Kuenzel, T., Borst, J. G., & van der Heijden, M.(2011). Factors controlling the input-output relationship of spherical bushy cells in the gerbil cochlear nucleus. *Journal of Neuroscience, 31*(11), 4260–4273.

Kuenzel, T., Nerlich, J., Wagner, H., Rubsamen, R., & Milenkovic, I. (2015). Inhibitory properties underlying non-monotonic input-output relationship in low-frequency spherical bushy neurons of the gerbil. *Front Neural Circuits, 9*, 14. doi:10.3389/fncir.2015.00014

Lee, D. J., Cahill, H. B., & Ryugo, D. K. (2003). Effects of congenital deafness in the cochlear nuclei of Shaker-2 mice: an ultrastructural analysis of synapse morphology in the endbulbs of Held. *Journal of Neurocytology, 32*(3), 229–243. doi:10.1023/B:NEUR.0000010082.99874.14

Liberman, M. C. (1978). Auditory-nerve response from cats raised in a low-noise chamber. *Journal of the Acoustical Society of America, 63*(2), 442–455.

Lorente de No, R. (1933). Anatomy of the eighth nerve. III. General plans of structure of the primary cochlear nuclei. *Laryngoscope, 43*, 327–350.

Lu, C. C., Appler, J. M., Houseman, E. A., & Goodrich, L. V. (2011). Developmental profiling of spiral ganglion neurons reveals insights into auditory circuit assembly. *Journal of Neuroscience, 31*(30), 10903–10918. doi:10.1523/Jneurosci.2358-11.2011

Lu, C. C., Cao, X. J., Wright, S., Ma, L., Oertel, D., & Goodrich, L. V. (2014). Mutation of Npr2 leads to blurred tonotopic organization of central auditory circuits in mice. *PLoS Genetics, 10*(12), e1004823. doi:10.1371/journal.pgen.1004823

Manis, P. B., & Marx, S. O. (1991). Outward currents in isolated ventral cochlear nucleus neurons. *Journal of Neuroscience, 11*(9), 2865–2880.

May, B. J., Prell, G. S., & Sachs, M. B. (1998). Vowel representations in the ventral cochlear nucleus of the cat: effects of level, background noise, and behavioral state. *Journal of Neurophysiology, 79*(4), 1755–1767.

McGinley, M. J., Liberman, M. C., Bal, R., & Oertel, D. (2012). Generating synchrony from the asynchronous: compensation for cochlear traveling wave delays by the dendrites of individual brainstem neurons. *Journal of Neuroscience, 32*(27), 9301–9311. doi:10.1523/JNEUROSCI.0272-12.2012

McGinley, M. J., & Oertel, D. (2006). Rate thresholds determine the precision of temporal integration in principal cells of the ventral cochlear nucleus. *Hearing Research, 216–217*, 52–63. doi:10.1016/j.heares.2006.02.006

Needham, K., & Paolini, A. G. (2003). Fast inhibition underlies the transmission of auditory information between cochlear nuclei. *Journal of Neuroscience, 23*(15), 6357–6361.

Nelken, I., & Young, E. D. (1994). Two separate inhibitory mechanisms shape the responses of dorsal cochlear nucleus type IV units to narrowband and wideband stimuli. *Journal of Neurophysiology, 71*(6), 2446–2462.

Oertel, D. (1983). Synaptic responses and electrical properties of cells in brain slices of the mouse anteroventral cochlear nucleus. *Journal of Neuroscience*, *3*(10), 2043–2053.

Oertel, D., Bal, R., Gardner, S. M., Smith, P. H., & Joris, P. X. (2000). Detection of synchrony in the activity of auditory nerve fibers by octopus cells of the mammalian cochlear nucleus. *Proceedings of the National Academy of Sciences USA*, *97*(22), 11773–11779. doi:10.1073/pnas.97.22.11773

Oertel, D., Cao, X. J., Ison, J. R., & Allen, P. D. (2017). Cellular computations underlying detection of gaps in sounds and lateralizing sound sources. *Trends in Neuroscience*, *40*(10), 613–624. doi:10.1016/j.tins.2017.08.001

Oertel, D., Wright, S., Cao, X. J., Ferragamo, M., & Bal, R. (2011). The multiple functions of T stellate/multipolar/chopper cells in the ventral cochlear nucleus. *Hearing Research*, *276*(1–2), 61–69. doi:10.1016/j.heares.2010.10.018

Oertel, D., Wu, S. H., Garb, M. W., & Dizack, C. (1990). Morphology and physiology of cells in slice preparations of the posteroventral cochlear nucleus of mice. *Journal of Comparative Neurology*, *295*(1), 136–154. doi:10.1002/cne.902950112

Oleskevich, S., Clements, J., & Walmsley, B. (2000). Release probability modulates short-term plasticity at a rat giant terminal. *Journal of Physiology-London*, *524*(2), 513–523. doi:DOI 10.1111/j.1469-7793.2000.00513.x

Oleskevich, S., & Walmsley, B. (2002). Synaptic transmission in the auditory brainstem of normal and congenitally deaf mice. *Journal of Physiology*, *540*(Pt 2), 447–455.

Oliver, D. L. (1987). Projections to the inferior colliculus from the anteroventral cochlear nucleus in the cat: possible substrates for binaural interaction. *Journal of Comparative Neurology*, *264*(1), 24–46. doi:10.1002/cne.902640104

Osen, K. K. (1969). Cytoarchitecture of the cochlear nuclei in the cat. *Journal of Comparative Neurology*, *136*(4), 453–484. doi:10.1002/cne.901360407

Ostapoff, E. M., & Morest, D. K. (1991). Synaptic organization of globular bushy cells in the ventral cochlear nucleus of the cat: a quantitative study. *Journal of Comparative Neurology*, *314*(3), 598–613. doi:10.1002/cne.903140314

Palmer, A. R., Jiang, D., & Marshall, D. H. (1996). Responses of ventral cochlear nucleus onset and chopper units as a function of signal bandwidth. *Journal of Neurophysiology*, *75*(2), 780–794.

Palombi, P. S., & Caspary, D. M. (1992). GABAA receptor antagonist bicuculline alters response properties of posteroventral cochlear nucleus neurons. *Journal of Neurophysiology*, *67*(3), 738–746.

Paolini, A. G., Clarey, J. C., Needham, K., & Clark, G. M. (2005). Balanced inhibition and excitation underlies spike firing regularity in ventral cochlear nucleus chopper neurons. *European Journal of Neuroscience*, *21*(5), 1236–1248. doi:10.1111/j.1460-9568.2005.03958.x

Paolini, A. G., & Clark, G. M. (1999). Intracellular responses of onset chopper neurons in the ventral cochlear nucleus to tones: evidence for dual-component processing. *Journal of Neurophysiology*, *81*(5), 2347–2359.

Pliss, L., Yang, H., & Xu-Friedman, M. A. (2009). Context-dependent effects of NMDA receptors on precise timing information at the endbulb of Held in the cochlear nucleus. *Journal of Neurophysiology*, *102*(5), 2627–2637. doi:10.1152/jn.00111.2009

Recio, A., & Rhode, W. S. (2000). Representation of vowel stimuli in the ventral cochlear nucleus of the chinchilla. *Hearing Research*, *146*(1–2), 167–184.

Rhode, W. S., & Greenberg, S. (1994a). Encoding of amplitude modulation in the cochlear nucleus of the cat. *Journal of Neurophysiology*, *71*(5), 1797–1825.

Rhode, W. S., & Greenberg, S. (1994b). Lateral suppression and inhibition in the cochlear nucleus of the cat. *Journal of Neurophysiology*, *71*(2), 493–514.

Rhode, W. S., Oertel, D., & Smith, P. H. (1983). Physiological response properties of cells labeled intracellularly with horseradish peroxidase in cat ventral cochlear nucleus. *Journal of Comparative Neurology*, *213*(4), 448–463. doi:10.1002/cne.902130408

Rhode, W. S., & Smith, P. H. (1985). Characteristics of tone-pip response patterns in relationship to spontaneous rate in cat auditory nerve fibers. *Hearing Research*, *18*(2), 159–168.

Rhode, W. S., & Smith, P. H. (1986). Encoding timing and intensity in the ventral cochlear nucleus of the cat. *Journal of Neurophysiology*, *56*(2), 261–286.

Rosen, S. (1992). Temporal information in speech: acoustic, auditory and linguistic aspects. *Philosophical Transactions of the Royal Society of London Ser. B Biological Science*, *336*(1278), 367–373. doi:10.1098/rstb.1992.0070

Ryugo, D. K., Pongstaporn, T., Huchton, D. M., & Niparko, J. K. (1997). Ultrastructural analysis of primary endings in deaf white cats: morphologic alterations in endbulbs of Held. *Journal of Comparative Neurology*, *385*(2), 230–244.

Schmidt, H., Stonkute, A., Juttner, R., Schaffer, S., Buttgereit, J., Feil, R., . . . Rathjen, F. G. (2007). The receptor guanylyl cyclase Npr2 is essential for sensory axon bifurcation within the spinal cord. *Journal of Cell Biology*, *179*(2), 331–340. doi:DOI 10.1083/jcb.200707176

Schneggenburger, R., Meyer, A. C., & Neher, E. (1999). Released fraction and total size of a pool of immediately available transmitter quanta at a calyx synapse. *Neuron*, *23*(2), 399–409. doi: 10.1016/S0896-6273(00)80789-8

Schofield, B. R. (1995). Projections from the cochlear nucleus to the superior paraolivary nucleus in guinea pigs. *Journal of Comparative Neurology*, *360*(1), 135–149. doi:10.1002/cne.903600110

Schofield, B. R., & Cant, N. B. (1997). Ventral nucleus of the lateral lemniscus in guinea pigs: cytoarchitecture and inputs from the cochlear nucleus. *Journal of Comparative Neurology*, *379*(3), 363–385.

Schofield, B. R., Mellott, J. G., & Motts, S. D. (2014). Subcollicular projections to the auditory thalamus and collateral projections to the inferior colliculus. *Frontiers in Neuroanatomy*, *8*, 70. doi:10.3389/fnana.2014.00070

Sento, S., & Ryugo, D. K. (1989). Endbulbs of Held and spherical bushy cells in cats: morphological correlates with physiological properties. *Journal of Comparative Neurology*, *280*(4), 553–562. doi:10.1002/cne.902800406

Shannon, R. V., Zeng, F. G., Kamath, V., Wygonski, J., & Ekelid, M. (1995). Speech recognition with primarily temporal cues. *Science*, *270*(5234), 303–304.

Silver, R. A., Momiyama, A., & Cull-Candy, S. G. (1998). Locus of frequency-dependent depression identified with multiple-probability fluctuation analysis at rat climbing fibre Purkinje cell synapses. *Journal of Physiology-London*, *510*(3), 881–902. doi:DOI 10.1111/j.1469-7793.1998.881bj.x

Smith, P. H., Joris, P. X., Banks, M. I., & Yin, T. C. T. (1993). Responses of cochlear nucleus cells and projections of their axons. In M. A. Merchan, J. M. Juiz, D. A. Godfrey, & E. Mugnaini (Eds.), *The Mammalian Cochlear Nuclei, Organization and Function* (Vol. 239, pp. 349–360). New York and London: Plenum Press. (Reprinted from: Not in File).

Smith, P. H., Joris, P. X., Carney, L. H., & Yin, T. C. (1991). Projections of physiologically characterized globular bushy cell axons from the cochlear nucleus of the cat. *Journal of Comparative Neurology*, *304*(3), 387–407. doi:10.1002/cne.903040305

Smith, P. H., Joris, P. X., & Yin, T. C. (1993). Projections of physiologically characterized spherical bushy cell axons from the cochlear nucleus of the cat: evidence for delay lines to the medial superior olive. *Journal of Comparative Neurology*, *331*(2), 245–260. doi:10.1002/cne.903310208

Smith, P. H., Massie, A., & Joris, P. X. (2005). Acoustic stria: anatomy of physiologically characterized cells and their axonal projection patterns. *Journal of Comparative Neurology*, *482*(4), 349–371. doi:10.1002/cne.20407

Smith, P. H., & Rhode, W. S. (1987). Characterization of HRP-labeled globular bushy cells in the cat anteroventral cochlear nucleus. *Journal of Comparative Neurology*, *266*(3), 360–375. doi:10.1002/cne.902660305

Smith, P. H., & Rhode, W. S. (1989). Structural and functional properties distinguish two types of multipolar cells in the ventral cochlear nucleus. *Journal of Comparative Neurology*, *282*(4), 595–616. doi:10.1002/cne.902820410

Spirou, G. A., Rager, J., & Manis, P. B. (2005). Convergence of auditory-nerve fiber projections onto globular bushy cells. *Neuroscience*, *136*(3), 843–863.

Taberner, A. M., & Liberman, M. C. (2005). Response properties of single auditory nerve fibers in the mouse. *Journal of Neurophysiology*, *93*(1), 557–569. doi:10.1152/jn.00574.2004

Taschenberger, H., Scheuss, V., & Neher, E. (2005). Release kinetics, quantal parameters and their modulation during short-term depression at a developing synapse in the rat CNS. *Journal of Physiology*, *568*(Pt 2), 513–537. doi:10.1113/jphysiol.2005.093468

Ter-Avetisyan, G., Rathjen, F. G., & Schmidt, H. (2014). Bifurcation of axons from cranial sensory neurons is disabled in the absence of Npr2-Induced cGMP signaling. *Journal of Neuroscience*, *34*(3), 737–747. doi:10.1523/Jneurosci.4183-13.2014

Thompson, A. M., & Thompson, G. C. (1991). Posteroventral cochlear nucleus projections to olivocochlear neurons. *Journal of Comparative Neurology*, *303*(2), 267–285. doi:10.1002/cne.903030209

Tolbert, L. P., Morest, D. K., & Yurgelun-Todd, D. A. (1982). The neuronal architecture of the anteroventral cochlear nucleus of the cat in the region of the cochlear nerve root: horseradish peroxidase labelling of identified cell types. *Neuroscience*, *7*(12), 3031–3052.

Trussell, L. O., Zhang, S., & Raman, I. M. (1993). Desensitization of AMPA receptors upon multiquantal neurotransmitter release. *Neuron*, *10*(6), 1185–1196. doi: 10.1016/0896-6273(93)90066-Z

Tsuji, J., & Liberman, M. C. (1997). Intracellular labeling of auditory nerve fibers in guinea pig: central and peripheral projections. *Journal of Comparative Neurology*, *381*(2), 188–202.

Wang, X., & Sachs, M. B. (1992). Coding of envelope modulation in the auditory nerve and anteroventral cochlear nucleus. *Philosophical Transactions of the Royal Society of London Ser. B, Biological Science*, *336*(1278), 399–402. doi:10.1098/rstb.1992.0074

Wang, Y., & Manis, P. B. (2008). Short-term synaptic depression and recovery at the mature mammalian endbulb of Held synapse in mice. *Journal of Neurophysiology*, *100*(3), 1255–1264. doi:10.1152/jn.90715.2008

Wang, Y., Ren, C., & Manis, P. B. (2010). Endbulb synaptic depression within the range of presynaptic spontaneous firing and its impact on the firing reliability of cochlear nucleus bushy neurons. *Hearing Research*, *270*(1–2), 101–109. doi:10.1016/j.heares.2010.09.003

Wenthold, R. J. (1987). Evidence for a glycinergic pathway connecting the two cochlear nuclei: an immunocytochemical and retrograde transport study. *Brain Research, 415*(1), 183–187.

Wickesberg, R. E. (1996). Rapid inhibition in the cochlear nuclear complex of the chinchilla. *Journal of the Acoustical Society of America, 100*(3), 1691–1702.

Wickesberg, R. E., & Oertel, D. (1990). Delayed, frequency-specific inhibition in the cochlear nuclei of mice: a mechanism for monaural echo suppression. *Journal of Neuroscience, 10*(6), 1762–1768.

Wickesberg, R. E., Whitlon, D., & Oertel, D. (1994). In vitro modulation of somatic glycine-like immunoreactivity in presumed glycinergic neurons. *Journal of Comparative Neurology, 339*(3), 311–327. doi:10.1002/cne.903390302

Winter, I. M., & Palmer, A. R. (1990). Responses of single units in the anteroventral cochlear nucleus of the guinea pig. *Hearing Research, 44*(2–3), 161–178.

Wright, S., Hwang, Y., & Oertel, D. (2014). Synaptic transmission between end bulbs of Held and bushy cells in the cochlear nucleus of mice with a mutation in Otoferlin. *Journal of Neurophysiology, 112*(12), 3173–3188. doi:10.1152/jn.00522.2014

Wu, S. H., & Oertel, D. (1984). Intracellular injection with horseradish peroxidase of physiologically characterized stellate and bushy cells in slices of mouse anteroventral cochlear nucleus. *Journal of Neuroscience, 4*(6), 1577–1588.

Wu, S. H., & Oertel, D. (1986). Inhibitory circuitry in the ventral cochlear nucleus is probably mediated by glycine. *Journal of Neuroscience, 6*(9), 2691–2706.

Wu, S. H., & Oertel, D. (1987). Maturation of synapses and electrical properties of cells in the cochlear nuclei. *Hearing Research, 30*(1), 99–110.

Xie, R., & Manis, P. B. (2017). Intrinsic excitability and synaptic properties of auditory nerve input of radiate and planar multipolar neurons in the mouse anteroventral cochlear nucleus. *Frontiers in Neural Circuits*. doi:10.3389/fncir.2017.00077

Yang, H., & Xu-Friedman, M. A. (2008). Relative roles of different mechanisms of depression at the mouse endbulb of Held. *Journal of Neurophysiology, 99*(5), 2510–2521. doi:10.1152/jn.01293.2007

Yang, H., & Xu-Friedman, M. A. (2009). Impact of synaptic depression on spike timing at the endbulb of Held. *Journal of Neurophysiology, 102*(3), 1699–1710. doi:10.1152/jn.00072.2009

Yang, H., & Xu-Friedman, M. A. (2015). Skipped-stimulus approach reveals that short-term plasticity dominates synaptic strength during ongoing activity. *Journal of Neuroscience, 35*(21), 8297–8307. doi:10.1523/Jneurosci.4299-14.2015

Yang, Y., Ramamurthy, B., Neef, A., & Xu-Friedman, M. A. (2016). Low somatic sodium conductance enhances action potential precision in time-coding auditory neurons. *Journal of Neuroscience, 36*(47), 11999–12009. doi:10.1523/JNEUROSCI.1475-16.2016

Yin, T. C. T. (2002). Neural mechanisms of encoding binaural localization cues in the auditory brainstem. In D. Oertel, R. R. Fay, & A. N. Popper (Eds.), *Integrative Functions in the Mammalian Auditory Pathway* (15th ed., pp. 99–159). New York: NY: Springer. (Reprinted from: Not in File).

Young, E. D., Robert, J. M., & Shofner, W. P. (1988). Regularity and latency of units in ventral cochlear nucleus: implications for unit classification and generation of response properties. *Journal of Neurophysiology, 60*, 1–29.

Zeng, F. G., Kong, Y. Y., Michalewski, H. J., & Starr, A. (2005). Perceptual consequences of disrupted auditory nerve activity. *Journal of Neurophysiology, 93*(6), 3050–3063. doi:10.1152/jn.00985.2004

Zeng, F. G., Oba, S., Garde, S., Sininger, Y., & Starr, A. (1999). Temporal and speech processing deficits in auditory neuropathy. *Neuroreport*, *10*, 3429–3435.

Zhuang, X., Sun, W., & Xu-Friedman, M. A. (2017). Changes in properties of auditory nerve synapses following conductive hearing loss. *Journal of Neuroscience*, *37*(2), 323–332. doi:10.1523/JNEUROSCI.0523-16.2016

CHAPTER 5

IN VITRO STUDIES OF NEUROMODULATION AND PLASTICITY IN THE DORSAL COCHLEAR NUCLEUS

LAURENCE O. TRUSSELL

Abstract

The dorsal cochlear nucleus (DCN), a division of the cochlear nuclear complex, has been the subject of intense interest for its role in auditory processing and hearing disorders. The tonotopic layout of DCN principal cells and the refinement of processing of auditory signals by interneurons are together thought to permit encoding of sound source elevation. However, the many cell types and complex connectivity of the DCN suggest more diverse functions than localization. A prominent non-auditory input to the DCN has been proposed to assist in such functions as orienting to sounds of interest, detecting moving sounds, or cancelling self-generated sounds. Synaptic plasticity in the DCN may be essential for dynamic tuning of non-auditory input. Indeed, long-term changes in synaptic or membrane properties could underlie tinnitus, which is associated with hyperactivity in the DCN in some animal models. Finally, the DCN is invested with wide-ranging neuromodulatory mechanisms, suggesting that changes in the behavioral state of animals associated with such neuromodulatory systems might alter sensory processing at the earliest stages of the auditory pathway. This review will focus on studies that have utilized the in vitro brain slice approach to identify basic mechanisms of synaptic plasticity and neuromodulation in the DCN.

Keywords: cochlear nucleus, sound localization, synaptic plasticity, synapses, inhibition, modulation, tinnitus

THE dorsal cochlear nucleus (DCN) is a mammalian-specific structure that has long fascinated auditory physiologists due to its rich cellular diversity, the striking nonlinearity of its neural responses, and its highly complex circuitry. Detailed reviews of the structure of the DCN and its function in hearing are available (Trussell & Oertel, 2018; Young & Davis, 2002; Young & Oertel, 2010), so only a brief overview will be presented here to provide context for a discussion of plasticity and modulation. Mammals feature higher-frequency hearing than birds, reptiles, and turtles, and meet the attendant challenges to encoding high-frequency sounds with unique circuitry. Brain regions like the lateral superior olive and medial nucleus of the trapezoid body may use high-frequency binaural cues like interaural level and amplitude modulation phase differences to localize azimuthal sound sources. By contrast, the DCN is a monaural processing region that appears to take advantage of the pinna's remarkable capacity to create sound source–dependent filtering of signals before they reach the eardrum, particularly for higher-frequency sounds. A prominent feature of this so-called "head related transfer function," is the presence of spectral notches whose position in the sound spectrum is highly dependent on the location of the sound source, particularly in elevation (Rice, May, Spirou, & Young, 1992). Accordingly, principal cells of the DCN are quite sensitive to these notches, and thus may encode elevation cues (Nelken & Young, 1994).

The cellular basis of this sensitivity centers on the connectivity of principal cells and a set of inhibitory interneurons (Trussell & Oertel, 2018; Young & Davis, 2002). The DCN is a layered structure, with a superficial molecular layer that lies against the ependymal layer of the brainstem, followed by a cell body layer and finally a deep layer (Brawer, Morest, & Kane, 1974; Osen, 1969; Wickesberg & Oertel, 1988). Figure 5.1 illustrates the cell types of the DCN and their synaptic innervation. The primary principal cell of the DCN is the fusiform cell (also called pyramidal cell), whose soma is situated in the cell body layer, and whose dendrites extend basally to the deep layer, and apically to the molecular layer. Auditory nerve fibers tuned to different sound frequencies innervate the array of fusiform cells on their basal dendrites, and thereby form a frequency map (Wickesberg & Oertel, 1988). Acoustic responses of fusiform cell from auditory nerve inputs may be reinforced or modified by additional tonotopic inputs from excitatory T-stellate neurons of the ventral cochlear nucleus (Oertel, Wright, Cao, Ferragamo, & Bal, 2011). Fusiform cells in turn project to the central nucleus of the inferior colliculus, contributing to the frequency map at that midbrain station. Auditory-evoked fusiform cell activity is tempered by two types of glycinergic interneuron. Vertical cells (also called tuberculoventral cells) of the deep layer contact the soma and basal dendrites of fusiform cells (Rubio & Juiz, 2004). These cells are narrowly tuned, possibly to frequencies just below the best frequency of the fusiform cell they innervate (Young & Voigt, 1982). Further inhibition of fusiform cells is made by the broadly tuned D-stellate of the ventral cochlear nucleus (Nelken & Young, 1994). Together, the threshold and tuning characteristics of these inhibitory cells are believed to contribute to the complex response profiles observed in fusiform cells (Young & Davis, 2002).

In addition to the auditory input to DCN, there also exists multimodal input that terminates on auditory granule cells, excitatory neurons whose axons form the parallel fibers of the DCN molecular layer and innervate the apical dendrites of fusiform cells (Trussell & Oertel, 2018). Parallel fibers also activate two types of interneurons, the cartwheel cell and the superficial stellate cell, whose dendrites ramify in the molecular layer,

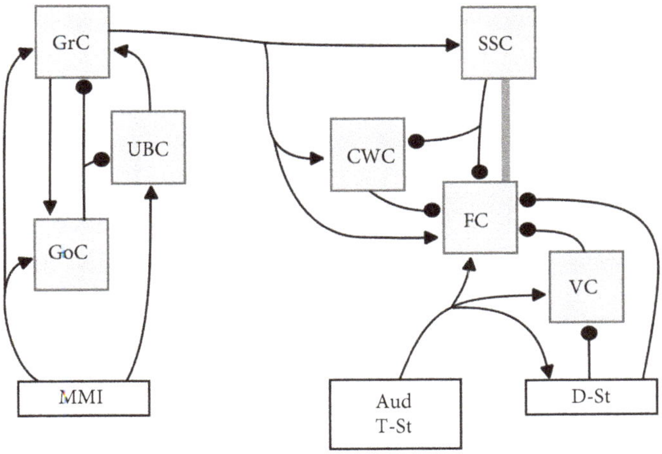

FIGURE 5.1. Schematic of microcircuitry of the DCN. Left side of figure shows the granule cell domain, including the multimodal input and its preprocessing circuitry. Right side shows multisensory integration domain. Labeled gray boxes indicate cell types, open boxes indicate extrinsic inputs. Arrowheads are excitatory synapses, filled circles are inhibitory synapses, and grey line is an electrical (gap junction mediated) synapse. Abbreviations: Aud, auditory nerve; CWC, cartwheel cell; D-St, D-stellate cell; FC, fusiform cell; GoC, Golgi cell; GrC, granule cell; MMI, multimodal inputs; SSC, superficial stellate cell; T-St, T-stellate cell; UBC, unipolar brush cell; VC, vertical cell.

and whose axon terminals inhibit the fusiform cell by co-releasing GABA and glycine. Given these two categories of input, auditory and multimodal, one view of the DCN is that it acts as a "multisensory" integrator, with apical and basal dendrites responsible for receiving multimodal and auditory input, respectively.

However, this simple view must be weighted by an appreciation of the cellular components of the auditory granule cell domain and molecular layer of the DCN, which closely resemble the circuitry of the cerebellar cortex. Auditory granule cells are distributed in up to seven regions in and around the entire cochlear nuclear complex, all feeding their axons into the DCN molecular layer through different routes (Mugnaini, Warr, & Osen, 1980). The inputs to the granule cells originate from across the central nervous system and comprise cortical, pontine, collicular, vestibular, proprioceptive fibers, as well as the fine, type II auditory nerve fibers (Shore & Zhou, 2006). These fibers form bouton or mossy endings onto granule cell dendrites. In addition, multimodal inputs also terminate on excitatory unipolar brush cells (UBCs), which in turn activate granule cells via an intrinsic mossy fiber ending (Mugnaini, Diño, & Jaarsma, 1997). Inhibitory Golgi cells receive both auditory and parallel fiber input and terminate on granule cells and UBCs (Yaeger & Trussell, 2015). Accordingly, the signals transmitted in the molecular layer are both highly diverse and highly preprocessed at this stage.

This brief overview of DCN circuitry will be revisited in later sections, particularly with respect to modulation and plasticity. However, it should be emphasized that significant features of the circuitry remain to be clarified, and this gap in knowledge limits our understanding of the significance of plasticity in the DCN. For example, it is not known whether specific modalities are conveyed to parallel fibers as a "labeled line" or whether granule cells integrate multiple modalities, as in the cerebellar cortex (Arenz, Bracey, & Margrie, 2009; Huang et al., 2013). Moreover, it remains unclear whether molecular layer interneurons serve as feedforward inhibitors of fusiform cell activity, or whether these cell types receive different afferent signals, setting the stage for lateral inhibition (Roberts & Trussell, 2010). Also unclear is whether molecular layer interneurons act purely within isofrequency laminae of the fusiform cell array, or act across best-frequency borders. Circuit-level questions like these are helpful to keep in mind when reflecting on the functional impact of modulation and plasticity.

Short-Term Plasticity

Short-term plasticity refers to use-dependent changes in synaptic strength that last for tens of milliseconds to seconds (Zucker & Regehr, 2002). Examples to be explored here include synaptic facilitation, synaptic depression, post-tetanic potentiation, and, as described in a later section, depolarization-induced suppression of release (Lovinger, 2008; Zucker & Regehr, 2002). With some exceptions, these forms of plasticity are interpreted as changes in the amount of neurotransmitter released. The topic is of considerable interest because of the potential for short-term plasticity to contribute to the response profile of neurons when activated by different patterns of acoustic stimuli in vivo. For example, a transient response to sound might reflect depression, while a "build-up" response could, in principle, reflect facilitation, and these purely synaptic phenomena would then be integrated with the intrinsic properties of the neuron to determine the in vivo response, as characterized, for example, in a post stimulus time histogram (Zhou, Li, Yuan, Tao, & Zhang, 2015). Indeed, an important future area of work will be to find ways to untangle the synaptic and intrinsic contributions to the classical response types of auditory neurons.

Synaptic Depression

Depression has been analyzed primarily using in vitro brain slice preparations, and these studies universally describe profound synaptic depression at auditory nerve terminals in the VCN (Wang & Manis, 2008; Xie & Manis, 2017; Yang & Xu-Friedman, 2009). In DCN, EPSCs recorded in fusiform or vertical cells exhibited depression when fibers in the deep layer were stimulated (Kuo, Lu, & Trussell, 2012; Sedlacek & Brenowitz, 2014; Tang & Trussell, 2017). There is some uncertainty regarding whether this kind of stimulation activates primary afferents or collaterals of T-stellate cells, and likely both contribute to the responses. Regardless of the types of fibers contributing to the EPSC in fusiform and vertical cells, their depression has consequences for synaptic inhibition of fusiform cells. Inhibitory synapses between vertical and fusiform cells exhibit little short-term plasticity (Kuo et al., 2012; Sedlacek & Brenowitz, 2014). However, when vertical cells are driven by depressing excitatory inputs, the resulting EPSPs gradually fall subthreshold, and resulting in an apparent depression of the feed forward inhibition to the fusiform cell (Sedlacek & Brenowitz, 2014). This result illustrates how short-term plasticity may have consequences to downstream responses in a circuit.

Brain slices and the solutions in which they are bathed clearly do not mimic normal tissues and their environment. Does depression occur in vivo or only in the in vitro brain slice preparation? In fact, enormous differences in the extent of depression in vivo versus in vitro were documented at the auditory nerve—VCN bushy cell synapse. Kuenzel et al. (Kuenzel, Borst, & van der Heijden, 2011), using juxtacellular recordings in guinea pig VCN, demonstrated a complete absence of short term EPSP depression in vivo. This study carefully discussed the possible reasons for this discrepancy between preparations—including differences in extracellular Ca^{2+}, presence of neuromodulators, and the effects of spontaneous activity of auditory nerve fibers—concluding that all three factors could be important. For example, depression is reduced when presynaptic release probability is lowered by lowering extracellular Ca^{2+} from the ~2 mM typical of many brain slice studies to the ~1–1.5 mM level found in brain extracellular fluid (Borst, 2010). Potential additional effects of anesthesia during recordings in vivo may also contribute to these differences. However, the studies of Kuenzel et al. (2011) were made with juxtacellular recording of axosomatic end-bulb synapses, and it remains unclear what is the level of synaptic depression exhibited by synapses made by afferents to dendrites of neurons in DCN. Presumably, if there is depression, the added excitatory influence of T-stellate cells recruited during a stimulus might mitigate a decline in afferent synaptic strength.

Prominent depression has also been described for inhibitory postsynaptic currents (IPSCs) generated by cartwheel cell synapses on fusiform cells or on other cartwheel cells (Mancilla & Manis, 2009; Roberts, Bender, & Trussell, 2008). Notably, depression was observed even when bath Ca^{2+} was reduced to in vivo levels. Depression was effectively modeled by assuming that synapses have two pools of vesicles which differ in their release probability (Pr) (Lu & Trussell, 2016). High-Pr vesicles are readily depleted and therefore account for depression of IPSCs, while low-Pr vesicles serve to maintain sustained inhibition to target cells. Interestingly, since cartwheel cells are spontaneously active in vitro and in vivo, it is likely that their synapses operate under a continual state of depression. As described in the section Neuromodulation, changes in spontaneous firing provides a mechanism for controlling synaptic strength and the level of inhibition provided to postsynaptic neurons. A smaller degree of depression was found for synapses made by inhibitory Golgi cells of the DCN and granule cell regions, when simulated with high-frequency trains (Yaeger & Trussell, 2015).

Desensitization

Desensitization is a form of synaptic depression in which postsynaptic transmitter-gated ion channels close despite the continued presence of the transmitter. In the DCN, profound desensitization occurs at synapses between mossy fibers and UBCs (Lu, Balmer, Romero, & Trussell, 2017). Two subtypes of UBC are found in the DCN: ON UBCs are excited by glutamate released from mossy fiber stimulation while OFF UBCs are inhibited. Transmission at the mossy fiber to the ON UBC synapse employs an odd form of depression that results in sustained transmission rather than loss of transmission. Repeated stimuli of presynaptic mossy fibers results in complete depression of the fast EPSC. Upon cessation of synaptic stimulation, a slow EPSC gradually rises over 100–200 ms and then decays over a 1-second period. This slow EPSC is sufficient to drive the majority of the excitatory response of the UBC. Slow EPSCs result from an unusual response of the AMPA receptors of UBCs, in which synaptic glutamate initially desensitizes the receptors (accounting for depression), but then allows reactivation of receptors as glutamate is slowly cleared from the synaptic cleft. This feature of the AMPA receptors requires co-expression of the γ2 transmembrane AMPA receptor regulatory protein (TARP) (Lu et al., 2017).

Synaptic Facilitation

Facilitation of EPSCs is characteristic of parallel fiber synapses made by auditory granule cells firing at rates between 10–100 Hz, and has been described for synapses onto Golgi, cartwheel, fusiform, and superficial stellate cells in vitro (Apostolides & Trussell, 2014; Manis, 1989; Roberts & Trussell, 2010; Yaeger & Trussell, 2015). The mechanism of facilitation was explored by making paired recordings between single granule and Golgi cells (Yaeger & Trussell, 2015). Spikes triggered in the granule cell led to EPSCs in Golgi cell whose mean amplitude facilitated by 250% over 5 stimuli at 90 Hz. Because the number of synapses and their release probability were small, it was possible to detect failures of transmission and ascribe them to failure to release transmitter (rather than to a stimulus failure). The fraction of failures could then be used to determine changes in release probability. This analysis clearly showed that facilitation was associated with a matching increase in release probability at the parallel fiber synapse. While the mechanism of this enhancement is not clear, it may reflect buildup of residual Ca^{2+} in terminals, saturation of presynaptic Ca^{2+} buffers, or binding of Ca^{2+} to a vesicle release protein that can augment exocytosis. A recent study of facilitation at cerebellar parallel fiber synapses showed that like many brain synapses, facilitation partially depends on the presynaptic protein synaptotagmin 7, but also requires as yet unknown factors (Turecek & Regehr, 2018). The physiological function of facilitation remains unexplored in the DCN at this time. However, given the multimodal flavor of the mossy fiber/parallel fiber pathway in DCN, facilitation may represent a way to provide a short-term strengthening or "reward" to parallel fibers that convey a particular modality. Alternatively, facilitation may be a mechanism for tuning parallel fiber synapses to particular patterns of activity rather than merely duration of activity: since the facilitated state activates over a few spikes, and lasts typically for less than 100 ms, repeated, brief bursts of spikes might represent an ideal mode of parallel fiber transmission. Such bursts are observed in granule cells of the cerebellar cortex in response to sensory stimuli in vivo (Chadderton, Margrie, & Häusser, 2004).

Long-Term Plasticity

Long-term plasticity in the DCN was proposed based on the close parallels between DCN circuitry and that of other cerebellum like structures. For example, plasticity is thought to underlie cerebellum-dependent motor learning and electrosensory lobe (ELL)-dependent cancellation of signals associated with self-generated electrical fields (Bell, Han, & Sawtell, 2008).

The starting point for exploring the possibility of such plasticity in the DCN is found in a study by Fujino & Oertel (2003). Using mouse brain slices, the authors recorded either from fusiform cells or cartwheel cells with patch pipettes and stimulated either auditory afferents or parallel fibers while monitoring EPSC amplitudes. Two induction protocols based on studies in hippocampus were explored: pairing of high-frequency synaptic stimuli (100 Hz) with a lengthy postsynaptic depolarization to −30 mV versus low-frequency stimuli (1 Hz) paired with briefer postsynaptic depolarization also to −30 mV. Several important conclusions came from this analysis. Both cell types responded to the high-frequency stimulation of parallel fibers with a long-term (> 1 hr) potentiation (LTP) of EPSC amplitude, and both responded to the low-frequency stimuli of parallel fibers with a long-term depression (LTD) of EPSC amplitude. Moreover, in both cells, plasticity was reversible, such that by changing stimulus protocols, LTP and LTD could be quickly expunged. Most interestingly, when the same protocol was applied to fusiform cells with stimulation of auditory afferents instead of parallel fibers, no plasticity was observed. Thus, both inhibitory and excitatory neurons could exhibit bidirectional plasticity, and in the case of the fusiform cell, the plasticity was input specific. Since cartwheel cells do not receive direct auditory afferents, the question of input specificity for those cells could not be addressed. In any case, the results clearly demonstrated that the multimodal signaling to the DCN was subject to prominent use-dependent plasticity, whereas auditory inputs were not.

The fact that auditory input was not plastic might suggest a presynaptic mechanism of LTP/LTD induction or expression, that is, a change in the parallel fiber terminals. However, further experiments by Fujino and Oertel (2003) indicated that the plasticity they documented could be inhibited by alterations in postsynaptic signaling pathways. In cartwheel and fusiform cells, LTP and LTD were reduced by inhibition of NMDA and metabotropic glutamate receptors (mGluRs). Both of these receptors appeared to contribute to EPSPs (see section on neuromodulation below). Moreover, depleting internal Ca^{2+} stores by including thapsigargin and caffeine in the patch pipette completely prevented plasticity. These results suggest that the activation of synaptic receptors and voltage dependent Ca^{2+} channels during the induction protocol led to activation of LTP and LTD pathways in a Ca^{2+}-dependent manner. Presumably, the two protocols led to different levels of intracellular Ca^{2+} and thus different synaptic outcomes (Lisman, 1989). However, these manipulations do not clarify what specific pathways are required. For example, Ca^{2+} spikes occurring during the release of Ca^{2+} induced by caffeine prior to induction might itself have interfered with plasticity mechanisms. Moreover, it is not clear from this work whether subtle or even naturally occurring patterns of signals might activate the cells in a manner that could lead to plasticity.

Other potential mechanisms of DCN plasticity were suggested by Tagoe, Deeping, & Hamann (2017). Field potential recordings from rat DCN slices before and after tetanic stimulation of parallel fibers revealed that LTP was associated with an apparent decrease in release probability, as estimate by paired-pulse ratios. This aspect of LTP was reverse upon application of an NMDA receptor antagonist. Moreover, LTP could not be induced if the slices were bathed in a high-Ca^{2+} solution, suggesting that release probability at parallel fiber synapses must be low to permit expression of LTP. Patch clamp recordings on identified cell types suggested that this effect was seen in fusiform cells; it remains possible that cartwheel cells also exhibit this dependence on release probability.

Spike Timing Dependent Plasticity

Previous work on rodent cerebellum and electrosensory lobe (ELL) of mormyrid electric fish had suggested the presence of spike timing dependent plasticity (STDP; Han, Grant, & Bell, 2000). This form of plasticity differs from that described earlier in that it is dependent not merely on postsynaptic depolarization but on postsynaptic spikes, and specifically the precise timing of those spikes in relation to the synaptic stimulus. In different preparations, the timing dependence could lead to LTP or LTD, and have timing requirements in the range of milliseconds to hundreds of milliseconds. In ELL, medium ganglion cells exhibit LTD of parallel fiber evoked EPSPs following a pairing protocol in which parallel fiber stimuli arise 5–30 ms before evoking a broad, Ca^{2+}-dependent spike in the ganglion cell. Other timing relationships, either positive or negative, resulted only in a weak non-associative LTP. Cartwheel cells in the DCN circuit are similar to medium ganglion cells of the ELL, as both are inhibitory, feature Ca^{2+}-dependent spikes, and have as their synaptic target a principal cell that receives afferent input as well as parallel fiber input. Given that the Fujino and Oertel study had found similar forms of plasticity in both excitatory and inhibitory neurons, it was important to determine whether differences in the synaptic responses in the two cell types might be revealed using the more subtle STDP analyses. Tzounopulos and colleagues (Tzounopoulos, Kim, Oertel, & Trussell, 2004) explored whether cartwheel cells could exhibit STDP by pairing parallel fiber stimuli with postsynaptic complex spikes. LTD was only observed when the spike was triggered 5 ms after the EPSP for modest (10 Hz) stimulus rates. Higher-frequency (40 Hz) pairings resulted in LTP with little timing dependence. Fusiform cells also exhibited STDP but with a very different timing profile: the same protocol that led to LTD in the cartwheel cell caused LTP in the fusiform cell, and reversing the timing relationship caused fusiform cell LTD. One interpretation then is that when spikes follow parallel fiber EPSPs, plasticity enhances the excitation of the fusiform cells and reduces its likelihood of inhibition.

How does this kind of LTP/LTD associated with STDP compare to that described by Fujino and Oertel (2003) in terms of site of expression and signaling mechanisms? These questions are difficult to address without side-by-side experimental analysis, but it is probable that they differ considerably. Tzounopoulos, Rubio, Keen, & Trussell (2007) explored the sites of expression and signaling pathways for fusiform and cartwheel cell STDP. LTP in fusiform cells was expressed as an enhancement of postsynaptic AMPA receptors, and required activation of NMDA receptors, intracellular Ca^{2+}, and activity of calcium-calmodulin dependent protein kinase II (CAMKII). STDP in cartwheel cells was much more complex in its signaling requirements. LTD, induced by the 5-ms delayed EPSP-complex spike sequence, was expressed presynaptically as reduced glutamate release, and required postsynaptic NMDA receptor activation and an intracellular Ca^{2+} rise. Unlike plasticity with the strong pairing protocols used in Fujino and Oertel's work, mGluRs were not required for STDP.

These results in cartwheel cells indicated the presence of a retrograde messenger. Indeed, LTD in cartwheel cells triggered with the STPD protocol was converted to LTP upon blocking endocannabinoid receptors (CB1R). This "revealed" LTP was expressed postsynaptically and had a mechanism similar to that of fusiform cell LTP. Apparently, the shape of the timing plot for STPD in cartwheel cells represented the summation of pre- and postsynaptic plasticity mechanisms with slightly different timing requirements. Immuno-electron microscopic analysis of CB1R distribution showed that CB1R are found on parallel fiber terminals apposing cartwheel cell spines but less so on terminals apposed to fusiform cell spines. Thus, synapse specific expression of CB1R is part of a mechanism to endow the inhibitory and excitatory neurons with distinct forms of STDP.

NEUROMODULATION

The DCN is invested with catecholaminergic, serotonergic and cholinergic fibers (Klepper & Herbert, 1991; Mellott, Motts, & Schofield, 2011; Thompson & Thompson, 2001). In vitro studies have shown that the transmitters associated with these fibers modify the activity of the DCN in remarkably diverse ways that go beyond simple alterations of excitability; indeed, these modulators differentially affect multiple aspects of neuronal circuitry, and thus could control the output of the DCN. This discussion will focus on effects of neuromodulators on in vitro slice preparations, primarily because their cellular mechanisms are most readily worked out in vitro. Our definition of neuromodulator is intentionally broad: a compound that is released at synapses, besides the conventional fast-acting transmitters, that alters the function of circuits. By this definition, substances such as Zn^{2+} or endocannabinoids, released by neurons whose cell bodies are within the DCN, also serve as neuromodulators. As will be seen, modulation impacts all levels of DCN function, and thus cannot be considered separately from either baseline function of the DCN circuit, or from the DCN while undergoing long-term plasticity. However, a significant caveat for in vitro studies of modulation, particularly for studies of modulators released by extrinsic inputs to DCN, is that the effects are generally studied by bath application of compounds to the brain slice bathing solution. Synaptic release of endogenous neuromodulators, the "real thing," could potentially result in different effects than those studied in vitro, depending on the location of sites of release, the modulators' concentration, and their receptors' distribution.

Noradrenaline

In recordings of IPSCs in fusiform cells, bath application noradrenaline was observed to have paradoxical effects (Kuo & Trussell, 2011). On the one hand, spontaneous IPSCs originating from spontaneously firing cartwheel cells were nearly eliminated in the presence of noradrenaline, suggesting presynaptic inhibition by the modulator. However, when cartwheel cells were electrical stimulated, the resulting evoked IPSCs were significantly enhanced by noradrenaline. These seemingly opposing effects were mediated by alpha-2 noradrenergic receptors. This paradox was resolved by the discovery that, rather than suppressing the synapses of cartwheel cells, noradrenaline suppresses their spontaneous action potentials. As noted previously, cartwheel cells are prone to synaptic depression. Thus, by tuning down spontaneous firing, cartwheel terminals recovered from depression and thus release more transmitter. Moreover, because spontaneous IPSCs in the fusiform cells were reduced in frequency, the "signal to noise" of inhibition was increased several fold. An additional outcome of this modulation was also described. Multiple cartwheel cells converge onto each fusiform cell, and effective postsynaptic inhibition requires a critical number of synchronously active inhibitory neurons. By using a combination of electrophysiological and optogenetic approaches, Lu & Trussell (2016) showed that under control conditions, that critical number was four cartwheel cells, whereas in the presence of noradrenaline a single cartwheel provided enough inhibition to block spiking in the fusiform cell. Thus, noradrenaline alters the effective size of the inhibitory microcircuit. If these different cartwheel cells were activated by different subsets of parallel fibers, then noradrenaline's actions could be seen as enhancing the salience of individual modalities, as reflected in their ability to control the fusiform cell's output.

Dopamine

The action of dopamine on cartwheel cells is completely different from that of noradrenaline (Bender, Ford, & Trussell, 2010; Bender, Uebele, Renger, & Trussell, 2012). Spontaneous action potentials in cartwheel cells appear as either simple Na^+-based spikes or as complex spikes, a mixture of Na^+ spikelets riding on a slower T-type Ca^{2+} channel dependent depolarization (Golding & Oertel, 1997; Kim & Trussell, 2007; Manis, Spirou, Wright, Paydar, & Ryugo, 1994). Application of dopamine activated the D3 receptor and transformed spontaneous spiking from mixtures of simple and complex spikes to all simple spikes (Bender et al., 2012). Moreover, dopamine resulted in elevation of threshold for evoking a complex spike. By reducing complex spike activation, inhibitory synaptic events at cartwheel cell terminals appeared more in isolation rather than as a cluster, reducing the potency of inhibitory signals in the fusiform cell (Bender et al., 2010). Again, a paradox was presented, as dopamine's effects were similar to that produced by pharmacologically blocking T-type Ca^{2+} channels, even though the somatically recorded T-type current was not inhibited by dopamine. In this case, it was discovered that dopamine selectively inhibited the T-type channels of the axon initial segment, and it was specifically this restricted population of channels that was responsible for originating the complex spike. Importantly, similar effects were obtained by driving release of dopamine from dopaminergic fibers. Thus, two catecholamines, dopamine and noradrenaline, both target cartwheel cell and influence their spike activity, but in totally different ways and with very different outcomes for synaptic inhibition.

Serotonin

The action of serotonin has have been explored extensively in the auditory system (see chapter by Hurley, this volume), yet until recently the effects of this compound had not been investigated in the DCN. Tang & Trussell (2015) showed that serotonin enhanced spontaneous firing in fusiform cells and increased fusiform cell sensitivity to electrical stimulation. This effect was mediated by 5HT2A and 5HT7 receptors, which enhanced the so-called I_H current carried by HCN (hyperpolarization and cyclic-nucleotide gated) channels. The interaction between receptor and channel required cAMP and Src kinase signaling pathways. In an in vivo context, this mechanism would be expected to enhance background signaling from the DCN and reduce the threshold for acoustic responses. However, a second study (Tang & Trussell, 2017) suggested a much more complex effect of serotonin in DCN. In this work, the authors systematically examined serotonin effects on granule, vertical, cartwheel and fusiform cells, and their respective synaptic contacts. They discovered very selective targets of serotonin. Granule and cartwheel cells and their synapses were unaffected. Vertical cells, which mediate feedforward inhibition of fusiform cells and are excited by auditory afferent fibers, had a response to serotonin identical to that of fusiform cells. Finally, auditory afferent input to fusiform cells was inhibited. The outcome of these multiple effects was striking: responses in fusiform cells to stimulation of auditory fibers were inhibited by serotonin, a consequence of suppression of auditory synapses on fusiform cells, and of recruitment of more inhibitory vertical cells. By contrast, parallel fiber EPSPs were more effective in bringing the fusiform cells to spike threshold due to the effects on HCN just described. Thus, serotonin appears to shift the balance of input between the two sensory streams, favoring the multimodal signals carried through the granule cell system.

Endocannabinoids

Endocannabinoids are neuromodulators that are produced intrinsically within the DCN rather than from extrinsic sources, unlike as serotonin or catecholamines. Besides their role in STDP described previously, endocannabinoids also play a role in a short-term plasticity called depolarization induced suppression of excitation (DSE). Here, a period of strong postsynaptic depolarization results in a depression of EPSP amplitude lasting about 10 seconds. In DCN, prominent DSE is seen for parallel fiber to cartwheel cell synapses, but less so for parallel fiber-fusiform synapses, and it is absent at auditory nerve-fusiform synapses (Zhao, Rubio, & Tzounopoulos, 2009). DSE is blocked by the CB1 receptor antagonist AM-251 and is mediated by 2-arachidonoylglycerol (2-AG), an endocannabinoid synthesized by diacylglycerol lipase alpha and beta (DGLα and DGLβ). Accordingly, these enzymes are localized specifically to cartwheel cell spines.

The depolarizing stimuli used in revealing DSE are severe, and therefore one may ask whether normal patterns of postsynaptic spiking could drive sufficient endocannabinoid release to mediate DSE. This was examined by Sedlacek, Tipton, & Brenowitz (2011), who monitored postsynaptic spikes, EPSPs in cartwheel cells, and found that ongoing spike activity could generate a "tonic" endocannabinoid dependent DSE proportional to spike rate. Interestingly, these investigators also monitored intracellular Ca^{2+}, and discovered that the Ca^{2+} requirements for this more physiological DSE were lower than that of DSE induced by strong stimuli. Together these results suggest that endocannabinoid signaling serves not only to guide long term plasticity but also to set synaptic strength of parallel fibers on an ongoing basis.

Acetylcholine

Cholinergic fibers in the DCN likely originate as either collaterals of cochlear efferent fibers originating in the superior olive, or projections from the pedunculopontine nuclei (Mellott et al., 2011). Two notable studies have examined cholinergic modulation and its interaction with plasticity mechanisms in the DCN. In recordings of cartwheel cells, He and colleagues simultaneously monitored both glutamatergic EPSPs and synaptic spine Ca^{2+} changes following from parallel fiber activation (He, Wang, Petralia,

& Brenowitz, 2014). The muscarinic acetylcholine receptor agonist oxotremorine-m increased both EPSPs and spine Ca^{2+}. The mechanism of this effect was quite complex. Spine Ca^{2+} increases were due to the activation of NMDA receptors during the EPSP depolarization, which caused relief of Mg^{2+} block of the receptors. However, the EPSP also activated L-type Ca^{2+} channels, and Ca^{2+} flux through these channels activated BK-type K^+ channels, which then opposed the EPSP, repolarizing the membrane. Blockade of BK channels or L-type Ca^{2+} channels enhanced EPSPs and spine Ca^{2+}. He et al. (2014) found that muscarinic receptors inhibited the L-type channels through a PKA dependent mechanism, thereby reducing BK activation and allowing a greater depolarization and NMDA receptor activation.

Very different functions of muscarinic receptors in DCN were described in Zhao & Tzounopoulos (2011). The inhibitory analog of DSE, depolarization induced suppression of inhibition (DSI), is normally absent for inhibitory inputs to fusiform cells. However, application of oxotremorine-M revealed a latent endocannabinoid-dependent DSI at these inputs. Moreover, the agonist also enhanced DSE onto fusiform cells. This regulation of short-term plasticity by cholinergic receptors illustrates how extrinsic and intrinsic neuromodulator systems may interact to shape circuit activity.

As already described, fusiform cells exhibit Hebbian synaptic plasticity, with STDP protocols producing anti-Hebbian plasticity (i.e., plasticity induced by a spike-EPSP timing relation opposite to that of Hebbian plasticity) in cartwheel cells and not fusiform cells. Zhao & Tzounopoulos (2011) found that when the agonist oxotremorine-m was applied during the STDP stimulus protocol, the fusiform cell now exhibited anti-Hebbian plasticity. This effect was NMDA receptor and postsynaptic Ca^{2+} dependent. The authors inferred that the muscarinic receptor agonist led to phospholipase C activation and consequent release of endocannabinoids. Endocannabinoids would then act on the presynaptic parallel fiber terminals to inhibit glutamate release in a manner analogous to the mechanism described for cartwheel cells, despite the reduced expression of CB1 receptors on terminals ending on fusiform cells as compared to cartwheel cells (Tzounopoulos et al., 2007). This confound notwithstanding, the study of Zhou et al. (2015) is significant as it raises the possibility that "learning rules" that guide plasticity in the auditory system are themselves plastic, and can be modified by neuromodulators such as acetylcholine that are associated with changes in the behavioral state of animals.

Zinc

Zn^{2+} ions are densely accumulated at parallel fiber terminals of the cochlear nucleus (Frederickson, Howell, Haigh, & Danscher, 1988; Rubio & Juiz, 1998). Indeed, their concentration at those synapses is one of the clearest factors that differentiates auditory from cerebellar granule cells, as the latter do not accumulate Zn^{2+}. Tzounopoulos and colleagues have published a series of studies that explored the remarkably complex effects of Zn^{2+} in the DCN, taking advantage of new reagents for selective buffering or detection of Zn^{2+}, as well as mouse lines with genetic deletion of the requisite Zn^{2+} receptors and transporters.

A common approach in the study of synaptic Zn^{2+} is to compare the physiological responses of synapses before and after chelation of Zn^{2+}. Brain slice recordings in which fusiform cells are patch clamped and parallel fibers are stimulated revealed that chelation of Zn^{2+} by the novel, high-affinity chelator ZX1 enhanced the amplitude of both AMPA and NMDA receptor mediated synaptic responses (Anderson et al., 2015; Kalappa, Anderson, Goldberg, Lippard, & Tzounopoulos, 2015). These and other experiments indicated that endogenous Zn^{2+}, released during synaptic transmission, directly inhibits glutamate receptor function. These effects were absent in mice lacking the presynaptic zinc transporter ZnT3, supporting the notion that ZX1 was indeed inhibiting a response to endogenous Zn^{2+}. However, additional inhibition of NMDA receptor occurred from ambient Zn^{2+}, whose source was not determined.

Consistent with the idea that endogenous Zn^{2+} is contained in vesicles, fluorescent reporters of Zn^{2+} showed bright labeling in the DCN molecular layer, and this fluorescent signal was absent in the ZnT3 KO mice (Kalappa et al., 2015). Stimulation of parallel fibers led to an increase in extracellular zinc-dependent fluorescence when detected with a cell-impermeable probe. Surprisingly, both of these Zn^{2+} signals were reduced in mice that had been noise exposed, indicating that damage to the auditory system can impact multimodal integration in the auditory granule cell system.

Other, more complex effects of Zn^{2+} were observed in the DCN. Perez-Rosello et al. (2013) showed that bath application of exogenous Zn^{2+} decreased EPSC amplitude, an effect that required expression of a postsynaptic metabotropic Zn^{2+} receptor, mZnR. This effect had a surprising mechanism: the Zn^{2+} binding to mZnR promoted release of the endocannabinoid 2-arachidonoylglycerol and presynaptic inhibition of glutamate release. This effect is distinct from the direct effect of Zn^{2+} on postsynaptic receptors described earlier. Pre- and postsynaptic effects of Zn^{2+} were further revealed by Kalappa & Tzounopoulos (2017). These authors found that high-frequency stimulation of parallel fibers in elevated bath Ca^{2+} (2.4 mM) led to facilitation, and this facilitation was reduced after chelation of Zn^{2+} by ZX1. Facilitation in physiological Ca^{2+} was less sensitive to ZX1. The authors proposed that Zn^{2+} release and subsequent suppression of glutamate release through retrograde transmission of endocannabinoids normally allows parallel fiber terminals to facilitate to a greater extent without vesicle depletion. However, other interpretations could be considered: endocannabinoids might directly modify the facilitation mechanism, or potentiate a distinct subpopulation of synaptic vesicles that enables transmission during high-frequency stimuli (Lu & Trussell, 2016).

Summary

The microcircuits of the DCN are distinguished by their sensitivity to use-dependent plasticity and to neuromodulators. These effects are remarkably interactive: modulators can affect both short and long-term plasticity, while plasticity can impact the release of intrinsic neuromodulators, and perhaps also extrinsic neuromodulators. Defining this playing field for fine control of DCN function invites deeper investigation. For example, it is highly unlikely that the host of neuromodulators described here act independently. Not only could multiple compounds be released at once, but these may involve overlapping sets of intracellular transduction pathways. Any proposed effect of a neuromodulator must eventually be confirmed by demonstrating effects of endogenously released neuromodulators, perhaps using optogenetic methods. Synaptic plasticity mechanisms must be demonstrated using activity patterns in cell populations like those in vivo, if they are to be relevant to auditory function. Indeed, such studies have been performed, although using paradigms conceptually quite different from the in vitro models. Lastly, it will be important to further examine synaptic plasticity and modulation following noise induced hearing loss or in tinnitus animal models, to assess how pathological changes in auditory function are due to changes at the level of the synapse.

Acknowledgments

I would like to thank Tavita Garrett for helpful comments on the manuscript. My work was supported by NIH grants DC004450 and NS028901.

References

Anderson, C. T., Radford, R. J., Zastrow, M. L., Zhang, D. Y., Apfel, U.-P., Lippard, S. J., & Tzounopoulos, T. (2015). Modulation of extrasynaptic NMDA receptors by synaptic and tonic zinc. *Proceedings of the National Academy of Sciences of the United States of America*, *112*(20), E2705–2714. https://doi.org/10.1073/pnas.1503348112

Apostolides, P. F., & Trussell, L. O. (2014). Chemical synaptic transmission onto superficial stellate cells of the mouse dorsal cochlear nucleus. *Journal of Neurophysiology*, *111*(9), 1812–1822. https://doi.org/10.1152/jn.00821.2013

Arenz, A., Bracey, E. F., & Margrie, T. W. (2009). Sensory representations in cerebellar granule cells. *Current Opinion in Neurobiology*, *19*(4), 445–451. https://doi.org/10.1016/j.conb.2009.07.003

Bell, C. C., Han, V., & Sawtell, N. B. (2008). Cerebellum-like structures and their implications for cerebellar function. *Annual Review of Neuroscience*, *31*, 1–24. https://doi.org/10.1146/annurev.neuro.30.051606.094225

Bender, K. J., Ford, C. P., & Trussell, L. O. (2010). Dopaminergic modulation of axon initial segment calcium channels regulates action potential initiation. *Neuron*, *68*(3), 500–511. https://doi.org/10.1016/j.neuron.2010.09.026

Bender, K. J., Uebele, V. N., Renger, J. J., & Trussell, L. O. (2012). Control of firing patterns through modulation of axon initial segment T-type calcium channels. *The Journal of Physiology*, *590*(1), 109–118. https://doi.org/10.1113/jphysiol.2011.218768

Borst, J. G. G. (2010). The low synaptic release probability in vivo. *Trends in Neurosciences*, *33*(6), 259–266. https://doi.org/10.1016/j.tins.2010.03.003

Brawer, J. R., Morest, D. K., & Kane, E. C. (1974). The neuronal architecture of the cochlear nucleus of the cat. *The Journal of Comparative Neurology*, *155*(3), 251–300. https://doi.org/10.1002/cne.901550302

Chadderton, P., Margrie, T. W., & Häusser, M. (2004). Integration of quanta in cerebellar granule cells during sensory processing. *Nature*, *428*(6985), 856–860. https://doi.org/10.1038/nature02442

Frederickson, C. J., Howell, G. A., Haigh, M. D., & Danscher, G. (1988). Zinc-containing fiber systems in the cochlear nuclei of the rat and mouse. *Hearing Research*, *36*(2–3), 203–211.

Fujino, K., & Oertel, D. (2003). Bidirectional synaptic plasticity in the cerebellum-like mammalian dorsal cochlear nucleus. *Proceedings of the National Academy of Sciences of the United States of America*, *100*(1), 265–270. https://doi.org/10.1073/pnas.0135345100

Golding, N. L., & Oertel, D. (1997). Physiological identification of the targets of cartwheel cells in the dorsal cochlear nucleus. *Journal of Neurophysiology*, *78*(1), 248–260.

Han, V. Z., Grant, K., & Bell, C. C. (2000). Reversible associative depression and nonassociative potentiation at a parallel fiber synapse. *Neuron*, *27*(3), 611–622.

He, S., Wang, Y.-X., Petralia, R. S., & Brenowitz, S. D. (2014). Cholinergic modulation of large-conductance calcium-activated potassium channels regulates synaptic strength and spine calcium in cartwheel cells of the dorsal cochlear nucleus. *Journal of Neuroscience*, *34*(15), 5261–5272. https://doi.org/10.1523/JNEUROSCI.3728-13.2014

Huang, C.-C., Sugino, K., Shima, Y., Guo, C., Bai, S., Mensh, B. D., . . . Hantman, A. W. (2013). Convergence of pontine and proprioceptive streams onto multimodal cerebellar granule cells. *ELife*, *2*, e00400. https://doi.org/10.7554/eLife.00400

Kalappa, B. I., Anderson, C. T., Goldberg, J. M., Lippard, S. J., & Tzounopoulos, T. (2015). AMPA receptor inhibition by synaptically released zinc. *Proceedings of the National Academy of Sciences of the United States of America*, *112*(51), 15749–15754. https://doi.org/10.1073/pnas.1512296112

Kalappa, B. I., & Tzounopoulos, T. (2017). Context-dependent modulation of excitatory synaptic strength by synaptically released zinc. *ENeuro*, *4*(1). https://doi.org/10.1523/ENEURO.0011-17.2017

Kim, Y., & Trussell, L. O. (2007). Ion channels generating complex spikes in cartwheel cells of the dorsal cochlear nucleus. *Journal of Neurophysiology*, *97*(2), 1705–1725. https://doi.org/10.1152/jn.00536.2006

Klepper, A., & Herbert, H. (1991). Distribution and origin of noradrenergic and serotonergic fibers in the cochlear nucleus and inferior colliculus of the rat. *Brain Research*, *557*(1–2), 190–201.

Kuenzel, T., Borst, J. G. G., & van der Heijden, M. (2011). Factors controlling the input-output relationship of spherical bushy cells in the gerbil cochlear nucleus. *Journal of Neuroscience*, *31*(11), 4260–4273. https://doi.org/10.1523/JNEUROSCI.5433-10.2011

Kuo, S. P., Lu, H.-W., & Trussell, L. O. (2012). Intrinsic and synaptic properties of vertical cells of the mouse dorsal cochlear nucleus. *Journal of Neurophysiology*, *108*(4), 1186–1198. https://doi.org/10.1152/jn.00778.2011

Kuo, S. P., & Trussell, L. O. (2011). Spontaneous spiking and synaptic depression underlie noradrenergic control of feed-forward inhibition. *Neuron*, *71*(2), 306–318. https://doi.org/10.1016/j.neuron.2011.05.039

Lisman, J. (1989). A mechanism for the Hebb and the anti-Hebb processes underlying learning and memory. *Proceedings of the National Academy of Sciences of the United States of America*, *86*(23), 9574–9578.

Lovinger, D. M. (2008). Presynaptic modulation by endocannabinoids. *Handbook of Experimental Pharmacology*, *184*, 435–477. https://doi.org/10.1007/978-3-540-74805-2_14

Lu, H.-W., Balmer, T. S., Romero, G. E., & Trussell, L. O. (2017). Slow AMPAR synaptic transmission is determined by stargazin and glutamate transporters. *Neuron*, *96*(1), 73–80.e4. https://doi.org/10.1016/j.neuron.2017.08.043

Lu, H.-W., & Trussell, L. O. (2016). Spontaneous activity defines effective convergence ratios in an inhibitory circuit. *Journal of Neuroscience*, *36*(11), 3268–3280. https://doi.org/10.1523/JNEUROSCI.3499-15.2016

Mancilla, J. G., & Manis, P. B. (2009). Two distinct types of inhibition mediated by cartwheel cells in the dorsal cochlear nucleus. *Journal of Neurophysiology*, *102*(2), 1287–1295.

Manis, P. B. (1989). Responses to parallel fiber stimulation in the guinea pig dorsal cochlear nucleus in vitro. *Journal of Neurophysiology*, *61*(1), 149–161.

Manis, P. B., Spirou, G. A., Wright, D. D., Paydar, S., & Ryugo, D. K. (1994). Physiology and morphology of complex spiking neurons in the guinea pig dorsal cochlear nucleus. *The Journal of Comparative Neurology*, *348*(2), 261–276. https://doi.org/10.1002/cne.903480208

Mellott, J. G., Motts, S. D., & Schofield, B. R. (2011). Multiple origins of cholinergic innervation of the cochlear nucleus. *Neuroscience*, *180*, 138–147. https://doi.org/10.1016/j.neuroscience.2011.02.010

Mugnaini, E., Diño, M. R., & Jaarsma, D. (1997). The unipolar brush cells of the mammalian cerebellum and cochlear nucleus: Cytology and microcircuitry. *Progress in Brain Research*, *114*, 131–150.

Mugnaini, E., Warr, W. B., & Osen, K. K. (1980). Distribution and light microscopic features of granule cells in the cochlear nuclei of cat, rat, and mouse. *Journal of Comparative Neurology*, *191*(4), 581–606.

Nelken, I., & Young, E. D. (1994). Two separate inhibitory mechanisms shape the responses of dorsal cochlear nucleus type IV units to narrowband and wideband stimuli. *Journal of Neurophysiology*, *71*(6), 2446–2462.

Oertel, D., Wright, S., Cao, X.-J., Ferragamo, M., & Bal, R. (2011). The multiple functions of T stellate/multipolar/chopper cells in the ventral cochlear nucleus. *Hearing Research*, *276*(1–2), 61–69. https://doi.org/10.1016/j.heares.2010.10.018

Osen, K. K. (1969). Cytoarchitecture of the cochlear nuclei in the cat. *The Journal of Comparative Neurology*, *136*(4), 453–484. https://doi.org/10.1002/cne.901360407

Perez-Rosello, T., Anderson, C. T., Schopfer, F. J., Zhao, Y., Gilad, D., Salvatore, S. R., . . . Tzounopoulos, T. (2013). Synaptic Zn2+ inhibits neurotransmitter release by promoting endocannabinoid synthesis. *Journal of Neuroscience*, *33*(22), 9259–9272. https://doi.org/10.1523/JNEUROSCI.0237-13.2013

Rice, J. J., May, B. J., Spirou, G. A., & Young, E. D. (1992). Pinna-based spectral cues for sound localization in cat. *Hearing Research*, *58*(2), 132–152.

Roberts, M. T., Bender, K. J., & Trussell, L. O. (2008). Fidelity of complex spike-mediated synaptic transmission between inhibitory interneurons. *The Journal of Neuroscience: The Official Journal of the Society for Neuroscience*, *28*(38), 9440–9450. https://doi.org/10.1523/JNEUROSCI.2226-08.2008

Roberts, M. T., & Trussell, L. O. (2010). Molecular layer inhibitory interneurons provide feedforward and lateral inhibition in the dorsal cochlear nucleus. *Journal of Neurophysiology*, *104*(5), 2462–2473. https://doi.org/10.1152/jn.00312.2010

Rubio, M. E., & Juiz, J. M. (1998). Chemical anatomy of excitatory endings in the dorsal cochlear nucleus of the rat: Differential synaptic distribution of aspartate aminotransferase, glutamate, and vesicular zinc. *Journal of Comparative Neurology*, *399*(3), 341–358.

Rubio, M. E., & Juiz, J. M. (2004). Differential distribution of synaptic endings containing glutamate, glycine, and GABA in the rat dorsal cochlear nucleus. *Journal of Comparative Neurology*, *477*(3), 253–272. https://doi.org/10.1002/cne.20248

Sedlacek, M., & Brenowitz, S. D. (2014). Cell-type specific short-term plasticity at auditory nerve synapses controls feed-forward inhibition in the dorsal cochlear nucleus. *Frontiers in Neural Circuits*, *8*, 78. https://doi.org/10.3389/fncir.2014.00078

Sedlacek, M., Tipton, P. W., & Brenowitz, S. D. (2011). Sustained firing of cartwheel cells in the dorsal cochlear nucleus evokes endocannabinoid release and retrograde suppression of parallel fiber synapses. *Journal of Neuroscience*, *31*(44), 15807–15817. https://doi.org/10.1523/JNEUROSCI.4088-11.2011

Shore, S. E., & Zhou, J. (2006). Somatosensory influence on the cochlear nucleus and beyond. *Hearing Research*, *216–217*, 90–99. https://doi.org/10.1016/j.heares.2006.01.006

Tagoe, T., Deeping, D., & Hamann, M. (2017). Saturation of long-term potentiation in the dorsal cochlear nucleus and its pharmacological reversal in an experimental model of tinnitus. *Experimental Neurology*, *292*, 1–10. https://doi.org/10.1016/j.expneurol.2017.02.011

Tang, Z.-Q., & Trussell, L. O. (2015). Serotonergic regulation of excitability of principal cells of the dorsal cochlear nucleus. *Journal of Neuroscience*, *35*(11), 4540–4551. https://doi.org/10.1523/JNEUROSCI.4825-14.2015

Tang, Z.-Q., & Trussell, L. O. (2017). Serotonergic modulation of sensory representation in a central multisensory circuit is pathway specific. *Cell Reports*, *20*(8), 1844–1854. https://doi.org/10.1016/j.celrep.2017.07.079

Thompson, A. M., & Thompson, G. C. (2001). Serotonin projection patterns to the cochlear nucleus. *Brain Research*, *907*(1–2), 195–207.

Trussell, L. O., & Oertel, D. (2018). Microcircuits of the dorsal cochlear nucleus. In D. L. Oliver, N. B. Cant, R. R. Fay, & A. N. Popper (Eds.), *The Mammalian Auditory Pathways: Synaptic Organization and Microcircuits* (Vol. 65, pp. 73–99). New York, NY: Springer-Verlag.

Turecek, J., & Regehr, W. G. (2018). Synaptotagmin 7 Mediates Both Facilitation and Asynchronous Release at Granule Cell Synapses. *Journal of Neuroscience*, *38*(13), 3240–3251. https://doi.org/10.1523/JNEUROSCI.3207-17.2018

Tzounopoulos, T., Kim, Y., Oertel, D., & Trussell, L. O. (2004). Cell-specific, spike timing-dependent plasticities in the dorsal cochlear nucleus. *Nature Neuroscience*, *7*(7), 719–725. https://doi.org/10.1038/nn1272

Tzounopoulos, T., Rubio, M. E., Keen, J. E., & Trussell, L. O. (2007). Coactivation of pre- and postsynaptic signaling mechanisms determines cell-specific spike-timing-dependent plasticity. *Neuron*, *54*(2), 291–301. https://doi.org/10.1016/j.neuron.2007.03.026

Wang, Y., & Manis, P. B. (2008). Short-term synaptic depression and recovery at the mature mammalian endbulb of Held synapse in mice. *Journal of Neurophysiology*, *100*(3), 1255–1264. https://doi.org/10.1152/jn.90715.2008

Wickesberg, R. E., & Oertel, D. (1988). Tonotopic projection from the dorsal to the anteroventral cochlear nucleus of mice. *The Journal of Comparative Neurology*, *268*(3), 389–399. https://doi.org/10.1002/cne.902680308

Xie, R., & Manis, P. B. (2017). Radiate and planar multipolar neurons of the mouse anteroventral cochlear nucleus: Intrinsic excitability and characterization of their auditory nerve input. *Frontiers in Neural Circuits*, *11*, 77. https://doi.org/10.3389/fncir.2017.00077

Yaeger, D. B., & Trussell, L. O. (2015). Single granule cells excite Golgi cells and evoke feedback inhibition in the cochlear nucleus. *Journal of Neuroscience*, *35*(11), 4741–4750. https://doi.org/10.1523/JNEUROSCI.3665-14.2015

Yang, H., & Xu-Friedman, M. A. (2009). Impact of synaptic depression on spike timing at the endbulb of Held. *Journal of Neurophysiology*, *102*(3), 1699–1710. https://doi.org/10.1152/jn.00072.2009

Young, E. D., & Davis, K. A. (2002). Circuitry and function of the dorsal cochlear nucleus. In D. Oertel, R. R. Fay, & A. N. Popper (Eds.), *Integrative Functions in the Mammalian Auditory Pathway* (Vol. *15*, pp. 160–206). New York, NY: Springer.

Young, E. D., & Oertel, D. (2010). Cochlear nucleus. In G. M. Shepherd & S. Grillner (Eds.), *Handbook of Brain Microcircuits* (pp. 215–223). New York, NY: Oxford University Press.

Young, E. D., & Voigt, H. F. (1982). Response properties of type II and type III units in dorsal cochlear nucleus. *Hearing Research*, *6*(2), 153–169.

Zhao, Y., Rubio, M. E., & Tzounopoulos, T. (2009). Distinct functional and anatomical architecture of the endocannabinoid system in the auditory brainstem. *Journal of Neurophysiology*, *101*(5), 2434–2446. https://doi.org/10.1152/jn.00047.2009

Zhao, Y., & Tzounopoulos, T. (2011). Physiological activation of cholinergic inputs controls associative synaptic plasticity via modulation of endocannabinoid signaling. *Journal of Neuroscience*, *31*(9), 3158–3168. https://doi.org/10.1523/JNEUROSCI.5303-10.2011

Zhou, M., Li, Y.-T., Yuan, W., Tao, H. W., & Zhang, L. I. (2015). Synaptic mechanisms for generating temporal diversity of auditory representation in the dorsal cochlear nucleus. *Journal of Neurophysiology*, *113*(5), 1358–1368. https://doi.org/10.1152/jn.00573.2014

Zucker, R. S., & Regehr, W. G. (2002). Short-term synaptic plasticity. *Annual Review of Physiology*, *64*, 355–405. https://doi.org/10.1146/annurev.physiol.64.092501.114547

CHAPTER 6

MOLECULAR AND STRUCTURAL CHANGES IN THE COCHLEAR NUCLEUS IN RESPONSE TO HEARING LOSS

MARIA E. RUBIO

Abstract

Hearing loss is the third most common health problem in the United States. It can affect the quality of life and relationships. About 48 million Americans have lost some hearing. Age, illness, and genetics contribute to the generation of hearing loss. During development, auditory synaptic circuitries are highly plastic and able to adapt to fluctuations in auditory experience. Whether this is so for mature auditory nerve synapses and circuitries within nuclei along the central auditory pathway is less understood. Daily fluctuations in auditory experience can lead to hearing deficits, including hearing loss and/or deafness, Therefore, understanding the cellular mechanisms that occur in mature central auditory synaptic circuitries that lead and/or contribute to hearing loss is important. This chapter focuses on published studies using animal models describing structural and molecular changes that occur in the cochlear nucleus in response to hearing loss, the first gateway of sound processing in the brain.

Keywords: cochlear nucleus, hearing loss, cellular mechanisms, deafening, presynaptic, postsynaptic

Introduction to the Cochlear Nucleus: Anatomy and Function

The cochlear nucleus is located in the lower brainstem in the angle formed by the lower pons, upper medulla, and the cerebellum (angle ponto-medular-cerebellosum), and it is composed of two main regions: the ventral cochlear nucleus (VCN) and dorsal cochlear nucleus (DCN). The auditory nerve (the central branch of spiral ganglion neurons) enters into the brainstem and divides the VCN in two additional regions: the anteroventral (AVCN) and posteroventral (PVCN) cochlear nucleus. The myelinated Type I auditory nerve fibers are the major source of excitation to the cochlear nucleus, carrying information from inner hair cells of the cochlea and innervating principal neurons in each of the regions (Figure 6.1; Lorente de Nó, 1981). The neurons of the cochlear nucleus are the first central processors of auditory information, and they provide inputs to all the major brainstem and midbrain auditory nuclei. The VCN represents the beginning of the binaural pathway through its projections to the superior olivary complex in the lower medulla. The synaptic circuitry of the VCN specializes in the precise and rapid representation of the incoming signals from the cochlear afferents (Young & Oertel, 2003, 2010). The DCN initiates the monaural pathway through its projections to the inferior colliculus in the midbrain and is key for up and down (vertical) sound processing. Apart from the primary sensory axons, the cochlear nucleus receives afferents from other auditory sources, among them the contralateral cochlear nucleus (Alibardi, 1998; Cant & Benson, 2003), as well as important modulatory inputs via descending projections from upper auditory regions, including the superior olivary complex (Cant & Benson, 2003), the inferior colliculus (Shore et al., 1991), and the auditory cortex (Meltzer & Ryugo, 2006), but also from non-auditory regions (somatosensory nuclei; Haenggeli et al., 2005; Shore et al., 2000; Heeringa et al., 2018). There exists an extended intrinsic synaptic circuitry in the cochlear nucleus complex not discussed in this chapter (see for details Cant, 1992; Rubio, 2018; Trussell & Oertel, 2018).

In the cochlear nucleus, there is an additional layer, the granular cell domain (GCD) that is an external shell of small neurons and neuropil that surrounds the magnocellular regions of the VCN (Figure 6.1; Osen, 1969). The GCD is not a major target of Type I auditory nerve fibers, although it does receive terminal branches of low spontaneous rate auditory nerve fibers (Liberman, 1991; Ryugo, 2008), as well as unmyelinated Type II auditory nerve fibers, that carry information from outer hair cells of the cochlea (Benson & Brown, 2004; Brown et al., 1988a;). This region is the target for a variety of nonprimary inputs (superior olivary complex; inferior colliculus; auditory cortex) (Brown et al., 1988b; Caicedo & Herbert, 1993; Saldaña, 1993) and nonauditory projections from somatosensory nuclei (cuneate: Weinberg & Rustioni, 1989; trigeminal nuclei: Itoh et al., 1987; Shore et al., 2000; vestibular organ: Burian & Goesttner, 1988; Kevetter & Parachio, 1989). Neurons within the GCD are in a position to integrate a wide spectrum of information carrying cues about attention, head position, sound localization, or sound recognition (Shore et al., 2000). Granule cell axons project into the superficial layer of the DCN (Rubio & Wenthold, 1997; Waterlood & Mugnaini, 1984).

The cochlear nucleus represents the first station of sound processing in the brainstem. Therefore, it is important to understand the cellular mechanisms in the neurons within the cochlear nucleus that lead and/or contribute to hearing loss. This book chapter will focus on the structural and molecular changes in the cochlear nucleus in response to hearing loss. For functional aspects of hearing loss in the cochlear nucleus, see chapter 7 by Manis in this volume.

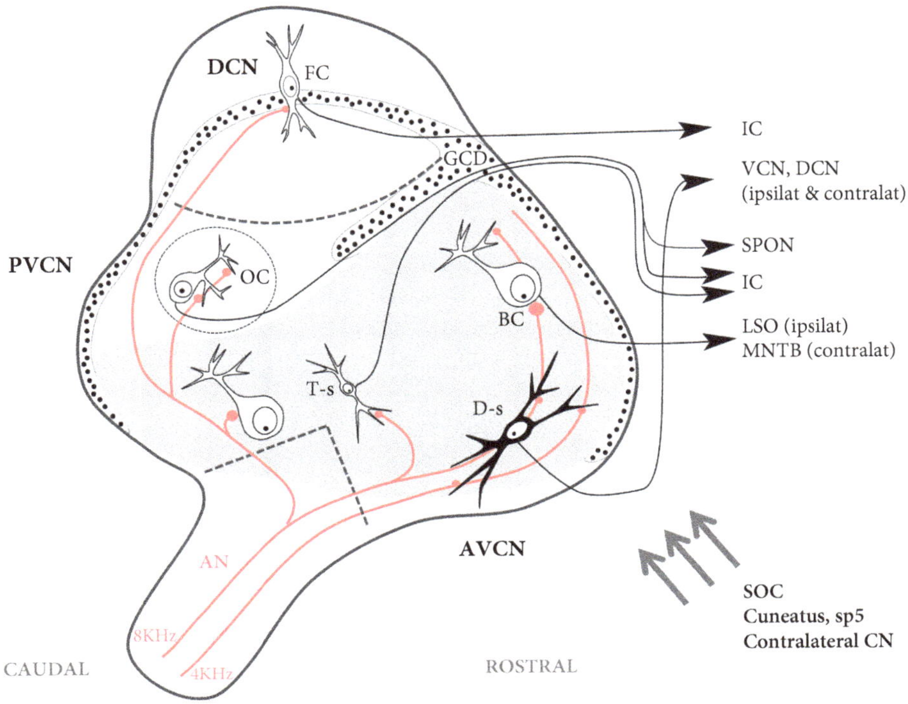

FIGURE 6.1. Schematic of three main subdivisions of the cochlear nucleus (*CN*) and principal neurons [bushy cells (*BC*), T stellate cells (*T-s*), and D stellate cells (*D-s*), within the anteroventral cochlear nucleus (*AVCN*) and the anterior posteroventral cochlear nucleus (*PVCN*); octopus cells (OC) within the posterior PVCN; and fusiform cells (FC) within the dorsal cochlear nucleus (DCN)]. The *pale gray* background represents the area of the ventral cochlear nucleus (*VCN*): the AVCN and anterior PVCN. Axonal projections from the principal cells and their targets are represented. The auditory nerve (*AN*) is represented entering the cochlear nucleus and dividing into descending and ascending branches. Middle frequency fibers (8 KHz) have a more caudal location within the AN, whereas lower frequency fibers (4 KHz) are more rostral. The extrinsic inputs to the AVCN from the superior olivary complex (*SOC*), cuneatus, spinal trigeminal nucleus (*sp5*), and contralateral cochlear nucleus are represented with three arrows. (*GCD*, granular cell domain; *IC*, inferior colliculus; *LSO*, lateral superior olive; *MNTB*, medial nucleus of the trapezoid body; *SPON*: superior olivary nucleus).

The Effect of Cochlear Synaptic Activity on the Gross Anatomy of the Cochlear Nucleus and Neuronal Death

The volume and number of neurons in the cochlear nucleus depend on input from the auditory nerve for survival during the critical period of development (usually before or at postnatal day 9) in a variety of vertebrate species (see for review, Harris & Rubel, 2006; Tierney et al., 1997). Removing afferent input by ablating peripheral sensory receptors (deafferentation) in embryonic or young animals before hearing onset results in a variety of changes, including a reduced size of the cochlear nucleus, largely due to fast and dramatic degeneration of auditory nerve fibers and death of target neurons. In contrast, peripheral deafferentation after the onset of hearing does not lead to a major decrease in the size of the cochlear nucleus or to neuronal death (Tierney et al., 1997); apoptotic markers show up only in microglial cells (Campos Torres et al., 1999). One study used microarray technology to survey for differences in baseline gene expression over three postnatal ages that define a critical period of afferent-dependent neuron survival in the mouse cochlear nucleus (Harris et al., 2005). In this study, findings support the concept that multiple neuroprotective mechanisms increase and pro-apoptotic factors decrease over development to protect mature neurons from stressful insults, thus making them less dependent on afferent input for survival. More studies are needed to underpin the cellular mechanisms that occur during maturation to render cochlear nucleus neurons less susceptible to loss of afferent input. Nonsyndromic deafness studies in animals have shown that spontaneous synaptic activity in hair cells of the organ of Corti in the cochlea before onset of hearing affects the size of the cochlear nuclei. In these animals, death of principal neurons has not been reported (Lee et al., 2003; Ryugo et al., 1997; Seal et al., 2008; Youssoufian et al., 2008), but it is likely that there was death that caused the shrinkage. The topographic organization of auditory nerve axons and those intrinsic within the cochlear nucleus are well organized in the deaf otoferlin mice as compared to normal-hearing mice (Wright et al., 2014), indicating that at least in the cochlear nucleus of mice, the gross topographic organization develops independently of activity before and after the onset of hearing. In contrast, studies of neonatal deafness in cats (Leake et al., 2006), together with findings in the superior olivary complex using acetylcholine receptor α9 knockout mice (Clause et al., 2014), argue that the precise temporal pattern of spontaneous activity before hearing onset is crucial for establishment of precise tonotopy.

Hearing loss mainly occurs in adulthood and during aging, with the exception of nonsyndromic deafness. The following sections focus on the structural and molecular effects of hearing loss in animal models when synaptic circuitries in the cochlear nucleus are mature as well as during ageing.

Hearing Loss: Structural and Molecular Presynaptic Effects in the Cochlear Nucleus

Hearing loss after the onset of hearing leads to a decrease in the number of afferent synapses on inner hair cells, which alters auditory transmission from the inner ear to the cochlear nucleus. The auditory nerve makes synaptic contact on principal neurons of the VCN, including bushy, stellate, and octopus cells. In the DCN, the auditory nerve innervates fusiform and multipolar cells (Figure 6.1). The synapse of the auditory nerve on principal neurons is a secure and strong glutamatergic synapse. For these reasons and in contrast to excitatory synapses in other parts of the central nervous system, auditory nerve synapses lack the classical activity-dependent synaptic plasticity mechanisms (Fujino & Oertel, 2003; Zhao et al., 2011). This raises the question of whether mature auditory nerve synapses are able to adapt to changes in auditory experience. Studies have reported structural and molecular changes at auditory nerve endings in response to hearing loss. The effects are considered a response to a decrease in auditory nerve activity, although it is unclear whether the response of cochlear nucleus neurons is compensatory or pathological.

The first evidence of the existence of structural plasticity at auditory nerve synapses was reported in studies from congenital deaf white cats and mice (Baker et al., 2010; Redd et al., 2002; Ryugo et al., 2005; O'Neil et al., 2010) and more recently from otoferlin knockout mice (Wright et al., 2014). Although in these studies it is not easy to distinguish developmental effects from those that occur at a later age, they did show that in congenital deafness the auditory nerve terminals including the endbulb of Held in the VCN shrunk. Moreover, after cochlear implant and electrical stimulation of 3-month-old white deaf cats for 3 months, the size of the endbulbs recovers (Ryugo et al., 2005; O'Neil et al., 2010), thus suggesting that auditory nerve activity maintains the size of endbulb terminals. These results may have clinical relevance because they suggest that reestablishing auditory nerve activity after prolonged deafness may restore the presynaptic terminal of the auditory nerve, which may lead to a recovery of function. However, it remains unclear whether the smaller size of endbulb endings of congenital deaf animals is totally or partially due to developmental effects or to a lack of synaptic activity of the auditory nerve at more mature stages. A decrease in size of endbulb endings was also observed in animal models with an early onset of hearing loss and during aging (Frisina & Walton, 2006; McGuire et al., 2015; Connelly et al., 2017). On the other hand, a decrease in size of endbulb endings was not observed in rodents when hearing loss occurs after hearing onset and in response to milder forms of hearing loss such as conductive hearing loss (Clarkson et al., 2016).

Few studies have addressed the molecular changes of auditory nerve endings following hearing loss. Studies focused on determining changes in excitatory (glutamate) neurotransmitters in the cochlear nucleus after cochlear ablation or after middle ear ossicle removal in rodents (Godfrey et al., 2015; Suneja et al., 1998). The auditory nerve is a glutamatergic synapse, thus the general thought was that finding a decrease or increase in glutamate concentration could reflect a change in the demands for synaptic transmission at the auditory nerve in response to cochlear deafferentation and hearing loss. In general, these biochemical studies showed a decrease in glutamate concentration in the cochlear nucleus. If glutamate was located exclusively at synaptic auditory nerve endings, the most logical conclusion from these studies would be that an intact cochlea is needed to maintain normal levels of glutamate at auditory nerve endings. However, there are intrinsic (i.e., parallel fibers from the granule cells) as well as other extrinsic (i.e., mossy fibers from somatosensory origin) inputs within the cochlear nucleus where synaptic endings contain and release glutamate (Gómez-Nieto & Rubio, 2009; Manis, 1989; Rubio & Juiz, 1998, 2004; Rubio et al., 2008). In addition, glutamate is an amino acid that is widely expressed in all-neuronal types (excitatory and inhibitory), as well as in glial cells (Zhou & Danbolt, 2014). Therefore, a decrease in glutamate may not directly reflect a decrease of glutamate concentration in auditory nerve terminals.

More recent studies used other markers for glutamate release such as vesicular glutamate transporters 1 and/or 2 (vGluT1, vGluT2), which fill synaptic vesicles with glutamate (Takamori et al., 2002; Weston et al., 2011). Mature auditory nerve endings contain only vGluT1 (Zhou et al., 2007; Gómez-Nieto & Rubio, 2009; Fyk-Kolodziej et al., 2011). Following reports in the brain (Erickson et al., 2006; Liguz-Lecznar & Skangiel-Kramska, 2007), vGluT1 expression levels could reflect the average presynaptic activity of auditory nerve endings. Evidence has shown that deafening after peripheral damage or kanamycin injection, the expression levels of vGluT1 at auditory nerve endings decreased when compared to non-deafened animals (Fyk-Kolodziej et al., 2011; Zeng et al., 2009). A similar decrease was also observed in milder forms of hearing loss such as unilateral and bilateral conductive hearing loss (Clarkson et al., 2016; Zhuang et al., 2017). Ultrastructurally, the decrease in vGluT1 expression correlated with a decrease in synaptic vesicle size and volume but not in the surface area of auditory nerve terminals, thus indicating that conductive hearing loss reduces the number of glutamate molecules per synaptic vesicle, which is likely to lead to a decrease in vesicular glutamate release (Clarkson et al., 2016; Herman et al., 2014). However, other studies investigating the effects of hearing loss on auditory nerve synapses in the cochlear nucleus reported contradictory results. For example, one study found an increase in vGluT1 expression levels (Ngodup et al., 2015), while in another study from a different research group, a decrease in vGluT1 expression was observed (Kurioka et al., 2016). In both studies, a broadband noise was used to inflict cochlear damage, so it is unclear whether the difference in these results is due to the duration of the noise exposure, the different strain or age of mice, and/or the time of analysis after noise exposure. A decrease in vGluT1 expression in the cochlear nucleus was also reported after acoustic overstimulation (Barker et al., 2012). Morphological results from various laboratories suggest either up- or down-regulation of glutamate release, which may reflect that the auditory nerve reacts differently to various forms of deafening. Further functional studies are needed to determine whether the changes in vGluT1 expression at auditory nerve endings in response to hearing loss correlate with physiological responses at the synapse.

Contrary to the auditory nerve endings and the endings of the parallel fibers of the granule cells, the extrinsic glutamatergic inputs from somatosensory origin within the cochlear nucleus contains vGluT2 (Zhou et al., 2007). Remarkably, after cochlear deafferentation or noise-induced hearing loss, vGluT2 expression levels increases in the GCD region (Barker et al., 2012; Zeng et al., 2009). What triggers this upregulation of vGluT2, together with its functional consequences, remains to be determined. In the DCN, it is well established that fusiform cells integrate auditory information through its basal dendrites and somatosensory information through its apical dendrites via the granule cells within the GCD (Fujino & Oertel, 2003; Kanold et al., 2011). Neural hyperactivity is induced in fusiform cells of the DCN following intense sound exposure. Researchers suggest that fusiform cells may be implicated as major generators of noise-induced tinnitus (see for review, Kaltenbach, 2007; Wu et al., 2016). Furthermore, new evidence shows that somatosensory signals influence auditory processing in the VCN. This appears to occur in the GCD, the major target region of somatosensory inputs and type II auditory nerve fibers, and also within the core, where collaterals of somatosensory axons distribute on principal neurons receiving Type I cochlear afferents (Heeringa et al., 2018). To understand the putative convergence of cochlear and somatosensory information within the GCD and the core of the VCN requires a better understanding of the role of the GCD in auditory processing. In addition, it requires the identification of the neuronal targets and the role of Type II unmyelinated auditory nerve fibers within the VCN, as well as determining the subset of principal neurons that receive both cochlear and somatosensory inputs. This convergence of auditory and somatosensory inputs in the VCN is of relevance, considering new evidence in animal models after noise exposure (Heeringa et al., 2018; Vogler et al., 2011) and clinical studies in humans (Gu et al., 2012) indicating that in addition to the DCN, the VCN is involved in the genesis of tinnitus.

Hearing loss has been suggested to unbalance the ratio of excitation and inhibition in the cochlear nucleus and along the auditory pathway. However, contrary to the glutamatergic synapses, we know less of the molecular and structural effects of hearing loss in presynaptic inhibitory endings. Biochemical and immunohistochemical studies after peripheral damage focused on investigating the effects of hearing loss in glycine and GABA (gamma-amino-butyric-acid) neurotransmitter content in the cochlear nucleus of the same side (Lee & Godfrey, 2014; Suneja et al., 1998). These studies showed a decrease in glycine but not in GABA concentration. Further studies need to focus in determining the structural and molecular effects of hearing loss in identified inhibitory inputs within the cochlear nucleus. It would be worthy to investigate whether hearing loss alters the expression levels of vesicular inhibitory neurotransmitter transporters, as a putative indication of changes in glycine release.

Hearing Loss: Structural and Molecular Postsynaptic Effects in the Cochlear Nucleus

In addition to presynaptic responses, studies in animals after deafening and with hearing loss have shown structural effects on the postsynaptic principal neurons within the VCN (bushy cells) and DCN (fusiform cells). Remarkably, these responses have been found in the same side of the deafening as well as in the contralateral side. The models of hearing loss used to study postsynaptic changes include congenital deafness, peripheral deafferentation, and conductive hearing loss. Structural and/or molecular responses of the other principal neurons of the cochlear nucleus (stellate and octopus cells in the VCN, and multipolar cells in the DCN) have not been performed.

Ultrastructural studies of congenitally deaf white cats and mice showed hypertrophy of the postsynaptic density (PSD) of bushy cells in apposition to auditory nerve endings (Lee et al. 2003; Redd et al., 2000; Ryugo et al. 1997). Interestingly, after cochlear implant and electrical stimulation for 3 months, the hypertrophy reversed and the postsynaptic densities were similar to those of normal-hearing cats (Ryugo et al. 2005; O'Neil et al. 2010). Deafening can have fast-acting consequences. After only 4 hours of peripheral deafening and before visible structural signs of degeneration at auditory nerve endings and synapses, the PSD of fusiform cells basal dendrites apposed to auditory nerve endings becomes thicker (Rubio, 2006). This, together with others reports in other systems (see for review Dosemeci et al., 2016) suggest that the PSD is a highly plastic structure strongly influenced by presynaptic activity (Gulley et al., 1977; Dosemeci et al., 2001). Biochemical binding studies have shown that the absence of auditory nerve inputs affects the amount and activity of glutamate receptors in the cochlear nucleus (Suneja et al., 2000). In addition, in vitro electrophysiological recordings reported larger excitatory postsynaptic current (EPSC) amplitude in bushy cells of congenitally deaf mice than in those with normal-hearing (Oleskevich & Walmsley, 2002). These two lines of evidence suggest, that the number and/or subunit composition of glutamate receptors at the auditory nerve synapse is altered in response to peripheral damage or congenital deafening. After peripheral damage and before subcellular signs of degeneration, one ultrastructural study showed that at the synapse of auditory nerve on fusiform cells basal dendrites, there was a redistribution of the GluA2, GluA3 and GluA4 subunits of the AMPA glutamate receptors (Rubio, 2006). Although these results are remarkable and suggest a fast response of the postsynaptic neurons to hearing loss, these effects in AMPA receptors expression were observed after peripheral cochlear damage. In this situation, it is difficult to separate the effects of damaging the nerve from those related to a decrease in the sensory input.

Milder forms of hearing loss also affect principal neurons receiving auditory nerve synapses. Sound reduction by unilateral conductive hearing loss (ossicle removal) alters the neuronal metabolic rates and protein synthesis in principal neurons of the ipsilateral VCN (Tucci et al., 1999; Huston et al., 2007). Transient unilateral conductive hearing loss (ear plugging) for one day led to a reversible increase in hearing thresholds and to reversible synaptic up-regulation of GluA3 AMPA receptors at the synapse of the auditory nerve on bushy cells in the VCN and fusiform cells in the DCN. The same neurons showed a down regulation of the α1 subunit of the glycine receptor (GlyR α1) at inhibitory synapses that also reversed once hearing levels were restored (Whiting et al., 2009), suggesting the existence of a homeostatic response to compensate for reduced acoustic stimulation. Longer periods (more than one week) of transient conductive hearing loss by unilateral ear plugging altered the cytoplasmic receptor pool of excitatory and inhibitory receptors in those same neuronal types (Wang et al., 2011). This study showed an increase in the expression of the GluA3 subunit of the AMPA receptors, and a decrease in the GlyR α1 subunit on the cell bodies of bushy cells and fusiform cells of the ipsilateral ventral and dorsal cochlear nucleus, respectively. On the other hand, the cytoplasmic expression levels of $GABA_A$ β2/3 subunits were unchanged (Wang et al., 2011). This up-regulation of GluA3 and down-regulation of GlyR α1 observed at the cell bodies, is similar to the synaptic changes mentioned previously after one-day ear plugging (Whiting et al., 2009). At the synaptic level, unilateral ear plugging for more than one week showed long lasting post-synaptic structural and molecular effects at the endbulb of the Held synapse, including larger postsynaptic densities and a sustained up-regulation of synaptic GluA3 (Clarkson et al., 2016). The same study showed that conductive hearing loss led to an increase in the central gain upstream the cochlear nucleus at level of the lateral lemniscus. This suggests that upper auditory nuclei compensate for the decrease signal from the cochlear nucleus. All together, these findings show that sensory dependent evoked plasticity is more complex than what might be predicted from experiments in reduced systems such as neuronal cultured cells or brain slices (see for review, Turrigiano, 2011). Future studies could investigate in the adult, long-term hearing sensitivities following conductive hearing loss, which is prevalent in children. Such studies will settle the central mechanisms of deficits in auditory perception, language acquisition or educational disabilities that occur after inadequate or abnormal sensory experience.

Hearing Loss Effects in the Contralateral Side

Reports exist of molecular effects of conductive hearing loss in neurons of the cochlear nucleus of the contralateral side to the affected ear. In particular, contralateral neurons of the cochlear nucleus have increased metabolic rates and protein synthesis (Hutson et al., 2007; Tucci et al., 1999). In addition, by immunohistochemistry at the light and electron microscopy level it has been reported that conductive hearing loss alters synaptic proteins. Bushy cells and fusiform cells of the contralateral side up-regulate the GluA3 subunits of AMPA receptors while they down-regulate the GlyRα1 in response unilateral conductive hearing loss (Wang et al., 2011; Whiting et al., 2009,), changes similar to what has been observed in the ipsilateral cochlear nucleus (Wang et al., 2011; Whiting et al., 2009). The pathways by which changes in neuronal activity in one cochlear nucleus influence activity in the other cochlear nucleus is still an open question. The cochlear nucleus complex is the first site at which binaural information converses in the CNS (for review, see Cant & Benson, 2003). Communication between cochlear nuclei can occur through glutamatergic and glycinergic commissural projections (Alibardi, 1998, 2000, 2003; Bledsoe et al., 2009; Shore et al., 2003) or via descending inputs from upper auditory nuclei, particularly descending cholinergic inputs (Darrow et al., 2006; Liberman & Brown, 1986; Spangler et al., 1987; Shore et al., 1991; Warren & Liberman, 1989a, b). Functional connections between the cochlear nuclei have been also shown (Davis, 2005; Ingham et al., 2006; Needham & Paolini, 2006; Shore et al., 2003; Sumner et al., 2005). Thus, unilateral conductive hearing loss could create an imbalance in the neuronal synaptic circuitry of the contralateral cochlear nucleus through two pathways—the commissural fibers and descending cholinergic inputs. More efforts are needed to determine the contribution of each pathway in normal hearing and in response to hearing loss.

Age-Related Hearing Loss: Structural and Molecular Changes

Prebycussis (age-related-hearing loss) is a widespread communication disorder and chronic medical condition in our aged population. Relatively few studies have examined age-related structural and molecular changes in the cochlear nucleus. The neurophysiological studies are very few and suggest a decline in glutamate and glycine-mediated excitation and inhibition, respectively (see for details chapter 7 by Manis in this volume). Biochemical studies of glycine inhibition in the cochlear nucleus are consistent with age-related functional declines of this neurotransmitter system that affect complex sound processing (Mildbrandt & Caspary, 1995). Biochemical studies investigating the effect of aging in glutamatergic synapses are also lacking.

Gross Morphological and Structural Changes during Aging

Studies investigating a population of young, middle, and old C57BL/J6 (C57) and CBA/CaJ (CBA) mice revealed changes in the dimensions and volumes of the AVCN as well as the number, density, and size of neurons (Frisina & Walton, 2006; Willot et al., 1987). The idea was to compare these parameters in a mouse strain with an early onset of hearing loss (C57) with those of CBA mice that have a "normal" age-induced hearing loss. The authors found that AVCN volumes did not change significantly with age in either strain. However, neuron number and density declined in C57s during the first 7 months, but they remained stable thereafter. In CBAs, reductions in neuron number and packing were not observed until the second year. Changes in neuronal sizes were observed but varied depending on the neuronal type and strain. Aging affected principally the caudal (high-frequency) area of the AVCN. DBA mice exhibit similar changes as C57s even if this strain exhibits a congenital accelerated, high-frequency cochlear hearing loss occurring at a rate even faster than C57s. Ultrastructurally, principal neurons in the AVCN (bushy cells and multipolar cells) displayed an increase in the incidence of heterochromatic nuclei and in the percentage of the soma occupied by lipofuscin, indicating an aging process (Briner & Willott, 1989). Additionally, multipolar cells showed a decrease in roundness and an increase in the number of nuclear invaginations. The PVCN, the area of octopus cells, decreased in overall volume, number of octopus cells, neuron size, and dendrite number and size. Interestingly, there was an increase in glial cell density. In the DCN of C57s and CBA mice, and unlike the AVCN, the nucleus volume, cell number, and size declined with age for C57s, particularly in deep layers. In CBA mice, the volume of the DCN increased in the first years and declined in old age. Taken together, these studies show that in aged mice the VCN is more affected than DCN, perhaps because the VCN has a higher proportion of direct inputs from the cochlea than the DCN, and the cochlear inputs show declines with age, especially in C57 mice due to their early onset of hearing loss.

Molecular Changes during Aging

Previous research has shown that the rat cochlear nucleus undergoes several molecular changes during aging. There are significant reductions in the levels of glutamate and glycine, without similar changes in the level of GABA (Banay-Schwartz et al., 1989a,b). GABA or any enzyme or protein involved in the synthesis of GABA remained stable with age in the cochlear nucleus. Biochemical studies showed a decline in glycine receptor binding in DCN and VCN of aged Fisher-344 rats (Milbrandt & Caspary, 1995); the decrease was due to an age-related decline in the number of binding sites, with little change in affinity. mRNA studies showed that GlyR α1 and β1 declined in AVCN of old rats, while subunit GlyR α2 increased (Krenning et al., 1998). The results from the rat DCN were confirmed in old C57, but not in middle age C57 or old CBA mice (Willott et al., 1997). Further studies are needed to tease apart the effects of species, hearing loss, and age and their impact in the cochlear nucleus regions.

Ultrastructural Synaptic Changes during Aging and in Mouse Models with an Early Onset of Hearing Loss

Only few studies determined how aging affects the number and ultrastructure of synapses in the cochlear nucleus (Fisher-344 rats: Helfert et al., 2003; CBA/Ca, heterozygous *shaker*-$2^{+/-}$, homozygous *shaker*-$2^{-/-}$, and DBA/2 mice: Connelly et al., 2017; DBA/J2 mice: McGuire et al., 2015). All these studies focused on the AVCN, where no synapse losses were observed in either rats or mice. This is in contrast with a dramatic degeneration of synaptic endings and dendrites in the inferior colliculus (Helfert et al., 1999). In rat AVCN, a decrease in size of synaptic endings of putative inhibitory and excitatory inputs was observed on dendrites that were < 2 μm in diameter (Helfert et al., 2003). The studies in mice investigated ultrastructural changes in the glutamatergic synapses of the auditory nerve (endbulb of Held) on bushy cells. Apart from a decrease in size of the endbulbs of mice with early onset of hearing loss (DBA/J2 and *shaker*-$2^{-/-}$mice), no dramatic ultrastructural changes were observed in the mitochondria fraction and postsynaptic density size (Connelly et al., 2017; McGuire et al., 2015). The reduction in the neurotransmitter glutamate and glycine found in aged rodents surprisingly contrast with no major ultrastructural changes at endbulb synapses on bushy cell bodies or putative glycinergic endings on dendrites. Synaptic replacement may occur during aging through the collaterization by neighboring axons or endings; these new endings may be smaller in size and could therefore contain less neurotransmitter. Alternatively, synaptic vesicles could be smaller, and/or the expression of presynaptic calcium channels could decrease during aging. Additional anatomical, molecular, and functional studies are needed to elucidate the presynaptic and postsynaptic cellular mechanisms underlying the age-related changes in the AVCN, as well the other regions of the cochlear nucleus.

Protective Mechanisms in the Cochlear Nucleus to Hearing Loss via Descending Inputs

There is increasing interest in determining whether the descending projections to the cochlear nucleus have a protective role in response to hearing loss (Kirk & Smith, 2003; Reiter & Liberman, 1995). In contrast to the ascending auditory pathway, less is known about the anatomy and function of the descending auditory pathways in the normal-hearing and in the hearing impaired. Immunohistochemical studies one week after cochlear ablation showed a massive increase in growth-associated protein 43 (GAP-43) expression levels in the VCN of the side of the lesion. GAP-43 immunoreactivity was found in axons and synaptic endings that made synaptic contacts with glutamatergic and glycinergic neurons. These endings had their origin in the contralateral ventral superior olive (VSO) in the lower brainstem (Hildebrandt et al., 2011; Illing & Resich, 2006; Meidinger et al., 2006). Neurons in the VSO, including the medial olivocochlear neurons, employ acetylcholine as a neurotransmitter (Vetter et al., 1991; Yao & Godfrey, 1996). Studies after noise-induced hearing loss have also reported that over time (8 months) after noise exposure, auditory nerve synapses degenerate, but in addition there is rewiring of the VCN synaptic circuitry (Kim et al. 2004). It is still undetermined what this rewiring means in terms of VCN function, and whether this rewiring correlates with new cholinergic endings from the VSO or other descending inputs from upper auditory nuclei.

Summary

Normal auditory nerve activity is key for maintaining fundamental structural, molecular, and functional parameters of auditory nerve synapses, as well as the postsynaptic excitatory or inhibitory neurons within the cochlear nucleus, and that hearing deficits alter those parameters. The studies summarized in this in chapter show that there are multiple ways through which neurons in the cochlear nucleus respond to fluctuations in their inputs and that probably these responses relate to the etiology of hearing loss. Studies of different models of hearing loss are necessary to underpin the cellular mechanisms, as well as determining common features, that will help us to understand whether the synaptic modifications compensate for the hearing deficits or represent pathological responses to hearing loss. However, it is also important to study the same model of hearing loss by a variety of approaches. Most of the anatomical and molecular studies are performed in mature animals, whereas most of the in vitro electrophysiological studies have been performed at early ages. For this reason, anatomical and molecular studies lack functional studies and, vice versa electrophysiological studies lack of anatomical and molecular verification. Progress of the field would thus profit from closer interactions between anatomists, electrophysiologists, and molecular biologists.

Acknowledgments

Support was provided by the National Institute for Deafness and Other Communication Disorders (grant DC013048).

Author Note

Maria E. Rubio declares that she has no conflict of interest.

References

Alibardi, L. (1998). Ultrastructural and immunocytochemical characterization of commissural neurons in the ventral cochlear nucleus of the rat. *Annals of Anatomy, 180*(5), 427–438.

Alibardi, L. (2000). Cytology, synaptology and immunocytochemistry of commissural neurons and their putative axonal terminals in the dorsal cochlear nucleus of the rat. *Annals of Anatomy, 182*, 207–220.

Alibardi, L. (2003). Ultrastructural immunocytochemistry for glycine in neurons of the dorsal cochlear nucleus of the guinea pig. *Journal of Submicroscopy Biology, 5*(4), 373–387.

Baker, C. A., Montey, K. L., Pongstapom, T., & Ryugo, D. K. (2010). Postnatal development of the endbulb of Held in congenitally deaf cats. *Frontiers in Neuroanatomy, 4*, 19.

Banay-Schwartz, M., Lajhta, A., & Palovits, M. (1989a). Changes with aging in the levels of amino acids in rat CNS structural elements I. Glutamate and related amino acids. *Neurochemical Research, 14*, 555–562.

Banay-Schwartz, M., Lajhta, A., & Palovits, M. (1989b). Changes with aging in the levels of amino acids in rat CNS structural elements. II. Taurine and small neutral amino acids. *Neurochemical Research, 14*, 563–570.

Barker, M., Solinski, H. J., Hashimoto, H., Tagoe, T., Pilati, N., & Hamann, M. H. (2012). Acoustic overexposure increases the expression of VGLUT-2 mediated projections from the lateral vestibular nucleus to the dorsal cochlear nucleus. *PlosOne*, https://doi.org/10.1371/journal.pone.0035955.

Benson, T. E., & Brown, M. C. (2004). Postsynaptic targets of type II auditory nerve fibers in the cochlear nucleus. *Journal of the Association for Research in Otolaryngology*, *5*(2), 111–125.

Bledsoe, S. C., Jr., Koehler, S., Tucci, D. L., Zhou, J., Le Prell, C., & Shore, S. E. (2009). Ventral cochlear nucleus responses to contralateral sound are mediated by commissural and olivocochlear pathways. *Journal of Neurophysiology*, *102*(2), 886–900.

Briner W., & Willott J. F. (1989). Ultrastructural features of neurons in the C57BL/6J mouse anteroventral cochlear nucleus: Young mice versus old mice with chronic presbycusis. *Neurobiology of Aging*, *10*(4), 295–303.

Brown, M. C., Berglund, A. M., Kiang, N. Y., & Ryugo, D. K. (1988a). Central trajectories of type II spiral ganglion neurons. *Journal of Comparative Neurology*, *278*(4), 581–590.

Brown, M. C., Liberman, M. C., Benson T. E., & Ryugo, D. K. (1988b). Brainstem branches from olivocochlear axons in cats and rodents. *Journal of Comparative Neurology*, *278*(4), 591–603.

Burian, M., & Goesttner, W. (1988). Projection of primary vestibular afferent fibres to the cochlear nucleus in the guinea pig. *Neuroscience Letters*, *84*(1), 13–17.

Caicedo, A., & Herbert, H. (1993). Topography of descending projections from the inferior colliculus to auditory brainstem nuclei in the rat. *Journal of Comparative Neurology*, *328*(3), 377–392.

Campos Torres, A., Vidal, P. P., & de Waele, C. (1999). Evidence for microglial reaction within the vestibular and cochlear nuclei following inner ear lesion in the rat. *Neuroscience*, *92*, 1475–1490.

Cant, N. B. (1992). The cochlear nucleus: Neural types and *their* synaptic organization. In D. B. Webster, A. N. Popper, & R. R. Fay (Eds.), *The mammalian auditory pathway: Neuroanatomy* (pp.66–116). New York, NY: Springer.

Cant, N. B., & Benson, C. G. (2003). Parallel auditory pathways: Projection patterns of the different neuronal populations in the dorsal and ventral cochlear nuclei. *Brain Research Bulletin*, *60*(5–6), 457–474.

Clarkson, C., Antunes, F., Rubio, M. E. (2016). Conductive hearing loss has long-lasting structural and molecular effects on pre- and post-synaptic structures of the auditory nerve in the cochlear nucleus. *Journal of Neuroscience*, *36*(39), 10214–10227.

Clause, A., Kim, G., Sonntag, M., Weisz, C. J. C., Vetter, D. E., Rübsamen, R., & Kandler, K. (2014). The precise temporal pattern of prehearing spontaneous activity is necessary for tonotopic map refinement. *Neuron*, *82*, 822–835.

Connelly, C. J., Ryugo, D. K., & Muniak, M. A. (2017). The effect of progressive hearing loss on the morphology of endbulbs of Held and bushy cells. *Hearing Research*, *343*, 14–33.

Darrow, K. N., Maison, S. F., & Liberman, M.C. (2006). Cochlear efferent feedback balances interaural sensitivity. *Nature Neuroscience*, *9*(12), 1474–1476.

Davis, K. A. (2005). Contralateral effects and binaural interactions in dorsal cochlear nucleus. *Journal of the Association in Research in Otolaryngology*, *6*, 280–296.

Dosemeci, A., Tao-Cheng, J. H., Vinade, L., Winters, C. A., Pozzo-Miller, L., & Reese, T. S. (2001). Glutamate-induced transient modification of the postsynaptic density. *Proceedings National Academy Sciences U S A*, *98*(18), 10428–10432.

Dosemeci, A., Weinberg, R. J., Reese, T. S., & Tao-Cheng, J-H. (2016) The postsynaptic density: There is more than meets the eye. *Frontiers in Synaptic Neuroscience, 8*, 23.

Erickson J. D., De Gois S., Varoqui H., Schafer M. K., & Weihe, E. (2006). Activity-dependent regulation of vesicular glutamate and GABA transporters: A means to scale quantal size. *Neurochemistry International, 48*(6–7), 643–649. Review.

Frisina, R. D., & Walton, J. P. (2006). Age-related structural and functional changes in the cochlear nucleus. Hearing Research, *216–217*, 216–223.

Fujino, K., & Oertel, D. (2003). Bidirectional synaptic plasticity in the cerebellum-like mammalian dorsal cochlear nucleus. *Proceedings of the National Academy of Sciences of the United States of America, 100*(1), 265–270.

Fyk-Kolodziej, B., Shimano, T., Gong, T. W., & Holt, A. G. (2011). Vesicular glutamate transporters: Spatio-temporal plasticity following hearing loss. *Neuroscience, 178*, 218–239.

Gómez-Nieto, R., Rubio, & M. E. (2009). A bushy cell network in the rat ventral cochlear nucleus. *Journal of Comparative Neurology, 516*(4), 241–263.

Godfrey, D. A., Chen, K., Godfrey, M. A., Lee, A. C., Crass, S. P., Shipp, D., Simo, H., & Robinson, K. T. (2015). Cochlear ablation effects on amino acid levels in the chinchilla cochlear nucleus. *Neuroscience, 297*, 137–159.

Gu, J. W., Hermann, B. S., Levine, R. A., & Melcher, J. R. (2012). Brainstem auditory evoked potentials suggest a role for the ventral cochlear nucleus in tinnitus. *Journal of the Association for Research in Otolaryngology, 13*(6), 819–833.

Gulley, R. L., Wenthold, R. J., Neises, G. R. (1977). Remodeling of neuronal membranes as an early response to deafferentation. A freeze-fracture study. *Journal Cell Biology, 75*(3), 837–850.

Haenggeli, C. A., Pongstaporn, T., Doucet, J. R., & Ryugo, D. K. (2005). Projections from the spinal trigeminal nucleus to the cochlear nucleus in the rat. *Journal of Comparative Neurology, 484*(2), 191–205.

Harris, J. A., Hardie, N. A., Bermingham-McDonogh, O., & Rubel, E. W. (2005). Gene expression differences over a critical period of afferent-dependent neuron survival in the mouse auditory brainstem. *Journal of Comparative Neurology, 491*, 460–474.

Harris, J. A., & Rubel, E. W. (2006). Afferent regulation of neuron number in the cochlear nucleus: Cellular and molecular analysis of a critical period. *Hearing Research, 216–2017*, 127–137.

Heeringa, A. N., Wu, W., & Shore, S. E. (2018). Multisensory integration enhances temporal coding in the ventral cochlear nucleus. *Journal of Neuroscience, 38*(11), 2832–2843.

Herman, M. A., Ackermann, F., Trimbuch, T., & Rossenmund, C. (2014). Vesicular glutamate transporter expression levels affects synaptic release probability at hippocampal synapses in culture. *Journal of Neuroscience, 34*(35), 11781–11791.

Helfert, R. H., Krenning, J., Wilson, T. S., & Hughes, L. F. (2003). Age-related synaptic changes in the anteroventral cochlear nucleus of Fisher-344 rats. *Hearing Research, 183*, 18–28.

Helfert, R. H., Sommer, T. J., Meeks, J., Hofstetter, P., & Hughes, L. F. (1999). Age-related synaptic changes in the central nucleus of the inferior colliculus of the Fisher-344 rat. *Journal of Comparative Neurology, 406*, 285–298.

Hildebrandt, H., Hoffmann, N. A., & Illing, R. B. (2011). Synaptic reorganization in the adult rat's ventral cochlear nucleus following its total sensory deafferentation. *PlosOne, 6*(8), e23686.

Hutson, K. A., Durham, D., & Tucci, D. L. (2007). Consequences of unilateral hearing loss: Time dependent regulation of protein synthesis in auditory brainstem nuclei. *Hearing Research, 233*(1–2), 124–134.

Illing R. B., & Resich, A. (2006). Specific plasticity responses to unilaterally decreased or increased hearing intensity in the adult cochlear nucleus and beyond. *Hearing Research, 216–217*, 189–197.

Ingham, N. J., Bleeck, S., & Winter, I. M. (2006). Contralateral inhibitory and excitatory frequency response maps in the mammalian cochlear nucleus. *European Journal of Neuroscience, 24*, 2515–2529.

Itoh, K., Kamiya, H., Mitani, A., & Yasui, Y. (1987). Direct projections from the dorsal column nuclei and the spinal trigeminal nuclei to the cochlear nuclei in the cat. *Brain Research, 400*(1), 145–150.

Kaltenbach, J. A. (2007). The dorsal cochlear nucleus as a contributor to tinnitus: Mechanisms underlying the induction of hyperactivity. *Progress in Brain Research, 166*, 89–106.

Kanold, P., Davis, K. A., & Young, E. (2011). Somatosensory context alters auditory responses in the cochlear nucleus. *Journal of Neurophysiology, 105*(3): 1063–1070.

Kevetter, G. A., & Parachio, A. A. (1989). Projections from the saccules to the cochlear nuclei in the Mongolian gerbil. *Brain, Behavior and Evolution, 34*(4), 193–200.

Kim, J. J., Gross, S. J., Potashner, S. J., & Morest, D. K. (2004). Fine structure of long-term changes in the cochlear nucleus after acoustic overstimulation: Chronic degeneration and new growth of synaptic endings. *Journal of Neuroscience Research, 77*(6), 817–828.

Kirk, E. C., & Smith, D. W. (2003). Protection from acoustic trauma is not a primary function of the medial olivocochlear efferent system. *Journal of the Association for Research in Otolaryngology, 4*, 445–465.

Krenning, J., Hughes, L. F., Caspary, D. M., & Helfert, R. H. (1998). Age-related glycine receptor subunit changed in the cochlear nucleus of Fisher-344 rats. *Laryngoscope, 108*, 26–31.

Kurioka, T., Lee, M. Y., Heeringa, A. N., Beyer, L. A., Swiderski, D. L., Kanicki, A. C., . . . Raphael, Y. (2016). Selective hair cell ablation and noise exposure lead to different patterns of changes in the cochlea and the cochlear nucleus. *Neuroscience, 332*, 242–257.

Leake, P. A., Hradek, G. T., Chair, L., & Snyder, R. L. (2006). Neonatal deafness results in degraded topographic specificity of auditory nerve projections to the cochlear nucleus in cats. *Journal of Comparative Neurology, 497*(1), 13–31.

Lee, A. C., Godfrey, D. A. (2014). Cochlear damage affects neurotransmitter chemistry in the central auditory system. *Frontiers in Neurology, 5*, 227. doi: 10.3389/fneur.2014.00227

Lee, D. J., Cahill, H. B., & Ryugo, D. K. (2003). Effects of congenital deafness in the cochlear nuclei of Shaker-2 mice: An ultrastructural analysis of synapse morphology in the endbulbs of Held. *Journal of Neurocytology, 32*(3), 229–243.

Liberman, M. C. (1991). Central projections of auditory-nerve fibers of differing spontaneous rate. I. Anteroventral cochlear nucleus. *The Journal of Comparative Neurology, 313*(2), 240–258.

Liberman, M. C., & Brown, C. (1986). Physiology and anatomy of single olivocochlear neurons in the cat. *Hearing Research, 24*(1), 17–36.

Liguz-Lecznar M., & Skangiel-Kramska J. (2007). Vesicular glutamate transporters (VGLUTs): The three musketeers of glutamatergic system. *Acta Neurobiologiae Experimentalis 67*(3): 207–218. Review.

Lorente de Nó, R. (1981). *The primary acoustic nuclei.* New York, NY: Raven Press.

Manis, P. B. (1989). Responses to parallel fiber stimulation in the guinea pig dorsal cochlear nucleus in vitro. *Journal of Neurophysiology, 61*, 149–161.

McGuire, B., Fiorillo B., Ryugo, D. K., & Lauer, A. M. (2015). Auditory nerve synapses persist in ventral cochlear nucleus after loss of acoustic input in mice with early-onset progressive hearing loss. *Brain Research, 1605*, 22–30.

Meidinger, M. A., Hidebrandt-Schoenfeld, H., & Illing R. B. (2006). Cochlear damage induces GAP-43 expression in cholinergic synapses of the cochlear nucleus in the adult rat: a light and electron micriscipy study. *European Journal of Neuroscience, 23*, 3187–3199.

Meltzer, N. E., & Ryugo, D. K. (2006). Projections from auditory cortex to cochlear nucleus: A comparative analysis of rat and mouse. *The Anatomical Record. Discoveries in Molecular Cellular Evolutionary Biology, 288*, 397–408.

Milbrandt, J. C., & Caspary, D. M. (1995). Age-related reduction of [3H]strychnine binding sites in the cochlear nucleus of the Fisher 344 rat. *Neuroscience, 67*(3), 713–719.

Needham, K., & Paolini, A. G. (2006). Neural timing, inhibition and the nature of stellate cell interaction in the ventral cochlear nucleus. *Hearing Research, 216*, 31–42.

Ngodup, T., Goetz, J. A., McGuire, B. C., Sun, W., Lauer, A. M., & Xu-Friedman, M. A. (2015). Activity-dependent, homeostatic regulation of neurotransmitter release from auditory nerve fibers. *Proceedings of the National Academy of Sciences USA, 112*, 6479–6484.

Oleskevich, S., & Walmsley, B. (2002). Synaptic transmission in the auditory brainstem of normal and congenitally deaf mice. *Journal of Physiology, 540*(2), 447–455.

O'Neil, J. N., Limb, C. J., Baker, C. A., & Ryugo, D. K. (2010). Bilateral effects of unilateral cochlear implantation in congenitally deaf cats. *Journal of Comparative Neurology, 518*(12), 2382–23404.

Osen, K. K. (1969). Cytoarchitecture of the cochlear nuclei in the cat. *Journal of Comparative Neurology, 136*(4), 453–484.

Redd, E. E., Cahill, Pongstaporn, T., & Ryugo, D. K. (2002). The effects of congenital deafness on auditory nerve synapses: Type I and Type II multipolar cells in the anteroventral cochlear nucleus of cats. *Journal of the Association for Research in Otolaryngology, 3*, 403–417.

Redd, E. E., Pongstaporn, T., & Ryugo, D. K. (2000). The effects of congenital deafness on auditory nerve synapses and globular bushy cells in cats. *Hearing Research, 147*, 160–174.

Reiter, E. R., & Liberman, M. C. (1995). Efferent-mediated protection from acoustic overexposure: Relation to slow effects of olivocochlear stimulation. *Journal of Neurophysiology, 73*(2), 506–514.

Rubio, M. E. (2006). Redistribution of synaptic AMPA receptors at glutamatergic synapses in the dorsal cochlear nucleus as an early response to cochlear ablation in the rat. *Hearing Research, 216–217*, 154–167.

Rubio, M. E. (2018). Microcircuits of the anteroventral cochlear nucleus. In D. L. Oliver et al. (Eds.), *Springer handbook of auditory research*. The mammalian auditory pathways (65, 41–71). New York, NY: Springer International Publishing AG 2018 41. https://doi.org/10.1007/978-3-319-71798-2_3

Rubio, M. E., Gudsnuk K. A., Smith Y., & Ryugo D. K. (2008). Revealing the molecular layer of the primate dorsal cochlear nucleus. *Neuroscience, 154*, 99–113.

Rubio, M. E., & Juiz, J. M. (1998). Chemical anatomy of excitatory endings in the dorsal cochlear nucleus: Synaptic distribution of aspartate amino-transferase, glutamate and zinc. *Journal of Comparative Neurology, 399*, 341–358.

Rubio, M. E., & Juiz, J. M. (2004). Differential distribution of synaptic endings containing glutamate, glycine, and GABA in the rat dorsal cochlear nucleus. *Journal of Comparative Neurology, 477*(3), 253–272.

Rubio, M. E., & Wenthold, R. J. (1997). Glutamate receptors are selectively targeted to postsynaptic sites in neurons. *Neuron, 18*(6), 939–950.

Ryugo, D. K. (2008). Projections of low spontaneous rate, high threshold auditory nerve fibers to the small cell cap of the cochlear nucleus in cats. *Neuroscience, 154*(1), 114–126.

Ryugo, D. K., Kretzmer, E. A., & Niparko, J. K. (2005). Restoration of auditory nerve synapses in cats by cochlear implants. *Science, 310*(5753), 1490–1492.

Ryugo, D. K., Pongstaporn, T., Huchton, D. M., & Niparko, J. K. (1997). Ultrastructural analysis of primary endings in deaf white cats: Morphologic alterations in endbulbs of Held. *The Journal of Comparative Neurology, 385*(2), 230–244.

Saldaña, E. (1993). Descending projections from the inferior colliculus to the cochlear nuclei in mammals. In M. A. Merchán, J. M. Juiz, D. A. Godfrey, & E. Mugnaini (Eds.), *The mammalian cochlear nuclei: Organization and function* (pp. 153–165). New York, NY: Plenum Publishing Corporation.

Seal, P. A., Akil, O., Yi, E., Weber, C. M., Grant, L., Yoo, J., . . . Edwards, R. H. (2008). Sensorineural deafness and seizures in mice lacking vesicular glutamate transporter 3. *Neuron, 57*(2), 263–275.

Shore, S. E., El Kashlan, H., & Lu, J. (2003). Effects of trigeminal ganglion stimulation on unit activity of ventral cochlear nucleus neurons. *Neuroscience, 119*, 1085–1101.

Shore, S. E., Helfert, R. H., Bledsoe, S. C. Jr., Altschuler, R. A., & Godfrey, D. A. (1991). Descending projections to the ventral and dorsal divisions of the cochlear nucleus in guinea pig. *Hearing Research, 52*, 255–268.

Shore, S. E., Vass, Z., Wys, N. L., & Altschuler, R. A. (2000). Trigeminal ganglion innervates the auditory brainstem. *Journal of Comparative Neurology, 419*(3), 271–285.

Spangler, K. M., Cant, N. B., Henkel, C.K., Farley, G.R., & Warr, W. B. (1987). Descending projections from the superior olivary complex to the cochlear nucleus of the cat. *The Journal of Comparative Neurology, 259*(3), 452–465.

Sumner, C. J., Tucci, D. L., & Shore, S. E. (2005). Responses of the ventral cochlear nucleus to contralateral sound following conductive hearing loss. *Journal of Neurophysiology, 94*, 4234–4343.

Suneja, S. K., Potashner, S. J., & Benson, C. G. (1998). Plastic changes in glycine and GABA release and uptake in adult brain stem auditory nuclei after unilateral middle ear ossicle removal and cochlear ablation. *Experimental Neurology, 151*, 273–288.

Suneja, S. K., Potashner, S. J., & Benson, C. G. (2000). AMPA receptor binding in adult guinea pig brain stem after unilateral ablation. *Experimental Neurology, 165*, 355–389.

Takamori, S., Malherbe, P., Broger, C., & Jahn, R. (2002). Molecular cloning and functional characterization of human vesicular glutamate transporter 3. *EMBO Reports, 3*(8), 798–803.

Tierney, T. S., Russell, F. A., & Moore, D. R. (1997). Susceptibility of developing cochlear nucleus neurons to deafferentation-induced death abruptly ends just before the onset of hearing. *Journal of Comparative Neurology, 378*, 295–306.

Trussell, L. O., & Oertel, D. (2018). Microcircuits of the dorsal cochlear nucleus. In D. L. Oliver et al. (Eds.), The mammalian auditory pathways, *Springer handbook of auditory research* (65, pp.73–99). New York, NY: Springer International Publishing AG 2018 41.

Tucci, D. L., Cant, N. B., & Durham, D. (1999). Conductive hearing loss results in a decrease in central auditory system activity in the young gerbil. *Laryngoscope, 109*(9), 1359–1371.

Turrigiano, G. (2011). Too many cooks? Intrinsic and synaptic homeostatic mechanisms in cortical circuit refinement. *Annual Review in Neuroscience, 34*, 89–103.

Vetter, D. E., Adams, J. C., & Mugnaini, E. (1991). Chemically distinct rat olivocochlear neurons. *Synapse, 7*, 21–43.

Vogler, D. P., Roberston, D., & Mulders, W. H. A.M. (2011). Hyperactivity in the ventral cochlear nucleus after cochlear trauma. *Journal of Neuroscience, 31*(18), 6639–6645.

Wang, H., Yin, G., Rogers, K., Miralles, C., De Blas, A. L., & Rubio, M. E. (2011). Monaural conductive hearing loss alters the general expression of the GluA3 AMPA and glycine receptor α1 subunits in bushy and fusiform cells of the cochlear nucleus. *Neuroscience, 199*, 438–451.

Warren, E. H. 3rd, & Liberman, M. C. (1989a). Effects of contralateral sound on auditory-nerve responses. I. Contributions of cochlear efferents. Hearing Research, 37(2), 89–104.

Warren, E. H. 3rd., & Liberman, M. C. (1989b). Effects of contralateral sound on auditory-nerve responses. II. Dependence on stimulus variables. Hearing Research, 37(2), 105–121.

Waterlood, F. G., & Mugnaini, E. (1984). Cartwheel neurons of the dorsal cochlear nucleus: A Golgi-electron microscopic study in rat. *Journal of Comparative Neurology, 227*(1), 136–157.

Weinberg, R. J., & Rustioni, A. (1989). Brainstem projections to the rat cuneate nucleus. *Journal of Comparative Neurology, 282*(1), 142–156.

Weston, M.C., Nehring, R. B., Wojcik, S. M., & Rosendmund C. (2011). Interplay between VGLUT isoforms and endophilin A1 regulates neurotransmitter release and short-term plasticity. *Neuron, 69*, 1147–1159.

Whiting, B., Moiseff, A., & Rubio, M. E. (2009). Cochlear nucleus neurons redistribute synaptic AMPA and glycine receptors in response to monaural conductive hearing loss. *Neuroscience, 163*(4), 1264–1276.

Willott J. F., Milbrandt, J. C., Bross, L. S., & Caspary, D. M. (1997). Glycine immunoreactivity and receptor binding in the cochlear nucleus of C57BL/6J and CBA/CaJ mice: effects of cochlear impairment and aging. *Journal of Comparative Neurology, 385*, 405–414.

Willot, J. F., Parham, K., & Hunter, P. K. (1987). Comparison of the auditory sensitivity of neurons of the ventral cochlear nucleus and inferior colliculus of young and aging C57/BL and CBA/J mice. *Hearing Research, 53*, 78–94.

Wright, S., Hwang, Y., & Oertel, D. (2014). Synaptic transmission between end bulbs of Held and bushy cells in the cochlear nucleus of mice with a mutation in Otoferlin. *Journal of Neurophysiology, 112*(12), 3173–3188.

Wu, C., Martel, D. T., & Shore, S. E. (2016). Increased synchrony and bursting of dorsal cochlear nucleus fusiform cells correlate with tinnitus. *Journal of Neuroscience, 36*(6), 2068–2073.

Yao, W., & Godfrey, D.A. (1996). Autoradiographic distribution of muscarinic acetylcholine receptor subtypes in rat cochlear nucleus. *Auditory Neuroscience, 2*, 241–255.

Young, E. D., & Oertel, D. (2003). Cochlear nucleus. In G. M. Shepherd (Ed.), *The synaptic organization of the brain* (5th ed., ch. 4, pp.125–163). Oxford, England: Oxford University Press.

Young, E. D., Oertel, D. (2010). Cochlear nucleus. In G. M. Shepherd & S. Grillner (Eds.), *Handbook of Brain Microcircuits* (pp. 215–223). New York, NY: Oxford.

Youssoufian, M., Oleskevich, S., & Walmsley, B. (2008). Maturation of auditory brainstem projections and calyces in the congenitally deaf (dn/dn) mouse. *The Journal of Comparative Neurology, 506*(3), 442–451.

Zhao, Y., Rubio, M. E., & Tzounopoulos, T. (2011). Mechanisms underlying input-specific synaptic plasticity in the dorsal cochlear nucleus. *Hearing Research, 279*(1–2), 67–73.

Zeng, C., Nannapaneni, N., Zhou, J., Hughes, L. F., & Shore, S. (2009). Cochlear damage changes the distribution of vesicular glutamate transporters associated with auditory and nonauditory inputs to the cochlear nucleus. *Journal of Neuroscience, 29*(13), 4210–4217.

Zhou, J., Nannapaneni, N., & Shore, S. (2007). Vessicular glutamate transporters 1 and 2 are differentially associated with auditory nerve and spinal trigeminal inputs to the cochlear nucleus. *Journal of Comparative Neurology*, *500*(4), 777–787.

Zhou, Y., & Danbolt, N. C. (2014). Glutamate as a neurotransmitter in the healthy brain. *Journal of Neural Transmission*, *121*(8), 799–817.

Zhuang, X., Sun, W., & Xu-Friedman, M. A. (2017). Changes in properties of auditory nerve synapses following conductive hearing loss. *Journal of Neuroscience*, *37*(2), 323–332.

CHAPTER 7

AGE-RELATED AND NOISE-INDUCED HEARING LOSS

Central Consequences in the Ventral Cochlear Nucleus

RUILI XIE, TESSA-JONNE F. ROPP, MICHAEL R. KASTEN, AND PAUL B. MANIS

Abstract

Hearing loss generally occurs in the auditory periphery but leads to changes in the central auditory system. Noise-induced hearing loss (NIHL) and age-related hearing loss (ARHL) affect neurons in the ventral cochlear nucleus (VCN) at both the cellular and systems levels. In response to a decrease in auditory nerve activity associated with hearing loss, the large synaptic endings of the auditory nerve, the endbulbs of Held, undergo simplification of their structure and the volume of the postsynaptic bushy neurons decreases. A major functional change shared by NIHL and ARHL is the development of asynchronous transmitter release at endbulb synapses during periods of high afferent firing. Compensatory adjustements in transmitter release, including changes in release probability and quantal content, have also been reported. The excitability of the bushy cells undergoes subtle changes in the long-term, although short-term, reversible changes in excitability may also occur. These changes are not consistently observed across all models of hearing loss, suggesting that the time course of hearing loss, and potential developmental effects, may influence endbulb transmission in multiple ways. NIHL can alter the representation of the loudness of tonal stimuli by VCN neurons and is accompanied by changes in spontaneous activity in VCN neurons. However, little is known about the representation of more complex stimuli. The relationship between mechanistic changes in VCN neurons with noise-induced or age-related hearing loss, the accompanying change in sensory coding, and the reversibility of changes with the reintroduction of auditory nerve activity are areas that deserve further thoughtful exploration.

Keywords: hearing, cochlear nucleus, synaptic transmission, spontaneous activity, aging, noise-induced hearing loss, genetic hearing loss

THE cochlear nuclear complex (CNC) is the sole target of the auditory nerve. The CNC performs the initial computations that transform auditory information into separate representational streams, or distinct "parallel" pathways (Cant & Benson, 2003). These initial computations depend on auditory nerve targets, local circuit innervation patterns, and the physiological properties of different cell types across the CNC. Specific processing mechanisms within the CNC are in turn essential for the other centers of the ascending auditory pathways to precisely and effectively perform their sensory integration tasks. The processing mechanisms at each stage, including in the CNC, are also sensitive to the status of the auditory periphery as it is modified by noise-induced hearing loss (NIHL) or age-related hearing loss (ARHL). Hearing-loss induces changes in excitatory and inhibitory synaptic function, network structure, and the intrinsic electrical excitability of neurons.

The pathology of the auditory system that leads to hearing loss has been most extensively studied in the auditory periphery. Damage to the peripheral end organ, the cochlea, can affect the functional organization of the central auditory system by altering the activity patterns in the auditory nerve. Changes in central function include the organization of central neural circuits, the dynamic operation of synapses, and the excitability of cells. All of these contribute to how sensory stimuli are represented in the spike firing population code in terms of both rate and timing. Synapses in the CNC are the first in the central auditory pathway to experience anatomical and physiological changes, and activity-dependent changes in their function can degrade the information available to the rest of the central auditory system. For this reason, the response of the central auditory system to peripheral auditory pathology, including auditory neuropathies (Moser & Starr, 2016) is now recognized as an important consideration when evaluating and treating hearing loss (Atcherson, Nagaraj, Kennett, & Levisee, 2015; Moore et al., 2014).

In this chapter, we focus on the consequences of noise-induced and age-related hearing loss, and some select preclinical genetic deafness models, on processing in one region of the CNC, the ventral cochlear nucleus (VCN). We discuss the consequences of hearing loss for target neurons that form the major output pathways of the ventral cochlear nucleus (VCN). A particular focus of the existing literature is on the consequences for the specialized synapses of the auditory nerve, the endbulbs of Held (Manis, Xie, Wang, Marrs, & Spirou, 2012), that terminate on VCN bushy neurons. This chapter considers how the total loss of auditory nerve input affects VCN neurons; outlines potential and distinct consequences of peripheral hearing loss that may influence how VCN cells respond to that loss; reviews studies that have examined the consequences of noise-induced hearing loss (NIHL) and age-related hearing loss (ARHL) at both the systems and cellular levels; and reviews studies of hearing loss resulting from genetic causes, at the cellular level. Other kinds of hearing loss, such as caused by ototoxic drugs and conductive mechanism failures, are not discussed, but it is important to recognize that these types of loses are likely to involve related mechanistic changes in the central auditory system.

Cells of the VCN

Bushy (BCs) and planar multipolar cells (pMCs, also known as "T-stellate cells") are two of the four neuronal types that project from the VCN to other auditory centers (Cant & Benson, 2003). BCs project to the superior olivary complex, where they innervate cells involved in binaural processing and facilitate sound localization. BCs can be divided into two major populations based on the shape of their soma and on their projections: spherical bushy cells (sBCs) and globular bushy cells (gBCs). sBCs receive synaptic input from 2–4 auditory nerve fibers via large endings called endbulbs of Held (Manis et al., 2012). Each endbulb has up to 100 individual release sites. This synaptic configuration facilitates strong and very rapid release of neurotransmitter for each spike in the presynaptic auditory nerve fiber. sBCs project to the lateral superior olive and, in animals with good low-frequency hearing, to the medial superior olive. It is unclear whether the sBCs are present in mice (Lauer, Connelly, Graham, & Ryugo, 2013). gBCs receive convergent input from 10 to 70 auditory nerve fibers (ANFs) in cat (Liberman, 1991; Spirou, Rager, & Manis, 2005) and project to the lateral superior olive, as well as the medial nucleus of the trapezoid body. All bushy cell types spike precisely in response to rapid fluctuations in sound intensity at low frequencies (in cells with characteristic frequencies (CF) up to 3 kHz in cats and guinea pigs), and can report the phase of a tone with high temporal precision. Very low frequency bushy cells (CF < 500 Hz) can improve the temporal precision of spiking relative to auditory nerve fibers (Joris, Carney, Smith, & Yin, 1994). Consequently, the bushy cell pathways are important for both azimuthal sound localization (which depends on temporal differences between the ears) and for pitch discrimination (which depends on frequency-specific firing to a sound). When representing higher frequencies, bushy cells convey other kinds of temporal cues, including onsets and envelope information and may provide information useful for aspects of auditory scene analysis (Keine, Rubsamen, & Englitz, 2017).

The other major cell population in the VCN, the pMCs ("T-stellate cells"), project to the inferior colliculus (Adams, 1983) and additionally have collaterals in the VCN and the dorsal cochlear nucleus (DCN; Doucet & Ryugo, 1997; Oertel, Wu, Garb, & Dizack, 1990). pMCs encode acoustic cues, such as sound intensity and amplitude modulation, in their firing rate and spike timing (Frisina, Smith, & Chamberlain, 1990; Rhode & Greenberg, 1994). Like BCs, pMCs receive strong direct AN input, but pMCs have poor temporal firing precision relative to the fine structure of the acoustic waveform. pMCs are also thought to be part of a pathway that is involved in early stages of analyzing narrow-band signals embedded in wideband maskers (Pressnitzer, Meddis, Delahaye, & Winter, 2001; Xie & Manis, 2013b), a process known as comodulation masking release (Hall, Haggard, & Fernandes, 1984).

Two other smaller populations of cells found in the CNC are the octopus and radiate multipolar cells (rMC, also known as "D-stellate cells"). Both of these cell types receive convergent input from auditory nerve fibers representing a wide range of cochlear locations by virtue of the orientation of their dendrites (Oertel, Bal, Gardner, Smith, & Joris, 2000; Oertel et al., 1990; Xie & Manis, 2017a), and thus have very broad sensitivity to sound frequency (Godfrey, Kiang, & Norris, 1975; Jiang, Palmer, & Winter, 1996; Palmer, Jiang, & Marshall, 1996; Rhode & Smith, 1986; Ritz & Brownell, 1982). The octopus cells are found in the posteroventral cochlear nucleus and are highly specialized to provide detection of coincident activity across a population of auditory nerve fibers (McGinley, Liberman, Bal, & Oertel, 2012; Spencer, Grayden, Bruce, Meffin, & Burkitt, 2012). They respond transiently with an "onset" response to tones, but can represent low-frequency pitch information with high precision (Rhode, 1998). The rMCs are inhibitory neurons that project widely within the CNC (Arnott, Wallace, Shackleton, & Palmer, 2004; Doucet, Ross, Gillespie, & Ryugo, 1999; Oertel et al., 1990), and also to the contralateral CNC (Doucet & Ryugo, 2006; Schofield & Cant, 1996; Smith, Massie, & Joris, 2005). For these two cell types, there is a very limited literature about the consequences of hearing loss on their responses to sound.

Physiological and Anatomical Changes in Following Total Loss of AN Activity

Long-term damage to auditory structures causes pronounced changes in VCN cellular and anatomical properties. To understand the role of auditory nerve spike activity in the auditory nerve, two different approaches are taken to abolish responses to sound. The most direct is cochlear ablation, where the cochlea is removed, destroying the dendrites (and often somas, depending on the technique used) of the spiral ganglion cells (SGCs). Loss of the cochlea and SGC dendrites silences the activity of the auditory nerve, leaving spontaneous and trophic activity intact; death of SGC somas destroys the auditory nerve eliminating even spontaneous and trophic activity. The other approach is to apply tetrodotoxin (TTX) to block voltage-gated sodium channels. TTX silences the spiking activity of the nerve, eliminating all but spontaneous quantal release of neurotransmitter and trophic signaling at central ANF terminals.

Similar to TTX, cochlear ablation in cats immediately decreases the spontaneous firing rates of VCN neurons, but not dorsal cochlear nucleus neurons (Koerber, Pfeiffer, Warr, & Kiang, 1966). Spontaneous rates in the VCN do not recover up to 77 days after cochlear destruction. Both cochlear ablation and TTX application to the cochlea cause rapid compensatory changes in VCN neurons within hours after cessation of auditory nerve activity (Pasic, Moore, & Rubel, 1994; Pasic & Rubel, 1989; Sie & Rubel, 1992). Unilateral cochlear removal in p7 mouse and gerbil results in quantitative neuronal cell loss in the anterior VCN (aVCN) within 48 hours, while in mouse, TUNEL labeling (indicative of apoptosis) is seen as soon as 12 hours after cochlea removal. In older animals, cochlear ablation after a "critical period" (about p7 in rodents), leads to no neuronal cell loss (Hashisaki & Rubel, 1989; Mostafapour, Cochran, Del Puerto, & Rubel, 2000); however, neuronal cell size in aVCN is reduced after cochlear removal in older mice (Pasic et al., 1994; Pasic & Rubel, 1989). Decreases in aVCN cell size, but not in number, are seen when inner hair cells are acutely ablated in genetically engineered adult mice with a diphtheria toxin receptor (Tong et al., 2015). Overall, these studies are consistent in observing that acute loss of auditory nerve activity causes neuronal apoptosis in aVCN in animals before the onset of hearing, whereas older animals demonstrate changes in aVCN morphology and physiology.

Many neurons, including those in the auditory pathways, undergo homeostatic adjustments in their excitability in response to long-term synaptic input and firing changes (Desai, Rutherford, & Turrigiano, 1999; Kotak et al., 2005; Leao, Berntson, Forsythe, & Walmsley, 2004; Ngodup et al., 2015; Rao et al., 2010). In general, long-term decreases in excitatory synaptic drive lead to increased electrical excitability. In chickens, cochlear ablation leads to a transient decrease in immunoreactivity for Kv1.1 and Kv3.1 potassium channels, but protein levels of both channels recover to near normal levels by 2 weeks (Lu, Monsivais, Tempel, & Rubel, 2004). In rats, a short-term block of auditory nerve activity by TTX results in a loss of immunoreactivity for presynaptic KCNQ5 (a ligand-regulated voltage-sensitive potassium conductance (Schroeder, Hechenberger, Weinreich, Kubisch, & Jentsch, 2000)) in endbulbs within 2 hours (Caminos, Garcia-Pino, & Juiz, 2015); whether this is a persistent or transient loss is not clear. In order to determine whether destruction of the SGCs and removal of the ANF input also affects the electrical excitability of aVCN neurons, Francis and Manis (2000) performed bilateral cochlear ablations in 4-week old rats, including a substantial invasion of the modiolus to remove the SGCs. The intrinsic excitability of VCN neurons (including both BCs and MCs) showed only modest changes two weeks after the ablation. Presumed BCs, specifically those showing only single spike responses to depolarizing current injection, were slightly depolarized, had smaller action potentials with smaller spike after-hyperpolarizations, and had shorter membrane time constants. The population of BCs that fired 2–3 spikes in response to intracellular current injection were not significantly affected. Presumed MCs (largely pMCs) nearly doubled their input resistance on average but showed no other changes.

Taken together, these results indicate that in adult animals after loss of peripheral activity and input, not only do VCN cells survive, but they also largely retain their fundamental physiological identities.

Noise-Induced Hearing Loss

Overexposure to noise, particularly at extreme loudness or for a prolonged time, can severely injure the auditory periphery (D'Sa, Gross, Francone, & Morest, 2007; Feng,

Bendiske, & Morest, 2012; Guthrie, 2017; Valero et al., 2017; Wang, Hirose, & Liberman, 2002) and lead to permanent noise-induced hearing loss (NIHL). The consequences of NIHL are complex and depend on the level, duration, and pattern of exposure (Wang et al., 2002). Thus, it is difficult to assign a single consequence for central processing to NIHL. However, consideration of the types of peripheral pathology induced by noise can help to set the conceptual framework for studying central consequences of NIHL. Intense noise exposure can damage hair cell stereocilia, resulting in elevated thresholds at the level of the ANF, but responses to sound can still occur (Liberman, 1987; Liberman & Dodds, 1984). Modest noise can also eliminate the response to sound in individual ANFs by damaging the inner hair cells or the SGC terminals (Kujawa & Liberman, 2009). More extensive damage to cochlear structures can reduce the sensory response by damaging the lateral wall of the cochlea (Wang et al., 2002). If damaged inner hair cells remain functionally connected to SGCs, the auditory nerve can still possess spontaneous activity, because the spontaneous firing is driven by vesicular (quantal) release from inner hair cells (Chapochnikov et al., 2014; Kiang, Liberman, & Levine, 1976; Rutherford, Chapochnikov, & Moser, 2012; Siegel, 1992). However, damage to inner hair cell synaptic mechanisms, the SGC afferent synapses or dendrites, or to the stria vascularis can lead to silencing of the auditory nerve or death of nerve fibers. The integrity of the stereocilary bundle may determine whether there is any sensory activity in an individual auditory nerve. Damage to the reticular lamina, tectorial membrane, or the stria vascularis may affect large numbers of ANFs. In many studies of NIHL, sound responses are not completely abolished, but individual ANFs may exhibit high thresholds and low average firing rates for the same sound intensity (Heinz, Issa, & Young, 2005; Heinz & Young, 2004), while other ANFs may be silent. The recognition that the high-threshold, low-spontaneous population of ANFs is particularly vulnerable to noise damage (Furman, Kujawa, & Liberman, 2013; Kujawa & Liberman, 2006, 2009) and aging (Sergeyenko, Lall, Liberman, & Kujawa, 2013) increases the complexity of interpreting central responses to hearing loss. All of these factors need to be considered when evaluating the effects of NIHL on VCN neurons.

NIHL: VCN Neuroanatomy

Extremely loud noise damages the peripheral auditory system leading to hearing loss and degeneration of synapses and neurons in the CNC (D'Sa et al., 2007; Feng et al., 2012; Kim, Gross, Morest, & Potashner, 2004; Kim, Gross, Potashner, & Morest, 2004a, 2004b; Sekiya et al., 2012). In adult mice (F1 C57BL/6J X CBA), 6 hours of exposure to broadband noise at 115 dB SPL destroys essentially all outer hair cells, and damages a majority of the inner hair cells and auditory nerve fibers (Feng et al 2012). The exposure results in a decrease in the synaptic vesicle protein SV2 in synapses in the posteroventral cochlear nucleus (PVCN) and a reduction of the total volume of the PVCN, as measured eight weeks after exposure. In adult Sprague-Dawley rats, a one-minute exposure to an octave-band noise centered at 4 kHz at 137 dB SPL produced similar damage in the cochlea but only a selective loss of neurons in aVCN (Sekiya et al., 2012).

The damaging effect of a single traumatic noise exposure can be long lasting in the VCN and may be followed by a period of axonal sprouting and re-innervation from non-cochlear sources. In chinchillas exposed to 108 dB SPL octave-band noise for 3 hours (Kim, Gross, Morest et al., 2004; Kim, Gross et al., 2004a, 2004b), there was long-term neurodegeneration with substantial loss of axons and synaptic terminals in the first 16–24 weeks after exposure. The degenerated VCN synapses included excitatory endings belonging to both the auditory nerve, and endings that are presumably local collaterals between VCN neurons (Kim, Gross, Morest et al., 2004; Kim, Gross et al., 2004a).

Following the noise exposure, the number of synapses in the VCN recovers, apparently by new growth of synaptic endings as observed at 24–32 weeks after noise exposure. The recovery was more pronounced for excitatory synapses, possibly as an adaptive compensation for decreased auditory nerve inputs (Kim, Gross, Morest et al., 2004). Some of the new synapses, including axo-somatic terminals onto gBCs, appear to come from central neurons instead of the terminals from the SGCs, suggesting a dynamic reorganization of synaptic connections following NIHL (Kim, Gross, Morest et al., 2004; Kim, Gross et al., 2004b). Indeed, following noise exposure, the expression of growth-associated protein 43 (GAP-43), a protein found in neuronal growth cones (Skene, 1989) and in synapses undergoing remodeling (Holahan, 2017), is increased in the VCN (Kraus et al., 2011; Michler & Illing, 2002).

While the precise origin of these new synapses is unclear, cochlear ablation experiments suggest these synapses might be collaterals of olivocochlear fibers (Meidinger, Hildebrandt-Schoenfeld, & Illing, 2006). In rats, cholinergic inputs to the VCN are thought to arise from collaterals of the olivocochlear system (~20%), from small neurons in the ventral nucleus of the trapezoid body (~65%), and from sources within the CNC (~15%; Jin, Godfrey, & Sun, 2005). Consistent with new or additional innervation by a cholinergic component of the olivocochlear system, there is an increase in the activity of ChAT, the synthetic enzyme for acetylcholine, in the VCN following cochlear ablation (Jin et al., 2005). Two other potential sources of non-cholinergic terminals are the pMCs, which normally have collaterals within the VCN (Oertel et al., 1990) and trigeminal ganglion afferents, which also sparsely innervate the central VCN (Shore, Vass, Wys, & Altschuler, 2000). Overall, these results suggest that the loss of auditory nerve input to the VCN may be associated with a compensatory innervation by other central auditory, and potentially non-auditory, pathways that already project into the VCN. However, whether this also occurs with NIHL or aging is not yet certain.

NIHL: System-Level Functional Studies

Acoustic trauma has immediate effect on the response properties of VCN cells. Boettcher and Salvi (1993) recorded peristimulus histograms (PSTH) before and after an acute exposure in rats. The exposure stimulus was a three to five-minute continuous tone at 90–105 dB SPL, positioned a half-octave above the unit characteristic frequency (CF). Noise exposure increased compound action potential thresholds above the exposure frequency by ~15 dB. Although there were no clear changes in the PSTH patterns, they found that the effect of the tone exposure varied within the response area of the cell. For cells whose spontaneous activity was inhibited by the sound exposure (27% of recorded cells), suppression of inhibition was seen, and most (64%) cells also exhibited increased firing at CF. In the remainder of the cells, overt inhibition was not observed at or near the frequency of the exposure stimulus. However, most (66%) of these cells showed a broadening of tuning with increased sound level concurrent with a general decrease in firing rate. The decrease in firing rate was observed independently at CF or above CF, or both at and above CF, in 66% of the recorded cells. Interestingly, spontaneous rates of most of the cells remained largely unchanged after the noise exposure, although a subset of cells showed changes in spontaneous rate despite no overt evidence for a change in inhibition. The mechanisms underlying these changes are not entirely clear. Some of the effects can be explained by the increase in thresholds in the cochlear region affected by the tone exposure, but some of the effects may result from a short-term suppression of excitability of local inhibitory neurons or depression of inhibitory synapses. It is unclear whether these short-term effects are reversible.

Cai, Ma, and Young (2009) examined long-term changes in the response properties of cells in the VCN after noise exposure. Measurements were made between 33 and 121 days after exposing cats to a narrowband noise centered at 2 kHz at 111–112 dB SPL for four hours. This exposure paradigm produces a permanent threshold shift across low frequencies, while maintaining relatively normal thresholds in the high frequency response areas. Although individual VCN units mirrored the effects of the cochlear threshold shift, the general physiological response characteristics across units were similar to those seen in unexposed animals. All of the expected response patterns, including primary-like, primary-like with notch and choppers were observed. Measures of discharge regularity and first spike latency were also not different between normal and exposed cats; however, neurons with chopper PSTHs (from pMCs; (Rhode, Oertel, & Smith, 1983; Rouiller & Ryugo, 1984; Smith & Rhode, 1989)) exhibited increased firing rates for suprathreshold sounds, even though their thresholds were elevated. In contrast, neurons with primary-like and primary-like with notch responses (BCs) had lower firing rates to BF tones, more closely reflecting the pattern of activity in the noise-impaired auditory nerve (Heinz et al., 2005; Heinz & Young, 2004). Neurons in noise-exposed animals also tended to have broader tuning, as determined by smaller Q10 values relative to normal units, irrespective of PSTH shape. The mechanism that causes the increase in firing rates of MCs is not clear, although weakened inhibition from the two main inhibitory sources, the tuberculoventral cells or the rMP cells, are prime candidates.

Vogler, Robertson, and Mulders (2011) compared the effects of a sham noise exposure, a mechanical lesion of the basal cochlear region, and acoustic trauma from a 10 kHz, 124 dB SPL tone for 2 hours in adult guinea pigs. Recordings were made 2 weeks after exposure. All PSTH types (primary-like, chopper and onset) could be identified in the noise exposed and mechanical trauma animals, and the frequency of occurrence was not different from the sham exposure animals. Neurons from both the low and high frequency regions of the VCN showed increased spontaneous firing, although this was most pronounced in the primary-like and onset cells, and less clear in the chopper class (although the transient choppers appeared to show a larger increase in spontaneous firing than the sustained choppers). Rate-intensity functions were not reported in this study.

These studies differ considerably in their noise exposure paradigms, species and recovery times. However, they are consistent in noting that NIHL does not substantially affect the fundamental response properties of VCN neurons of different classes, in that all of the expected PSTH patterns are present in similar proportions as in control subjects. Thresholds increase in parallel with threshold shifts in auditory nerve. In terms of possibly pathological changes in the VCN, NIHL induced by intense stimuli appears to increase spontaneous firing rates, at least in some cell populations, and selectively increases the steepness of the tone rate-intensity function in MCs, which may contribute to loudness recruitment.

NIHL: Synaptic Changes in the CN

In addition to the well documented anatomical changes across CN synapses and cells after NIHL, notable changes in synaptic physiology were also observed in mature animals. Synaptic transmission was studied at the endbulb of Held in mature CBA/CaJ mice at 2–4 months of age, under normal hearing and NIHL (Xie & Manis, 2012). NIHL was induced by a 2-hour exposure to 8-16kHz band noise at 106 dB SPL at postnatal day 25. As shown in Figure 7.1A, auditory nerve stimulation evoked EPSCs in BCs of normal hearing mice throughout the 400 Hz stimulus train, with reliable synchronous EPSCs during the latter half of the train (inset). In age-matched young mice with NIHL, the EPSCs were similar only during the initial phase of the train. EPSCs deteriorated in the second half of the train, showing long-lasting asynchronous EPSCs and reduced peak amplitude (Figure 7.1B). The results indicate that synaptic transmission at the endbulb of Held is compromised during high rate activity after NIHL. In a separate study (Rich, Xie, & Manis, 2010), synaptic quantal release frequency and amplitude were increased at auditory nerve synapses onto VCN stellate neurons (mostly pMCs) in mice with a permanent NIHL produced by octave band noise exposure for 2 hours at 114 dB SPL. A more modest exposure (98 dB SPL) that produced a temporary threshold shift only increased event frequency, but not amplitude. It is unclear whether the increased frequency is a consequence of additional innervation in response to cochlear damage or represents a compensatory response of synaptic release mechanisms.

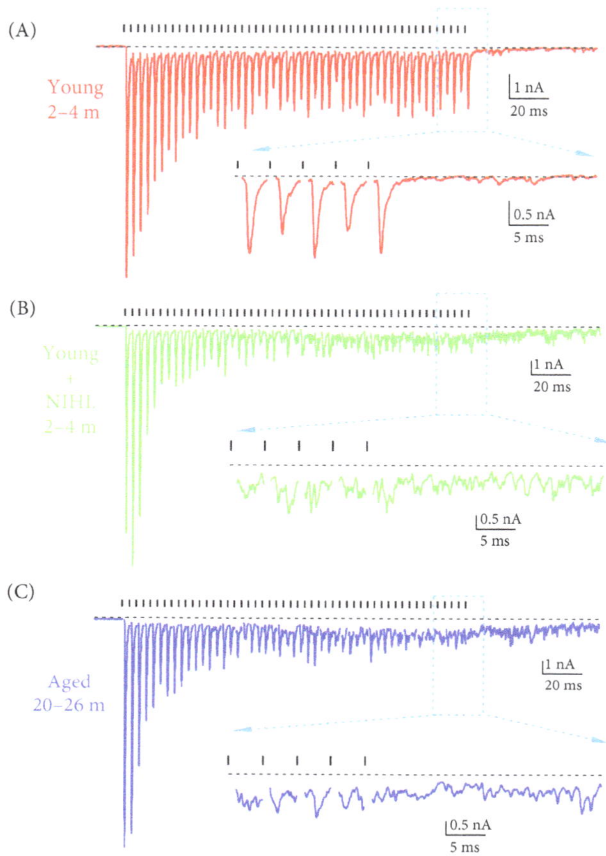

FIGURE 7.1. Synaptic transmission at the endbulb of Held deteriorates similarly in young mice with noise-induced hearing loss (NIHL) and aged mice with age-related hearing loss (ARHL). **A**: Example EPSCs evoked by auditory nerve stimulation at 400 Hz in normal hearing young mice (2–4 months). Ticks on top mark the onset of the stimuli in the 400 Hz train. Insets show the last 5 stimuli. **B**: Example EPSCs in age-matched young mice with NIHL, which was induced by noise exposure to a 8–16kHz band noise at 106 dB SPL for 2 hours at the age of 25 days. Notice the reduced EPSC peak amplitude and the increased asynchronous release (EPSC responses that are not timely are locked to the stimulus inputs) during the late stage of the trains. **C**: Example EPSCs in aged mice with ARHL. Notice the reduced EPSC amplitudes and increased asynchronous release similar to **B**. This reduction suggests that the physiological function of the endbulb of Held synapses changes during hearing loss.

Sources: A and C are modified with permission of John Wiley and Sons from Figure 4 in Xie and Manis, 2017, *Journal of Physiology*; NIHL trace in **B** is unpublished data by Xie and Manis.

NIHL: Synaptic Changes in the CN after "Benign" Noise Exposure

The intense, long duration noise exposures described earlier are not commonly encountered in the environment. Recent studies on NIHL have focused on noise exposure at moderate levels that only cause temporary threshold-shift in hearing, as evaluated by auditory brainstem response measurements. Surprisingly, Kujawa and Liberman (2009) found that exposure to noise at moderate levels can cause permanent cochlear synaptopathy, involving damage of the synapses between the inner hair cells and the peripheral terminal of the SGCs, even while the inner hair cells remain intact. SGC somata can survive for a long time after such deafferentation (Kujawa & Liberman, 2009) and the same is likely true for SGC central branches (the auditory nerve) and the synaptic terminals in CNC. The degeneration of endbulb and other CNC synapses seen after intense noise trauma (Kim, Gross, Morest et al., 2004; Kim, Gross et al., 2004a, 2004b) has not been reported following exposure to noise at moderate levels.

Physiologically, moderate noise exposure modifies sensory inputs to CN and leads to homeostatic regulation of vesicle release at CN synapses (Ngodup et al., 2015; Rich et al., 2010). At the endbulb of Held synapse, the high release probability of the synaptic transmission measured in normal hearing CBA/Caj mice was reduced after the mice were reared between 6 and 50 days in noise (1.6–39 kHz) at 90-94 dB SPL (Ngodup et al., 2015). The number of release sites at the endbulb of Held was significantly increased in noise-reared mice, which is consistent with larger vesicular glutamate transporter type 1 (vGluT1) labeled puncta at the terminals. The decreased release probability recovered to normal levels after the noise-reared mice were returned to quiet, suggesting that there is a homeostatic regulation of vesicle release at the endbulb of Held that relies on the activity levels of the auditory nerve input. Interestingly, in these experiments, the intrinsic excitability of the BCs as reflected by spike threshold, action potential height, and action potential width, showed small but significant changes. These results suggest that noise exposure, even if it is not overtly damaging, can dynamically adjust the operating points of central synapses and cells.

Age-Related Hearing Loss

When considering the effects of age, it is important to recognize that the majority of SGCs survive throughout the lifetime of the organism (Makary, Shin, Kujawa, Liberman, & Merchant, 2011; Sergeyenko et al., 2013; Sha et al., 2008). The integrity and functionality of SGC central synapses in the CNC will therefore play an essential role in the development of ARHL. Indeed, during aging SGC synapses show anatomical and physiological modifications that could contribute to ARHL.

AHRL: System Level Functional Studies

There are surprisingly few studies of the effects of aging on the responses of VCN neurons in vivo. The progression of hearing loss in 7–12 month old C57BL/6J mice (Willott, Parham, & Hunter, 1991) in part replicates the age-related cochlear pathology that often accompanies aging. The peripheral loss of high frequency hearing is also reflected in the sensitivity of neurons in the VCN. Single unit and multi-unit recordings in C57BL/6J mice, 7–12 months old, show an elevation in thresholds in the VCN with age as compared to young mice of the same strain or CBA/J mice (which show a much slower ARHL) of the same age. Multi-unit recordings suggest a loss of neurons with high frequency tuning, as no neurons were responsive to frequencies above 32 kHz in aged mice. This is accompanied by an increase in neurons with BFs between 8 and 32 kHz. Surprisingly, these elevations in threshold in the C57BL/6J mice are not as pronounced in recordings from the dorsal cochlear nucleus and inferior colliculus in the same strain, suggesting compensatory mechanisms downstream of the VCN. Although no differentiation of unit types by PSTH or regularity was attempted, the results in the VCN suggest that BCs and MCs likely have similar patterns of threshold shifts. Frisina and Walton (2006) reported that there is little change in gap duration recovery curves using near-field evoked potentials in the VCN of old (24 mo) as compared to young (7 mo) CBA mice.

ARHL: Synaptic Changes

In normal aging CBA/J mice, the aVCN cell number and packing density remains stable in the first year of life but shows a reduction during the second year of life (Willott, Jackson, & Hunter, 1987). The densities and the numbers of synaptic terminals in aVCN did not change with age in Fischer-344 rats up to 28 months (Helfert, Krenning, Wilson, & Hughes, 2003); however, aged rats demonstrated reduced synaptic terminal size that may reflect a reduction in neurotransmitter levels (Banay-Schwartz, Lajtha, & Palkovits, 1989a, 1989b). In a separate study, VCN synapses in 25–26 month Fischer-344 rats showed more complex endings than young rats, indicative of possible collateralization of CN neuronal processes to offset degenerative losses of SGC terminals (Keithley & Croskrey, 1990). In 18–20 month-old Wistar rats, VCN synapses showed significant decline in the immunostaining of both VGluT1 and VGAT synaptic markers, consistent with an overall decline in both excitatory and inhibitory synaptic endings during aging (Alvarado, Fuentes-Santamaria, Gabaldon-Ull, Blanco, & Juiz, 2014).

The extension of brain slice methods to record from increasingly older mice has enabled more precise analysis of synaptic transmission and excitability, revealing how specific cellular mechanisms are affected by ARHL. During ARHL, the physiological function of VCN synapses declines. In 20–26 month-old CBA/CaJ mice (Xie & Manis, 2017b), synaptic transmission at the endbulb of Held synapse was compromised by decreased synchronous release with a simultaneous increase in asynchronous release during the later phase of the 400 Hz stimulus train. In aged mice, auditory nerve stimulation evoked spikes in postsynaptic BCs with a significantly higher failure rate and decreased temporal precision (Figure 7.2). This suggests that endbulb of Held synapses cannot effectively and faithfully transmit sound information from the periphery to the VCN in aged mice (Xie, 2016). Both studies reveal two functionally important findings about the synaptic changes under ARHL (Xie, 2016; Xie & Manis, 2017b). First, synaptic transmission at the endbulb of Held in aged mice was found to be relatively normal during the onset phase of the stimulus train, but the synapses were unable to sustain ongoing activity during prolonged trains of stimulation. This finding predicts that the hearing of these aged mice with ARHL would be relatively normal for brief sound signals but may be challenged to carry information for long-duration or ongoing sounds, especially in the presence of background noise. These observations provide an additional predicted neural explanation for "hidden hearing loss," in which responses would be similar to those in normal hearing to traditional brief tone burst assessments (which rely predominantly on the early part of the stimulus), but would reveal deficits during complex auditory tasks that depend more on sustained responses (Xie, 2016). Second, deterioration of synaptic transmission with ARHL was more profound for high rates of ANF firing (400 Hz stimulation) than for low rates (100 Hz stimulation). This indicates that aged VCN synapses are functionally challenged when processing high rate auditory nerve inputs. For example, cochlear implants can stimulate the auditory nerve at rates up to and beyond 300 Hz, and the failure of high-rate stimuli to further improve temporal pitch discrimination (Shannon, 1983; Zeng, 2002) might partly be due to these limitations of synaptic transmission. From a mechanistic standpoint, the degradation of synaptic release at high rates appears to be linked to abnormal calcium signaling in the endbulb of Held terminals in aged mice during high rate activities, as the age effect could be largely reversed by acute addition of an exogenous calcium buffer (Xie & Manis, 2017b). Whether this reflects a change in overall cell calcium handling (such as by mitochondrial uptake, calcium binding proteins or plasma membrane pumps) or an age-related change in the calcium-dependent mechanisms involved in transmitter release (Foster, 2007) remains unclear.

In studies of ARHL, it is often hard to differentiate contributions that are due to normal aging versus those that are due to hearing loss. Phenomenologically similar changes in sustained synaptic transmission are evident at the endbulb of Held in NIHL at 2–4 months of age (Figure 7.1B), in ARHL at 25–30 months of age (Figure 7.1C), and in dn/dn mice at ~13 days of age (Oleskevich & Walmsley, 2002), consistent with the idea that the compromised synaptic transmission is a pathological response to the change in ANF activity associated with hearing loss. However, "normal" aging of the auditory system almost never exists because of the continuous exposure to environmental sounds throughout life. In this sense, ARHL might be better described as the result of a lifetime accumulation of "noise" exposure. Indeed, hearing loss early in life due to noise exposure accelerates the aging of the auditory system in mice (Fernandez, Jeffers, Lall, Liberman, & Kujawa, 2015; Kujawa & Liberman, 2006). In summary, noise exposure

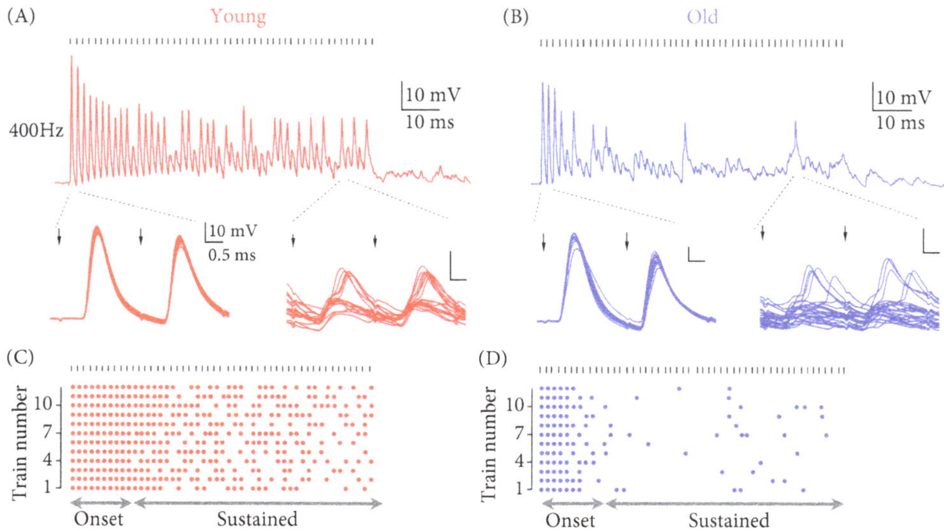

FIGURE 7.2. Encoding of auditory information decreases in firing rate and temporal precision in bushy neurons in aged CBA/CaJ mice. **A–B**: Current clamp responses of bushy neurons to 400 Hz train stimulation at the auditory nerve in young (**A**) and aged (**B**) mice. Insets show magnified view of two stimuli at the onset (left) and during the sustained phase of the train (right). Notice that old bushy neuron fired fewer spikes during the sustained phase, and the evoked spikes showed prominent temporal jitter (**B**, bottom right panel). Ticks on top mark the timing of stimulation. **C–D**: Raster plot of spikes evoked by the train in **A** and **B**. Onset: the first 10 stimuli of the train; sustained: the last 40 stimuli of the train. Each dot represents a single spike.

Modified with permission of The American Physiological Society from Figure 5 in Xie, 2016, *Journal of Neurophysiology*.

and aging are intermingled in the development of ARHL, and more carefully controlled experiments are required to parse out these two factors.

Synaptic Changes in the CN during Hearing Loss Related to Genetic Causes

Besides NIHL and ARHL, hearing loss is also frequently observed in the form of congenital deafness or other early onset progressive hearing losses that associate with genetic causes (Angeli, Lin, & Liu, 2012). These hearing impairments can lead to substantial anatomical and physiological changes at CN synapses. In particular these impairments may affect normal cochlear development and affect early activity-dependent development and refinement of central connections. At the endbulb of Held, the generalized response to genetic deafness often consists of synaptic atrophy and a compensatory enhancement in synaptic transmission that promotes increased central gain. Here we consider selected studies that have examined the effects of congenital deafness and early onset deafness.

In congenitally deaf white cats, the CN is 50% smaller in volume than that of hearing cats (Saada, Niparko, & Ryugo, 1996), accompanied by reduced synaptic size and branching of the endbulb of Held synapses, increased synaptic vesicle density, and elongated postsynaptic density (Baker, Montey, Pongstaporn, & Ryugo, 2010; Ryugo, Pongstaporn, Huchton, & Niparko, 1997). The synaptic pathology could be rescued by stimulating the congenitally deaf cats with cochlear implants for three months (Ryugo, Kretzmer, & Niparko, 2005), consistent with the idea that the morphological changes of CN synapses are significantly influenced by auditory nerve activity (Ryugo, Rosenbaum, Kim, Niparko, & Saada, 1998). Similar patterns of morphological changes of the endbulb of Held synapse were also observed in congenital deaf *shaker-2* mice (Connelly, Ryugo, & Muniak, 2017; Limb & Ryugo, 2000).

In congenitally deaf *dn/dn* mouse, the volume of aVCN endbulb of Held synapses was significantly smaller than normal mouse (Youssoufian, Couchman, Shivdasani, Paolini, & Walmsley, 2008), consistent with synaptic atrophy due to sensory inactivity of the auditory nerve. The synaptic transmission at the endbulb of Held was enhanced in deaf *dn/dn* mouse, showing increased transmitter release probability and larger evoked EPSCs, possibly as a compensatory mechanism to the reduced activity (Oleskevich & Walmsley, 2002). This study also showed the presence of asynchronous release at the endbulb synapse, similar to what is seen in NIHL and ARHL. Interestingly, spontaneous activity was recorded from unidentified cells in the CNC in these mice, indicating that the prolonged absence of sound-evoked activity in the nerve does not necessarily lead to an electrically silent central system (Youssoufian et al., 2008). Notably, no anatomical change was found in the downstream calyx of Held synapses in the nucleus of the trapezoid body of the same *dn/dn* mouse. Unlike the endbulb of Held, synaptic transmission at the calyx of Held in the MNTB showed no differences between normal hearing and deaf *dn/dn* mouse (Oleskevich, Youssoufian, & Walmsley, 2004; Youssoufian, Oleskevich, & Walmsley, 2005), although acute manipulations have revealed alterations in calyx function (Weatherstone et al., 2017).

In congenitally deaf mice that carry a mutation in otoferlin, which is an essential protein in the transmitter release process in hair cells (Michalski et al., 2017; Roux et al., 2006), the volume of the VCN was decreased by 46%, with smaller endbulb of Held synapses than hearing mice (Wright, Hwang, & Oertel, 2014). Postsynaptic bushy neurons in deaf mice receive more auditory nerve terminals, with increased amplitude of both quantal and evoked EPSCs (Wright et al., 2014). Similarly, in congenitally deaf jerker mice the cochlear nucleus is smaller in size, but develops normal topography in its auditory nerve innervation (Cao, McGinley, & Oertel, 2008). Endbulb of Held synapses near the nerve root in jerker mice were smaller than in hearing mice. The light-microscopic morphology of synaptic terminals in PVCN multipolar and octopus cell areas was not different between jerker and hearing mice. However, the deaf jerker mice showed an increased spontaneous event frequency and enhanced synaptic depression as measured onto both octopus and T-stellate neurons (Cao et al., 2008).

DBA/2j mice carry multiple recessive alleles of hearing loss genes (Erway, Willott, Archer, & Harrison, 1993; Johnson, Longo-Guess, Gagnon, Yu, & Zheng, 2008) and develop early onset progressive hearing loss starting at 3 weeks of age and reach nearly complete deafness by 7 months (McGuire, Fiorillo, Ryugo, & Lauer, 2015; Willott & Erway, 1998; Xie & Manis, 2013a; Zheng, Johnson, & Erway, 1999). No significant changes were found in VCN volume, number of neurons or VGluT1-positive auditory nerve terminals between two age groups of DBA/2j mice at 1–2 months and 9–10 months (McGuire et al., 2015). However, endbulb of Held synapses were smaller in DBA/2j mice at 9–10 months (McGuire et al., 2015). Synaptic transmission at the endbulb of Held was significantly modified during the early stage of hearing loss in these mice (Wang & Manis, 2005). Compared to young DBA/2j mice at 22 days, quantal synaptic transmission in the high frequency region of the aVCN in 45-day-old mice was smaller in amplitude and decreased in frequency, and the release probability of evoked synaptic transmission was significantly reduced. Surprisingly, evoked glycinergic inhibition from the DCN onto BCs was transiently enhanced during the onset of the hearing loss at 20–35 days in DBA/2j mice, becoming weaker and unreliable by 6–7 months of age, when the mice exhibit a profound hearing loss (Xie & Manis, 2013a).

Changes of synaptic transmission at the endbulb of Held are also widely reported during hearing loss caused by other genetic mutations. In BCs from hearing impaired CPX-I (Complexin I; a protein involved in synaptic vesicle fusion with the presynaptic membrane) knockout mice, the resting release probability was significantly reduced, facilitation was increased, release was delayed, EPSC jitter was increased, and tone evoked steady-state (adapted) firing rates were increased (Strenzke et al., 2009). Mice with a targeted deletion of the CACNA2D3 gene, which encodes the auxiliary subunit $\alpha_2\delta 3$ of the voltage gated calcium channels, show distorted ABR waveforms and compromised temporal processing (Pirone et al., 2014). Endbulb of Held synapses were smaller in $\alpha_2\delta 3^{-/-}$ mice and synaptic transmission was impaired with reduced firing rate and increased first spike latency in response to tones in postsynaptic bushy neurons (Pirone et al., 2014). Mice with deletion of exons 4 and 5 of the Bassoon gene show reduced auditory nerve sensory inputs in the aVCN (Jing et al., 2013) without affecting the endbulb of Held synaptic structure (Mendoza Schulz et al., 2014); however, the readily releasable vesicle pool and vesicle replenishment were decreased at the endbulb. Compensation for these deficiencies include increased postsynaptic densities, quantal size and vesicular release probability, resulting in unaltered EPSC amplitude (Mendoza Schulz et al., 2014). Deletion of AMPA glutamate receptor subunit GluA3 impaired the hearing of mice without changing the ending profile area of the endbulb of Held synapse, but reduced the number and size of postsynaptic density in BCs (Garcia-Hernandez, Abe, Sakimura, & Rubio, 2017).

SUMMARY

VCN synapses undergo both anatomical and physiological changes in response to noise-induced hearing loss and aging. These changes are generally considered to be secondary to degeneration of cochlear structure and reduced peripheral activity, but they have additional functional consequences for the representation of sound in the brain. Structurally, volume changes in postsynaptic cells and simplification of the structure of the surviving, activity deprived endbulbs are frequently associated with hearing loss. A major functional change shared by noise-induced hearing loss and aging is the development of asynchronous transmitter release at endbulb synapses during periods of high afferent firing, and this is also seen in at least one genetic model of hearing loss. In some cases, there appear to be compensatory responses in transmitter release, including changes in release probability and in the quantal content. These are not consistently observed across all models of hearing loss, suggesting that the time course of hearing loss and potential developmental effects may influence endbulb transmission in multiple ways. The electrical excitability of postsynaptic cells appears to undergo subtle changes, at least in the long-term, although studies that have examined ion channel expression in the VCN suggest that short-term, reversible changes in excitability may also occur. There is far less information about synaptic function and excitability of the pMCs and octopus cells, and none regarding the rMCs, in spite of their potentially critical role as providing inhibition to many principal cell types in the CNC (Arnott et al., 2004; Nelken & Young, 1994). Finally, there are clear indications that inhibition onto BCs and pMCs is reduced after hearing loss, although in most studies the exact sources of inhibition (rMCs, DCN vertical cells, or descending inputs from the olivary complex) are not clear. Overall, the relationship between the cellular and network changes and the consequences for auditory information processing are still unclear. The systems-level studies that have been done in the VCN with respect to hearing loss are limited.

A major question is whether changes in synaptic transmission or excitability in the VCN following NIHL or ARHL are reversible with the introduction of peripheral stimulation, as occurs when people are fitted with cochlear implants after a period of hearing loss, or which might occur with peripheral regeneration. So far this has only been studied in terms of the morphology of endbulbs of Held after electrical stimulation in two different models of deafness (Ryugo et al., 2010; Ryugo et al., 2005), with slightly different results. Whether other functional changes in synaptic transmission also occur, such as a reduction of the asynchronous release, and whether normalization of spontaneous rates and inhibitory tone can occur, could be important factors in designing effective stimulation patterns.

The relationship between the mechanistic changes and sensory coding by VCN neurons is an area that deserves further exploration. The studies we have discussed indicate that hearing loss is likely to alter how the loudness of tonal stimuli is represented centrally. Whether there are significant changes in coding for more complex stimuli, or for stimuli embedded in broadband sounds typical of many acoustic environments is not clear. Future studies should employ a careful categorization of cell types according to established criteria and should explore population responses to more naturalistic stimuli that better engage the networks of other excitatory and inhibitory cells that influence the firing of the principal neurons. In addition, such studies would benefit from an evaluation of the functional and morphological status of the auditory periphery in the same experimental subjects, to clarify the status of activity in the nerve.

Acknowledgments

This work was supported by NIDCD grants R01DC004551 to PBM, and R03DC013396 and R01DC016037 to RX. TFR was supported by T32DC005360.

References

Adams, J. C. (1983). Multipolar cells in the ventral cochlear nucleus project to the dorsal cochlear nucleus and the inferior colliculus. *Neuroscience Letters*, *37*(3), 205–208.

Alvarado, J. C., Fuentes-Santamaria, V., Gabaldon-Ull, M. C., Blanco, J. L., & Juiz, J. M. (2014). Wistar rats: A forgotten model of age-related hearing loss. *Frontiers in Aging Neuroscience*, *6*, 29. doi:10.3389/fnagi.2014.00029

Angeli, S., Lin, X., & Liu, X. Z. (2012). Genetics of hearing and deafness [Special Issue: The Anatomy and Biology of Hearing and Balance]. *Anatomical Record*, *295*(11), 1812–1829. doi:10.1002/ar.22579

Arnott, R. H., Wallace, M. N., Shackleton, T. M., & Palmer, A. R. (2004). Onset neurones in the anteroventral cochlear nucleus project to the dorsal cochlear nucleus. *Journal of the Association of Research Otolaryngology*, *5*(2), 153–170. doi:10.1007/s10162-003-4036-8

Atcherson, S. R., Nagaraj, N. K., Kennett, S. E., & Levisee, M. (2015). Overview of central auditory processing deficits in older adults. *Seminars in Hearing*, *36*(3), 150–161. doi:10.1055/s-0035-1555118

Baker, C. A., Montey, K. L., Pongstaporn, T., & Ryugo, D. K. (2010). Postnatal development of the endbulb of held in congenitally deaf cats. *Frontiers in Neuroanatomy*, *4*, 19. doi:10.3389/fnana.2010.00019

Banay-Schwartz, M., Lajtha, A., & Palkovits, M. (1989a). Changes with aging in the levels of amino acids in rat CNS structural elements. I. Glutamate and related amino acids. *Neurochemical Research*, *14*(6), 555–562.

Banay-Schwartz, M., Lajtha, A., & Palkovits, M. (1989b). Changes with aging in the levels of amino acids in rat CNS structural elements. II. Taurine and small neutral amino acids. *Neurochemical Research*, *14*(6), 563–570.

Boettcher, F. A., & Salvi, R. J. (1993). Functional changes in the ventral cochlear nucleus following acute acoustic overstimulation. *Journal of the Acoustical Society of America*, *94*(4), 2123–2134.

Cai, S., Ma, W. L., & Young, E. D. (2009). Encoding intensity in ventral cochlear nucleus following acoustic trauma: implications for loudness recruitment. *Journal of the Association of Research Otolaryngology, 10*(1), 5–22. doi:10.1007/s10162-008-0142-y

Caminos, E., Garcia-Pino, E., & Juiz, J. M. (2015). Loss of auditory activity modifies the location of potassium channel KCNQ5 in auditory brainstem neurons. *Journal of Neuroscience Research, 93*(4), 604–614. doi:10.1002/jnr.23516

Cant, N. B., & Benson, C. G. (2003). Parallel auditory pathways: projection patterns of the different neuronal populations in the dorsal and ventral cochlear nuclei. *Brain Research Bulletin, 60*(5–6), 457–474.

Cao, X. J., McGinley, M. J., & Oertel, D. (2008). Connections and synaptic function in the posteroventral cochlear nucleus of deaf jerker mice. *Journal of Comparative Neurology, 510*(3), 297–308. doi:10.1002/cne.21788

Chapochnikov, N. M., Takago, H., Huang, C. H., Pangrsic, T., Khimich, D., Neef, J., . . . Moser, T. (2014). Uniquantal release through a dynamic fusion pore is a candidate mechanism of hair cell exocytosis. *Neuron, 83*(6), 1389–1403. doi:10.1016/j.neuron.2014.08.003

Connelly, C. J., Ryugo, D. K., & Muniak, M. A. (2017). The effect of progressive hearing loss on the morphology of endbulbs of Held and bushy cells. *Hearing Research, 343*, 14–33. doi:10.1016/j.heares.2016.07.004

Desai, N. S., Rutherford, L. C., & Turrigiano, G. G. (1999). Plasticity in the intrinsic excitability of cortical pyramidal neurons. *Nature Neuroscience, 2*(6), 515–520. doi:10.1038/9165

Doucet, J. R., Ross, A. T., Gillespie, M. B., & Ryugo, D. K. (1999). Glycine immunoreactivity of multipolar neurons in the ventral cochlear nucleus which project to the dorsal cochlear nucleus. *Journal of Comparative Neurology, 408*(4), 515–531. doi:10.1002/(SICI)1096-9861(19990614)408:4

Doucet, J. R., & Ryugo, D. K. (1997). Projections from the ventral cochlear nucleus to the dorsal cochlear nucleus in rats. *Journal of Comparative Neurology, 385*(2), 245–264. doi:10.1002/(SICI)1096-9861(19970825)385:2<245::AID-CNE5>3.0.CO;2-1 [pii]

Doucet, J. R., & Ryugo, D. K. (2006). Structural and functional classes of multipolar cells in the ventral cochlear nucleus. *Anatomical Record Part A: Discoveries in Molecular, Cellular, and Evolutionary Biology, 288*(4), 331–344. doi:10.1002/ar.a.20294

D'Sa, C., Gross, J., Francone, V. P., & Morest, D. K. (2007). Plasticity of synaptic endings in the cochlear nucleus following noise-induced hearing loss is facilitated in the adult FGF2 overexpressor mouse. *European Journal of Neuroscience, 26*(3), 666–680. doi:10.1111/j.1460-9568.2007.05695.x

Erway, L. C., Willott, J. F., Archer, J. R., & Harrison, D. E. (1993). Genetics of age-related hearing loss in mice: I. Inbred and F1 hybrid strains. *Hearing Research, 65*(1–2), 125–132.

Feng, J., Bendiske, J., & Morest, D. K. (2012). Degeneration in the ventral cochlear nucleus after severe noise damage in mice. *Journal of Neuroscience Research, 90*(4), 831–841. doi:10.1002/jnr.22793

Fernandez, K. A., Jeffers, P. W., Lall, K., Liberman, M. C., & Kujawa, S. G. (2015). Aging after noise exposure: Acceleration of cochlear synaptopathy in "recovered" ears. *Journal of Neuroscience 35*(19), 7509–7520. doi:10.1523/JNEUROSCI.5138-14.2015

Foster, T. C. (2007). Calcium homeostasis and modulation of synaptic plasticity in the aged brain. *Aging Cell, 6*(3), 319–325. doi:10.1111/j.1474-9726.2007.00283.x

Francis, H. W., & Manis, P. B. (2000). Effects of deafferentation on the electrophysiology of ventral cochlear nucleus neurons. *Hearing Research, 149*(1–2), 91–105.

Frisina, R. D., Smith, R. L., & Chamberlain, S. C. (1990). Encoding of amplitude modulation in the gerbil cochlear nucleus: I. A hierarchy of enhancement. *Hearing Research*, *44*(2–3), 99–122.

Frisina, R. D., & Walton, J. P. (2006). Age-related structural and functional changes in the cochlear nucleus. *Hearing Research*, *216–217*, 216–223. doi:10.1016/j.heares.2006.02.003

Furman, A. C., Kujawa, S. G., & Liberman, M. C. (2013). Noise-induced cochlear neuropathy is selective for fibers with low spontaneous rates. *Journal of Neurophysiology*, *110*(3), 577–586. doi:10.1152/jn.00164.2013

Garcia-Hernandez, S., Abe, M., Sakimura, K., & Rubio, M. E. (2017). Impaired auditory processing and altered structure of the endbulb of Held synapse in mice lacking the GluA3 subunit of AMPA receptors. *Hearing Research*, *344*, 284–294. doi:10.1016/j.heares.2016.12.006

Godfrey, D. A., Kiang, N. Y., & Norris, B. E. (1975). Single unit activity in the posteroventral cochlear nucleus of the cat. *Journal of Comparative Neurology*, *162*(2), 247–268. doi:10.1002/cne.901620206

Guthrie, O. W. (2017). Noise induced DNA damage within the auditory nerve. *Anatomical Record (Hoboken)*, *300*(3), 520–526. doi:10.1002/ar.23494

Hall, J. W., Haggard, M. P., & Fernandes, M. A. (1984). Detection in noise by spectro-temporal pattern analysis. *Journal of the Acoustical Society of America*, *76*(1), 50–56.

Hashisaki, G. T., & Rubel, E. W. (1989). Effects of unilateral cochlea removal on anteroventral cochlear nucleus neurons in developing gerbils. *Journal of Comparative Neurology*, *283*(4), 5–73.

Heinz, M. G., Issa, J. B., & Young, E. D. (2005). Auditory-nerve rate responses are inconsistent with common hypotheses for the neural correlates of loudness recruitment. *Journal of the Association of Research Otolaryngology*, *6*(2), 91–105. doi:10.1007/s10162-004-5043-0

Heinz, M. G., & Young, E. D. (2004). Response growth with sound level in auditory-nerve fibers after noise-induced hearing loss. *Journal of Neurophysiology*, *91*(2), 784–795. doi:10.1152/jn.00776.2003

Helfert, R. H., Krenning, J., Wilson, T. S., & Hughes, L. F. (2003). Age-related synaptic changes in the anteroventral cochlear nucleus of Fischer-344 rats. *Hearing Research*, *183*(1–2), 18–28. doi:S0378595503001941 [pii]

Holahan, M. R. (2017). A shift from a pivotal to supporting role for the growth-associated protein (GAP-43) in the coordination of axonal structural and functional plasticity. *Frontiers in Cellular Neuroscience*, *11*, 266. doi:10.3389/fncel.2017.00266

Jiang, D., Palmer, A. R., & Winter, I. M. (1996). Frequency extent of two-tone facilitation in onset units in the ventral cochlear nucleus. *Journal of Neurophysiology*, *75*(1), 380–395. doi:10.1152/jn.1996.75.1.380

Jin, Y. M., Godfrey, D. A., & Sun, Y. (2005). Effects of cochlear ablation on choline acetyltransferase activity in the rat cochlear nucleus and superior olive. *Journal of Neuroscience Research*, *81*(1), 91–101. doi:10.1002/jnr.20536

Jing, Z., Rutherford, M. A., Takago, H., Frank, T., Fejtova, A., Khimich, D., . . . Strenzke, N. (2013). Disruption of the presynaptic cytomatrix protein bassoon degrades ribbon anchorage, multiquantal release, and sound encoding at the hair cell afferent synapse. *Journal of Neuroscience*, *33*(10), 4456–4467. doi:10.1523/JNEUROSCI.3491-12.2013

Johnson, K. R., Longo-Guess, C., Gagnon, L. H., Yu, H., & Zheng, Q. Y. (2008). A locus on distal chromosome 11 (ahl8) and its interaction with Cdh23 ahl underlie the early onset, age-related hearing loss of DBA/2J mice. *Genomics*, *92*(4), 219–225. doi:10.1016/j.ygeno.2008.06.007

Joris, P. X., Carney, L. H., Smith, P. H., & Yin, T. C. (1994). Enhancement of neural synchronization in the anteroventral cochlear nucleus. I. Responses to tones at the characteristic frequency. *Journal of Neurophysiology*, *71*(3), 1022–1036.

Keine, C., Rubsamen, R., & Englitz, B. (2017). Signal integration at spherical bushy cells enhances representation of temporal structure but limits its range. *Elife*, *6*. doi:10.7554/eLife.29639

Keithley, E. M., & Croskrey, K. L. (1990). Spiral ganglion cell endings in the cochlear nucleus of young and old rats. *Hearing Research*, *49*(1–3), 169–177.

Kiang, N. Y., Liberman, M. C., & Levine, R. A. (1976). Auditory-nerve activity in cats exposed to ototoxic drugs and high-intensity sounds. *Annals of Otology, Rhinology, and Laryngology*, *85*(6 PT. 1), 752–768. doi:10.1177/000348947608500605

Kim, J. J., Gross, J., Morest, D. K., & Potashner, S. J. (2004). Quantitative study of degeneration and new growth of axons and synaptic endings in the chinchilla cochlear nucleus after acoustic overstimulation. *Journal of Neuroscience Research*, *77*(6), 829–842. doi:10.1002/jnr.20211

Kim, J. J., Gross, J., Potashner, S. J., & Morest, D. K. (2004a). Fine structure of degeneration in the cochlear nucleus of the chinchilla after acoustic overstimulation. *Journal of Neuroscience Research*, *77*(6), 798–816. doi:10.1002/jnr.20213

Kim, J. J., Gross, J., Potashner, S. J., & Morest, D. K. (2004b). Fine structure of long-term changes in the cochlear nucleus after acoustic overstimulation: Chronic degeneration and new growth of synaptic endings. *Journal of Neuroscience Research*, *77*(6), 817–828. doi:10.1002/jnr.20212

Koerber, K. C., Pfeiffer, R. R., Warr, W. B., & Kiang, N. Y. (1966). Spontaneous spike discharges from single units in the cochlear nucleus after destruction of the cochlea. *Experimental Neurology*, *16*(2), 119–130.

Kotak, V. C., Fujisawa, S., Lee, F. A., Karthikeyan, O., Aoki, C., & Sanes, D. H. (2005). Hearing loss raises excitability in the auditory cortex. *Journal of Neuroscience* *25*(15), 3908–3918. doi:10.1523/JNEUROSCI.5169-04.2005

Kraus, K. S., Ding, D., Jiang, H., Lobarinas, E., Sun, W., & Salvi, R. J. (2011). Relationship between noise-induced hearing-loss, persistent tinnitus and growth-associated protein-43 expression in the rat cochlear nucleus: Does synaptic plasticity in ventral cochlear nucleus suppress tinnitus? *Neuroscience*, *194*, 309–325. doi:10.1016/j.neuroscience.2011.07.056

Kujawa, S. G., & Liberman, M. C. (2006). Acceleration of age-related hearing loss by early noise exposure: Evidence of a misspent youth. *Journal of Neuroscience* *26*(7), 2115–2123. doi:10.1523/JNEUROSCI.4985-05.2006

Kujawa, S. G., & Liberman, M. C. (2009). Adding insult to injury: Cochlear nerve degeneration after "temporary" noise-induced hearing loss. *Journal of Neuroscience* *29*(45), 14077–14085. doi:10.1523/JNEUROSCI.2845-09.2009

Lauer, A. M., Connelly, C. J., Graham, H., & Ryugo, D. K. (2013). Morphological characterization of bushy cells and their inputs in the laboratory mouse (Mus musculus) anteroventral cochlear nucleus. *PLoS One*, *8*(8), e73308. doi:10.1371/journal.pone.0073308

Leao, R. N., Berntson, A., Forsythe, I. D., & Walmsley, B. (2004). Reduced low-voltage activated K+ conductances and enhanced central excitability in a congenitally deaf (dn/dn) mouse. *Journal of Physiology*, *559*(Pt 1), 25–33. doi:10.1113/jphysiol.2004.067421

Liberman, M. C. (1987). Chronic ultrastructural changes in acoustic trauma: Serial-section reconstruction of stereocilia and cuticular plates. *Hearing Research*, *26*(1), 65–88.

Liberman, M. C. (1991). Central projections of auditory-nerve fibers of differing spontaneous rate. I. Anteroventral cochlear nucleus. *Journal of Comparative Neurology, 313*(2), 240–258. doi:10.1002/cne.903130205

Liberman, M. C., & Dodds, L. W. (1984). Single-neuron labeling and chronic cochlear pathology. III. Stereocilia damage and alterations of threshold tuning curves. *Hearing Research, 16*(1), 55–74.

Limb, C. J., & Ryugo, D. K. (2000). Development of primary axosomatic endings in the anteroventral cochlear nucleus of mice. *Journal of the Association of Research Otolaryngology, 1*(2), 103–119.

Lu, Y., Monsivais, P., Tempel, B. L., & Rubel, E. W. (2004). Activity-dependent regulation of the potassium channel subunits Kv1.1 and Kv3.1. *Journal of Comparative Neurology, 470*(1), 93–106. doi:10.1002/cne.11037

Makary, C. A., Shin, J., Kujawa, S. G., Liberman, M. C., & Merchant, S. N. (2011). Age-related primary cochlear neuronal degeneration in human temporal bones. *Journal of the Association of Research Otolaryngology, 12*(6), 711–717. doi:10.1007/s10162-011-0283-2

Manis, P. B., Xie, R., Wang, Y., Marrs, G. S., & Spirou, G. A. (2012). The endbulbs of Held. In L. O. Trussell, A. N. Popper, & R. R. Fay (Eds.), *Synaptic Mechanisms in the Auditory System* (Vol. 41, pp. 61–93). New York, NY: Springer.

McGinley, M. J., Liberman, M. C., Bal, R., & Oertel, D. (2012). Generating synchrony from the asynchronous: compensation for cochlear traveling wave delays by the dendrites of individual brainstem neurons. *Journal of Neuroscience, 32*(27), 9301–9311. doi:10.1523/JNEUROSCI.0272-12.2012

McGuire, B., Fiorillo, B., Ryugo, D. K., & Lauer, A. M. (2015). Auditory nerve synapses persist in ventral cochlear nucleus long after loss of acoustic input in mice with early-onset progressive hearing loss. *Brain Research, 1605*, 22–30. doi:10.1016/j.brainres.2015.02.012

Meidinger, M. A., Hildebrandt-Schoenfeld, H., & Illing, R. B. (2006). Cochlear damage induces GAP-43 expression in cholinergic synapses of the cochlear nucleus in the adult rat: a light and electron microscopic study. *European Journal of Neuroscience Journal of Neuroscience 23*(12), 3187–3199. doi:10.1111/j.1460-9568.2006.04853.x

Mendoza Schulz, A., Jing, Z., Sanchez Caro, J. M., Wetzel, F., Dresbach, T., Strenzke, N., . . . Moser, T. (2014). Bassoon-disruption slows vesicle replenishment and induces homeostatic plasticity at a CNS synapse. *EMBO Journal, 33*(5), 512–527. doi:10.1002/embj.201385887

Michalski, N., Goutman, J. D., Auclair, S. M., Boutet de Monvel, J., Tertrais, M., Emptoz, A., . . . Petit, C. (2017). Otoferlin acts as a Ca(2+) sensor for vesicle fusion and vesicle pool replenishment at auditory hair cell ribbon synapses. *Elife, 6*. doi:10.7554/eLife.31013

Michler, S. A., & Illing, R. B. (2002). Acoustic trauma induces reemergence of the growth- and plasticity-associated protein GAP-43 in the rat auditory brainstem. *Journal of Comparative Neurology, 451*(3), 250–266. doi:10.1002/cne.10348

Moore, D. R., Edmondson-Jones, M., Dawes, P., Fortnum, H., McCormack, A., Pierzycki, R. H., & Munro, K. J. (2014). Relation between speech-in-noise threshold, hearing loss and cognition from 40-69 years of age. *PLoS One, 9*(9), e107720. doi:10.1371/journal.pone.0107720

Moser, T., & Starr, A. (2016). Auditory neuropathy—neural and synaptic mechanisms. *Nature Reviews Neurology, 12*(3), 135–149. doi:10.1038/nrneurol.2016.10

Mostafapour, S. P., Cochran, S. L., Del Puerto, N. M., & Rubel, E. W. (2000). Patterns of cell death in mouse anteroventral cochlear nucleus neurons after unilateral cochlea removal. *Journal of Comparative Neurology, 426*(4), 561–571.

Nelken, I., & Young, E. D. (1994). Two separate inhibitory mechanisms shape the responses of dorsal cochlear nucleus type IV units to narrowband and wideband stimuli. *Journal of Neurophysiology, 71*(6), 2446–2462.

Ngodup, T., Goetz, J. A., McGuire, B. C., Sun, W., Lauer, A. M., & Xu-Friedman, M. A. (2015). Activity-dependent, homeostatic regulation of neurotransmitter release from auditory nerve fibers. *Proceedings of the National Academy of Sciences USA, 112*(20), 6479–6484. doi:10.1073/pnas.1420885112

Oertel, D., Bal, R., Gardner, S. M., Smith, P. H., & Joris, P. X. (2000). Detection of synchrony in the activity of auditory nerve fibers by octopus cells of the mammalian cochlear nucleus. *Proceedings of the National Academy of Sciences USA, 97*(22), 11773–11779. doi:10.1073/pnas.97.22.11773

Oertel, D., Wu, S. H., Garb, M. W., & Dizack, C. (1990). Morphology and physiology of cells in slice preparations of the posteroventral cochlear nucleus of mice. *Journal of Comparative Neurology, 295*(1), 136–154. doi:10.1002/cne.902950112

Oleskevich, S., & Walmsley, B. (2002). Synaptic transmission in the auditory brainstem of normal and congenitally deaf mice. *Journal of Physiology, 540*(Pt 2), 447–455.

Oleskevich, S., Youssoufian, M., & Walmsley, B. (2004). Presynaptic plasticity at two giant auditory synapses in normal and deaf mice. *Journal of Physiology, 560*(Pt 3), 709–719. doi:10.1113/jphysiol.2004.066662

Palmer, A. R., Jiang, D., & Marshall, D. H. (1996). Responses of ventral cochlear nucleus onset and chopper units as a function of signal bandwidth. *Journal of Neurophysiology, 75*(2), 780–794.

Pasic, T. R., Moore, D. R., & Rubel, E. W. (1994). Effect of altered neuronal activity on cell size in the medial nucleus of the trapezoid body and ventral cochlear nucleus of the gerbil. *Journal of Comparative Neurology, 348*(1), 111–120. doi:10.1002/cne.903480106

Pasic, T. R., & Rubel, E. W. (1989). Rapid changes in cochlear nucleus cell size following blockade of auditory nerve electrical activity in gerbils. *Journal of Comparative Neurology, 283*(4), 474–480. doi:10.1002/cne.902830403

Pirone, A., Kurt, S., Zuccotti, A., Ruttiger, L., Pilz, P., Brown, D. H., . . . Engel, J. (2014). alpha2delta3 is essential for normal structure and function of auditory nerve synapses and is a novel candidate for auditory processing disorders. *Journal of Neuroscience 34*(2), 434–445. doi:10.1523/JNEUROSCI.3085-13.2014

Pressnitzer, D., Meddis, R., Delahaye, R., & Winter, I. M. (2001). Physiological correlates of comodulation masking release in the mammalian ventral cochlear nucleus. *Journal of Neuroscience 21*(16), 6377–6386.

Rao, D., Basura, G. J., Roche, J., Daniels, S., Mancilla, J. G., & Manis, P. B. (2010). Hearing loss alters serotonergic modulation of intrinsic excitability in auditory cortex. *Journal of Neurophysiology, 104*(5), 2693–2703. doi:10.1152/jn.01092.2009

Rhode, W. S. (1998). Neural encoding of single-formant stimuli in the ventral cochlear nucleus of the chinchilla. *Hearing Research, 117*(1–2), 39–56.

Rhode, W. S., & Greenberg, S. (1994). Encoding of amplitude modulation in the cochlear nucleus of the cat. *Journal of Neurophysiology, 71*(5), 1797–1825.

Rhode, W. S., Oertel, D., & Smith, P. H. (1983). Physiological response properties of cells labeled intracellularly with horseradish peroxidase in cat ventral cochlear nucleus. *Journal of Comparative Neurology, 213*(4), 448–463. doi:10.1002/cne.902130408

Rhode, W. S., & Smith, P. H. (1986). Encoding timing and intensity in the ventral cochlear nucleus of the cat. *Journal of Neurophysiology, 56*(2), 261–286. doi:10.1152/jn.1986.56.2.261

Rich, A. W., Xie, R., & Manis, P. B. (2010). Hearing loss alters quantal release at cochlear nucleus stellate cells. *Laryngoscope, 120*(10), 2047–2053. doi:10.1002/lary.21106

Ritz, L. A., & Brownell, W. E. (1982). Single unit analysis of the posteroventral cochlear nucleus of the decerebrate cat. *Neuroscience, 7*(8), 1995–2010.

Rouiller, E. M., & Ryugo, D. K. (1984). Intracellular marking of physiologically characterized cells in the ventral cochlear nucleus of the cat. *Journal of Comparative Neurology, 225*(2), 167–186. doi:10.1002/cne.902250203

Roux, I., Safieddine, S., Nouvian, R., Grati, M., Simmler, M. C., Bahloul, A., . . . Petit, C. (2006). Otoferlin, defective in a human deafness form, is essential for exocytosis at the auditory ribbon synapse. *Cell, 127*(2), 277–289. doi:10.1016/j.cell.2006.08.040

Rutherford, M. A., Chapochnikov, N. M., & Moser, T. (2012). Spike encoding of neurotransmitter release timing by spiral ganglion neurons of the cochlea. *Journal of Neuroscience 32*(14), 4773–4789. doi:10.1523/JNEUROSCI.4511-11.2012

Ryugo, D. K., Baker, C. A., Montey, K. L., Chang, L. Y., Coco, A., Fallon, J. B., & Shepherd, R. K. (2010). Synaptic plasticity after chemical deafening and electrical stimulation of the auditory nerve in cats. *Journal of Comparative Neurology, 518*(7), 1046–1063. doi:10.1002/cne.22262

Ryugo, D. K., Kretzmer, E. A., & Niparko, J. K. (2005). Restoration of auditory nerve synapses in cats by cochlear implants. *Science, 310*(5753), 1490–1492. doi:10.1126/science.1119419

Ryugo, D. K., Pongstaporn, T., Huchton, D. M., & Niparko, J. K. (1997). Ultrastructural analysis of primary endings in deaf white cats: Morphologic alterations in endbulbs of Held. *Journal of Comparative Neurology, 385*(2), 230–244.

Ryugo, D. K., Rosenbaum, B. T., Kim, P. J., Niparko, J. K., & Saada, A. A. (1998). Single unit recordings in the auditory nerve of congenitally deaf white cats: Morphological correlates in the cochlea and cochlear nucleus. *Journal of Comparative Neurology, 397*(4), 532–548.

Saada, A. A., Niparko, J. K., & Ryugo, D. K. (1996). Morphological changes in the cochlear nucleus of congenitally deaf white cats. *Brain Research, 736*(1–2), 315–328.

Schofield, B. R., & Cant, N. B. (1996). Origins and targets of commissural connections between the cochlear nuclei in guinea pigs. *Journal of Comparative Neurology, 375*(1), 128–146. doi:10.1002/(SICI)1096-9861(19961104)375:1<128::AID-CNE8>3.0.CO;2-5

Schroeder, B. C., Hechenberger, M., Weinreich, F., Kubisch, C., & Jentsch, T. J. (2000). KCNQ5, a novel potassium channel broadly expressed in brain, mediates M-type currents. *Journal of Biological Chemistry, 275*(31), 24089–24095. doi:10.1074/jbc.M003245200

Sekiya, T., Viberg, A., Kojima, K., Sakamoto, T., Nakagawa, T., Ito, J., & Canlon, B. (2012). Trauma-specific insults to the cochlear nucleus in the rat. *Journal of Neuroscience Research, 90*(10), 1924–1931. doi:10.1002/jnr.23093

Sergeyenko, Y., Lall, K., Liberman, M. C., & Kujawa, S. G. (2013). Age-related cochlear synaptopathy: An early-onset contributor to auditory functional decline. *Journal of Neuroscience 33*(34), 13686–13694. doi:10.1523/JNEUROSCI.1783-13.2013

Sha, S. H., Kanicki, A., Dootz, G., Talaska, A. E., Halsey, K., Dolan, D., . . . Schacht, J. (2008). Age-related auditory pathology in the CBA/J mouse. *Hearing Research, 243*(1–2), 87–94. doi:10.1016/j.heares.2008.06.001

Shannon, R. V. (1983). Multichannel electrical stimulation of the auditory nerve in man. I. Basic psychophysics. *Hearing Research, 11*(2), 157–189.

Shore, S. E., Vass, Z., Wys, N. L., & Altschuler, R. A. (2000). Trigeminal ganglion innervates the auditory brainstem. *Journal of Comparative Neurology, 419*(3), 271–285.

Sie, K. C., & Rubel, E. W. (1992). Rapid changes in protein synthesis and cell size in the cochlear nucleus following eighth nerve activity blockade or cochlea ablation. *Journal of Comparative Neurology, 320*(4), 501–508. doi:10.1002/cne.903200407

Siegel, J. H. (1992). Spontaneous synaptic potentials from afferent terminals in the guinea pig cochlea. *Hearing Research, 59*(1), 85–92.

Skene, J. H. (1989). Axonal growth-associated proteins. *Annual Review of Neuroscience, 12*, 127–156. doi:10.1146/annurev.ne.12.030189.001015

Smith, P. H., Massie, A., & Joris, P. X. (2005). Acoustic stria: Anatomy of physiologically characterized cells and their axonal projection patterns. *Journal of Comparative Neurology, 482*(4), 349–371. doi:10.1002/cne.20407

Smith, P. H., & Rhode, W. S. (1989). Structural and functional properties distinguish two types of multipolar cells in the ventral cochlear nucleus. *Journal of Comparative Neurology, 282*(4), 595–616. doi:10.1002/cne.902820410

Spencer, M. J., Grayden, D. B., Bruce, I. C., Meffin, H., & Burkitt, A. N. (2012). An investigation of dendritic delay in octopus cells of the mammalian cochlear nucleus. *Frontiers in Computational Neuroscience, 6*, 83. doi:10.3389/fncom.2012.00083

Spirou, G. A., Rager, J., & Manis, P. B. (2005). Convergence of auditory-nerve fiber projections onto globular bushy cells. *Neuroscience, 136*(3), 843–863. doi:10.1016/j.neuroscience.2005.08.068

Strenzke, N., Chanda, S., Kopp-Scheinpflug, C., Khimich, D., Reim, K., Bulankina, A. V., . . . Moser, T. (2009). Complexin-I is required for high-fidelity transmission at the endbulb of Held auditory synapse. *Journal of Neuroscience 29*(25), 7991–8004. doi:10.1523/JNEUROSCI.0632-09.2009

Tong, L., Strong, M. K., Kaur, T., Juiz, J. M., Oesterle, E. C., Hume, C., . . . Rubel, E. W. (2015). Selective deletion of cochlear hair cells causes rapid age-dependent changes in spiral ganglion and cochlear nucleus neurons. *Journal of Neuroscience 35*(20), 7878–7891. doi:10.1523/JNEUROSCI.2179-14.2015

Valero, M. D., Burton, J. A., Hauser, S. N., Hackett, T. A., Ramachandran, R., & Liberman, M. C. (2017). Noise-induced cochlear synaptopathy in rhesus monkeys (*Macaca mulatta*). *Hearing Research, 353*, 213–223. doi:10.1016/j.heares.2017.07.003

Vogler, D. P., Robertson, D., & Mulders, W. H. (2011). Hyperactivity in the ventral cochlear nucleus after cochlear trauma. *Journal of Neuroscience 31*(18), 6639–6645. doi:10.1523/JNEUROSCI.6538-10.2011

Wang, Y., Hirose, K., & Liberman, M. C. (2002). Dynamics of noise-induced cellular injury and repair in the mouse cochlea. *Journal of the Association of Research Otolaryngology, 3*(3), 248–268. doi:10.1007/s101620020028

Wang, Y., & Manis, P. B. (2005). Synaptic transmission at the cochlear nucleus endbulb synapse during age-related hearing loss in mice. *Journal of Neurophysiology, 94*(3), 1814–1824. doi:10.1152/jn.00374.2005

Weatherstone, J. H., Kopp-Scheinpflug, C., Pilati, N., Wang, Y., Forsythe, I. D., Rubel, E. W., & Tempel, B. L. (2017). Maintenance of neuronal size gradient in MNTB requires sound-evoked activity. *Journal of Neurophysiology, 117*(2), 756–766. doi:10.1152/jn.00528.2016

Willott, J. F., & Erway, L. C. (1998). Genetics of age-related hearing loss in mice. IV. Cochlear pathology and hearing loss in 25 BXD recombinant inbred mouse strains. *Hearing Research, 119*(1–2), 27–36.

Willott, J. F., Jackson, L. M., & Hunter, K. P. (1987). Morphometric study of the anteroventral cochlear nucleus of two mouse models of presbycusis. *Journal of Comparative Neurology, 260*(3), 472–480. doi:10.1002/cne.902600312

Willott, J. F., Parham, K., & Hunter, K. P. (1991). Comparison of the auditory sensitivity of neurons in the cochlear nucleus and inferior colliculus of young and aging C57BL/6J and CBA/J mice. *Hearing Research, 53*(1), 78–94.

Wright, S., Hwang, Y., & Oertel, D. (2014). Synaptic transmission between end bulbs of Held and bushy cells in the cochlear nucleus of mice with a mutation in Otoferlin. *Journal of Neurophysiology, 112*(12), 3173–3188. doi:10.1152/jn.00522.2014

Xie, R. (2016). Transmission of auditory sensory information decreases in rate and temporal precision at the endbulb of Held synapse during age-related hearing loss. *Journal of Neurophysiology, 116*(6), 2695–2705.

Xie, R., & Manis, P. B. (2012). *Changes in excitatory synaptic transmission to bushy cells following noise-induced hearing loss.* Paper presented at the Association for Research in Otolaryngology Midwinter Meeting Abstr., San Diego, CA.

Xie, R., & Manis, P. B. (2013a). Glycinergic synaptic transmission in the cochlear nucleus of mice with normal hearing and age-related hearing loss. *Journal of Neurophysiology*, doi: 10.1152/jn.00151.02013. doi:10.1152/jn.00151.2013

Xie, R., & Manis, P. B. (2013b). Target-specific IPSC kinetics promote temporal processing in auditory parallel pathways. *Journal of Neuroscience 33*(4), 1598–1614.

Xie, R., & Manis, P. B. (2017a). Radiate and planar multipolar neurons of the mouse anteroventral cochlear nucleus: Intrinsic excitability and characterization of their auditory nerve input. *Frontiers in Neural Circuits.* doi:10.3389/fncir.2017.00077

Xie, R., & Manis, P. B. (2017b). Synaptic transmission at the endbulb of Held deteriorates during age-related hearing loss. *Journal of Physiology, 595*(3), 919–934.

Youssoufian, M., Couchman, K., Shivdasani, M. N., Paolini, A. G., & Walmsley, B. (2008). Maturation of auditory brainstem projections and calyces in the congenitally deaf (dn/dn) mouse. *Journal of Comparative Neurology, 506*(3), 442–451. doi:10.1002/cne.21566

Youssoufian, M., Oleskevich, S., & Walmsley, B. (2005). Development of a robust central auditory synapse in congenital deafness. *Journal of Neurophysiology, 94*(5), 3168–3180. doi:10.1152/jn.00342.2005

Zeng, F. G. (2002). Temporal pitch in electric hearing. *Hearing Research, 174*(1–2), 101–106.

Zheng, Q. Y., Johnson, K. R., & Erway, L. C. (1999). Assessment of hearing in 80 inbred strains of mice by ABR threshold analyses. *Hearing Research, 130*(1–2), 94–107. doi:S0378-5955(99)00003-9 [pii]

CHAPTER 8

THE COCHLEAR NUCLEUS AS A GENERATOR OF TINNITUS-RELATED SIGNALS

JAMES A. KALTENBACH AND DONALD A. GODFREY

Abstract

Tinnitus most commonly begins with alterations of input from the ear resulting from cochlear trauma or overstimulation of the ear. Because the cochlear nucleus is the first processing center in the brain receiving cochlear input, it is the first brainstem station to adjust to this modified input from the cochlea. Research published over the last 30 years demonstrates changes in neural circuitry and activity in the cochlear nucleus that are associated with and may be the origin of the signals that give rise to tinnitus percepts at the cortical level. This chapter summarizes what is known about these disturbances and their relationships to tinnitus. It also summarizes the mechanisms that trigger tinnitus-related disturbances and the anatomical, chemical, neurophysiological, and biophysical defects that underlie them. It concludes by highlighting some major controversies that research findings have generated and discussing the clinical implications the findings have for the future treatment of tinnitus.

Keywords: cochlear nucleus, tinnitus, plasticity, tinnitus-signaling, tinnitus mechanisms, tinnitus origins

As a direct receiver of input from the auditory nerve, the cochlear nucleus is in a pivotal position to respond to the effects of altered input from the ear caused by tinnitus-producing manipulations such as intense sound and ototoxic drug exposure. Alterations of input from the ear caused by these manipulations can manifest as long-term readjustments in circuitry and biophysical properties of neurons, which can disturb the normal state of ongoing activity. As we will see in this chapter, a variety of disturbances relevant to tinnitus have been identified in the cochlear nucleus, and it is the purpose of this chapter to summarize what is known about these disturbances, their relationship to tinnitus, where they originate, and how they affect auditory centers beyond the cochlear nucleus. We will also summarize the current state of knowledge concerning the mechanisms that trigger these tinnitus-related disturbances and the nature of the anatomical, chemical, and biophysical defects that underlie them. Finally, we will discuss some of the major controversies that continue to cloud an understanding of the biological basis of tinnitus as related to the cochlear nucleus and then discuss some of the clinical implications of what is and is not known.

Changes in the Cochlear Nucleus Induced by Agents that Cause Tinnitus in Humans

Historically, the search for neural correlates of tinnitus focused on signals and signal patterns that mimic those evoked by sound. The reasoning was that if a resemblance to sound-evoked activity could be demonstrated, then it seemed likely that such signals carried the necessary information needed to encode the phantom sound percepts that underlie tinnitus. In this section, we will review the key changes in activity that are associated with tinnitus and possess the requisite signatures of sound-encoding signals. We will then examine the evidence supporting the belief that such changes are related to tinnitus.

Changes in Tonotopic Map Representation

Studies of tinnitus signaling in the cochlear nucleus developed as an offshoot of studies of neural plasticity, and particularly in understanding how the tonotopic map was affected by cochlear injury. It was just beginning to be known that the tonotopic map of the auditory cortex underwent a massive reorganization following injury to selected areas of the cochlea, induced by mechanical lesions. Specifically, when a selected frequency region within the cochlea was mechanically lesioned, the corresponding region of the tonotopic map of the auditory cortex neither degenerated nor lost its sensitivity to sound; instead, the tonotopic region affected by the cochlear lesion adopted new frequency tuning properties, expanding the representation of frequencies neighboring those affected by the lesion (Robertson & Irvine, 1989). The reorganized map is thought to have sound encoding potential because the pitch of sound percepts is determined by a "place" code, that is, the tonotopic locus where activity reaches a peak (Evans, 1978). Furthermore, similar changes have been found in the somatosensory cortex after peripheral damage and are believed to underlie phantom pain (Wall et al., 2002). The hypothesis that a similar reorganization might occur at the level of the cochlear nucleus was put to the test in the dorsal cochlear nucleus (DCN), where tonotopy was most easily mapped (Kaltenbach et al., 1996; Meleca et al., 1997). Contrary to expectation, those early studies failed to show any evidence of map reorganization following cochlear injury, such as found in the auditory cortex. Although the map representation included wider than normal areas in which neurons were most sensitive to border frequencies, the tuning properties in the expanded frequency region were all pathological, and the new "ectopic" or expanded frequency selectivity was found to be an artifact of downshifted characteristic frequencies caused by loss of the original tuning curve tip (Kaltenbach et al., 1996; Meleca et al., 1997); this phenomenon was described as a "pseudoplasticity" or "pseudoreorganization" of the tonotopic map (Kaltenbach et al., 1996) and seems unlikely to provide the information needed for the reorganization of the tonotopic map observed at the cortical level following cochlear injury (Eggermont, 2006; Komiya & Eggermont, 2000; Norena & Eggermont, 2005; Robertson & Irvine, 1989;).

Increases in Spontaneous Activity (Hyperactivity)

Manipulations that cause tinnitus have been found in many studies to raise the level of resting (spontaneous) activity in the cochlear nucleus. This was originally characterized in the DCN (based on multiunit and single unit recordings) using an intense tone as the inducing manipulation (Brozoski et al., 2002; Kaltenbach & McCaslin, 1996; Kaltenbach et al., 1998, 2000; Zhang & Kaltenbach, 1998), but later studies confirmed that a similar state of hyperactivity can be induced in the anteroventral cochlear nucleus (AVCN) by using intense noise (Vogler et al., 2011) and in the DCN by using the ototoxic drug cisplatin (Kaltenbach et al., 2002; Melamed et al., 2000; Rachel et al., 2002). Studies of the tonotopic distribution pattern of hyperactivity in the DCN originally showed a stereotypic profile of activity that follows a predictable time course: the hyperactivity emerged after several days of plastic readjustment following a period of 2–3 days when activity was reduced or unchanged (Kaltenbach et al., 1998, 2000). This progression is suggestive of a dynamic process, with hyperactivity spread broadly across the entire tonotopic map but gradually becoming more narrowly focused on the frequency region just above the frequency of the exposure sound (Figure 8.1). Hyperactivity in the DCN following cisplatin treatment was found to be correlated with the loss of outer hair cells (OHCs) (Kaltenbach et al., 2002), suggesting that the hyperactive state may be a secondary adjustment resulting from loss of primary afferent input from the type II spiral ganglion cells, which receive their synaptic input from OHCs. The induction of hyperactivity by manipulations that cause tinnitus has been demonstrated in numerous studies at both single unit and multiunit levels and now appears to be a general phenomenon that can be induced in various species, including hamster (Kaltenbach & Afman, 2000; Manzoor et al., 2012, 2013b), guinea pig (Shore et al., 2008), chinchilla (Brozoski et al., 2002), mouse (Li et al., 2013), and rat (Brozoski et al., 2013; Zhang & Kaltenbach, 1998) by a variety of manipulations that are tinnitus inducing in humans, including sound exposure (Brozoski et al., 2002; Kaltenbach & McCaslin, 1996), ototoxic drug treatment (Kaltenbach et al., 2002; Groschel et al., 2016), and cochlear ablation/eighth nerve deafferentation (Sasaki et al., 1980). Hyperactivity has been found in both dorsal and ventral subdivisions of the

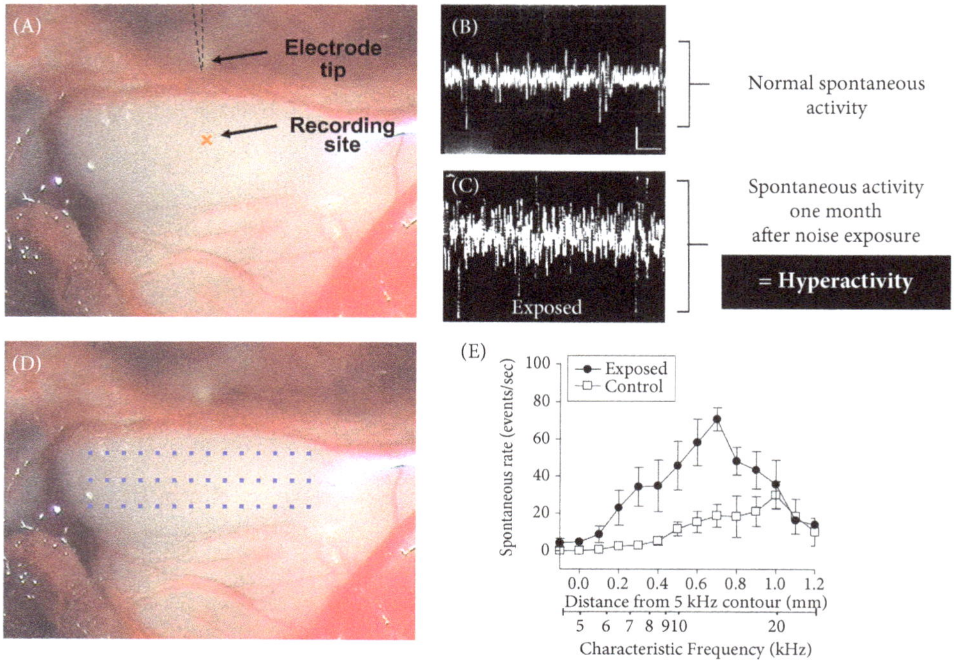

FIGURE 8.1. Intense sound exposure, which is one of the most common and powerful inducers of tinnitus, causes neurons in the DCN to develop hyperactivity. This hyperactivity is shown in this comparison of multiunit recordings from the DCN surface (site marked by X in panel A) of a normal hearing animal (B) with that from an animal that was exposed to an intense (127 dB SPL) 10 kHz tone a month earlier (C). The hyperactivity is apparent as increased spike frequency and amplitude. When this activity is mapped over the DCN surface (D), it shows a distribution pattern that is consistently higher across the tonotopic axis than control levels and shows a distinct peak in the high-frequency half of the tonotopic range (E).

Adapted from Kaltenbach and Godfrey (2008), with permission from the American Speech and Hearing Association (ASHA).

cochlear nuclei, although most studies have focused on the DCN. In the DCN, most evidence points to the fusiform cells as the main source of hyperactivity, although, as we shall discuss, some evidence suggests that DCN cartwheel cells may also be involved (Chang et al., 2002; Du et al., 2012). However, the time course of emergence of hyperactivity now appears to vary, depending on the intensity and duration of the inducing exposure sound (Gao et al., 2016). The relationship of hyperactivity to tinnitus will be addressed later in this chapter.

Increased Bursting Activity

Bursting activity is a form of neural discharge pattern in which spikes occur as couplets or in clusters or runs of 3 or more spikes separated by brief (< 10 ms) but similar intervals (Figure 8.2 B,C). Bursting activity is a characteristic of neuronal signaling at all levels of the auditory system, but its occurrence at the cochlear nucleus level is significant because action potentials concentrated in brief intervals can lead to postsynaptic depolarizations that can be temporally summated; these summated potentials are more powerful drivers of postsynaptic activity in the afferent pathway than are depolarizations that arise from inputs at more widely spaced intervals. Increases in bursting activity also contribute to the increase in firing rate and thus are a major factor underlying hyperactivity (Finlayson & Kaltenbach, 2009). The increases in bursting activity observed in animal models of noise-induced tinnitus have special significance in the context of tinnitus. Bursting activity could increase the salience of percepts. If the bursting activity is concentrated in a specific tonotopic frequency range, the percepts for that frequency range may become more salient. Previous studies showing that increased spontaneous activity is concentrated in the high-pitch region of the DCN (Finlayson & Kaltenbach, 2009) are consistent with this assertion. Bursting activity also promotes long term potentiation, which is widely believed to provide a neuronal substrate for memory (Thomas et al., 1998). Thus, increases in bursting could promote greater sensitivity in the response to ongoing activation, especially if that activation is increased. Finally, since bursting activity contains short interspike intervals, it provides a potential mechanism for representation of high-pitch sounds by periodicity coding (Evans, 1978). Any or all of these properties of bursting could contribute to or reinforce the perceptual impact of sounds arising from the altered activity.

Evidence that cochlear nucleus neurons develop enhanced bursting activity after noise exposure has been reported in several studies, both in vivo (Finlayson & Kaltenbach, 2009; Wu et al., 2016) and in vitro (Chang et al., 2002; Pilati et al., 2012). Evidence of increased bursting activity of DCN fusiform cells was observed in several ways in the in vivo study of Finlayson and Kaltenbach. The most obvious was an increase in the percentage of units displaying spike bursts (i.e., from 47% in controls to 56% in exposed animals; Figure 8.2D). Units in exposed animals also showed an increase in the proportion of spikes occurring in bursts (from 20% of spikes in controls to 28% in exposed animals). And lastly, the rate at which bursts occurred was found to be increased in exposed animals relative to those in controls for both couplets and runs. The changes were larger in the Chang et al. in vitro study: doubling of the occurrence of units with bursting activity in the exposed-side-DCN of brain slices from exposed rats.

Increased Neural Synchrony

The term "neural synchrony" refers to the presence of correlated firing such that impulses generated by one neuron occur simultaneously or synchronously with those from one or more other neuron(s). Under normal conditions, most auditory neurons fire in a quasi-random way, and the intervals between spikes are described by a Poisson

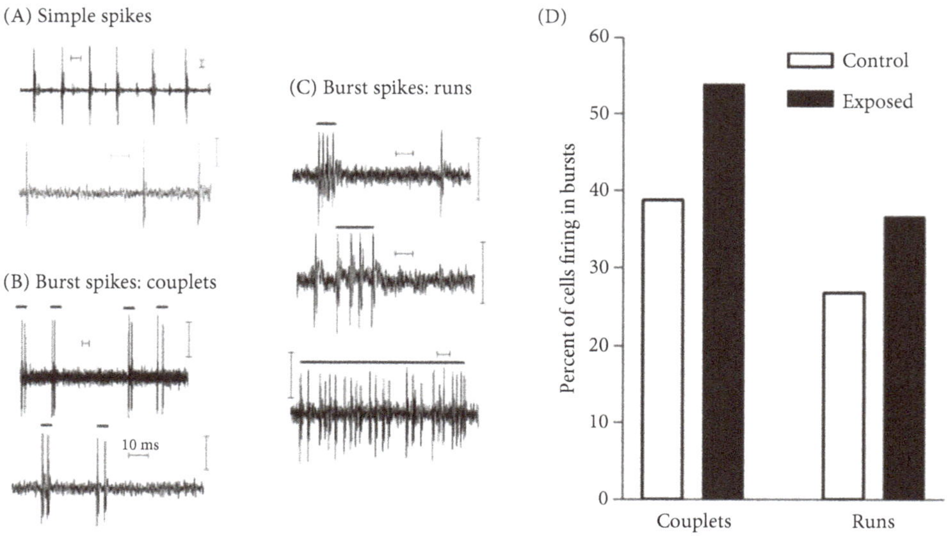

FIGURE 8.2. Bursting activity is increased in the DCN following noise exposure. Non-bursting or "simple" spikes (A) occur as regular or irregular trains of spikes and contrast with bursting activity, which can occur in different forms, including spike couplets (B) and runs (C). Intense sound exposure causes fusiform cells to develop more bursting activity as indicated by the higher prevalence of both spike couplets and runs (D).

Graphs adapted from Finlayson and Kaltenbach (2009).

distribution (Kiang et al., 1965). Stimulation has the effect of increasing the firing rates of neurons, which increases the probability that the different neurons will fire simultaneously. This leads to a shifting of the interval distribution toward shorter intervals, although the pattern of firing may remain similar (Pfeiffer & Kiang, 1965). One would expect that under conditions in which the neuronal firing rate increases as in the animal models of tinnitus, the interval histograms would show a similar tendency to fire with shorter interspike intervals and thus increased synchrony. Increases in synchrony could also be caused by changes in neural circuitry, as proposed by Wu et al. (2016). The reason that an increase in synchrony is important in the context of tinnitus is that synchronous discharges increase the probability that a postsynaptic cell will receive coincident inputs that will drive it to a higher state of depolarization by spatial summation, leading to an increase in its firing rate. Synchronously firing neurons thus have more driving power than asynchronously firing neurons. A second potentially significant feature of synchronous firing is that it could carry a code for sound percepts. This point has been argued previously in the context of tinnitus based on the notion that neurons firing synchronously will be more likely to produce a percept that has salience and therefore stands out above the general background of random activity (Chen & Jastreboff, 1995).

Changes in neural synchrony are often interpreted as putative correlates of tinnitus at cortical and subcortical levels of the auditory system, such as the auditory nerve

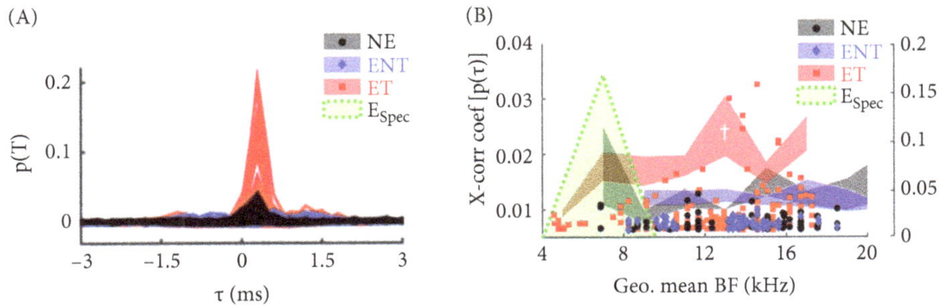

FIGURE 8.3. Synchronous firing between pairs of neurons is increased in animals that have been sound exposed and test positive for tinnitus. The increased synchrony is apparent in a cross correlation histogram (A), which plots the number of spikes that occur in one recorded neuron after a spike is generated in another recorded neuron. As can be seen, there is an increase in the number of spikes occurring at nearly the same time in the sound-exposed animals with tinnitus as compared to the unexposed control animals that do not have tinnitus. This increased synchrony is found across the entire recorded part of the tonotopic range in the exposed animals with tinnitus but reaches a peak between the 12 and 16 kHz loci (B) NE: Non-exposed sham, ENT: Exposed-no tinnitus, ET: Exposed-tinnitus, E-Exposed, E_{spec}: Noise exposure spectrum.

Graphs adapted from Wu et al. (2016), with permission from Elsevier.

and auditory cortex (Cazals et al., 1998; see review of Roberts et al., 2010). Increases in the 1 kHz spectral peak of electrocochlear ensemble activity in the absence of acoustic stimulation are induced in the guinea pig auditory nerve after several days of salicylate treatment, and these have been interpreted as evidence for increased synchronous firing across the eighth nerve fiber population (Cazals et al., 1998). Similar increases, although at lower spectral frequency, have also been observed following acute treatment with salicylate in cats by Martin et al. (1993) and Schreiner and Snyder (1987). Only recently has a concerted effort been made to systematically test whether increases in synchrony occur at the cochlear nucleus level. Wu et al. (2016) reported increased synchrony between fusiform cell pairs recorded in the DCN of their guinea pig model of chronic noise-induced tinnitus. Interestingly, the increases were highest in the 12–16 kHz tonotopic range (Figure 8.3A,B), which correlated with the frequency region over which behavioral evidence for tinnitus was strongest, supporting the hypothesis that the increased synchrony, either alone or in concert with other signal patterns, may represent a neural code for the pitch of tinnitus.

Do the Activity Changes in the Cochlear Nucleus Underlie Tinnitus?

The relevance of activity changes in the cochlear nucleus to tinnitus has been studied along two lines of inquiry. The first has examined how these activity changes compare with activity changes induced by sound stimulation, while the second has focused more on the question of whether the activity changes are associated with tinnitus percepts.

Comparison with Stimulus-Driven Activity

As described above, tonotopic mapping studies have revealed that animals treated with tinnitus inducing agents show elevations in spontaneous firing rate with a stereotypical profile characterized by an activity peak in the mid- to high-frequency region of the DCN (Kaltenbach et al., 2000). The activity peak, when averaged across animals, was found to resemble the multiunit activity profile obtained from normal animals responding to a high-frequency tone (Kaltenbach & Afman, 2000). This resemblance suggests that the DCN of tone exposed animals is behaving as though it is signaling the presence of a high pitch sound in the absence of a corresponding stimulus. Based on this tonotopic profile, one might infer that this hyperactive state represents a physiological model of tinnitus, which predicts that animals possessing such hyperactivity might experience tinnitus-like percepts. Much work, which will be discussed further, has been oriented toward the testing of this prediction.

Altered Activity and Tinnitus Percepts

The hypothesis that changes in neural activity are related to tinnitus has been addressed by testing whether animals showing any of the observed changes in activity following treatment with tinnitus inducing agents also show behavioral evidence of tinnitus percepts. Most such studies were modifications of the original test designed by Pawel Jastreboff et al. (1988). Jastreboff's test yielded results supporting the hypothesis that rats experience acute tinnitus following treatment with sodium salicylate. Jastreboff's lab also reported that neurons in the inferior colliculus of salicylate-treated rats show elevations of spontaneous firing rates (Jastreboff & Sasaki, 1986) as well as increases in bursting discharge patterns (Chen & Jastreboff, 1995). Subsequently, behavioral studies have reported evidence consistent with tinnitus induction following intense noise exposure in several other species, including hamsters (Heffner & Harrington, 2002), chinchillas (Brozoski et al., 2002), rats (Pace et al., 2016; Zhang et al., 2016), and mice (Middleton et al., 2011; Li et al., 2013). Other studies have shown that the DCN fusiform cells of animals with behavioral evidence of tinnitus exhibit elevated levels of spontaneous activity, bursting activity, and/or synchrony, whereas animals showing little or no behavioral evidence of tinnitus showed little or no increase in these properties (Brozoski et al., 2002; Cacace et al., 2014; Kaltenbach et al., 2004; Li et al., 2013; Luo et al., 2014; Middleton et al., 2011; Wu et al., 2016).

More recent work has provided further confirmation for the assertion that sound exposure conditions that cause both acute and chronic alterations of spontaneous activity in the DCN also cause animals to experience tinnitus-like percepts. This relationship has been tested with a variety of preparations and methods. Using manganese-enhanced magnetic resonance imaging (MEMRI), several studies have found evidence for increased activation states in both DCN and ventral cochlear nucleus (VCN) of noise-exposed (Brozoski et al., 2007, 2013) or blast-treated rats (Ouyang et al., 2017) that tested positive for tinnitus in behavioral tests. Luo et al. (2014) demonstrated immediate and sustained (up to 1 month) increases of spontaneous activity in the DCN of rats that correlated with behavioral evidence of tinnitus induced by exposure to blast noise. Wu et al. (2016) found that hyperactivity of DCN fusiform cells manifests as both increased spontaneous and sound evoked activity in noise-exposed guinea pigs that showed behavioral evidence of tinnitus based on the gap detection test. Using flavoprotein imaging as a measure of activation levels, Middleton et al., (2011) found evidence for increased resting activity in mice showing behavioral evidence of tinnitus in the gap detection test, while Li et al. (2013), using electrophysiological recordings in vitro, found spontaneous hyperactivity in the DCN of mice testing positive for tinnitus, again using the gap detection test. Most of these studies can be credited for removing the effects of hearing loss on the behavioral test by using animals that developed either no hearing loss or only a temporary hearing loss that recovered by the time the behavioral test was performed. One concern this raises is that they may model a form of tinnitus which is not associated with hearing loss, a condition that is not often found clinically (J. A. Henry, personal communication).

Wu et al (2016) found that the burst rate of DCN fusiform cells, the percentage time bursting activity was displayed, and the degree of synchronous firing by DCN fusiform cells correlated positively with tinnitus behavior, whereas burst duration was negatively correlated with tinnitus behavior.

Imaging Studies in Humans with Tinnitus

Owing to the invasiveness of recording activity from neurons in the human brain, knowledge of activation states in human subjects has come almost entirely from neuroimaging studies. While most of these studies have focused on cortical regions, a few have also examined activity at subcortical levels, and at least three of these have included analysis of the region thought to represent the cochlear nucleus (Lanting et al., 2010; Lockwood et al., 2001; Van Gendt et al., 2012). All three of these studies found increases in activity in the cochlear nucleus of subjects with tinnitus compared with those having no tinnitus. Efforts were made in two of these studies to remove the effects of hearing loss by examining patients with either gaze-evoked or somatically modulatable tinnitus. One of the studies interpreted the region of hyperactivation as representing the DCN (Lockwood et al., 2001). The results are generally consistent with the animal work described earlier showing increased DCN activation associated with tinnitus and somatic modulatability of activity in the DCN (see chapter by Shore, this volume).

Origin of Tinnitus-Related Activity and Its Relationship with Higher-Order Nuclei

Two fundamental issues that impact the significance of cochlear nucleus activity as it relates to tinnitus is where it originates and whether it influences activity elsewhere in the auditory system. The first of these issues concerns the question of whether the activity changes could be derived peripherally from the ear or auditory nerve or centrally from higher levels of the brain. The second concerns the question of whether the activity changes have impact on how neurons function at higher levels of the brain, which could account for the fact that tinnitus is a conscious percept requiring cortical functionality.

Does Tinnitus-Related Activity Originate in the Auditory Periphery?

Although changed activity in the cochlear nucleus results from peripheral damage, several independent lines of evidence suggest that the hyperactivity that develops in the cochlear nuclei after treatment with a tinnitus inducer does not originate in the auditory periphery. Previous studies have shown that acoustic or ototoxic injury to the cochlea results in reductions of spontaneous activity of auditory nerve fibers (Liberman & Dodds, 1984; Liberman & Kiang, 1978; Wang et al., 1997). Diminutions of spontaneous activity are found weeks to months following noise exposure (Liberman & Dodds, 1984). The reductions of activity show a tonotopic profile corresponding to the regions of noise-induced hair cell injury. Decreased activity was found to be maximal in the area with the greatest injury to the tallest row of inner hair cell stereocilia and sloped toward normal levels along the edges of the lesion (Liberman & Dodds, 1984). A second line of evidence is that noise-induced hyperactivity was found to persist in the DCN following both partial and complete ablation of the cochlear partition (Zacharek et al., 2002). These results are consistent with studies in humans reporting that tinnitus often develops secondarily following loss of input to the cochlear nucleus from the ear (Berliner et al., 1992; Fahy et al., 2002; House & Brackmann, 1981; Kameda et al., 2010). These findings converge to support the notion that the increased spontaneous activity of central auditory neurons is a manifestation of reduced or weakened input from the auditory nerve. Thus, deafferentation, whether anatomical or functional, may be one of several important triggers of tinnitus signal generation in the cochlear nuclei. The mechanisms by which this might occur are discussed in a later section. It is worth noting that increases in bursting activity have been observed in the auditory nerve of noise-exposed cats, although this bursting was not associated with increases in spontaneous firing rate (Liberman & Kiang, 1978). The possibility that increased burst firing in the auditory nerve after noise exposure could be relayed centrally and contribute to the increased bursting activity observed in the DCN cannot be ruled out.

Could the Changes in the Cochlear Nucleus Originate from Higher-Order Auditory Stations?

It has been suggested by some investigators that since hyperactivity, increased bursting or increased synchrony are found at the auditory cortical or subcortical forebrain areas of animals treated with tinnitus inducing agents, including noise (Kalappa et al., 2014; Norena & Eggermont, 2006; Seki & Eggermont, 2003;), quinine: (Eggermont & Kenmochi, 1998), or salicylate (Ochi & Eggermont, 1996; Eggermont & Kenmochi, 1998), this may be where the tinnitus-related changes observed in the cochlear nucleus originate. This "top-down" model, however, is inconsistent with the finding that hyperactivity induced in the DCN by noise exposure persists in the DCN even after input from all descending pathways from higher-order auditory centers has been removed (Zhang et al., 2006). This isolation preparation was achieved by transecting all the descending fiber tracts originating from outside the cochlear nucleus, including the dorsal and intermediate acoustic striae and the trapezoid body. This preparation would have removed descending inputs to the cochlear nuclei from the auditory cortex (Meltzer & Ryugo, 2006), inferior colliculus (Andersen et al., 1980; Caicedo & Herbert, 1993; Faye-Lund, 1986; Malmierca et al., 1996;) and superior olivary complex (Schofield, 2002; Spangler et al., 1987). The hyperactivity that persisted was no weaker than that present when the descending inputs were intact. This would seem to rule out a descending source for the maintenance of hyperactivity in the cochlear nuclei. A role of corticofugal pathways in the maintenance of hyperactivity also seems dubious in light of a study by Imig and Durham (2005), who found that removal of descending cortical input to the cochlear nucleus by surgical decortication produced an increase in metabolic activity of the DCN, indicating release from inhibition. Finally, two imaging studies conducted in human subjects with tinnitus using fMRI found elevated states of activation in the cochlear nucleus and inferior colliculus but not in the auditory cortex (Lanting et al., 2010; Van Gendt et al., 2012). This pattern would seem to contraindicate that the hyperactivity observed in the cochlear nucleus is derived from the cortex. These considerations lead to the view that the cochlear nucleus generates its own state of hyperactivity, independent of inputs from other sources, although it does not rule out the possibility that these changes might also be associated with changes in the level of activity or synaptic function in those descending inputs. As will be discussed later in this chapter and in the chapter by Shore (this volume), there is evidence for such changes in at least two of these descending pathways (the cholinergic system from the superior olivary complex and glutamatergic system from branches of the somatosensory pathway). Changes in descending pathways might be involved in establishing DCN hyperactivity, but they are not needed for maintaining it, as also evidenced by the finding that increased bursting activity and increased sensitivity of acetylcholine receptors occurs in slices of DCN, which have no external connections (Chang et al., 2002).

Do Activity Changes in the Cochlear Nuclei Drive Similar Changes at Higher Levels?

Each of the activity changes just described has counterparts in the inferior colliculus. Hyperactivity, bursting activity, and increased neural synchrony all occur in the inferior colliculus of animals that have been exposed to noise or a tinnitus-inducing drug and/or yielded positive evidence for tinnitus in behavioral tests (Bauer et al., 2008). The hyperactivity that occurs in the IC shows characteristics similar to hyperactivity in the DCN. For example, the peak of the hyperactivity profile occurs in roughly the same high-frequency region of the tonotopic map and follows a similar time course of development as hyperactivity in the DCN (Manzoor et al., 2012, 2013b). In addition, the hyperactivity induced in the IC can be abolished by ablating the contralateral DCN. Also, ablation of the DCN is sufficient to prevent induction of tinnitus in animals (Brozoski et al., 2012). These findings suggest that hyperactivity in the IC is derived from the DCN. A result that raises some question about this conclusion is that ablation of the DCN did not abolish behavioral signs of tinnitus once it was already induced (Brozoski & Bauer, 2005). It could be that hyperactivity in the DCN leads to hyperactivity in the IC, but once the IC hyperactivity has become established, it no longer depends on input from the DCN. This may mean that although the DCN may drive hyperactivity in the IC, the IC may compensate for loss of hyperactive input through homeostatic mechanisms. Further research is needed to clarify this issue

Mechanisms Underlying the Induction of Tinnitus-Related Signal Generation

Efforts to elucidate mechanisms of tinnitus induction have focused on the primary factors that are known to determine the rate and pattern of neural discharges. These include anatomical and chemical changes occurring at the synaptic level and changes that affect the biophysical properties of neurons (i.e., ion channels). Each of these are summarized below.

Synaptopathies

The hypothesis that has received the most attention concerning the mechanism underlying the generation of tinnitus-related activity is that it results from disturbance in the balance of excitation and inhibition. For example, the emergence of hyperactivity is conceptualized as the product of a shift of the balance toward the side of greater excitation, due either to a weakening of inhibition, a strengthening of excitation, or some combination of both. Studies providing support for this concept are reviewed below.

Anatomical changes in excitatory and inhibitory synapses

Anatomical studies bearing on the question of how the balance of excitatory and inhibitory synapses is affected following a tinnitus-inducing manipulation report evidence for degenerative, regenerative, and axonal sprouting (plasticity). Kim et al. (2004) quantified the occurrence of excitatory and inhibitory synapses in the posteroventral cochlear nucleus (PVCN) of chinchillas exposed to intense (108 dB SPL) noise for 3 hours. Synapses were differentiated using classical criteria: those containing pleomorphic (flat) vesicles and symmetrical junctions were interpreted as inhibitory, whereas those containing round vesicles with asymmetrical junctions were interpreted as excitatory. In their noise exposed animals, a progressive decline was found between the first and 24th week after exposure in the total number of both excitatory and inhibitory synapses in the PVCN; much of this decline reflected the loss of auditory nerve input or transneuronal degeneration of neurons in the PVCN. Over a period of a few additional weeks, the recovery was virtually complete for excitatory synapses but incomplete for inhibitory synapses. This was interpreted as evidence of a greater recovery of excitatory than inhibitory synapses, thus favoring a net shift towards stronger excitation, which could correlate with chronic tinnitus but not early onset tinnitus. A similar pattern was also observed on the globular bushy cells of the AVCN. Whether this pattern of recovery also occurs in the DCN was not reported. A later study by Du et al. (2012) found a decrease in immunohistochemically labeled synaptic terminals in the DCN fusiform soma layer of chinchillas 10 days after exposure to intense noise. Electron microscopic study showed evidence of degeneration of terminal endings on cartwheel cells, enlarged and misshaped pleomorphic/flattened vesicles in one of two previously described (Wouterlood & Mugnaini, 1984) synaptic terminal types. These changes occurred only in the middle frequency region of the DCN, which corresponded to the focus of energy in the spectrum of noise used to expose the animals. The investigators interpreted these results as suggesting a reduction of inhibitory input to cartwheel cells. The source of the inhibitory terminals was not identified but could possibly be other cartwheel cells. The authors expressed the possibility that, if so, the disinhibited cartwheel cells may themselves become hyperactive, or alternatively there may also be loss of inhibitory cartwheel cell terminals onto fusiform cells. This latter possibility could account for the increased fusiform cell activity that others have observed following noise exposure.

Chemical changes in inhibitory and excitatory synapses

Effects of cochlear damage on central auditory system chemistry have been recently reviewed (Gold & Bajo, 2014; Lee & Godfrey, 2014), so we will focus on the major changes in the cochlear nucleus that may underlie tinnitus symptoms. In addition to cochlear damage resulting from intense sound and ototoxic drugs, cochlear ablation is among the procedures that are likely to be tinnitus inducing since human subjects often develop tinnitus secondarily following eighth nerve resection (Berliner et al, 1992; Soussi & Otto, 1994; Kameda et al., 2010). Neural pathways that may be involved in the neurotransmitter changes described next are shown schematically in Figure 8.4.

Reductions in GABA receptor subunit α1 and glutamate decarboxylase messenger RNA expression have been measured in whole cochlear nucleus of guinea pigs a week after partial cochlear damage (Dong et al., 2009). After intense sound exposure, early decreases of these same molecules were followed by increases at 4 weeks survival (Dong et al., 2010), perhaps as a response of the cells to the early depletions. Decreases of GABA levels have been measured in the VCN of rats and chinchillas, although not to any great extent in the DCN, after cochlear ablation (Godfrey et al., 2014, 2015), and in the VCN and superficial DCN after treatment with the ototoxic drug carboplatin (Godfrey et al., 2005), but not after intense sound (Godfrey et al., 2012). Increases in GABA release and uptake were measured in the VCN but not in the DCN after cochlear ablation (Suneja et al., 1998b). After short-term conductive hearing loss, no change in expression of $GABA_A$ receptor subunits was found on fusiform cells of the DCN or bushy cells of the VCN (Wang et al., 2011). Overall, since messenger RNA expression does not always correlate well with protein expression (Wang et al., 2009), these results do not provide strong evidence that changes in GABA neurotransmission in the cochlear nucleus, particularly in the DCN, underlie tinnitus symptoms. However, a study on slices from mouse DCN provides evidence for involvement of decreased GABA neurotransmission in the activity of DCN neurons of mice with behavioral evidence of tinnitus (Middleton et al., 2011).

Evidence is stronger for involvement of glycine neurotransmission in DCN hyperactivity. At the whole cochlear nucleus level, a decrease in messenger RNA for glycine receptor subunit α1 was measured a week after partial cochlear damage in guinea pigs (Dong et al., 2009) and, as for GABA, an early decrease followed by increased expression of the same molecule at 4 weeks after intense sound exposure (Dong et al., 2010). Measurements of glycine levels have revealed small decreases in the DCN after cochlear ablation in rats and chinchillas or intense sound exposure in hamsters (Godfrey et al., 2012, 2014, 2015). Increases were measured in the chinchilla DCN after carboplatin treatment (Godfrey et al., 2005), but large decreases in glycine-immunoreactive puncta were measured on several rat cochlear nucleus cell types, including DCN fusiform cells, after treatment with a different ototoxic drug, neomycin (Asako et al., 2005). Decreased glycine release and increased uptake were measured in the guinea pig DCN after cochlear ablation (Suneja et al., 1998b), changes which may reflect decreased glycine neurotransmission. Strong evidence for glycine involvement has come from studies of glycine receptors. In chinchillas, there is evidence that fusiform cells, the major neuron type projecting from the DCN to the inferior colliculus, are sensitive to the actions of the glycine antagonist strychnine (Caspary et al., 1987). Fusiform cells receive some excitatory input from auditory nerve fibers and some from the parallel fiber axons of granule cells, whereas they receive inhibitory input especially from nearby cartwheel cells (Berrebi & Mugnaini, 1991; Godfrey et al., 1997; Mancilla & Manis, 2009; Oertel & Young, 2004;

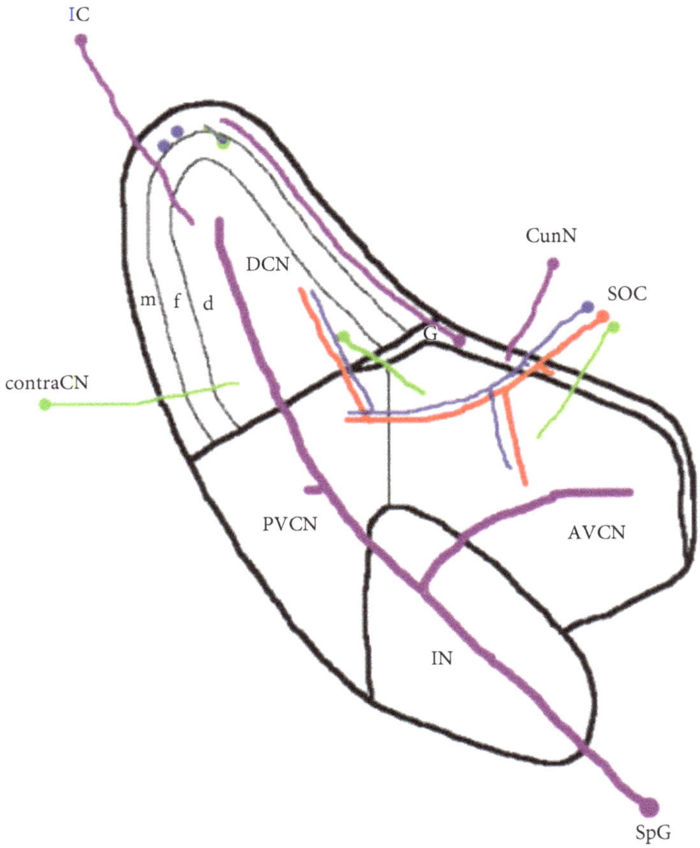

FIGURE 8.4. Diagrammatic representation of some of the pathways innervating cochlear nucleus neurons via 4 prominent neurotransmitters. Pathways likely using glutamate (purple) are based on Wenthold (1978), Oliver et al. (1983), Osen et al. (1995), Wright & Ryugo (1996), Godfrey et al. (1997, 2015), and Milinkeviciute et al. (2017). Pathways likely using acetylcholine (red) are based on Godfrey et al. (1987, 1990), Godfrey (1993), Vetter et al. (1993), Sherriff & Henderson (1994), and Mellott et al. (2011). Pathways likely using GABA (blue) are based on Davies (1981), Mugnaini (1985), Godfrey et al. (1988), Osen et al. (1990), Potashner et al. (1993), Saint Marie et al. (1993), and Apostolides and Trussell (2013). Pathways likely using glycine (green) are based on Wenthold (1987), Osen et al. (1990), Altschuler et al. (1993), Oertel & Wickesberg (1993), Potashner et al. (1993), Saint Marie et al. (1993), and Oertel and Young (2004). General origins of pathways (colored dots) are indicated, but exact terminations are not included and not always known. *Abbreviations*: AVCN, anteroventral cochlear nucleus; contraCN, contralateral cochlear nucleus; CunN, cuneate nucleus; DCN, dorsal cochlear nucleus, with molecular (m), fusiform soma (f), and deep (d) layers; IC, inferior colliculus; IN, interstitial nucleus (auditory nerve root); PVCN, posteroventral cochlear nucleus; SOC, superior olivary complex, with also pontomesencephalic tegmentum for acetylcholine; and SpG, spiral ganglion. Green dot in deep DCN represents tuberculoventral cells. Blue dots in molecular layer represent stellate and Golgi cells. Green dot in superficial DCN fusiform soma layer, with smaller blue superimposed, represents cartwheel cells, for which there is evidence for GABA as well as glycine as neurotransmitters.

Roberts & Trussell, 2010). The excitatory inputs employ glutamate as neurotransmitter, and the inhibitory inputs primarily use glycine (Oertel & Young, 2004), although GABA may also be involved (Apostolides & Trussell, 2013). A small but statistically significant decrease in glycine receptor binding was measured in guinea pig superficial DCN after cochlear ablation (Suneja et al., 1998a). Decreased expression of glycine receptor α1 subunit protein and decreased strychnine binding, indicative of decreased glycine receptor function, were found in the DCN fusiform cells of rats with behavioral evidence of tinnitus (Wang et al., 2009). Also, high, ototoxic, doses of salicylate have been reported to decrease the frequency of spontaneous inhibitory postsynaptic currents onto fusiform cells in rats, although there was no change in fusiform cell spontaneous activity (Zugaib et al., 2016). Arguing against a strong role of glycine, however, are the results of Middleton et al. (2011) mentioned previously: they did not find much difference in the effects of the glycine antagonist strychnine on DCN activity of mice with behavioral evidence of tinnitus, as compared to control mice. Together, the findings for GABA and glycine would seem to indicate that weakened inhibition of fusiform cells could be an important mechanism contributing to the emergence of hyperactivity in this cell type.

Related to inhibitory neurotransmission is a third amino acid, taurine, which has been found to be associated with GABA and glycine neurotransmission (Albrecht & Schousboe, 2005; Ottersen et al., 1988; Walberg et al., 1990). Taurine can act as an agonist at glycine and both $GABA_A$ and $GABA_B$ receptors (Albrecht & Schousboe, 2005) and may thereby promote inhibitory synaptic activity. Being also associated with glia (Hassel et al., 1995), taurine levels often increase in regions where nerve fibers are degenerating and gliosis is expected, such as the VCN after cochlear ablation (Godfrey et al., 2014) or treatment with carboplatin (Godfrey et al., 2005). However, after exposure to intense sound, small but consistent decreases in taurine levels were measured throughout the hamster central auditory system (Godfrey et al., 2012), possibly correlating with decreased inhibitory neurotransmission. Taurine is considered to be important in recovery from neural injury (Gupta et al., 2006), and there is evidence that adding it to the diet of rats can decrease behavioral evidence of tinnitus (Brozoski et al., 2010).

From a simpleminded point of view, if increased neural spontaneous activity underlies tinnitus, and decreased inhibitory neurotransmitter function is associated, one might expect an increase in excitatory neurotransmitter function to also possibly be involved. This does not seem to apply for the excitatory amino acids glutamate and aspartate after cochlear ablation or ototoxic drug treatment, since their levels, synthesis, release, uptake, and messenger RNA for AMPA and NMDA receptor subunits fairly consistently decrease in the cochlear nucleus following these manipulations (Dong et al., 2009; Godfrey et al., 2012, 2014, 2015; Potashner et al., 1997; Wenthold, 1978; Zeng et al., 2009). However, following intense sound exposure, after initial decreases, increases in messenger RNA for AMPA and NMDA receptor subunits were measured at 4 weeks survival for whole guinea pig cochlear nucleus (Dong et al., 2010), and many increases in glutamate AMPA-type receptor expression were measured in the chinchilla VCN, although not in the DCN, after noise trauma (Muly et al., 2004). Increased D-aspartate release and decreased uptake have also been reported in both VCN and DCN of chinchillas after noise trauma (Muly et al., 2004), changes that may be associated with increased excitatory neurotransmission. At 5 months after intense sound exposure, small but consistent increases in glutamate concentration were found throughout the hamster cochlear nucleus and larger increases for aspartate (Godfrey et al., 2012). Although evidence for a neurotransmitter function of aspartate is much less than for glutamate, the two amino acids are closely linked metabolically (Ross et al., 1995), so that increases in aspartate concentration could easily contribute to increased excitatory neurotransmission by increasing the supply of glutamate.

Most acetylcholine neurotransmission in the cochlear nucleus has been associated with centrifugal pathways to its various parts (Godfrey, 1985; Mellott et al., 2011). Acetylcholine can serve as either an excitatory or inhibitory neurotransmitter, depending on the nature of the postsynaptic channels at a particular synapse (Moises & Womble, 1995). In the cochlear nucleus, early in vivo studies found mainly excitatory effects of acetylcholine in the VCN and inhibitory effects in the DCN (Comis, 1970; Martin & Adams, 1979; Caspary et al., 1983; Godfrey, 1985), but more recent in vitro studies found predominantly excitatory muscarinic acetylcholine effects in the rat DCN (Chen et al., 1994, 1995). Cochlear ablation results in short-term increases in activity of the synthetic enzyme for acetylcholine, choline acetyltransferase, throughout the rat cochlear nucleus, but most of these increases are no longer present at 2 months after the lesion (Jin et al., 2005). Binding to muscarinic acetylcholine receptors also increases after cochlear ablation throughout the rat cochlear nucleus except for the DCN molecular layer, and continues to increase through 2 months after the lesion (Jin & Godfrey, 2006). After intense sound exposure, choline acetyltransferase activity increased in most hamster cochlear nucleus regions through 2 months after exposure (Jin et al., 2006), but the increase was sustained through 5 months only in the granular region adjacent to the AVCN (Godfrey et al., 2013). These results suggest an increase in acetylcholine function in the cochlear nucleus after types of cochlear damage that may result in tinnitus, especially in granular regions. Granule cells themselves do not appear to use acetylcholine as neurotransmitter, but they receive innervation that uses acetylcholine (Köszeghy et al., 2012), and themselves use glutamate as transmitter (Chen et al., 1999; Godfrey et al., 1997). Their axons mostly or entirely project to the superficial layers of the DCN to synapse on the dendrites of cartwheel and fusiform cells (Berrebi & Mugnaini, 1991; Godfrey et al., 1997; Mugnaini et al., 1980; Osen, 1988; Wouterlood and Mugnaini, 1984). There is evidence that, besides granule cells, cartwheel cells of mice have muscarinic acetylcholine receptors that affect glutamate neurotransmission from granule cells onto them (He et al., 2014) and that fusiform cells of rats also have such receptors (Chen et al., 1994, 1995; Pál et al., 2009). In addition, Golgi cells, which provide inhibitory input to granule cells, were hyperpolarized via muscarinic acetylcholine receptors in slices of mouse DCN (Irie et al., 2006), which could result in increased granule cell activity. A recent study reported that blocking muscarinic acetylcholine receptors affected spontaneous activity and stimulus timing-dependent plasticity in fusiform cells of guinea pigs (Stefanescu & Shore, 2017). These effects on long-term synaptic plasticity may be mediated through endocannabinoid signaling (Zhao & Tzounopoulos, 2011).

After intense tone exposure in rats, increased sensitivity to the non-selective acetylcholine agonist carbachol was found among bursting neurons, which could be cartwheel cells, or fusiform cells that had changed their firing patterns, or both, in the DCN of rat brain slices (Chang et al., 2002). As already mentioned, cartwheel cells provide inhibitory, glycinergic/GABAergic input to fusiform cells (Oertel & Young, 2004; Apostolides & Trussell, 2013), as well as to other cartwheel cells (Mancilla & Manis, 2009; Roberts & Trussell, 2010). On the other hand, an in vivo study found that the hyperactivity measured in hamsters previously exposed to an intense tone could be decreased by application of carbachol to the DCN (Manzoor et al., 2013b).

It is difficult to combine all the data on neurotransmitter-related changes following cochlear damage that may lead to tinnitus into a comprehensive understanding of what changes may underlie the tinnitus symptoms. This is partly because of the variety of animal models used in the studies, sometimes giving conflicting results, partly because of different survival times used in the various studies, which may only sample one or a few time points during the progression of changes that may underlie tinnitus, and partly because the various studies have measured only certain aspects of neurotransmitter chemistry. However, available data suggest that there may be an increase in acetylcholine function, mediated through muscarinic receptors in the granule cell—cartwheel cell—fusiform cell system, combined with increased excitation mediated by glutamate, and some decreased function of cartwheel cells and their inhibitory glycinergic (and possibly also GABAergic) neurotransmission onto fusiform cells. This could result in increased spontaneous activity of fusiform cells, because of direct cholinergic activation and increased granule cell activation, together with decreased cartwheel cell inhibition. If this is the case, then the suppression of DCN hyperactivity by application of 100 μM of the acetylcholine agonist carbachol to the DCN surface (Manzoor et al., 2013a) may result from a general delayed suppression of the circuitry by this high dose, such as by a long term depression mechanism. Alternatively, in view of the variety of neurotransmitter-related changes after cochlear damage, tinnitus may be a manifestation of any imbalance among neural activities in the central auditory system that may result from changes in the various neurotransmitter functions.

Channelopathies

The concept that tinnitus signal generation might arise as a result of changes in the intrinsic membrane properties of neurons is relatively more recent than the synaptopathy concept. The channelopathy theory is simple and intuitively appealing because ion channels largely control the base level of excitability of a cell, by changing the thresholds for action potential generation, the durations of action potentials, and/or the recovery times (refractory periods) following action potentials. The distribution and numbers of expressed ion channels in the somatic or dendritic membranes also determine the properties of spatial and temporal integration. All of these factors determine the rates and patterns of neuronal impulse generation, and thus a change in any of these features is a potential mechanism of tinnitus related activity. In practice, it is to some extent arbitrary to draw a line of separation between changes in neurotransmitter receptor expression and changes in ion channel expression as independent categories, since many receptors function as ligand-gated ion channels. Therefore, to differentiate this category from those of a more synaptic nature, the present subsection will examine only changes in channels that are not synaptic receptor channels (ionotropic). These include the voltage-gated ion channels and the non-voltage-gated ion channels and are discussed separately.

Changes in voltage-gated ion channels

Much less is known about the role of ion channels in tinnitus compared to synaptic anatomy and chemistry, and only a few studies concern the cochlear nucleus. The first hints of altered ion channel conductances were obtained from studies of brain slices of mice examined 2 weeks following bilateral cochlear ablations (Francis & Manis, 2000). Cells in the VCN showed smaller action potentials, more depolarization, and smaller afterhyperpolarizations with shorter membrane time constants compared to cells from unablated control mice. Some cells also showed evidence of increased input resistance.

Direct evidence for altered ion conductance that seems likely to be related to tinnitus has recently been reported by Pilati et al. (2012). They observed a decrease in high-voltage-activated (HVA) potassium currents in DCN fusiform cells exposed to intense sound 3–4 days earlier. This decrease was found to correlate with a shift from regular to burst firing (complex or irregular spiking) and longer duration action potentials of fusiform cells. Since increases in bursting activity were previously shown to contribute to the increase in overall discharge rate of fusiform cells (Finlayson & Kaltenbach, 2009), the findings of Pilati et al. may provide a mechanism underlying hyperactivity, with decreased HVA potassium conductances contributing to slower repolarization following action potential generation and the emergence of bursting activity.

Li et al. (2013) measured KCNQ2/3 (M) currents in DCN fusiform cells to investigate the role of Kv7.2/3 (KCNQ) channels as a possible substrate of noise-induced tinnitus. KCNQ channels function as brakes on action potential generation and therefore control the excitability of neurons (Delmas & Brown, 2005; Soldovieri et al., 2011). Decreases in their expression lead to hyperexcitability disorders such as epilepsy (Soldovieri et al., 2011). In the study by Li et al., KCNQ currents were found to be reduced in DCN fusiform cells of mice immediately after they tested positive for tinnitus 1 week after noise exposure. Such reductions were not found in unexposed control mice or in noise-exposed mice testing negative for tinnitus. The reduced KCNQ currents were observed in the hyperactive high-frequency half of the DCN, but not in the low frequency half, which was not hyperactive. Animals that had been pretreated with the anti-epileptic drug and KCNQ blocker, retigabine, did not show tinnitus, nor did they exhibit hyperactivity in the DCN. The authors inferred from their findings that KCNQ channel reduction is essential for the induction of tinnitus and tinnitus-related hyperactivity in the DCN following noise exposure. This reduced channel conductance could induce hyperactivity by shifting the voltage dependence of the channel to more positive voltages, pushing the cell closer to the threshold for action potential generation. Although retigabine has a number of serious side effects which limit its usefulness as a therapeutic agent, a more recent study has shown that a less toxic drug that also blocks KCNQ channels has a similar effect as retigabine on tinnitus and tinnitus-associated hyperactivity (Kalappa et al., 2015).

Non-voltage/non-ligand-gated ion channels

In the cochlear nucleus, changes in the expression/conductivity have also been observed in the two-pore-domain potassium channels (K_{2PD}) as well as in the expression of the inward-rectifier potassium channels. K_{2PD} channels are involved in setting resting membrane potentials via their role in regulating potassium ion leakage. These channels thus participate in the control of neuronal excitability. Holt and colleagues (2006) reported that decreases occur in the expression of multiple subunits of the K_{2PD} channel in the cochlear nucleus of rats following bilateral cochlear ablation. The timing of the decreases varied with subunits: some decreases occurred between 3 days and 3 months, while others were decreased only at the beginning or end of this post-ablation range. Since the decreases were found in whole cochlear nucleus homogenates, future studies will be required to pin down the distribution and degree of change in this channel in specific subdivisions. Nonetheless, the available results do suggest another potential mechanism that could contribute to the hyperactive state underlying tinnitus, since reductions in this channel's expression would be expected to become manifest as a decrease in potassium leakage, thus shifting the potential in the positive direction and making the cell more excitable.

Issues, Challenges, and Controversies

As the foregoing narrative has summarized, the concept that the cochlear nucleus plays a key role in the generation of tinnitus-related signals is supported by a substantial body of evidence. However, like many other concepts in neuroscience, this concept is complex and has elements that remain unclear or even controversial. Next we highlight the main issues that are most uncertain and provoke the most discussion and controversy:

1. *The neural correlate of tinnitus.* Although the three abnormal states of activity (hyperactivity, increased bursting, increased neural synchrony) that are associated with tinnitus have the hallmarks of sound encoding signals in terms of tonotopicity and timing (see previous discussion), it remains unclear which of these is necessary and sufficient for the generation of tinnitus percepts. Whether tinnitus is the product of one of these or instead results from a combination of these signals is an issue that needs further clarification.
2. *The trigger of tinnitus activity induction.* An issue that needs further elucidation is the precise change that triggers induction of the abnormal states of activity in the cochlear nuclei. What is the relative importance of inner versus outer hair cell

injury? Injury to either type of hair cell has been reported to trigger tinnitus related changes in activity in central auditory nuclei (Bauer et al., 2008; Kaltenbach et al., 2002), but there is also evidence that chronic increases in spontaneous activity and tinnitus can be induced by moderate sound exposure conditions (80 dB SPL) that do not cause chronic hearing loss and would seem to be below the intensity level needed to permanently damage either inner or outer hair cells (Brozoski et al., 2002; Kaltenbach et al., 2005). Thus, the common view that the abnormal activity is triggered by deafferentation caused by injury to the cochlea may be too simplistic. Indeed, recent evidence suggests that tinnitus related activity may be induced by other triggers such as activity-dependent (e.g., LTP/LTD) (Stefanescu & Shore, 2017) or homeostatic plasticity (Schaette & Kempter, 2006) and/or excitotoxic injury (Criddle et al., 2018), but the issue of the relative importance of each of these remains obscure. Perhaps all contribute to some degree as part of a complex equation of interacting factors.

3. *Mechanism of tinnitus signal induction*. Further work is needed to clarify the precise mechanism leading to these abnormal states. As we have described, both synaptic and non-synaptic mechanisms have received experimental support for a contributory role from careful in-depth studies, but more research is needed to determine which is more critical to the emergence of signals that are tinnitus producing.
4. *The role of descending pathways*. The role of upregulation of descending inputs (Godfrey et al., 2013; Lee & Godfrey, 2014) to the cochlear nucleus is unclear. It is possible that this up-regulation reflects a compensatory increase in central gain caused by the loss of normal input from the ear. This possibility is difficult to reconcile with the finding that hyperactivity persists in the cochlear nucleus even after all descending inputs from higher-order auditory nuclei have been removed, but the effects of descending pathway terminals may persist for several hours after their axons have been cut (Chen et al., 1998), longer than the post-surgery time in the Zhang et al. (2006) study. Perhaps the effects of the descending inputs are decreased as a secondary consequence of diminished input from the ear. Alternatively, upregulated inputs from descending pathways may play a role in triggering the induction of abnormal activity in the cochlear nucleus but may not be required for its maintenance. Yet another possibility is that the upregulation of the descending cholinergic system to the cochlear nucleus might also be an attempt by the CNS to compensate for or suppress the hyperactivity that develops in the cochlear nucleus after noise exposure.
5. *The role of dorsal versus ventral cochlear nuclei*. The relative roles of the dorsal and ventral subdivisions of the cochlear nucleus in driving activation states at higher levels of the auditory pathway where tinnitus-related signals are translated and interpreted as tinnitus percepts needs to be clarified. While fusiform cells in the DCN have been shown to be important, other studies suggest that cartwheel cells might also become hyperactive after noise exposure and that changes occur also in the VCN. Increased cartwheel cell activity needs to be reconciled with the

hyperactivation of fusiform cells as a driver of hyperactivity in the inferior colliculus, since cartwheel cells are inhibitory to fusiform cells.

6. Lastly, the link between these changes and the intracellular processes governing gene and protein expression that determine the level and pattern of firing by neurons has yet to be characterized.

In conclusion, while tinnitus research has provided a skeletal framework for understanding the early stages of tinnitus signal generation, many questions at the cellular, molecular and circuit levels remain to be clarified. It seems that the problems have reached a level of complexity that will require an extraordinary level of sophistication and coordination of complementary approaches and experimental design to clarify or resolve these issues. More pooling of resources and cooperation among laboratories may be needed than has been typical in the past.

Clinical Implications of Our Current Understanding of Tinnitus-Generating Mechanisms

The mechanisms of tinnitus generation are very complex, and the ability to treat this disorder will depend not only on knowledge of the locus and mechanisms of the underlying defects, but also on an ability to successfully correct those defects without producing untoward side effects. This is complicated by the fact that the receptors and ion channels that become disturbed in tinnitus are shared by numerous other cell populations, many of which are located in parts of the brain that control or affect vital functions. The ability to successfully target the tinnitus defects without disturbing those other functions is likely to be a challenge, but there are reasons to be optimistic that this goal is achievable. First, the brainstem auditory nuclei normally have high levels of spontaneous activity relative to other areas of the brain (Kilduff et al., 1982). If the elevations of activity that result in tinnitus generation raise the activation state into a range above the activation levels of other brainstem nuclei, this opens up the possibility that the cells that generate tinnitus signals would be more likely to respond to drugs that inhibit spontaneous activity without inhibiting brain areas involved in the control of vital functions. Second, recent studies have succeeded in demonstrating suppression of noise-induced hyperactivity in the DCN and IC using the Kv3 channel modulator, AUT00063 (Glait et al., 2018; Anderson et al. 2018). The suppression effects were achieved without affecting response thresholds and without affecting at least two vital functions (heart rate and breathing rate). Third, a recent study by Kalappa et al. (2015) reports development of a new drug, SF0034, that blocks KCNQ channels without causing severe side effects. When mice were pretreated with this drug before being exposed to intense noise, the mice did not develop hyperactivity in DCN fusiform cells and showed no behavioral signs of tinnitus after the noise exposure. Fourth, there are promising signs that cochlear nucleus stimulation using electrodes placed in or on the DCN results in suppression of tinnitus, both in rats and humans (Luo et al., 2012; Soussi & Otto, 1994; Behr et al., 2007; Roberts et al., 2017). And fifth, tinnitus loudness can be reduced in humans by applying electrical stimulus trains that are known to induce long term depression of DCN fusiform cells in animals (Marks et al., 2018). These are promising signs that the understanding of the role of the cochlear nucleus as a tinnitus generator site have begun to yield translational applications that may eventually prove to be the stepping stones to more effective anti-tinnitus therapies.

References

Albrecht, J., & Schousboe, A. (2005). Taurine interaction with neurotransmitter receptors in the CNS: an update. *Neurochemistry Research 30*(12), 1615–1621.

Altschuler, R. A., Juiz, J. M., Shore, S. E., Bledsoe, S. C., Helfert, R. H., & Wenthold, R. J. (1993). "Inhibitory amino acid synapses and pathways in the ventral cochlear nucleus." In M. A. Merchan, J. M. Juiz, D. A. Godfrey, & E. Mugnaini (Eds.), *The Mammalian Cochlear Nuclei: Organization and Function* (pp. 211–224). New York, NY: Plenum Press.

Andersen, R. A., Roth, G. L., Aitkin, L. M., & Merzenich, M. M. (1980). The efferent projections of the central nucleus and the pericentral nucleus of the inferior colliculus in the cat. *Journal of Comparative Neurology 194*(3), 649–662.

Anderson, L. A., Hesse, L. L., Pilati, N., Bakay, W. M. H., Alvaro, G., Large, C. H., McAlpine, D., Schaette, R., and Linden, J. F. (2018). Increased spontaneous firing rates in auditory midbrain following noise exposure are specifically abolished by a Kv3 channel modulator. *Hear. Res. 365*, 77–89.

Apostolides, P. F., & Trussell, L. O. (2013). Rapid, activity-independent turnover of vesicular transmitter content at a mixed glycine/GABA synapse. *Journal of Neuroscience 33*, 4768–4781.

Asako, M., Holt, A. G., Griffith, R. D., Buras, E. D., & Altschuler, R. A. (2005). Deafness-related decreases in glycine-immunoreactive labeling in the rat cochlear nucleus. *Journal of Neuroscience Research 81*(1), 102–109.

Bauer, C. A., Turner, J. G., Caspary, D. M., Myers, K. S., & Brozoski, T. J. (2008). Tinnitus and inferior colliculus activity in chinchillas related to three distinct patterns of cochlear trauma. *Journal of Neuroscience Research 86*, 2564–2578.

Behr, R., Müller, J., Shehata-Dieler, W., Schlake, H. P., Helms, J., Roosen, K., . . . Lorens, A. (2007). The high rate CIS auditory brainstem implant for restoration of hearing in NF-2 patients. *Skull Base 2007*(2), 91–107.

Berliner, K. I., Shelton, C., Hitselberger, W. E., & Luxford, W. M. (1992). Acoustic tumors: Effect of surgical removal on tinnitus. *American Journal of Otology 13*(1), 13–17.

Berrebi, A. S., & Mugnaini, E. (1991). Distribution and targets of the cartwheel cell axon in the dorsal cochlear nucleus of the guinea pig. *Anatomy and Embryology 183*(5), 427–454.

Brozoski, T. J., & Bauer, C. A. (2005). The effect of dorsal cochlear nucleus ablation on tinnitus in rats. *Hearing Research 206*(1–2), 227–236.

Brozoski, T. J., Bauer C. A., & Caspary D. M. (2002). Elevated fusiform cell activity in the dorsal cochlear nucleus of chinchillas with psychophysical evidence of tinnitus. *Journal of Neuroscience* 22(6), 2383–2390.

Brozoski, T. J., Caspary, D. M., Bauer, C. A., & Richardson, B. D. (2010). The effect of supplemental dietary taurine on tinnitus and auditory discrimination in an animal model. *Hearing Research* 270(1–2), 71–80.

Brozoski, T. J., Ciobanu, L., & Bauer, C. A. (2007). Central neural activity in rats with tinnitus evaluated with manganese-enhanced magnetic resonance imaging (MEMRI). *Hearing Research* 228(1–2), 168–179.

Brozoski, T. J., Wisner, K. W., Odintsov, B., & Bauer, C. A. (2013). Local NMDA receptor blockade attenuates chronic tinnitus and associated brain activity in an animal model. *PLoS One* 8(10), e77674.

Brozoski, T. J., Wisner, K. W., Sybert, L. T., & Bauer, C. A. (2012). Bilateral dorsal cochlear nucleus lesions prevent acoustic-trauma induced tinnitus in an animal model. *Journal of the Association for Research in Otolaryngology* 13(1), 55–66.

Cacace, A. T., Brozoski, T., Berkowitz, B., Bauer, C., Odintsov, B., Bergkvist, M., et al. (2014). Manganese enhanced magnetic resonance imaging (MEMRI): A powerful new imaging method to study tinnitus. *Hearing Research* 311, 49–62.

Caicedo, A., & Herbert, H. (1993). Topography of descending projections from the inferior colliculus to auditory brainstem nuclei in the rat. *Journal of Comparative Neurology* 328(3), 377–392.

Caspary, D. M., Havey, D. C., & Faingold, C. L. (1983). Effects of acetylcholine on cochlear nucleus neurons. *Experimental Neurology* 82(2), 491–498.

Caspary, D. M., Pazara, K. E., Kössl, M., & Faingold, C. L. (1987). Strychnine alters the fusiform cell output from the dorsal cochlear nucleus. *Brain Research* 417, 273–282.

Cazals, Y., Horner, K. C., & Huang, Z. W. (1998). Alterations in average spectrum of cochleoneural activity by longterm salicylate treatment in the guinea pig, a plausible index of tinnitus. *Journal of Neurophysiology* 80(4), 2113–2120.

Chang, H., Chen, K., Kaltenbach, J. A., Zhang, J., & Godfrey, D. A. (2002). Effects of acoustic trauma on dorsal cochlear nucleus neuron activity in slices. *Hearing Research* 164(1–2), 59–68.

Chen, G.-D., & Jastreboff, P. J. (1995). Salicylate-induced abnormal activity in the inferior colliculus of rats. *Hearing Research* 82(2), 158–178.

Chen K., Chang, H., Zhang, J., Kaltenbach, J. A., Godfrey, D. A. (1999). Altered spontaneous activity in rat dorsal cochlear nucleus following loud sound exposure. In J. Hazell (Ed.), *Proceedings of the Sixth International Tinnitus Seminar* (pp. 212–217). London, England: The Tinnitus and Hyperacusis Centre.

Chen, K., Waller, H. J., & Godfrey, D. A. (1994). Cholinergic modulation of spontaneous activity in rat dorsal cochlear nucleus. *Hearing Research* 77(1–2), 168–176.

Chen, K., Waller, H. J., Godfrey, D. A. (1995). Muscarinic receptor subtypes in rat dorsal cochlear nucleus. *Hearing Research* 89(1–2), 137–145.

Chen, K., Waller, H. J., & Godfrey, D. A. (1998). Effects of endogenous acetylcholine on spontaneous activity in rat dorsal cochlear nucleus slices. *Brain Research* 783(2), 219–226.

Comis, S. D. (1970). Centrifugal inhibitory processes affecting neurones in the cat cochlear nucleus. *Journal of Physiology* 210(3), 751–760.

Criddle, M. W., Godfrey, D. A., and Kaltenbach, J. A. (2018). Attenuation of noise-induced hyperactivity in the dorsal cochlear nucleus by pre-treatment with MK-801. *Brain Research 1682*, 71–77.

Davies, W. E. (1981). The effect of lesions of the dorsal acoustic stria on the levels of glutamic acid decarboxylase and GABA transaminase in the inferior colliculus and cochlear nucleus of the guinea-pig. *Neurochemistry International* 3(5), 343–347.

Delmas, P., & Brown, D. A. (2005). Pathways modulating neural KCNQ/M (Kv7) potassium channels. *Nature Reviews Neuroscience* 6(11), 850–862.

Dong, S., Mulders, W. H., Rodger, J., & Robertson, D. (2009). Changes in neuronal activity and gene expression in guinea-pig auditory brainstem after unilateral partial hearing loss. *Neuroscience 159*, 1164–1174.

Dong, S., Mulders, W. H. A. M., Rodger, J., Woo, W., & Robertson, D. (2010). Acoustic trauma evokes hyperactivity and changes in gene expression in guinea-pig auditory brainstem. *European Journal of Neuroscience 31*(9), 1616–1628.

Du, X., Chen K., Choi, C. H., Li, W., Cheng, W., Stewart, C., . . . Kopke, R. D. (2012). Selective degeneration of synapses in the dorsal cochlear nucleus of chinchilla following acoustic trauma and effects of antioxidant treatment. *Hearing Research 283*(1–2), 1–13.

Eggermont, J. J. (2006). Cortical tonotopic map reorganization and its implications for treatment of tinnitus. *Acta Otolaryngologica Supplement 556*, 9–12.

Eggermont, J. J., & Kenmochi, M. (1998). Salicylate and quinine selectively increase spontaneous firing rates in secondary auditory cortex. *Hearing Research 117*(1–2), 149–160.

Evans, E. F. (1978). Place and time coding of frequency in the peripheral auditory system: Some physiological pros and cons. *Audiology 17*(5), 369–420.

Fahy, C., Nikolopoulos, T. P., & O'Donoghue., G. M. (2002). Acoustic neuroma surgery and tinnitus. *European Archives of Otorhinolaryngology 259*(6), 299–301.

Faye-Lund, H. (1986). Projection from the inferior colliculus to the superior olivary complex in the albino rat. *Anatomy and Embryology (Berlin) 175*(1), 35–52.

Finlayson, P. G., & Kaltenbach, J. A. (2009). Alterations in the spontaneous discharge patterns of single units in the dorsal cochlear nucleus following intense sound exposure. *Hearing Research 256*,104–117.

Francis, H. W., & Manis, P. B. (2000). Effects of deafferentation on the electrophysiology of ventral cochlear nucleus neurons. *Hearing Research 149*(1–2), 91–105.

Gao, Y., Manzoor, N., Kaltenbach, J. A. (2016). Evidence of activity-dependent plasticity in the dorsal cochlear nucleus, *in vivo*, induced by brief sound exposure. *Hearing Research 341*, 31–42. doi:10.1016/j.heares.2016.07.011

Glait, L., Fan, W., Stillitano, G., Sandridge, S., Pilati, N., Large, C., Alvaro, G., and Kaltenbach, J. A. (2018). Effects of AUT00063, a Kv3.1 channel modulator, on noise-induced hyperactivity in the dorsal cochlear nucleus. *Hear. Res. 361*, 36–44.

Godfrey, D. A. (1985). Cholinergic neurotransmission in the cochlear nucleus. In D. G. Drescher (Ed.), *Auditory Biochemistry* (pp. 163–183). Springfield, IL: Charles C. Thomas.

Godfrey, D. A. (1993). Comparison of quantitative and immunohistochemistry for choline acetyltransferase in the rat cochlear nucleus. In M. A. Merchán, J. M. Juiz, D. A. Godfrey, & E. Mugnaini (Eds.), *The Mammalian Cochlear Nuclei: Organization and Function* (pp. 267–278). New York, NY: Plenum Publishing Corporation.

Godfrey, D. A., Beranek, K. L., Carlson, L., Parli, J. A., Dunn, J. D., & Ross, C. D. (1990). Contribution of centrifugal innervation to choline acetyl transferase activity in the cat cochlear nucleus. *Hearing Research 49*, 259–280.

Godfrey, D. A., Chen, K., Godfrey, M. A., Lee, A. C., Crass, S. P., Shipp, D., Simo, H., & Robinson, K. T. (2015) Cochlear ablation effects on amino acid levels in the chinchilla cochlear nucleus. *Neuroscience 297*, 137–159.

Godfrey, D. A., Kaltenbach, J. A., Chen, K., Ilyas, O., Liu, X., Licari F, et al. (2012). Amino acid concentrations in the hamster central auditory system and long-term effects of intense tone exposure. *Journal of Neuroscience Research 90*(11), 2214–2224.

Godfrey, D. A., Kaltenbach, J. A., Chen, K., Ilyas, O. (2013). Choline acetyltransferase activity in the hamster central auditory system and long-term effects of intense tone exposure. *Journal of Neuroscience Research 91*(7), 987–996.

Godfrey, D. A., Jin, Y. M., Liu, X., Godfrey, M. A. (2014). Effects of cochlear ablation on amino acid levels in the rat cochlear nucleus and superior olive. *Hearing Research 309*, 44–54.

Godfrey, D. A., Godfrey, M. A., Ding, D. L., Chen, K., & Salvi, R. J. (2005). Amino acid concentrations in chinchilla cochlear nucleus at different times after carboplatin treatment. *Hearing Research 206*(1–2), 64–73.

Godfrey, D. A., Godfrey, T. G., Mikesell, N. L., Waller, H. J., Yao, W., Chen, K., & Kaltenbach, J. A. (1997). Chemistry of granular and closely related regions of the cochlear nucleus. In J. Syka (Ed.), *Acoustical signal processing in the central auditory system* (pp. 139–153). New York, NY : Plenum Press.

Godfrey, D. A., Park-Hellendall, J. L., Dunn, J. D., & Ross, C. D. (1987). Effects of trapezoid body and superior olive lesions on choline acetyltransferase activity in the rat cochlear nucleus. *Hearing Research 28*, 253–270.

Godfrey, D. A., Parli, J. A., Dunn, J. D., & Ross, C. D. (1988). Neurotransmitter microchemistry of the cochlear nucleus and superior olivary complex. In J. Syka & R. B. Masterton (Eds.), *Auditory Pathway* (pp. 107–121). New York, NY: Plenum Publishing Corporation.

Gold, J. R., & Bajo, V. M. (2014). Insult-induced adaptive plasticity of the auditory system. *Frontiers in Neuroscience 8*, 110.

Gröschel, M., Götze, R., Müller, S., Ernst, A., & Basta, D. (2016). Central nervous activity upon systemic salicylate application in animals with kanamycin-induced hearing loss: A manganese-enhanced MRI (MEMRI) study. *PLoS One 11*(4), e0153386.

Gupta, R. C., Seki, Y., & Yosida, J. (2006). Role of taurine in spinal cord injury. *Current Neurovascular Research 3*(3), 225–235.

Hassel, B., Westergaard, N., Schousboe, A., & Fonnum, F. (1995). Metabolic differences between primary cultures of astrocytes and neurons from cerebellum and cerebral cortex. Effects of fluorocitrate. *Neurochemical Research 20*(4), 413–420.

He, S., Wang, Y. X., Petralia, R. S., & Brenowitz, S. D. (2014). Cholinergic modulation of large-conductance calcium-activated potassium channels regulates synaptic strength and spine calcium in cartwheel cells of the dorsal cochlear nucleus. *Neuroscience 34*(15), 5261–5272.

Heffner, H. E., & Harrington, I. A. (2002). Tinnitus in hamsters following exposure to intense sound. *Hearing Research 170*(1–2), 83–95.

Holt, A. G., Asako, M., Duncan, R. K., Lomax, C. A., Juiz, J. M., & Altschuler, R. A. (2006). Deafness associated changes in expression of two-pore domain potassium channels in the rat cochlear nucleus. *Hearing Research 216–217*, 146–153.

House, J. W., & Brackmann, D. E. (1981). Tinnitus: surgical treatment. *Ciba Foundation Symposium 85*, 204–216.

Imig, T. J., & Durham, D. (2005). Effect of unilateral noise exposure on the tonotopic distribution of spontaneous activity in the cochlear nucleus and inferior colliculus in the cortically intact and decorticate rat. *Journal of Comparative Neurology 490*(4), 391–413.

Irie, T., Fukui, I., & Ohmori, H. (2006). Activation of GIRK channels by muscarinic receptors and group II metabotropic glutamate receptors suppresses Golgi cell activity in the cochlear nucleus of mice. *Journal of Neurophysiology 96*, 2633–2644.

Jastreboff, P. J., & Sasaki, C. T. (1986). Salicylate-induced changes in spontaneous activity of single units in the inferior colliculus of the guinea pig. *Journal of the Acoustical Society of America 80*, 1384–1391.

Jastreboff, P. J., Brennan, J. F., Coleman, J. K., & Sasaki, C. T. (1988). Phantom auditory sensation in rats, an animal model for tinnitus. *Behavioral Neuroscience 102*, 811–822.

Jin, Y. M., & Godfrey, D. A. (2006). Effects of cochlear ablation on muscarinic acetylcholine receptor binding in the rat cochlear nucleus. *Journal of Neuroscience Research 83*(1), 157–166.

Jin, Y. M., & Godfrey, D. A., Sun, Y. (2005). Effects of cochlear ablation on choline acetyltransferase activity in the rat cochlear nucleus and superior olive. *Journal of Neuroscience Research 81*(1), 91–101.

Jin, Y. M., Godfrey, D. A., Wang, J., & Kaltenbach, J. A. (2006). Effects of intense tone exposure on choline acetyltransferase activity in the hamster cochlear nucleus. *Hearing Research 216–217*,168–175.

Kalappa, B. I., Brozoski, T. J., Turner, J. G., & Caspary, D. M. (2014). Single unit hyperactivity and bursting in the auditory thalamus of awake rats directly correlates with behavioural evidence of tinnitus. *Journal of Physiology 592*(22), 5065–5078.

Kalappa, B. I., Soh, H., Duignan, K. M., Furuya, T., Edwards, S., Tzingounis, A. V., Tzounopoulos, T. (2015). Potent KCNQ2/3-specific channel activator suppresses in vivo epileptic activity and prevents the development of tinnitus. *Journal of Neuroscience 35*(23), 8829–8842.

Kaltenbach, J. A., Godfrey, D. A. (2008). Dorsal cochlear nucleus hyperactivity and tinnitus: Are they related? *American Journal of Audiology 17*(2), S148–S161. doi:10.1044/1059-0889(2008/08-0004)

Kaltenbach, J. A., & Afman, C. E. (2000). Hyperactivity in the dorsal cochlear nucleus after intense sound exposure and its resemblance to tone-evoked activity: A physiological model for tinnitus. *Hearing Research 140*, 165–172.

Kaltenbach, J. A., & McCaslin, D. (1996). Increases in spontaneous activity in the dorsal cochlear nucleus following exposure to high intensity sound: A possible neural correlate of tinnitus. *Auditory Neuroscience 3*, 57–78.

Kaltenbach, J. A., Meleca, R., & Falzarano, P. R. (1996). Alterations in the tonotopic organization of the cochlear nucleus following cochlear lesions. In Salvi, R., Henderson, D., Fiorino, F., & Colletti, V. (Eds.), *Auditory System Plasticity and Regeneration* (pp. 317–332). New York, NY: Thieme Medical Publishers.

Kaltenbach, J. A., Godfrey, D. A., Neumann, J. B., McCaslin, D. L., Afman, C. E., Zhang, J. (1998). Changes in spontaneous neural activity in the dorsal cochlear nucleus following exposure to intense sound: relation to threshold shift. *Hearing Research 124*(1–2), 78–84.

Kaltenbach, J. A., Rachel, J. D., Mathog, T. A., Zhang, J. S., Falzarano, P. R., & Lewandowski, M. (2002). Cisplatin induced hyperactivity in the dorsal cochlear nucleus and its relation to outer hair cell loss: relevance to tinnitus. *Journal of Neurophysiology 88*, 699–714.

Kaltenbach, J. A., Zacharek, M. A., Zhang, J., & Frederick, S. S. (2004). Activity in the dorsal cochlear nucleus of hamsters previously tested for tinnitus following intense tone exposure. *Neuroscience Letters 355*(1–2), 121–125.

Kaltenbach, J. A., Zhang, J., & Finlayson, P. Tinnitus as a plastic phenomenon and its possible neural underpinnings in the dorsal cochlear nucleus. *Hearing Research 206*(1–2), 200–226.

Kaltenbach, J. A., Zhang, J., & Afman, C. E. (2000). Plasticity of spontaneous neural activity in the dorsal cochlear nucleus after intense sound exposure. *Hearing Research 147*(1–2), 282–292.

Kameda, K., Shono, T., Hashiguchi, K., Yoshida, F., & Sasaki, T. (2010). Effect of tumor removal on tinnitus in patients with vestibular schwannoma. *Journal of Neurosurgery 112*(1), 152–157.

Kiang, N. Y.-S., Watanabe, T., Thomas, E. C., & Clark, L. F. (1965). *Discharge patterns of single fibers in the cat's auditory nerve*. Research monograph no. 35. Cambridge, MA: MIT Press.

Kilduff, T. S., Sharp, F. R., & Heller, H. C. (1982). [14C]2-deoxyglucose uptake in ground squirrel brain during hibernation. *Journal of Neuroscience 2*(2), 143–157.

Kim, J. J., Gross, J., Morest, D. K., & Potashner, S. J. (2004). Quantitative study of degeneration and new growth of axons and synaptic endings in the chinchilla cochlear nucleus after acoustic overstimulation. *Journal of Neuroscience Research 77*(6), 829–842.

Komiya, H., & Eggermont, J. J. (2000). Spontaneous firing activity of cortical neurons in adult cats with reorganized tonotopic map following pure-tone trauma. *Acta Otolaryngologica 120*(6), 750–756.

Köszeghy, Á., Vincze, J., Rusznák, Z., Fu, Y., Paxinos, G., Csernoch, L., & Szücs, G. (2012). Activation of muscarinic receptors increases the activity of the granule neurones of the rat dorsal cochlear nucleus: A calcium imaging study. *Pflugers Archives: European Journal of Physiology 463*, 829–844.

Lanting, C. P., de Kleine, E., Eppinga, R. N., & van Dijk, P. (2010). Neural correlates of human somatosensory integration in tinnitus. *Hearing Research 267*(1–2), 78–88.

Lee, A. C., & Godfrey, D. A. (2014). Cochlear damage affects neurotransmitter chemistry in the central auditory system. *Frontiers in Neurology 5*, 227.

Li, S., Choi, V., & Tzounopoulos, T. (2013). Pathogenic plasticity of Kv7.2/3 channel activity is essential for the induction of tinnitus. *Proceedings of the National Academy of Science USA 110*(24), 9980–9985.

Liberman, M. C., & Dodds, L. W. (1984). Single-neuron labeling and chronic cochlear pathology. II. Stereocilia damage and alterations of spontaneous discharge rates. *Hearing Research 16*, 43–53.

Liberman, M. C., & Kiang, N. Y. (1978). Acoustic trauma in cats. Cochlear pathology and auditory-nerve activity. *Acta Otolaryngologica Supplement 358*, 1–63.

Lockwood, A. H., Wack, D. S., Burkard, R. F., Coad, M. L., Reyes, S. A., Arnold, S. A., & Salvi, R. J. (2001). The functional anatomy of gaze-evoked tinnitus and sustained lateral gaze. *Neurology 56*(4), 472–480.

Luo, H., Pace, E., Zhang, X., & Zhang, J. (2014). Blast-induced tinnitus and spontaneous firing changes in the rat dorsal cochlear nucleus. *Journal of Neuroscience Research 92*(11), 1466–1477.

Luo, H., Zhang, X., Nation, J., Pace, E., Lepczyk, L., & Zhang, J. (2012). Tinnitus suppression by electrical stimulation of the rat dorsal cochlear nucleus. *Neuroscience Letters 522*(1), 16–20.

Malmierca, M. S., Le Beau, F. E., & Rees, A. (1996). The topographical organization of descending projections from the central nucleus of the inferior colliculus in guinea pig. *Hearing Research 93*(1–2), 167–180.

Mancilla, J. G., & Manis, P. B. (2009). Two distinct types of inhibition mediated by cartwheel cells in the dorsal cochlear nucleus. *Journal of Neurophysiology 102*, 1287–1295.

Manzoor, N. F., Chen, G., & Kaltenbach, J. A. (2013a). Suppression of noise-induced hyperactivity in the dorsal cochlear nucleus following application of the cholinergic agonist, carbachol. *Brain Research 1523*, 28–36.

Manzoor, N. F., Gao, Y., Licari, F., & Kaltenbach, J. A. (2013b). Comparison and contrast of noise-induced hyperactivity in the dorsal cochlear nucleus and inferior colliculus. *Hearing Research* 295,114–123.

Manzoor, N. F., Licari, F. G., Klapchar, M., Elkin, R. L., Gao, Y., Chen, G., & Kaltenbach, J. A. (2012). Noise-induced hyperactivity in the inferior colliculus: its relationship with hyperactivity in the dorsal cochlear nucleus. *Journal of Neurophysiology 108*(4), 976–988.

Marks, K. L., Martel, D. T., Wu, C., Basura, G. J., Roberts, L. E., Schvartz-Leyzac, K. C., and Shore, S. E. (2018). Auditory-somatosensory bimodal stimulation desynchronizes brain circuitry to reduce tinnitus in guinea pigs and humans. *Sci. Transl. Med. 10*(422).

Martin, M. R., & Adams, J. C. (1979). Effects of DL-alpha-aminoadipate on synaptically and chemically evoked excitation of anteroventral cochlear nucleus neurons of the cat. *Neuroscience 4*(8), 1097–1105.

Martin, W. H., Schwegler, J. W., Scheibelhoffer, J., & Ronis, M. L. (1993). *Salicylate-induced changes in cat auditory nerve activity. Laryngoscope 103*, 600–604.

Melamed, S. B., Kaltenbach, J. A., Church, M. W., Burgio, D. L., & Afman, C. E. (2000). Cisplatin-induced increases in spontaneous neural activity in the dorsal cochlear nucleus and associated outer hair cell loss. *Audiology 39*, 24–29.

Meleca, R. J., Kaltenbach, J. A., & Falzarano, P. R. (1997). Changes in the tonotopic map of the dorsal cochlear nucleus in hamsters with hair cell loss and radial nerve bundle degeneration. *Brain Research 750*(1–2), 201–213.

Mellott, J. G., Motts, S. D., Schofield, B. R. (2011). Multiple origins of cholinergic innervation of the cochlear nucleus. *Neuroscience 180*,138–147.

Meltzer, N. E., & Ryugo, D. K. (2006). Projections from auditory cortex to cochlear nucleus: A comparative analysis of rat and mouse. *Anatomical Record Part A: Discoveries in Molecular, Cellular and Evolutionary Biology 288*(4), 397–408.

Middleton, J. W., Kiritani, T., Pedersen, C., Turner, J. G., Shepherd, G. M., & Tzounopoulos, T. (2011). Mice with behavioral evidence of tinnitus exhibit dorsal cochlear nucleus hyperactivity because of decreased GABAergic inhibition. *Proceedings of the National Academy of Science USA 108*(18), 7601–7606.

Milinkeviciute, G., Muniak, M. A., & Ryugo, D. K. (2017). Descending projections from the inferior colliculus to the dorsal cochlear nucleus are excitatory. *Journal of Comparative Neurology 525*(4), 773–793.

Moises, H. C., & Womble, M. D. 1995. Acetylcholine-operated ionic conductances in central neurons. In T. W. Stone (Ed.), *CNS Neurotransmitters and Neuromodulators. Acetylcholine* (pp.129–148). Boca Raton, FL: CRC Press.

Mugnaini, E. (1985). GABA neurons in the superficial layers of the rat dorsal cochlear nucleus: Light and electron microscopic immunocytochemistry. *Journal of Comparative Neurology 235*(1), 61–81.

Mugnaini, E., Warr, W. B., & Osen, K. K. (1980). Distribution and light microscopic features of granule cells in the cochlear nuclei of cat, rat, and mouse. *Journal of Comparative Neurology 191*(4), 581–606.

Muly, S. M., Gross, J. S., Potashner, S. J. (2004). Noise trauma alters D-[3H]aspartate release and AMPA binding in chinchilla cochlear nucleus. *Journal of Neuroscience Research 75*, 585–596.

Noreña, A. J., & Eggermont, J. J. (2005). Enriched acoustic environment after noise trauma reduces hearing loss and prevents cortical map reorganization. *Journal of Neuroscience 25*(3), 699–705.

Noreña, A. J., & Eggermont, J. J. (2006). Enriched acoustic environment after noise trauma abolishes neural signs of tinnitus. *Neuroreport, 17*(6), 559–563.

Ochi, K., & Eggermont, J. J. (1996). Effects of salicylate on neural activity in cat primary auditory cortex. *Hearing Research* 95(1–2), 63–76.

Oertel, D., & Wickesberg, R. E. (1993). Glycinergic inhibition in the cochlear nuclei: Evidence for tuberculoventral neurons being glycinergic. In M. A. Merchan, J. M. Juiz, D. A. Godfrey, & E. Mugnaini (Eds.), *The Mammalian Cochlear Nuclei: Organization and Function* (pp. 225–237). New York, NY: Plenum Press.

Oertel, D., & Young, E. D. (2004). What's a cerebellar circuit doing in the auditory system? *Trends in Neuroscience* 27(2), 104–110.

Oliver, D. L., Potashner, S. J., Jones, D. R., & Morest, D. K. (1983). Selective labeling of spiral ganglion and granule cells with D-aspartate in the auditory system of cat and guinea pig. *Journal of Neuroscience* 3(3), 455–472.

Osen, K. K. (1988). Anatomy of the mammalian cochlear nuclei: A review. In J. Syka & R. B. Masterton (Eds.), *Auditory Pathway* (pp. 65–75). New York, NY: Plenum Press.

Osen, K. K., Ottersen, O. P., & Storm-Mathisen, J. (1990). Colocalization of glycine-like and GABA-like immunoreactivities: A semiquantitative study of individual neurons in the dorsal cochlear nucleus of cat. In O. P. Ottersen & J. Storm-Mathisen (Eds.), *Glycine Neurotransmission* (pp. 417–451). Hoboken, NJ: John Wiley & Sons.

Osen, K. K., Storm-Mathisen, J., Ottersen, O. P., & Dihle, B. (1995). Glutamate is concentrated in and released from parallel fiber terminals in the dorsal cochlear nucleus: A quantitative immunocytochemical analysis in guinea pig. *Journal of Comparative Neurology* 357, 482–500.

Ottersen, O. P., Madsen, S., Storm-Mathisen, J., Somogyi, P., Scopsi, L., & Larsson, L. I. (1988). Immunocytochemical evidence suggests that taurine is colocalized with GABA in the Purkinje cell terminals, but that the stellate cell terminals predominantly contain GABA: A light- and electronmicroscopic study of the rat cerebellum. *Experimental Brain Research* 72(2), 407–416.

Ouyang, J., Pace, E., Lepczyk, L., Kaufman, M., Zhang, J., Perrine et al. (2017). Blast-induced tinnitus and elevated central auditory and limbic activity in rats: A manganese-enhanced MRI and behavioral study. *Science Reports* 7(1), 4852.

Pace, E., Luo, H., Bobian, M., Panekkad, A., Zhang, X., Zhang, H., et al. (2016) A conditioned behavioral paradigm for assessing onset and lasting tinnitus in rats. *PLoS One* 11(11), e0166346.

Pál, B., Köszeghy, Á., Pap, P., Bakondi, G., Pocsai, K., Szücs, G., & Rusznák, Z. (2009). Targets, receptors and effects of muscarinic neuromodulation on giant neurones of the rat dorsal cochlear nucleus. *European Journal of Neuroscience* 30(5), 769–782.

Pfeiffer, R. R., & Kiang, N. Y-S. (1965). Spike discharge patterns of spontaneous and continuously stimulated activity in the cochlear nucleus of anesthetized cats. *Biophysical Journal* 5 (3), 301–316.

Pilati, N., Large, C., Forsythe, I. D., & Hamann, M. (2012). Acoustic over-exposure triggers burst firing in dorsal cochlear nucleus fusiform cells. *Hearing Research* 283(1–2), 98–106.

Potashner, S. J., Benson, C. G., Ostapoff, E.-M., Lindberg, N., & Morest, D. K. (1993). Glycine and GABA: Transmitter candidates of projections descending to the cochlear nucleus. In M. A. Merchan, J. M. Juiz, D. A. Godfrey, & E. Mugnaini (Eds.), *The mammalian cochlear nuclei: Organization and function* (pp.195–210). New York, NY: Plenum Press.

Potashner, S. J., Suneja, S. K., & Benson, C. G. (1997). Regulation of D-aspartate release and uptake in adult brain stem auditory nuclei after unilateral middle ear ossicle removal and cochlear ablation. *Experimental Neurology* 148, 222–235.

Rachel, J. D., Kaltenbach, J. A., & Janisse, J. (2002). Increases in spontaneous neural activity in the hamster dorsal cochlear nucleus following cisplatin treatment: A possible basis for cisplatin-induced tinnitus. *Hearing Research 164*(1–2), 206–214.

Roberts, D. S., Otto, S., Chen, B., Peng, K. A., Schwartz, M. S., Brackmann, D. E., & House, J. W. (2017). Tinnitus suppression after auditory brainstem implantation in patients with neurofibromatosis type-2. *Otology and Neurotology 38*(1), 118–122.

Roberts, L. E., Eggermont, J. J., Caspary, D. M., Shore, S. E., Melcher, J. R., & Kaltenbach, J. A. (2010). Ringing ears: The neuroscience of tinnitus. *Journal of Neuroscience 30*(45), 14972–14979.

Roberts, M. T., & Trussell, L. O. (2010). Molecular layer inhibitory interneurons provide feed-forward and lateral inhibition in the dorsal cochlear nucleus. *Journal of Neurophysiology 104*, 2462–2473.

Robertson, D., & Irvine, D. R. (1989). Plasticity of frequency organization in auditory cortex of guinea pigs with partial unilateral deafness. *Journal of Comparative Neurology 282*(3), 456–471.

Ross, C. D., Parli, J. A., & Godfrey, D. A. (1995). Amino acid concentrations and selected enzyme activities in rat auditory, olfactory, and visual systems. *Neurochemical Research 20*, 1483–1490.

Saint Marie, R. L., Ostapoff, E.-M., Benson, C. G., Morest, D. K., & Potashner, S. J. (1993). Non-cochlear projections to the ventral cochlear nucleus: Are they mainly inhibitory? In M. A. Merchan, J. M. Juiz, D. A. Godfrey, & E. Mugnaini (Eds.), *The mammalian cochlear nuclei: organization and function* (pp. 121–131). New York, NY: Plenum Press.

Sasaki, C. T., Kauer, J. S., & Babitz, L. (1980). Differential [14C]2-deoxyglucose uptake after deafferentation of the mammalian auditory pathway—a model for examining tinnitus. *Brain Research 194*(2), 511–516.

Schaette, R., & Kempter, R. (2006). Development of tinnitus-related neuronal hyperactivity through homeostatic plasticity after hearing loss: a computational model. *European Journal of Neuroscience 23*(11), 3124–3138.

Schofield, B. R. (2002). Ascending and descending projections from the superior olivary complex in guinea pigs: Different cells project to the cochlear nucleus and the inferior colliculus. *Journal of Comparative Neurology 453*(3), 217–225.

Schreiner, C. E., & Snyder R. L. (1987). A physiological animal model of peripheral tinnitus. In Feldmann, H. (Ed.) *Proceedings of the Third International Tinnitus Seminar*, Muenster (pp. 100–106). Karlsuhe, Germany: Harsch Verlag.

Seki, S., & Eggermont, J. J. (2003). Changes in spontaneous firing rate and neural synchrony in cat primary auditory cortex after localized tone-induced hearing loss. *Hearing Research 180*, 28–38.

Sherriff, F. E., & Henderson, Z. (1994). Cholinergic neurons in the ventral trapezoid nucleus project to the cochlear nuclei in the rat. *Neuroscience 58*(3), 627–633.

Shore, S. E., Koehler, S., Oldakowski, M., Hughes, L. F., & Syed, S. (2008). Dorsal cochlear nucleus responses to somatosensory stimulation are enhanced after noise-induced hearing loss. *European Journal of Neuroscience 27*, 155–168.

Soldovieri, M. V., Miceli, F., & Taglialatela, M. (2011). Driving with no brakes: molecular pathophysiology of Kv7 potassium channels. *Physiology (Bethesda). 26*(5), 365–376.

Soussi, T., & Otto, S. R. (1994). Effects of electrical brainstem stimulation on tinnitus. *Acta Otolaryngologica 114*(2), 135–140.

Spangler, K. M., Cant, N. B., Henkel, C. K., Farley, G. R., & Warr, W. B. (1987). Descending projections from the superior olivary complex to the cochlear nucleus of the cat. *Journal of Comparative Neurology 259*(3), 452–465.

Stefanescu, R. A., & Shore, S. E. (2017). Muscarinic acetylcholine receptors control baseline activity and Hebbian stimulus timing-dependent plasticity in fusiform cells of the dorsal cochlear nucleus. *Journal of Neurophysiology 117*, 1229–1238.

Suneja, S. K., Benson, C. G., & Potashner, S. J. (1998a). Glycine receptors in adult guinea pig brain stem auditory nuclei: regulation after unilateral cochlear ablation. *Experimental Neurology 154*, 473–488.

Suneja, S. K., Potashner, S. J., & Benson, C. G. (1998b). Plastic changes in glycine and GABA release and uptake in adult brain stem auditory nuclei after unilateral middle ear ossicle removal and cochlear ablation. *Experimental Neurology 151*, 273–288.

Thomas, M. J., Watabe, A. M., Moody, T. D., Makhinson, M., & O'Dell, M. T. (1998). Postsynaptic complex spike bursting enables the induction of LTP by theta frequency synaptic stimulation. *Journal of Neuroscience 18*(18), 7118–7126.

Van Gendt, M. J., Boyen, K., de Kleine, E., Langers, D. R., & van Dijk, P. (2012). The relation between perception and brain activity in gaze-evoked tinnitus. *Journal of Neuroscience 32*(49), 17528–17539.

Vetter, D. E., Cozzari, C., Hartman, B. K., & Mugnaini, E. (1993). Choline acetyltransferase in the rat cochlear nuclei: Immunolocalization with a monoclonal antibody. In M. A. Merchan, J. M. Juiz, D. A. Godfrey, & E. Mugnaini (Eds.), *The Mammalian Cochlear Nuclei: Organization and Function* (pp. 279–290). New York, NY: Plenum Press.

Vogler, D. P., Robertson, D., & Mulders, W. H. (2011). Hyperactivity in the ventral cochlear nucleus after cochlear trauma. *Journal of Neuroscience 31*(18), 6639–6645.

Walberg, F., Ottersen, O. P., & Rinvik, E. (1990). GABA, glycine, aspartate, glutamate and taurine in the vestibular nuclei: an immunocytochemical investigation in the cat. *Experimental Brain Research 79*(3), 547–563.

Wall, J. T., Xu, J., & Wang, X. (2002). Human brain plasticity: An emerging view of the multiple substrates and mechanisms that cause cortical changes and related sensory dysfunctions after injuries of sensory inputs from the body. *Brain Research Reviews 39*(2–3), 181–215.

Wang, H., Brozoski, T. J., Turner, J. G., Ling, L., Parrish, J. L., Hughes, L. F., & Caspary, D. M. (2009). Plasticity at glycinergic synapses in dorsal cochlear nucleus of rats with behavioral evidence of tinnitus. *Neuroscience 164*, 747–759.

Wang, J., Powers, N. L., Hofstetter, P., Trautwein, P., Ding, D., & Salvi, R. (1997). Effects of selective inner hair cell loss on auditory nerve fiber threshold, tuning and spontaneous and driven discharge rate. *Hearing Research 107*(1–2), 67–82.

Wang, H., Yin, G., Rogers, K., Miralles, C., DeBlas, A. L., Rubio, M. E. (2011). Monaural conductive hearing loss alters the expression of the GluA3 AMPA and glycine receptor α1 subunits in bushy and fusiform cells of the cochlear nucleus. *Neuroscience 199*, 438–451.

Wenthold, R. J. (1978). Glutamic acid and aspartic acid in subdivisions of the cochlear nucleus after auditory nerve lesion. *Brain Research 143*(3), 544–548.

Wenthold, R. J. (1987). Evidence for a glycinergic pathway connecting the two cochlear nuclei: An immunocytochemical and retrograde transport study. *Brain Research 415*(1), 183–187.

Wouterlood, F. G., & Mugnaini, E. (1984). Cartwheel neurons of the dorsal cochlear nucleus: A Golgi-electron microscopic study in rat. *Journal of Comparative Neurology 227*, 136–157.

Wright, D. D., & Ryugo, D. K. (1996). Mossy fiber projections from the cuneate nucleus to the cochlear nucleus in the rat. *Journal of Comparative Neurology 365*, 159–172.

Wu, C., Martel, D. T., & Shore, S. E. (2016). Increased synchrony and bursting of dorsal cochlear nucleus fusiform cells correlate with tinnitus. *Journal of Neuroscience 36*(6), 2068–2073.

Zacharek, M. A., Kaltenbach, J. A., Mathog, T. A., & Zhang, J. (2002). Effects of cochlear ablation on noise induced hyperactivity in the hamster dorsal cochlear nucleus: Implications for the origin of noise induced tinnitus. *Hearing Research* 172(1–2), 137–143.

Zeng, C., Nannapaneni, N., Jianxun, Z., Hughes, L. F., & Shore, S. (2009). Cochlear damage changes the distribution of vesicular glutamate transporters associated with auditory and nonauditory inputs to the cochlear nucleus. *Journal of Neuroscience* 29, 4210–4217.

Zhang, J. S., Kaltenbach, J. A. (1998). Increases in spontaneous activity in the dorsal cochlear nucleus of the rat following exposure to high-intensity sound. *Neuroscience Letters* 250(3), 197–200.

Zhang, J. S., Kaltenbach, J. A., Godfrey, D. A., & Wang, J. (2006). Origin of hyperactivity in the hamster dorsal cochlear nucleus following intense sound exposure. *Journal of Neuroscience Research* 84(4), 819–831.

Zhang, J., Luo, H., Pace, E., Li, L., Liu, B. (2016). Psychophysical and neural correlates of noised-induced tinnitus in animals: Intra- and inter-auditory and non-auditory brain structure studies. *Hearing Research* 334, 7–19.

Zhao, Y., & Tzounopoulos, T. (2011). Physiological activation of cholinergic inputs controls associative synaptic plasticity via modulation of endocannabinoid signaling. *Journal of Neuroscience* 31(9), 3158–3168.

Zugaib, H., Ceballos, C. C., Leão, R. M. (2016). High doses of salicylate reduces glycinergic inhibition in the dorsal cochlear nucleus of the rat. *Hearing Research* 332, 188–198.

CHAPTER 9

MULTIMODAL INPUTS TO THE COCHLEAR NUCLEUS AND THEIR ROLE IN THE GENERATION OF TINNITUS

SUSAN E. SHORE AND DAVID T. MARTEL

Abstract

As the first brain station in the auditory neuraxis, the cochlear nucleus integrates information from the cochlea with multimodal information from somatosensory ganglia and brainstem nuclei, as well as motor systems. Fusiform cells in the dorsal division of the cochlear nucleus receive auditory nerve fiber synapses on their basal dendrites and multimodal synapses on their apical dendrites via granule-cell axons. Multimodal integration in fusiform cells is modified by inhibitory interneurons in a cerebellar-like arrangement. Like other cerebellar-like brain circuits, fusiform cells exhibit spike-timing-dependent plasticity, or STDP, which is reflected in vivo as stimulus-timing-dependent plasticity or StDP. This chapter describes how fusiform-cell circuitry uses STDP to process multisensory information. StDP disruption results in tinnitus, or phantom sound perception, which can be alleviated through circuit modulation to restore normal plasticity.

Keywords: tinnitus, stimulus-timing-dependent plasticity, STDP, cochlear nucleus, multisensory integration, vesicular glutamate transporter, long-term potentiation/depression, synchrony, SFR

MULTIMODAL INNERVATION OF THE COCHLEAR NUCLEUS

THE cochlear nucleus (CN) is the obligatory central site in the brain for all cochlear-auditory nerve synapses. It is also the first central auditory site for multimodal integration, receiving projections from non-auditory brain areas, including the trigeminal ganglion (Shore, 2005; Shore, Vass, Wys, & Altschuler, 2000), spinal trigeminal nucleus (Sp5), cuneate (cu) and gracile nuclei (C. A. Haenggeli, Pongstaporn, Doucet, & Ryugo, 2005; H. Li & Mizuno, 1997; Wright & Ryugo, 1996; Zhou & Shore, 2004), cervical nerves (Zhan, Pongstaporn, & Ryugo, 2006), vestibular afferents and nuclei (Bukowska, 2002; Burian & Gstoettner, 1988), and the pontine nuclei (PN; Babalian, 2005; Ohlrogge, Doucet, & Ryugo, 2001). Synapses from these regions project to the granule cell domain (GCD) and are primarily located on CN granule cells in the marginal area of ventral CN (VCN) and the dorsal CN (DCN), but can also be found on the cell bodies and dendrites of large cells in the magnocellular VCN (Alibardi, 2004; C. Haenggeli, Doucet, & Ryugo, 2002; Ohlrogge et al., 2001; Wright & Ryugo, 1996) as well as Golgi cells and unipolar brush cells in the deep layers of DCN (Mugnaini et al., 1980b; Mugnaini et al., 1980a; Dino and Mugnaini, 2008). Projections from the somatosensory ganglia and brainstem nuclei have primarily been studied using tract tracing but were identified as glutamatergic using electron microscopy and by co-labeling with vesicular glutamate transporters (VGluTs; Zhou & Shore, 2004). In contrast to the cochlear auditory nerve fibers, whose synaptic terminals co-label with the isoform VGluT1, multimodal synaptic terminals in the CN co-label primarily with VGluT2 (Zeng, Shroff, & Shore, 2011; Zhou, Zeng, Cui, & Shore, 2010).

Electrically stimulating multimodal projections, such as somatosensory nuclei/dorsal column nuclei/or the PN, activates granule cells via VGluT2 positive terminals (Barker et al., 2012; Burian & Gstoettner, 1988; Zhou, Nannapaneni, & Shore, 2007). The parallel-fiber axons of granule cells, in turn, depolarize the principal output neurons of DCN, the fusiform cells, as well as inhibitory interneurons, the cartwheel cell (Golding & Oertel, 1997), via their apical dendrites. In contrast, sound activates the VGluT1 positive auditory nerve fibers, which contact the basal dendrites of fusiform cells (Voigt & Young, 1988). Both sound and multimodal inputs activate cartwheel cell via presumed descending projections (Parham & Kim, 1995; Portfors & Roberts, 2007) and parallel-fiber inputs, respectively, to cartwheel-cell apical dendrites. Cartwheel cells provide feed-forward or lateral inhibition to fusiform cells (Roberts & Trussell, 2010). The DCN, thus is similar to cerebellar circuits by virtue of granule cell activation of parallel fiber inputs to apical dendrites of fusiform cell and cartwheel-cell apical dendrites, and the feed forward inhibition of fusiform cells by cartwheel cells (Oertel & Young, 2004). See Figure 9.1 for a schematic of multimodal inputs to the CN circuit.

Multimodal Inputs Induce Long-Term Plasticity in the DCN

Parallel-fiber axons of the CN granule cells thus transmit the bulk of multimodal information to DCN fusiform cells and their inhibitory interneurons, cartwheel cells (CWCs;

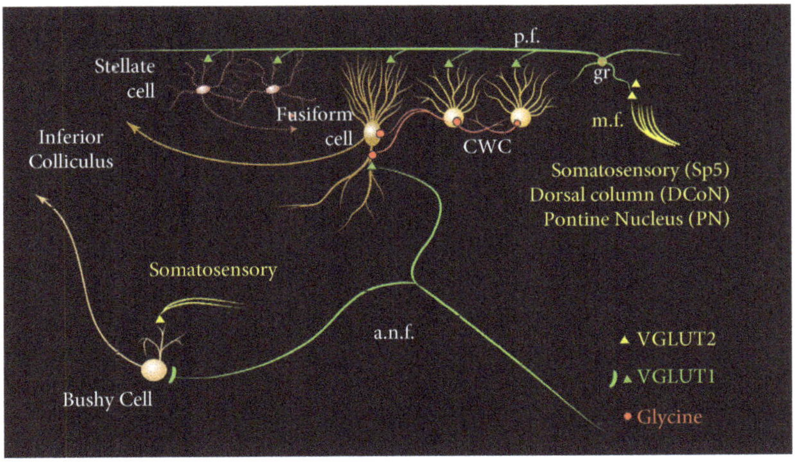

FIGURE 9.1. **Multimodal integration in cochlear nucleus circuitry**. Stimulation of multimodal projections (spinal trigeminal (Sp5); dorsal column (DCoN); pontine (PN)) activates granule cells (gr) via VGluT2+ terminals (yellow). Gr-pf axons depolarize fusiform cells and cartwheel cells via apical dendrites (plastic synapse). Sound activates fusiform cells via VGluT 1+ (green) auditory nerve fiber (ANF) contacts on basal dendrites (non-plastic synapse). Bimodal plasticity of fusiform cell spontaneous or sound-driven firing rates is achieved by integration of ANF and multimodal inputs through StDP. Synapses on cartwheel cells (CWCs) in vitro demonstrate STDP. Sound and multimodal inputs activate CWCs via presumed descending and gr-pf inputs, respectively, to CWC apical dendrites. CWCs provide feed forward or lateral inhibition to fusiform cells. Bushy cells are excited by sound via ANF-VGluT 1+ somatic inputs and Sp5/Cu/PN-VGluT 2+ somatic and dendritic inputs.

Dino & Mugnaini, 2008; Mugnaini, Osen, Dahl, Friedrich, & Korte, 1980; Mugnaini, Warr, & Osen, 1980). Synapses from parallel fibers onto the apical dendrites of fusiform and cartwheel cells exhibit Ca^{2+}-dependent long-term potentiation (LTP) and depression (LTD; Fujino & Oertel, 2003). But whether LTP or LTD occurs depends on spike timing (Tzounopoulos, Kim, Oertel, & Trussell, 2004) and can follow classical Hebbian or anti-Hebbian rules. In Hebbian plasticity, when presynaptic spikes are followed by postsynaptic spikes LTP occurs and conversely when postsynaptic spikes precede presynaptic spikes LTD occurs. In contrast, in anti-Hebbian plasticity, when presynaptic spikes precede postsynaptic spikes LTD occurs, and when postsynaptic spikes precede presynaptic spikes LTP follow. This process is termed spike-timing-dependent plasticity (STDP). Thus, STDP is a process whereby synapses are strengthened or weakened depending on the temporal pattern of pre- and postsynaptic events driving the cell (Bi & Poo, 1998; Tzounopoulos et al., 2004; Figure 9.2).

In vivo the macroscopic equivalent of STDP—*stimulus* timing dependent plasticity (StDP; S. D. Koehler & S. E. Shore, 2013a) —is elicited by electrically stimulating multimodal inputs that depolarize the parallel fiber synapses onto fusiform-cell apical dendrites, (the presynaptic events), in temporal proximity to sound stimulation, which

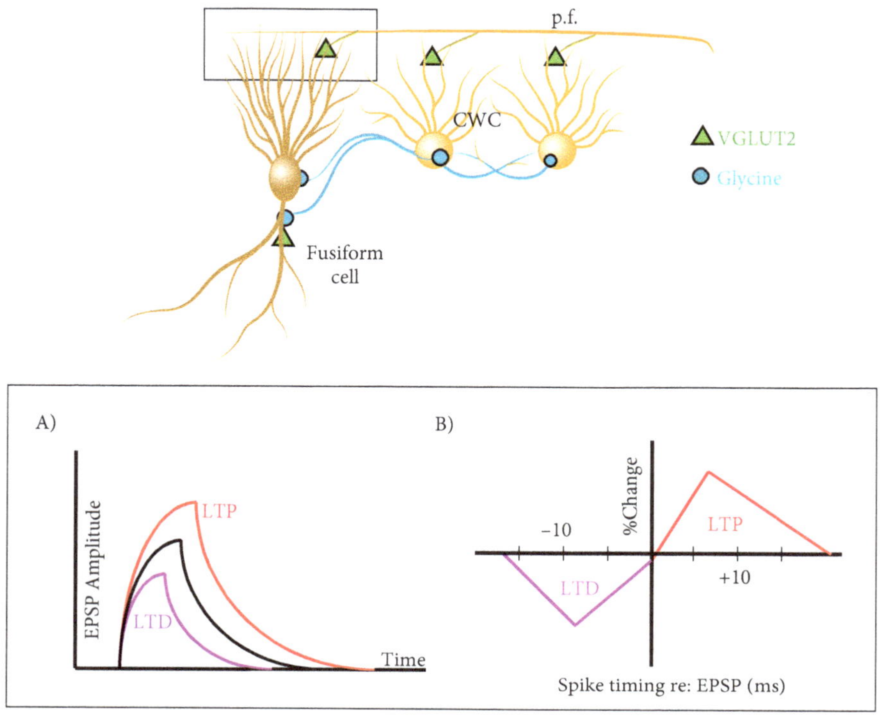

FIGURE 9.2. **Fusiform cells exhibit spike-timing-dependent plasticity (STDP) at their apical dendrites. A)** In fusiform cells, apical-fiber synapses that repetitively elicit a postsynaptic spike can enhance the amplitude of the resulting EPSP (red), a process termed long-term potentiation (LTP). In contrast, spikes that precede apical fiber input EPSPs l reduce the amplitude of resultant ESPSs (blue), a process termed long-term depression (LTD). **B)** Timing rules, or the percentage change in EPSP amplitude over a repeated EPSP-spike pairing, quantify STDP. Positive x-axis values indicate EPSPs before spikes and negative values indicate spikes before EPSPs.

activates spikes in the postsynaptic fusiform cell. A plot of changes in fusiform-cell firing rate after bimodal stimulation in which change in firing rate is plotted as a function of bimodal interval reveals the "learning rule." StDP manifests primarily as Hebbian plasticity across a population of fusiform cells (S. D. Koehler & S. E. Shore, 2013b). But it can also manifest as anti-Hebbian plasticity, either as "enhancing" (potentiating) plasticity, in which response rate is increased after bimodal stimulation at all bimodal intervals, or as "suppressing" (depressing) plasticity in which response rate is suppressed at all bimodal intervals (S. D. Koehler & S. E. Shore, 2013a), as shown in Figure 9.3. StDP can be achieved using deep brain stimulation of brainstem nuclei combined with auditory stimulation (Koehler & Shore, 2013), or trans-cutaneous stimulation of the cheek

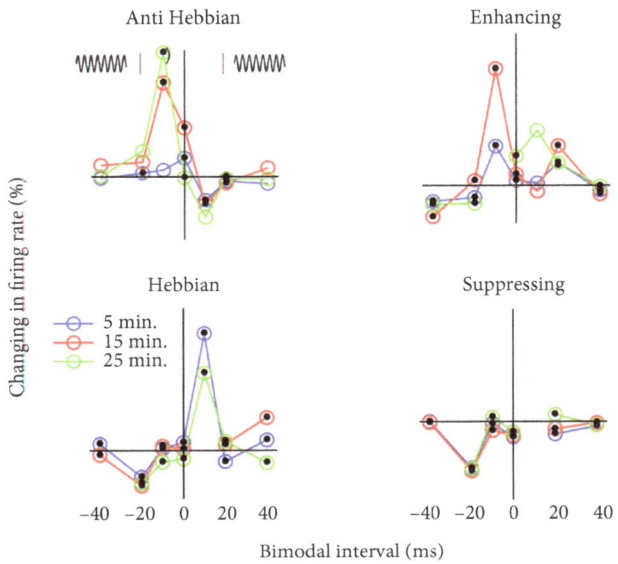

FIGURE 9.3. **Fusiform cells show variable individual timing rules in vivo.** Responses of fusiform cells to 50 ms BF tones before and 5, 15, or 25 min after bimodal stimulation (deep brain, Sp5+tone at BF). Change in firing rate (from before to after bimodal stimulation) is plotted for 4 different fusiform cells for 6 different bimodal intervals. Positive x-axis values indicate sound before somatosensory stimulation; negative values indicate somatosensory before sound stimulation. The bimodal interval (BI) was randomly varied from somatosensory preceding sound by 40 ms to somatosensory following the onset of sound by 40 ms. Examples show units with Hebbian-like or Anti-Hebbian-like stimulus-timing dependence, and enhancing-only or suppressing-only stimulus-timing dependence. Blue, red, and green lines indicate the change in firing rate 5, 15, and 25 minutes after bimodal stimulation, respectively.

Figure reproduced with permission from Koehler and Shore, 2013a.

overlying the trigeminal ganglion, or on the neck region above the C2 cervical ganglion, combined with sound (Wu, Martel, & Shore, 2015a; Figure 9.4). Interestingly, in vivo, whether Hebbian or anti-Hebbian plasticity arises also depends on tone duration (e.g., compare Figure 9.3, using 50 ms tones to Figure 9.4, using either 10 or 50 ms tones combined with electrical stimulation) demonstrating that fusiform-cell circuit plasticity exhibits context-dependence which could enhance or diminish the salience of multimodal stimuli. However, the observation that stimulation of fusiform cells with auditory stimuli alone does not result in long-term effects (Figure 9.4E, F), whereas unimodal somatosensory stimulation (deep brain and transdermal) do result in LTP (S. D. Koehler & S. E. Shore, 2013b; Wu et al., 2015a), is consistent with in vitro findings of plasticity at apical but not basal fusiform-cell dendrites (Fujino & Oertel, 2003). This

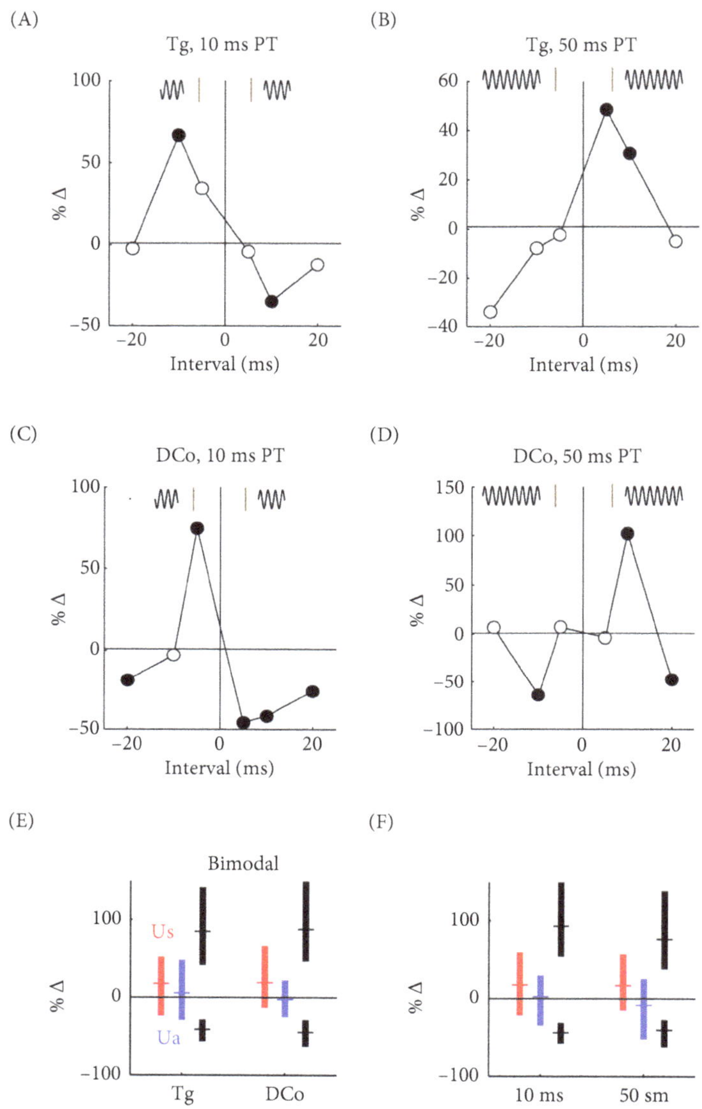

FIGURE 9.4. **Transdermal stimulation elicits StDP with context-dependent learning rules.** Trigeminal (Tg) stimulation in guinea pigs via a transdermal cheek electrode elicits anti-Hebbian learning rules following **A)** 10 ms pairing tone (PT) stimulation, or Hebbian learning rules following **B)** 50 ms pairing tone. Dorsal column (DCo) stimulation produces similar tone-duration-dependent learning rules (**C, D**). Regardless of somatosensory stimulation location **E)** or pairing-tone duration **F)**, unimodal somatosensory (red) and auditory (blue) stimulation did not produce significant changes in fusiform cell firing compared to baseline, but bimodal stimulation did (black).

Figure reproduced with permission from Wu et al., 2015a.

suggests that coding of unimodal auditory stimuli by the fusiform-cell circuit is not context-dependent.

Function of Multimodal Inputs to the Dorsal Cochlear Nucleus

As in other cerebellar-like circuits, the DCN is thought to adjust perception by incorporating predictive signals from the somatosensory system (Bell, Han, Sugawara, & Grant, 1997; Nelson, 2004). Internally generated sounds that arise from movement, as in head orientation, vocalization or chewing, recruit the somatosensory system, producing near-coincident auditory and somatosensory inputs to DCN. The circuit adaptively adjusts fusiform-cell output to amplify external (unpredicted) auditory cues while subtracting internally generated sounds. This process likely involves voluntary motor commands processed by the PN, which, in addition to relaying cortical motor efferent projections to the cerebellum, sends projections to the GCD (Babalian, 2005; Ohlrogge et al., 2001), thereby routing motor information to the DCN. Thus, the incorporation of motor as well as sensory information into this circuit may be fundamental for sound localization in the vertical plane (Davis, Ramachandran, & May, 2003; May, 2000) and for suppression of body-generated sounds, in addition to the acknowledged role of the trigeminal brainstem nucleus (Requarth & Sawtell, 2011; Singla, Dempsey, Warren, Enikolopov, & Sawtell, 2017).

Mechanisms Underlying StDP in DCN Fusiform Cells

StDP has been demonstrated in vivo in fusiform cells (S. D. Koehler & S. E. Shore, 2013a) using deep brain electrical-somatosensory stimulation combined with sound stimulation (Dehmel, Pradhan, Koehler, Bledsoe, & Shore, 2012; S. D. Koehler & S. E. Shore, 2013a), as well as transdermal electrical stimulation of the somatosensory system combined with sound stimulation (Wu et al., 2015a). In vitro, the development of STDP requires activation of NMDA and muscarinic cholinergic receptors as well as endocannabinoid receptors (Perez-Rosello et al., 2013; Sedlacek, Tipton, & Brenowitz, 2011; Zhao & Tzounopoulos, 2011). Likewise, in vivo studies show that blocking both AChRs and NMDARs (Stefanescu & Shore, 2015; Figure 9.5) results in significant alterations in the StDP "learning rules," which mimic learning rule changes after tinnitus-induction (see next section; S. D. Koehler & S. E. Shore, 2013b; Stefanescu, Koehler, & Shore, 2015; Wu et al., 2015a). NMDARs may be involved in limiting plasticity in response

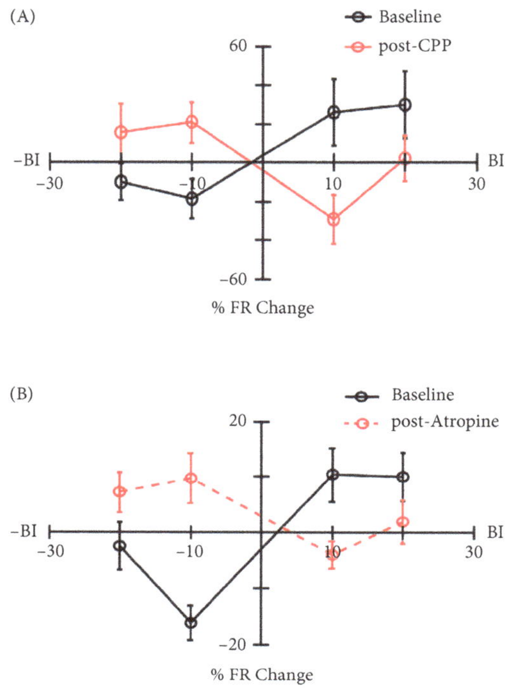

FIGURE 9.5. **Blocking NMDA and acetylcholine receptors alters StDP**. StDP timing rules were changed from Hebbian at baseline (black) to anti-Hebbian post-infusion (red) of **A)** CPP, an NMDA receptor antagonist, and **B)** atropine, an ACh receptor antagonist.

Figure reproduced with permission from Stefanescu and Shore, 2015.

to repeated unimodal stimulation because NMDAR antagonists unmask unimodal plasticity not previously observed in the normal animal (Stefanescu & Shore, 2015). While muscarinic AChR agonists might thus enhance bimodal plasticity, NMDAR antagonists could provide a way to induce plasticity with unimodal stimuli as well as bimodal stimuli.

The Role of Feed Forward Inhibition and Retrograde Signaling in STDP

As shown in vitro, Hebbian plasticity increases synapse strength when presynaptic EPSPs are paired with post-synaptic spikes, while anti-Hebbian plasticity reduces synapse strength (Abbott & Nelson, 2000; Markram, Lubke, Frotscher, & Sakmann, 1997; Tzounopoulos et al., 2004). Both Hebbian and anti-Hebbian plasticity likely enable the fusiform cells to alter synapse strength to adaptively enhance fusiform-cell responses to external sounds while decreasing synaptic strength to decrease responses to self-generated sounds, similar to the electric eel's electrosensory lobe (Bell, 1981; Bell et al., 1997; Singla et al., 2017).

Fusiform cells exhibiting Hebbian-like learning rules in vivo show predominantly excitatory receptive fields, while those with anti-Hebbian-like learning rules show more inhibition in their receptive fields (Koehler & Shore, 2013a; Koehler & Shore, 2013b). Computational models of cerebellar-like circuits, which are like the DCN fusiform-cell circuit, demonstrate that inhibition is essential for stabilizing network dynamics by preventing "run-away" excitation (Isaacson & Scanziani, 2011; Luz & Shamir, 2012; Moore, Carlen, Knoblich, & Cardin, 2010). The structural similarity of other cerebellar-like circuits to the DCN (Froemke, Letzkus, Kampa, Hang, & Stuart, 2010), including hippocampus (Magee & Johnston, 1997; Song, Miller, & Abbott, 2000), neocortex (Min & Nevian, 2012; Sarihi et al., 2008) and amygdala (Mahanty & Sah, 1998), suggests that inhibition could also influence STDP in these circuits.

In vitro, parallel-fiber inputs that trigger Ca^{2+} influx into the fusiform cell after post-synaptic NMDA-receptor activation elicit Hebbian plasticity in fusiform cells, but anti-Hebbian plasticity in cartwheel cells (Tzounopoulos et al., 2004; Tzounopoulos, Rubio, Keen, & Trussell, 2007). Differential expression of presynaptic neuromodulator receptors in cartwheel and fusiform cells can help explain these learning-rule differences. For example, endocannabinoid receptors that hyperpolarize pre-synaptic terminals are more numerous in parallel fiber terminals on cartwheel-cell dendrites than on fusiform-cell dendrites (Zhao, Rubio, & Tzounopoulos, 2011). Sustained parallel-fiber EPSPs, leading to post-synaptic Ca^{2+} release in fusiform cells, would tend to elicit Hebbian plasticity. However, in the cartwheel cell, sustained Ca^{2+} release coupled with muscarinic AChR activation retrogradely activates pre-synaptic endocannabinoid receptors on parallel fibers, thereby suppressing glutamate release from their synaptic terminals (Sedlacek et al., 2011) thus converting Hebbian plasticity into anti-Hebbian plasticity (Zhao & Tzounopoulos, 2011). By altering STDP timing rules through differential activation of these receptors, the fusiform-cell circuit exhibits input-selective gain-control. This gain-control process allows single fusiform cells to learn new stimulus representations through Hebbian plasticity, while anti-Hebbian plasticity attenuates circuit responses when external contexts change (S. D. Koehler & S. E. Shore, 2013a).

In vivo, fusiform cells exhibit a complex mixture of Hebbian and anti-Hebbian plasticity compared to in vitro preparations of isolated neural circuits (Figure 9.3; Koehler & Shore, 2013a; Wu, Martel, & Shore, 2015). In normal hearing animals, fusiform cells show predominantly Hebbian timing rules, although a sizeable fraction also undergoes anti-Hebbian rules. However, the proportions of learning-rule types can change depending on the environmental context, which influences differential activation of inhibition. For instance, tone duration can modulate whether a given fusiform cell exhibits Hebbian or anti-Hebbian plasticity. Short-duration tones elicit opposite learning rules to those elicited by long-duration tones (Wu, Martel & Shore, 2015). By activating feed-forward inhibition by cartwheel cells for a longer time, longer tones can result in delayed firing in fusiform cells. A similar firing delay occurs through inactivation of A-type potassium channels (Kanold & Manis, 1999; Manis, 1990). This in turn alters the timing of post-synaptic spikes relative to the presynaptic, parallel-fiber events. In visual cortex, feed forward inhibition of pyramidal neurons can also change plasticity from LTP to LTD, and vice-versa (Vogels et al., 2013; L. Wang, Fontanini, & Maffei, 2012). Switches between LTP and LTD require Ca^{2+} influx via NMDAR activation (Kurotani, Yamada, Yoshimura, Crair, & Komatsu, 2008), which then triggers retrograde co-activation of endocannabinoid receptors (Maejima, Hashimoto, Yoshida, Aiba, & Kano, 2001; Nevian & Sakmann, 2006; Rodriguez-Moreno & Paulsen, 2008; Sjostrom, Turrigiano, & Nelson, 2003), as in the fusiform-cell circuit.

Computational studies have shown that StDP-like learning rules can regulate responses of parallel arrays of neurons, through a process similar to classical lateral inhibition (Masquelier, Guyonneau, & Thorpe, 2009). Inputs that consistently trigger spikes from a specific neuron in an array strengthen that neuron's response (Hebbian plasticity). With lateral inhibition, the neuron's response becomes stronger compared to that of neighboring neurons. Thus, individual neurons in the array can *tune* their outputs to sharpen the output of the entire array in response to specific inputs. Repeating this process over the elements of the array allows the array to enhance the salience of many different stimuli, even in the presence of a noisy signal. By enhancing firing of information-conveying neurons and reducing activity of neighboring neurons, StDP-mediated lateral inhibition provides a mechanism for eliciting array responses tuned to specific stimuli (Cohen & Mizrahi, 2015). In the DCN, StDP-mediated lateral inhibition could sharpen responses of fusiform cell arrays to aid in the computation of spectral-notch information for sound localization, particularly during head motion relative to a sound source (Hofman, Van Riswick, & Van Opstal, 1998; Populin & Yin, 1998),

The fusiform-cell circuit also uses StDP in the suppression of self-generated sounds. To demonstrate this effect, Singla et al. (2017) recorded the activity of DCN fusiform cells and VCN cells while mice were licking from a water spout. When the mice were actively licking, DCN responses were dampened, while VCN responses remained robust. However, when the recorded "licking sound" was played back to the mice in the absence of licking behavior, responses in VCN and DCN responses to the sound both remained robust. Furthermore, blocking spinal trigeminal inputs to the CN with lidocaine resulted in significant increases in fusiform cell firing that correlated with lick-generated sounds. These findings demonstrate how the fusiform cells use multisensory information to adaptively cancel out self-generated sounds.

Alterations to the DCN Circuit in Tinnitus

Neural signatures of tinnitus include increased spontaneous firing rate (SFR), increased synchrony across fusiform cell pairs and increased bursting from individual fusiform cells with BFs in tinnitus frequency regions (Figure 9.6A–C). Furthermore,

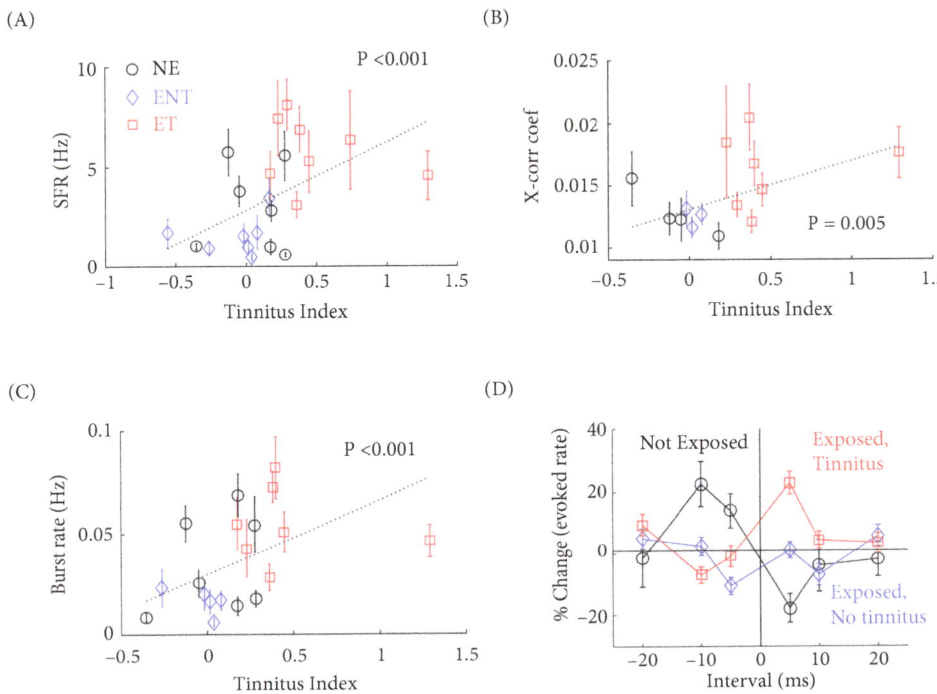

FIGURE 9.6. **Neural signatures of tinnitus in fusiform cells.** Compared to non-exposed controls (NE, black) and noise-overexposed no-tinnitus (ENT, blue) animals, noise-overexposed animals that develop tinnitus (ET, red) show increased tinnitus indices (TI) that correlate with **A)** spontaneous firing rates (SFR), **B)** pairwise-unit synchrony, and **C)** single-unit bursting. **D)** Percent change in fusiform-cell firing rate to a BF tone 15 min. after auditory-somatosensory bimodal stimulation as a function of bimodal interval. Negative intervals indicate auditory (sound) before somatosensory; positive intervals indicate somatosensory before auditory (sound) stimulation. Somatosensory stimulation was transdermal (200 μsec) with electrodes overlying the C2–4 vertebrae. Non-exposed control animals (N) had anti-Hebbian rules; exposed, tinnitus animals (ET) had Hebbian or enhancing rules (indicating a strengthened circuit). Exposed, no-tinnitus animals (ENT) had suppressing timing rules.

Figures reproduced with permission from Wu et al., 2016, and Koehler and Shore, 2013b.

fusiform cells from noise-exposed animals with behavioral signs of tinnitus exhibit broader StDP timing rules with more LTP-eliciting bimodal intervals (Koehler & Shore, 2013b; Figure 9.6D). In contrast, fusiform cells in noise-exposed animals that do not develop signs of tinnitus show more bimodal intervals eliciting LTD (Koehler & Shore, 2013b; Marks et al., 2018; Wu, Martel, & Shore, 2016). This pattern reflects a hyperexcitable CN circuit in animals with tinnitus compared to those in animals without tinnitus and normal hearing animals, a finding which has also been described by other studies (Dehmel et al., 2012; Li, Choi, & Tzounopoulos, 2013; Li, Kalappa, & Tzounopoulos, 2015; Middleton et al., 2011; Pilati, Large, Forsythe, & Hamann, 2012).

When the fusiform cell circuit is in a hyperexcitable and hypersynchronous state, spontaneous activity is theoretically "bound" into an auditory object that the brain interprets as a phantom sound (Singer, 1999). Tinnitus-related alterations in fusiform-cell multisensory integration predict a somatosensory element in tinnitus, consistent with observations that over two thirds of tinnitus sufferers can modulate the pitch and/or intensity of their tinnitus through muscular contractions (R. A. Levine, 1999; Levine, Nam, Oron, & Melcher, 2007; Wu, Stefanescu, Martel, & Shore, 2014). Interestingly, some humans without tinnitus can *induce* transient tinnitus through somatic manipulations of the head and neck (Abel & Levine, 2004). These findings suggest a fundamental role for the DCN fusiform-cell circuit role in the generation and ultimately treatment of tinnitus (Marks et al., 2018).

As the first obligatory central nucleus in the auditory pathway, increased and synchronous spontaneous activity in the fusiform cell circuit propagates up the ascending auditory pathway. Indeed, DCN ablation has been suggested to prevent noise-overexposure induced tinnitus (Brozoski, Wisner, Sybert, & Bauer, 2012). Thus, it would be expected that target nuclei in the auditory neuraxis would also show tinnitus-related increases in SFR and synchrony. This prediction is consistent with studies in the medial geniculate body (MGB; Kalappa, Brozoski, Turner, & Caspary, 2014) and auditory cortex (Engineer et al., 2011), which show that increased SFR, synchrony and behavioral measures of tinnitus are correlated. However, studies in the inferior colliculus (IC) complicate this picture. Several studies have shown that enhanced spontaneous activity does not appear to be directly related to noise- induced tinnitus (Berger, Coomber, Wells, Wallace, & Palmer, 2014; Mulders & Robertson, 2009; Ropp, Tiedemann, Young, & May, 2014). Other studies of IC neurons suggest that increased synchrony correlates with tinnitus only in the external nucleus (Bauer, Turner, Caspary, Myers, & Brozoski, 2008). Sturm, Zhang-Hooks, Roos, Nguyen, and Kandler (2017) showed that in tinnitus animals, changes in excitatory as well as inhibitory synaptic strength do occur in the central nucleus and that these magnitude and direction of these changes depend on whether the postsynaptic neuron is excitatory or inhibitory, leading to an overall increase in net excitation of the IC. Mere increased SFR in IC might reflect generalized hyperactivity that is a consequence of noise exposure (Ma, Hidaka, & May, 2006; Manzoor, Gao, Licari, & Kaltenbach, 2013), while tinnitus arises from pathological enhancement of spontaneous synchrony. These findings suggest that both increased SFR and synchrony across a population of neurons are necessary for tinnitus, and that the CN is a likely candidate for its generation.

Disinhibition-Mediated Synchrony

Other studies have shown that fusiform cells show altered glycine-receptor expression in animals with evidence of tinnitus (Wang et al., 2009), perhaps driving the circuit to produce more spikes. Increased fusiform-cell spiking increases the probability that a pre-synaptic event will correlate with a spike, thereby biasing the circuit toward LTP. This process is termed disinhibition-mediated LTP (Ormond & Woodin, 2009, 2011). Disinhibition-mediated LTP in the DCN circuit could strengthen LTP across groups of fusiform cells, producing the enhanced synchrony observed in tinnitus (Shore, Roberts, & Langguth, 2016; Wu et al., 2016). Similarly, in the hippocampus, a cerebellar-like circuit, disinhibition mediates LTP by rapidly activating NMDA receptors and upregulating pyramidal-cell firing before inhibition prevents EPSP generation (Ormond & Woodin, 2009, 2011). This process requires circuitry with coordinated regulation of excitatory/inhibitory plasticity. Like the hippocampus, the fusiform-cell-circuit parallel fibers concurrently activate fusiform cells and their inhibitory interneuron cartwheel cells (Oertel & Young, 2004; Tzounopoulos et al., 2004).

Multimodal Influences on Tinnitus Generation by CN Neurons

Following acoustic insult, auditory nerve input to CN is reduced by deafferentation (Zeng, Nannapaneni, Zhou, Hughes, & Shore, 2009), but central changes that result in physiological correlates of tinnitus—increased spontaneous activity (SA), synchrony and bursting—develop over time (Kaltenbach, Zhang, & Finlayson, 2005; Salvi, Wang, & Ding, 2000; Wu et al., 2016). The somatosensory system compensates for the reduced auditory nerve input to the cochlear nucleus by upregulating its excitatory input and altering StDP-mediated auditory- somatosensory plasticity in the DCN (Dehmel et al., 2012; S. D. Koehler & S. E. Shore, 2013b; Shore, Koehler, Oldakowski, Hughes, & Syed, 2008; Zeng, Yang, Shreve, Bledsoe, & Shore, 2012a), providing a physiological basis for "somatic" (Abel & Levine, 2004; R. Levine, 1999) and perhaps most forms of tinnitus. The upregulation of somatosensory projections from Sp5 and Cu to the CN (Shore & Zhou, 2006; Zeng et al., 2012a) as well as alterations in NMDA and ACh receptors (Stefanescu & Shore, 2015; Stefanescu & Shore, 2017) likely contribute to tinnitus development by altering fusiform cell StDP in the somatosensory -parallel-fiber circuits (Figure 9.2, Figure 9.5; Dehmel et al., 2012; S. D. Koehler & S. E. Shore, 2013b; Zeng et al., 2009; Zeng et al., 2012a). Clinical reports of additional tinnitus modulators such as eye gaze or balance (Said, Izita, Gonzalez, & Tovar, 2006; Wall, Rosenberg, & Richardson, 1987) also implicate the motor system, consistent with brain-imaging studies demonstrating motor system deficits in tinnitus subjects (Benninger et al., 2011). These cases suggest that the motor system may play a previously unappreciated role in mediating tinnitus, as a major recipient of PN output, the cerebellum, has been proposed as a putative tinnitus generation site (Bauer, Kurt, Sybert, & Brozoski, 2013).

What Happens to Fusiform Cells in an Animal Model of Tinnitus?

Terminal endings from Sp5 and Cu are increased in number after cochlear damage (Zeng, Yang, Shreve, Bledsoe, & Shore, 2012b). Vesicular glutamate transporter1 (Vglut1), which co-labels with AN terminals (Zhou et al., 2007), was decreased following cochlear damage, while Vglut2, which co-labels with somatosensory inputs (Zhou et al., 2010), was significantly increased in regions receiving somatosensory inputs in guinea pigs (Zeng et al., 2012a) and mice (Heeringa, Stefanescu, Raphael, & Shore, 2016). Four sources of Vglut2-positive inputs to the CN have been identified: Sp5 (Zhou et al., 2007); contralateral CN (Zhou et al., 2010), cu (Zeng et al., 2011) and PN (preliminary data). The increased number of somatosensory inputs to the granule-PF-fusiform cell circuit likely contributes to the alterations in StDP observed after noise induced tinnitus (Dehmel et al., 2012; S. Koehler & S. Shore, 2013) by differentially driving up EPSPs in fusiform-cell apical dendrites compared to cartwheel cell apical dendrites.

Reversing StDP, Synchrony and Spontaneous Rates to Treat Tinnitus

StDP inversions associated with tinnitus can be reversed by repeated daily stimulation with a bimodal stimulus shown to induce LTD in guinea pigs (Marks et al., 2018). In the study by Marks et al. (2018), the bimodal auditory-somatosensory stimulus was presented to guinea pigs with behavioral evidence of tinnitus under the assumption that repeated induction of LTD in the fusiform-cell circuit would reduce spontaneous rates and synchrony and lead to tinnitus reduction. The prediction was borne out and demonstrated that just 4 weeks of this specialized stimulation was sufficient to reduce tinnitus in all the animals. As predicted by the circuitry, unimodal auditory stimulation that activates the non-plastic basal dendrites of fusiform cells had no effect on spontaneous rates or tinnitus. Unimodal somatosensory stimulation predictably enhanced spontaneous rates and worsened tinnitus. Given the significant results of bimodal stimulation in the animal model, 20 human subjects with somatic tinnitus were treated with the same bimodal stimulus for 4 weeks with the same result: The bimodal stimulus resulted in significant and cumulative reductions in tinnitus loudness and discomfort in the human subjects, whereas the unimodal auditory stimulation had no effect. The unimodal somatosensory stimulation was not employed in the human study as it had been shown to have a deleterious effect in animals (Marks et al., 2018). This study demonstrates that systematic study of circuitry involved in generating tinnitus can lead to potential treatments for tinnitus in humans by reversing circuit plasticity through bimodal stimulation.

Concluding Remarks

This chapter has outlined how a complex cerebellar-like circuit, the fusiform-cell circuit in the DCN, is involved in fundamental processes for localizing sounds in space and suppression of self-generated signals, and how disruption of the circuit hampers function essential for survival. Through processes of multisensory integration and long-term plasticity, the circuit dampens internally generated sounds, thereby enhancing the salience of sounds. When normal auditory processing is disrupted by deafferentation, the fusiform-cell circuit undergoes homeostatic plasticity that interacts with underlies timing-dependent plasticity to render the circuit hyperexcitable and leads to the development of tinnitus. Remarkably, the same plastic mechanisms that drive tinnitus can be reversed to treat this debilitating condition.

References

Abbott, L. F., & Nelson, S. B. (2000). Synaptic plasticity: Taming the beast. *Nature Neuroscience, 3 Suppl*, 1178–1183. doi:10.1038/81453

Abel, M. D., & Levine, R. A. (2004). Muscle contractions and auditory perception in tinnitus patients and nonclinical subjects. *Cranio, 22*(3), 181–191.

Alibardi, L. (2004). Mossy fibers in granule cell areas of the rat dorsal cochlear nucleus from intrinsic and extrinsic origin innervate unipolar brush cell glomeruli. *Journal of Submicroscopic Cytology and Pathology, 36*(2), 193–210.

Babalian, A. L. (2005). Synaptic influences of pontine nuclei on cochlear nucleus cells. *Experimental Brain Research, 167*(3), 451–457. doi:10.1007/s00221-005-0178-8

Barker, M., Solinski, H. J., Hashimoto, H., Tagoe, T., Pilati, N., & Hamann, M. (2012). Acoustic overexposure increases the expression of VGLUT-2 mediated projections from the lateral vestibular nucleus to the dorsal cochlear nucleus. *PLoS One, 7*(5), e35955. doi:10.1371/journal.pone.0035955 PONE-D-11-18058 [pii]

Bauer, C. A., Kurt, W., Sybert, L. T., & Brozoski, T. J. (2013). The cerebellum as a novel tinnitus generator. *Hearing Research, 295*, 130–139.

Bauer, C. A., Turner, J. G., Caspary, D. M., Myers, K. S., & Brozoski, T. J. (2008). Tinnitus and inferior colliculus activity in chinchillas related to three distinct patterns of cochlear trauma. *Journal of Neuroscience Research, 86*(11), 2564–2578. doi:10.1002/jnr.21699

Bell, C. C. (1981). An efference copy which is modified by reafferent input. *Science, 214*(4519), 450–453.

Bell, C. C., Han, V. Z., Sugawara, Y., & Grant, K. (1997). Synaptic plasticity in a cerebellum-like structure depends on temporal order. *Nature, 387*(6630), 278–281. doi:10.1038/387278a0

Benninger, D. H., Berman, B. D., Houdayer, E., Pal, N., Luckenbaugh, D. A., Schneider, L., . . . Hallett, M. (2011). Intermittent theta-burst transcranial magnetic stimulation for treatment of Parkinson disease. *Neurology, 76*(7), 601–609. doi:10.1212/WNL.0b013e31820ce6bb 76/7/601 [pii]

Berger, J. I., Coomber, B., Wells, T. T., Wallace, M. N., & Palmer, A. R. (2014). Changes in the response properties of inferior colliculus neurons relating to tinnitus. *Frontiers in Neurology, 5*, 203. doi:10.3389/fneur.2014.00203

Bi, G. Q., & Poo, M. M. (1998). Synaptic modifications in cultured hippocampal neurons: Dependence on spike timing, synaptic strength, and postsynaptic cell type. *Journal of Neuroscience, 18*(24), 10464–10472.

Brozoski, T. J., Wisner, K. W., Sybert, L. T., & Bauer, C. A. (2012). Bilateral dorsal cochlear nucleus lesions prevent acoustic-trauma induced tinnitus in an animal model. *Journal of the Association for Research in Otolaryngology, 13*(1), 55–66. doi:10.1007/s10162-011-0290-3

Bukowska, D. (2002). Morphological evidence for secondary vestibular afferent connections to the dorsal cochlear nucleus in the rabbit. *Cells, Tissues, Organs, 170*(1), 61–68. doi:47921 [pii] 47921

Burian, M., & Gstoettner, W. (1988). Projection of primary vestibular afferent fibres to the cochlear nucleus in the guinea pig. *Neuroscience Letters, 84*(1), 13–17. doi:0304-3940(88)90329-1 [pii]

Cohen, L., & Mizrahi, A. (2015). Plasticity during motherhood: Changes in excitatory and inhibitory layer 2/3 neurons in auditory cortex. *Journal of Neuroscience, 35*(4), 1806–1815. doi:10.1523/JNEUROSCI.1786-14.2015

Davis, K. A., Ramachandran, R., & May, B. J. (2003). Auditory processing of spectral cues for sound localization in the inferior colliculus. *Journal of the Association for Research Otolaryngologists, 4*(2), 148–163. doi:10.1007/s10162-002-2002-5

Dehmel, S., Pradhan, S., Koehler, S., Bledsoe, S., & Shore, S. (2012). Noise overexposure alters long-term somatosensory-auditory processing in the dorsal cochlear nucleus—possible basis for tinnitus-related hyperactivity? *Journal of Neuroscience, 32*(5), 1660–1671. doi:10.1523/JNEUROSCI.4608-11.2012

Dino, M. R., & Mugnaini, E. (2008). Distribution and phenotypes of unipolar brush cells in relation to the granule cell system of the rat cochlear nucleus. *Neuroscience*. doi:S0306-4522(08)00108-5 [pii] 10.1016/j.neuroscience.2008.01.035

Engineer, N. D., Riley, J. R., Seale, J. D., Vrana, W. A., Shetake, J. A., Sudanagunta, S. P., . . . Kilgard, M. P. (2011). Reversing pathological neural activity using targeted plasticity. *Nature, 470*(7332), 101–104. doi:nature09656 [pii] 10.1038/nature09656

Froemke, R. C., Letzkus, J. J., Kampa, B. M., Hang, G. B., & Stuart, G. J. (2010). Dendritic synapse location and neocortical spike-timing-dependent plasticity. *Frontiers in Synaptic Neuroscience, 2*, 29. doi:10.3389/fnsyn.2010.00029

Fujino, K., & Oertel, D. (2003). Bidirectional synaptic plasticity in the cerebellum-like mammalian dorsal cochlear nucleus. *Proceedings of the National Academy of Sciences of the United States of America, 100*(1), 265–270.

Golding, N. L., & Oertel, D. (1997). Physiological identification of the targets of cartwheel cells in the dorsal cochlear nucleus. *Journal of Neurophysiology, 78*(1), 248–260.

Haenggeli, C., Doucet, J., & Ryugo, D. (2002). Trigeminal projections to the cochlear nucleus in rats. *Abstracts for the Association for Research in Otolaryngology, 25*, 7.

Haenggeli, C. A., Pongstaporn, T., Doucet, J. R., & Ryugo, D. K. (2005). Projections from the spinal trigeminal nucleus to the cochlear nucleus in the rat. *Journal of Comparative Neurology, 484*(2), 191–205. doi:10.1002/cne.20466

Heeringa, A., Stefanescu, R. A., Raphael, Y., & Shore, S. (2016). Altered vesicular glutamate transporter distributions in the mouse cochlear nucleus following cochlear insult. *Neuroscience,325*, 119.

Hofman, P. M., Van Riswick, J. G., & Van Opstal, A. J. (1998). Relearning sound localization with new ears. *Nature Neuroscience, 1*(5), 417–421. doi:10.1038/1633

Isaacson, J. S., & Scanziani, M. (2011). How inhibition shapes cortical activity. *Neuron, 72*(2), 231–243. doi:10.1016/j.neuron.2011.09.027

Kalappa, B. I., Brozoski, T. J., Turner, J. G., & Caspary, D. M. (2014). Single unit hyperactivity and bursting in the auditory thalamus of awake rats directly correlates with behavioural evidence of tinnitus. *Journal of Physiology, 592*(Pt 22), 5065–5078. doi:10.1113/jphysiol.2014.278572

Kaltenbach, J. A., Zhang, J., & Finlayson, P. (2005). Tinnitus as a plastic phenomenon and its possible neural underpinnings in the dorsal cochlear nucleus. *Hearing Research, 206*(1–2), 200–226. doi:S0378-5955(05)00078-X [pii] 10.1016/j.heares.2005.02.013

Kanold, P. O., & Manis, P. B. (1999). Transient potassium currents regulate the discharge patterns of dorsal cochlear nucleus pyramidal cells. *Journal of Neuroscience, 19*(6), 2195–2208.

Koehler, S., & Shore, S. (2013). Stimulus timing-dependent plasticity in dorsal cochlear nucleus is altered in tinnitus. *Journal of Neuroscience, 33*(50), 19647–19656.

Koehler, S. D., & Shore, S. E. (2013a). Stimulus-timing dependent multisensory plasticity in the guinea pig dorsal cochlear nucleus. *PLoS One, 8*(3), e59828. doi:10.1371/journal.pone.0059828

Koehler, S. D., & Shore, S. E. (2013b). Stimulus timing-dependent plasticity in dorsal cochlear nucleus is altered in tinnitus. *Journal of Neuroscience, 33*(50), 19647–19656. doi:10.1523/JNEUROSCI.2788-13.2013 33/50/19647 [pii]

Kurotani, T., Yamada, K., Yoshimura, Y., Crair, M. C., & Komatsu, Y. (2008). State-dependent bidirectional modification of somatic inhibition in neocortical pyramidal cells. *Neuron, 57*(6), 905–916. doi:10.1016/j.neuron.2008.01.030

Levine, R. (1999). Somatic modulation of tinnitus appears to be a fundamental attribute of tinnitus. *Proceedings of the 6th International Tinnitus Seminar, Cambridge England, 1*, 93–197.

Levine, R. A. (1999). Somatic (craniocervical) tinnitus and the dorsal cochlear nucleus hypothesis. *American Journal of Otolaryngology, 20*(6), 351–362.

Levine, R. A., Nam, E. C., Oron, Y., & Melcher, J. R. (2007). Evidence for a tinnitus subgroup responsive to somatosensory based treatment modalities. *Progress in Brain Research, 166*, 195–207. doi:S0079-6123(07)66017-8 [pii] 10.1016/S0079-6123(07)66017-8

Li, H., & Mizuno, N. (1997). Single neurons in the spinal trigeminal and dorsal column nuclei project to both the cochlear nucleus and the inferior colliculus by way of axon collaterals: A fluorescent retrograde double-labeling study in the rat. *Neuroscience Research, 29*, 135–142.

Li, S., Choi, V., & Tzounopoulos, T. (2013). Pathogenic plasticity of Kv7.2/3 channel activity is essential for the induction of tinnitus. *Proceedings of the National Academy of Sciences of the United States, 110*(24), 9980–9985. doi:10.1073/pnas.1302770110 1302770110 [pii]

Li, S., Kalappa, B. I., & Tzounopoulos, T. (2015). Noise-induced plasticity of KCNQ2/3 and HCN channels underlies vulnerability and resilience to tinnitus. *Elife, 4*. doi:10.7554/eLife.07242

Luz, Y., & Shamir, M. (2012). Balancing feed-forward excitation and inhibition via Hebbian inhibitory synaptic plasticity. *PLoS Computational Biology, 8*(1), e1002334. doi:10.1371/journal.pcbi.1002334

Ma, W. L., Hidaka, H., & May, B. J. (2006). Spontaneous activity in the inferior colliculus of CBA/J mice after manipulations that induce tinnitus. *Hearing Research*, *212*(1–2), 9–21. doi:S0378-5955(05)00303-5 [pii] 10.1016/j.heares.2005.10.003

Maejima, T., Hashimoto, K., Yoshida, T., Aiba, A., & Kano, M. (2001). Presynaptic inhibition caused by retrograde signal from metabotropic glutamate to cannabinoid receptors. *Neuron*, *31*(3), 463–475.

Magee, J. C., & Johnston, D. (1997). A synaptically controlled, associative signal for Hebbian plasticity in hippocampal neurons. *Science*, *275*(5297), 209–213.

Mahanty, N. K., & Sah, P. (1998). Calcium-permeable AMPA receptors mediate long-term potentiation in interneurons in the amygdala. *Nature*, *394*(6694), 683–687. doi:10.1038/29312

Manis, P. B. (1990). Membrane properties and discharge characteristics of guinea pig dorsal cochlear nucleus neurons studied in vitro. *Journal of Neuroscience*, *10*(7), 2338–2351.

Manzoor, N. F., Gao, Y., Licari, F., & Kaltenbach, J. A. (2013). Comparison and contrast of noise-induced hyperactivity in the dorsal cochlear nucleus and inferior colliculus. *Hearing Research*, *295*, 114–123. doi:10.1016/j.heares.2012.04.003 S0378-5955(12)00089-5 [pii]

Markram, H., Lubke, J., Frotscher, M., & Sakmann, B. (1997). Regulation of synaptic efficacy by coincidence of postsynaptic APs and EPSPs. *Science*, *275*(5297), 213–215.

Marks, K. L., Martel, D. T., Wu, C., Basura, G. J., Roberts, L. E., Schvartz-Leyzac, K. C., & Shore, S. E. (2018). Auditory-somatosensory bimodal stimulation desynchronizes brain circuitry to reduce tinnitus in guinea pigs and humans. *Science Translational Medicine*, *10*(422). doi:10.1126/scitranslmed.aal3175

Masquelier, T., Guyonneau, R., & Thorpe, S. J. (2009). Competitive STDP-based spike pattern learning. *Neural Computation*, *21*(5), 1259–1276. doi:10.1162/neco.2008.06-08-804

May, B. J. (2000). Role of the dorsal cochlear nucleus in the sound localization behavior of cats. *Hearing Research*, *148*(1–2), 74–87.

Middleton, J. W., Kiritani, T., Pedersen, C., Turner, J. G., Shepherd, G. M., & Tzounopoulos, T. (2011). Mice with behavioral evidence of tinnitus exhibit dorsal cochlear nucleus hyperactivity because of decreased GABAergic inhibition. *Proceedings of the National Academy of Sciences of the United States of America*, *108*(18), 7601–7606. doi:10.1073/pnas.1100223108 1100223108 [pii]

Min, R., & Nevian, T. (2012). Astrocyte signaling controls spike timing-dependent depression at neocortical synapses. *Nature Neuroscience*, *15*(5), 746–753. doi:10.1038/nn.3075

Moore, C. I., Carlen, M., Knoblich, U., & Cardin, J. A. (2010). Neocortical interneurons: from diversity, strength. *Cell*, *142*(2), 189–193. doi:10.1016/j.cell.2010.07.005

Mugnaini, E., Osen, K. K., Dahl, A. L., Friedrich, V. L., Jr., & Korte, G. (1980a). Fine structure of granule cells and related interneurons (termed Golgi cells) in the cochlear nuclear complex of cat, rat and mouse. *Journal of Neurocytology*, *9*(4), 537–570.

Mugnaini, E., Warr, W. B., & Osen, K. K. (1980b). Distribution and light microscopic features of granule cells in the cochlear nuclei of cat, rat, and mouse. *Journal of Comparative Neurology*, *191*(4), 581–606.

Mulders, W. H., & Robertson, D. (2009). Hyperactivity in the auditory midbrain after acoustic trauma: Dependence on cochlear activity. *Neuroscience*, *164*(2), 733–746. doi:S0306-4522(09)01395-5 [pii] 10.1016/j.neuroscience.2009.08.036

Nelson, S. B. (2004). Hebb and anti-Hebb meet in the brainstem. *Nature Neuroscience*, *7*(7), 687–688. doi:10.1038/nn0704-687 nn0704-687 [pii]

Nevian, T., & Sakmann, B. (2006). Spine Ca2+ signaling in spike-timing-dependent plasticity. *Journal of Neuroscience*, *26*(43), 11001–11013. doi:10.1523/JNEUROSCI.1749-06.2006

Oertel, D., & Young, E. D. (2004). What's a cerebellar circuit doing in the auditory system? *Trends in Neuroscience*, *27*(2), 104–110. doi:10.1016/j.tins.2003.12.001

Ohlrogge, M., Doucet, J. R., & Ryugo, D. K. (2001). Projections of the pontine nuclei to the cochlear nucleus in rats. *Journal of Comparative Neurology*, *436*(3), 290–303.

Ormond, J., & Woodin, M. A. (2009). Disinhibition mediates a form of hippocampal long-term potentiation in area CA1. *PLoS One*, *4*(9), e7224. doi:10.1371/journal.pone.0007224

Ormond, J., & Woodin, M. A. (2011). Disinhibition-mediated LTP in the hippocampus is synapse specific. *Frontiers in Cellular Neuroscience*, *5*, 17. doi:10.3389/fncel.2011.00017

Parham, K., & Kim, D. O. (1995). Spontaneous and sound-evoked discharge characteristics of complex-spiking neurons in the dorsal cochlear nucleus of the unanesthetized decerebrate cat. *Journal of Neurophysiology*, *73*(2), 550–561.

Perez-Rosello, T., Anderson, C. T., Schopfer, F. J., Zhao, Y., Gilad, D., Salvatore, S. R., . . . Tzounopoulos, T. (2013). Synaptic Zn2+ inhibits neurotransmitter release by promoting endocannabinoid synthesis. *Journal of Neuroscience*, *33*(22), 9259–9272. doi:10.1523/JNEUROSCI.0237-13.2013 33/22/9259 [pii]

Pilati, N., Large, C., Forsythe, I. D., & Hamann, M. (2012). Acoustic over-exposure triggers burst firing in dorsal cochlear nucleus fusiform cells. *Hearing Research*, *283*(1–2), 98–106. doi:10.1016/j.heares.2011.10.008 S0378-5955(11)00262-0 [pii]

Populin, L. C., & Yin, T. C. (1998). Pinna movements of the cat during sound localization. *Journal of Neuroscience*, *18*(11), 4233–4243.

Portfors, C. V., & Roberts, P. D. (2007). Temporal and frequency characteristics of cartwheel cells in the dorsal cochlear nucleus of the awake mouse. *Journal of Neurophysiology*, *98*(2), 744–756.

Requarth, T., & Sawtell, N. B. (2011). Neural mechanisms for filtering self-generated sensory signals in cerebellum-like circuits. *Current Opinion in Neurobiology*, *21*(4), 602–608. doi:S0959-4388(11)00099-7 [pii] 10.1016/j.conb.2011.05.031

Roberts, M. T., & Trussell, L. O. (2010). Molecular layer inhibitory interneurons provide feedforward and lateral inhibition in the dorsal cochlear nucleus. *Journal of Neurophysiology*, *104*(5), 2462–2473. doi:jn.00312.2010 [pii] 10.1152/jn.00312.2010

Rodriguez-Moreno, A., & Paulsen, O. (2008). Spike timing-dependent long-term depression requires presynaptic NMDA receptors. *Nature Neuroscience*, *11*(7), 744–745. doi:10.1038/nn.2125

Ropp, T. J., Tiedemann, K. L., Young, E. D., & May, B. J. (2014). Effects of unilateral acoustic trauma on tinnitus-related spontaneous activity in the inferior colliculus. *Journal of the Association for Research Otolaryngology*, *15*(6), 1007–1022. doi:10.1007/s10162-014-0488-2

Said, J., Izita, A., Gonzalez, A. L., & Tovar, E. (2006). Comparative results of craniocorpography and the test of balance in tinnitus and vertigo patients. *International Tinnitus Journal*, *12*(2), 179–183.

Salvi, R. J., Wang, J., & Ding, D. (2000). Auditory plasticity and hyperactivity following cochlear damage. *Hearing Research*, *147*(1–2), 261–274. doi:S0378-5955(00)00136-2 [pii]

Sarihi, A., Jiang, B., Komaki, A., Sohya, K., Yanagawa, Y., & Tsumoto, T. (2008). Metabotropic glutamate receptor type 5-dependent long-term potentiation of excitatory synapses on fast-spiking GABAergic neurons in mouse visual cortex. *Journal of Neuroscience*, *28*(5), 1224–1235. doi:10.1523/JNEUROSCI.4928-07.2008

Sedlacek, M., Tipton, P. W., & Brenowitz, S. D. (2011). Sustained firing of cartwheel cells in the dorsal cochlear nucleus evokes endocannabinoid release and retrograde suppression of parallel fiber synapses. *Journal of Neuroscience, 31*(44), 15807–15817. doi:10.1523/JNEUROSCI.4088-11.2011 31/44/15807 [pii]

Sefanescu, R., & Shore, S. (2015). NMDA receptors mediate stimulus timing dependent plasticity and neural synchrony in dorsal cochlear nucleus. *Frontiers in Neural Circuits* 9:75. doi: 10.3389/fncir.2015.00075

Shore, S. E. (2005). Multisensory integration in the dorsal cochlear nucleus: Unit responses to acoustic and trigeminal ganglion stimulation. *European Journal of Neuroscience, 21*(12), 3334–3348. doi:EJN4142 [pii] 10.1111/j.1460-9568.2005.04142.x

Shore, S. E., Koehler, S., Oldakowski, M., Hughes, L. F., & Syed, S. (2008). Dorsal cochlear nucleus responses to somatosensory stimulation are enhanced after noise-induced hearing loss. *European Journal of Neuroscience, 27*(1), 155–168. doi:10.1111/j.1460-9568.2007.05983.x

Shore, S. E., Roberts, L. E., & Langguth, B. (2016). Maladaptive plasticity in tinnitus: Triggers, mechanisms and treatment. *Nature Review Neurology, 12*(3), 150–160. doi:10.1038/nrneurol.2016.12

Shore, S. E., Vass, Z., Wys, N. L., & Altschuler, R. A. (2000). Trigeminal ganglion innervates the auditory brainstem. *Journal of Comparative Neurology, 419*(3), 271–285. doi:10.1002/(SICI)1096-9861(20000410)419:3<271::AID-CNE1>3.0.CO;2-M [pii]

Shore, S. E., & Zhou, J. (2006). Somatosensory influence on the cochlear nucleus and beyond. *Hearing Research, 216–217*, 90–99. doi:S0378-5955(06)00009-8 [pii] 10.1016/j.heares.2006.01.006

Singer, W. (1999). Neuronal synchrony: A versatile code for the definition of relations? *Neuron, 24*(1), 49–65, 111–125.

Singla, S., Dempsey, C., Warren, R., Enikolopov, A. G., & Sawtell, N. B. (2017). A cerebellum-like circuit in the auditory system cancels responses to self-generated sounds. *Nature Neuroscience, 20*(7), 943–950. doi:10.1038/nn.4567

Sjostrom, P. J., Turrigiano, G. G., & Nelson, S. B. (2003). Neocortical LTD via coincident activation of presynaptic NMDA and cannabinoid receptors. *Neuron, 39*(4), 641–654.

Song, S., Miller, K. D., & Abbott, L. F. (2000). Competitive Hebbian learning through spike-timing-dependent synaptic plasticity. *Nature Neuroscience, 3*(9), 919–926. doi:10.1038/78829

Stefanescu, R. A., Koehler, S. D., & Shore, S. E. (2015). Stimulus-timing-dependent modifications of rate-level functions in animals with and without tinnitus. *Journal of Neurophysiology, 113*(3), 956–970. doi:10.1152/jn.00457.2014

Stefanescu, R. A., & Shore, S. E. (2017). Muscarinic acetylcholine receptors control baseline activity and Hebbian stimulus timing-dependent plasticity in fusiform cells of the dorsal cochlear nucleus. *Journal of Neurophysiology, 117*, 1229–1238.

Stefanescu, R. A., & Shore, S. E. (2015). NMDA receptors mediate stimulus-timing-dependent plasticity and neural synchrony in the dorsal cochlear nucleus. *Frontiers in Neural Circuits, 9*, 75. doi:10.3389/fncir.2015.00075

Sturm, J. J., Zhang-Hooks, Y. X., Roos, H., Nguyen, T., & Kandler, K. (2017). Noise trauma-induced behavioral gap detection deficits correlate with reorganization of excitatory and inhibitory local circuits in the inferior colliculus and are prevented by acoustic enrichment. *Journal of Neuroscience, 37*(26), 6314–6330. doi:10.1523/JNEUROSCI.0602-17.2017

Tzounopoulos, T., Kim, Y., Oertel, D., & Trussell, L. O. (2004). Cell-specific, spike timing-dependent plasticities in the dorsal cochlear nucleus. *Nature Neuroscience, 7*(7), 719–725. doi:10.1038/nn1272 nn1272 [pii]

Tzounopoulos, T., Rubio, M. E., Keen, J. E., & Trussell, L. O. (2007). Coactivation of pre- and postsynaptic signaling mechanisms determines cell-specific spike-timing-dependent plasticity. *Neuron*, *54*(2), 291–301. doi:S0896-6273(07)00249-8 [pii] 10.1016/j.neuron.2007.03.026

Vogels, T. P., Froemke, R. C., Doyon, N., Gilson, M., Haas, J. S., Liu, R., . . . Sprekeler, H. (2013). Inhibitory synaptic plasticity: spike timing-dependence and putative network function. *Front Neural Circuits*, *7*, 119. doi:10.3389/fncir.2013.00119

Voigt, H. F., & Young, E. D. (1988). Neural correlations in the dorsal cochlear nucleus: Pairs of units with similar response properties. *Journal of Neurophysiology*, *59*(3), 1014–1032.

Wall, M., Rosenberg, M., & Richardson, D. (1987). Gaze-evoked tinnitus. *Neurology*, *37*(6), 1034–1036.

Wang, H., Brozoski, T. J., Turner, J. G., Ling, L., Parrish, J. L., Hughes, L. F., & Caspary, D. M. (2009). Plasticity at glycinergic synapses in dorsal cochlear nucleus of rats with behavioral evidence of tinnitus. *Neuroscience*, *164*(2), 747–759. doi:10.1016/j.neuroscience.2009.08.026 S0306-4522(09)01383-9 [pii]

Wang, L., Fontanini, A., & Maffei, A. (2012). Experience-dependent switch in sign and mechanisms for plasticity in layer 4 of primary visual cortex. *Journal of Neuroscience*, *32*(31), 10562–10573. doi:10.1523/JNEUROSCI.0622-12.2012

Wright, D. D., & Ryugo, D. K. (1996). Mossy fiber projections from the cuneate nucleus to the cochlear nucleus in the rat. *Journal of Comparative Neurology*, *365*(1), 159–172. doi:10.1002/(SICI)1096-9861(19960129)365:1<159::AID-CNE12>3.0.CO;2-L [pii] 10.1002/(SICI)1096-9861(19960129)365:1<159::AID-CNE12>3.0.CO;2-L

Wu, C., Martel, D. T., & Shore, S. E. (2015a). Transcutaneous induction of stimulus-timing-dependent plasticity in dorsal cochlear nucleus. *Frontiers in Systems Neuroscience*, *9*, 116. doi:10.3389/fnsys.2015.00116

Wu, C., Martel, D. T., & Shore, S. E. (2015b). Transcutaneous induction of stimulus-timing-dependent plasticity in dorsal cochlear nucleus. *Frontiers in Systems Neuroscience*. doi:10.3389/fnsys.2015.00116

Wu, C., Martel, D. T., & Shore, S. E. (2016). Increased synchrony and bursting of dorsal cochlear nucleus fusiform cells correlate with tinnitus. *Journal of Neuroscience*, *36*(6), 2068–2073. doi:10.1523/JNEUROSCI.3960-15.2016

Wu, C., Stefanescu, R. A., Martel, D. T., & Shore, S. E. (2014). Listening to another sense: Somatosensory integration in the auditory system. *Cell and Tissue Res*. doi:10.1007/s00441-014-2074-7

Zeng, C., Nannapaneni, N., Zhou, J., Hughes, L. F., & Shore, S. (2009). Cochlear damage changes the distribution of vesicular glutamate transporters associated with auditory and nonauditory inputs to the cochlear nucleus. *Journal of Neuroscience*, *29*(13), 4210–4217. doi:29/13/4210 [pii] 10.1523/JNEUROSCI.0208-09.2009

Zeng, C., Shroff, H., & Shore, S. E. (2011). Cuneate and spinal trigeminal nucleus projections to the cochlear nucleus are differentially associated with vesicular glutamate transporter-2. *Neuroscience*, *176*, 142–151. doi:10.1016/j.neuroscience.2010.12.010

Zeng, C., Yang, Z., Shreve, L., Bledsoe, S., & Shore, S. (2012a). Somatosensory projections to cochlear nucleus are upregulated after unilateral deafness. *Journal of Neuroscience*, *32*(45), 15791–15801. doi:10.1523/JNEUROSCI.2598-12.2012

Zeng, C., Yang, Z., Shreve, L., Bledsoe, S., & Shore, S. (2012b). Somatosensory projections to cochlear nucleus are upregulated after unilateral deafness. *Journal of Neuroscience*, *32*(45), 15791–15801. doi:10.1523/JNEUROSCI.2598-12.2012

Zhan, X., Pongstaporn, T., & Ryugo, D. K. (2006). Projections of the second cervical dorsal root ganglion to the cochlear nucleus in rats. *Journal of Comparative Neurology*, *496*(3), 335–348.

Zhao, Y., Rubio, M., & Tzounopoulos, T. (2011). Mechanisms underlying input-specific expression of endocannabinoid-mediated synaptic plasticity in the dorsal cochlear nucleus. *Hearing Research*, *279*(1–2), 67–73. doi:10.1016/j.heares.2011.03.007 S0378-5955(11)00078-5 [pii]

Zhao, Y., & Tzounopoulos, T. (2011). Physiological activation of cholinergic inputs controls associative synaptic plasticity via modulation of endocannabinoid signaling. *Journal of Neuroscience*, *31*(9), 3158–3168. doi:10.1523/JNEUROSCI.5303-10.2011 31/9/3158 [pii]

Zhou, J., Nannapaneni, N., & Shore, S. (2007). Vessicular glutamate transporters 1 and 2 are differentially associated with auditory nerve and spinal trigeminal inputs to the cochlear nucleus. *Journal of Comparative Neurology*, *500*(4), 777–787. doi:10.1002/cne.21208

Zhou, J., & Shore, S. (2004). Projections from the trigeminal nuclear complex to the cochlear nuclei: A retrograde and anterograde tracing study in the guinea pig. *Journal of Neuroscience Research*, *78*(6), 901–907. doi:10.1002/jnr.20343

Zhou, J., Zeng, C., Cui, Y., & Shore, S. (2010). Vesicular glutamate transporter 2 is associated with the cochlear nucleus commissural pathway. *Journal of the Association for Research Otolaryngology*, *11*(4), 675–687. doi:10.1007/s10162-010-0224-5

CHAPTER 10

PERINATAL DEVELOPMENT OF THE MEDIAL NUCLEUS OF THE TRAPEZOID BODY

SHOBHANA SIVARAMAKRISHNAN, ASHLEY BRANDEBURA, PAUL HOLCOMB, DANIEL HELLER, DOUGLAS KOLSON, DAKOTA JACKSON, PETER H. MATHERS, AND GEORGE A. SPIROU

Abstract

Bushy cells (BC) of the cochlear nucleus mono-innervate their target neuron, the principal cell of the medial nucleus of the trapezoid body (MNTB), via the calyx of Held (CH) terminal, which is a typically mammalian structure and perhaps the largest nerve terminal in the brain. CH:MNTB innervation has become an attractive model to study neural circuit formation because it forms quickly, passing through stages of competition in mice within 2–4 days. BCs innervate MNTB neurons by E17, but CHs do not begin to grow for another five days (P3). Progress has been made to identify molecular factors for axon guidance, CH growth, and physiological maturation of synaptic partners, but important details remain to be discovered. We summarize key events in CH formation and highlight unresolved issues in molecular and physiological signaling, roles for non-neural cells, and the nature of competition during the first postnatal week.

Keywords: MNTB, calyx of Held, gene expression, synaptic transmission, synaptogenesis, pruning

The calyx of Held (CH) was first described by Hans Held in 1893, and has since figured prominently in key discoveries about nervous system function. The large size of the CH made it amenable to early study using the light microscope, and its appearance was used as justification for and against the Neuron Doctrine (Ramon y Cajal, 1995; von Gersdorff & Borst, 2002). It is a typically mammalian structure and, despite early controversy (Moore & Moore, 1971; Richter et al., 1983), is now an accepted structure in humans (Kulesza, 2008; Kulesza & Grothe, 2015). The CH is perhaps the largest nerve terminal in the mammalian brain, and has more active zones by species than the cerebellar mossy fiber rosette (CH: 554 in postnatal day (P)9 rat, Satzler et al., 2002; 678 in P14 rat, Taschenberger et al., 2002; 2400 in adult cat, Rowland et al., 2000; mossy fiber rosette: 191–424 in P18 rat, Xu-Friedman & Regehr, 2003; 42–243 in P21 mouse, Kim et al., 2013). The CH, which originates from globular bushy cells (GBC) of the ventral cochlear nucleus (VCN) and forms a 1:1 innervation of principal neurons in the medial nucleus of the trapezoid body (MNTB; Friauf & Ostwald, 1988; Smith et al., 1991; Spirou et al., 1990; Tolbert et al., 1982;), is a key component of binaural convergence in the superior olivary complex (Harrison & Warr, 1962; van Noort, 1969; Warr, 1972). The CH functions at the synaptic level as a reliable and temporally precise relay of neural activity in vivo (Guinan & Li, 1990) with modification of postsynaptic activity likely by inhibitory inputs (Kopp-Scheinpflug et al., 2003, 2008; Awatramani et al., 2004, 2005). The fast and precise excitatory input provided by the CH to MNTB principal neurons translates into system-level function by driving inhibition in binaural circuits, since the postsynaptic MNTB principal cells are glycinergic (Campistron et al., 1986; Finlayson & Caspary, 1989). The main targets of the MNTB are the medial superior olive (MSO), lateral superior olive (LSO) and the superior paraolivary nucleus (SPN), where neuronal activity is based on time of arrival of excitatory and inhibitory inputs (Boudreau & Tsuchitani, 1968; Brand et al., 2002; Felix & Magnusson, 2016; Goldberg & Brown, 1969; Kuwada & Batra, 1999; Yin & Chan, 1990). We and others established the CH:MNTB system as a powerful model for neural circuit formation, due to the rapid pace of transition from small terminal to the readily measured end point of 1:1 innervation onto most neurons in just 3–4 days (Hoffpauir et al., 2006; Holcomb et al., 2013; Kandler & Friauf, 1993). In this review we focus on the timeline for CH:MNTB innervation and highlight important unsolved mysteries.

Embryology

The embryonic origins of the MNTB are poorly understood. MNTB neurons are born in the mouse hindbrain between embryonic day (E)11 and E12 (Figure 10.1; Pierce, 1973) and the rat hindbrain between E13 and E16 (Kudo et al., 2000). Altman and Bayer (1980) postulated the rhombic lip as the site of MNTB origin, as the rhombic lip is the primary proliferative zone in the hindbrain. However, if this postulate is true, the MNTB must arise from an Atoh1-negative region of the rhombic lip, as the MNTB is not fate-mapped in the *Atoh1-Cre* lineage (Maricich et al., 2009). The MNTB is derived from progenitor cells in rhombomeres 4 and 5, as it is lineage-labeled with the *Hoxb1-Cre* (rhombomere 4) and the *Egr2-Cre* (rhombomeres 3 and 5) transgenic lines (Maricich et al., 2009; Marrs et al., 2013).

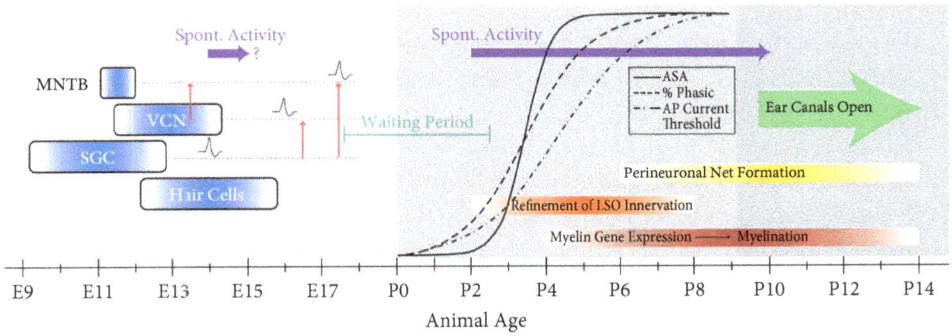

FIGURE 10.1. Temporal correlation of CH and MNTB neuron maturation. Trapezoid fiber inputs to the MNTB are observed by E17.5. However, there is a waiting period before rapid CH growth begins. Rapid CH growth, measured by an increase in its apposed surface area, occurs between P2–P4 (solid line). During this period, innervation of MNTB neurons by multiple protocalyceal inputs changes to a single large CH. The intrinsic response of MNTB neurons to current injection changes from tonic firing to one or a few spikes at the onset of the current step (phasic firing). Postsynaptic spike threshold also increases during this time, accompanied by an increase in input resistance. By P8, mono-innervation is almost complete and, in parallel, postsynaptic spike thresholds stabilize and intrinsic firing in most MNTB neurons is phasic. Spontaneous activity has been clearly demonstrated in the early postnatal period, but may also be important in establishing brainstem circuitry before E15. Depicted on the left are developmental milestones at different points in the brainstem auditory circuit. Dates of neurogenesis are shown in blue. The age of measurable connectivity between regions is shown with red arrows. Action potential waveforms indicate the first age at which activity was recorded in each region. Refinement of MNTB projections to the LSO occurs from P2 to P8. Expression of genes for myelination can be detected at P4 and myelination of bushy cell axons occurs by P9. PNNs can be detected around MNTB neurons as early as P6 but continue to refine their structure through P14. Most of these developmental milestones occur before the onset of hearing at P10. SGC: spiral ganglion cells, VCN: ventral cochlear nucleus; ASA: apposed surface area.

Modified from Marrs and Spirou, 2012; Hoffpauir et al., 2010.

The earliest (though not specific) marker for MNTB principal cells is the En1 transcription factor (Altieri et al., 2015; Jalabi et al., 2013; Marrs et al., 2013). Using the *En1-Cre* strain for lineage tracing, presumptive MNTB neurons can be identified near the ventral edge of the brainstem at E12.5, though they are clustered laterally along with cells that will give rise to other superior olivary nuclei (Altieri et al., 2015; Marrs et al., 2013). The MNTB cells appear to migrate medially from this lateral location, and the nucleus becomes morphologically distinct in its medial position around E17.5 (Marrs et al., 2013). The importance of En1 for MNTB development is highlighted by *En1* conditional deletion studies, in which the nucleus forms but is not maintained in postnatal mice (Altieri et al., 2015; Jalabi et al., 2013). In addition, En1 expression is necessary for activation of another MNTB transcription factor, FoxP1 (Altieri et al., 2015; Marrs et al., 2013). A third transcription factor likely to be important for MNTB formation is Ptf1a, which is required for formation of inhibitory interneurons in other neural circuits (Fujiyama et al., 2009; Jusuf et al., 2011). It is unclear if or where Ptf1a fits into the genetic hierarchy of En1 and FoxP1 expression in the developing MNTB.

Although the primary growth period of the calyx occurs postnatally, the initial wiring is established before birth. The VCN is derived from progenitor cells in rhombomeres 2–4 (Farago et al., 2006). Birth of GBC neurons in the VCN peaks at E12 in mouse, whereas the peak birth of the spiral ganglion cells occurs at E11 (Figure 10.1; Pierce, 1973). GBC axons extend across the midline by E13.5 into the region where the MNTB will form (Howell et al., 2007; Kandler & Friauf, 1993), though the migration of MNTB neurons is not complete until E17.5 (Marrs et al., 2013). Although MNTB cells are functionally innervated by GBCs as early as E17.5 (Hoffpauir et al., 2010), rapid growth of the calyx does not initiate until P2 after a 4-day waiting period has ensued (Holcomb et al., 2013; Kandler & Friauf, 1993). Whether contacts exist between GBCs and MNTB principal cells prior to E17.5 has yet to be determined, though it is conceivable that the arrival of MNTB neurons through medial migration initiates collateral branching of the ventral acoustic stria axons to form calyceal connections (Kandler & Friauf, 1993).

Axonal projections from the GBC to the MNTB require the netrin-DCC signaling pathway as a midline attractant, as germline mutations in either *netrin1* or *DCC* genes alter axonal outgrowth from the VCN and prevent midline crossing of this contralateral projection (Howell et al., 2007). Likewise, the midline repulsive slit-Robo signaling pathway helps regulate midline crossing. Conditional mutations in *Robo3*, which are normally permissive for midline crossing, prevent contralateral projection of the ventral acoustic stria and result in aberrant ipsilateral connections when *Robo3* is deleted using the *Egr2-Cre* driver line (Michalski et al., 2013; Renier et al., 2010).

Formation of a Calyx of Held

GBC axons that have arrived within the MNTB during embryonic ages branch profusely and collectively and form 5–20 small contacts on somata of MNTB neurons by P2 (Holcomb et al., 2013). Volume electron microscopy in mice at 1-day intervals, beginning at P2, reveals the emergence of large terminals (>35μm^2 of apposed surface area, ASA) onto nearly half the cells by P3, and onto nearly all cells by P4. About 60% of cells receiving large inputs at P3 are contacted by more than one large input, suggesting competition between inputs (Figure 10.2; panel D). By P6, about 75% of all cells have resolved to mono-innervation via a large CH and, by P9, this number reaches 88% (Holcomb et al., 2013). These two phases of strengthening and pruning are similar to refinement of innervation at the neuromuscular junction (Tapia et al., 2012) except that the time frame at the CH:MNTB is compressed. This short time frame entails rapid assembly of active zones, whereby several hundred are assembled over a time frame of days (Hoffpauir et al., 2006).

As CHs grow, they extend many collateral processes. These collaterals are sometimes tipped with growth cones and the longest collaterals extend >75 μm from the edges of

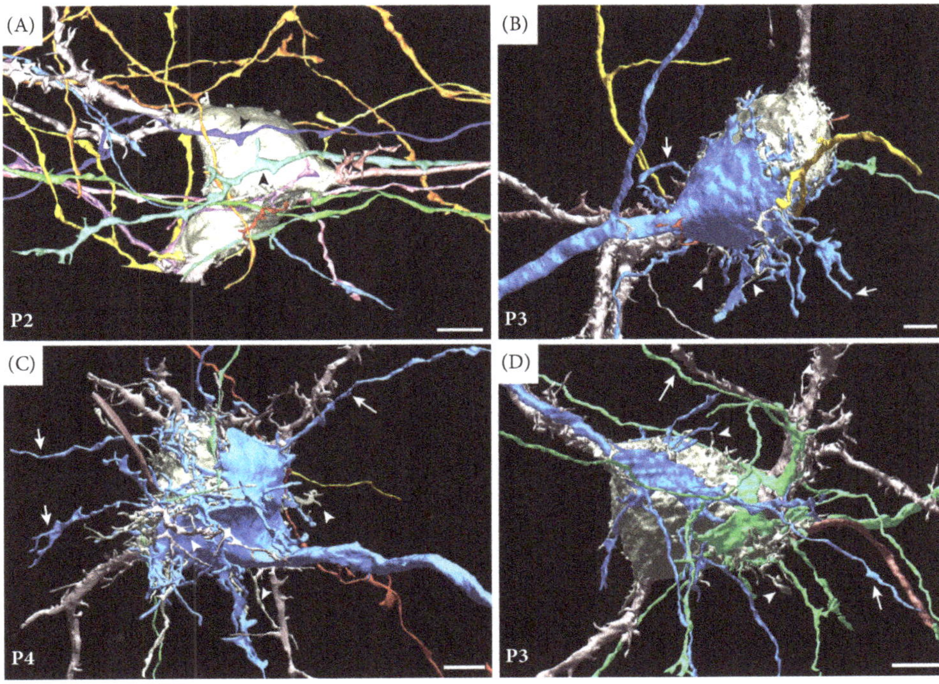

FIGURE 10.2. Growth of the Calyx of Held.
(A) At P2, MNTB principal cell bodies (tan) are relatively smooth, with multiple axons (assorted colors) making contact in an *en passant* fashion (black arrowheads). No protocalyces are evident at this age. (B) At P3, principal cells have begun to form both short and long projections (white arrowheads). Many inputs have been removed, leaving only a few larger inputs including one solid, cup-like protocalyx (blue) with a few collateral projections (white arrows). (C) By P4, the protocalyx has spread to occupy substantial somatic surface area. Longer collateral projections have formed from both the principal cell (white arrowheads) and protocalyx (white arrows). (D) Similarly sized competing protocalyces (blue, green) occupy distinct territories on the principal cell surface, and both produce collateral projections (white arrows). Collaterals can also be seen from the principal cell (white arrowheads). Scale bars: 5μm.

Modified from Holcomb et al., 2013, with permission.

the apposed terminal (Holcomb et al., 2013; Kandler & Friauf, 1993; Morest, 1968). The presence of growth cone-tipped collaterals and high variability in collateral length could suggest that these collaterals undergo dynamic motility. More recent in vivo two photon experiments performed in perinatal rat pups reported many calyx collaterals exhibit high levels of turnover during one-hour imaging sessions and, further, that these collateral structures can form functional synaptic contacts with off-target principal cells (Rodríguez-Contreras et al., 2008). Collectively, these collateral arbors may aid in the selection of appropriate synaptic partners. Interestingly, significant postsynaptic reorganization parallels the initial growth of the CH. By P2 in rodents, only small terminals are found along the soma of each principal neuron and the neurons are densely packed together within the MNTB (Figure 10.2, panel A). As protocalyces form over the next two days, the principal cells begin to separate from one another and extend many collateral structures, termed somatic spicules (Figure 10.2; Holcomb et al., 2013). The function and dynamics of these structures has yet to be explored.

Each principal neuron in the MNTB is surrounded by specialized lattice-like structures of extracellular matrix, known as perineuronal nets (PNNs: see chapter by Morawski and colleagues for greater detail). PNNs begin forming during the first postnatal week (Blosa et al., 2013; Kolson et al., 2016). They are composed mostly of chondroitin sulfate proteoglycans (such as aggrecan and brevican), hyaluronan, Hapln linker proteins, and tenascin-R (reviewed by Wang & Fawcett, 2012). Their exact functions are still being investigated, but they are involved in the control of synaptic plasticity and regulation of synaptic activity (Balmer, 2016; Carulli et al., 2010; reviewed by Sorg et al., 2016). In the visual cortex, *Hapln1* knockout mice demonstrate a functional gain in the ability to compensate for loss of connectivity following denervation (Carulli et al., 2010). This study suggests that the formation of PNNs serves to limit synaptic plasticity after a critical period. Thus, it is intriguing to think that PNNs in the MNTB may cement and stabilize the large CH terminal and inhibit multi-innervation at more mature ages. Microarray analysis detects significantly changing transcript levels for three main PNN components (aggrecan, brevican and Hapln1), all of which increase between P0 and P6 when the CH is growing and refining to mono-innervation (Kolson et al., 2016). Immunofluorescence shows the linker protein, Hapln1, is visible as early as P0 in the MNTB. However, there is a delay between protein expression of the linker protein and the other PNN components because brevican and aggrecan are not detectable until after P6 (Figure 10.1; Kolson et al., 2016). *Brevican* knockout mice show a delay in synaptic transmission between the CH and principal neurons along with prolonging of action potentials when compared to wildtype controls at P23–31, but these mice have not been evaluated at early developmental ages (Blosa et al., 2015). Although the overall structure of the PNNs is comparable between the *brevican* knockout and wildtype mice (Blosa et al., 2015), other components of the PNNs, such as aggrecan, still are present in the knockouts and may suggest redundant function. However, more extensive perturbations, such as double and triple knockouts, or knockout of the linker protein, Hapln1, and their effects on CH refinement to mono-innervation remain to be investigated.

Cell Signaling in MNTB Development

The CH terminal grows to its large size in synchrony with biophysical maturation of the principal neuron and an increase in principal neuron size (Hoffpauir et al., 2006, 2010; Rusu & Borst, 2011; see later section in this review). The contralateral CH projection to principal neurons is also tonotopically organized (reviewed by Kandler et al., 2009). Notably, MNTB innervation of LSO transitions from a relatively broad territory along the tonotopic axis at P2 to a narrowed territory by P8 (Figure 10.1; Kim & Kandler, 2003), suggesting that the MNTB-LSO connection sharpens in parallel with maturation of the CH and principal neuron. This coordinated maturation of pre- and postsynaptic partners and functional refinement of synaptic projections to LSO suggests mechanisms of cell signaling to regulate maturation of the systems. Genetic perturbation studies are a useful means of testing the functionality of such signaling interactions. This section provides a review of genetic perturbations that affect early development of either the GBC or the principal neuron and their effects on CH-principal neuron connectivity, morphology and size.

The *Fmr1* gene is associated with fragile X syndrome (FXS) and autism spectrum disorder (ASD; Hagerman et al., 2010). Interestingly, patients with FXS and ASD present with abnormal auditory brainstem responses (ABRs; Roth et al., 2012). *Fmr1* knockouts have been used to model these disorders and examine effects in the MNTB (Rotschafer et al., 2015; Ruby et al., 2015). Compared to their wildtype counterparts, the ABRs of *Fmr1*$^{-/-}$ mice have elevated thresholds and smaller amplitudes of waves I and III, indicating both peripheral and central deficits. Neuronal cell size is reduced in both bushy cells and principal neurons, and there is an increase in the number of VGAT^{+} punctae in the MNTB, suggesting an altered excitatory:inhibitory synaptic balance (Rotschafer et al., 2015). A similar phenotype is observed in *Fmr1*$^{-/-}$ rats, which have smaller principal neurons and fewer calyces (Ruby et al., 2015). The protein product of the *Fmr1* gene, FMRP (Fragile X mental retardation) negatively regulates mRNA translation and binds Kv3.1b mRNA in the brainstem (Strumbos et al., 2010). Kv3.1b is normally expressed along a tonotopic gradient in MNTB, with the highest expression in the medial MNTB (Li et al., 2001). *Fmr1*$^{-/-}$ mice have disrupted Kv3.1b tonotopy and do not show the increase in Kv3.1b expression following high-frequency stimulation that is found in controls (Strumbos et al., 2010). An intriguing hypothesis is that the disruption of ion channel distribution along the tonotopic gradient affects neural activity, which in turn may be related to the decrease in cell size. In wild-type mice, the lateral low-frequency encoding neurons are larger than their medial counterparts (Weatherstone et al., 2017). Similar to *Fmr1*$^{-/-}$ rodents, in Deafwaddler mice, which have a spontaneous mutation in the *Pmca2* (plasma membrane calcium ATPase 2) gene, the neuronal size gradient is disrupted across the tonotopic axis. It is noteworthy that the phenotype of decreased cell size is also observed in human patients with ASD (Lukose et al., 2015).

Many signaling pathways regulate different steps in CH formation, including where a calyx projects (ipsilateral vs. contralateral), how large and complex the terminal grows, and the subsequent refinement to mono-innervation. The GBC normally projects its axon to form the CH in the contralateral MNTB (Cant & Casseday, 1986). In addition to the netrin-DCC and slit-Robo signaling pathways mentioned earlier, an important signaling component mediating this projection pattern is the interaction of the Eph receptor tyrosine kinase family with Ephrin ligands. The Eph signaling pathway is unique in that both traditional forward signaling, initiated from the ligand and processed through the receptor, and reverse signaling, which involves signaling initiated by the extracellular domain of the receptor and processed through the membrane-bound ligand, can occur. In a series of knockout and dominant negative overexpression experiments, a 10% increase in ipsilateral calyx formation was seen in EphB2/EphB3 double knockout mice. Furthermore, reverse signaling through EphB2-EphrinB2 promotes contralateral calyx formation and inhibits ipsilateral sprouting, because ephrin-B2^{lacZ} mice, where the cytoplasmic domain of Ephrin-B2 is replaced by β-galactosidase, exhibited a significant increase in ipsilateral calyx formation (Hsieh et al., 2010). EphrinB2 is not expressed in the principal neurons until after E17 when the initial synaptogenesis has already occurred (Hsieh et al., 2010; Marrs & Spirou, 2012) and therefore does not seem to be acting as a typical guidance factor. Rather, EphrinB2 seems to act as a repulsive signal to inhibit ipsilateral sprouting of an axon that has already crossed the midline, possibly interacting with developing PNNs to limit ipsilateral connections postnatally (Blosa et al., 2013; Kolson et al., 2016).

The contactin superfamily consists of a group of cell adhesion molecules whose expression is enriched in the developing nervous system (reviewed by Shimoda & Watanabe, 2009). Expression of *Cntn5* (contactin 5) is important for mediating adhesion of the calyceal contact with the principal neuron rather than a role in axon migration because the mRNA is not expressed until after P1, when initial synaptogenesis has already occurred. Whereas nearly all principal neurons are contacted by a large CH terminal at P6 in wildtype mice (Holcomb et al., 2013; Toyoshima et al., 2009), 8% of principal neurons lack a CH terminal in *Cntn5*$^{-/-}$ mice. The neurons that lack calyceal innervation later undergo apoptosis due to lack of innervation (Toyoshima et al., 2009).

Several signaling pathways affect calyx size, morphology and refinement to mono-innervation, but most perturbations yield an incomplete and often mild phenotype, suggesting that formation of the large CH terminals is a robust process. The Sad-A and Sad-B kinases are a pair of serine/threonine kinases that localize within the CH terminal. Double conditional knockout mice, where Cre expression is driven by the *Parvalbumin* promoter, which is expressed both presynaptically at birth and postsynaptically by the end of the first postnatal week, have significantly smaller CH terminals when evaluated at P24 (Lilley et al., 2014). Genetic conditional deletion of two receptors for Bmp signaling, Bmpr1a/b, results in smaller terminal size and an almost 40% reduction in the number of mono-innervated principal neurons at P7–10 (Xiao et al., 2013). Electrophysiological studies show that the timing of synaptic transmission is impaired in the Bmpr1 knockout mice. Smaller excitatory postsynaptic currents (EPSCs) in the knockout mice correspond with delays in the rise time of the excitatory postsynaptic potentials (EPSPs) and action potentials, which occur with long delays. However, the first phenotypic differences cannot be observed until P3, suggesting that initial synaptogenesis of small glutamatergic inputs is not altered in these knockout mice (Xiao et al., 2013). These data suggest that Bmp signaling is required for the initial stage of growth of large terminals and that further growth and competition are inter-related processes that establish mono-innervation.

Further evidence supporting the idea that fast neurotransmission drives CH growth is demonstrated through *Egr2*-driven conditional knockout of the dynamin family of GTPases that are required for clathrin-mediated endocytosis, *Dnm1/3* (Fan et al.,

2016). Similar to the Bmp conditional knockout, initial synaptogenesis is not affected in the *Dnm1/3* conditional knockout mice. Wild-type mice demonstrate a significant functional maturation in the kinetics of spontaneous EPSCs (sEPSCs) across development, but the knockout mice do not display this developmental transformation in fast firing properties, and sEPSCs have slower rise and decay times. Additionally, the principal neurons in the knockout mice display more immature biophysical properties, including a higher membrane excitability and frequency of spontaneous action potentials. However, in stark contrast to most of the previously listed genetic perturbations, the *Dnm1/3* conditional knockout mice have a severe phenotype, with a lack of initial growth of terminals into the protocalyx phase and accumulating degeneration of MNTB neurons (Fan et al., 2016). The drastic phenotypes seen in this knockout model may be due to deficits in the balance of exo- and endocytosis, and suggest that a minimal level of endocytosis is required for CH growth. Alternatively, generalized effects on cell signaling could account for this extreme phenotype. It is worth noting that in both the Bmpr and Dyn1/3 cKO mice, both presynaptic and postsynaptic gene expression was affected, so that altered function in both synaptic partners could underlie alterations in CH maturation.

Functional Maturation of Synaptic Partners

Functional synaptic input to the MNTB from VCN begins during embryonic ages. By E15.5 in mice, both auditory nerve and VCN neurons can generate action potentials (AP), and by E16.5, APs can be reliably evoked in VCN neurons by auditory nerve fiber stimulation. At E17.5, the earliest age at which the MNTB is recognizable in tissue sections, a single stimulus pulse initiates a series of subthreshold inputs of varying latency that can generate spikes in the MNTB principal cell (Hoffpauir et al., 2010; Marrs & Spirou, 2012). In response to direct activation of VCN inputs to the MNTB, synaptic latencies shorten during the first postnatal week, postsynaptic spikes increase in height and decrease in duration, and tonic firing changes to an adult-like phasic response (Figure 10.3; Hoffpauir et al., 2010; Sierksma et al., 2017).

Spontaneous Activity during the Period of CH Growth

Since formation of the CH occurs before the ear canals open, this process is considered to be independent of environmental sound, given the caveat that pups may self-stimulate their cochlea by vocalization. Spontaneous activity has been demonstrated in the MNTB, but its role in CH formation is debatable. Blockade of inner hair cell activation and synaptic transmission by genetic deletion of *Cacna1d* ($Ca_V1.3$) yields

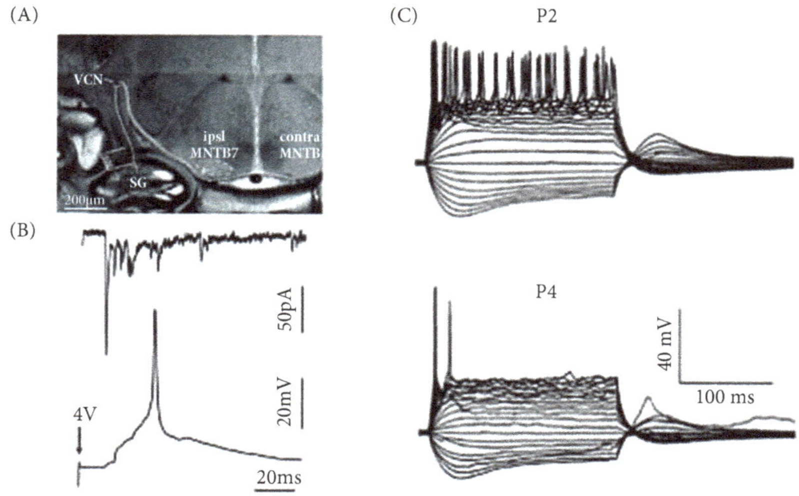

FIGURE 10.3. Physiological responses in the MNTB during embryonic and early postnatal ages. (A, B) Activation of the contralateral MNTB by auditory nerve stimulation at E17. (A) Whole-head mouse slice illustrating the auditory brainstem circuit from the spiral ganglion to the MNTB. The auditory nerve is stimulated at the base of the cochlea and recordings are made from principal cells in the contralateral MNTB. SG: spiral ganglion; VCN: ventral cochlear nucleus; ipsi: ipsilateral; contra: contralateral. (B) Responses in an MNTB principal cell at E17 evoked by auditory nerve stimulation. Top trace: synaptic currents recorded under voltage-clamp to a single shock delivered to the auditory nerve. Bottom trace: Changes in membrane potential recorded under current clamp to the same auditory nerve stimulus. Synaptic currents show multiple components. An initial rapid current of ~150 pA is followed by several smaller currents (~50 pA), suggesting multiple presynaptic inputs on the principal cell. The principal cell responds to synaptic input with a delayed spike that is evoked by EPSP summation. (C) MNTB principal neurons transition from tonic to phasic firing during the period of rapid CH growth. Intrinsic firing to somatic current injection is illustrated at P2 and P4. At P2, depolarizing current steps evoke sustained firing while, at P4, phasic firing occurs at the onset of the current pulse at all depolarizations. Hyperpolarizing currents evoke a sag in membrane potential at P2 that continues to occur at P4. Current steps are 200 ms long.

Modified from Hoffpauir et al., 2010; Marrs and Spirou, 2012.

a smaller MNTB with 1/3 fewer neurons (and similar changes across the superior olivary complex; Hirtz et al., 2011) but with, at best, subtle effects on CH formation and neurotransmission onto the remaining neurons (Erazo-Fisher et al., 2007). *Slc17a8* (vesicular glutamate transporter 3) knockout does not alter the biophysical properties of MNTB neurons or their excitability by glutamate photo-uncaging and, similar to *otoferlin* knockout, does not alter innervation of LSO by MNTB (Noh et al., 2010), suggesting little effect of cochlear silencing on CH formation. Likewise, CHs form and mature normally by P20 in dn/dn mice, which lack auditory nerve spontaneous activity (Leao et al., 2006b; Youssoufian et al., 2005). However, these mice exhibit reduced but present spontaneous activity, thus GBCs may generate activity in the absence of cochlear input.

Spiral ganglion neurons are spontaneously active in vitro at embryonic ages (earliest age tested, E14), (Marrs and Spirou, 2012), suggesting that synaptic connections, functional from auditory nerve to MNTB by E17.5, permit a flow of spontaneous activity through these neural circuits beginning in the embryo. Starting at about P2, characteristic bursts (~10 Hz) and minibursts (~100 Hz) of spontaneous activity, which are likely of cochlear origin, can be recorded from GBC axons and MNTB neurons (Clause et al., 2014; Sierksma et al., 2017; Tritsch et al., 2007; Tritsch & Bergles, 2010). Simulations of the contributions of intrinsic and synaptic conductances to burst firing suggest that activation of NMDA receptors on principal neurons increases both the number of spikes as well as spike frequencies within minibursts, but not bursts, relative to GBC input (Sierksma et al., 2017). NMDA receptors are predicted to have a stronger effect on bursting at P3 than at P5 or P6 (Sierksma et al., 2017), which agrees well with the measured decline in the NMDA contribution to EPSCs during the early postnatal period, and the shift in balance towards a more rapidly decaying AMPA-centric synaptic response (Hoffpauir et al., 2010; Joshi & Wang, 2002). Taken together, the early postnatal presence of bursting spontaneous activity in the MNTB and the embryonic presence of spontaneous spiking in spiral ganglion cells suggest that early spontaneous activity in the pathway between the spiral ganglion and MNTB may create a state of activity-dependent homeostatic regulation of CH:MNTB innervation. Clause et al. (2014) demonstrated that altering spontaneous firing in the spiral ganglion does not affect the average rate of spontaneous firing in the MNTB, but changes its temporal pattern, without effect on CH morphology. Patterned spontaneous activity shapes neuronal maps by pruning extensive branching of afferent axons (Shatz, 1996). The formation of functional pre-calyx contacts onto MNTB neurons in the *Dnm1/3* knockout does not preclude roles for spontaneous activity in this step of maturation, especially if vesicle fusion rates are low (Fan et al., 2016). The possibility remains, then, that spontaneous activity plays roles in maintaining bouton-like synaptic contacts measured from E17.5, transition to the protocalyx stage, and resolving competition among supernumerary inputs.

NMDA-dependent bursting may strengthen activity in the immature CH:MNTB synapse through activation of small conductance apamin-sensitive, Ca^{++}-dependent K^+ channels (S_K channels). S_K channels are activated by bursts of spikes in MNTB neurons that produce calcium sparks, and by calcium influx through NMDA receptors. They give rise to spontaneous outward currents that regulate the resting membrane conductance and the resting potential of MNTB neurons. The number of MNTB neurons that exhibit calcium sparks and S_K-dependent transient outward currents gradually increases from P6 (40%) to hearing onset around P10 (~90%), and then decreases by P14 (5%), suggesting that this temporary feature is pertinent to synapse maturation (Zhang & Huang, 2017) and perhaps the initial stages of CH formation. Embryonic and early postnatal spontaneous activity may therefore regulate ion channel expression through NMDA receptor activation in the developing MNTB well before sound-induced cochlear drive becomes established. In addition to spontaneously active VCN inputs, MNTB neurons at embryonic and early postnatal ages also receive tonic and phasic depolarizing GABAergic and glycinergic inputs that regulate membrane excitability (Hoffpauir et al., 2010; Awatramani et al., 2005).

Changes in Postsynaptic Excitability during CH Growth

CH growth and presynaptic pruning are accompanied by a reduction in postsynaptic excitability. Small currents of ~30 pA can evoke APs at E17.5–P2, but these values rapidly increase nearly tenfold by P4 (Hoffpauir et al., 2010). During this time frame, CHs grow from bouton size into cup-shaped terminals up to 400 μm^2 in ASA with the postsynaptic cell (Holcomb et al., 2013). By P4, postsynaptic membrane resistance decreases and low-threshold K^+ subunits, hyperpolarization-activated cation channels and leak channels are upregulated (Berntson & Walmsley, 2008; Hoffpauir et al., 2010; Leao et al., 2005a; Leao et al., 2005b; Leao et al., 2006a; Sierksma & Borst, 2017; Sierksma et al., 2017). Consequently, sustained spiking during current injection changes to an adult-like phasic response (Figure 10.3). Developmental increases in the peak Na^+ current and its faster inactivation, and increases in the magnitude of delayed rectifier K^+ currents (Elezgarai et al., 2003; Ishikawa et al., 2003; Leao et al., 2005a) are confirmed by upregulation of *Kcna* gene family expression (*Kcna2, Kcnab3*) and of the *Scn1a* gene expression between P0-P6 (Kolson et al., 2016).

Increases in EPSC amplitude occur along with changes in postsynaptic input resistance. Between P3-P6, EPSC amplitudes gradually increase from the pA to nA range (Hoffpauir et al., 2010; Iwasaki & Takahashi, 1998). Using minimal stimulation of the trapezoid fiber bundle in slices containing the MNTB, Hoffpauir et al. (2010) showed that ~50% of principal neurons between E18 and P0 are driven by small inputs. At P1, this percentage decreases to 33% and by P3, there are no principal neurons driven by small inputs. Even at more mature CH:MNTB synapses (P16–19), spike failure in the MNTB during repeated stimulation occurs when EPSCs become smaller than ~300 pA (Grande & Wang, 2011). Thus, at these early ages, MNTB neurons are unable to follow repeated input. Both short-term synaptic facilitation and depression are present to varying degrees at early postnatal ages and modulate the ability of MNTB neurons to follow trapezoid fiber stimulus rates (reviewed by Borst & van Hoeve, 2012). Nonetheless, the ability of the postsynaptic response to follow CH input increases as the synapse matures towards hearing onset, with the principal neuron achieving a 90% success rate in following trapezoid fiber stimulation by the end of the second postnatal week (Wu & Kelly, 1991).

The improved ability of the MNTB neuron to follow input is also illustrated by a decrease in its input resistance during the embryonic and early postnatal period. Input resistances, which are as high as 1 GΩ at E17, decrease to ~200 MΩ by P6, after which they do not change. Age-dependent decreases in postsynaptic excitability are also illustrated by the finding that, at E17, the maximum slope resistance occurs at membrane potentials more hyperpolarized than the resting membrane potential, whereas by P6, maximum slope resistances are observed at resting potentials (Hoffpauir et al., 2010). Pre- and postsynaptic changes during early development therefore appear to be remarkably well-orchestrated.

Regulation of Calcium during CH Growth

As a general feature of synaptic development, correlated pre-and postsynaptic maturation and the refinement of developing synaptic connections by spontaneous activity are strongly linked to calcium signaling. The temporal dynamics and mode of calcium entry into developing nerve terminals and their postsynaptic counterparts confer specificity to downstream events such as synaptic pruning and dendritic arborization (reviewed by Rosenberg & Spitzer, 2011), and are critical to the rate of outgrowth of the presynaptic growth cone (Gomez & Spitzer, 1999; Vonhoff & Keshishian, 2017). The spatiotemporal calcium profile in the developing CH is therefore likely to be a crucial factor in the early establishment of mono-innervation in the MNTB.

The class of presynaptic Ca^{++} channels triggering transmitter release from the CH switches early in postnatal development, suggesting spatiotemporal changes in the presynaptic calcium profile during and immediately following establishment of the 1:1 CH:MNTB connection. At P6, a third of the presynaptic Ca^{++} current flows through high-threshold N-type Ca^{++} channels sensitive to ωCgTx GVIA, and the P/Q type Ca^{++} channel blocker ωAga-IVA blocks most of the remaining current. By P8, the N-type Ca^{++} channel contributes to only 10%, and the P/Q channel to most, of the remaining presynaptic Ca^{++} current (Iwasaki et al., 2000; Iwasaki & Takahashi, 1998). There is a general decrease in expression of Ca^{++} channel genes in the MNTB during this time (*Cacna1b, Cacna1e, Cacna1g, Cacnb3*; Kolson et al., 2016), which may indicate an overall refinement of calcium channel subtypes in principal neurons (Bollmann et al., 1998) and other cells, including glia. Given the likely importance of early presynaptic calcium profiles in establishing monoinnervation in the MNTB, presynaptic Ca^{++} currents at ages younger than P4, which have not been measured, will provide valuable information about developmental changes in CH Ca^{++} channel subtypes.

The shift from multiple Ca^{++} channels to a single class of channels in the CH accompanies a shortening of the distance between Ca^{++} channels and Ca^{++} sensors and the formation of Ca^{++} nanodomains (Wang et al., 2008; Kochubey et al., 2009). Nanodomain formation, which is mediated by septin 5 and SNARE proteins (Yang et al., 2010), preserves temporal precision across the synapse (Yang et al., 2014). The finding that Ca^{++} sensor sensitivity is lower at P9 than at P16 (K_D values of ~80 μM and 120 μM, respectively; Kochubey et al., 2009; Wang et al., 2008) suggests, by extrapolation, that Ca^{++} channels are not tightly coupled to Ca^{++}-sensors during the first postnatal week, but this has yet to be determined. The slow Ca^{++} buffer EGTA is more effective at attenuating transmitter release at P8 than at P16, and Ca^{++} cooperativity values are higher in younger CHs (Fedchyshyn & Wang, 2005). This finding supports poorer spatial coupling between Ca^{++} channels and Ca^{++} sensors, as well as the requirement for a higher number of Ca^{++} channels to trigger transmitter release during early development. Computer simulations demonstrate that tight Ca^{++} channel-Ca^{++} sensor coupling almost doubles the Ca^{++} concentration seen by the Ca^{++} sensor (Naraghi & Neher, 1997; Schneggenburger & Neher, 2000). Thus, as the synapse matures during the second postnatal week, fewer Ca^{++} channels are needed to trigger transmitter release and endogenous Ca^{++} buffering is less likely to saturate with high-frequency stimulation. The early establishment of Ca^{++} nanodomains might therefore factor into the development of the low Ca-affinity of the transmitter release process at this synapse.

Fast endogenous calcium buffering in CH terminals becomes more prevalent with age and appears to be specific to the type of calcium binding protein. Between P3 and P6, parvalbumin forms the primary calcium buffer, and is present in almost all CHs as measured by immunohistochemistry (Felmy & Schneggenburger, 2004; Kolson et al., 2016). This fraction remains constant with further development (Felmy & Schneggenburger, 2004), suggesting that presynaptic calcium buffering is established as CHs complete their phase of most rapid growth. In contrast, calretinin is expressed in very few CHs at P6 (~5%) and in an only slightly larger fraction after hearing onset (P14; 18%). Furthermore, calretinin content appears to be highly variable in the CH population at P6, with calretinin-negative and -positive CHs interspersed (Felmy & Schneggenburger, 2004). Since presynaptic calcium transients at P6 decay much slower than those at P11 (2.5 s and 0.9 s, respectively; Chuhma & Ohmori, 2001), calcium extrusion rates are critical at early postnatal ages. The slow rate of calcium buffering by parvalbumin makes it effective on intracellular calcium transients after an action potential, with a primary influence on short-term plasticity (Caillard et al., 2000). Calretinin, in contrast, with a fast buffering capacity similar to that of BAPTA, regulates fast transmission evoked by single spikes (Schwaller, 2014). Its buffering is also more highly activity-dependent than that of parvalbumin (Schwaller, 2010). Thus differences in the prevalence of parvalbumin and calretinin in young CHs, and the heterogenous distribution of calretinin, suggest that co-localization of presynaptic fast and slow calcium buffers would differentially affect calcium extrusion rates in the CH population and may have a proportionally larger role in CH:MNTB development during the first postnatal week. Interestingly, decreases in noradrenaline sensitivity of presynaptic calcium currents point to a developmental shift in the regulation of presynaptic calcium channels by inhibitory G-protein pathways (Leao & von Gersdorff, 2002).

Glia in MNTB Development

Neuroglia in the MNTB, as in other brain regions, serve a diverse and important array of functions. As in the cerebral cortex (Parnavelas, 1999) and cerebellum (Buffo & Rossi, 2013), glial cells in the brainstem are believed to be derived from the ventricular neuroepithelium, from which radial glial processes project to create a "scaffold" that may be the basis for later neural organization (van Hartesveldt et al., 1986; Gomez et al., 1990). Both astrocytes and oligodendrocytes are present in the MNTB as early as P0 in mice and rats, with microglia appearing in substantial numbers only after P6 (Dinh et al., 2014; Saliu et al., 2014). Using EdU injections of pregnant rat dams, Saliu et al (2014) showed that glial progenitor cells in the rat MNTB begin to divide prenatally (E19 or earlier), rapidly increase their rate of division until around the onset of hearing (approximately P12), and then slow their division exponentially until barely distinguishable at P18. EdU-labeled cells later stain positive for the commonly used astrocyte marker, S100β. This timeline of glial proliferation occurs in synchrony with the developmental timeline of the CH terminal (Saliu et al., 2014). Although S100ß is often used as a marker for astrocytes, this protein is also expressed in NG2$^+$ oligodendrocyte precursor cells (OPCs; Hachem et al., 2005). Therefore, proliferating glia in the MNTB may potentially assume either an oligodendrocytic or astrocytic fate (Buffo & Rossi, 2013; Hamori et al., 1997).

Both astrocytes and OPCs participate in a multi-partite synaptic system in the MNTB that is only partially understood. Light and ultrastructural analyses of the developing MNTB have shown that vellous processes, either from astrocytes or OPCs, occupy non-innervated territory on the principal cell surface, surround growing terminals, and interpose between the principal cell and terminals (Dinh et al., 2014; Elezgarai et al., 2001; Holcomb et al., 2013; Reyes-Haro et al., 2010). Dinh et al. (2014) showed that vellous processes, present as early as P0, express S100ß, aldehyde dehydrogenase 1 family member L1 (ALDH1L1), or glial fibrillary acidic protein (GFAP), though the pattern of expression differs for each protein. From P0 to at least P23, ALDH1L1$^+$ glial processes associate with MNTB principal neurons and, later in development, the growing calyx. Processes expressing S100ß are similarly associated with these structures, though the processes were found to be more homogenously distributed throughout the MNTB. GFAP shows no expression within the MNTB at P0 and expression only in glial processes within the MNTB from P6 to P24. No GFAP$^+$ cell bodies are found present in the MNTB at any age studied (Dinh et al., 2014). However, the extent of overlap in expression of these proteins in these processes has yet to be determined. A single astrocyte or OPC may also contact multiple principal cells, opening the possibility for regulation of network-level organization by these cells. In some cases, vellous processes can completely block processes filled with vesicles (presumably calyceal projections) near the principal cell surface from establishing contact, suggesting they may play a direct physical role in competition during calyx development (Holcomb et al., 2013). Additionally, these vellous processes contain metabotropic glutamate receptors (mGluR2/3, P0-24 rats, P6–18 mice) and transporters (EAAT1[GLAST], EAAT2[GLT-1], P10–15 rats), allowing them to respond to glutamate release from the CH, take up excess glutamate, and prevent glutamate receptor saturation in the immature calyx (Elezgarai et al., 2001; Renden et al., 2005; Uwechue et al., 2012). As the calyx matures and fenestrates (P16 and later), the risk of receptor saturation decreases, glutamate uptake by glial cells is less necessary, and expression of mGluR2/3 decreases in these processes (Elezgarai et al.,

2001; Renden et al., 2005). Astrocytes may also influence synaptic refinement through gliotransmission and the induction of neuronal slow inward currents (nSICs); repeated stimulation of midline axons causes astrocytes to release both glutamate and D-serine that, together, co-activate NMDA receptors on the principal cell and induce nSICs (Reyes-Haro et al., 2010). In contrast, direct, AMPA receptor-mediated synaptic connections are established between the CHs and OPCs, allowing these cells to receive synchronized input (Müller et al., 2009). Glutamatergic input to $NG2^+$ OPCs has generally been shown to inhibit differentiation of these cells into more mature oligodendrocytes (Gallo et al., 1996 Karadottir & Attwell, 2007; Yuan et al., 1998). However, it has been demonstrated more recently in the rat corpus callosum that the frequency of stimulation has a direct influence on OPC proliferation and differentiation, with 5 Hz stimulation increasing OPC differentiation and 25 Hz and 300 Hz stimulation increasing OPC proliferation (Nagy et al., 2017). As activity can influence both GBC axon diameter and myelin thickness (Sinclair et al., 2017), it is intriguing to think that changes in firing patterns may allow terminals to regulate their own oligodendrocyte differentiation and, therefore, their own axon myelination. The studies of both astrocyte gliotransmission and CH:OPC synapses were performed in 8–10 day old mice, after monoinnervation has already been established. Future studies will need to focus on earlier postnatal time points to elucidate the reciprocal effects that neuron-glial interactions may have on development of the MNTB.

Myelination

Wrapping of axons by myelin sheaths provides an electrically insulating layer that allows the rapid and temporally precise propagation of action potentials. Functionally, the integration of binaural signals and regulation of conduction timing is controlled through the morphological characteristics of axon diameter, myelin thickness, node formation and localization of ion channels (Ford et al., 2015, Seidl & Rubel, 2016; Xu et al., 2017). Myelination in the MNTB, as detectable by immunohistochemistry, begins by P9, when most MNTB principal neurons are monoinnervated by CHs (Saliu et al., 2014). A noticeable increase in myelination is evident around the time of ear canal opening at P10–12, with the developmental growth of axon diameter, increase in myelin thickness, and associated conduction velocity, increasing until P25 and P35, respectively (Sinclair et al., 2017). Myelin wraps leave axon membrane exposed at nodes of Ranvier and at heminodes leading into the nerve terminal. $Na_v1.6$, $Na_v\beta4$, and $K_v3.1$ channels are concentrated at the heminode leading into the CH, with fewer channels in the nerve terminal proper (Berret et al., 2016; Leao et al., 2005a). Na_v channel clusters at the CH axon heminode in rats are not detectable by IHC at P6. Broad expression of Na_v channels begins at P8, and complete clustering at the heminode occurs by P16 (Xu et al., 2017). $Na_v1.2$-mediated Na^+ currents and the expression of functional AMPA receptors allow a subpopulation of excitable, immature pre-myelinating oligodendrocytes to generate action potentials in response to current injections. Following knockdown of $Na_V1.2$ channels in immature oligodendrocytes, the expression of myelin basic protein decreases, suggesting a functional role for excitable oligodendrocytes in forming compact myelin (Berret et al., 2017). Computer simulations utilizing morphological measurements of internode length, internode axon diameter, and node diameter predict that the differences associated with tonotopic arrangement of the MNTB adjust the conduction velocity and timing of action potentials for sound localization (Ford et al., 2015).

Specifying CH Competition and Growth

Despite much progress in specifying features and factors in CH growth and MNTB maturation in general, a close view of the earliest steps and mechanisms for these events remains to be worked out. For example, a common theme in neural development is exuberant innervation of a postsynaptic territory, followed by selective strengthening of some inputs and pruning of others. Perhaps the best studied example is the neuromuscular junction (NMJ), which undergoes two phases of strengthening and pruning. At birth, motor end plates are innervated by 10 to 20 small inputs (Tapia et al., 2012). Two or three of these inputs enlarge as the others are pruned. These remaining inputs vie for territory on the motor end plate through a process that can extend for longer than one week. This latter process defines a second phase of strengthening and pruning that resolves to mono-innervation (Balice-Gordon & Lichtman, 1993; Walsh & Lichtman, 2003).

The CH innervation of MNTB neurons in adults resembles the NMJ in that multiple (up to about 20) small inputs innervate the MNTB cell body prior to CH growth, and a single CH mono-innervates its target neuron in adults. However, there is not yet a clear picture of the transition from multiple small inputs to mono-innervation. This lack of clarity is due in part to the speed of CH growth, which was estimated to be, at minimum, the addition of 200 μm^2 of ASA per day (Holcomb et al., 2013). Kandler and Friauf (1993), in their classical study using tract-tracing techniques, did not find a single instance of dual innervation of an MNTB neuron by growing CHs. More recently, in vivo juxtacellular and whole-cell electrophysiological recording of MNTB neurons shows evidence for dual innervation in at most 3/132 cells (2%) at P3 and P4 (Sierksma et al., 2017). In contrast, minimal stimulation in vitro yields a higher percentage of multiply innervated cells (4/29 (13%) at P4; Hoffpauir et al., 2006) and at P7–12 (6/101 (6%); Bergsman et al., 2004). Since in vitro recordings represent an underestimate due to sectioning of many fibers at the tissue surface near the recording, the results from Bergsman et al. (2004) in older animals imply that a small percentage of MNTB neurons may be multiply innervated around hearing onset.

As a more objective means of assessing multiple inputs, Holcomb et al. (2013) employed volume electron microscopy across a unique time series of images, covering daily intervals at P2–4. Animals were carefully timed at one half day resolution relative to birth. At P2, large diameter fibers branch profusely, yielding 5–20 small, but no large, inputs onto MNTB cell bodies. Just 24 hours later, 43% (16/37) of MNTB cells are contacted by large terminals, and over one-half of these (56%, 9/16) are contacted by two, and in one instance three large nerve terminals. These data from P3 are instructive since they capture the CH growth process on its first day, and they indicate a large percentage of MNTB neurons with competing inputs (Figure 10.3). Knockout of Bmp1 receptors delays CH growth and a majority (~3/4) of MNTB cells are multi-innervated when tested at P14-16 (Xiao et al., 2013). The most parsimonious interpretation is that competition failed to resolve onto these neurons, although supernumerary innervation could have been induced by the genetic manipulation. Resolution of these EM images, in vitro physiology and genetic manipulation data with other experiments may lie in the fact that competition seems to occur when inputs are still early in their growth phase (Hoffpauir et al., 2006; Holcomb et al., 2013). Most competing inputs at P3 and P4 in these studies were less than 100 μm^2 (ASA), and more than one-half of these were less than 50 μm^2. Both inputs onto the same cell exceeded 100 μm^2 in only one case at each of P3 and P4. These smaller inputs may have eluded detection as contacting the same cell in light microscopy studies, or had too small a physiological signature to be differentiated, especially given the unreliability of linking large postsynaptic currents in vivo to prepotentials. Small inputs also may exhibit less spontaneous activity and be more difficult to detect (Sierksma et al., 2017). Furthermore, volume EM shows that, beyond a size threshold at each age older than P3, the largest inputs all mono-innervate their targets (Hoffpauir et al., 2006; Holcomb et al., 2013).

Summary

In recent years, studies of neural development have revealed new roles for both neurons and glia in formation of neural circuits. In the MNTB, the route from multiple small inputs to monoinnervation is faster than in other mammalian systems, achieving >80% completion within four days. Associated with this transition are birth and death of glia, pruning of inputs, growth and rearrangement of principal MNTB neurons and refinement of their projections to the LSO. Partially overlapping, but largely following from these events, are other steps in maturation such as completion of the formation of perineuronal nets and myelination of CH axons. An overall picture of tissue transformation emerges with likely undiscovered types of cellular and molecular communication among all constituent cell types. The coming years will be exciting as these mechanisms are revealed at a systems level of action and interaction.

Acknowledgments

This work was supported by NIH grants R01 DC007695 (GS), F31 DC014393 (PH) and CoBRE GM103503.

References

Altieri, S. C., Jalabi, W., Zhao, T., Romito-DiGiacomo, R. R., & Maricich, S. M. (2015). En1 directs superior olivary complex neuron positioning, survival, and expression of FoxP1. *Developmental Biology*, *408*(1), 99–108.

Altman, J., & Bayer, S. A. (1980). Development of the brain stem in the rat. III. Thymidine-radiographic study of the time of origin of neurons of the vestibular and auditory nuclei of the upper medulla. *Journal of Comparative Neurology*, *194*(4), 877–904.

Awatramani, G. B., Turecek, R., & Trussell, L. O. (2004). Inhibitory control at a synaptic relay. *Journal of Neuroscience*, *24*(11), 2643–2647.

Awatramani, G. B., Turecek, R., & Trussell, L. O. (2005). Staggered development of GABAergic and glycinergic transmission in the MNTB. *Journal of Neurophysiology*, *93*(2), 819–828.

Balice-Gordon, R. J., & Lichtman, J. W. (1993). In vivo observations of pre- and postsynaptic changes during the transition from multiple to single innervation at developing neuromuscular junctions. *Journal of Neuroscience*, *13*(2), 834–855.

Balmer, T. S. (2016). Perineuronal nets enhance the excitability of fast-spiking neurons. *eNeuro*, *3*(4).

Bergsman, J. B., De Camilli, P., & McCormick, D. A. (2004). Multiple large inputs to principal cells in the mouse medial nucleus of the trapezoid body. *Journal of Neurophysiology*, *92*(1), 545–552.

Berntson, A. K., & Walmsley, B. (2008). Characterization of a potassium-based leak conductance in the medial nucleus of the trapezoid body. *Hearing Research*, *244*(1–2), 98–106.

Berret, E., Barron, T., Xu, J., Debner, E., Kim, E. J., & Kim, J. H. (2017). Oligodendroglial excitability mediated by glutamatergic inputs and Nav1.2 activation. *Nature Communications*, *8*(1), 557.

Berret, E., Kim, S. E., Lee, S. Y., Kushmerick, C., & Kim, J. H. (2016). Functional and structural properties of ion channels at the nerve terminal depends on compact myelin. *Journal of Physiology*, *594*(19), 5593–5609.

Blosa, M., Sonntag, M., Bruckner, G., Jager, C., Seeger, G., Matthews, R. T., . . . Morawski, M. (2013). Unique features of extracellular matrix in the mouse medial nucleus of trapezoid body: Implications for physiological functions. *Neuroscience*, *228*, 215–234.

Blosa, M., Sonntag, M., Jager, C., Weigel, S., Seeger, J., Frischknecht, R., . . . Morawski, M. (2015). The extracellular matrix molecule brevican is an integral component of the machinery mediating fast synaptic transmission at the calyx of Held. *Journal of Physiology*, *593*(19), 4341–4360.

Bollmann, J. H., Helmchen, F., Borst, J. G., & Sakmann, B. (1998). Postsynaptic Ca^{2+} influx mediated by three different pathways during synaptic transmission at a calyx-type synapse. *Journal of Neuroscience*, *18*(24), 10409–10419.

Borst, J. G., & van Hoeve, J. S. (2012). The calyx of Held synapse: From model synapse to auditory relay. *Annual Review of Physiology*, *74*, 199–224.

Boudreau, J. C., & Tsuchitani, C. (1968). Binaural interaction in the cat superior olive S segment. *Journal of Neurophysiology*, *31*(3), 442–454.

Brand, A., Behrend, O., Marquardt, T., McAlpine, D., & Grothe, B. (2002). Precise inhibition is essential for microsecond interaural time difference coding. *Nature*, *417*(6888), 543–547.

Buffo, A., & Rossi, F. (2013). Origin, lineage and function of cerebellar glia. *Progress in Neurobiology*, *109*, 42–63.

Caillard, O., Moreno, H., Schwaller, B., Llano, I., Celio, M. R., & Marty, A. (2000). Role of the calcium-binding protein parvalbumin in short-term synaptic plasticity. *Proceedings of the National Academy of Sciences USA*, *97*(24), 13372–13377.

Cajal, S. R.-y. (1995). *Histology of the nervous system of man and vertebrates* (Vol. 1). Oxford, England: Oxford University Press.

Campistron, G., Buijs, R. M., & Geffard, M. (1986). Glycine neurons in the brain and spinal cord. Antibody production and immunocytochemical localization. *Brain Research*, *376*(2), 400–405.

Cant, N. B., & Casseday, J. H. (1986). Projections from the anteroventral cochlear nucleus to the lateral and medial superior olivary nuclei. *Journal of Comparative Neurology*, *247*(4), 457–476.

Carulli, D., Pizzorusso, T., Kwok, J. C., Putignano, E., Poli, A., Forostyak, S., . . . Fawcett, J. W. (2010). Animals lacking link protein have attenuated perineuronal nets and persistent plasticity. *Brain*, *133*(Pt 8), 2331–2347.

Chuhma, N., & Ohmori, H. (2001). Differential development of Ca^{2+} dynamics in presynaptic terminal and postsynaptic neuron of the rat auditory synapse. *Brain Research*, *904*(2), 341–344.

Clause, A., Kim, G., Sonntag, M., Weisz, C. J., Vetter, D. E., Rubsamen, R., & Kandler, K. (2014). The precise temporal pattern of prehearing spontaneous activity is necessary for tonotopic map refinement. *Neuron*, *82*(4), 822–835.

Dinh, M. L., Koppel, S. J., Korn, M. J., & Cramer, K. S. (2014). Distribution of glial cells in the auditory brainstem: Normal development and effects of unilateral lesion. *Neuroscience*, *278*, 237–252.

Elezgarai, I., Bilbao, A., Mateos, J. M., Azkue, J. J., Benitez, R., Osorio, A., . . . Grandes, P. (2001). Group II metabotropic glutamate receptors are differentially expressed in the medial nucleus of the trapezoid body in the developing and adult rat. *Neuroscience*, *104*(2), 487–498.

Elezgarai, I., Diez, J., Puente, N., Azkue, J. J., Benitez, R., Bilbao, A., . . . Grandes, P. (2003). Subcellular localization of the voltage-dependent potassium channel Kv3.1b in postnatal and adult rat medial nucleus of the trapezoid body. *Neuroscience*, *118*(4), 889–898.

Erazo-Fischer, E., Striessnig, J., & Taschenberger, H. (2007). The role of physiological afferent nerve activity during in vivo maturation of the calyx of Held synapse. *Journal of Neuroscience*, *27*(7), 1725–1737.

Fan, F., Funk, L., & Lou, X. (2016). Dynamin 1- and 3-mediated endocytosis is essential for the development of a large central synapse in vivo. *Journal of Neuroscience*, *36*(22), 6097–6115.

Farago, A. F., Awatramani, R. B., & Dymecki, S. M. (2006). Assembly of the brainstem cochlear nuclear complex is revealed by intersectional and subtractive genetic fate maps. *Neuron*, *50*(2), 205–218.

Fedchyshyn, M. J., & Wang, L. Y. (2005). Developmental transformation of the release modality at the calyx of Held synapse. *Journal of Neuroscience*, *25*(16), 4131–4140.

Felix, R. A., 2nd, & Magnusson, A. K. (2016). Development of excitatory synaptic transmission to the superior paraolivary and lateral superior olivary nuclei optimizes differential decoding strategies. *Neuroscience*, *334*, 1–12.

Felmy, F., & Schneggenburger, R. (2004). Developmental expression of the Ca^{2+}-binding proteins calretinin and parvalbumin at the calyx of Held of rats and mice. *European Journal of Neuroscience*, *20*(6), 1473–1482.

Finlayson, P. G., & Caspary, D. M. (1989). Synaptic potentials of chinchilla lateral superior olivary neurons. *Hearing Research*, *38*(3), 221–228.

Ford, M. C., Alexandrova, O., Cossell, L., Stange-Marten, A., Sinclair, J., Kopp-Scheinpflug, C., . . . Grothe, B. (2015). Tuning of Ranvier node and internode properties in myelinated axons to adjust action potential timing. *Nature Communications*, *6*, 8073.

Friauf, E., & Ostwald, J. (1988). Divergent projections of physiologically characterized rat ventral cochlear nucleus neurons as shown by intra-axonal injection of horseradish peroxidase. *Experimental Brain Research*, *73*(2), 263–284.

Fujiyama, T., Yamada, M., Terao, M., Terashima, T., Hioki, H., Inoue, Y. U., . . . Hoshino, M. (2009). Inhibitory and excitatory subtypes of cochlear nucleus neurons are defined by distinct bHLH transcription factors, Ptf1a and Atoh1. *Development*, *136*(12), 2049–2058.

Gallo, V., Zhou, J. M., McBain, C. J., Wright, P., Knutson, P. L., & Armstrong, R. C. (1996). Oligodendrocyte progenitor cell proliferation and lineage progression are regulated by glutamate receptor-mediated K+ channel block. *Journal of Neuroscience*, *16*(8), 2659–2670.

Goldberg, J. M., & Brown, P. B. (1969). Response of binaural neurons of dog superior olivary complex to dichotic tonal stimuli: some physiological mechanisms of sound localization. *Journal of Neurophysiology*, *32*(4), 613–636.

Gomez, L. A., Brusco, A., & Saavedra, J. P. (1990). Immunocytochemical study of S-100 positive glial cells in the brainstem and spinal cord of the rat embryo. *International Journal of Developmental Neuroscience*, *8*(1), 55–64.

Gomez, T. M., & Spitzer, N. C. (1999). In vivo regulation of axon extension and pathfinding by growth-cone calcium transients. *Nature*, *397*(6717), 350–355.

Grande, G., & Wang, L. Y. (2011). Morphological and functional continuum underlying heterogeneity in the spiking fidelity at the calyx of Held synapse in vitro. *Journal of Neuroscience*, *31*(38), 13386–13399.

Guinan, J. J., Jr., & Li, R. Y. (1990). Signal processing in brainstem auditory neurons which receive giant endings (calyces of Held) in the medial nucleus of the trapezoid body of the cat. *Hearing Research*, *49*(1–3), 321–334.

Hachem, S., Aguirre, A., Vives, V., Marks, A., Gallo, V., & Legraverend, C. (2005). Spatial and temporal expression of S100B in cells of oligodendrocyte lineage. *Glia*, *51*(2), 81–97.

Hagerman, R., Hoem, G., & Hagerman, P. (2010). Fragile X and autism: Intertwined at the molecular level leading to targeted treatments. *Molecular Autism*, *1*(1), 12.

Hamori, J., Jakab, R. L., & Takacs, J. (1997). Morphogenetic plasticity of neuronal elements in cerebellar glomeruli during deafferentation-induced synaptic reorganization. *Journal of Neural Transplantation & Plasticity*, *6*(1), 11–20.

Harrison, J. M., & Warr, W. B. (1962). A study of the cochlear nuclei and ascending auditory pathways of the medulla. *Journal of Comparative Neurology*, *119*, 341–379.

Held, H. (1893). Die Centrale Gehorleitung. *Archives* of *Anatomy and Physiology Abstracts*, *17:201–248*.

Hirtz, J. J., Boesen, M., Braun, N., Deitmer, J. W., Kramer, F., Lohr, C., . . . Friauf, E. (2011). Cav1.3 calcium channels are required for normal development of the auditory brainstem. *Journal of Neuroscience, 31*(22), 8280–8294.

Hoffpauir, B. K., Grimes, J. L., Mathers, P. H., & Spirou, G. A. (2006). Synaptogenesis of the calyx of Held: Rapid onset of function and one-to-one morphological innervation. *Journal of Neuroscience, 26*(20), 5511–5523.

Hoffpauir, B. K., Kolson, D. R., Mathers, P. H., & Spirou, G. A. (2010). Maturation of synaptic partners: Functional phenotype and synaptic organization tuned in synchrony. *Journal of Physiology, 588*(Pt 22), 4365–4385.

Holcomb, P. S., Hoffpauir, B. K., Hoyson, M. C., Jackson, D. R., Deerinck, T. J., Marrs, G. S., . . . Spirou, G. A. (2013). Synaptic inputs compete during rapid formation of the calyx of Held: A new model system for neural development. *Journal of Neuroscience, 33*(32), 12954–12969.

Howell, D. M., Morgan, W. J., Jarjour, A. A., Spirou, G. A., Berrebi, A. S., Kennedy, T. E., & Mathers, P. H. (2007). Molecular guidance cues necessary for axon pathfinding from the ventral cochlear nucleus. *Journal of Comparative Neurology, 504*(5), 533–549.

Hsieh, C. Y., Nakamura, P. A., Luk, S. O., Miko, I. J., Henkemeyer, M., & Cramer, K. S. (2010). Ephrin-B reverse signaling is required for formation of strictly contralateral auditory brainstem pathways. *Journal of Neuroscience, 30*(29), 9840–9849.

Ishikawa, T., Nakamura, Y., Saitoh, N., Li, W. B., Iwasaki, S., & Takahashi, T. (2003). Distinct roles of Kv1 and Kv3 potassium channels at the calyx of Held presynaptic terminal. *Journal of Neuroscience, 23*(32), 10445–10453.

Iwasaki, S., Momiyama, A., Uchitel, O. D., & Takahashi, T. (2000). Developmental changes in calcium channel types mediating central synaptic transmission. *Journal of Neuroscience, 20*(1), 59–65.

Iwasaki, S., & Takahashi, T. (1998). Developmental changes in calcium channel types mediating synaptic transmission in rat auditory brainstem. *Journal of Physiology, 509 (Pt 2)*, 419–423.

Jalabi, W., Kopp-Scheinpflug, C., Allen, P. D., Schiavon, E., DiGiacomo, R. R., Forsythe, I. D., & Maricich, S. M. (2013). Sound localization ability and glycinergic innervation of the superior olivary complex persist after genetic deletion of the medial nucleus of the trapezoid body. *Journal of Neuroscience, 33*(38), 15044–15049.

Joshi, I., & Wang, L. Y. (2002). Developmental profiles of glutamate receptors and synaptic transmission at a single synapse in the mouse auditory brainstem. *Journal of Physiology, 540*(Pt 3), 861–873.

Jusuf, P. R., Almeida, A. D., Randlett, O., Joubin, K., Poggi, L., & Harris, W. A. (2011). Origin and determination of inhibitory cell lineages in the vertebrate retina. *Journal of Neuroscience, 31*(7), 2549–2562.

Kandler, K., Clause, A., & Noh, J. (2009). Tonotopic reorganization of developing auditory brainstem circuits. *Nature Neuroscience, 12*(6), 711–717.

Kandler, K., & Friauf, E. (1993). Pre- and postnatal development of efferent connections of the cochlear nucleus in the rat. *Journal of Comparative Neurology, 328*(2), 161–184.

Karadottir, R., & Attwell, D. (2007). Neurotransmitter receptors in the life and death of oligodendrocytes. *Neuroscience, 145*(4), 1426–1438.

Kim, G., & Kandler, K. (2003). Elimination and strengthening of glycinergic/GABAergic connections during tonotopic map formation. *Nature Neuroscience, 6*(3), 282–290.

Kim, H. W., Kim, N., Kim, K. W., & Rhyu, I. J. (2013). Three-dimensional imaging of cerebellar mossy fiber rosettes by ion-abrasion scanning electron microscopy. *Microscopy and Microanalysis, 19 Suppl 5*, 172–177.

Kochubey, O., Han, Y., & Schneggenburger, R. (2009). Developmental regulation of the intracellular Ca^{2+} sensitivity of vesicle fusion and Ca^{2+}-secretion coupling at the rat calyx of Held. *Journal of Physiology*, *587*(Pt 12), 3009–3023.

Kolson, D. R., Wan, J., Wu, J., Dehoff, M., Brandebura, A. N., Qian, J., . . . Spirou, G. A. (2016). Temporal patterns of gene expression during calyx of held development. *Developmental Neurobiology*, *76*(2), 166–189.

Kopp-Scheinpflug, C., Dehmel, S., Tolnai, S., Dietz, B., Milenkovic, I., & Rubsamen, R. (2008). Glycine-mediated changes of onset reliability at a mammalian central synapse. *Neuroscience*, *157*(2), 432–445.

Kopp-Scheinpflug, C., Lippe, W. R., Dorrscheidt, G. J., & Rubsamen, R. (2003). The medial nucleus of the trapezoid body in the gerbil is more than a relay: Comparison of pre- and postsynaptic activity. *Journal of the Association of Research Otolaryngology*, *4*(1), 1–23.

Kudo, M., Sakurai, H., Kurokawa, K., & Yamada, H. (2000). Neurogenesis in the superior olivary complex in the rat. *Hearing Research*, *139*(1–2), 144–152.

Kulesza, R. J., Jr. (2008). Cytoarchitecture of the human superior olivary complex: Nuclei of the trapezoid body and posterior tier. *Hearing Research*, *241*(1–2), 52–63.

Kulesza, R. J., Jr., & Grothe, B. (2015). Yes, there is a medial nucleus of the trapezoid body in humans. *Frontiers in Neuroanatomy*, *9*, 35.

Kuwada, S., & Batra, R. (1999). Coding of sound envelopes by inhibitory rebound in neurons of the superior olivary complex in the unanesthetized rabbit. *Journal of Neuroscience*, *19*(6), 2273–2287.

Leao, K. E., Leao, R. N., Sun, H., Fyffe, R. E., & Walmsley, B. (2006). Hyperpolarization-activated currents are differentially expressed in mice brainstem auditory nuclei. *Journal of Physiology*, *576*(Pt 3), 849–864.

Leao, R. M., Kushmerick, C., Pinaud, R., Renden, R., Li, G. L., Taschenberger, H., . . . von Gersdorff, H. (2005). Presynaptic Na+ channels: locus, development, and recovery from inactivation at a high-fidelity synapse. *Journal of Neuroscience*, *25*(14), 3724–3738.

Leao, R. M., & Von Gersdorff, H. (2002). Noradrenaline increases high-frequency firing at the calyx of Held synapse during development by inhibiting glutamate release. *Journal of Neurophysiology*, *87*(5), 2297–2306.

Leao, R. N., Naves, M. M., Leao, K. E., & Walmsley, B. (2006). Altered sodium currents in auditory neurons of congenitally deaf mice. *European Journal of Neuroscience*, *24*(4), 1137–1146.

Leao, R. N., Svahn, K., Berntson, A., & Walmsley, B. (2005). Hyperpolarization-activated (I) currents in auditory brainstem neurons of normal and congenitally deaf mice. *European Journal of Neuroscience*, *22*(1), 147–157.

Li, W., Kaczmarek, L. K., & Perney, T. M. (2001). Localization of two high-threshold potassium channel subunits in the rat central auditory system. *Journal of Comparative Neurology*, *437*(2), 196–218.

Lilley, B. N., Krishnaswamy, A., Wang, Z., Kishi, M., Frank, E., & Sanes, J. R. (2014). SAD kinases control the maturation of nerve terminals in the mammalian peripheral and central nervous systems. *Proceedings of the National Academy of Sciences USA*, *111*(3), 1138–1143.

Lukose, R., Beebe, K., & Kulesza, R. J., Jr. (2015). Organization of the human superior olivary complex in 15q duplication syndromes and autism spectrum disorders. *Neuroscience*, *286*, 216–230.

Maricich, S. M., Xia, A., Mathes, E. L., Wang, V. Y., Oghalai, J. S., Fritzsch, B., & Zoghbi, H. Y. (2009). Atoh1-lineal neurons are required for hearing and for the survival of neurons in the spiral ganglion and brainstem accessory auditory nuclei. *Journal of Neuroscience*, *29*(36), 11123–11133.

Marrs, G. S., Morgan, W. J., Howell, D. M., Spirou, G. A., & Mathers, P. H. (2013). Embryonic origins of the mouse superior olivary complex. *Developmental Neurobiology, 73*(5), 384–398.

Marrs, G. S., & Spirou, G. A. (2012). Embryonic assembly of auditory circuits: Spiral ganglion and brainstem. *Journal of Physiology, 590*(10), 2391–2408.

Michalski, N., Babai, N., Renier, N., Perkel, D. J., Chedotal, A., & Schneggenburger, R. (2013). Robo3-driven axon midline crossing conditions functional maturation of a large commissural synapse. *Neuron, 78*(5), 855–868. doi: 10.1016/j.neuron.2013.04.006

Moore, J. K., & Moore, R. Y. (1971). A comparative study of the superior olivary complex in the primate brain. *Folia Primatologica (Basel), 16*(1), 35–51.

Morest, D. K. (1968). The collateral system of the medial nucleus of the trapezoid body of the cat, its neuronal architecture and relation to the olivo-cochlear bundle. *Brain Research, 9*(2), 288–311.

Muller, J., Reyes-Haro, D., Pivneva, T., Nolte, C., Schaette, R., Lubke, J., & Kettenmann, H. (2009). The principal neurons of the medial nucleus of the trapezoid body and NG2(+) glial cells receive coordinated excitatory synaptic input. *Journal of General Physiology, 134*(2), 115–127.

Nagy, B., Hovhannisyan, A., Barzan, R., Chen, T. J., & Kukley, M. (2017). Different patterns of neuronal activity trigger distinct responses of oligodendrocyte precursor cells in the corpus callosum. *PLoS Biology, 15*(8), e2001993.

Naraghi, M., & Neher, E. (1997). Linearized buffered Ca2+ diffusion in microdomains and its implications for calculation of [Ca2+] at the mouth of a calcium channel. *Journal of Neuroscience, 17*(18), 6961–6973.

Noh, J., Seal, R.P., Garver, J.A., Edwards, R.H., & Kandler, K. (2010). Glutamate co-release at GABA/glycinergic synapses is crucial for the refinement of an inhibitory map. *Nature Neuroscience, 13*(2), 232–238.

Parnavelas, J. G. (1999). Glial cell lineages in the rat cerebral cortex. *Experimental Neurology, 156*(2), 418–429.

Pierce, E. T. (1973). Time of origin of neurons in the brain stem of the mouse. *Progress in Brain Research, 40*(0), 53–65.

Renden, R., Taschenberger, H., Puente, N., Rusakov, D. A., Duvoisin, R., Wang, L. Y., . . . von Gersdorff, H. (2005). Glutamate transporter studies reveal the pruning of metabotropic glutamate receptors and absence of AMPA receptor desensitization at mature calyx of Held synapses. *Journal of Neuroscience, 25*(37), 8482–8497.

Renier, N., Schonewille, M., Giraudet, F., Badura, A., Tessier-Lavigne, M., Avan, P., . . . Chedotal, A. (2010). Genetic dissection of the function of hindbrain axonal commissures. *PLoS Biology, 8*(3), e1000325.

Reyes-Haro, D., Muller, J., Boresch, M., Pivneva, T., Benedetti, B., Scheller, A., . . . Kettenmann, H. (2010). Neuron-astrocyte interactions in the medial nucleus of the trapezoid body. *Journal of General Physiology, 135*(6), 583–594.

Richter, E. A., Norris, B. E., Fullerton, B. C., Levine, R. A., & Kiang, N. Y. (1983). Is there a medial nucleus of the trapezoid body in humans? *American Journal of Anatomy, 168*(2), 157–166.

Rodriguez-Contreras, A., van Hoeve, J. S., Habets, R. L., Locher, H., & Borst, J. G. (2008). Dynamic development of the calyx of Held synapse. *Proceedings of the National Academy of Sciences USA, 105*(14), 5603–5608.

Rosenberg, S. S., & Spitzer, N. C. (2011). Calcium signaling in neuronal development. [Review]. *Cold Spring Harbor Perspectives in Biology, 3*(10), a004259.

Roth, D. A., Muchnik, C., Shabtai, E., Hildesheimer, M., & Henkin, Y. (2012). Evidence for atypical auditory brainstem responses in young children with suspected autism spectrum disorders. *Developmental Medicine and Child Neurology*, *54*(1), 23–29.

Rotschafer, S. E., Marshak, S., & Cramer, K. S. (2015). Deletion of Fmr1 alters function and synaptic inputs in the auditory brainstem. *PLoS One*, *10*(2), e0117266.

Rowland, K. C., Irby, N. K., & Spirou, G. A. (2000). Specialized synapse-associated structures within the calyx of Held. *Journal of Neuroscience*, *20*(24), 9135–9144.

Ruby, K., Falvey, K., & Kulesza, R. J. (2015). Abnormal neuronal morphology and neurochemistry in the auditory brainstem of Fmr1 knockout rats. *Neuroscience*, *303*, 285–298.

Rusu, S. I., & Borst, J. G. (2011). Developmental changes in intrinsic excitability of principal neurons in the rat medial nucleus of the trapezoid body. *Developmental Neurobiology*, *71*(4), 284–295.

Saliu, A., Adise, S., Xian, S., Kudelska, K., & Rodriguez-Contreras, A. (2014). Natural and lesion-induced decrease in cell proliferation in the medial nucleus of the trapezoid body during hearing development. *Journal of Comparative Neurology*, *522*(5), 971–985.

Satzler, K., Sohl, L. F., Bollmann, J. H., Borst, J. G., Frotscher, M., Sakmann, B., & Lubke, J. H. (2002). Three-dimensional reconstruction of a calyx of Held and its postsynaptic principal neuron in the medial nucleus of the trapezoid body. *Journal of Neuroscience*, *22*(24), 10567–10579.

Schneggenburger, R., & Neher, E. (2000). Intracellular calcium dependence of transmitter release rates at a fast central synapse. *Nature*, *406*(6798), 889–893.

Schwaller, B. (2010). Cytosolic Ca2+ buffers. *Cold Spring Harbor Perspectives in Biology*, *2*(11), a004051.

Schwaller, B. (2014). Calretinin: from a "simple" Ca(2+) buffer to a multifunctional protein implicated in many biological processes. *Frontiers in Neuroanatomy*, *8*, 3.

Seidl, A. H., & Rubel, E. W. (2016). Systematic and differential myelination of axon collaterals in the mammalian auditory brainstem. *Glia*, *64*(4), 487–494.

Shatz, C. J. (1996). Emergence of order in visual system development. *Journal of Physiology Paris*, *90*(3–4), 141–150.

Shimoda, Y., & Watanabe, K. (2009). Contactins: Emerging key roles in the development and function of the nervous system. *Cell Adhesion and Migration*, *3*(1), 64–70.

Sierksma, M. C., & Borst, J. G. G. (2017). Resistance to action potential depression of a rat axon terminal in vivo. *Proceedings of the National Academy of Sciences USA*, *114*(16), 4249–4254.

Sierksma, M. C., Tedja, M. S., & Borst, J. G. (2017). In vivo matching of postsynaptic excitability with spontaneous synaptic inputs during formation of the rat calyx of Held synapse. *Journal of Physiology*, *595*(1), 207–231.

Sinclair, J. L., Fischl, M. J., Alexandrova, O., Hebeta, M., Grothe, B., Leibold, C., & Kopp-Scheinpflug, C. (2017). Sound-evoked activity influences myelination of brainstem axons in the trapezoid body. *Journal of Neuroscience*, *37*(34), 8239–8255.

Smith, P. H., Joris, P. X., Carney, L. H., & Yin, T. C. (1991). Projections of physiologically characterized globular bushy cell axons from the cochlear nucleus of the cat. *Journal of Comparative Neurology*, *304*(3), 387–407.

Sorg, B. A., Berretta, S., Blacktop, J. M., Fawcett, J. W., Kitagawa, H., Kwok, J. C., & Miquel, M. (2016). Casting a wide net: Role of perineuronal nets in neural plasticity. *Journal of Neuroscience*, *36*(45), 11459–11468.

Spirou, G. A., Brownell, W. E., & Zidanic, M. (1990). Recordings from cat trapezoid body and HRP labeling of globular bushy cell axons. *Journal of Neurophysiology*, *63*(5), 1169–1190.

Strumbos, J. G., Brown, M. R., Kronengold, J., Polley, D. B., & Kaczmarek, L. K. (2010). Fragile X mental retardation protein is required for rapid experience-dependent regulation of the potassium channel Kv3.1b. *Journal of Neuroscience*, *30*(31), 10263–10271.

Tapia, J. C., Wylie, J. D., Kasthuri, N., Hayworth, K. J., Schalek, R., Berger, D. R., . . . Lichtman, J. W. (2012). Pervasive synaptic branch removal in the mammalian neuromuscular system at birth. *Neuron*, *74*(5), 816–829.

Taschenberger, H., Leao, R. M., Rowland, K. C., Spirou, G. A., & von Gersdorff, H. (2002). Optimizing synaptic architecture and efficiency for high-frequency transmission. *Neuron*, *36*(6), 1127–1143.

Tolbert, L. P., Morest, D. K., & Yurgelun-Todd, D. A. (1982). The neuronal architecture of the anteroventral cochlear nucleus of the cat in the region of the cochlear nerve root: horseradish peroxidase labelling of identified cell types. *Neuroscience*, *7*(12), 3031–3052.

Toyoshima, M., Sakurai, K., Shimazaki, K., Takeda, Y., Shimoda, Y., & Watanabe, K. (2009). Deficiency of neural recognition molecule NB-2 affects the development of glutamatergic auditory pathways from the ventral cochlear nucleus to the superior olivary complex in mouse. *Developmental Biology*, *336*(2), 192–200.

Tritsch, N. X., & Bergles, D. E. (2010). Developmental regulation of spontaneous activity in the Mammalian cochlea. *Journal of Neuroscience*, *30*(4), 1539–1550.

Tritsch, N. X., Yi, E., Gale, J. E., Glowatzki, E., & Bergles, D. E. (2007). The origin of spontaneous activity in the developing auditory system. *Nature*, *450*(7166), 50–55.

Uwechue, N. M., Marx, M. C., Chevy, Q., & Billups, B. (2012). Activation of glutamate transport evokes rapid glutamine release from perisynaptic astrocytes. *Journal of Physiology*, *590*(10), 2317–2331.

Van Hartesveldt, C., Moore, B., & Hartman, B. K. (1986). Transient midline raphe glial structure in the developing rat. *Journal of Comparative Neurology*, *253*(2), 174–184.

van Noort, J. (1969). The anatomical basis for frequency analysis in the cochlear nuclear complex. *Psychiatria, Neurologia, Neurochirurgia*, *72*(1), 109–114.

von Gersdorff, H., & Borst, J. G. (2002). Short-term plasticity at the calyx of Held. *Nature Reviews: Neuroscience*, *3*(1), 53–64.

Vonhoff, F., & Keshishian, H. (2017). In vivo calcium signaling during synaptic refinement at the drosophila neuromuscular junction. *Journal of Neuroscience*, *37*(22), 5511–5526.

Walsh, M. K., & Lichtman, J. W. (2003). In vivo time-lapse imaging of synaptic takeover associated with naturally occurring synapse elimination. *Neuron*, *37*(1), 67–73.

Wang, D., & Fawcett, J. (2012). The perineuronal net and the control of CNS plasticity. [Review]. *Cell and Tissue Research*, *349*(1), 147–160.

Wang, L. Y., Neher, E., & Taschenberger, H. (2008). Synaptic vesicles in mature calyx of Held synapses sense higher nanodomain calcium concentrations during action potential-evoked glutamate release. *Journal of Neuroscience*, *28*(53), 14450–14458.

Warr, W. B. (1972). Fiber degeneration following lesions in the multipolar and globular cell areas in the ventral cochlear nucleus of the cat. *Brain Research*, *40*(2), 247–270.

Weatherstone, J. H., Kopp-Scheinpflug, C., Pilati, N., Wang, Y., Forsythe, I. D., Rubel, E. W., & Tempel, B. L. (2017). Maintenance of neuronal size gradient in MNTB requires sound-evoked activity. *Journal of Neurophysiology*, *117*(2), 756–766.

Wu, S. H., & Kelly, J. B. (1991). Physiological properties of neurons in the mouse superior olive: Membrane characteristics and postsynaptic responses studied in vitro. *Journal of Neurophysiology*, *65*(2), 230–246.

Xiao, L., Michalski, N., Kronander, E., Gjoni, E., Genoud, C., Knott, G., & Schneggenburger, R. (2013). BMP signaling specifies the development of a large and fast CNS synapse. *Nature Neuroscience, 16*(7), 856–864.

Xu-Friedman, M. A., & Regehr, W. G. (2003). Ultrastructural contributions to desensitization at cerebellar mossy fiber to granule cell synapses. *Journal of Neuroscience, 23*(6), 2182–2192.

Xu, J., Berret, E., & Kim, J. H. (2017). Activity-dependent formation and location of voltage-gated sodium channel clusters at a CNS nerve terminal during postnatal development. *Journal of Neurophysiology, 117*(2), 582–593.

Yang, Y. M., Fedchyshyn, M. J., Grande, G., Aitoubah, J., Tsang, C. W., Xie, H., . . . Wang, L. Y. (2010). Septins regulate developmental switching from microdomain to nanodomain coupling of Ca(2+) influx to neurotransmitter release at a central synapse. *Neuron, 67*(1), 100–115.

Yang, Y. M., Wang, W., Fedchyshyn, M. J., Zhou, Z., Ding, J., & Wang, L. Y. (2014). Enhancing the fidelity of neurotransmission by activity-dependent facilitation of presynaptic potassium currents. *Nature Communications, 5*, 4564.

Yin, T. C., & Chan, J. C. (1990). Interaural time sensitivity in medial superior olive of cat. *Journal of Neurophysiology, 64*(2), 465–488.

Youssoufian, M., Oleskevich, S., & Walmsley, B. (2005). Development of a robust central auditory synapse in congenital deafness. *Journal of Neurophysiology, 94*(5), 3168–3180.

Yuan, X., Eisen, A. M., McBain, C. J., & Gallo, V. (1998). A role for glutamate and its receptors in the regulation of oligodendrocyte development in cerebellar tissue slices. *Development, 125*(15), 2901–2914.

Zhang, Y., & Huang, H. (2017). SK channels regulate resting properties and signaling reliability of a developing fast-spiking neuron. *Journal of Neuroscience, 37*(44), 10738–10747.

CHAPTER 11

EXTRACTION OF AUDITORY INFORMATION BY MODULATION OF NEURONAL ION CHANNELS

LEONARD K. KACZMAREK

Abstract

All neurons express a subset of over seventy genes encoding potassium channel subunits. These channels have been studied in auditory neurons, particularly in the medial nucleus of the trapezoid body. The amplitude and kinetics of various channels in these neurons can be modified by the auditory environment. It has been suggested that such modulation is an adaptation of neuronal firing patterns to specific patterns of auditory inputs. Alternatively, such modulation may allow a group of neurons, all expressing the same set of channels, to represent a variety of responses to the same pattern of incoming stimuli. Such diversity would ensure that a small number of genetically identical neurons could capture and encode many aspects of complex sound, including rapid changes in timing and amplitude. This review covers the modulation of ion channels in the medial nucleus of the trapezoid body and how it may maximize the extraction of auditory information.

Keywords: potassium channel, MNTB, medial nucleus of the trapezoid body, ion channels, firing patterns, sound localization

Introduction

It has been known since the 1970s that the excitability of neurons is not fixed. Fundamental characteristics of a neuron, such as the height and width of its action potentials, firing rate and the absence or presence of adaptation to a maintained synaptic barrage, can be altered in response to synaptic or hormonal stimulation. Most commonly such changes are brought about by posttranslational modifications such as phosphorylation of ion channels in the plasma membrane, or by the acute insertion or removal of channels from the membrane. In many cases, particularly in well-studied invertebrate models, the biological significance of such modulation is apparent. For example, changes in potassium and calcium currents that alter transmitter release at sensory neurons underlie behavioral phenomena such as habituation and sensitization (Kandel & Schwartz, 1982). In other neurons, similar stimulation-induced changes in potassium, calcium and non-selective cation channels trigger a prolonged period of spontaneous firing that causes a series of reproductive behaviors lasting many hours (Conn & Kaczmarek, 1989).

The need for such modulation of ion channels in neurons of the central auditory system is, at first glance, less apparent. Many auditory neurons, particularly in brainstem nuclei, fire at rates of up to many hundreds of Hz and lock their action potentials to auditory events with microsecond precision (Joris, 1996; Joris & Yin, 1995; Kopp-Scheinpflug, Tolnai, Malmierca, & Rubsamen, 2008). Such high rates and temporal precision are required for the transmission of auditory information and for the detection of small differences in pitch and location of sounds. One might imagine that accurate detection of such nuances in sensory information would be best achieved by having neurons that are invariant in their response properties, and that modulation of ion channels over time could alter firing patterns and introduce errors that degrade the signal. It is known, however, that that many of the ion channels in auditory brainstem nuclei are regulated by second messenger pathways and that rapid changes in phosphorylation state, current amplitude, and rates of channel synthesis and transcription are produced by auditory stimulation.

This review will describe the modulation of several types of ion channels in auditory brainstem nuclei, particularly in the medial nucleus of the trapezoid body (MNTB), a nucleus that participates in circuits for the localization of sounds in space, and in which there have been many studies of channel modulation. Rather than focus on the mechanisms by which modulation occurs, which have been described in other reviews (Gan & Kaczmarek, 1998; Johnston, Forsythe, & Kopp-Scheinpflug, 2010; Kaczmarek, 2017; Kaczmarek et al., 2005; Schneggenburger & Forsythe, 2006; Taschenberger & von Gersdorff, 2000), the emphasis will be on the potential biological implication of such modulation and on the potential benefits for auditory processing of allowing individual neurons to take on a variety of electrophysiological personalities.

The MNTB and Binaural Processing

Figure 11.1 shows a schematic diagram of auditory brainstem circuits that underlie the detection of interaural differences in timing and levels of incoming sounds. Bushy cells in anterior cochlear nucleus receive inputs from the ipsilateral cochlea. Information from these cells is communicated to the medial and lateral olivary nuclei (MSO and

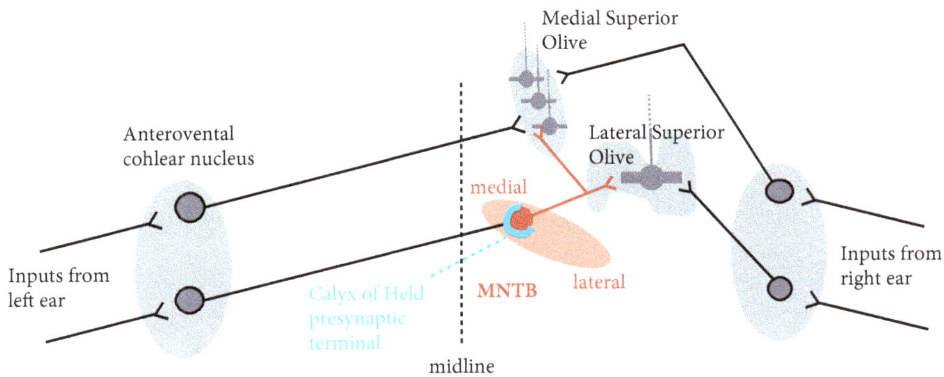

FIGURE 11.1. A schematic diagram of auditory brainstem circuits that underlie the detection of interaural differences in timing and levels of incoming sounds

LSO) where inputs from the two ears are compared directly. An intermediate nucleus in this network is the MNTB. The glycinergic neurons in this nucleus receive strong excitatory input from the bushy cells and relay this in the form of inhibition to both the MSO and LSO. These inhibitory inputs are required for the determination of differences in both the level and timing of sounds received by the two ears (Grothe, 2003).

The synaptic drive from the bushy cells to the principal neurons of the MNTB is provided by the very large calyx of Held presynaptic terminals (Schneggenburger & Forsythe, 2006). These provide very secure and very precisely timed excitation at the somata of the MNTB neurons, allowing MNTB neurons to lock their action potentials to the phase of sound stimuli of frequencies up to 2000 Hz or more, and also to the envelope of higher-frequency sounds that are amplitude-modulated at frequencies up to ~2000 Hz (Joris, 1996; Joris & Yin, 1995). The firing rate of MNTB neurons, however, is dependent on the amplitude, as well as the frequency, of incoming sounds. Even in silence, MNTB neurons are driven to fire at rates from 10 to >200 Hz by the level of spontaneous transmitter release from hair cells that occurs even in the absence of auditory stimulation (Kopp-Scheinpflug et al., 2008). As the amplitude of sounds is increased, the firing rate of MNTB neurons can be pushed to over 800 Hz. Thus these neurons respond to changes in the timing and amplitude of auditory stimuli.

Potassium Channels Operate in Different Voltage Ranges

While the excitability of all neurons is determined by several types of ion channels, including those selective for sodium, calcium and chloride, as well as by non-selective cation channels, the greatest diversity is provided by potassium channels. There are over seventy different genes that encode subunits of K^+ channels, and many of these can combine to form heteromeric channels. This, coupled with the existence of different channel isoforms produced by alternative splicing, provides an immeasurable number of potential different K^+ channels. Figure 11.2B lists the potassium channel subunits that are currently known and categorizes them by the mechanism for their activation. Also indicated are the subset of potassium channels that have been localized in the MNTB. These are marked in bold and color. The general properties of these channels will be described in a later section.

One way that K^+ channels differ from each other is in the range of voltages in which they operate (Figure 11.2A). Some K^+ channels are already open near the resting potential of a neuron (~−65 mV for an MNTB neuron). These include leak channels that are open at all voltages, and so-called low-threshold or low-voltage activated channels that are open close to the resting potential and that increase their open probability with small depolarizations from rest (Figure 11.2A). In contrast, high-threshold voltage-dependent K^+ channels typically open only when the membrane potential becomes more positive than about −15 mV. Under physiological conditions, such positive membrane potentials are only encountered during an action potential, and the primary role of these channels is to provide rapid repolarization of action potentials. Although, strictly speaking, the activation of a channel has no fixed threshold, the terms *low threshold* and *high threshold* are useful in that they refer to potentials at which measurable currents can first be detected in voltage clamp experiments.

Altering Potassium Channels Alters the Type of Information Extracted from Synaptic Inputs

Before describing the types of channels in MNTB neurons in more detail, we will discuss how differences in the voltage-dependence of K^+ currents influence firing patterns using a simple computational model. Figure 11.3 shows the response of model neurons to trains of synaptic inputs. The voltage-dependent K^+ current in the model in Figure 11.3A is a high-threshold current that provides very rapid repolarization of action potentials. As the amplitude of the synaptic currents applied to these neurons is increased, the rate of firing of the neurons increases. The timing of most of the action potentials during the synaptic depolarization is independent of the precise timing of the synaptic inputs. As a result, such a neuron provides a code in which the firing rate of the neurons encodes the amplitude of the synaptic stimulus train.

In Figure 11.3B, the total level of potassium conductance in the model neuron is the same as that in Figure 11.3A, and the other parameters are identical. The voltage-dependence of the potassium current has, however, been altered so that it now activates

(A)

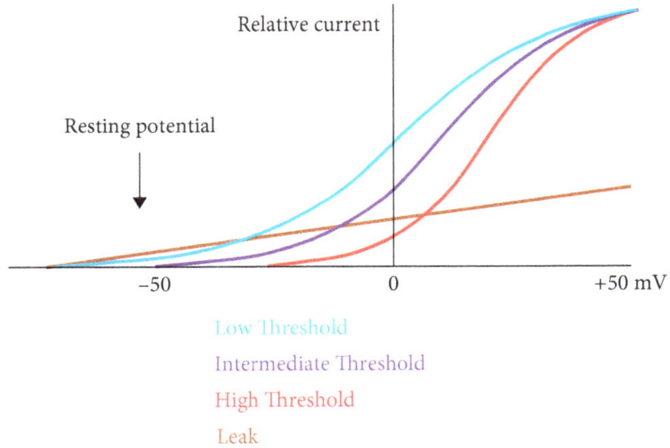

(B)

Voltage-dependent K⁺ channel subunits

Kv1.1, 1.2, 1.3, 1.4, 1.5, 1.6, 1.7, 1.8
Kv2.1, 2.2
Kv3.1, 3.2, 3.3, 3.4
Kv4.1, 4.2, 4.3
Kv5.1
Kv6.1, 6.2, 6.3, 6.4
Kv7.1 (LQT1), 7.2, 7.3, 7.4, 7.5
Kv8.1, 8.2
Kv9.1, 9.2, 9.3
Kv10.1, 10.2
Kv11.1, 11.2, 11.3 (HERG)
Kv12.1, 12.2, 12.3

Low Threshold
Intermediate Threshold
High Threshold
A-current
Leak

Ca^{2+}-dependent K⁺ channel subunits

KCa1.1 (Slo)
KCa2.1 (SK1)
KCa2.2 (SK2)
KCa2.3 (SK3)
KCa3.1 (SK4)

Na^+-dependent K⁺ channel subunits

KNa1.1 (Slack)
KNa1.2 (Slick)

Inward rectifier K⁺ subunits

Kir1.1
Kir2.1, 2.2, 2.3, 2.4
Kir3.1, 3.2, 3.3, 3.4
Kir4.1, 4.2
Kir5.1
Kir6.1, 6.2
Kir7.1

Two pore domain K⁺ channel subunits

K2P1.1
K2P2.1
K2P3.1
K2P4.1
K2P5.1
K2P6.1
K2P7.1
K2P9.1
K2P10.1
K2P12.1
K2P13.1
K2P15.1
K2P16.1
K2P17.1
K2P18.1

FIGURE 11.2. K^+ channels differ from each other in the range of voltages in which they operate. A. Schematic diagram illustrating the range of voltages at which low-, intermediate-, and high-threshold and leak K^+ channels activate. B. A list of known K^+ channel genes. Those marked in color have been found to be expressed in the MNTB.

at more negative potentials, close to the resting membrane potential. This has the effect of decreasing the membrane time constant and increasing the threshold for triggering an action potential. A train of synaptic stimuli similar to that in Figure 11.3A now evokes a very different response. Once the threshold for triggering an action potential is reached, each synaptic potential within the train triggers only a single action potential, and this is now independent of the amplitude of the stimulus (Figure 11.3B). Such a neuron therefore encodes only the timing, but not the amplitude of the synaptic stimulus.

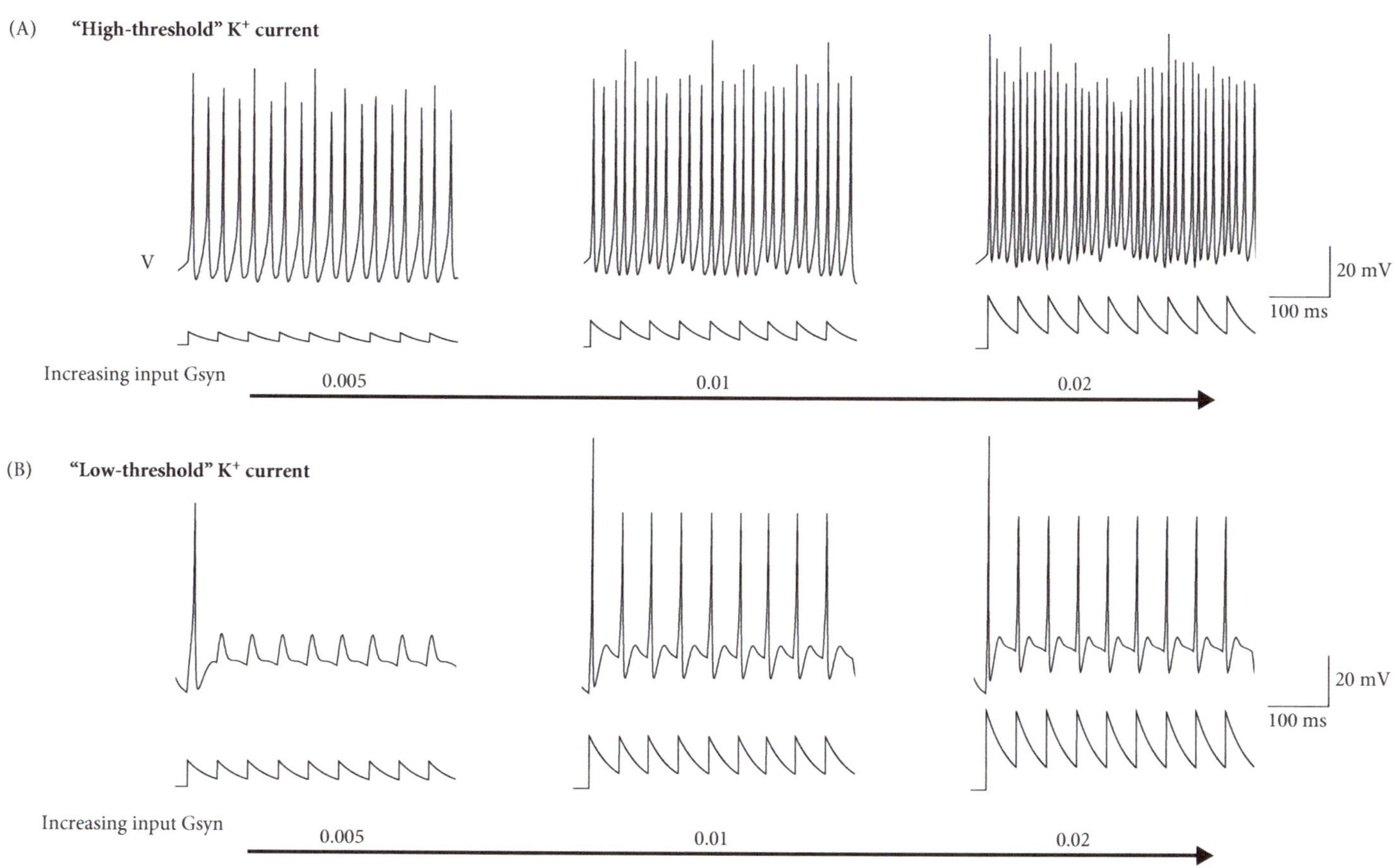

FIGURE 11.3. Computed responses of model neurons to trains of synaptic inputs. A. Neurons with only a high-threshold K^+ current respond to changes in the amplitude of the stimulus. B. Neurons with only a low-threshold K^+ current lock their action potentials faithfully to the onset of all suprathreshold synaptic inputs (Chambers et al., 2017).

Firing patterns such as those in Figure 11.3 have been extensively characterized in auditory brainstem nuclei. For example, stellate cells of the ventral cochlear nucleus have firing patterns similar to those of Figure 11.3A, and these are sometimes termed chopper patterns (Oertel, Wright, Cao, Ferragamo, & Bal, 2011), while bushy cells in the anteroventral cochlear nucleus, as well as the principal neurons of the MNTB phase-lock their action potentials to sound stimuli and have firing pattern that more closely resemble those of Figure 11.3B (Manis & Marx, 1991; Trussell, 1999).

In contrast to the simple model of Figure 11.3, all neurons express the genes for more than one type of potassium channel. The vast majority of neurons, including those that primarily encode amplitude or timing information, have multiple components of potassium currents that activate at both positive and negative potentials. The ratios of such components, however, differ in the different cell types such that each neuron in an auditory nucleus expresses a slightly different blend of channels. The most common distribution, and one that is found for many of the channels in Figure 11.2B, is a tonotopic gradient along the tonotopic axis. As one example, the high-threshold Kv3.1 potassium channel is expressed at highest levels at the medial, high frequency aspect of the MNTB and other auditory nuclei (Brew & Forsythe, 2005; Li, Kaczmarek, & Perney, 2001; Figure 11.4). In contrast, as will be described later, some channels are expressed in a gradient in the opposite direction, with highest levels in the lateral, low-frequency part of the MNTB. Note from Figure 11.4 that, although the existence of the tonotopic gradient is obvious, it is not a smooth gradient, and that some cells with low levels of Kv3.1 can be found at the medial end, while a few neurons in the lateral region also appear to have a high level of Kv3.1.

How Does Diversity of Ion Channel Expression Arise?

How do gradients, in which neighboring neurons express slightly different levels of potassium channels from their immediate neighbors, come about? The topographic organization of axons and synaptic connections from the cochlea through to all auditory brainstem nuclei is already present very early in development. At least in part, this may arise from the action of growth factors and other morphogens such as ephrins, which that may be secreted preferentially from cells beyond the medial or lateral aspects of the nucleus (Cramer, 2005; Cramer & Miko, 2016). The connections are then refined before the onset of hearing by patterns of spontaneous activity that are generated in cochlear hair cells and then propagated to brainstem nuclei (Clause et al., 2014; Kandler, Clause, & Noh, 2009).

At least some of the same factors that contribute to the topographic pattern of connectivity may also influence the levels of potassium channels in brainstem neurons. Nevertheless, the existence of gradients in potassium channels depends on ongoing

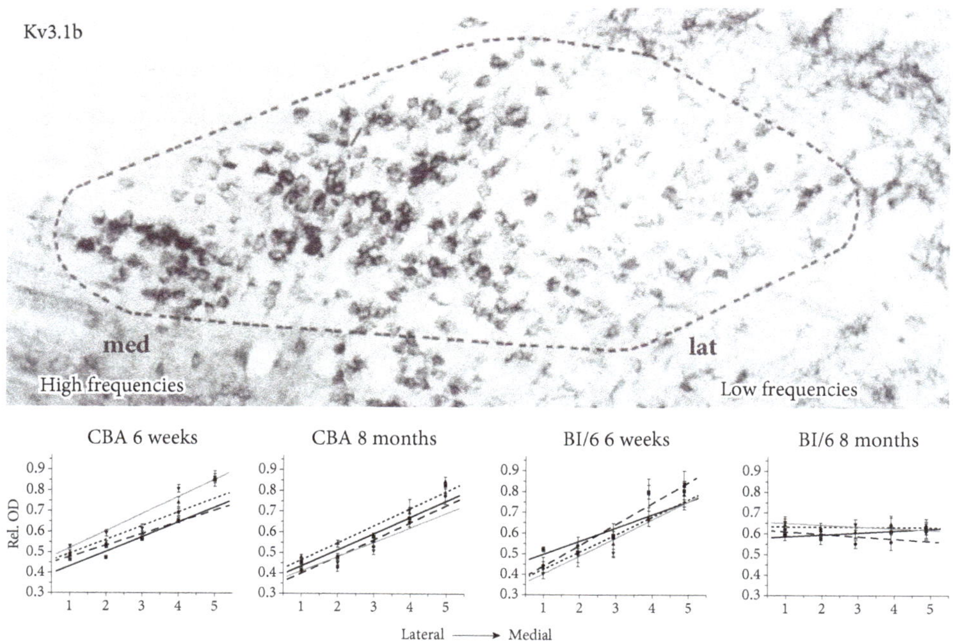

FIGURE 11.4. Gradient of immunostaining for the Kv3.1b K+ channel subunit along the tonotopic axis of the MNTB (Li et al., 2001). Graphs at bottom show quantification of this gradient for young (6 weeks) and old (8 months) mice of CBA and Bl/6 mice. Bl/6 mice have normal hearing at 6 weeks but are hearing impaired at 8 months, while CBA mice maintain normal hearing over this time span (von Hehn et al., 2004).

neuronal activity, even in adults. For example, strains of mice that have normal hearing throughout their lifespan maintain normal tonotopic gradients of Kv3.1, whereas those that undergo hearing loss with age progressively lose this gradient (Figure 11.4; von Hehn, Bhattacharjee, & Kaczmarek, 2004). Gradients of channel expression and activity are absent in congenitally deaf mice (Leao et al., 2006).

It is well established that gradients, as well as more complex spatiotemporal patterns, can be generated in an ensemble of originally identical cells, provided the individual cells interact with their neighbors to influence the synthesis of components in nearby cells (Nicolis & Prigogine, 1977). A change in the level of a component in one unit, brought about by a transient external stimulus, results in the self-organization of the entire group of cells into a gradient or other spatiotemporal pattern. The hypothesis advanced in this article is that such interactions between nearby neurons in auditory nuclei such as the MNTB result in the establishment of tonotopic gradients in potassium channels and other components. Specifically, an elevation in levels of one type of potassium channel subunit in a neuron produces a decrease in expression of the same subunit in neighboring neurons. This alone could be responsible for establishing a gradient.

The consequences of such "lateral inhibition" of channel expression go beyond simply establishing a gradient. They may enhance the amount of information propagated through the nucleus. Take the simple hypothetical example of two identical neurons both of which are exposed to the same complex stimulus pattern (Figure 11.5). If the potassium conductance of these neurons is dominated by high-threshold

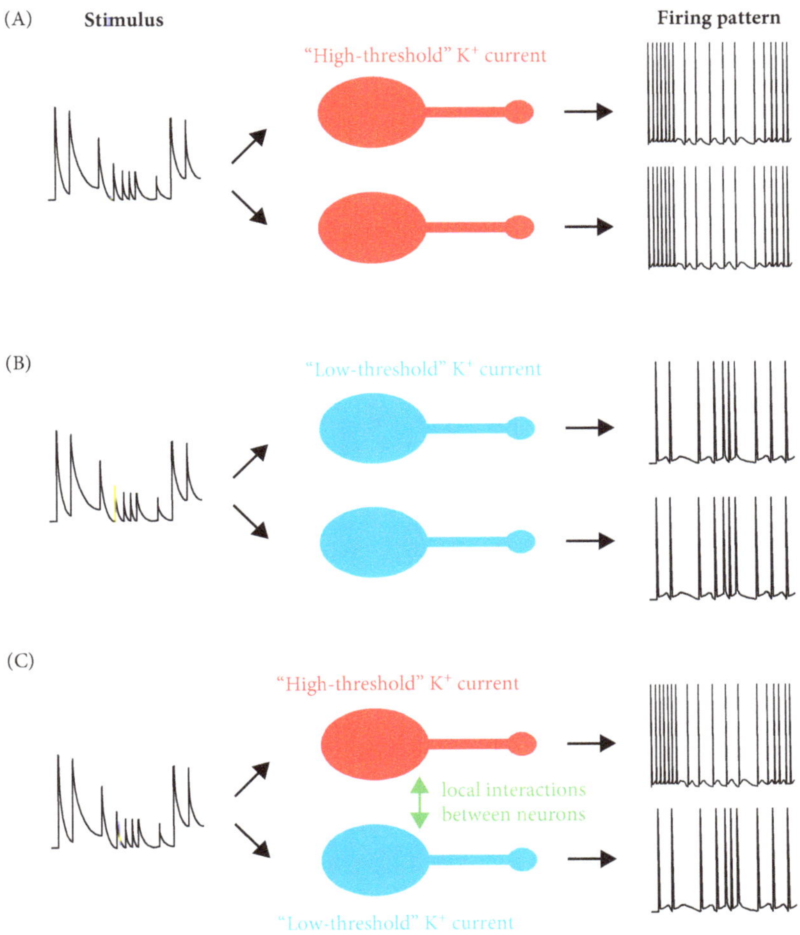

FIGURE 11.5. Diagram illustrating the hypothesis that lateral interactions that produce diversity in K^+ channels in neighboring cells increase the amount of information transmitted through an auditory nucleus. A. If the K^+ conductance of two neurons is uniform and composed of high-threshold channels, both neurons fire with an identical pattern that reflects changes in stimulus amplitude. B. If the K^+ conductance is uniform and dominated low-threshold channels, the two neurons fire action potentials that are phase-locked to the onset of synaptic depolarizations. C. If interactions between the two neurons lead to high-threshold currents in one of the neurons and low-threshold currents in the other, the output of the two-neuron ensemble includes both amplitude and timing information.

currents, such as those of Kv3 family channels, the action potentials will reflect primarily changes in stimulus amplitude (Figure 11.5A). Conversely, if the potassium conductance of these neurons is dominated by low-threshold currents, such as those of Kv1 family channels, the neurons will fire with action potentials that are phase-locked to the onset of transients in the stimulus (Figure 11.5B). In this case, the output of the neurons will contain little information about changes in signal amplitude during the stimulus. If, however, the two neurons interact laterally, a stimulation-induced increase in high-threshold current in one neurons could trigger a decrease in the same current in its neighbor. Assuming there exist mechanisms to maintain total levels of potassium current constant, these interactions will result in a two-neuron "gradient" with one neuron faithfully tracking timing information and the second monitoring stimulus amplitude (Figure 11.5C). This will, of course, greatly increase the amount of information being transmitted over what is possible with identical neurons.

Diversity of K^+ Conductance Enhances Throughput of Information in a Network

The hypothetical model in Figure 11.5 is clearly an extreme example, and it is perhaps unlikely that two neighboring neurons would come to encode such different aspect of a stimulus. Whatever the mechanism for generating diversity, however, even small differences in the intrinsic excitability of different neurons in a network can dramatically enhance the ability of that network to extract the maximal information about the amplitude and timing of its synaptic inputs. This can readily be demonstrated in numerical computations of MNTB-like neurons. Figure 11.6 shows the response of each neuron in an ensemble of 50 neurons to stimulation at 700 Hz (Kaczmarek, 2012). The firing pattern of each neuron is shown as a raster plot under the stimuli. The neuronal units in this ensemble are unable to follow 700 Hz but respond to the stimulus with a lower rate of firing. Also shown in the figure is a color-coded adjusted phase vector strength, which is calculated by determining the accuracy with which individual units are locked in time to the stimuli, as well as the degree of entrainment to the stimulus train (Kaczmarek, 2012). This is calculated for individual units (convergence of units =1) as well as the output of the entire network (convergence of inputs = 50). When all units are identical, there is no additional information in the output of the ensemble over that in a single cell, and the adjusted phase vector strength is the same for single neurons and the entire network (Figure 11.6, *top*). Introducing diversity in the levels of a high-threshold K^+ current substantially increases the information encoded in the output of the ensemble over that in individual neurons (Figure 11.6, *center*).

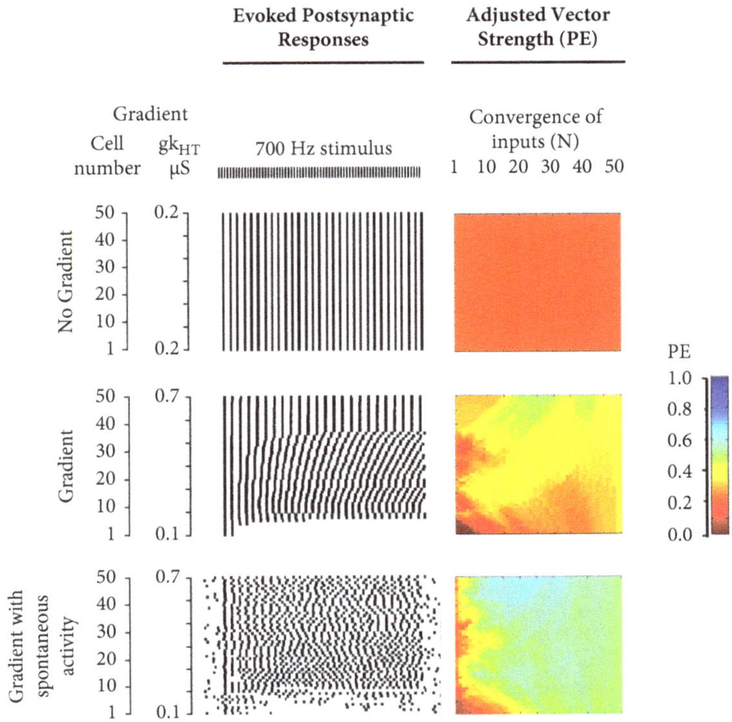

FIGURE 11.6. Gradients and diversity in amplitude of a high-threshold K^+ channel enhance information output in an ensemble of 50 model MNTB neurons. Left panels show raster plots for the timing of the peaks of postsynaptic output of 50 individual neurons receiving an identical 700 Hz stimulus. Each peak that follows a stimulus pulse is represented as a short vertical line, and these are aligned vertically for the 50 neurons in a linear ensemble. Right panels show a color-coded representation of a parameter PE that quantifies both the accuracy of phase-locking and entrainment to the stimulus (Kaczmarek, 2012). This is shown for linear combinations of the output from 1 to 50 of the neurons in the ensemble. Top panels show results for an ensemble with no channel gradient. Center panels show results for a gradient in high-threshold K^+ current. Lower panels show the effect of increasing diversity in response by introducing random spontaneous activity in the stimulus.

Counterintuitively, introducing even more diversity by simply allowing spontaneous random firing of the input results in an even further increase in overall accuracy of the output of the ensemble (Figure 11.6, *bottom*). This is because the spontaneous activity alters the intrinsic excitability of different units at the time of arrival of phase-locked information in the inputs.

Even though random spontaneous perturbations improve the accuracy of an ensemble, this does not mean that randomizing the expression of levels of ion channel subunits is a useful strategy for optimal accuracy. Computations similar to those in figure 6 have demonstrated that maximal information can be propagated through the ensemble if the levels of conductance in different neurons can specifically be adjusted to the pattern of synaptic inputs (Kaczmarek, 2012). As with the hypothetical case shown in Figure 11.5, if such adjustments are made in real auditory nuclei such as the MNTB, they are likely to involve lateral interactions between individual neurons.

Types of Potassium Channels in the MNTB

This section will provide more molecular details of the types of potassium channels expressed in MNTB neurons.

Low-Threshold Potassium Channels

The Kv1 subfamily of potassium channel subunits are the prototypical low-threshold channels. At least four members of this group (Kv1.1, Kv1.2, Kv1.3. and Kv1.6) have been found within the MNTB (Brew & Forsythe, 1995; Brew, Hallows, & Tempel, 2003; Dodson, Barker, & Forsythe, 2002; Dodson et al., 2003; Gazula et al., 2010; Grigg, Brew, & Tempel, 2000; Johnston et al., 2010; Kopp-Scheinpflug, Fuchs, Lippe, Tempel, & Rubsamen, 2003). The voltage-dependence of these is such that they open at or near the resting potential of MNTB neurons and are strongly activated by small depolarizations from rest. In principal neurons of the MNTB, this has the effect of limiting firing to a single action potential at the onset of an excitatory synaptic input or of a sustained depolarization. The opening of Kv1 channels near the resting potential also provides neurons with a short membrane time constant. These features provide neurons with the ability to lock their action potentials to incoming stimuli with high temporal accuracy. This role for low-threshold potassium currents was first described in bushy cells of the cochlear nucleus (Manis & Marx, 1991).

The different Kv1 family subunits are localized in different compartments of the MNTB. Kv1.1/Kv1.2 heteromeric channels are localized to the initial segment of the axon of postsynaptic neurons, but are absent from the presynaptic calyx of Held terminal and from the postsynaptic cell bodies of MNTB neurons (Dodson et al., 2002). Kv1.2 homomers as well as Kv1.1/1.2 heteromers exist on presynaptic axons coming from the cochlear nucleus, but are absent from the membrane of the presynaptic terminal itself (Dodson et al., 2003). In contrast Kv1.3 channels are found selectively in the plasma membrane of the presynaptic terminal and on intracellular vesicles within the terminal (Gazula et al., 2010).

Low-threshold K^+ currents and Kv1 family channel subunits have been found to be expressed along a tonotopic gradient in the MNTB and in other auditory nuclei in different species (Adamson, Reid, Mo, Bowne-English, & Davis, 2002; Barnes-Davies, Barker, Osmani, & Forsythe, 2004; Brew & Forsythe, 2005; Fukui & Ohmori, 2004; Gazula et al., 2010; Leao et al., 2006; Walmsley, Berntson, Leao, & Fyffe, 2006). In the MNTB, Kv1.1 and Kv1.3 have been found to be expressed at highest levels in lateral low-frequency neurons (Gazula et al., 2010; Leao et al., 2006). As with the Kv3.1b channel, levels of low-threshold K^+ currents are reduced and corresponding tonotopic gradients are abolished in deaf animals (Leao, Berntson, Forsythe, & Walmsley, 2004; Leao et al., 2006).

Two other subunits of the voltage-dependent channel family, Kv11.1 and Kv11.3 (ERG1 and ERG3), also contribute to the low-threshold currents that activate near rest in MNTB neurons of mice, but not of rats (Hardman & Forsythe, 2009). In addition, Na^+-activated K^+ channel subunits, $K_{Na}1.1$ and $K_{Na}1.2$ (Slack and Slick), are expressed in MNTB neurons (Bhattacharjee, Gan, & Kaczmarek, 2002; Bhattacharjee, von Hehn, Mei, & Kaczmarek, 2005). Like Kv1 and Kv11 subfamily channels, these channels open near the resting potential, and their activity is further increased by elevations of cytoplasmic Na^+ levels (Kaczmarek, 2013; Kaczmarek et al., 2017). Pharmacological activation of these channels increases the temporal accuracy of firing of firing of MNTB neurons in brainstem slices (Yang, Desai, & Kaczmarek, 2007).

Despite our knowledge about the types of low-threshold channels in the MNTB, there is little information about what regulates the levels of these channels. It is also not known if rapid changes in current amplitude are produced by stimulation of synaptic inputs. In particular, the molecular mechanisms that regulate the expression or modulation of Kv1 family channels in MNTB neurons are not yet well understood. As in other neurons, the activity of K_{Na} channels is expected to be increased by Na^+ entry during high frequency activity, and these channels are potently regulated by protein kinase C activation (Barcia et al., 2012; Santi et al., 2006). The role of their phosphorylation in MNTB neurons has not yet been investigated.

Leak K^+ Channels

A leak conductance is defined as one that has no time dependence and little or no voltage dependence. Technically, therefore, a leak conductance would be open at rest and contribute to setting the resting potential, the time constant and the threshold for action potential generation. Such a leak K^+ conductance, which is typically produced by members of the two pore domain K_{2P} channel family, has been characterized in MNTB neurons (Berntson & Walmsley, 2008). Messenger RNA for $K_{2P}1.1$ (also known as TWIK) is strongly expressed in MNTB neurons (Kaczmarek et al., 2005), and the leak current in these currents is generally consistent with the properties of $K_{2P}1.1$ currents (Berntson & Walmsley, 2008). As for the low-threshold channels, there have been no studies of mechanisms that determine expression levels of leak channels in the MNTB.

"Intermediate Threshold" Potassium Channels

The Kv2.2 potassium channel is expressed in a tonotopic gradient in the MNTB, with highest levels found at the axon hillock of neurons within the medial, high frequency end of the nucleus (Johnston, Griffin, Baker, Skrzypiec et al., 2008; Tong et al., 2013). Unlike the channels listed in the preceding two sections, Kv2.2 channels are not open at typical resting potentials (~ –65 mV) but begin to activate with depolarizations to ~ –40 mV and are half-activated by ~ –10 mV. Their activation with voltage is relatively slow. As a result, they do not contribute significantly to the onset or shape of a single evoked action potential, but contribute to the hyperpolarization between action potentials during repetitive firing (Johnston, Griffin, Baker, Skrzypiec et al., 2008; Tong et al., 2013). Elimination of Kv2.2 currents reduces the number of action potentials that can be evoked during trains of high frequency stimuli.

Levels of Kv2.2 currents in MNTB neurons do not remain constant over time. Spontaneous neurotransmitter release from cochlear hair cells in vivo drives the synaptic input to MNTB neurons at rates of 10 Hz up to 150 Hz or more even in the absence of auditory stimulation (Brownell, 1975; Kopp-Scheinpflug, Lippe, Dorrscheidt, & Rubsamen, 2003). In MNTB neurons within brain slices, the amplitude of Kv2.2 currents in MNTB neurons is increased by prolonged stimulation of synaptic inputs at such low rates (~10 Hz for 1 hour; Steinert et al., 2011). Such low-frequency stimulation is therefore likely be represent the default situation in quiet environments, suggesting Kv2.2 channels contribute to repolarization in this situation. The increase in Kv2.2 currents is produced by the release of the volume transmitter nitric oxide (NO) during low frequency stimulation (to be discussed further) and the activity of both the cyclic GMP-dependent protein kinase and protein kinase C (Steinert et al., 2011).

High-Threshold Potassium Channels

The Kv3 family of K^+ subunits is required for many neurons in the nervous system to fire at high rates (Kaczmarek & Zhang, 2017). This family also regulates the repolarization of action potentials in many presynaptic terminals, controlling the amount of neurotransmitter release during the action potential. The canonical high-threshold K^+ channel in the MNTB is Kv3.1b, which is expressed in the soma of the postsynaptic principal MNTB neurons as well as in the calyx of Held presynaptic terminals (Figure 11.4; Elezgarai et al., 2003; Li et al., 2001; Macica & Kaczmarek, 2001; Song et al., 2005). Under normal conditions, Kv3.1b channels do not begin to activate until the membrane potential reaches about –15 to –10 mV and half-maximal activation occurs at ~ +15 mV (Brown et al., 2016; Luneau et al., 1991). Kv3.3 channels have properties similar to those of Kv3.1 (Kaczmarek & Zhang, 2017), but are localized primarily to the membrane of the presynaptic terminals (Zhang et al., 2016). Elimination of Kv3 currents by pharmacological agents or deletion of the Kv3.1 gene impairs the ability of MNTB neurons to follow stimulation at rates greater than 200 Hz (Macica et al., 2003; Wang, Gan, Forsythe, & Kaczmarek, 1998)

Both the activity and synthesis of Kv3.1b channels are altered in response to changes in the auditory environment. One mechanism that can rapidly alter Kv3.1b currents is changes in its phosphorylation state. In rats, serine residue 503 in the cytoplasmic C-terminus of the channel can be phosphorylated by PKC, which produces a partial suppression of high-threshold current (Kanemasa, Gan, Perney, Wang, & Kaczmarek, 1995; Macica et al., 2003; Song & Kaczmarek, 2006). In vivo, in a quiet environment, the serine 503 site is basally phosphorylated, but physiological increases in sound levels for only five minutes or less activate a phosphatase that rapidly dephosphorylates the channel (Figure 11.7A; Song et al., 2005). Similar dephosphorylation of Kv3.1b occurs in brain slices of the MNTB in response to stimulation of the presynaptic input at 600 Hz, increasing Kv3.1b current and allowing neurons to maintain firing at high rates of stimulation (Song et al., 2005). Conversely, stimulation at much lower frequencies (10–100 Hz) for up to an hour suppresses Kv3.1 currents, an effect that is mediated by synthesis and release of NO and resultant changes in phosphorylation, although direct links to the serine 503 site have not been established (Steinert et al., 2008; Steinert et al., 2011).

In intact animals, auditory stimulation similar to that which causes dephosphorylation of Kv3.1b, but for a slightly longer time (30 minutes or more), produces increases in levels of Kv3.1b protein in both mice and rats (Figure 11.7B; Leão et al., 2010; Strumbos, Brown, Kronengold, Polley, & Kaczmarek, 2010; Strumbos, Polley, & Kaczmarek, 2010). This produces a further increase in high-threshold K^+ current and increased repolarization of action potentials (Leão et al., 2010). The greatest increases occur in neurons along the tonotopic axis corresponding to the frequency of the auditory stimulus (Figure 11.7C; Strumbos, Polley et al., 2010). Interestingly, levels of Kv3.1b in neurons in regions of the MNTB not expected to be activated by the sound stimulus appear to decrease (Strumbos, Polley et al., 2010), a finding consistent with some form of lateral inhibition of channel synthesis across the nucleus.

The mechanism by which auditory stimulation increases levels of Kv3.1b protein involves the regulation of translation of mRNA by the Fragile X Mental Retardation Protein FMRP, an RNA-binding protein that directly binds Kv3.1b mRNA (Darnell et al., 2001; Strumbos, Brown et al., 2010). In mice lacking FMRP, auditory stimulation fails to produce any increase in level of the channel, and the normal tonotopic gradient of Kv3.1 protein in the MNTB is absent (Strumbos, Brown et al., 2010).

Finally, long-term changes in the production of Kv3.1b channels in the MNTB and other nuclei are regulated by alterations in the rate of transcription of the *Kv3.1* gene. As will be described later, the transcription of Kv3.1, and likely of other channels such as Kv3.3, is regulated by the transcription factor CREB (cAMP response element-binding protein; Gan & Kaczmarek, 1998; Gan, Perney, & Kaczmarek, 1996; Tong et al., 2010).

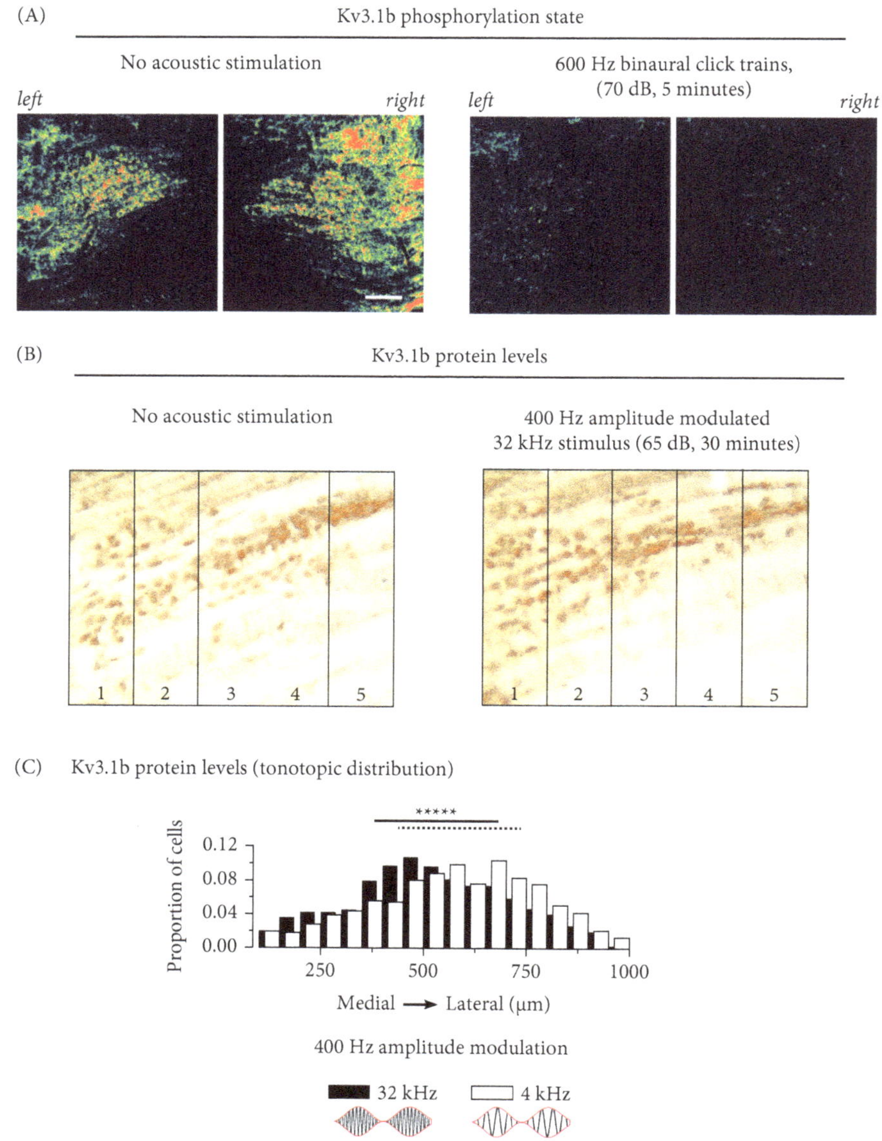

FIGURE 11.7. Acoustic stimulation alters the phosphorylation state and synthesis of Kv3.1b channels in the MNTB. A. Pseudocolor images of levels of Kv3.1b phosphorylation state by immunostaining using an anti-phosphoserine-503-specific antibody (red = high phosphorylation, blue = low phosphorylation. Five minutes of physiological sound stimulation greatly reduces phosphorylation, increasing Kv3.1 current (Song et al., 2005). B. Immunostaining for total levels of Kv3.1b in the MNTB of mice. Levels of the channel are increased by exposure of mice to a physiological stimulus that drives neurons at 400 Hz compared to those in mice maintained in a soundproof room for the same duration (Strumbos, Brown et al., 2010). C. Differences in the distribution of levels of Kv3.1b along the tonotopic axis of the MNTB of rats exposed for 30 minutes to a 32 kHz sound stimulus versus a 4 kHz stimulus. Both stimuli were amplitude modulated at 400 Hz (Strumbos, Polley et al., 2010).

Transient A-Type Potassium Channels

Once activated by depolarization, a subset of voltage-dependent K^+ channels rapidly inactivate if the depolarization is maintained. The currents of such channels are termed A-currents (Connor & Stevens, 1971b). In addition to contributing to the repolarization of action potentials, A-currents have two major functions: (1) regulating the rate of repetitive firing and (2) introducing a delay between the time that a neuron receives an excitatory stimulus and the onset on firing (Byrne, 1980; Connor & Stevens, 1971a; Strong & Kaczmarek, 1986). Because timing delays play a key role in the discrimination of interaural timing and level differences (Brand, Behrend, Marquardt, McAlpine, & Grothe, 2002; Grothe, 2003), A-currents could potentially play an important role in the processing of information through the MNTB. Currents corresponding to the Kv4.3 A-type K^+ channel subunit, as well as Kv4.3 immunoreactivity have been found in MNTB neurons of mice but not rats (Johnston, Griffin, Baker, & Forsythe, 2008). Numerical simulations suggest that this current may influence the response of the neurons to small excitatory inputs such as those from non-calyceal inputs (Johnston, Griffin, Baker, & Forsythe, 2008), but the precise role of these channels, and whether they undergo regulation in MNTB neurons is not known.

Immunoreactivity for another A-type channel, Kv3.4, is present in the calyx of Held presynaptic terminals (Ishikawa et al., 2003). This high-threshold K^+ channel subunit typically inactivates rapidly (within 10–15 msec) at positive potentials, a process that is regulated by PKC phosphorylation of residues in the cytoplasmic N-terminal domain (Beck, Sorensen, Slater, & Covarrubias, 1998; Covarrubias, Wei, Salkoff, & Vyas, 1994). As with Kv4.3, the modulation and physiological significance of Kv3.4 channels in the presynaptic terminals is not yet understood. No gradients in either A-type currents or in Kv3.4 immunoreactivity has been found along the medio-lateral axis of the MNTB (Leao et al., 2006). It is possible that Kv3.4 subunits play a role in development and the establishment of synaptic contacts, because they are expressed abundantly in most fiber tracts and their growth cones during pathfinding (Huang, Chu, Hwang, & Tsaur, 2012).

Evidence for Lateral Interactions among MNTB Neurons

Volume Transmitter Signaling Through Nitric Oxide

Direct evidence that a signal can spread laterally within the MNTB has been obtained by Steinert, Forsythe and their colleagues (Steinert et al., 2008; Steinert et al., 2011). Stimulation of the presynaptic input at a relatively low rate (100 Hz, for ~ 60 sec, or 10 Hz for 1 hour, comparable to spontaneous in vivo rates of firing in the absence of sound stimuli) causes an increase in levels of NO and cyclic GMP in the principal

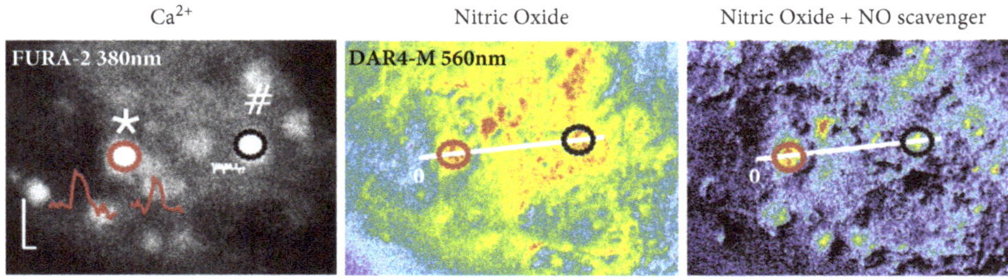

FIGURE 11.8. Spread of nitric oxide through the MNTB during synaptic stimulation of brainstem slices. Left image shows images of cellular calcium levels and transients detected using the calcium indicator Fura-2 after a train of 100 Hz stimuli. Only the neuron marked with a red circle received a direct synaptic input. The center panel shows an image of NO levels in response to the same stimulus using a fluorescent probe to detect NO (DAR-4M). Elevation of NO is detected throughout a wide area. The right panel shows changes in NO in response to a second synaptic stimulus after application of an extracellular scavenger of NO. In the presence of the scavenger, the elevation in NO levels is confined to the neurons receiving the direct synaptic input.

Modified from Steinert et al., 2008.

neurons (Steinert et al., 2008; Steinert et al., 2011). These increases occur both in the neurons that receive a direct synaptic input, and in those that are located in adjacent regions but which are not stimulated synaptically. Extracellular application of an NO scavenger does not block the increase in neurons that receive the synaptic input, but completely prevents it in neurons not receiving a direct input (Figure 11.8). These and other experiments have established that, once generated by a synaptic stimulus, NO acts as volume transmitter that diffuses throughout the MNTB to influence the properties of neighboring neurons (Steinert et al., 2008).

As stated earlier, two of the effects of NO on MNTB neurons are to reduce Kv3.1b potassium currents and to increase Kv2 potassium currents (Steinert et al., 2008; Steinert et al., 2011). These actions are believed to act primarily through dephosphorylation of the channels or related components following activation of a PP2A-like protein phosphatase, most likely mediated by a NO-dependent activation of PKG, the cyclic GMP-dependent protein kinase (Moreno, Vega-Saenz de Miera, Nadal, Amarillo, & Rudy, 2001). Such mechanisms could also therefore contribute much longer-term changes in channel expression.

Transcription Is Coordinated in Groups of Adjacent MNTB Neurons

The promoter that regulates the transcription of the *Kv3.1* channel gene contains a cyclic AMP/Ca^{2+}-response element (CRE; Gan & Kaczmarek, 1998; Gan et al., 1996). This element is activated on binding phosphorylated transcription factor CREB (cAMP response element-binding protein). Phosphorylation of CREB occurs during stimulation that elevates intracellular cyclic AMP or Ca^{2+} levels, leading to synthesis of messenger RNA encoding Kv3.1 (Gan et al., 1996). Immunostaining for phosphorylated CREB (pCREB) in the MNTB therefore provides a picture of which cells are likely to be actively transcribing CRE-regulated genes such as that for Kv3.1.

Levels of CREB do not vary significantly across the medial-lateral tonotopic axis of the MNTB (von Hehn et al., 2004). Phosphorylation of CREB, however, appears to be an "all or none" event in the nucleus of each neuron. In some neurons, nuclei are heavily stained for pCREB, while others have no detectable phosphorylation of this transcription factor. In animals with normal hearing, however, neurons with high pCREB are found adjacent to each other. One or more large clusters pCREB-positive neurons are found along the tonotopic axis, separated by regions devoid of pCREB staining (Figure 11.9A). An interesting aspect of these pCREB-positive clusters is that they can be found in different locations along the tonotopic axis even in animals maintained in similar auditory environments. The lower panels in Figure 11.9A show examples of immunostaining, represented as "bar codes," in which the major clusters of pCREB-positive neurons are found in the lateral, central or medial aspects of the MNTB.

The clustering of pCREB-positive neurons along the tonotopic axis depends on ongoing activity in the auditory system (von Hehn et al., 2004). In the BL/6 strain of mice, which lose hearing after several months of age, the clusters are present at 6 weeks of age, but at 8 months immunostaining occurs apparently randomly across the tonotopic axis (Figure 11.9B, C) and this is correlated with the disappearance of the gradient in the Kv3.1 channel itself (see Figure 11.4; von Hehn et al., 2004).

The simplest explanation for the existence of pCREB-positive clusters of neurons in the MNTB is that these are produced by lateral interactions between MNTB neurons and that these are shaped by synaptic inputs, which regulate the transcription of mRNA for Kv3.1 in adjacent set of neurons. The fact that these clusters are found in different places along the tonotopic axis in different animals suggests that they represent an ongoing adaptation to the auditory environment.

What Are Potential Mechanisms for Interactions among MNTB Neurons that Establish Levels of K^+ Channels?

1. *Local release of transmitter and other components:* As shown in Figure 11.8, there is good evidence that at least one substance, NO, acts as a local volume transmitter in the MNTB to modulate potassium channels in adjacent neurons (Steinert et al., 2008; Steinert et al., 2011). In addition, it is known that, during development,

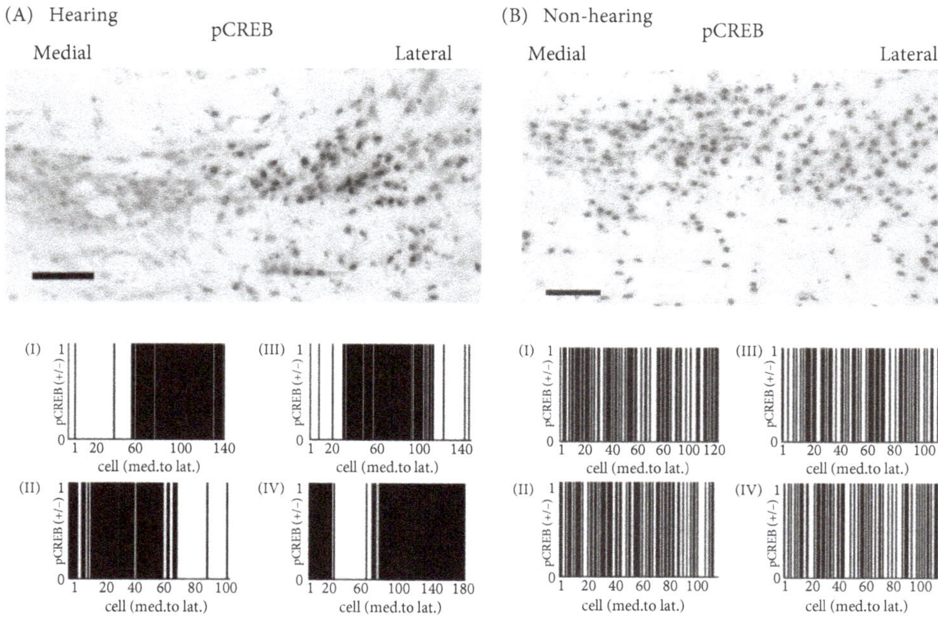

FIGURE 11.9. Patterns of immunostaining for phospho-CREB in the MNTB of mice with normal hearing and those with impaired hearing. A. A coronal section showing pCREB staining in the MNTB of a mouse with normal hearing (8-month-old CBA strain) stained for pCREB. Lower graphs show the distribution of pCREB staining across the medial-lateral axis for four different animals. Scale bar, 250µm. B. As for A, but for 8-month-old BL/6 mice, which, at this age, have impaired hearing (von Hehn et al., 2004).

neurotransmitter released at the terminals of MNTB neurons can spillover to act on the axons of adjacent MNTB neurons, providing another potential way for these cells to communicate with each other directly (Weisz, Rubio, Givens, & Kandler, 2016). Recent studies have also demonstrated that cells are capable of releasing many other substances in the external medium. These include exosomes, which are extracellular vesicles that are first formed as multivesicular bodies within the cytoplasm and then ejected from the cell (Edgar, 2016). These exosomes can be taken up by other cells and they provide a mechanism for the transfer or proteins, lipids, mRNAs and other large molecules from one cell to its neighbors. As of now, the existence of this mechanism has not be tested in the MNTB.

2. *Direct synaptic connections*: A proportion of MNTB neurons have recurrent collateral axons that branch off the main axon near its target in the LSO, and project back to the MNTB (Dondzillo, Thompson, & Klug, 2016; Kuwabara & Zook, 1991). These fibers terminate near the dendrites of the same cells but also provide inhibitory input to nearby principal neurons. It has been estimated that up to one third of MNTB neurons have such collateral fibers (Dondzillo et al., 2016). Such

lateral inhibition could provide side band inhibition that would enhance the frequency tuning of MNTB neurons. If such glycinergic inhibition is also coupled to mechanisms that modulate the synthesis or activity of K^+ channels, however, this would provide the needed transfer of information to establish gradients or other patterns of channel expression across the nucleus.

In theory, other inputs to the MNTB, such as glycinergic inputs from the ventral nucleus of the trapezoid body (Albrecht, Dondzillo, Mayer, Thompson, & Klug, 2014; Mayer, Albrecht, Dondzillo, & Klug, 2014), perhaps shaped by inputs from higher centers, could also mediate lateral interactions between neurons in the MNTB to influence channel expression.

3. *Neuron-glial cell interactions:* At least two types of glial cells in the MNTB are influenced by synaptic inputs. The cell bodies of the principal neurons of the MNTB, and the presynaptic calyces of Held are surrounded by astrocytes, which may completely envelop these presynaptic terminals (Reyes-Haro et al., 2010). Stimulation of the presynaptic fibers evokes inward currents these glial cells, and can elevate internal Ca^{2+} levels. The processes of astrocytes make contact with several different MNTB principal neurons, and spontaneous calcium transients in the astrocytes produce slow NMDA-mediated inward currents in the neurons (Reyes-Haro et al., 2010). A second type of glial cell, characterized by its expression of the proteoglycan NG2, receives direct AMPA receptor-mediated synaptic inputs from the calyx of Held presynaptic terminals, and these inputs are synchronized in time to the neuronal inputs (Muller et al., 2009). Thus glial cell-mediated interactions provide a potential mechanism for mediating local interactions in the MNTB.

Conclusion

Neurons in the MNTB, as well as the presynaptic terminals that contact them, express a variety of different types of K^+ channel subunits. The level of any specific subunit varies from neuron to neuron, and, for many of the subunits, a tonotopic gradient of expression exists within the nucleus. As a result, some MNTB neurons have a complement of subunits that favors rapid firing with lower temporal accuracy, while the mix of channels in other neurons favors accurate phase-locking. The activity of different channel subunits is, however, subject to very rapid modulation by auditory stimuli. The rate at which different channels are synthesized is also regulated by the auditory environment. These findings indicate that modulation of K^+ channels in individual neurons will alter specific aspects of a sound stimulus to which the neuron responds. If such modulation were to be coordinated among groups of MNTB neurons, through direct or indirect lateral interactions between the neurons, this would allow the ensemble of neurons to extract the maximal amount of information about the timing and intensity of auditory stimuli. Similar modulation of ion channels is likely to play a role at all levels of auditory processing.

References

Adamson, C. L., Reid, M. A., Mo, Z. L., Bowne-English, J., & Davis, R. L. (2002). Firing features and potassium channel content of murine spiral ganglion neurons vary with cochlear location. *Journal of Comparative Neurology*, *447*(4), 331–350. doi:10.1002/cne.10244

Albrecht, O., Dondzillo, A., Mayer, F., Thompson, J. A., & Klug, A. (2014). Inhibitory projections from the ventral nucleus of the trapezoid body to the medial nucleus of the trapezoid body in the mouse. *Front Neural Circuits*, *8*, 83. doi:10.3389/fncir.2014.00083

Barcia, G., Fleming, M. R., Deligniere, A., Gazula, V. R., Brown, M. R., Langouet, M., . . . Nabbout, R. (2012). De novo gain-of-function KCNT1 channel mutations cause malignant migrating partial seizures of infancy. *Nature Genetics*, *44*(11), 1255–1259. doi:10.1038/ng.2441

Barnes-Davies, M., Barker, M. C., Osmani, F., & Forsythe, I. D. (2004). Kv1 currents mediate a gradient of principal neuron excitability across the tonotopic axis in the rat lateral superior olive. *European Journal of Neuroscience*, *19*(2), 325–333.

Beck, E. J., Sorensen, R. G., Slater, S. J., & Covarrubias, M. (1998). Interactions between multiple phosphorylation sites in the inactivation particle of a K+ channel. Insights into the molecular mechanism of protein kinase C action. *Journal of General Physiology*, *112*(1), 71–84.

Berntson, A. K., & Walmsley, B. (2008). Characterization of a potassium-based leak conductance in the medial nucleus of the trapezoid body. *Hearing Research*, *244*(1–2), 98–106. doi:10.1016/j.heares.2008.08.003

Bhattacharjee, A., Gan, L., & Kaczmarek, L. K. (2002). Localization of the Slack potassium channel in the rat central nervous system. *Journal of Comparative Neurology*, *454*(3), 241–254. doi:10.1002/cne.10439

Bhattacharjee, A., von Hehn, C. A., Mei, X., & Kaczmarek, L. K. (2005). Localization of the Na+-activated K+ channel Slick in the rat central nervous system. *Journal of Comparative Neurology*, *484*(1), 80–92. doi:10.1002/cne.20462

Brand, A., Behrend, O., Marquardt, T., McAlpine, D., & Grothe, B. (2002). Precise inhibition is essential for microsecond interaural time difference coding. *Nature*, *417*(6888), 543–547. doi:10.1038/417543a

Brew, H. M., & Forsythe, I. D. (1995). Two voltage-dependent K+ conductances with complementary functions in postsynaptic integration at a central auditory synapse. *Journal of Neuroscience*, *15*(12), 8011–8022.

Brew, H. M., & Forsythe, I. D. (2005). Systematic variation of potassium current amplitudes across the tonotopic axis of the rat medial nucleus of the trapezoid body. *Hearing Research*, *206*(1–2), 116–132. doi:10.1016/j.heares.2004.12.012

Brew, H. M., Hallows, J. L., & Tempel, B. L. (2003). Hyperexcitability and reduced low threshold potassium currents in auditory neurons of mice lacking the channel subunit Kv1.1. *Journal of Physiology*, *548*(Pt 1), 1–20.

Brown, M. R., El-Hassar, L., Zhang, Y., Alvaro, G., Large, C. H., & Kaczmarek, L. K. (2016). Physiological modulators of Kv3.1 channels adjust firing patterns of auditory brainstem neurons. *Journal of Neurophysiology*, jn 00174 02016. doi:10.1152/jn.00174.2016

Brownell, W. E. (1975). Organization of the cat trapezoid body and the discharge characteristics of its fibers. *Brain Research*, *94*(3), 413–433.

Byrne, J. H. (1980). Analysis of ionic conductance mechanisms in motor cells mediating inking behavior in Aplysia californica. *Journal of Neurophysiology*, *43*(3), 630–650.

Chambers, A.R., Pilati, N., Large, C.H., Kaczmarek, L.K., & Polley, D.B. (2017). Pharmacological modulation of Kv3.1 mitigates auditory midbrain temporal processing deficits following auditory nerve damage. *Scientific Reports*, *7*. doi: 10.1038/s41598-017-17406-x

Clause, A., Kim, G., Sonntag, M., Weisz, C. J., Vetter, D. E., Rubsamen, R., & Kandler, K. (2014). The precise temporal pattern of prehearing spontaneous activity is necessary for tonotopic map refinement. *Neuron*, *82*(4), 822–835. doi:10.1016/j.neuron.2014.04.001

Conn, P. J., & Kaczmarek, L. K. (1989). The bag cell neurons of Aplysia. A model for the study of the molecular mechanisms involved in the control of prolonged animal behaviors. *Molecular Neurobiology*, *3*(4), 237–273. doi:10.1007/BF02740607

Connor, J. A., & Stevens, C. F. (1971a). Prediction of repetitive firing behaviour from voltage clamp data on an isolated neurone soma. *Journal of Physiology*, *213*(1), 31–53.

Connor, J. A., & Stevens, C. F. (1971b). Voltage clamp studies of a transient outward membrane current in gastropod neural somata. *Journal of Physiology*, *213*(1), 21–30.

Covarrubias, M., Wei, A., Salkoff, L., & Vyas, T. B. (1994). Elimination of rapid potassium channel inactivation by phosphorylation of the inactivation gate. *Neuron*, *13*(6), 1403–1412.

Cramer, K. S. (2005). Eph proteins and the assembly of auditory circuits. *Hearing Research*, *206*(1–2), 42–51. doi:10.1016/j.heares.2004.11.024

Cramer, K. S., & Miko, I. J. (2016). Eph-ephrin signaling in nervous system development. *F1000Res*, *5*. doi:10.12688/f1000research.7417.1

Darnell, J. C., Jensen, K. B., Jin, P., Brown, V., Warren, S. T., & Darnell, R. B. (2001). Fragile X mental retardation protein targets G quartet mRNAs important for neuronal function. *Cell*, *107*(4), 489–499.

Dodson, P. D., Barker, M. C., & Forsythe, I. D. (2002). Two heteromeric Kv1 potassium channels differentially regulate action potential firing. *Journal of Neuroscience*, *22*(16), 6953–6961.

Dodson, P. D., Billups, B., Rusznak, Z., Szucs, G., Barker, M. C., & Forsythe, I. D. (2003). Presynaptic rat Kv1.2 channels suppress synaptic terminal hyperexcitability following action potential invasion. *Journal of Physiology*, *550*(Pt. 1), 27–33.

Dondzillo, A., Thompson, J. A., & Klug, A. (2016). Recurrent inhibition to the medial nucleus of the trapezoid body in the Mongolian gerbil (Meriones unguiculatus). *PloS One*, *11*(8), e0160241. doi:10.1371/journal.pone.0160241

Edgar, J. R. (2016). Q&A: What are exosomes, exactly? *BMC Biology*, *14*, 46. doi:10.1186/s12915-016-0268-z

Elezgarai, I., Díez, J., Puente, N., Azkue, J. J., Benítez, R., Bilbao, A., . . . Grandes, P. (2003). Subcellular localization of the voltage-dependent potassium channel Kv3.1b in postnatal and adult rat medial nucleus of the trapezoid body. *Neuroscience*, *118*(4), 889–898. doi:http://dx.doi.org/10.1016/S0306-4522(03)00068-X

Fukui, I., & Ohmori, H. (2004). Tonotopic gradients of membrane and synaptic properties for neurons of the chicken nucleus magnocellularis. *Journal of Neuroscience*, *24*(34), 7514–7523. doi:10.1523/JNEUROSCI.0566-04.2004

Gan, L., & Kaczmarek, L. K. (1998). When, where, and how much? Expression of the Kv3.1 potassium channel in high-frequency firing neurons. *Journal of Neurobiology*, *37*(1), 69–79.

Gan, L., Perney, T. M., & Kaczmarek, L. K. (1996). Cloning and characterization of the promoter for a potassium channel expressed in high frequency firing neurons. *Journal of Biological Chemistry*, *271*(10), 5859–5865.

Gazula, V. R., Strumbos, J. G., Mei, X., Chen, H., Rahner, C., & Kaczmarek, L. K. (2010). Localization of Kv1.3 channels in presynaptic terminals of brainstem auditory neurons. *Journal of Comparative Neurology*, *518*(16), 3205–3220. doi:10.1002/cne.22393

Grigg, J. J., Brew, H. M., & Tempel, B. L. (2000). Differential expression of voltage-gated potassium channel genes in auditory nuclei of the mouse brainstem. *Hearing Research*, *140*(1–2), 77–90.

Grothe, B. (2003). New roles for synaptic inhibition in sound localization. *Nature Reviews: Neuroscience*, *4*(7), 540–550. doi:10.1038/nrn1136

Hardman, R. M., & Forsythe, I. D. (2009). Ether-a-go-go-related gene K+ channels contribute to threshold excitability of mouse auditory brainstem neurons. *Journal of Physiology*, *587*(Pt. 11), 2487–2497.

Huang, C.-Y., Chu, D., Hwang, W.-C., & Tsaur, M.-L. (2012). Coexpression of high-voltage-activated ion channels Kv3.4 and Cav1.2 in pioneer axons during pathfinding in the developing rat forebrain. *Journal of Comparative Neurology*, *520*(16), 3650–3672. doi:10.1002/cne.23119

Ishikawa, T., Nakamura, Y., Saitoh, N., Li, W.-B., Iwasaki, S., & Takahashi, T. (2003). Distinct roles of Kv1 and Kv3 potassium channels at the calyx of Held presynaptic terminal. *Journal of Neuroscience*, *23*(32), 10445–10453.

Johnston, J., Forsythe, I. D., & Kopp-Scheinpflug, C. (2010). Going native: Voltage-gated potassium channels controlling neuronal excitability. *Journal of Physiology*, *588*(Pt 17), 3187–3200. doi:10.1113/jphysiol.2010.191973

Johnston, J., Griffin, S. J., Baker, C., & Forsythe, I. D. (2008). Kv4 (A-type) potassium currents in the mouse medial nucleus of the trapezoid body. *European Journal of Neuroscience*, *27*(6), 1391–1399. doi:10.1111/j.1460-9568.2008.06116.x

Johnston, J., Griffin, S. J., Baker, C., Skrzypiec, A., Chernova, T., & Forsythe, I. D. (2008). Initial segment Kv2.2 channels mediate a slow delayed rectifier and maintain high frequency action potential firing in medial nucleus of the trapezoid body neurons. *Journal of Physiology*, *586*(14), 3493–3509.

Joris, P. X. (1996). Envelope coding in the lateral superior olive. II. Characteristic delays and comparison with responses in the medial superior olive. *Journal of Neurophysiology*, *76*(4), 2137–2156.

Joris, P. X., & Yin, T. C. (1995). Envelope coding in the lateral superior olive. I. Sensitivity to interaural time differences. *Journal of Neurophysiology*, *73*(3), 1043–1062.

Kaczmarek, L. K. (2012). Gradients and modulation of K(+) channels optimize temporal accuracy in networks of auditory neurons. *PLoS Computational Biology*, *8*(3), e1002424. doi:10.1371/journal.pcbi.1002424

Kaczmarek, L. K. (2013). Slack, slick and sodium-activated potassium channels. *ISRN Neuroscience*, *2013*(2013). doi:10.1155/2013/354262

Kaczmarek, L. K. (2017). Tuning neuronal potassium channels to the auditory environment. *Auditory Development and Plasticity*, *64*, 133–159.

Kaczmarek, L. K., Aldrich, R. W., Chandy, K. G., Grissmer, S., Wei, A. D., & Wulff, H. (2017). International Union of Basic and Clinical Pharmacology. C. Nomenclature and properties of calcium-activated and sodium-activated potassium channels. *Pharmacological Reviews*, *69*(1), 1–11. doi:10.1124/pr.116.012864

Kaczmarek, L. K., Bhattacharjee, A., Desai, R., Gan, L., Song, P., von Hehn, C. A., . . . Yang, B. (2005). Regulation of the timing of MNTB neurons by short-term and long-term modulation of potassium channels. *Hearing Research, 206*(1–2), 133–145.

Kaczmarek, L. K., & Zhang, Y. (2017). Kv3 Channels: Enablers of rapid firing, neurotransmitter release, and neuronal endurance. *Physiological Reviews, 97*(4), 1431–1468. doi:10.1152/physrev.00002.2017

Kandel, E. R., & Schwartz, J. H. (1982). Molecular biology of learning: modulation of transmitter release. *Science, 218*(4571), 433–443.

Kandler, K., Clause, A., & Noh, J. (2009). Tonotopic reorganization of developing auditory brainstem circuits. *Nature Neuroscience, 12*(6), 711–717. doi:10.1038/nn.2332

Kanemasa, T., Gan, L., Perney, T. M., Wang, L. Y., & Kaczmarek, L. K. (1995). Electrophysiological and pharmacological characterization of a mammalian Shaw channel expressed in NIH 3T3 fibroblasts. *Journal of Neurophysiology, 74*(1), 207–217.

Kopp-Scheinpflug, C., Fuchs, K., Lippe, W. R., Tempel, B. L., & Rubsamen, R. (2003). Decreased temporal precision of auditory signaling in Kcna1-null mice: An electrophysiological study in vivo. *Journal of Neuroscience, 23*(27), 9199–9207.

Kopp-Scheinpflug, C., Lippe, W. R., Dorrscheidt, G. J., & Rubsamen, R. (2003). The medial nucleus of the trapezoid body in the gerbil is more than a relay: Comparison of pre- and postsynaptic activity. *Journal of the Association of Research Otolaryngology, 4*(1), 1–23. doi:10.1007/s10162-002-2010-5

Kopp-Scheinpflug, C., Tolnai, S., Malmierca, M. S., & Rubsamen, R. (2008). The medial nucleus of the trapezoid body: comparative physiology. *Neuroscience, 154*(1), 160–170. doi:10.1016/j.neuroscience.2008.01.088

Kuwabara, N., & Zook, J. M. (1991). Classification of the principal cells of the medial nucleus of the trapezoid body. *Journal of Comparative Neurology, 314*(4), 707–720. doi:10.1002/cne.903140406

Leão, K. E., Leão, R. N., Deardorff, A. S., Garrett, A., Fyffe, R., & Walmsley, B. (2010). Sound stimulation modulates high-threshold K+ currents in mouse auditory brainstem neurons. *European Journal of Neuroscience, 32*(10), 1658–1667. doi:10.1111/j.1460-9568.2010.07437.x

Leao, R. N., Berntson, A., Forsythe, I. D., & Walmsley, B. (2004). Reduced low-voltage activated K+ conductances and enhanced central excitability in a congenitally deaf (dn/dn) mouse. *Journal of Physiology, 559*(Pt 1), 25–33. doi:10.1113/jphysiol.2004.067421

Leao, R. N., Sun, H., Svahn, K., Berntson, A., Youssoufian, M., Paolini, A. G., . . . Walmsley, B. (2006). Topographic organization in the auditory brainstem of juvenile mice is disrupted in congenital deafness. *Journal of Physiology, 571*(Pt 3), 563–578. doi:10.1113/jphysiol.2005.098780

Li, W., Kaczmarek, L. K., & Perney, T. M. (2001). Localization of two high-threshold potassium channel subunits in the rat central auditory system. *Journal of Comparative Neurology, 437*(2), 196–218.

Luneau, C. J., Williams, J. B., Marshall, J., Levitan, E. S., Oliva, C., Smith, J. S., . . . et al. (1991). Alternative splicing contributes to K+ channel diversity in the mammalian central nervous system. *Proceedings of the National Academy of Sciences, 88*(9), 3932–3936.

Macica, C. M., & Kaczmarek, L. K. (2001). Casein kinase 2 determines the voltage dependence of the Kv3.1 channel in auditory neurons and transfected cells. *Journal of Neuroscience, 21*(4), 1160–1168.

Macica, C. M., von Hehn, C. A., Wang, L. Y., Ho, C. S., Yokoyama, S., Joho, R. H., & Kaczmarek, L. K. (2003). Modulation of the Kv3.1b potassium channel isoform adjusts the fidelity of the firing pattern of auditory neurons. *Journal of Neuroscience, 23*(4), 1133–1141.

Manis, P. B., & Marx, S. O. (1991). Outward currents in isolated ventral cochlear nucleus neurons. *Journal of Neuroscience, 11*(9), 2865–2880.

Mayer, F., Albrecht, O., Dondzillo, A., & Klug, A. (2014). Glycinergic inhibition to the medial nucleus of the trapezoid body shows prominent facilitation and can sustain high levels of ongoing activity. *Journal of Neurophysiology, 112*(11), 2901–2915. doi:10.1152/jn.00864.2013

Moreno, H., Vega-Saenz de Miera, E., Nadal, M. S., Amarillo, Y., & Rudy, B. (2001). Modulation of Kv3 potassium channels expressed in CHO cells by a nitric oxide-activated phosphatase. *Journal of Physiology, 530*(Pt 3), 345–358.

Muller, J., Reyes-Haro, D., Pivneva, T., Nolte, C., Schaette, R., Lubke, J., & Kettenmann, H. (2009). The principal neurons of the medial nucleus of the trapezoid body and NG2(+) glial cells receive coordinated excitatory synaptic input. *Journal of General Physiology, 134*(2), 115–127. doi:10.1085/jgp.200910194

Nicolis, G., & Prigogine, I. (1977). *Self-organization in nonequilibrium systems.* New York, NY: John Wiley & Sons.

Oertel, D., Wright, S., Cao, X. J., Ferragamo, M., & Bal, R. (2011). The multiple functions of T stellate/multipolar/chopper cells in the ventral cochlear nucleus. *Hearing Research, 276*(1–2), 61–69. doi:10.1016/j.heares.2010.10.018

Reyes-Haro, D., Muller, J., Boresch, M., Pivneva, T., Benedetti, B., Scheller, A., . . . Kettenmann, H. (2010). Neuron-astrocyte interactions in the medial nucleus of the trapezoid body. *Journal of General Physiology, 135*(6), 583–594. doi:10.1085/jgp.200910354

Santi, C. M., Ferreira, G., Yang, B., Gazula, V. R., Butler, A., Wei, A., . . . Salkoff, L. (2006). Opposite regulation of Slick and Slack K+ channels by neuromodulators. *Journal of Neuroscience, 26*(19), 5059–5068. doi:10.1523/JNEUROSCI.3372-05.2006

Schneggenburger, R., & Forsythe, I. D. (2006). The calyx of Held. *Cell and Tissue Research, 326*(2), 311–337. doi:10.1007/s00441-006-0272-7

Song, P., & Kaczmarek, L. K. (2006). Modulation of Kv3.1b potassium channel phosphorylation in auditory neurons by conventional and novel protein kinase C isozymes. *Journal of Biological Chemistry, 281*(22), 15582–15591.

Song, P., Yang, Y., Barnes-Davies, M., Bhattacharjee, A., Hamann, M., Forsythe, I. D., . . . Kaczmarek, L. K. (2005). Acoustic environment determines phosphorylation state of the Kv3.1 potassium channel in auditory neurons. *Nature Neuroscience, 8*(10), 1335–1342.

Steinert, J. R., Kopp-Scheinpflug, C., Baker, C., Challiss, R. A. J., Mistry, R., Haustein, M. D., . . . Forsythe, I. D. (2008). Nitric oxide is a volume transmitter regulating postsynaptic excitability at a glutamatergic synapse. *Neuron, 60*(4), 642–656. doi:http://dx.doi.org/10.1016/j.neuron.2008.08.025

Steinert, J. R., Robinson, S. W., Tong, H., Haustein, M. D., Kopp-Scheinpflug, C., & Forsythe, I. D. (2011). Nitric oxide is an activity-dependent regulator of target neuron intrinsic excitability. *Neuron, 71*(2), 291–305. doi:http://dx.doi.org/10.1016/j.neuron.2011.05.037

Strong, J. A., & Kaczmarek, L. K. (1986). Potassium currents that regulate action potentials and repetitive firing. In L. K. Kaczmarek & I. B. Levitan (Eds.), *Neuromodulation: The Biochemical Control of Neuronal Excitability* (pp. 119 137). New York, NY: Oxford University Press.

Strumbos, J. G., Brown, M. R., Kronengold, J., Polley, D. B., & Kaczmarek, L. K. (2010). Fragile X mental retardation protein is required for rapid experience-dependent regulation of the potassium channel Kv3.1b. *Journal of Neuroscience, 30*(31), 10263–10271. doi:10.1523/JNEUROSCI.1125-10.2010

Strumbos, J. G., Polley, D. B., & Kaczmarek, L. K. (2010). Specific and rapid effects of acoustic stimulation on the tonotopic distribution of Kv3.1b potassium channels in the adult rat. *Neuroscience, 167*(3), 567–572.

Taschenberger, H., & von Gersdorff, H. (2000). Fine-tuning an auditory synapse for speed and fidelity: Developmental changes in presynaptic waveform, EPSC kinetics, and synaptic plasticity. *Journal of Neuroscience, 20*(24), 9162–9173.

Tong, H., Kopp-Scheinpflug, C., Pilati, N., Robinson, S. W., Sinclair, J. L., Steinert, J. R., . . . Forsythe, I. D. (2013). Protection from noise-induced hearing loss by Kv2.2 potassium currents in the central medial olivocochlear system. *Journal of Neuroscience, 33*(21), 9113–9121. doi:10.1523/JNEUROSCI.5043-12.2013

Tong, H., Steinert, J. R., Robinson, S. W., Chernova, T., Read, D. J., Oliver, D. L., & Forsythe, I. D. (2010). Regulation of Kv channel expression and neuronal excitability in rat medial nucleus of the trapezoid body maintained in organotypic culture. *Journal of Physiology, 588*(Pt 9), 1451–1468. doi:10.1113/jphysiol.2009.186676

Trussell, L. O. (1999). Synaptic mechanisms for coding timing in auditory neurons. *Annual Review of Physiology, 61*, 477–496. doi:10.1146/annurev.physiol.61.1.477

von Hehn, C. A., Bhattacharjee, A., & Kaczmarek, L. K. (2004). Loss of Kv3.1 tonotopicity and alterations in cAMP response element-binding protein signaling in central auditory neurons of hearing impaired mice. *Journal of Neuroscience, 24*(8), 1936–1940.

Walmsley, B., Berntson, A., Leao, R. N., & Fyffe, R. E. (2006). Activity-dependent regulation of synaptic strength and neuronal excitability in central auditory pathways. *Journal of Physiology, 572*(Pt 2), 313–321. doi:10.1113/jphysiol.2006.104851

Wang, L. Y., Gan, L., Forsythe, I. D., & Kaczmarek, L. K. (1998). Contribution of the Kv3.1 potassium channel to high-frequency firing in mouse auditory neurones. *Journal of Physiology, 509*(Pt 1), 183–194.

Weisz, C. J., Rubio, M. E., Givens, R. S., & Kandler, K. (2016). Excitation by axon terminal GABA spillover in a sound localization circuit. *Journal of Neuroscience, 36*(3), 911–925. doi:10.1523/JNEUROSCI.1132-15.2016

Yang, B., Desai, R., & Kaczmarek, L. K. (2007). Slack and slick K(Na) channels regulate the accuracy of timing of auditory neurons. *Journal of Neuroscience, 27*(10), 2617–2627.

Zhang, Y., Zhang, X. F., Fleming, M. R., Amiri, A., El-Hassar, L., Surguchev, A. A., . . . Kaczmarek, L. K. (2016). Kv3.3 channels bind hax-1 and arp2/3 to assemble a stable local actin network that regulates channel gating. *Cell, 165*(2), 434–448. doi:10.1016/j.cell.2016.02.009

CHAPTER 12

THE MEDIAL SUPERIOR OLIVARY NUCLEUS

Meeting the Need for Speed

BENEDIKT GROTHE, CHRISTIAN LEIBOLD, AND MICHAEL PECKA

Abstract

It doesn't get any more precise than this: Neurons in the medial superior olive (MSO) in many mammals, including humans, are sensitive to temporal differences between their synaptic inputs of only a few microseconds. These neurons are the basis for our ability to resolve even a 5-μs disparity in the time of arrival of a sound at each ear. This capacity enables humans to discriminate between temporally overlapping sounds based on spatial segregation, as for instance, at a cocktail party or a poster session at a scientific conference. This chapter aims at providing a comprehensive summary on the current state of research regarding the MSO, ranging from cellular and circuit anatomy to subcellular and channel physiology to spatial coding and perception. Consequently, the chapter is subdivided according to these thematic aspects. Nonetheless, while such subdivisions are helpful for providing structure to the reader, they can also convey the inter-dependencies between these topics: for example, when studying the spatial sensitivity of MSO neurons on the mechanistic level, it is crucial to also consider its anatomical specializations (on the subcellular and circuit level), as well as corresponding perceptional phenomena. Finally, the chapter suggests a complete picture of the MSO only emerges by including evolutionary considerations, that is, the phylogenetic origin of the many fascinating specializations that can be observed within the MSO circuit.

Keywords: coincidence detection, ITD, neuronal population code, SPN, adaptation, glycine, spatial hearing, context-dependent sound localization, ultrafast neural processing

Preface: Definition and Computations

Traditionally, neuronal structures are defined as regions or nuclei that can be anatomically delineated and, ideally, unambiguously recognized in all species of a clade (here: in all mammals). Usually, it is irrelevant whether the structure in question contains different neuronal types and/or serves one or more functions. The cochlear nucleus (CN), for instance, contains multiple neuronal types that clearly serve different functions, but these cell types can be identified in all mammals and always permit unambiguous delineation of the CN. In the case of the MSO, matters are more complex, and its delimitation has been guided largely by the morphology of a specific cell type, which is arranged in a particular way and performs an explicit function, rather than by comparative means. Specifically, the textbook definition of the MSO is as follows: A structure that consists of bipolar neurons whose somata are located in one parasagittal plane, whose dendrites are oriented orthogonally to this plane, point medially and laterally, and serve only one function. This "defining" function is the detection of microsecond differences in the time of arrival of inputs from the two ears (interaural time difference, ITD), which allows differences in the bilateral time of arrival of sounds to be utilized for sound localization in the horizontal plane. This straight-forward view of the MSO goes back to early studies in carnivores (e.g., cats and dogs), animals in which the MSO attracted attention because of the sheer beauty of its unique anatomical organization (Goldberg & Brown, 1969; Ramón y Cajal, 1909; Figure 12.1). Moreover, the MSOs of dogs and cats were among the first shown to be sensitive to ITDs (Caird & Klinke, 1983; Goldberg & Brown, 1969; Yin & Chan, 1990). Although its cytoarchitecture (Kapfer et al., 2002; Rautenberg, Grothe, & Felmy, 2009) and its ITD sensitivity (Brand et al., 2002; Franken, Bremen, & Joris, 2014; Pecka et al., 2008; Spitzer & Semple, 1995; van der Heijden et al., 2013) have since been confirmed in other ITD-using mammals, reducing the MSO to a single neuron type and a single function is problematic for the following reasons:

1. The MSO includes neurons that deviate from the strictly bipolar type and their unique biophysical properties (Smith, 1995).
2. Even the predominant bipolar neurons are not always arranged within one parasagittal plane, as they are in dogs, cats, or gerbils. In small mammals that do not use ITDs for sound localization, like various bats (reviewed in Grothe, 2000), mice (Fischl et al., 2016), rats, and short-tailed opossums (Kapfer et al., 2002), these cells are distributed within a more spherical MSO. Indeed, this diversity has given rise to the erroneous claim that the MSO is missing in these mammals.
3. Synaptic input patterns of MSO bipolar neurons differ across mammals, although they receive the same set of inputs from both sides of the brain (to be discussed in "The MSO Circuit and Anatomical Adaptations for Speed"). In mammals that

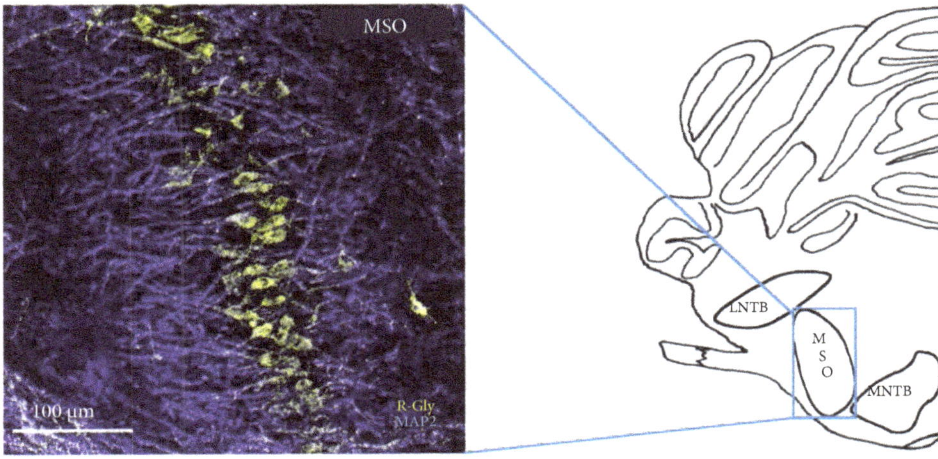

FIGURE 12.1. **The MSO.** The position of the MSO deep in the brainstem is shown in a coronal section (right side). Glycine receptors (yellow; left side) are restricted to the area of the cell bodies of MSO cells, which are arranged in a sagittal plane, with dendrites pointing medially and laterally (blue).

Reproduced from Kapfer et al. (2002), with permission.

use ITDs, such as cats, gerbils, and chinchillas, the four major axonal projections to MSO are arranged in an orderly fashion, with ipsilateral glutamatergic inputs targeting only lateral, and contralateral glutamatergic inputs targeting only medial dendrites. In addition, glycinergic inputs from both sides synapse only in the somatic region of these neurons (Clark, 1969; Kapfer et al., 2002; Kuwabara & Zook, 1992; Perkins, 1973; Stotler, 1953; Werthat et al., 2008). In contrast, in mammals that do not exploit ITDs, the inhibitory and excitatory inputs are intermingled along the somata and among the dendrites (Kapfer et al., 2002).

4. Finally, bipolar neurons in the MSO of bats can be highly sensitive to temporal features of sounds (like amplitude modulations; Grothe, 1994), but their ITD sensitivity seems to be too crude to serve sound localization for these small animals (Grothe & Park, 1998; Harnischfeger, Neuweiler, & Schlegel, 1985) or show predominantly monaural response properties (Covey, Vater, & Casseday, 1991; Grothe et al., 1992).

A phylogenetic framework that can explain these differences may be found in Grothe (2000) and Grothe & Pecka, (2014). In this chapter, we follow a strategy that avoids problems relating to the anatomical delineation of nuclei/structures and simplifies matters, without losing sight of the organizational and functional variations found across different species. This can be done by simply addressing specific cell types with definable functional and/or computational properties independently of their exact location or arrangement within the Superior Olivary Complex (SOC), rather than focusing on structures that contain multiple neuronal types. Emphasizing cell identity is the only way to disentangle complexities associated with the definition of a nucleus across species, and it may also help clarify the definitions of the superior periolivary/paraolivary nucleus (SPN/SPON); for example, with regard to the OFF cells that have been assigned to different nuclei in different species (compare to chapter by Magnusson & Gómez-Álvarez, this volume; see also Behrend et al., 2002).

With regard to MSO cell types, rather little is known about the properties of the "non-principal" neurons, except that they are multipolar, exhibit low thresholds, and fire repetitively upon current injections in vitro, which contrasts with the high threshold phasic responses seen in bipolar neurons (Smith, 1995). Nothing is known about their responses or function in vivo. We will therefore focus on the principal MSO neurons in ITD-using mammals only. These neurons are tuned for execution of the temporally most precise computations known in mammals, which rely on their anatomical and synaptic arrangement, as well as on some peculiar features of their inputs and their rather unique biophysical properties.

We will address and summarize in turn (1) the anatomical arrangement of principal cells, including synaptic inputs and the morphological adaptations for speed; (2) their biophysical properties, which permit processing of information on microsecond scales; (3) the computational tasks involved in ITD processing; and (4) the functional significance of the coding properties of these cells and their implications for auditory spatial perception.

The MSO Circuit and Anatomical Adaptations for Speed

A major feature of the MSO and its input pathways in mammals that use ITDs (Figure 12.2) is the structural organization that enables accurate registration of the arrival times of inputs. The specializations begin at the level of the two classes of bushy cells and their inputs (see chapter by Oertel, Cao, & Recio-Spinoza, this volume), which provide precise information relating to the temporal features of stimuli, such as envelope onsets and the fine structure of ongoing components (e.g., phase-locking to low-frequency sounds). Spherical bushy cells (SBCs) on both sides provide the binaural excitatory, glutamatergic inputs to the MSO, with ipsilateral inputs targeting the lateral and contralateral inputs the medial dendrites. Hence, as first described in detail by Stotler (1953), ipsi- and contralateral inputs are kept spatially separated at the level of the MSO neurons. It follows that owing to the longer path length, excitation from the contralateral side arrives slightly later than that from the ipsilateral ear. Because spike generation by the MSO neurons

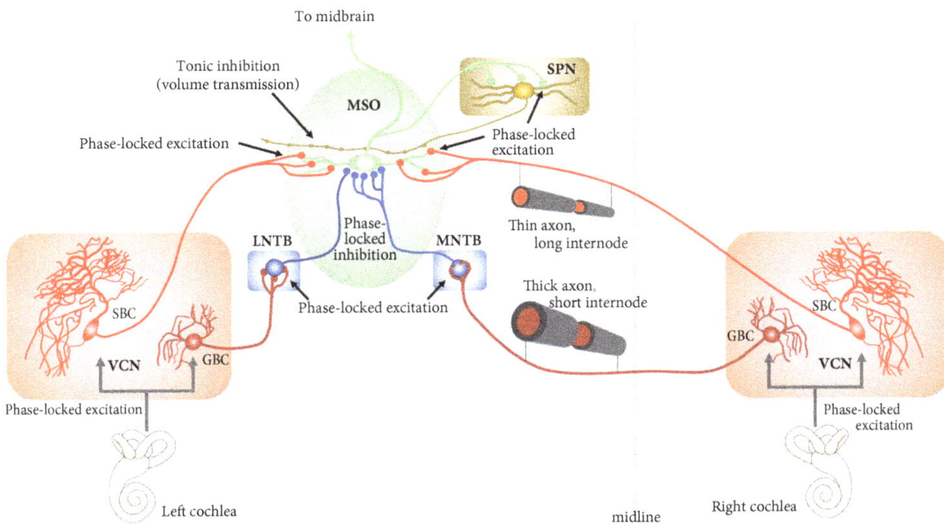

FIGURE 12.2. **The MSO circuit.** MSO neurons receive excitatory inputs from SBCs in both the ipsi- and contralateral VCN. SBC fibers target MSO dendrites. Bushy cells are driven by the auditory nerve. GBCs in the ipsilateral VCN excite ipsilateral LNTB neurons via large endbulb-of-Held-like synapses. GBCs from the contralateral side make contact with ipsilateral MNTB neurons via the calyx of Held synapse. GBC fibers projecting to low-frequency MNTB neurons have large axon diameters but unusually short internodes. SBC fibers are much thinner but have longer internodes. MNTB and LNTB neurons are glycinergic (inhibitory) and target MSO cell bodies and proximal dendrites. MSO cells send their main output to the inferior colliculus (auditory midbrain). Collaterals from this projection synapse on GABAergic neurons in the SPN. These SPN neurons provide feedback into the MSO via slow volume transmission targeting presynaptic $GABA_B$ receptors. All connections except the SPN-MSO projection are phase-locked to low-frequency sounds and time-locked to sound envelope.

GBC = globular bushy cell; SPC = spherical bushy cell; LNTB = lateral nucleus of the trapezoid body; MNTB = medial nucleus of the trapezoid body; MSO = medial superior olive; SPN = superior paraolivary nucleus; VCN = ventral cochlear nucleus.

depends on coincidence detection (see under the following heading, "Biophysical Properties"), this configuration of inputs may itself generate a "preferred ITD"; that is, provide an external delay between incoming signals from the two ears that precisely offsets the difference in axonal path length between the excitatory inputs from the two sides. This "preferred delay" corresponds to an ITD that favors sounds from the contralateral hemisphere, since slightly earlier arrival of the sound at the contralateral ear will compensate for the internal delay. Indeed, this slight contralateral bias has been experimentally observed in the MSO (Brand et al., 2002; Franken, Bremen, & Joris, 2014; Pecka et al., 2008; to be discussed in "The Nature of Internal Delays" and Figure 12.6c).

In contrast to its avian analogue the nucleus laminaris (Seidl, Rubel, & Harris, 2010), in which the excitatory inputs are arranged as delay lines that provide different combinations of internal delays to different binaural neurons (in accordance with the scenario proposed by L. Jeffress [Jeffress, 1948]), there is no evidence for systematic variation in axonal length in the MSO inputs (Grothe, 2000; Karino et al., 2011).

In addition to bilateral excitation, the MSO receives bilateral inhibitory synaptic inputs and at least one additional inhibitory feedback input that acts via volume transmission (Figure 12.2). The latter originates from a monosynaptic MSO-SPN-MSO feedback loop. We will address the function of this volume transmission later on in the section "The Nature of the Spatial Code and Dynamics of Spatial Processing". The direct synaptic inhibition is glycinergic (Grothe & Sanes 1993, 1994) and comes from the medial and, less prominently, from the lateral nucleus of the trapezoid body (MNTB, LNTB, respectively; Kuwabara & Zook, 1992; Spirou & Berrebi, 1997; Spirou, Rowland, & Berrebi, 1998). In contrast to the case in other mammals, in which these inputs target both dendrites and somata of MSO neurons, experience-dependent developmental pruning of glycinergic inputs from the dendrites takes place in ITD-using mammals, which restricts large inhibitory synapses to the somata and the most proximal dendrites (Couchman, Grothe, & Felmy, 2012; Kapfer et al., 2002; Werthat et al., 2008; Figure 12.3). This arrangement correlates with the fact that strong inhibitory currents can be elicited by only a small number of input fibers (Couchman, Grothe, & Felmy, 2010). Perturbation of this developmental removal of dendritic inhibitory inputs (Kapfer et al., 2002) disrupts the normal development of ITD tuning in gerbils (Seidl & Grothe, 2005). How such inhibition may alter ITD tuning will be discussed as well.

The inhibitory pathway starts with globular bushy cells (GBCs), which excite a monaural (ipsilateral) subpopulation of LNTB neurons (Roberts, Seeman, & Golding, 2014)

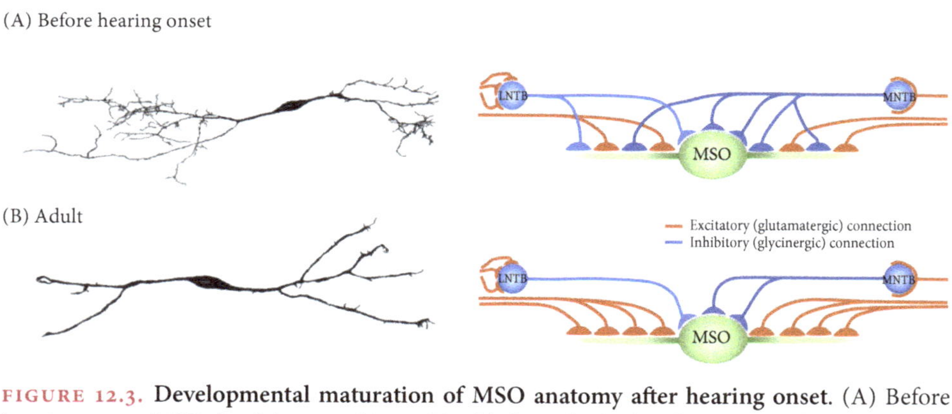

FIGURE 12.3. **Developmental maturation of MSO anatomy after hearing onset.** (A) Before hearing onset, MSO dendrites are thin and highly branched. The glycinergic inhibitory inputs from MNTB and LNTB are targeted to dendrites and cell somata. (B) One week after hearing onset, the MSO dendrites are thicker and less tufted. The inhibitory inputs are now confined to the cell somata and proximal dendrites.

via large endbulb of Held-like synapses (Spirou, Rowland, & Berrebi, 1998) and (contralateral) MNTB neurons via the extensively studied calyx of Held synapse (Borst & Soria van Hoeve, 2012). LNTB and, more prominently, MNTB then provide glycine-mediated hyperpolarizing inhibition to the MSO somata (Grothe & Sanes, 1993; Kapfer et al., 2002; Roberts, Seeman, & Golding, 2014).

The GBC-MNTB-MSO pathway in particular exhibits unique adaptations for fast conduction of action potentials and temporally precise transmission. First, GBCs receive strong synaptic inputs from auditory nerve (AN) fibers (Xu-Friedman & Regehr, 2005; see Oertel et al., this volume) that cause action potentials to follow the temporal structure of inputs with the highest possible temporal precision. For instance, the precision of phase-locking in GBCs surpasses that of single AN fibers, as shown for cats and gerbils (Joris et al., 1994; Wei et al., 2017). Second, GBC fibers have the largest axon diameter known in the auditory brainstem (Ford et al., 2015; Morest, 1968), which partly explains their higher conduction velocity. Moreover, GBC axons tuned to low frequencies have recently been shown to exhibit a unique myelination pattern: although they are even thicker than GBCs tuned to higher frequencies (and much thicker than SBC axons), their internodes are significantly shorter. Although at first sight paradoxical, this pattern in fact results in an even higher conduction velocity (Ford et al., 2015; Figure 12.2, Figure 12.6B). Notably, this unusual myelination pattern is not found on GBC axons of mice, which do not utilize ITDs; hence, it appears to be specifically related to ITD processing (Stange-Marten et al., 2017). Third, each MNTB neuron receives input from a GBC fiber via a single calyx of Held synapse, a type known for its exceptional speed and reliability (Borst & Soria van Hoeve, 2012). Fourth, as has recently been shown in gerbils, a significant proportion of such synapses tuned to low sound frequencies do not prolong synaptic delays during ongoing activity, a feature that is highly unusual for chemical synapses (Stange-Marten et al., 2017). Hence, the additional synapse not only expedites conduction speed, but in these cases also ensures absolute time constancy despite the additional synapse. Finally, the inputs are restricted to the MSO cell somata (Clark, 1969; Kapfer et al., 2002), which results in precise and strong inhibition (Couchman, Grothe, & Felmy, 2012; Grothe & Sanes, 1994; Roberts, Seeman, & Golding, 2013).

These unusual properties of the main inhibitory pathway to the MSO relate to a number of indirect and direct observations that demonstrate that this inhibition, despite the additional synapse in the MNTB, precedes the direct excitation from contralateral SBGs (Brand et al., 2002; Goldwyn et al., 2017; Grothe & Pecka, 2014; Roberts, Seeman, & Golding, 2013) and acts in a phase-locked manner (Pecka et al., 2008; see also figure 12.1d in Franken et al., 2015; compare figures 12.2 and 12.5 in Goldwyn et al., 2017). Less is known about the weaker LNTB-mediated inhibition, but in vitro recordings suggest that its timing may be less reliable than that of MNTB-driven inhibition (Roberts, Seeman, & Golding, 2014). Since strong inhibitory input is consistently found in in vitro MSO preparations, it is clear that inhibition at least contributes to cellular ITD processing. Its particular role is nonetheless still under debate, as we will discuss. But first we turn to biophysical aspects of cellular coincidence detection of excitatory and inhibitory inputs.

Biophysical Properties

To achieve cycle-by-cycle ITD sensitivity of their phase-locked inputs, MSO neurons must be able to limit temporal integration of synaptic currents to the oscillation period of the fine structure of their bushy cell inputs. For example, if we assume the phase-locking limit of bushy cells to be about 2 kHz, the memory time scale of the coincidence mechanism must be at most 1/(2 kHz) = 500 μs or lower. Such microsecond-scale operation places strong constraints on the biophysical properties of the neural elements involved, including dendritic filtering, synaptic dynamics, and transmembrane channel kinetics. In the following paragraphs, we will review these aspects in the mature MSO cell and consider how they contribute to ITD processing.

Dendrite Morphology and Synaptic Distributions

As mentioned earlier, a defining anatomical property of MSO principal neurons is their bipolar form, with one lateral and one medial dendrite originating from the soma (Henkel & Brunso-Bechtold, 1990; Kiss & Majorossy, 1983; Rautenberg, Grothe, & Felmy, 2009; Stotler, 1953). The two major dendrites are relatively thick (~4 μm diameter) close to the soma, such that the border between soma and dendrite is not clearly demarcated anatomically, and is largely a matter of definition (Rautenberg, Grothe & Felmy, 2009). The primary dendrites are relatively short (100 to 150 μm) and tapered, terminating in filopodia-like structures. Often one also observes dendrites branching at an intermediate distance from the soma and leading to two major dendritic trunks. The marked bipolar morphology serves two major functional purposes:

1. Excitatory synaptic inputs from the two input pathways remain anatomically segregated, with inhibitory synapses from either hemisphere being restricted to the soma (Clark, 1969; Kapfer et al., 2002; Kuwabara & Zook, 1992; Stotler, 1953).
2. Owing to the thickness of the proximal dendrite its axial resistance is very low, and it therefore has little temporal filtering capacity. The dendrites also act as large current sinks, which results in additional leakage from the soma (Rall, 1962; Agmon-Snir, Carr, & Rinzel, 1998; Dasika, White, & Colburn, 2007). The relatively small diameters of the distal dendrites result in locally higher input resistances and thereby amplify voltage responses to distal inputs relative to more proximal inputs (Mathews et al., 2010).

It has been argued that the separation of inputs on dendrites facilitates binaural coincidence detection via a ceiling effect imposed by the synaptic reversal potential (Agmon-Snir, Carr, & Rinzel, 1998; Dasika, White, & Colburn, 2007), which leads to an effective reduction of the threshold conductance for binaural inputs relative to monaural inputs. This threshold effect, however, is particularly strong for thin dendrites and might thus be more relevant to the avian binaural coincidence detector in the nucleus laminaris (Smith & Rubel, 1979) than to the mammalian MSO with its thick dendrites.

Thus, despite the clear anatomical allocation of the binaural input pathways to the lateral and medial dendrites first described by Stotler (1953), its functional role remains unclear. It may have an important developmental function, for example in selecting the composition of inputs that provide precise ipsi- or contralateral excitation/inhibition appropriately tuned to the timing of the other inputs. In this context, a detailed description of how individual fibers make synaptic contacts along the dendrite is of the utmost importance, because this pattern defines the temporal profile of dendritic depolarization upon unilateral excitation. Unfortunately, very little is known about the properties of single fibers. Based on single-fiber stimulation, Couchman et al. (2010) estimated that only 1 or 2 active excitatory SBC fibers per cochlear nucleus are necessary to evoke an action potential from the resting state. However, this result was obtained using single stimuli applied to slices during blockade of inhibitory inputs. When repetitive stimulation (pulse trains of few hundred Hz) is employed under similar conditions, these numbers increase by more than twofold due to synaptic adaptation (N. Kladisios and F. Felmy, personal communication, January 26, 2018). But even the latter figures are surprisingly small, given the large number of excitatory synaptic contacts that have been described anatomically (Stotler, 1953). The available evidence thus suggests that individual fibers may make multiple contacts on one dendrite. An anatomical verification of this assertion is, however, still lacking.

Synaptic Kinetics and Integration

Synaptic transmission at MSO cells mainly relies on two ligand-gated ion channels, amino-3-hydroxyl-5-methyl-4-isoxazole propionate (AMPA) receptor-mediated excitation and glycine receptor-mediated inhibition. Only a relatively small (< 5%) N-methyl-D-aspartate (NMDA) receptor-mediated current has been reported to contribute to excitatory postsynaptic currents (EPSCs) in the adult MSO (Couchman, Grothe, & Felmy, 2010; Smith, Owens, & Forsythe, 2000). MSO AMPA signaling is spectacularly fast. In contrast to the AMPA decay time constants of sometimes 10 and more milliseconds known from cortical synapses (see e.g., Salin et al., 1996), voltage clamp recordings from MSO neurons reveal decay time constants of about 250 μs (Couchman, Grothe, & Felmy, 2010; Figure 12.4A). At least synaptically, these short decay time constants would allow to detect the coincidence of excitatory currents for inputs up to about 4 kHz at least. Synaptic inhibition on the other hand exhibits much slower kinetics, decaying within about 1.5 ms (Couchman, Grothe, & Felmy, 2010; Myoga et al.,

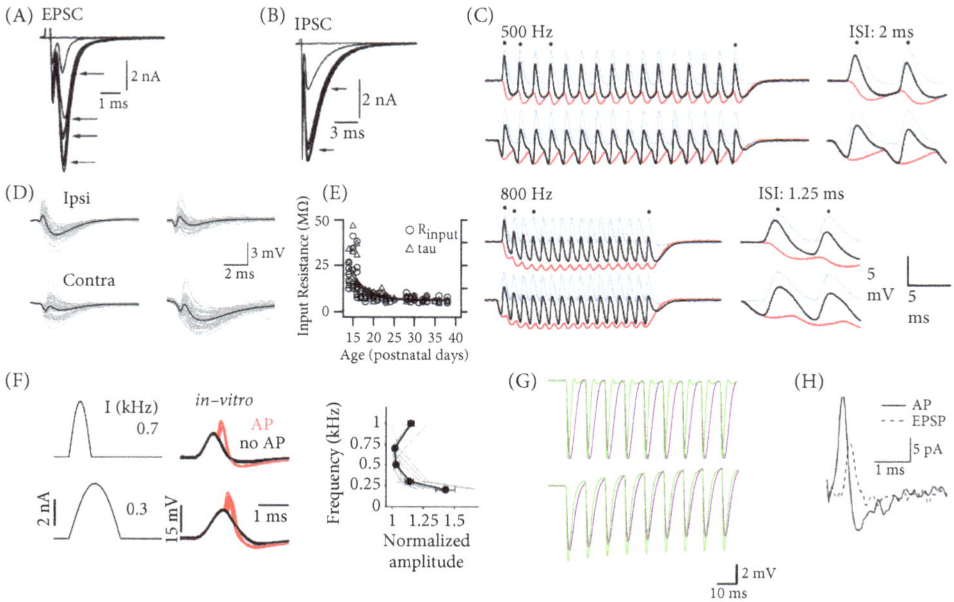

FIGURE 12.4. Synaptic and membrane properties.

(A) Intracellularly recorded EPSCs evoked by local stimulation. Arrows mark jumps in amplitude evoked by increasing stimulation strengths.

(B) Same as A for IPSCs. A & B taken from Couchman et al. (2010), with permission.

(C) Intracellular membrane potential recordings for simulated trains (conductance clamp) of excitatory and inhibitory synaptic conductances (black) of 500 Hz (top) and 800 Hz (bottom). For each stimulus frequency, the pair of traces corresponds to inhibition lagging excitation by 0.1 ms (upper traces) and inhibition leading excitation by 0.6 ms (lower traces). Blue and red traces, respectively, depict results for simulated excitatory and inhibitory conductances only. Black dots mark peaks of the blue traces that are delayed with respect to the peaks of the black traces depending on the relative inhibitory lag/lead. From Myoga et al., (2014) with permission.

(D) Intracellularly recorded compound postsynaptic potentials evoked by distal auditory nerve stimulations in vitro. Note that EPSP components lag behind IPSP components. From Roberts et al. (2013), with permission.

(E) Input resistance and membrane time constant decrease by an order of magnitude during early postnatal development. From Scott et al. (2005), with permission.

(F) Left: Intracellular recording of action potentials evoked by half-sine current stimulations. APs (red) have low amplitudes. Right: The AP threshold is frequency dependent. Ordinate depicts the frequencies used to generate half sine wave stimuli (inverse period length). The threshold amplitudes (abscissa) are normalized to the minimum of each cell. From Lehnert et al. (2014), with permission.

(G) Computationally simulated membrane voltages for fast (active) Kv1 conductances (top) and slow, effectively passive leak conductances (bottom) for 100 Hz stimulations with inhibitory conductances. The conductance amplitude was adjusted to yield the same input resistance for both model variants (fast and slow conductances). Particularly for strong HCN currents (green), Kv1 decreases half-widths of IPSPs substantially. The purple trace was obtained for weak HCN currents. From Baumann et al. (2013), with permission.

(H) On-cell recording demonstrating stronger after-hyperpolarization after an action potential than after an EPSP. From Couchman et al. (2010), with permission.

EPSC/P= excitatory postsynaptic current/potential; IPSC/P = inhibitory postsynaptic current/potential; AP = action potential; HCN = hyperpolarization-activated cyclic nucleotide–gated.

2014). Based on these studies, combined with other in vitro and in vivo data (Grothe & Sanes, 1994; Myoga et al., 2014; Pecka et al., 2008), the cycle-by-cycle action of inhibition is assumed to be restricted to frequencies up to approximately 1000 Hz (Figure 12.4B, C).

The mechanism of integration of the four synaptic input pathways has been controversially discussed in the literature, particularly with regard to the ability of the glycinergic currents to contribute to cycle-by-cycle coincidence detection (Franken et al., 2015; Myoga et al., 2014; Pecka et al., 2008; Roberts, Seeman, & Golding, 2013). There is general agreement that excitatory coincidence detection constitutes the backbone of ITD processing (Franken et al., 2015; Jeffress, 1948; Joris, Smith, & Yin, 1998; Leibold, 2010; Myoga et al., 2014; Pecka et al., 2008) and also that the spike rate of MSO cells can largely be accounted for by a linear combination of the binaural inputs (Joris et al., 2006; van der Heijden et al., 2013; Plauška, Borst, & van der Heijden, 2016); but see Franken et al., 2015. However, both the anatomical evidence for strong and relatively fast-acting (Figure 12.4B) and temporally preceding (Figure 12.4D) glycinergic inhibitory synapses (see section 1) and the effects of pharmacological blockade of glycinergic signaling on ITD tuning (Brand et al., 2002; Pecka et al., 2008) suggest a fundamental role of the two inhibitory pathways in shaping the ITD tuning curves, particularly in determining the position of the preferred ITD (Figure 12.4C). Explaining such inhibition-induced peak shifts in models in which inhibitory and excitatory currents act on the same time scale is quite straightforward (Brand et al., 2002; Leibold & van Hemmen, 2005), if the contralateral inhibition precedes excitation. Incorporation of the measured, slower inhibitory synaptic kinetics generally does not produce shifts in the preferred ITD (Day & Semple, 2011; Leibold & van Hemmen, 2005; Roberts, Seeman, & Golding, 2013; Zhou, Carney, & Colburn, 2005) for all delays between contralateral excitation and inhibition, but nevertheless shows such effects for a wide range of delays (Leibold, 2010; Myoga et al., 2014). The question of the functional role of inhibition for ITD processing will be discussed in detail later.

Subthreshold Channels

The main determinant of the short memory time scale of MSO neurons is their short membrane time constant of 300 μs and sometimes even less (Couchman, Grothe, & Felmy, 2010), which is attained during early development (Figure 12.4E). For comparison, typical membrane time constants of cortical neurons are in the range of 10 milliseconds (Stuart & Sakmann, 1995). Apart from the anatomical leakage contribution imposed by the thick proximal dendrites as described earlier, the time constant is mainly determined by the fact that transmembrane channels continue to conduct at rest. Two such channels have been described in great detail in the literature: (1) a hyperpolarization-activated, cyclic nucleotide-gated (HCN) channel (Baumann et al., 2013; Khurana et al., 2011), which generates a cationic inward current, and (2) a dendrotoxin (DTX)-sensitive voltage-gated potassium (Kv1) channel (Mathews et al., 2010; Svirskis et al., 2002), which generates an outward current. The two channels balance each other and thereby fix both the resting potential at about −67 mV (Couchman, Grothe, & Felmy, 2010) and the input resistance of 2–8 MOhm in mature neurons (Couchman, Grothe, & Felmy, 2010; Scott, Mathews, & Golding, 2005;). Apart from their directionality, the channels mainly differ in their time constants. Kv1 channels are fast opening ($\tau \sim 1.5$ ms), whereas the HCN channel kinetics is much slower, with a reaction time of ~100 ms, far longer than the dynamics typically induced by the fine structure of the stimulus.

Functionally, the fast Kv1 kinetics has been shown to shorten EPSPs (Mathews et al., 2010; Scott, Mathews, & Golding, 2005; Svirskis et al., 2002; Svirskis, Dodla, & Rinzel, 2003), thereby further reducing the time window for coincidence detection of the AMPA-mediated synaptic potentials. The same argument, however, also applies to the additional sharpening of glycine-mediated inhibitory potentials (Baumann et al., 2013). Furthermore, sharpening can be achieved not only by fast Kv1 kinetics, but also by the HCN reversal potential of about −35 mV, which speeds up the decay of IPSPs (Baumann et al., 2013). Thus, the membrane potential dynamics results from an intricate non-linear interplay between all synaptic and channel kinetics.

In addition to temporal sharpening, fast Kv1 activation has been shown to underlie membrane potential resonances in MSO cells (Remme et al., 2014; Mikiel-Hunter, Kotak, & Rinzel, 2016; Fischer, Leibold, & Felmy, 2018), which would amplify input fine structure in the range of several hundred Hz. The functional role of these resonances is not fully understood. Modeling and in vitro physiology suggest that these resonances permit a frequency-dependent reduction of the spike threshold (Lehnert et al., 2014; Remme et al., 2014; Figure 12.4F).

The Kv1 kinetics has also been shown to affect preferred ITDs in vitro (Myoga et al., 2014) and in modeling studies (Jercog et al., 2010; Myoga et al., 2014). Since Kv1 opens with a short time constant of only ~1.5 ms, it will be sensitive to the slope of the subthreshold postsynaptic currents (PSCs). Fast-rising PSCs will not be affected by Kv1 opening, whereas slow depolarization will be counterbalanced by Kv1 opening. This effective high-pass filtering will differentially affect the inputs from the two ears (and hence shift preferred ITD) if they have different slopes, either because of differential temporal jitter or differences in the relative delay between excitation and inhibition (Jercog et al., 2010; Myoga et al., 2014).

Based on computational modeling, Kv1 and HCN1 channels have been proposed to be non-isotropically distributed along the dendrites, exhibiting a higher density at the soma (Mathews et al., 2010). However, antibody staining of HCN also shows strong immunofluorescence at the dendrites (Khurana et al., 2011). The putative somatic colocalization of Kv1 channels and glycinergic synapses argues in favor of a functional role for both currents (Figure 12.4G) rather than cooperation between Kv1 channels and (spatially segregated) glutamatergic synapses (Baumann et al., 2013; Myoga et al., 2014). Moreover, since Myoga et al. (2014) have shown that temporal broadening of the EPSPs by adding jitter actually amplifies inhibition-induced peak shifts, the idea that Kv1 mainly sharpens the already ultrabrief EPSCs would not seem necessary, at least from the perspective of the inhibition model.

While bath application of DTX suppresses a large fraction of the potassium currents, a background of DTX-insensitive outward currents with slower kinetics still remains (Scott, Mathews and Golding, 2005), which argues for the presence of additional yet unidentified potassium channels with as yet unknown functional roles.

Action Potential Generation

MSO cells exhibit unusually small action potential (AP) amplitudes of 10 mV or less (Yin & Chan, 1990; Scott, Hage, & Golding, 2007; Couchman, Grothe, & Felmy, 2010; Figure 12.4F, H). For practical reasons, it has even been argued that in vitro APs can be more reliably detected by measuring the associated after-hyperpolarization (Figure 12.4H) rather than their upstroke and peak (Couchman, Grothe, & Felmy, 2010). The large somatic leak currents described in the previous section are the most obvious reason for tiny APs. But if most of the synaptic currents leave the cell through subthreshold channels, how can a sufficiently large proportion of the remaining ions actually reach the spike-generating zone of the thin axon and sustain excitability? In a modeling study based on measured axonal morphology, Lehnert et al. (2014) showed that the large somatic leak may indeed prevent the initiation of APs in the axon initial segment in response to fast fluctuating inputs, and shift the spike initiation zone to the proximal nodes of Ranvier. This result is consistent with the finding that sodium channels in the axons of high-frequency neurons of the avian nucleus laminaris are located further distally than those in low-frequency neurons (Kuba, Ishii, & Ohmori, 2006). Thus, the initial portion of the axon isolates the somatic leak from the spike-generating zone and the efficacy of the isolation needs to be larger the higher the input frequency, that is, the more difficult it is for the stimulus to elicit an AP.

In addition to the many circuit, synapse and membrane elements and mechanisms that have been proposed to determine the optimal ITD of a neuron (reviewed earlier), asymmetries in axonal morphology have also been considered. If the axon originates from the lateral dendrite, somatic inhibition would effectively delay the contralateral input, leading to contralaterally leading best ITDs (Zhou, Carney, & Colburn, 2005). Anatomical evidence for systematic axonal asymmetry, however, is absent (Rautenberg, Grothe, & Felmy, 2009).

Modulatory Influences

Since changes in ITD of only 10 μs have marked effects on MSO response rates, biophysical processes occurring on scales longer than about 5 ms cannot directly interact with the mechanism for coincidence detection of features in the fine structure of the stimulus. Nevertheless, such slow pathways have been described for MSO cells and play a role in controlling the excitability of the neuron.

HCN channels found in the axon initial segment decrease MSO spiking probability by adding a leak current (Ko et al., 2016). Serotonin released during states of increased attention shifts the membrane potential required for half-maximum activation of HCN to more negative voltages, thereby reducing leak and increasing spike probability (Ko et al., 2016).

Presynaptic gamma-aminobutyric acid $(GABA)_B$ receptors reduce the transmission of both the glutamatergic and the glycinergic MSO inputs (Stange et al., 2013). The GABA is supplied by a feedback loop which includes GABAergic neurons in the superior periolivary nucleus that are driven by the MSO, project back to it, and release GABA from extrasynaptic varicosities. Implications of this negative feedback on ITD encoding will be discussed next.

The Computation of Interaural Time Differences

As we have seen, principal MSO neurons fundamentally serve as coincidence detectors for their binaural inputs and each responds maximally to a specific range of ITDs. Although some MSO neurons are responsive (i.e., fire action potentials) to monaural stimulation of either ear alone, the sum of the two monaurally evoked responses is generally far below the response to binaural stimulation at favorable ITDs. Moreover, the preferred ITD can be predicted from the phase delay between the two monaural responses (Yin & Chan, 1990). Thus, to achieve maximal coincidence between ipsi- and contralateral inputs, the external delay (i.e., ITD) must be compensated for by the internal delay within the brain. Conversely, the effective internal delay determines the preferred ITD and thus the range of sensitivity (i.e., ITD tuning) of a given MSO neuron (and for a given stimulation frequency to be further discussed under "The Nature of Internal Delays").

Generally, MSO neurons are very broadly tuned; that is, response rates are modulated over a large range of ITDs that exceeds the range of ITDs that are generated by the shape of the skull under anechoic conditions, the so-called "physiological range" (Figure 12.5). For the majority of recorded ITD functions—irrespective of species—the highest neuronal spatial sensitivity (the slope of the ITD rate function that conveys most information about changes in location) is positioned around the midline (Harper & McAlpine, 2004), and preferred ITDs mostly correspond to contralateral positions at the edge or even outside of the physiological range. More specifically, the preferred ITD of a cell depends on the best frequency (BF), irrespective of the head size of the species studied, and on average preferred ITDs increase with decreasing BF (Figure 12.5) (Middlebrooks et al., 1994; McAlpine, Jiang, & Palmer, 2001; Hancock & Delgutte, 2004; Pecka et al., 2008; Werner-Reiss & Groh, 2008). These data thus refuted the long-standing idea of the MSO as a distributed labeled-line encoder of azimuthal space (as had been found in

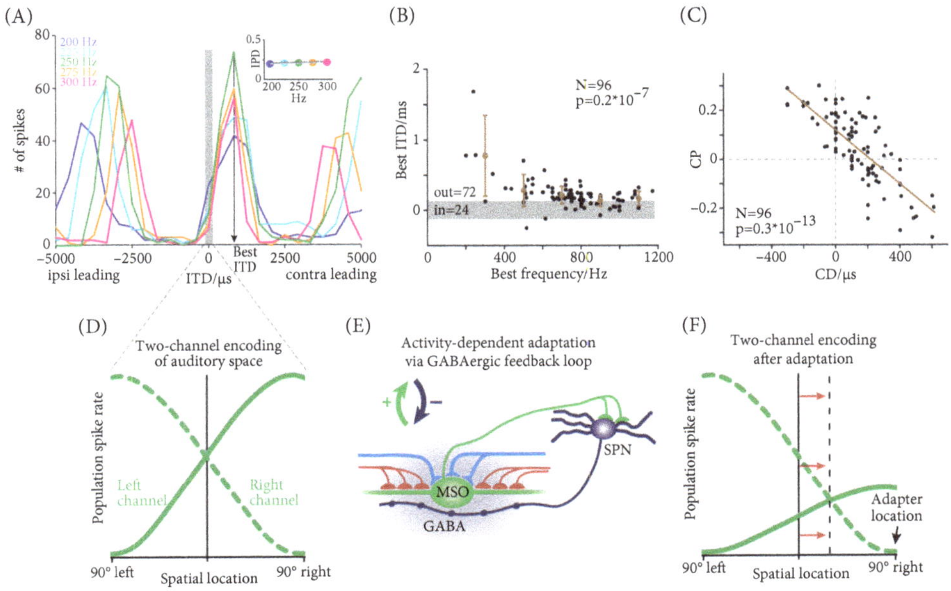

FIGURE 12.5. Coding of ITDs in the MSO.

(A) Extracellular recording of a gerbil MSO neuron (from Pecka et al., 2008, figure 12.1). ITD response functions were obtained at five different pure tone frequencies (color-coded, BF = 250 Hz). The gray area demarcates the physiological range of ITDs, that is, range of ITDs generated by the inter-ear distance. The inset shows the corresponding frequency-phase plot for this neuron, from which CD ("characteristic delay," the slope of the function) and CP ("characteristic phase," the phase intercept of the function at 0 Hz) can be obtained.

(B) Best ITDs (peak of the ITD response function at BF) of gerbil MSO neurons lie predominately outside the physiological range and are negatively correlated with BF. The data shown is for 96 MSO neurons (pooled from Pecka et al., 2008; Stange et al., 2013; Dietz et al., 2014) and reveals a highly significant dependency of best ITD upon BF, with 75% of best ITDs lying outside the physiological range. Single-neuron data are shown in black, while mean values (±SD) within 200 Hz wide bins are given in brown.

(C) CP and CD of MSO neurons are significantly negatively correlated. Data are from the same neurons as in B. This correlation can potentially be exploited for the coding of sound source locations at the population level.

(D) Since the slopes of ITD functions from all neurons within an MSO typically exceed the physiological range of ITDs (a consequence of the dependency of best ITDs on BF, see panel B), left and right MSOs can be regarded as two oppositely tuned hemispheric channels for the coding of auditory space, in which the laterality of a sound source is defined by the relative activity levels of the two channels.

(E) A negative feedback loop between the MSO and the SPN causes a slow-acting, long-lasting reduction in the response of MSO neurons, which is proportional to their prior activity level (Stange et al., 2013). This response modulation is mediated by volume transmission of GABA onto the MSO, where it acts on $GABA_B$ receptors (mostly pre-synaptically).

(F) This activity-dependent adaptation introduces an asymmetry into hemispheric population coding, as strongly lateralized sound sources will induce adaptation of the contralateral channel only. This hemispheric asymmetry can be observed both at the level of MSO neurons and in the perception of human listeners (e.g., shifts in the perceived location of midline, red arrows, and dashed vertical line).

CD = characteristic delay; CP = characteristic phase; BF = best frequency; GABA = gamma-aminobutyric acid.

owls and chicks) in which preferred ITDs in each frequency band are distributed within the physiological range (or even clustered around the midline).

What then is the nature of the neuronal ITD code—and hence of the internal delay—that underlies the BF dependency of ITD tuning in MSO neurons? In vivo recordings from the MSO are technically very challenging, and these questions are thus still subject of ongoing debate and investigation. A number of recent studies have included enormously difficult experiments that yielded exciting, but unfortunately contradictory, findings regarding the mechanism(s) used to create internal delays. We will first briefly review the current hypotheses in light of the known anatomy and physiology of the MSO circuit, and then turn to recent advances in our understanding of spatial coding in the MSO and mammals in general.

The Nature of Internal Delays

Important insights into possible mechanisms for the generation of internal delays come from the tuning of MSO neurons for sound frequency: by definition, the highest spike rates (and the greatest modulation of the response) are evoked by pure tones presented at a neuron's BF. Shifting the pure-tone frequency away from the BF in either direction results in a systematic reduction in the maximum spike rates elicited, and in a reduction in the dynamic range of the spike rate elicited by different ITDs (Figure 12.5). More importantly, by testing ITD sensitivity in MSO neurons at multiple frequencies (or using broadband noise) one can determine their characteristic delay (CD), that is, the ITD for which the relative discharge rate is identical for different stimulus frequencies. Theoretically, for neurons with a pure axonal conduction delay from one or both ears (i.e., a pure time delay as generated by delay lines), the CD corresponds to the ITD at which response peaks are aligned for all stimulus frequencies to which the neuron is sensitive. As mentioned before, the observed dependency of best ITDs on BF (i.e., internal delays) in the MSO rules out a Jeffress-like topographic arrangement of best ITDs. Nonetheless, theoretically this BF dependency could still be achieved by systematic pattern of variation of axonal length from the two ears, analogous to the delay-line system found in birds (compare Figure 12.6). However, while the inhibitory pathway within the MSO circuit indeed exhibits anatomical adaptations to achieve superior conduction speed and timing relative to excitation (see first section and Figure 12.6), current anatomical data do not support the existence of any systematic arrangement of axon length within the excitatory inputs themselves (Karino et al., 2011). Moreover, CDs of MSO neurons are typically not found at response peaks, but tend to align along the slopes of the ITD functions. This suggests that ITD sensitivity in these neurons is not generated by a simple time delay mechanism and that some form of phase delay must be present ("CP," the characteristic phase).

Given the anatomical and physiological evidence for inhibitory inputs to MSO neurons, it may not be surprising that CPs are indeed observed. In fact, it is well

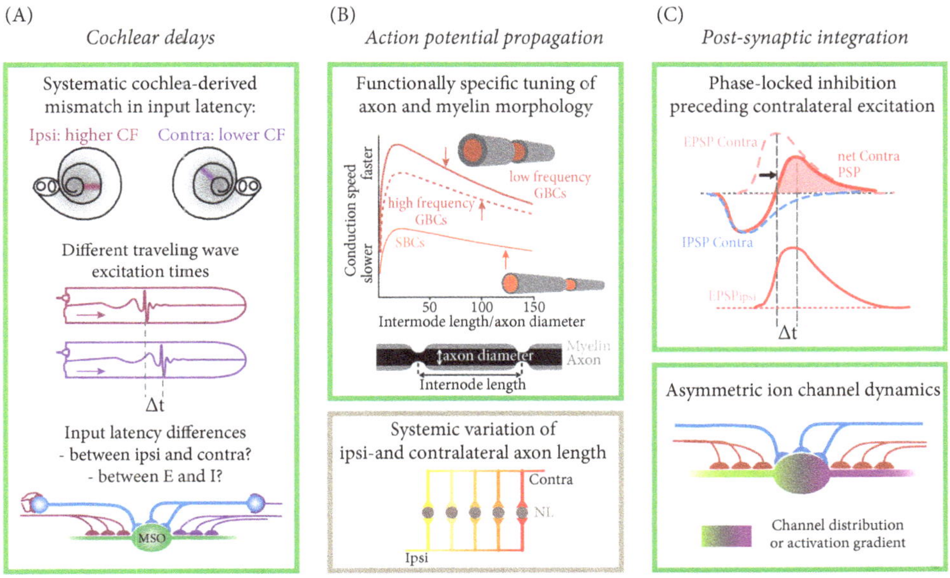

FIGURE 12.6. Complementary mechanisms that (potentially) contribute to the internal delay in circuits for ITD computation.

Mechanisms suggested or established for the mammalian MSO (green boxes) and avian NL (brown boxes).

(A) Cochlear delays: The traveling wave of the cochlear basilar membrane excites basal regions earlier than apical regions. This mechanical delay of excitation could potentially be exploited by a systematic mismatch in CF of inputs from the two ears to the MSO (Schroeder, 1977; Shamma et al., 1989). However, while discrepancies in frequency tuning between ipsi- and contralateral MSO inputs have been reported, no *systematic* mismatch has been found (Plauška et al., 2017). An as yet unexplored variation of this hypothesis posits a systematic mismatch between excitatory and inhibitory inputs from the same ear, which—in addition to differences in axon morphology (see panel B)—could contribute to the observed temporal precedence of inhibition (see Figure 12.4)

(B) Action potential propagation: Both in mammalian and avian ITD detector circuits, axon morphology contributes to the tuning of input times, albeit in distinct ways. In the MSO circuit (green box), axon diameter and myelination vary between inputs. The graph shows computer simulations of the dependence of conduction velocity upon the ratio of internode length to axon diameter in low-frequency GBCs (solid red line), high-frequency GBCs (dashed red line), and SBC axons (orange line). Arrows denote the ratios found in the gerbil. SBCs that provide the contralateral excitatory input to the MSO have thinner axons and larger internode lengths than the axons of GBCs that innervate the contralateral MNTB (and thus are part of the inhibitory MSO input). Notably, the ratios for low-frequency GBCs (but not high-frequency GBCs) deviate significantly from the canonical value of 100 because of the unusually short intermodal length given the axonal diameter. This extraordinary patterning of myelination is restricted to low-frequency GBCs and is associated with a further increase in conduction speed, suggesting a specific morphological adaptation of the contralateral inhibitory pathway for fast AP conduction for ITD processing (see also Stange-Marten et al., 2017). Graph re-drawn and modified from Ford et al. (2015). Additionally, axons of SBCs exhibit differential myelination and variation in axon caliber depending on whether they terminate on the ipsilateral or the contralateral MSO (Seidl & Rubel, 2016).

established that the constellation of ipsilateral excitation and contralateral inhibition from the MNTB for coincidence detection in the lateral superior olive (LSO) results in a CP of half a cycle. It is further well documented that the temporal sensitivity for the input timing between inhibition and excitation in the LSO lies in the range of tens to hundreds of microseconds (Tollin, 2003; Tollin & Yin, 2005; Beiderbeck et al., 2018). Inhibition is therefore likely to contribute to tuning internal delays to the relevant ITDs (Brand et al., 2002; Seidl & Grothe, 2005), reviewed in Grothe, Pecka, & McAlpine (2010). This, however, does not mean that other factors like axonal length are not important. It only means that there is no indication for systematic variations in other parameters and that such factors on their own cannot explain overall delays (see Figure 12.6).

Nevertheless, phase delays could also be generated by other mechanisms. Two recent studies were able to obtain in vivo whole-cell recordings from MSO cells, thus enabling direct examination of the changes in membrane polarization in MSO neurons during ITD processing.

Based on data from whole-cell and attached-cell recordings, van der Heijden and colleagues (2013) concluded that inhibition is not detectable during—and hence does not contribute to—ITD tuning of MSO cells. This apparent lack of discernible inhibition may be due to the fixed temporal relationship between contralateral excitation and inhibition, resulting in a net PSP which, at least without further manipulations, may not always allow one to disentangle the different synaptic components. Physiological studies of the MNTB-derived inhibitory input, however, have consistently found that contralateral inhibition precedes contralateral excitation (Roberts, Seeman, & Golding, 2013; Goldwyn et al., 2017; see Figure 12.4) and thereby changes the timing of the composite contralateral input (Myoga et al., 2014). Anatomical findings of thicker axons and unusual myelination geared for fast conduction times specifically within the inhibitory pathway to the MSO support these physiological results (Ford et al., 2015; Stange-Marten et al., 2017) that were already predicted based on theoretical considerations (Brand et al. 2002). Another in vivo whole-cell study of the MSO carried out additional pharmacological interventions during recordings, a feat requiring utmost technical ability (Franken et al., 2015). Unlike van der Heijden and colleagues (2013), these authors indeed observed prominent inhibition in their MSO recordings, albeit not consistently

---

In the avian nucleus laminaris (NL, brown box), internal delays are generated via axonal delay lines, that is, systematic variation of axonal length and caliber (and myelination) to equalize conduction times between ipsi- and contralateral inputs (Jeffress, 1948; Seidl et al., 2014).

(C) Post-synaptic integration: Upper box: Internal delays in the MSO could be created by the observed temporal precedence of contralateral inhibition relative to contralateral excitation, which may result in a delayed net contralateral post-synaptic potential (Pecka et al., 2008; Myoga et al., 2014). Lower box: Alternatively or additionally, asymmetries in the distribution of activation dynamics of somatic ion channels (such as low-threshold potassium channels) could induce asymmetries in temporal filtering that would result in an effective internal delay (Jercog et al., 2010; Franken et al., 2015).

in all cells (which could be related to the relatively high CFs of the recorded neurons). Interestingly, they also consistently observed phasic hyperpolarizations prior to suprathreshold excitatory events. The authors concluded that this hyperpolarization might be caused by the action of additional, excitatory inputs that inactivate low-threshold potassium channels (Franken et al., 2015). However, the origin of this additional input is unclear.

Another, perhaps complementary, hypothesis for the generation of internal delays is based on the possible presence of small differences in spectral tuning between inputs from the two ears, and has been investigated in two other recent studies. The so-called stereausis hypothesis arose from the application of theories developed to account for binaural pitch detection based on coincidence detection (Loeb, White, & Merzenich, 1983) and later adapted for sound localization (Shamma, Shen, & Gopalaswamy, 1989). Analyses of monaural spike trains from auditory nerve recordings confirm the feasibility of this scenario (Joris et al., 2006), and one study indicates that such a mechanism may contribute to ITD tuning under some conditions involving complex stimuli (Benichoux et al., 2015). In contrast, studies using simple dichotic stimuli indicate no or, at best, only a minor and non-systematic contribution of stereausis to ITD tuning (Pecka et al., 2008; Plauška, van der Heijden, & Borst, 2017).

In summary, the nature of the internal delay in MSO neurons is still not clear. Quite possibly, many, if not all of the mechanisms mentioned previously (including conduction delay) may contribute. Nonetheless, one factor often neglected in considerations of the role of inhibitory inputs is the intriguing possibility that the characteristic delay is adjusted and/or refined during ontogeny. Anatomical refinement of glycinergic inhibition has been shown to be at least partially dependent on auditory experience during early development, and auditory deprivation can alter the distribution of best ITDs. Thus, while other mechanisms (axonal length, cochlear delays etc.) can establish an approximate ITD early in development, an experience-dependent process could selectively optimize inhibitory inputs following the onset of hearing to achieve and maintain the desired tuning.

The Nature of the Spatial Code and Dynamics of Spatial Processing

The fact that ITD functions of MSO neurons show very broad tuning (essentially linear modulation between -90° and 90°) that is stereotypical within a given spectral band stimulated the idea of hemispheric, oppositely coding channels on each side of the brain that might be compared at later stages of the pathway (Figure 12.5) (McAlpine, Jiang, & Palmer, 2001; Stecker & Middlebrooks, 2003; Hancock & Delgutte, 2004; Harper & McAlpine, 2004). This concept relies on the idea that similar activity levels in both channels should encode sound-source position at the midline, such that a relative increase in activity in one of the brain hemispheres would indicate a corresponding contralateral location with respect to the more active brain hemisphere. This strategy might well optimize coding efficiency in animals with small head sizes, but might be sub-optimal for animals with larger heads and high frequency hearing, owing to the increasing ambiguity of spike-rate-to-ITD mapping (Harper & McAlpine, 2004; Lüling et al., 2011; Goodman, Benichoux, & Brette, 2013; Harper et al., 2014). Such ambiguity could, however, be eliminated by making use of additional information from other ITD-sensitive channels (such as the low-frequency neurons in the LSO, see next paragraph) during the decoding (Lingner et al., 2018). One interesting observation in this regard is that CD and BF, as well as CD and CP, are negatively correlated (Figure 12.5); (Agapiou & McAlpine, 2008; Lüling et al., 2011). This correlation could be neuronally exploited to acquire frequency-invariant information about ITDs, either in the context of population average coding (Lüling et al., 2011) or a pattern recognition approach (Goodman, Benichoux, & Brette, 2013; Benichoux et al., 2015).

While the models for possible ITD representation are manifold (see preceding discussion and Day & Delgutte, 2013), elegant adaptation paradigms with human subjects not only strongly imply that a population code underlies sound localization in humans/primates, but have also highlighted the fact that prior stimulation influences subsequent spatial perception (Phillips & Hall, 2005; Vigneault-MacLean, Hall, & Phillips, 2007). Traditionally, such adaptive coding strategies have not been associated with sound localization, yet recent findings from both human psychophysics (Getzmann, 2004; Phillips & Hall, 2005; Vigneault-MacLean, Hall, & Phillips, 2007; Maier et al., 2009; Dahmen et al., 2010; Lingner et al., 2018) and animal physiology (Magnusson et al., 2008; Park et al., 2008; Dahmen et al., 2010; Stange et al., 2013) have clearly demonstrated a dependency of spatial tuning, and even spatial perception, on the preceding stimulus (specifically, on the properties of the stimulus and their temporal profile). It has become apparent that dynamic adaptation mechanisms act on spatial processing in the brainstem, including the MSO and LSO (Magnusson et al., 2008; Stange et al., 2013). The response levels of individual neurons are negatively correlated with their prior spiking activity, which is typical of gain modulation. Notably, this modulation, which acts on time scales of tens of milliseconds and can last for seconds, is mediated by $GABA_B$ receptor signaling, even though MSO cells are not themselves GABAergic. Instead, as already described, a di-synaptic feedback-loop exists, with MSO neurons innervating GABAergic neurons in the nearby SPN, which subsequently feed back onto the MSO (Figure 12.5; Stange et al., 2013).

The resulting activity-dependent rate adaptations do not shift the preferred ITDs of MSO neurons directly; that is, best ITDs are not altered. However, these modulations have significant consequences at the level of hemispheric population coding, because of the activity-dependent nature of the adaptation. For example, a strongly lateralized sound source will generate unequal adaptation in the two hemispheres, with pronounced rate adaptation only in the contralateral channel. Accordingly, this hemispheric asymmetry should shift the perceived location of a subsequently presented sound source (Figure 12.5). As noted earlier, Phillips and colleagues first tested this hypothesis in a number of psychophysical paradigms, and were able to demonstrate a pronounced shift in the perceived location of sound sources after prior presentation of a lateralized adapter in human listeners (Phillips & Hall, 2005; Vigneault-MacLean, Hall, & Phillips, 2007). Stange et al. (2013) have demonstrated that $GABA_B$-mediated rate adaptation in the MSO is sufficient to explain these shifts in human perception. Moreover, we have recently developed a new decoding model in which sound location is initially computed in both brain hemispheres independently between MSO and LSO and then combined to yield a hemispherically balanced code. This model not only closely captures the observed absolute localization errors caused by stimulus history, but also predicts a selective dilation and compression of perceptional space (Lingner et al., 2018). These model predictions are confirmed by improvement and degradation of spatial resolution in human listeners showing that the primary function of these perceptual shifts seems to be the relative segregation of the adapting and the subsequent sound source. Specifically, as the reported shifts in location are directed away from the adapter location, the perceived distance between the sound sources is increased relative to the actual distance (Lingner et al., 2018).

Taken together, these findings suggest that ITD coding in the MSO serves to encode the relative separation of concurrent or subsequent sound sources, rather than to provide an absolute representation of position in space.

References

Agapiou, J. P., & McAlpine, D. (2008). Low-frequency envelope sensitivity produces asymmetric binaural tuning curves. *Journal of Neurophysiology*, *100*(4), 2381–2396. doi: 10.1152/jn.90393.2008.

Agmon-Snir, H., Carr, C. E., & Rinzel, J. (1998). The role of dendrites in auditory coincidence detection. *Nature*, *393*(6682), 268–272. doi: 10.1038/30505.

Baumann, V. J. et al. (2013) Tonotopic organization of the hyperpolarization-activated current (Ih) in the mammalian medial superior olive. *Frontiers in Neural Circuits*, *7*, 117. doi: 10.3389/fncir.2013.00117.

Behrend, O. et al. (2002). Auditory response properties in the superior paraolivary nucleus of the gerbil. *Journal of Neurophysiology*, *87*(6), 2915–2928. doi: 10.1152/jn.2002.87.6.2915.

Beiderbeck, B. et al. (2018). Precisely timed inhibition facilitates action potential firing for spatial coding in the auditory brainstem. *Nature Communications*, *9*(1), 1771. doi: 10.1038/s41467-018-04210-y.

Benichoux, V. et al. (2015). Neural tuning matches frequency-dependent time differences between the ears. *eLife*, *4*. doi: 10.7554/eLife.06072.

Borst, J. G. G., & Soria van Hoeve, J. (2012). The calyx of Held synapse: From model synapse to auditory relay. *Annual Review of Physiology*, *74*, 199–224. doi: 10.1146/annurev-physiol-020911-153236.

Brand, A. et al. (2002). Precise inhibition is essential for microsecond interaural time difference coding. *Nature*, *417*(6888), 543–547. doi: 10.1038/417543a.

Caird, D., & Klinke, R. (1983). Processing of binaural stimuli by cat superior olivary complex neurons. *Experimental Brain Research*, *52*(3), 385–399.

Clark, G. M. (1969). Vesicle shape versus type of synapse in the nerve endings of the cat medial superior olive. *Brain Research*, *15*(2), 548–551.

Couchman, K., Grothe, B., & Felmy, F. (2010). Medial superior olivary neurons receive surprisingly few excitatory and inhibitory inputs with balanced strength and short-term dynamics. *Journal of Neuroscience*, *30*(50), pp. 17111–17121. doi: 10.1523/JNEUROSCI.1760-10.2010.

Couchman, K., Grothe, B., & Felmy, F. (2012). Functional localization of neurotransmitter receptors and synaptic inputs to mature neurons of the medial superior olive. *Journal of Neurophysiology*, *107*(4), 1186–1198. doi: 10.1152/jn.00586.2011.

Covey, E., Vater, M., & Casseday, J. H. (1991). Binaural properties of single units in the superior olivary complex of the mustached bat. *Journal of Neurophysiology*, *66*(3), 1080–1094. doi: 10.1152/jn.1991.66.3.1080.

Dahmen, J. C. et al. (2010). Adaptation to stimulus statistics in the perception and neural representation of auditory space. *Neuron*, *66*(6), 937–948. doi: 10.1016/j.neuron.2010.05.018.

Dasika, V. K., White, J. A., & Colburn, H. S. (2007). Simple models show the general advantages of dendrites in coincidence detection." *Journal of Neurophysiology*, *97*(5), 3449–3459. doi: 10.1152/jn.00669.2005.

Day, M. L., & Delgutte, B. (2013). Decoding sound source location and separation using neural population activity patterns. *Journal of Neuroscience*, *33*(40), 15837–15847. doi: 10.1523/JNEUROSCI.2034-13.2013.

Day, M. L., & Semple, M. N. (2011). Frequency-dependent interaural delays in the medial superior olive: Implications for interaural cochlear delays. *Journal of Neurophysiology*, *106*(4), 1985–1999. doi: 10.1152/jn.00131.2011.

Dietz, M., Marquardt, T., Stange, A., Pecka, M., Grothe, B., & McAlpine, D. (2014) Emphasis of spatial cues in the temporal fine structure during the rising segments of amplitude-modulated sounds II: single-neuron recordings. *Journal of Neurophysiology*, *111*(10), 1973–1985. doi: 10.1152/jn.00681.2013.

Fischer, L., Leibold, C., & Felmy, F. (2018). Resonance properties in auditory brainstem neurons. *Frontiers in Cellular Neuroscience*, *12*, 8. doi: 10.3389/fncel.2018.00008.

Fischl, M. J. et al. (2016). Physiology and anatomy of neurons in the medial superior olive of the mouse. *Journal of Neurophysiology*, *116*(6), 2676–2688. doi: 10.1152/jn.00523.2016.

Ford, M. C. et al. (2015). Tuning of Ranvier node and internode properties in myelinated axons to adjust action potential timing. *Nature Communications*, *6*, 8073. doi: 10.1038/ncomms9073.

Franken, T. P. et al. (2015). In vivo coincidence detection in mammalian sound localization generates phase delays. *Nature Neuroscience*, *18*(3), 444–452. doi: 10.1038/nn.3948.

Franken, T. P., Bremen, P., Joris, P. X. (2014). Coincidence detection in the medial superior olive: mechanistic implications of an analysis of input spiking patterns. *Frontiers in Neural Circuits*, *8*, 42. doi: 10.3389/fncir.2014.00042.

Getzmann, S. (2004). Spatial discrimination of sound sources in the horizontal plane following an adapter sound. *Hearing Research*, *191*(1–2), 14–20. doi: 10.1016/j.heares.2003.12.020.

Goldberg, J. M., & Brown, P. B. (1969). Response of binaural neurons of dog superior olivary complex to dichotic tonal stimuli: Some physiological mechanisms of sound localization. *Journal of Neurophysiology*, *32*(4), 613–636.

Goldwyn, J. H. et al. (2017). Signatures of somatic inhibition and dendritic excitation in auditory brainstem field potentials. *Journal of Neuroscience*, *37*(43), 10451–10467. doi: 10.1523/JNEUROSCI.0600-17.2017.

Goodman, D. F., Benichoux, V., & Brette, R. (2013). Decoding neural responses to temporal cues for sound localization. *eLife*, *2*, e01312. doi: 10.7554/eLife.01312.

Grothe, B. (1994). Interaction of excitation and inhibition in processing of pure tone and amplitude-modulated stimuli in the medial superior olive of the mustached bat. *Journal of Neurophysiology*, *71*(2), 706–721.

Grothe, B. (2000). The evolution of temporal processing in the medial superior olive, an auditory brainstem structure. *Progress in Neurobiology*, *61*(6), 581–610.

Grothe, B. et al. (1992). Monaural interaction of excitation and inhibition in the medial superior olive of the mustached bat: an adaptation for biosonar. *Proceedings of the National Academy of Sciences of the United States of America*, *89*(11), 5108–5112.

Grothe, B., & Park, T. J. (1998). Sensitivity to interaural time differences in the medial superior olive of a small mammal, the Mexican free-tailed bat." *Journal of Neuroscience*, *18*(16), 6608–6622.

Grothe, B., & Pecka, M. (2014). The natural history of sound localization in mammals—a story of neuronal inhibition. *Frontiers in Neural Circuits*, *8*, 116. doi: 10.3389/fncir.2014.00116.

Grothe, B., Pecka, M., & McAlpine, D. (2010). Mechanisms of sound localization in mammals. *Physiological Reviews*, *90*(3), 983–1012. doi: 10.1152/physrev.00026.2009.

Grothe, B., & Sanes, D. H. (1993). Bilateral inhibition by glycinergic afferents in the medial superior olive. *Journal of Neurophysiology*, *69*(4), 1192–1196.

Grothe, B., & Sanes, D. H. (1994). Synaptic inhibition influences the temporal coding properties of medial superior olivary neurons: An in vitro study. *The Journal of Neuroscience*, *14*(3 Pt. 2), 1701–1709.

Hancock, K. E., & Delgutte, B. (2004). A physiologically based model of interaural time difference discrimination. *Journal of Neuroscience*, *24*(32), 7110–7117. doi: 10.1523/JNEUROSCI.0762-04.2004.

Harnischfeger, G., Neuweiler, G., & Schlegel, P. (1985). Interaural time and intensity coding in superior olivary complex and inferior colliculus of the echolocating bat *Molossus ater*. *Journal of Neurophysiology*, *53*(1), 89–109.

Harper, N. S. et al. (2014). The neural code for auditory space depends on sound frequency and head size in an optimal manner. *PloS One*, *9*(11), p. e108154. doi: 10.1371/journal.pone.0108154.

Harper, N. S., & McAlpine, D. (2004). Optimal neural population coding of an auditory spatial cue. *Nature*, *430*(7000), 682–686. doi: 10.1038/nature02768.

van der Heijden, M. et al. (2013). Directional hearing by linear summation of binaural inputs at the medial superior olive." *Neuron*, *78*(5), 936–948. doi: 10.1016/j.neuron.2013.04.028.

Henkel, C. K., & Brunso-Bechtold, J. K. (1990). Dendritic morphology and development in the ferret medial superior olivary nucleus. *Journal of Comparative Neurology*, *294*(3), 377–388. doi: 10.1002/cne.902940307.

Jeffress, L. A. (1948). A place theory of sound localization. *Journal of Comparative and Physiological Psychology*, *41*(1), 35–39.

Jercog, P. E. et al. (2010). Asymmetric excitatory synaptic dynamics underlie interaural time difference processing in the auditory system. *PLoS Biology*, *8*(6), e1000406. doi: 10.1371/journal.pbio.1000406.

Joris, P. X. et al. (1994). Enhancement of neural synchronization in the anteroventral cochlear nucleus. I. Responses to tones at the characteristic frequency. *Journal of Neurophysiology*, *71*(3), 1022–1036.

Joris, P. X. et al. (2006). Binaural and cochlear disparities. *Proceedings of the National Academy of Sciences of the United States of America*, *103*(34), 12917–12922. doi: 10.1073/pnas.0601396103.

Joris, P. X., Smith, P. H., & Yin, T. C. (1998). Coincidence detection in the auditory system: 50 years after Jeffress. *Neuron*, *21*(6), 1235–1238.

Kapfer, C. et al. (2002). Experience-dependent refinement of inhibitory inputs to auditory coincidence-detector neurons. *Nature Neuroscience*, *5*(3), 247–253. doi: 10.1038/nn810.

Karino, S. et al. (2011). Axonal branching patterns as sources of delay in the mammalian auditory brainstem: a re-examination. *Journal of Neuroscience*, *31*(8), 3016–3031. doi: 10.1523/JNEUROSCI.5175-10.2011.

Khurana, S. et al. (2011). Dynamic interaction of Ih and IK-LVA during trains of synaptic potentials in principal neurons of the medial superior olive. *Journal of Neuroscience*, *31*(24), 8936–8947. doi: 10.1523/JNEUROSCI.1079-11.2011.

Kiss, A., & Majorossy, K. (1983). Neuron morphology and synaptic architecture in the medial superior olivary nucleus. Light- and electron microscope studies in the cat. *Experimental Brain Research*, *52*(3), 315–327.

Ko, K. W. et al. (2016). Serotonin modulates spike probability in the axon initial segment through HCN channels. *Nature Neuroscience*, *19*(6), 826–834. doi: 10.1038/nn.4293.

Kuba, H., Ishii, T. M., & Ohmori, H. (2006). Axonal site of spike initiation enhances auditory coincidence detection. *Nature*, *444*(7122), 1069–1072. doi: 10.1038/nature05347.

Kuwabara, N., & Zook, J. M. (1992). Projections to the medial superior olive from the medial and lateral nuclei of the trapezoid body in rodents and bats. *Journal of Comparative Neurology*, *324*(4), 522–538. doi: 10.1002/cne.903240406.

Lehnert, S. et al. (2014). Action potential generation in an anatomically constrained model of medial superior olive axons. *Journal of Neuroscience*, *34*(15), 5370–5384. doi: 10.1523/JNEUROSCI.4038-13.2014.

Leibold, C. (2010). Influence of inhibitory synaptic kinetics on the interaural time difference sensitivity in a linear model of binaural coincidence detection. *Journal of the Acoustical Society of America*, *127*(2), 931–942. doi: 10.1121/1.3282997.

Leibold, C., & van Hemmen, J. L. (2005). Spiking neurons learning phase delays: How mammals may develop auditory time-difference sensitivity. *Physical Review Letters*, *94*(16), 168102. doi: 10.1103/PhysRevLett.94.168102.

Lingner, A. et al. (2018). .A novel concept for dynamic adjustment of auditory space. *Scientific Reports*, *8*(1), 8335. doi: 10.1038/s41598-018-26690-0.

Loeb, G. E., White, M. W., & Merzenich, M. M. (1983). .Spatial cross-correlation: A proposed mechanism for acoustic pitch perception. *Biological Cybernetics*, *47*(3), 149–163.

Lüling, H. et al. (2011). Frequency-invariant representation of interaural time differences in mammals. *PLoS Computational Biology*, *7*(3), e1002013. doi: 10.1371/journal.pcbi.1002013.

Magnusson, A. K. et al. (2008). Retrograde GABA signaling adjusts sound localization by balancing excitation and inhibition in the brainstem. *Neuron*, *59*(1), 125–137. doi: 10.1016/j.neuron.2008.05.011.

Maier, J. K. et al. (2009). Context effects in the discriminability of spatial cues. *Journal of the Association for Research in Otolaryngology*, *11*(2), 319–328. doi: 10.1007/s10162-009-0200-0.

Mathews, P. J. et al. (2010). Control of submillisecond synaptic timing in binaural coincidence detectors by K(v)1 channels. *Nature Neuroscience*, *13*(5), 601–609. doi: 10.1038/nn.2530.

McAlpine, D., Jiang, D., Palmer, A. R. (2001). A neural code for low-frequency sound localization in mammals. *Nature Neuroscience*, *4*(4), 396–401. doi: 10.1038/86049.

Middlebrooks, J. C. et al. (1994). A panoramic code for sound location by cortical neurons. *Science*, *264*(5160), 842–844.

Mikiel-Hunter, J., Kotak, V., & Rinzel, J. (2016). High-Frequency Resonance in the Gerbil Medial Superior Olive. *PLoS Computational Biology*, *12*(11), e1005166. doi: 10.1371/journal.pcbi.1005166.

Morest, D. K. (1958). The collateral system of the medial nucleus of the trapezoid body of the cat, its neuronal architecture and relation to the olivo-cochlear bundle. *Brain Research*, *9*(2), 288–311.

Myoga, M. H. et al. (2014). Glycinergic inhibition tunes coincidence detection in the auditory brainstem. *Nature Communications*, *5*, 3790. doi: 10.1038/ncomms4790.

Park, T. J. et al. (2008). Dynamic changes in level influence spatial coding in the lateral superior olive. *Hearing Research*, *238*(1–2), 58–67. doi: 10.1016/j.heares.2007.10.009.

Pecka, M. et al. (2008). Interaural Time Difference Processing in the Mammalian Medial Superior Olive: The Role of Glycinergic Inhibition. *Journal of Neuroscience.*, *28*(27), 6914–6925. doi: 10.1523/JNEUROSCI.1660-08.2008.

Perkins, R. E. (1973). An electron microscopic study of synaptic organization in the medial superior olive of normal and experimental chinchillas. *The Journal of Comparative Neurology*, *148*(3), pp. 387–415. doi: 10.1002/cne.901480306.

Phillips, D. P., & Hall, S. E. (2005). Psychophysical evidence for adaptation of central auditory processors for interaural differences in time and level. *Hearing Research*, *202*(1–2), 188–199. doi: 10.1016/j.heares.2004.11.001.

Plauška, A., Borst, J. G., & van der Heijden, M. (2016). Predicting binaural responses from monaural responses in the gerbil medial superior olive. *Journal of Neurophysiology*, *115*(6), 2950–2963. doi: 10.1152/jn.01146.2015.

Plauška, A., van der Heijden, M., & Borst, J. G. G. (2017). A test of the stereausis hypothesis for sound localization in mammals. *Journal of Neuroscience*, *37*(30), 7278–7289. doi: 10.1523/JNEUROSCI.0233-17.2017.

Rall, W. (1962). Theory of physiological properties of dendrites. *Annals of the New York Academy of Sciences*, *96*, 1071–1092.

Ramón y Cajal, S. (1909). *Histologie du système nerveux de l'homme & des vertébrés.* Paris, France: Maloine. Available at: http://archive.org/details/histologiedusyst01ram (Accessed: 30 May 2018).

Rautenberg, P. L., Grothe, B. and Felmy, F. (2009). Quantification of the three-dimensional morphology of coincidence detector neurons in the medial superior olive of gerbils during late postnatal development. *The Journal of Comparative Neurology*, *517*(3), 385–396. doi: 10.1002/cne.22166.

Remme, M. W. H. et al. (2014). Subthreshold resonance properties contribute to the efficient coding of auditory spatial cues. *Proceedings of the National Academy of Sciences of the United States of America*, *111*(22), E2339–2348. doi: 10.1073/pnas.1316216111.

Roberts, M. T., Seeman, S. C., & Golding, N. L. (2013). A mechanistic understanding of the role of feedforward inhibition in the mammalian sound localization circuitry. *Neuron*, *78*(5), 923–935. doi: 10.1016/j.neuron.2013.04.022.

Roberts, M. T., Seeman, S. C., & Golding, N. L. (2014). The relative contributions of MNTB and LNTB neurons to inhibition in the medial superior olive assessed through single and paired recordings. *Frontiers in Neural Circuits*, *8*, 49. doi: 10.3389/fncir.2014.00049.

Salin, P. A. et al. (1996). Distinct short-term plasticity at two excitatory synapses in the hippocampus. *Proceedings of the National Academy of Sciences of the United States of America*, *93*(23), 13304–13309.

Schroeder, M. R. (1977). New viewpoints in binaural interactions. In: E. F. Evans, J. P. Wilson, (Eds), *Psychophysics and physiology of hearing*. New York: Academic Press; 455–467.

Scott, L. L., Hage, T. A., & Golding, N. L. (2007). Weak action potential backpropagation is associated with high-frequency axonal firing capability in principal neurons of the gerbil medial superior olive. *Journal of Physiology*, *583*(Pt 2), 647–661. doi: 10.1113/jphysiol.2007.136366.

Scott, L. L., Mathews, P. J., & Golding, N. L. (2005). Posthearing developmental refinement of temporal processing in principal neurons of the medial superior olive. *Journal of Neuroscience*, *25*(35), 7887–7895. doi: 10.1523/JNEUROSCI.1016-05.2005.

Seidl, A. H., & Grothe, B. (2005). Development of sound localization mechanisms in the Mongolian gerbil is shaped by early acoustic experience. *Journal of Neurophysiology*, *94*(2), 1028–1036. doi: 10.1152/jn.01143.2004.

Seidl, A. H., Rubel, E. W., & Harris, D. M. (2010). Mechanisms for adjusting interaural time differences to achieve binaural coincidence detection. *Journal of Neuroscience*, *30*(1), 70–80. doi: 10.1523/JNEUROSCI.3464-09.2010.

Seidl, A. H., & Rubel, E. W. (2016). "Systematic and differential myelination of axon collaterals in the mammalian auditory brainstem," *Glia*, *64*(4), 487–494. doi: 10.1002/glia.22941.

Shamma, S. A., Shen, N. M., & Gopalaswamy, P. (1989). Stereausis: Binaural processing without neural delays. *Journal of the Acoustical Society of America*, *86*(3), 989–1006.

Smith, A. J., Owens, S., & Forsythe, I. D. (2000). Characterisation of inhibitory and excitatory postsynaptic currents of the rat medial superior olive. *Journal of Physiology*, *529*(Pt 3), 681–698.

Smith, D. J., & Rubel, E. W. (1979). Organization and development of brain stem auditory nuclei of the chicken: Dendritic gradients in nucleus laminaris. *Journal of Comparative Neurology*, *186*(2), 213–239. doi: 10.1002/cne.901860207.

Smith, P. H. (1995). Structural and functional differences distinguish principal from nonprincipal cells in the guinea pig MSO slice. *Journal of Neurophysiology*, *73*(4), 1653–1667. doi: 10.1152/jn.1995.73.4.1653.

Spirou, G. A., & Berrebi, A. S. (1997). Glycine immunoreactivity in the lateral nucleus of the trapezoid body of the cat. *Journal of Comparative Neurology*, *383*(4), 473–488.

Spirou, G. A., Rowland, K. C., & Berrebi, A. S. (1998). Ultrastructure of neurons and large synaptic terminals in the lateral nucleus of the trapezoid body of the cat. *Journal of Comparative Neurology*, *398*(2), 257–272.

Spitzer, M. W., & Semple, M. N. (1995). Neurons sensitive to interaural phase disparity in gerbil superior olive: Diverse monaural and temporal response properties. *Journal of Neurophysiology*, *73*(4), 1668–1690. doi: 10.1152/jn.1995.73.4.1668.

Stange, A. et al. (2013). Adaptation in sound localization: From GABAB receptor-mediated synaptic modulation to perception. *Nature Neuroscience*, *16*(12), 1840–1847. doi: 10.1038/nn.3548.

Stange-Marten, A. et al. (2017). Input timing for spatial processing is precisely tuned via constant synaptic delays and myelination patterns in the auditory brainstem." *Proceedings of the National Academy of Sciences of the United States of America*. *114*(24), E4851–E4858. doi: 10.1073/pnas.1702290114.

Stecker, G. C., & Middlebrooks, J. C. (2003). Distributed coding of sound locations in the auditory cortex. *Biological Cybernetics*, *89*(5), 341–349. doi: 10.1007/s00422-003-0439-1.

Stotler, W. A. (1953). An experimental study of the cells and connections of the superior olivary complex of the cat. *Journal of Comparative Neurology*, *98*(3), 401–431.

Stuart, G., & Sakmann, B. (1995). Amplification of EPSPs by axosomatic sodium channels in neocortical pyramidal neurons. *Neuron*, *15*(5), 1065–1076.

Svirskis, G. et al. (2002). Enhancement of signal-to-noise ratio and phase locking for small inputs by a low-threshold outward current in auditory neurons. *Journal of Neuroscience*, *22*(24), 11019–11025.

Svirskis, G., Dodla, R., & Rinzel, J. (2003). Subthreshold outward currents enhance temporal integration in auditory neurons. *Biological Cybernetics*, *89*(5), pp. 333–340. doi: 10.1007/s00422-003-0438-2.

Tollin, D. J. (2003). The lateral superior olive: A functional role in sound source localization. *Neuroscientist*, 9(2),. 127–143.

Tollin, D. J., & Yin, T. C. T. (2005). Interaural phase and level difference sensitivity in low-frequency neurons in the lateral superior olive. *Journal of Neuroscience*, 25(46), 10648–10657. doi: 10.1523/JNEUROSCI.1609-05.2005.

Vigneault-MacLean, B. K., Hall, S. E., & Phillips, D. P. (2007). The effects of lateralized adaptors on lateral position judgements of tones within and across frequency channels. *Hearing Research*, *224*(1–2), 93–100. doi: 10.1016/j.heares.2006.12.001.

Wei, L. et al. (2017). Enhancement of phase-locking in rodents. I. An axonal recording study in gerbil. *Journal of Neurophysiology*, *118*(4), 2009–2023. doi: 10.1152/jn.00194.2016.

Werner-Reiss, U., & Groh, J. M. (2008). A rate code for sound azimuth in monkey auditory cortex: Implications for human neuroimaging studies. *Journal of Neuroscience*, *28*(14), 3747–3758. doi: 10.1523/JNEUROSCI.5044-07.2008.

Werthat, F. et al. (2008). Experience-dependent refinement of the inhibitory axons projecting to the medial superior olive. *Developmental Neurobiology*, *68*(13), 1454–1462. doi: 10.1002/dneu.20660.

Xu-Friedman, M. A., & Regehr, W. G. (2005). Dynamic-clamp analysis of the effects of convergence on spike timing. II. Few synaptic inputs. *Journal of Neurophysiology*, *94*(4), 2526–2534. doi: 10.1152/jn.01308.2004.

Yin, T. C., & Chan, J. C. (1990). Interaural time sensitivity in medial superior olive of cat. *Journal of Neurophysiology*, *64*(2), 465–488.

Zhou, Y., Carney, L. H., & Colburn, H. S. (2005). A model for interaural time difference sensitivity in the medial superior olive: interaction of excitatory and inhibitory synaptic inputs, channel dynamics, and cellular morphology. *Journal of Neuroscience*, 25(12), pp. 3046–3058. doi: 10.1523/JNEUROSCI.3064-04.2005.

CHAPTER 13

LATERAL SUPERIOR OLIVE

Organization, Development, and Plasticity

ECKHARD FRIAUF, ELISA G. KRÄCHAN, AND NICOLAS I.C. MÜLLER

Abstract

Auditory neurons in the mammalian brainstem are involved in several basic computation processes essential for survival; for example, sound localization. Differences in sound intensity between the two ears, so-called interaural level differences (ILDs), provide important spatial cues for localizing sound in the horizontal plane, particularly for animals with high-frequency hearing. The earliest center of ILD detection is the lateral superior olive (LSO), a prominent component of the superior olivary complex (SOC) in the medulla oblongata. LSO neurons receive input from both ears of excitatory and inhibitory nature and perform a subtraction-like process. The LSO has become a model system for studies addressing inhibitory synapses, map formation, and neural plasticity. This review aims to provide an overview of several facets of the LSO, focusing on its functional and anatomical organization, including development and plasticity. Understanding this important ILD detector is fundamental in multiple ways—among others, to analyze central auditory processing disorders and central presbyacusis.

Keywords: activity-dependent processes, auditory brainstem, excitatory neurotransmission, inhibitory neurotransmission, interaural level differences, map formation, sound localization, synaptic fidelity, synaptic plasticity, synaptic refinement

Organization of the Lateral Superior Olive

The lateral superior olive (LSO) is a conspicuous structure in the medullary brainstem of mammals and a principal component of the superior olivary complex (SOC), the first major site of input convergence from both ears. The SOC consists of three principal nuclei, namely the LSO, the medial superior olive (MSO), and the medial nucleus of the trapezoid body (MNTB). LSO neurons play a distinct role in binaural hearing (Boudreau & Tsuchitani, 1968). They are involved in sound source localization (Tollin, 2003; Tollin & Yin, 2002), which, according to the classic Duplex theory (Rayleigh, 1907), employs time differences in incoming sound of low frequency and intensity differences of high-frequency sound (Casseday & Neff, 1973; Middlebrooks, 2015). LSO neurons compute intensity differences occurring at the two tympanic membranes (eardrums; Figure 13.1A; Irvine, 1992; Masterton, Jane, & Diamond, 1967; Tsuchitani & Johnson, 1991). For interaural level difference (ILD) coding beyond the LSO, see Yin & Kuwada (2010). Neurons in the anatomically adjacent MSO are thought to exploit interaural time differences (ITD; see chapter by Grothe et al., this volume).

An animal's ability to determine the position of a sound source is a crucial step in auditory scene analysis and toward appropriate behavior. The sound shadow cast by an animal's head leads to a situation in which the sound at the shadowed ear is less intense than the sound arriving at the tympanic membrane of the other ear (Figure 13.1B). ILDs are detected by the auditory hindbrain via binaural processing mechanisms. This greatly facilitates localization of the direction of sound sources. When a sound source is positioned at an angle of ~90° from the midline, the ILD in humans amounts to 3 dB and 35 dB for frequencies of 200 Hz and 10 kHz, respectively (Middlebrooks, Makous, & Green, 1989; Shaw & Vaillancourt, 1985). The threshold of human listeners for ILD detection in high-frequency tones is ~1 dB (Middlebrooks & Green, 1991). In general, the ILD is larger when the sound is of higher than lower frequency. High-frequency sound signals have short waves, and obstacles, such as the head, reflect these waves rather than diffracting them.

The human head size relates to an interaural distance (distance between the two ears) of ~20 cm. In small mammals, such as rats, mice, or bats, the interaural distance can be < 2 cm. Acoustic shadowing becomes effective if the wavelength (λ) of a sound signal is shorter than the head size. For an interaural distance of 2 cm, the sound frequency (f) must therefore be above 17 kHz to generate analyzable ILDs ($f = v / \lambda$; $v = 340$ m/s). The aforementioned small animals encounter ILDs as large as 40 dB for sound stimuli in the 10–90 kHz range (Figure 13.1C; Greene, Anbuhl, Williams, & Tollin, 2014; Grothe & Pecka, 2014; Harnischfeger, Neuweiler, & Schlegel, 1985; Koka, Read, & Tollin, 2008; Maki & Furukawa, 2005). Noticeably, such ultrasound frequencies are physiological stimuli for small animals, because evolutionary pressure has favored small head size with high-frequency hearing (Heffner, Koay, & Heffner, 2001). Studies of the spatial cues employed by mice for sound localization are rare and have not focused on ILD (Chen, Cain, & Jen, 1995). This is somewhat surprising because, with the multitude of available (deaf) mutants, mice have become a key species in hearing research over the past two decades or so (Malmierca & Ryugo, 2012).

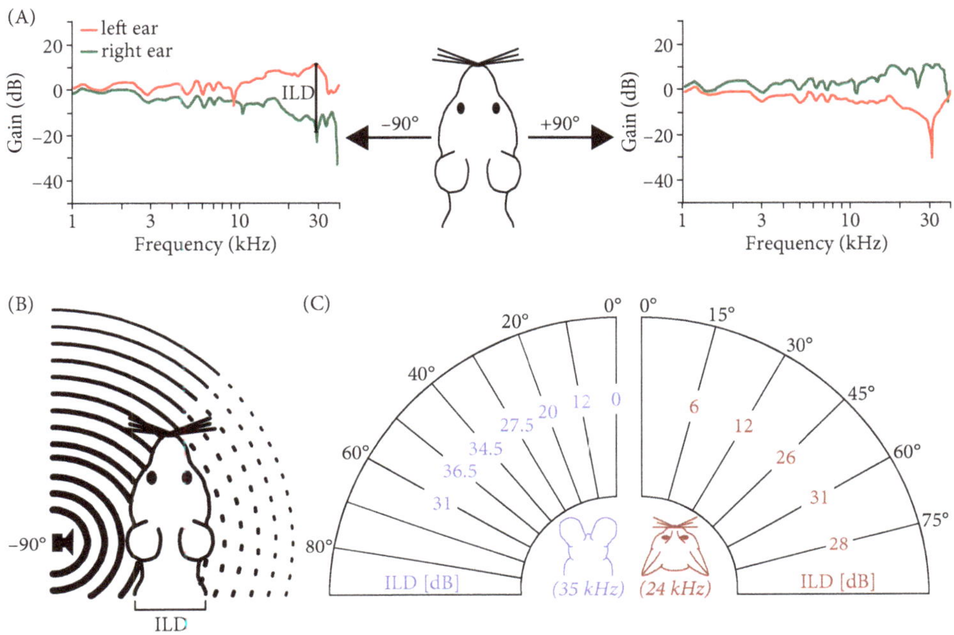

FIGURE 13.1. ILDs are the physical basis for localizing high-frequency sound sources. **A.** Head-related transfer functions (HRTFs) in a rat for left (red) and right ear (green) when stimulated with a loudspeaker mounted at −90° (left) or +90° (right) azimuth. ILDs are substantial at high frequencies, amounting to > 20 dB. For HRTFs in a cat, see Musicant et al. (1990). **B.** ILDs originate from the sound shadow casted by the animal's head. C ILDs for various azimuthal angles obtained in a bat (left) and a cat (right) for a 35 kHz tone and a 24 kHz tone, respectively.

Besides the acoustic shadowing effect of the head, the dimension, shape, and position of the pinnae contribute substantially to ILD (Chen et al., 1995). Interestingly, and in contrast to humans, many mammalian species feature vigorous pinnae movements. By changing pinna directionality, they can actively modulate ILDs, thereby optimizing listening conditions (Friauf & Herbert, 1985; Populin & Yin, 1998; Ruhland, Jones, & Yin, 2015; Walker, Peremans, & Hallam, 1998; Young, Rice, & Tong, 1996). Mice can resolve differences of ~15° at 15 kHz, which corresponds to an ILD of < 1 dB (Chen et al., 1995; Ehret & Dreyer, 1984; Walker et al., 1998). Thus, their ILD hearing capability is very well established.

Anatomical Organization of the LSO

Virtually every mammal possesses an LSO (well, in fact, two LSOs), but the size and the shape vary considerably across species (Figure 13.2). Across 53 species analyzed (Glendenning & Masterton, 1998), the volume of the LSO, in relation to the whole brain size, ranges from 0.8% in mice (0.32 mm^3/0.4 g) to 0.00026% in humans (3.22 mm^3/ 1,240 g). Neuron numbers differ more than 7-fold across species, from less than 1,000 in hamsters and squirrels to more than 7,000 in the orangutan (Hilbig, Beil, Hilbig, Call, & Bidmon, 2009; Irving & Harrison, 1967). The LSO of cats, rats, and mice comprises about 3,400, 1,400, and 1,200–1,600 neurons, respectively (Casey, 1990; Hirtz et al., 2011; Irving & Harrison, 1967; Satheesh et al., 2012). The human LSO is composed of ~2,000 neurons (Hilbig et al., 2009).

In transverse brainstem sections, the LSO of lower eutherian mammals is easily recognizable by its distinctive convoluted, convexo-concaved S-shape (cat, chinchilla, dog, mouse, rat; Table 13.1). In cats and dogs, the lateral limb extends dorsally, whereas the medial limb extends ventrally. The opposite holds for rats. In some species, authors have attributed a U-shape to the LSO (gerbil, guinea pig, mouse: Bazwinsky-Wutschke, Härtig, Kretzschmar, & Rübsamen, 2016; Hirtz et al., 2012; Nothwang, 2016; Rosengauer et al., 2012; Sanes, Merickel, & Rubel, 1989; Sterenborg et al., 2010), an N-shape (hamster: Reuss et al., 2009), a W-shape (ferret: Moore, Russell, & Cathcart, 1995), or a drop-shape (opossum: Bazwinsky-Wutschke et al., 2016; Willard & Martin, 1983). In the galago, a lemuriform monkey and extant example of the lowest level of primate organization, the LSO is small and not S-shaped. Instead, it is ovoid with indistinct convolutions (Moore, 2000). In the common marmoset, a more advanced simian monkey, the LSO is an irregularly oval nucleus with some indication of convolutions (Illing, Kraus, & Miçhler, 2000; Moore, 2000). The LSO of the rhesus macaque, another simian monkey, is not clearly S-shaped (Harrison & Irving, 1966; Hilbig et al., 2009); however, it is described to be more convoluted than that of non-primates (Bazwinsky, Bidmon, Zilles, & Hilbig, 2005). In the gibbon, an ape, the LSO is small and indistinct (Moore, 2000), and similar findings were made in bonobos, chimpanzees, and orangutans (Hilbig et al., 2009). With its reduced size, the LSO of these apes is very similar to the human LSO, which is also small and roughly oval or h-shaped in some cases (Kulesza, 2007; Moore, 2000).

Cytology of the LSO

The LSO of placental mammals is composed of a variety of neuronal classes. Overall, up to seven cell types have been described (Rietzel & Friauf, 1998). By far the most dominant class are principal neurons, which comprise ~75% of the population (Helfert & Schwartz, 1987). These neurons have fusiform somata and eccentric nuclei (Figure 13.3). Primary dendrites emerge from the two somatic poles and, in the coronal plane, tend to be oriented at right angles to the tonotopic axis (Cant, 1984; Helfert & Schwartz, 1987;

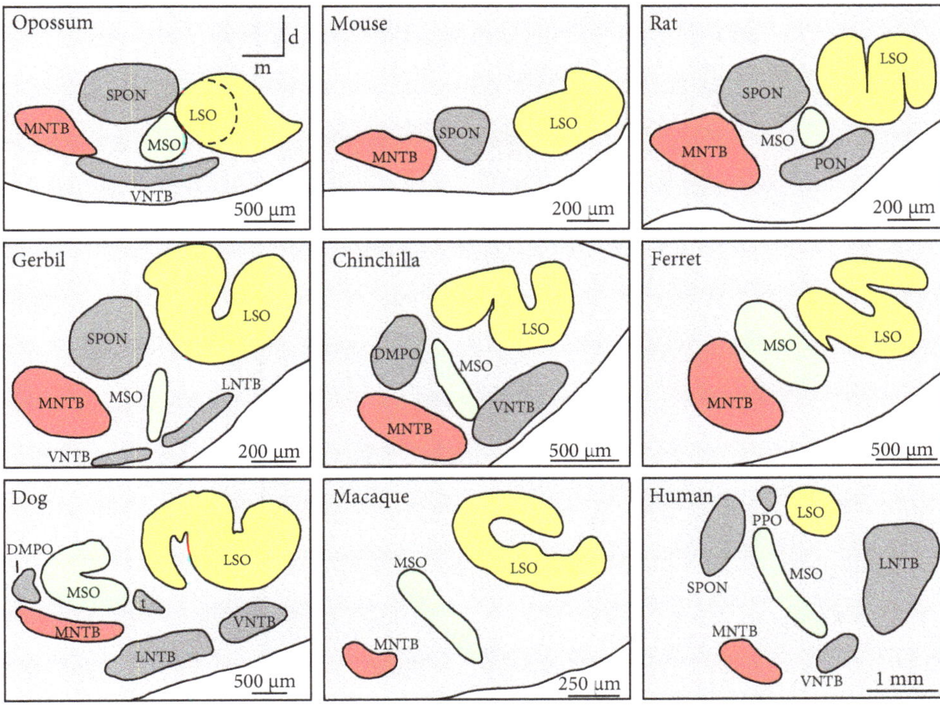

FIGURE 13.2. Anatomical organization of LSO, depicting the heterogeneity in shape and size across species. Schematic overview of SOCs in transverse brainstem sections from nine mammals. Principal nuclei are LSO (yellow), MNTB (red), and MSO (green).

Redrawn from: opossum (Willard & Martin, 1983), Copyright © 1983, with permission from Elsevier; mouse (Hirtz et al., 2011); rat (Srinivasan, Friauf, & Löhrke, 2004), Copyright © 2004, with permission from Elsevier; gerbil, reprinted by permission from Springer Nature (Bazwinsky-Wutschke, Härtig, Kretzschmar, & Rübsamen, 2016), Copyright © 2016; chinchilla (Azeredo et al., 1999), Copyright © 1999, with permission from Elsevier; ferret, reprinted by permission from Springer Nature (Henkel & Gabriele, 1999), Copyright © 2016; dog (Fech, Calderon-Garciduenas, & Kulesza, 2017), Copyright © 2017, with permission from Elsevier; macaque (Hilbig, Beil, Hilbig, Call, & Bidmon, 2009); human (Kulesza, 2008), Copyright © 2008, with permission from Elsevier.

Ollo & Schwartz, 1979; Rietzel & Friauf, 1998; Schofield & Cant, 1991). These dendrites branch extensively and extend over a substantial rostro-caudal distance, resulting in disc-shaped dendritic trees in parasagittal or horizontal sections (Helfert & Schwartz, 1986; Pickles, 1982; Scheibel & Scheibel, 1974).

Axon terminals on LSO principal neurons are in the form of conventional boutons whose size is quite large. Electron microscopy studies have shown that, on average, 74% of the somatic surface are apposed to such bouton-type synaptic endings (Helfert & Schwartz, 1986) and that these perisomatic terminals contain flattened synaptic vesicles and form symmetric synaptic contacts, indicative of an inhibitory transmitter phenotype (Brunso-Bechtold, Linville, & Henkel, 1994; Cant, 1984). Indeed, immunocytochemistry employing antibodies against glycine has demonstrated punctate labeling on LSO neurons, suggestive of immunopositive presynaptic terminals

Table 13.1. **Comparison of LSO size, contour, and highest audible frequency across a variety of species**

Species	LSO Size	LSO Contour in Transverse Sections	References	HAF @ 60 dB SPL* [kHz]
Bat (several species)	Large	S-shaped V-shaped	Grothe & Park, 2000; Harrison & Irving, 1966	64–120
Bonobo	Small	Oval	Hilbig et al., 2009	?
Cat	Large	S-shaped	Goldberg & Brown, 1968; Greene, Lomakin, & Davis, 2010; Grothe & Park, 2000; Hackney, 1987; Helfert & Schwartz, 1986; Moore, 2000; Scheibel & Scheibel, 1974; Tollin, 2003; Tsuchitani & Boudreau, 1966	79
Chimpanzee	Small	Elongated	Hilbig et al., 2009	25
Chinchilla	Large	W-shaped	Harrison & Irving, 1966	32.5
Dog	Large	S-shaped	Goldberg & Brown, 1968	45
Dolphin (porpoise)	Large	W-shaped	Harrison & Irving, 1966	136 (in H_2O)
Ferret	Large	S-shaped V-shaped	Moore et al., 1995; Rooney, Kavanagh, & Kelly, 1991	44
Galago	Small	Ovoid	Moore, 2000	68
Gerbil	Large	U-shaped	Bazwinsky-Wutschke et al., 2016; Fukui & Raphael, 2013; Nordeen, Killackey, & Kitzes, 1983; Radtke-Schuller, Seeler, & Grothe, 2015; Sanes et al., 1989	58

Table 13.1. **Continued**

Species	LSO Size	LSO Contour in Transverse Sections	References	HAF @ 60 dB SPL* [kHz]
Gibbon	Small/large	Indistinct	Hilbig et al., 2009; Moore, 2000	?
Guinea pig	Large	U-shaped	Harrison & Irving, 1966; Nothwang, 2016	49
Hamster	Large	N-shaped	Reuss et al., 2009	46.5
Hedgehog	Large	U-shaped	Harrison & Irving, 1966	59
Human	Small	roughly oval, h-shaped	Hilbig et al., 2009; Kulesza, 2007; Moore, 2000; Weinrich, Sonntag, Arendt, & Morawski, 2018	18
Macaque	Small/large	Unclear	Harrison & Irving, 1966; Moore, 2000; Hilbig et al., 2009	34.5
Marmoset		Oval	Moore, 2000	36
Mouse	large	S-shaped U-shaped	Harrison & Irving, 1966; Hirtz et al., 2012; McCullagh, Salcedo, Huntsman, & Klug, 2017; Nothwang, 2016; Ollo & Schwartz, 1979; Rosengauer et al., 2012; Sterenborg et al., 2010	88-92
Opossum (2 species)	Large	drop-shaped	Bazwinsky-Wutschke et al., 2016; Brownell, Manis, & Ritz, 1979	68, 76
Orangutan	Large	Roughly oval	Hilbig et al., 2009	?

(*continued*)

Table 13.1. **Continued**

Species	LSO Size	LSO Contour in Transverse Sections	References	HAF @ 60 dB SPL* [kHz]
Rat	Large	S-shaped	Grothe & Park, 2000; Harrison & Irving, 1966; Gillespie, Kim, & Kandler, 2005; Harrison & Warr, 1962; Kraus & Illing, 2004; Löhrke, Srinivasan, Oberhofer, Doncheva, & Friauf, 2005; Saldana & Berrebi, 2000; Vitten, Reusch, Friauf, & Löhrke, 2004	68

HAF = highest audible frequency at 60 dB_{SPL}. *Values summarized in Koay, Heffner, & Heffner, 1998, Heffner & Heffner, 2010, and Osmanski & Wang, 2011.

(Helfert, Bonneau, Wenthold, & Altschuler, 1989; Wenthold, Huie, Altschuler, & Reeks, 1987), and immunogold labeling has confirmed a glycinergic phenotype in terminals containing flattened vesicles (Helfert et al., 1992). In contrast, terminals with round synaptic vesicles contact relatively thin and distal dendrites via asymmetric synaptic junctions and are associated with glutamate. A glycinergic phenotype has also been demonstrated in quantitative autoradiography studies that revealed very heavy ^{3}H-strychnine binding in the LSO (Glendenning & Baker, 1988), with ~4-fold higher labeling in the high-frequency than in the low-frequency region (Sanes, Geary, Wooten, & Rubel, 1987). Immunohistochemistry has demonstrated the presence of glycine receptors (GlyRs), which densely encrust the somata and proximal dendrites of adult LSO principal cells (Friauf, Hammerschmidt, & Kirsch, 1997; Sato, Shiraishi, Nakagawa, Kuriyama, & Altschuler, 2000).

Another protein characteristic at glycinergic synapses, the glycine transporter 2 (GlyT2), is also abundant in the LSO (Friauf, Aragon, Löhrke, Westenfelder, & Zafra, 1999). Regarding the excitatory input to the LSO, high transcript levels of the glutamate receptor subunits GluA3 and $GluA4_{flop}$ have been described (Caicedo & Eybalin, 1999; Schmid, Guthmann, Ruppersberg, & Herbert, 2001). These subunits provide very rapid kinetics as well as high Ca^{2+} permeability to glutamate receptors of the AMPA (α-amino-3-hydroxy-5-methyl-4-isoxazolepropionic acid) type (Raman, Zhang, & Trussell, 1994).

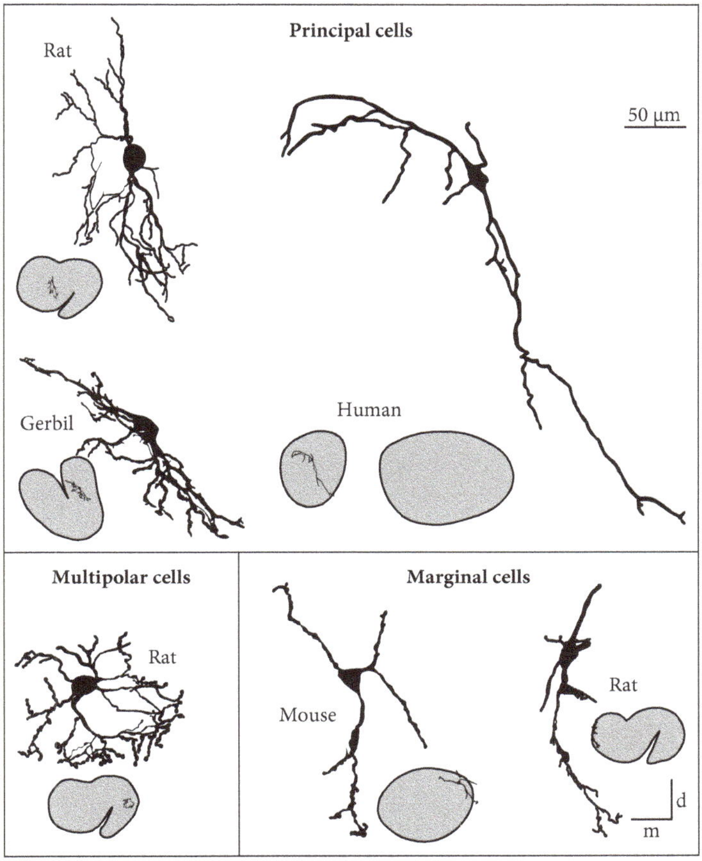

FIGURE 13.3. Cytology of LSO neurons in different species. Soma-dendritic reconstructions of three major cell types, illustrating differences in soma shape and dendritic arbors. Insets depict position and orientation of each neuron in the respective LSO.

Redrawn from: rat (Rietzel & Friauf, 1998), Copyright © 1998 Wiley-Liss, Inc.; mouse (Ollo & Schwartz, 1979), Copyright © 1979 Wiley-Liss, Inc.; gerbil (Sanes, Song, & Tyson, 1992), Copyright © 1992, with permission from Elsevier; human (Kulesza, 2007), Copyright © 2007, with permission from Elsevier.

Various subunits of N-methyl-D-aspartate receptors (NMDARs) are abundant in the LSO, namely GluN1 (Nakagawa, Sato, Shiraishi, Kuriyama, & Altschuler, 2000) and GluN2A-2D (Munemoto et al., 1998; Sato, Nakagawa, Kuriyama, & Altschuler, 1999). NMDARs assemble as heteromers endowed with distinct properties, are developmentally regulated, and play crucial roles in synaptic plasticity (Alexander et al., 2017; Paoletti, Bellone, & Zhou, 2013). Together, LSO principal cells are equipped with fast gating receptors that render them suited to preserving timing information (Rothman & Manis, 2003). Moreover, the diversity in NMDAR subunits predicts considerable pharmacological differences.

The glycinergic and glutamatergic inputs to LSO principal cells are also demonstrated by immunofluorescence studies employing a variety of presynaptic (e.g., vesicular glutamate transporters VGluT1 and VGluT3, GlyT2) and postsynaptic marker proteins (e.g., GlyRα1). The intensity of the immunosignals, together with the perisomatic location of the glycinergic axon terminals, is indicative of powerful synaptic strength. Serial block face scanning electron microscopy has shown that MNTB axon terminals contacting the soma of a single LSO neuron, presumably a principal cell, have several large boutons (diameter 3.7 μm), most of which contain several (up to 11) active zones (Gjoni, Aguet, Sahlender, Knott, & Schneggenburger, 2018). These large and multi-active-zone boutons probably provide the ultrastructural basis for strong inhibition caused by the MNTB-LSO synapses. Concerning the transmitter phenotype of LSO principal cells, the neurons are equipped with glutamate and glycine (Altschuler & Shore, 2010). Glutamatergic LSO neurons tend to project into the contralateral inferior colliculus (IC), whereas glycinergic neurons project into the ipsilateral IC (details in the section "Efferent Projections from the LSO").

Multipolar and marginal cells represent the other two major cell types in the LSO (Majorossy & Kiss, 1990). Multipolar neurons (~11% of the population) have round somata and 3–6 primary dendrites that can originate from all parts of the soma and branch repetitively, giving rise to 3-dimensional stellate dendritic trees (Figure 13.3). Marginal cells are the largest type, composing ~4% of the population (Helfert & Schwartz, 1986), and are primarily located along the border of the LSO (Figure 13.3). Synaptic terminals around their somata are similar in number and type to those found at principal neurons. Despite the peripheral location of their somata, their dendrites appear to stay within the nuclear area (Ollo & Schwartz, 1979; Rietzel & Friauf, 1998). Both γ-amino butyric acid (GABA) and glycine have been identified in somata of marginal cells (Korada & Schwartz, 1999), implying that many, if not all, of them are inhibitory neurons. Whereas physiological studies have concentrated on LSO principal cells, we know relatively little about the functional properties of the other types.

The LSO also contains neurons that send descending projections into the cochlea via the olivo-cochlear bundle (Warr & Boche, 2003). Because of their lateral location in the SOC, they belong to the lateral olivo-cochlear complex (LOC), which shows some interspecies differences (Aschoff & Ostwald, 1987; Warr, Beck Boche, Ye, & Kim, 2002). In rodents, the somata of LOC neurons are scattered in and around the LSO. Those located within the LSO are spherical, and their dendrites are oriented perpendicular to the curvature of the nucleus, similar to LSO principal cells (Vetter & Mugnaini, 1992). In "Functional Properties of LSO Neurons in Vitro" we will show that the LSO principal cells and LOC neurons are also physiologically distinct.

Effects of aging on the cytoarchitecture of the LSO have been analyzed in Fischer 344 rats, which, like most humans, slowly lose their hearing with age. In these animals, the LSO maintains a stable neuron number between 3 and 30 months of age, although there is a significant reduction of the neuron number in the MNTB (Casey, 1990). In Sprague-Dawley rats, loss of MNTB principal cells is even more severe than in Fisher 344 rats (34% vs. 8%; Casey & Feldman, 1982). As the LSO has remained unaddressed in this strain, whether massive cell loss in an input nucleus would affect the aging LSO remains an open question.

Afferent Projections to the LSO

The right half of Figure 13.4A depicts a general summary of the axonal projections into the LSO. From the cochlear nuclear complex (CNC), LSO principal neurons receive excitatory (glutamatergic) input from spherical bushy cells (SBCs) located in the ipsilateral anteroventral cochlear nucleus (AVCN). LSO principal neurons also receive inhibitory (glycinergic) input from principal cells of the ipsilateral MNTB (Bledsoe et al., 1990; Moore & Caspary, 1983; Sommer, Lingenhöhl, & Friauf, 1993; Spangler, Warr, & Henkel, 1985), which receive excitatory input from globular bushy cells (GBCs) of the contralateral AVCN (Figure 13.4B). Thus, inputs from the ipsilateral and the contralateral ear converge on single LSO neurons. In all mammals investigated, these inputs show a systematic medial-to-lateral, high-to-low best frequency arrangement termed cochleotopy or tonotopy (Figure 13.4B). The area devoted to high frequencies is disproportionately large in the LSO. The AVCN and MNTB afferents to the LSO display no polarity; rather, they terminate on both sides of the spindle-shaped somata (Glendenning, Hutson, Nudo, & Masterton, 1985). This is in contrast to the MSO, where the binaural inputs show a sharp polarity by terminating on homolateral dendrites (afferents from the right AVCN form synapses with laterally oriented dendrites in the ipsilateral MSO and with medially oriented dendrites in the contralateral MSO).

Aside from the elegant yet simplistic ipsilateral-excitatory (EI)/contralateral-inhibitory input scheme underlying ILD sensitivity (Figure 13.4B), LSO neurons receive inputs from cells other than SBCs and MNTB principal neurons. These inputs are provided by GBCs (Friauf & Ostwald, 1988; Kuwabara & Zook, 1991; Smith, Joris, Carney, & Yin, 1991) and by planar multipolar neurons (Darrow, Benson, & Brown, 2012; Doucet & Ryugo, 2003, 2006), residing in the ipsilateral ventral cochlear nucleus (VCN; Figure 13.4A). Projections from the ipsilateral posteroventral cochlear nucleus (PVCN) are tonotopically organized (Thompson & Thompson, 1987). LOC neurons receive excitatory and inhibitory inputs, but with longer latencies and slower kinetics than LSO principal cells (Adam, Finlayson, & Schwarz, 2001; Adam, Schwarz, & Finlayson, 1999; Fujino, Koyano, & Ohmori, 1997; Sterenborg et al., 2010). It is assumed that the excitatory input is preferentially provided by planar multipolar neurons in the cochlear nucleus (CN), which have relatively thin axons (Gomez-Alvarez & Saldana, 2016; Oertel, Wright, Cao, Ferragamo, & Bal, 2011; see also chapter by Oertel et al., this volume). There is no evidence for intrinsic connections within the LSO (G. Kim & Kandler, 2003).

Small multipolar neurons in the contralateral ventral nucleus of the trapezoid body (VNTB; Gomez-Alvarez & Saldana, 2016; Gomez-Nieto, Rubio, & Lopez, 2008; Warr & Beck, 1996) and posteroventral aspects of the ipsilateral lateral nucleus of the trapezoid body (LNTB) also project into the LSO (Glendenning, Masterton, Baker, & Wenthold, 1991). In the LNTB-LSO projection, axons terminate perisomatically (Kuwabara & Zook, 1992), and the projection is most likely glycinergic (Spirou & Berrebi, 1997). It is unclear whether an LNTB-LSO projection exists in rodents (Franken, Smith, & Joris, 2016). Finally, there are descending projections into the LSO that originate directly in

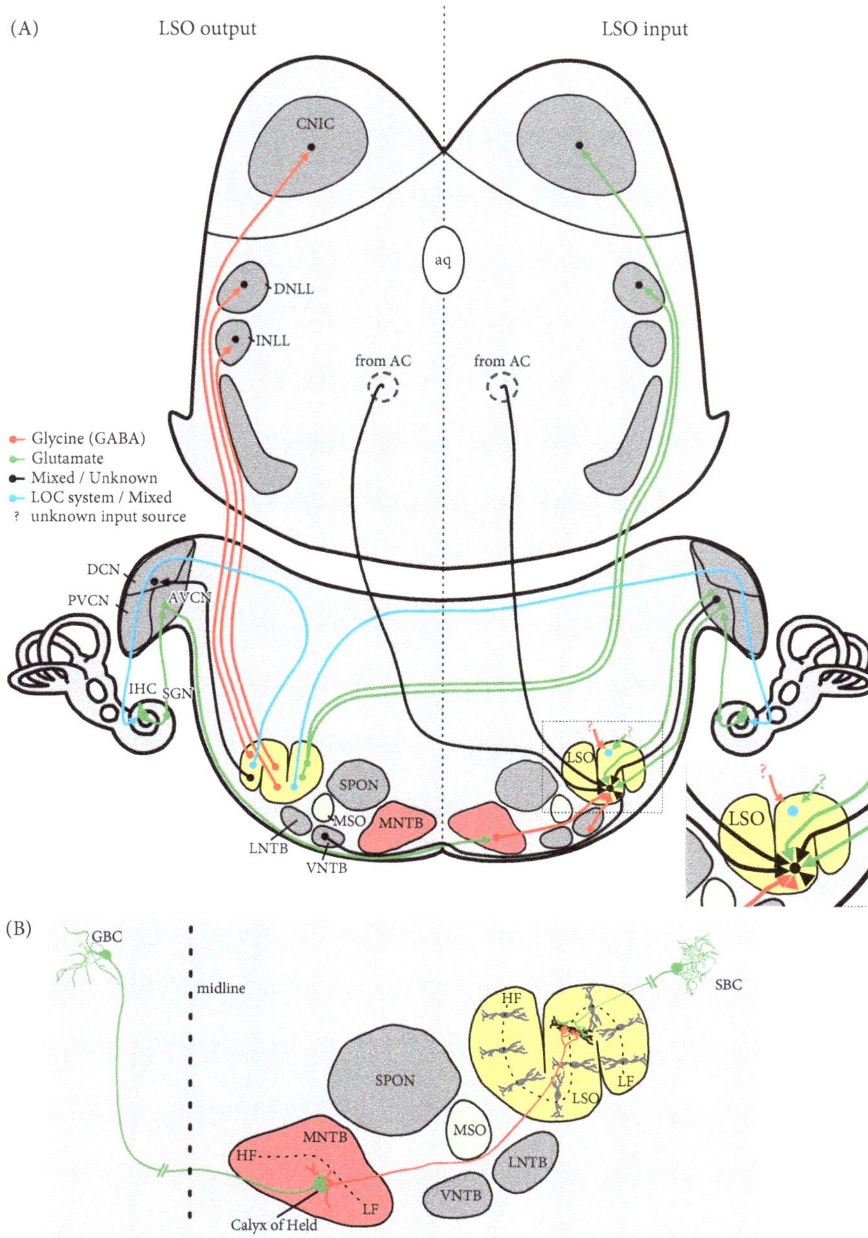

FIGURE 13.4. Afferents to and efferents from the LSO. **A.** Semi-schematic drawings of cross sections with overview of LSO inputs (= afferents; left) and outputs (= efferents; right). The transmitter type is marked with color. **B.** Close-up of the ILD brainstem circuit. Dotted lines indicate the tonotopic axis in MNTB and LSO.

the primary auditory cortex (AC) of both hemispheres (Coomes & Schofield, 2004; Feliciano, Saldaña, & Mugnaini, 1995). The cortico-olivary axons are thin, and some terminate on somata of LSO neurons that project into the IC (Coomes Peterson & Schofield, 2007). In summary, the basic connectivity of the LSO appears solved, but future research is needed to address interspecies differences. Moreover, several open questions concern the fine structure of connectivity. For example, the type of target neuron in the LSO and the transmitter phenotype are still unclear for several afferents (Gomez-Alvarez & Saldana, 2016). Likewise, the projection pattern of LSO neurons has not been clearly associated with biophysical response patterns and the transmitter repertoire that is present in the input-output microcircuits.

Efferent Projections from the LSO

The left half of Figure 13.4A depicts a general summary of the axonal projections emerging from the LSO. Principal neurons are a major source of ascending projections to the auditory midbrain (pioneer papers are summarized in Cant, 1984). They give rise to ipsilateral projections terminating in the intermediate nucleus of the lateral lemniscus (INLL), dorsal nucleus of the lateral lemniscus (DNLL), and IC, as well as to contralateral projections terminating in the DNLL and IC (Kelly, Liscum, van Adel, & Ito, 1998; Kelly, van Adel, & Ito, 2009; Malmierca & Hackett, 2010; Shneiderman, Stanforth, Henkel, & Saint Marie, 1999). Both types of projection appear to contribute relatively equally. Only a small portion (< 5%, cats) of LSO neurons project bilaterally via axon collaterals (Glendenning & Masterton, 1983). Ipsilateral projections are mainly inhibitory and glycinergic, whereas contralateral projections are excitatory and glutamatergic (Altschuler & Shore, 2010; Glendenning, Baker, Hutson, & Masterton, 1992; Ito & Oliver, 2010; Saint Marie & Baker, 1990; Saint Marie, Ostapoff, Morest, & Wenthold, 1989; Schofield, 2010). The olivo-collicular projections are tonotopically organized and terminate in laminae in the IC (Oliver, 2000). Among the glutamatergic neurons projecting contralaterally, ~6% are reportedly also glycinergic in rats, and among the glycinergic neurons projecting ipsilaterally, ~60% are also glutamatergic (Fredrich, Reisch, & Illing, 2009). Thus, at least four types of LSO neurons appear to exist concerning outputs to the (rat) IC. The functional implications of the two-transmitter scenario are unknown. At least in rats, all LSO neurons projecting into the IC are positive for the Ca^{2+}-binding protein parvalbumin (Fredrich et al., 2009). Since parvalbumin-expressing cells play a role in action potential (AP)–dependent homeostasis (Xue & Liu, 2014), these neurons may mediate the relationship between synaptic excitation and inhibition in an activity-dependent manner and participate in the formation of EI balance.

In addition to ascending projections, the LSO provides descending projections to the cochlea (Schofield, 2010; Warr, 1992) and, to a much smaller extent, to all three subdivisions of the ipsilateral CNC, predominantly the dorsal cochlear nucleus (DCN; Covey, Jones, & Casseday, 1984; Winter, Robertson, & Cole, 1989). LSO neurons projecting into the ipsilateral VCN are small, having a mean soma diameter of ~5 µm

(Fredrich et al., 2009). The projections into the cochlea are part of the LOC system (Warr & Boche, 2003). LOC cells are chemically distinct and provide cholinergic, GABAergic, dopaminergic, and peptidergic feedback to the cochlea (Vetter, Adams, & Mugnaini, 1991). Robust glutamate decarboxylase (GAD67) messenger ribonucleic acid (mRNA) levels characterize the GABAergic portion of the adult LOC system (Jenkins & Simmons, 2006). Functionally, LOC cells may provide a binaural adjustment required for accurate sound localization (Darrow, Maison, & Liberman, 2006). We will discuss further functional differences between LSO principal neurons and LOC neurons in the section, "Functional Properties of LSO Neurons in Vitro."

Functional Properties of LSO Neurons in Vivo

As stated previously, LSO neurons extract and encode ILDs. Accordingly, most LSO neurons are EI units, that is, their response type is ipsilateral excitatory and contralateral inhibitory (classification scheme after Goldberg & Brown, 1969). Notice that the inverse sequence, namely IE = contralateral-inhibitory; ipsilateral-excitatory, is also used by some authors; for example, Tollin & Yin, 2002. The existence of EI units is in perfect harmony with the converging contralateral glycinergic and ipsilateral glutamatergic inputs (cf. the section, "Afferent Projections to the LSO"). As mentioned already, there are species-specific peculiarities in the anatomical organization of the LSO (Figure 13.2). Despite these peculiarities, electrophysiological studies have revealed many general similarities of LSO neurons across species. For example, one major similarity is the tonotopic organization (bat: Covey, Vater, & Casseday, 1991; Harnischfeger et al., 1985; cat: Caird & Klinke, 1983; Guinan, Norris, & Guinan, 1972; chinchilla: Caspary & Faingold, 1989; Caspary & Finlayson, 1991; Finlayson & Caspary, 1989; Moore & Caspary, 1983; dog: Tsuchitani, 1988a, 1988b; Tsuchitani & Boudreau, 1966, 1967; gerbil: Sanes & Rubel, 1988).

Basically, LSO neurons perform a subtraction-like process. Upon ipsilateral stimulation with tone bursts, typical peri-stimulus time histograms (PSTHs), which provide information about the spiking pattern before, during, and after a stimulus, are sustained (Figure 13.5B), chopper-like, or primary-like (like in [primary] auditory nerve (AN) fibers). Such PSTHs demonstrate a robust on response with low variability in timing, which is followed by a tonic plateau discharge (Caird & Klinke, 1983; Joris, 1996; Tsuchitani, 1977, 1988a). Higher sound pressure levels (SPLs) decrease the first spike latency and increase the firing rate. Frequency tuning of LSO neurons is sharp as indicated by narrow V-shaped tuning curves (Figure 13.5A left). For a given neuron, tuning curves obtained upon contralateral stimulation are similarly sharp and display the highest sensitivity at the same tone frequency as those after ipsilateral stimulation, except that spontaneous activity is efficiently blocked throughout the stimulus duration (Figure 13.5A right). In other words, characteristic frequencies (CF) for ipsi- and contralateral inputs match very well, and the response area for the contralateral inhibition is a horizontal mirror image of the ipsilateral excitatory response area. Therefore, ipsilaterally

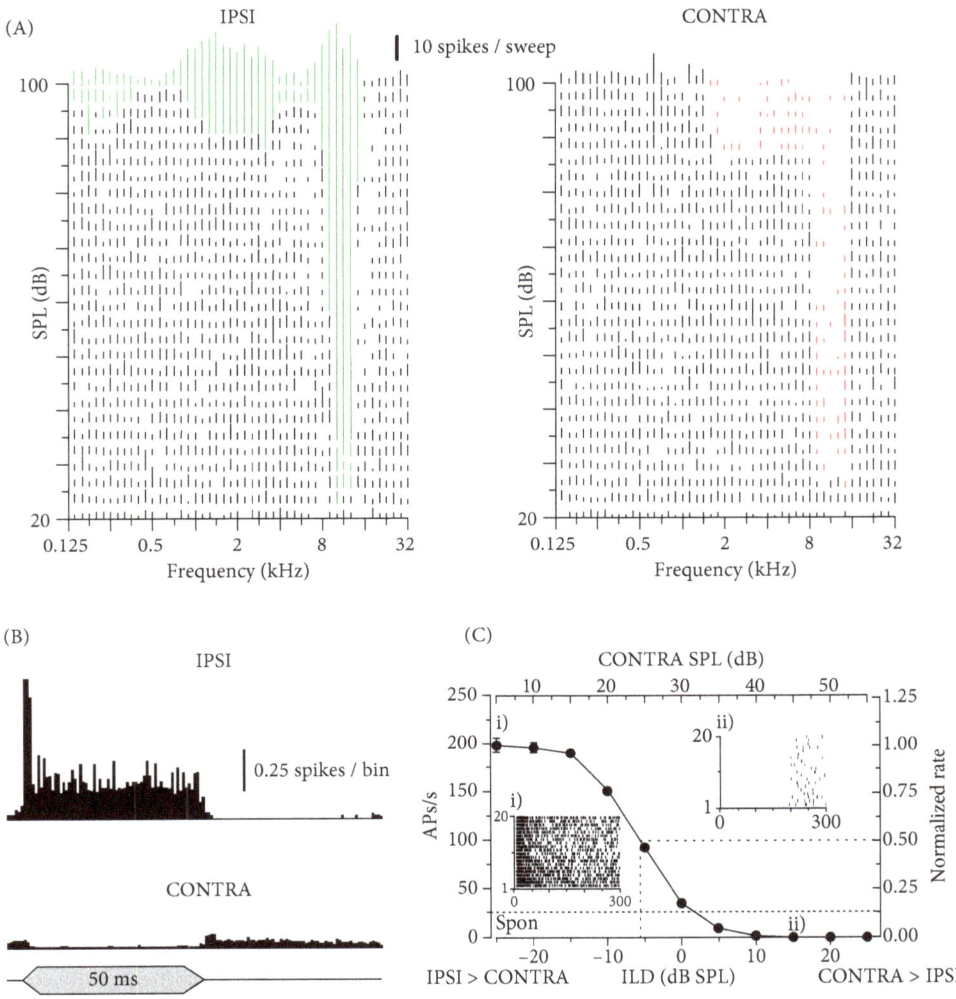

FIGURE 13.5. ILD coding of LSO neurons. **A.** Frequency-response plot of an ILD-sensitive LSO neuron in a cat. Stimulation of the ipsilateral (left) or contralateral (right) ear evokes excitatory (green) or inhibitory (red) responses, respectively. Vertical black bars show the spontaneous activity. **B.** PSTH of the neuron shown in **A** (50-ms tone bursts, 11.3 kHz, 80 dB SPL). Calibration bar shows the average number of APs per bin. **C.** Spatial receptive field of an ILD-sensitive LSO neuron. Plotted is the average firing rate in response to 300-ms ipsilateral tones at 30 dB SPL, as a function of increasing tone levels presented to the contralateral ear. Upper x-axis indicates sound level at contralateral ear; right y-axis shows normalized AP rate. Dashed lines mark ILD level at half-maximal firing rate (–6 dB). Dotted line shows level of spontaneous activity (Spon). Insets i and ii are raster plots of the neuronal firing at ILDs of –25 dB and 15 dB, respectively (x-axis: peri-stimulus time in ms; y-axis: trial #).

evoked excitation is matched by contralateral inhibition in both tonotopicity and efficacy. When stimulated binaurally, LSO EI cells generate APs when the sound at the ipsilateral ear is louder than the sound present at the contralateral ear (Figure 13.5C; Park, Monsivais, & Pollak, 1997). With increasing levels of the contralateral stimulus, the spike rate becomes more and more depressed, and the majority of EI cells are completely inhibited when the contralateral stimulus is 10 dB louder than the ipsilateral. Therefore, LSO neurons have spatial receptive fields in the ipsilateral sound field and sigmoid spike rate–ILD functions. Via the aforementioned projection pattern into the midbrain, namely excitatory output to the contralateral IC and inhibitory input to the ipsilateral IC (cf. section "Efferent Projections from the LSO"), LSO neurons set up the representation of space in the contralateral cerebral neocortex, which is characteristic for all sensory systems. In in vivo patch-clamp recordings, the first of this kind in the LSO, morphologically identified principal neurons did not respond with a phasic-tonic spike pattern to ipsilaterally presented 25-ms tones, but rather with an onset spike (Franken, Joris, & Smith, 2018). In contrast, non-principal LSO neurons fired throughout the stimulus. The authors proposed a revision of the prevailing notion of the LSO as a high-frequency nucleus integrating auditory information over time to send ILD cues to higher brain centers. Rather, they suggested that LSO principal cells are temporal differentiators and more akin to MSO cells in that they are also involved in temporal processing. The suggestion goes along with an earlier report stating that time and intensity are processed together in both the LSO and the MSO (Grothe & Park, 1995).

Iontophoretic application of glycine onto LSO neurons during ipsilateral acoustic stimulation mimics the inhibition obtained with contralateral stimulation (Moore & Caspary, 1983). Both contralaterally evoked inhibitory responses and the effects of iontophoretically applied glycine are abolished by strychnine, a GlyR antagonist. The results are corroborated by the presence of adult-type, strychnine-sensitive GlyRs containing ligand-binding $\alpha 1$ subunits. These subunits provide GlyRs with both short open and short decay times, thereby ensuring brief inhibitory postsynaptic potentials (IPSPs; Takahashi, Momiyama, Hirai, Hishinuma, & Akagi, 1992).

In intracellular in vivo recordings from EI LSO neurons of chinchillas (Finlayson & Caspary, 1989), stimulation with 3-ms tone pips evokes robust IPSPs and excitatory postsynaptic potentials (EPSPs) from the contralateral and ipsilateral ear, respectively, which have similar onset latencies (Figure 13.6B). AP bursts sit on top of the EPSPs. When the tone stimuli are presented simultaneously, the IPSP appears to be the dominant response, demonstrating its robustness.

The ipsilateral and contralateral pathways to the LSO vary in terms of axon length and number of synaptic relays (Figure 13.6A). Nevertheless, latency differences between ipsilateral inputs and contralateral inputs, which are also called characteristic delay (Yin & Kuwada, 1983), are remarkably small (Joris, 1996), indicating faster conduction velocity contralaterally than ipsilaterally. In cat LSO neurons, the latency differences average < 200 μs (Joris & Yin, 1998; Tollin & Yin, 2005). Several elements of the ILD pathway to the LSO are morphologically special. This holds for the endbulbs of Held on GBCs (Ryugo & Fekete, 1982) and the thick (5 μm) and heavily myelinated

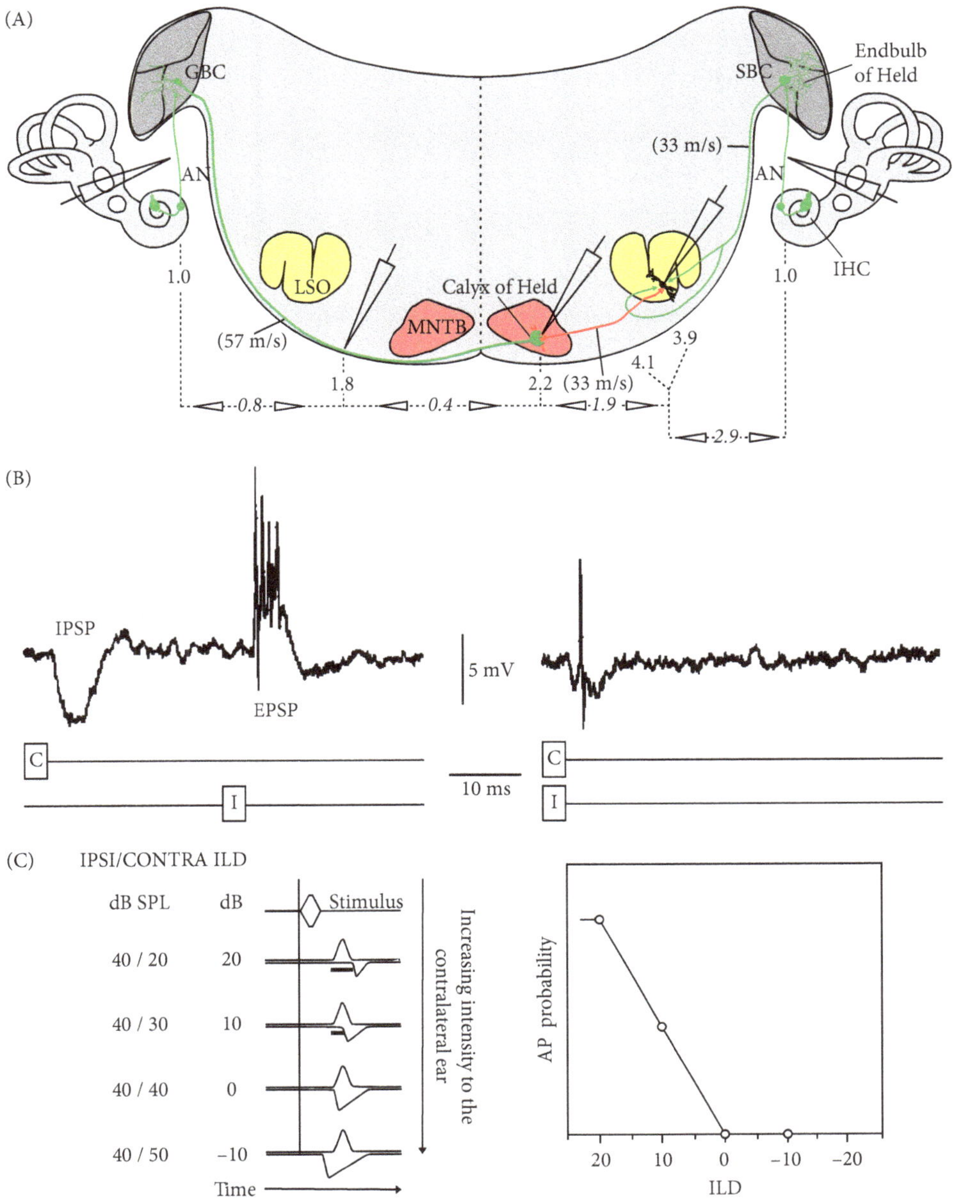

FIGURE 13.6. LSO inputs in vivo. **A** Semi-schematic drawing illustrating transmission delays along the ILD pathway. Delays were determined from extracellular in vivo recordings. Recording sites are marked with electrodes. Italic numbers indicate delays between two recording sites. Numbers in parentheses are approximate values for axon conduction velocities. **B** Intracellular recording from an ILD-sensitive LSO neuron to ipsilateral (I), contralateral (C) or binaural CF tones (3 ms unramped). **C.** Hypothetical EPSPs and IPSPs from an ILD-sensitive LSO neuron (left) and corresponding ILD function (right). ILDs are generated by increasing the sound level to the contralateral ear. Bars below PSPs indicate time window during which APs can be evoked.

Panel **A** redrawn from Joris and Yin (1998), with permission of The American Physiological Society; Panel **B** reprinted from *Hearing Research*, 3(8), Finlayson & Caspary, Synaptic potentials of chinchilla lateral superior olivary neurons, 221–228, Copyright © 1989, with permission from Elsevier; Panel C redrawn from Park et al. (1996), with permission from *Journal of Neuroscience*. Numbers for conduction velocities are from Tsuchitani and Johnson (1991).

axons of GBCs (Malmierca & Ryugo, 2012; Moritz, Eckstein, Tenzer, & Friauf, 2015) that give rise to a calyx of Held on MNTB principal cells (Borst & Soria van Hoeve, 2012; Schneggenburger & Forsythe, 2006; von Gersdorff & Borst, 2002). Even in the neuropil of the LSO, myelinated axons are abundant and non-myelinated fibers are almost absent (Cant, 1984). In addition, MNTB-LSO synapses release synaptic vesicles reliably and with high temporal precision, even at high frequency (Krächan, Fischer, Franke, & Friauf, 2017). All these features suggest that LSO inputs are also designed to process timing information (Figure 13.6C). Indeed, LSO neurons, especially low-frequency ones with a CF < 3 kHz, are sensitive to interaural phase differences, implying ITD sensitivity to the fine structure of sound (Finlayson & Caspary, 1991). Moreover, LSO neurons can be sensitive to ILDs in the envelopes of amplitude-modulated high-frequency tones (Batra, Kuwada, & Fitzpatrick, 1997a, 1997b; Joris & Yin, 1995). Inhibition is maximal when one presents stimuli to the ears in-phase (Tollin & Yin, 2005). When an ipsilateral stimulus lags the contralateral stimulus by the characteristic delay, excitatory and inhibitory postsynaptic inputs arrive coincidentally at the LSO neuron, resulting in maximal inhibition. The temporal integration of excitatory and inhibitory inputs does not only lead to spike suppression, but it can also promote spike generation. Microsecond-precise arrival differences of inhibition, relative to excitation, facilitate spiking in LSO neurons, thus increasing the separability of ILDs for faint sounds (Beiderbeck et al., 2018).

Rats with unilateral kainic acid lesions restricted to the LSO are impaired in localizing a noise burst (van Adel & Kelly, 1998). Such neurotoxic lesions destroy somata while sparing fibers of passage, and axon terminals. The destruction of the rat LSO by itself is sufficient to produce sound localization deficits similar in severity to those caused by complete unilateral destruction of the whole SOC. These results reflect the importance of the LSO circuitry for processing binaural cues, particularly ILDs. Surprisingly, and in some contrast, conditional genetic ablation of MNTB neurons in *Egr2;En1*^{cko} mice affects the ability of binaural sound localization only subtly (Jalabi et al., 2013). Furthermore, functional glycinergic innervation of the LSO remains substantial in such mice. One possible explanation for these unexpected results is the existence of a parallel glycinergic input to the LSO that is obscured in normal mice because glycinergic MNTB inputs dominate.

Relatively few aging studies have been performed in the SOC, and even fewer in the LSO (Frisina, 2010). Significant age-related functional deficits have been reported for LSO neurons in 20–23-month-old Fischer 344 rats, in which thresholds of both inhibitory and excitatory responses are elevated by 15–20 dB, particularly in LSO neurons with CFs > 8 kHz (Finlayson & Caspary, 1993). However, rate-level functions, maximal discharge rates, threshold-adjusted conduction latencies, and maximal inhibition are all unchanged between young and aged rats. Therefore, it is likely that the threshold shifts occur peripherally to the LSO. The resistibility of LSO neurons to age-related deterioration is surprising in light of the fact that MNTB neurons are selectively lost in Fischer 344 rats after 2 to 3 months (Casey & Feldman, 1985). It is possible that homeostatic plasticity, that is, compensatory changes in response to deafferentation, render

LSO neurons able to perform efficiently in the relatively narrow operating range of excitation and inhibition (Caspary, Ling, Turner, & Hughes, 2008). The mechanisms for such compensations are completely unknown. In Sprague-Dawley rats, where massive age-related decreases occur in the number of MNTB neurons, this cell loss is not reflected in a change in LSO function (Finlayson, 1995). The lack of age-related changes in inhibitory responses of LSO neurons in Sprague-Dawley rats is unexpected, and increased innervation from other MNTB neurons may compensate for the lost inhibitory inputs. Alternatively, but less likely, the excitatory innervation may become decreased.

Studies in other species (mice, gerbils) have also found relatively modest, if any, age-related changes in the SOC (Gleich, Weiss, & Strutz, 2004; O'Neill, Zettel, Whittemore, & Frisina, 1997). For example, calbindin immunoreactivity does not change in any obvious way with age in the LSO in C57 and CBA mouse strains, whereas it declines in the MNTB of C57 mice (Caspary et al., 2008). Similar to Fischer 344 rats, C57 mice are a well-established model for studying progressive hearing loss, because they share the same pattern of hearing loss as humans suffering from presbyacusis (Willott, 1997).

Functional Properties of LSO Neurons in Vitro

The ILD pathways converging on the LSO provide a favorable system to analyze neurotransmission of both excitatory and inhibitory nature and are characterized by high-frequency signaling, temporal precision, and robustness. Because MNTB projection neurons are much more accessible for experimental manipulations than local interneurons from which inhibitory inputs often arise, the MNTB-LSO projection in particular is suitable for studying inhibitory synapses. Moreover, the fact that the projection is maintained in transverse brainstem slices renders it amenable to in vitro experiments, which reveal mechanisms of synaptic performance, for example, during sustained synaptic activity, that cannot be revealed through in vivo experiments.

Earliest electrophysiological experiments employing LSO slices go back to the 1990s (Kandler & Friauf, 1995b; Sanes, 1990; Wu & Kelly, 1991). They confirmed the EI characteristics of LSO neurons by demonstrating graded EPSPs and IPSPs upon electrical activation of afferent fibers from the ipsilateral AVCN and the MNTB, respectively (Figure 13.7A). The latency of these EPSPs and IPSPs is similarly short (~1.1 ms vs. 1.3 ms), thus implying fast synaptic transmission, and their AMPA/glutamatergic and glycinergic nature was demonstrated in pharmacological blocking experiments (Kandler & Friauf, 1995b; Kotak, Korada, Schwartz, & Sanes, 1998; Wu & Kelly, 1991, 1992b, 1995). EPSPs last 1.5 ms, IPSPs last 3.2 ms (Sanes, 1990), and decay kinetics of both evoked excitatory (EPSCs) and inhibitory postsynaptic currents (IPSCs) are fast, displaying time constants of less than 1 ms (Figure 13.11B; Pilati et al., 2016). Whereas unitary EPSCs are relatively weak, unitary IPSCs are strong (mean conductances 0.7

nS vs. 9 nS), and there is a ~10-fold variability across separate inhibitory inputs onto a given LSO neuron (Gjoni, Zenke, Bouhours, & Schneggenburger, 2018). In terms of EI integration, these features are possibly key determinants of the spontaneous firing properties of LSO neurons, and the weak excitatory inputs, which converge from SBCs, appear to filter out the relatively high spontaneous AP activity of these cells (Gjoni, Zenke, et al., 2018). Indeed, whereas spontaneous firing of bushy cells averages ~30 APs/s in vivo (Kopp-Scheinpflug, Fuchs, Lippe, Tempel, & Rübsamen, 2003), it is almost absent in LSO neurons and averages only 2.5 APs/s in cells that are spontaneously active (Karcz et al., 2011; Tsuchitani & Boudreau, 1966). In order to suppress AP firing, inhibition needs to be ~2-fold stronger than excitation, which can be achieved by few, but strong unitary IPSPs.

During brief stimulus trains, APs are faithfully elicited when only the ipsilateral input is activated, and concurrent activation of the contralateral input blocks preferably the latter-occurring APs (Figure 13.7B; Sanes, 1990). In vitro experiments also show sensitivity of LSO neurons to bilateral time differences (Figure 13.7C; Wu & Kelly, 1992a), thus confirming data from in vivo studies. Upon repetitive activation of the afferent fibers from the ipsilateral AVCN (10 pulses), an average LSO neuron can fire APs with ~90% fidelity when stimulated at 125 Hz (Wu & Kelly, 1993). The failure rate increases with the pulse number, indicating short-term plasticity (STP) in form of short-term depression (STD) at SBC-LSO synapses in the range of tens of milliseconds. A 90% fidelity at 125 Hz is remarkable, yet GBC-MNTB synapses do even better and are able to fire with 90% fidelity to a much higher stimulation frequency, up to 677 Hz (Wu & Kelly, 1993). Noticeably, one must consider that GBC-MNTB synapses employ calyces of Held, whereas AVCN-LSO and MNTB-LSO synapses employ conventional axon boutons. During prolonged stimulation periods (40 s), MNTB-LSO connections sustain virtually failure-free transmission up to frequencies of 100 Hz (Kramer et al., 2014). A high quantal content (i.e., number of vesicles released with a single AP) and effective vesicle replenishment form the basis for this synaptic reliability (Krächan et al., 2017). Two Ca^{2+} sensors, the synaptotagmin (Syt) proteins Syt1 and Syt2, mediate synaptic vesicle fusion at the fast-releasing MNTB-LSO synapses (Bouhours, Gjoni, Kochubey, & Schneggenburger, 2017). Syt2 is generally regarded as the main fast Ca^{2+} sensor (Chen, Arai, Satterfield, Young, & Jonas, 2017) and is more abundant than Syt1 in the LSO (Cooper & Gillespie, 2011). However, analysis of conditional Syt1-Syt2 single and double knockout (KO) mice at P12–15 has demonstrated a redundant cooperation of Syt2 with Syt1 at MNTB-LSO synapses (Bouhours et al., 2017). In this context, it is remarkable that excitatory calyces of Held undergo a change from Syt1 to Syt2 between P3 and P14 (Kochubey, Babai, & Schneggenburger, 2016). Whether a similar shift occurs in inhibitory MNTB axons after P15 or whether the Sy1/Syt2 redundancy lasts into adulthood remains to be shown.

An interesting aspect revealed by in vitro recordings is that the balance between excitation and inhibition in the LSO can be achieved via feedback signaling

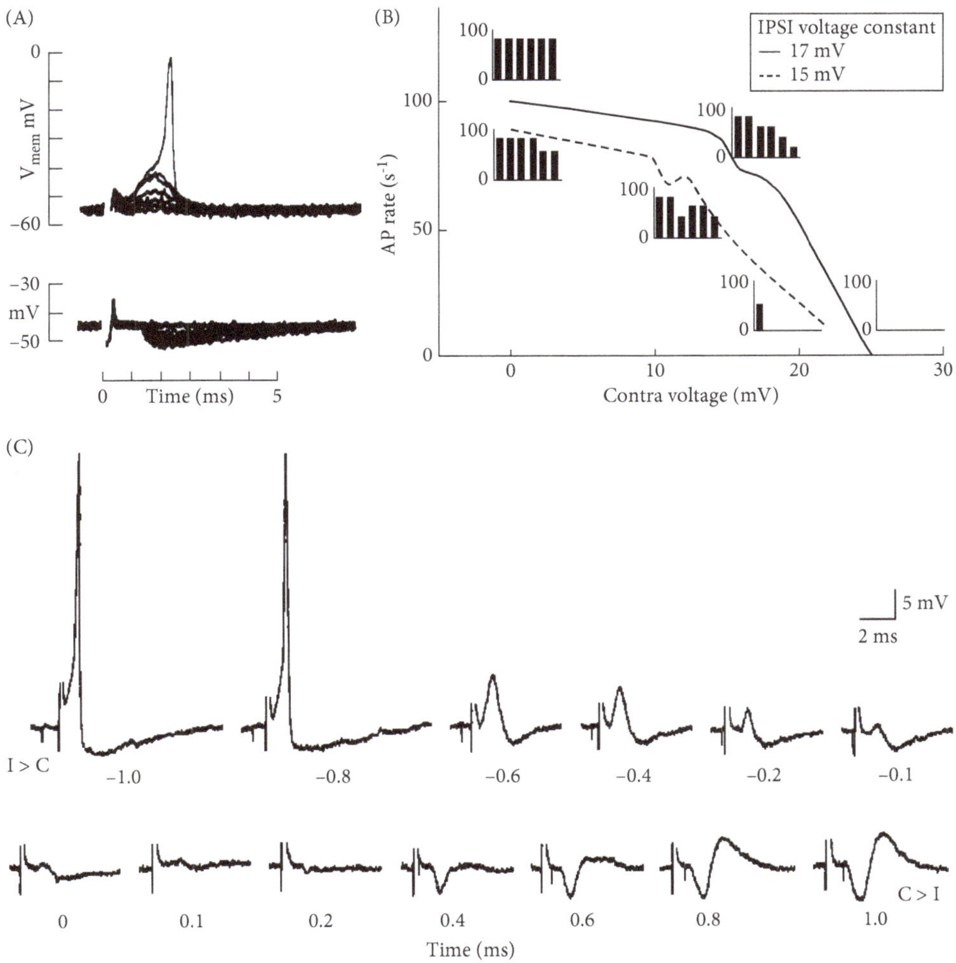

FIGURE 13.7. ITD and ILD sensitivity of LSO principal neurons in vitro. **A.** EPSPs (upper panel) and IPSPs (lower panel) upon electrical stimulation of the trapezoid body lateral to the SOC and the midline trapezoid body, respectively. Superimposed traces obtained at various stimulation intensities. **B.** Discharge rates of an LSO neuron upon stimulation of afferent fibers from the CN and the MNTB (6 pulses at 100 Hz). Stimulation intensities for CN fibers were constant (17 mV, solid line; 15 mV, dotted line), but intensities for MNTB fibers varied (Contra voltage). Insets: population AP rates to all 6 pulses at three Contra voltages. **C.** Voltage changes in a LSO neuron upon fiber stimulation from CN and MNTB. I > C and negative values: ipsilateral stimulation leads contralateral stimulation.

Panel **A** modified from Wu and Kelly (1991), with permission of The American Physiological Society; Panel **B** modified from Sanes (1990), with permission from *Journal of Neuroscience*; Panel **C** modified from Wu and Kelly (1992), with permission of The American Physiological Society.

(Magnusson, Park, Pecka, Grothe, & Koch, 2008). The retrograde process involves GABA release from LSO neurons during AP firing activity and the activation of $GABA_B$ receptors on excitatory and inhibitory terminals. It may put the LSO neurons into a position to rapidly fine-tune their sound localization sensitivity in an activity-dependent manner.

In vitro recordings have also contributed substantially to our knowledge about biophysical properties of LSO neurons, which are very difficult to obtain through in vivo experiments (see, however, Franken et al., 2018). In response to sustained depolarizing current pulses, the majority of LSO principal neurons fires a single short latency AP (Figure 13.8A left; Barnes-Davies, Barker, Osmani, & Forsythe, 2004; Sterenborg et al., 2010). By contrast, LOC neurons display a delayed 1st AP and tonic firing behavior (Figure 13.8A right; Fujino et al., 1997; Sterenborg et al., 2010). In response to depolarizing voltage pulses, principal LSO neurons exhibit a fast-activating Na^+ current (Na^+ fast) and a sustained K^+ current (K^+ sust; Figure 13.8B left). Moreover, they show a slowly activating inward current in response to hyperpolarization (I_h), which is mediated through hyperpolarization-activated and cyclic nucleotide-gated (HCN) channels (Figure 13.8C left; Leao, Leao, Sun, Fyffe, & Walmsley, 2006; Sterenborg et al., 2010). I_h controls the resting potential, dampens dendritic excitability, and temporal AP acuity (He, Chen, Li, & Hu, 2014; Rothman & Manis, 2003). In contrast to principal cells, LOC neurons exhibit a prominent, rapidly inactivating outward K^+ current of the A-type (I_A) when depolarized, yet lack the I_h current when hyperpolarized (Figure 13.8B,C right). Thus, one can physiologically distinguish principal and LOC neurons by their differences in voltage-gated currents. The firing pattern and channel properties of LSO neurons also correlate with the input resistance (R_{in}); low and high R_{in} are associated with single and multiple firing patterns, respectively. In the rat LSO, single-spiking neurons appear to be more abundant in the low-frequency region, whereas multiple-spiking neurons predominate in the high-frequency region (Barnes-Davies et al., 2004). The first group shows higher levels of a low-threshold K^+ current (I_{LT}). Blocking I_{LT} with α-dendrotoxin converts the single-firing pattern into a multiple-firing one, which is indicative of the presence of voltage-gated potassium 1 (K_v1) channels, which play important roles in determining the latency of the 1st AP and AP repolarization (Fischl et al., 2016; Kole, Letzkus, & Stuart, 2007). Indeed, immunolabeling has demonstrated the presence of $K_v1.1$ in the rat LSO (Barnes-Davies et al., 2004), but the subcellular location and the development (Kim & Rutherford, 2016) have not been revealed. It is interesting that the LSO of naked mole rats, which live in subterranean habitats and have poor sound localization capabilities (Heffner & Heffner, 1993), lacks HCN channels (Gessele, Garcia-Pino, Omerbasic, Park, & Koch, 2016). The functional significance of I_A has been described in a variety of neurons displaying repetitive firing (Rudy, 1988). Being an outward current, I_A counteracts depolarizing effects of excitatory synapses and modulates the rate of such repetitive firing (Manis, 2008; Rothman

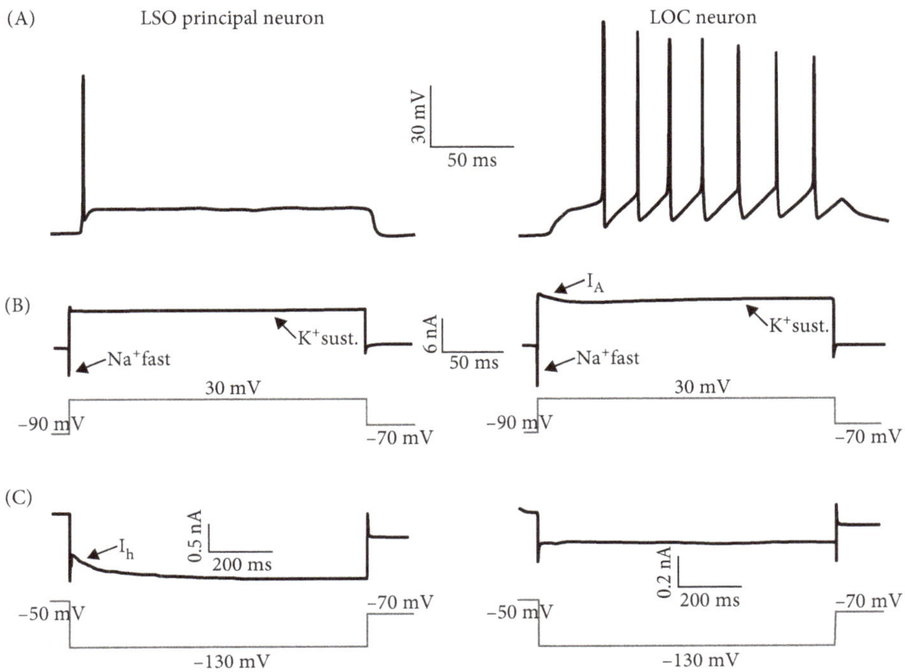

FIGURE 13.8. Firing behavior and voltage-activated currents of LSO principal and LOC neurons in vitro. **A.** AP response of a principal neuron (left) and a LOC neuron (right) upon current injection (0.1 nA). **B.** Current responses to a depolarizing voltage step (grey). **C.** As **B,** but for a hyperpolarizing voltage step (grey).

Reprinted from *Hearing Research, 270*(1–2), Sterenborg et al., Lateral olivocochlear (LOC) neurons of the mouse LSO receive excitatory and inhibitory synaptic inputs with slower kinetics than LSO principal neurons, 119–126, Copyright © 2010, with permission from Elsevier.

& Manis, 2003). Taken together, I_{LT} and I_A may act in concert to modulate the rate of repetitive firing in LOC neurons.

Fetal Development of the LSO

Neurogenesis, cell fate determination, axon outgrowth, and target finding are major steps in early circuit assembly. To yield a functional ILD circuit, the generation of proper input circuits (MNTB-LSO; CN-LSO) and output circuits (LSO-IC) is crucial. In this chapter, we summarize both normal and disturbed fetal development of the LSO. As most studies focused on rodents, particularly mice, we also focus on these species in the following discussion.

Neurogenesis and Differentiation of LSO Neurons

During fetal development, the hindbrain becomes segregated in morphologically defined bulges along the antero-posterior axis (Kiecker & Lumsden, 2005; Lumsden & Krumlauf, 1996). These bulges appear as spatially distinct segments or compartments (rhombomeres) and contain progenitor cells (Figure 13.9A; Schneider-Maunoury, Gilardi-Hebenstreit, & Charnay, 1998). Segmentation genes, that is, genes whose inactivation results in the elimination of hindbrain territories or a modification of their extent, govern the process of segment formation and encode transcription factors. Overlapping or nested patterns of gene expression in the prospective hindbrain provide environmental signals that lead to the unique characteristics of individual rhombomeres and ultimately determines cell fate.

Eight rhombomeres (r1–8) give rise to different cell lineages and cell fates in rodents (Figure 13.9B; Kiecker & Lumsden, 2005). Auditory brainstem neurons are derived from progenitor cells of the lower rhombic lip, a structure located at the dorsal portion of the hindbrain that spans the whole antero-posterior hindbrain axis (Wullimann et al., 2011). AVCN neurons are mainly derived from r3 and partially from r2 (Farago, Awatramani, & Dymecki, 2006). In contrast, LSO neurons are derived from r5, while MNTB principal neurons are derived from r3 and r5 (Marrs, Morgan, Howell, Spirou, & Mathers, 2013). LOC neurons are derived from r4 (Di Bonito et al., 2013; Karis et al., 2001). VCN neurons are born between embryonic days (E) 11 and 14 (Altman & Bayer, 1980; Farago et al., 2006; Pierce, 1967; Willaredt, Schluter, & Nothwang, 2015). MNTB neurons are born during a very brief period from E11–12 (Kudo, Sakurai, Kurokawa, & Yamada, 2000; Willaredt et al., 2015), whereas LSO neurons are born over a longer period, namely from E9–16 (Figure 13.9C; Kudo, Kitao, Okoyama, Moriya, & Kawano, 1996; Kudo et al., 2000; Willaredt et al., 2015).

What are the underlying mechanisms that identify these cells as "auditory neurons" specific for their target region? Key regulators in this process are the transcription factors encoded by the genes *Egr2* (*Krox20*) and *Mafb* (*Kreisler*). In r5, expression of these transcription factors begins at early embryonic stages (*Egr2*: E8; *MafB*: E9; Figure 13.9C; Willaredt et al., 2015). *Egr2* encodes a zinc finger transcription factor, which is specifically expressed in areas that later coincide with r3 and r5 (Chavrier et al., 1990; Gilardi, Schneider-Maunoury, & Charnay, 1991; Wilkinson, Bhatt, Chavrier, Bravo, & Charnay, 1989). Accordingly, genetic deletion of *Egr2* eliminates r3 and r5 (Figure 13.9B; Schneider-Maunoury et al., 1993). *Mafb* is expressed in r5 and r6 (Willaredt et al., 2015) and encodes a basic leucine zipper transcription factor (Cordes & Barsh, 1994). Similar to *Egr2* deletion, *Mafb* KO leads to an abnormal shape of the hindbrain, especially to a loss of rhombomeric segmentation (r4–r7) and missing r5 and r6 (Figure 13.9B; McKay et al., 1994).

Atoh1 (*Math1*) is a basic helix-loop-helix transcription factor, which is involved in neuronal specification of cell derivatives from the rhombic lip (Ben-Arie et al., 1996). Conditional deletion of *Atoh1* from r3 and r5 results in nearly complete neuronal loss in

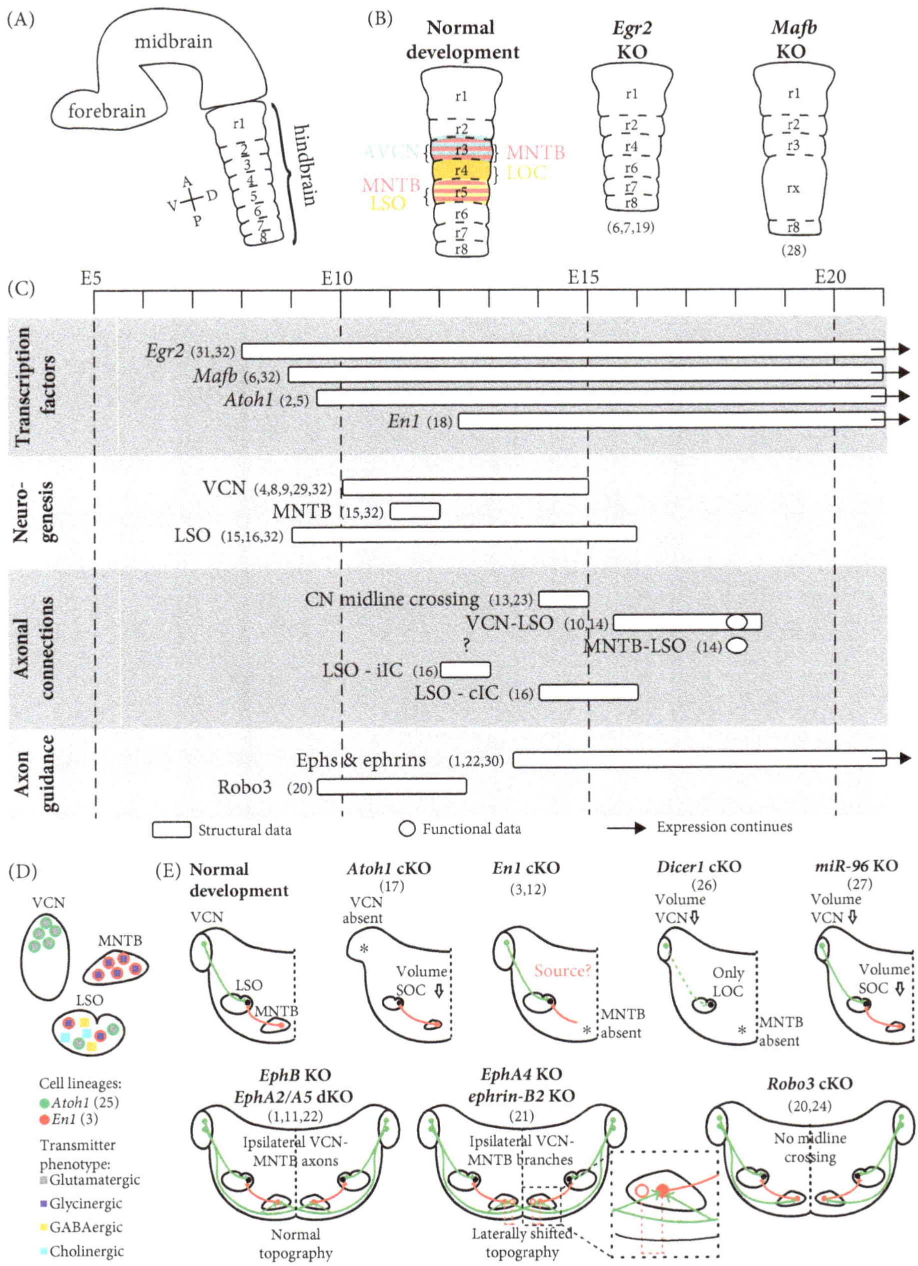

FIGURE 13.9. Fetal development of the rodent ILD pathway. **A.** Sagittal scheme of a fetal rodent brain, in which eight rhombomeres (r1–8) form spatially segregated hindbrain segments. A, anterior; P, posterior; V, ventral; D, dorsal. **B.** Origin of AVCN, LSO, LOC, and MNTB cells during normal development and upon genetic ablation of segmental genes *Egr2* or *Mafb*. **C.** Timeline depicting presence of transcription factors, neurogenesis, formation of initial axonal connections,

the AVCN and subsequently in the MNTB and LSO, likely due to a lack of trophic support (Figure 13.9E; Maricich et al., 2009).

Whereas the *Atoh1* lineage gives rise to excitatory neurons (Rose, Ahmad, Thaller, & Zoghbi, 2009), the cell lineage of the transcription factor Engrailed 1 (*En1*) is required for normal positioning and survival of glycinergic MNTB and LSO neurons (Figure 13.9D, E; Altieri, Jalabi, Zhao, Romito-DiGiacomo, & Maricich, 2015; Jalabi et al., 2013). As expected, sound source localization performance is impaired in *En1* cKOs although functional glycinergic input to the remaining LSO neurons was still observed. The source of this inhibition is unclear. Taken together, the data demonstrate the importance of *En1* for the survival of glycinergic MNTB and LSO neurons.

Even more severe disruption of SOC nuclei occurs in *Dicer1* cKOs (Rosengauer et al., 2012). *Dicer1* is involved in the generation of mature microRNAs, which are involved in translational repression (Bernstein, Caudy, Hammond, & Hannon, 2001; Song & Rossi, 2017). *Dicer1* cKOs display severely disrupted microRNA pathways, resulting in complete neuron loss in the MNTB and dramatic neuron loss in the VCN and LSO, in which principal cells are completely absent and only LOC cells persist (Rosengauer et al., 2012). This argues for a critical involvement of microRNAs in the histogenesis of SOC nuclei, further underlined in *mir96*—null mice, showing a 35% reduced volume in the VCN, MNTB, and LSO (Figure 13.9E; Schlüter et al., 2018).

Circuit Formation

Little is known about the spatiotemporal migration patterns after neurons of the ILD circuit are born. Cells of the *Atoh1* lineage migrate superficially from the rhombic lip to their target region (Rose et al., 2009; Wang, Rose, & Zoghbi, 2005). For the VCN, cells

---

and axon guidance molecules. **D.** *Atoh1* (green) and *En1* cell lineages (red) in the respective nuclei. Cell lineage and transmitter phenotype of various LSO neuron types and their input neurons. **E.** Fetal ILD pathway in normal development and upon knockout of several proteins that are critical for proper establishment of the ILD pathway. Numbers in parentheses refer to (1) Abdul-Latif, Salazar, Marshak, Dinh, & Cramer (2015); (2) Akazawa, Ishibashi, Shimizu, Nakanishi, & Kageyama (1995); (3) Altieri, Jalabi, Zhao, Romito-DiGiacomo, & Maricich (2015); (4) Altman & Bayer (1980); (5) Ben-Arie et al. (1996); (6) Cordes & Barsh (1994); (7) Deol (1964); (8) Farago, Awatramani, & Dymecki (2006); (9) Friauf & Kandler (1993); (10) Howell et al. (2007); (11) Hsieh et al. (2010); (12) Jalabi et al. (2013); (13) Kandler & Friauf (1993); (14) Kandler & Friauf (1995b); (15) Kudo, Sakurai, Kurokawa, & Yamada (2000); (16) Kudo, Kitao, Okoyama, Moriya, & Kawano (1996); (17) Maricich et al. (2009); (18) Marrs, Morgan, Howell, Spirou, & Mathers (2013); (19) McKay et al. (1994); (20) Michalski et al. (2013); (21) Miko, Nakamura, Henkemeyer, & Cramer (2007); (22) Nakamura, Hsieh, & Cramer (2012); (23) Niblock, Brunso-Bechtold, & Henkel (1995); (24) Renier et al. (2010); (25) Rose, Ahmad, Thaller, & Zoghbi (2009); (26) Rosengauer et al. (2012); (27) Schlüter et al. (2018); (28) Schneider-Maunoury et al. (1993); (29) Pierce (1967); (30) Wallace, Harris, Brubaker, Klotz, & Gabriele (2016); (31) Wilkinson, Bhatt, Chavrier, Bravo, & Charnay (1989); (32) Willaredt, Schluter, & Nothwang (2015).

mainly migrate tangentially between E11–15 (Hossain, D'Sa, & Morest, 2006; Wang et al., 2005), indicating that migration starts soon after neurons are born, since timeframes of neurogenesis and migration overlap. The MNTB and the LSO emerge between E16.5–17.5 (Marrs et al., 2013). At E17.5, both nuclei can be identified as a cell dense structure by marker labeling. Diffuse labeling is already apparent at E14.5, suggesting that migration has already started earlier. Hence, MNTB and LSO migration presumably occurs between E14–E18. Detailed spatiotemporal migration patterns for MNTB and LSO cells are yet to be resolved.

After neurogenesis and migration, neurons grow out axons to their target regions. In the auditory brainstem, axon outgrowth begins very shortly after neurons are born (Howell et al., 2007; Kandler & Friauf, 1993; Niblock, Brunso-Bechtold, & Henkel, 1995). Already at E13, rat CN axons grow along the ventral edge of the brainstem anlage (Niblock et al., 1995). At this time, only a few axons have crossed the midline and growth cones (axon endpoints) have a simple structure, lacking filopodia. Two days later, midline crossing is frequent and growth cones do contain several filopodia (Figure 13.9C; Kandler & Friauf, 1993; Niblock et al., 1995). CN axons innervate the ipsilateral LSO as early as E15.5, shown by the formation of axon branches (Howell et al., 2007). Functional CN-LSO and MNTB-LSO connectivity exist at E18, the earliest age examined (Kandler & Friauf, 1995b). LSO-IC axons grow out between E12–16 (Kudo et al., 1996). Interestingly, LSO axons innervate the contralateral IC about two days earlier than the ipsilateral IC (E12–13 vs. E14–16; Figure 13.9C).

Strikingly, VCN-LSO and MNTB-LSO projections are topographically organized already at postnatal day (P)0 and P2, respectively (Kil, Kageyama, Semple, & Kitzes, 1995; Sanes & Siverls, 1991). What might be the molecules involved in early circuit assembly and topographic organization in the auditory brainstem? We know from the topographical retino-geniculate projection that Eph receptors and their ephrin ligands play a critical role in establishing topographic maps (Triplett & Feldheim, 2012). One key function of Eph/ephrin signaling is axon guidance by forward and reverse signaling, providing attractive or repulsive cues (Cramer & Gabriele, 2014). Indeed, several Ephs and ephrins are expressed in the SOC from E13.5 until early postnatal stages (Abdul-Latif, Salazar, Marshak, Dinh, & Cramer, 2015; Nakamura, Hsieh, & Cramer, 2012), a period which largely coincides with the time window of axonal outgrowth from SOC nuclei (Figure 13.9C). Reverse signaling mediated through EphB2/EphB3-ephrin-B2 interaction is crucial for the normal development of the VCN-MNTB circuit (Hsieh et al., 2010; Nakamura et al., 2012). EphB2 KOs, EphB3 KOs, and ephrin-B2 KOs project a subset of VCN axons collaterals to the ipsilateral MNTB, resulting in a miswired VCN-MNTB circuitry virtually never observed in normal development. A similar phenotype exists in Ephrin-A2 or Ephrin-A5 single KOs, and Ephrin-A2/A5 double KOs, which all show aberrant ipsilateral VCN-MNTB axon collaterals. Interestingly, topographic wiring is unaffected in these KOs, both in normal contralateral axons and in miswired ipsilateral axons (Figure 13.9E; Abdul-Latif et al., 2015), indicating that different molecules regulate midline crossing and topographic organization. Indeed, VCN-MNTB axons in EphA4 and Ephrin-B2 KOs are laterally shifted compared to wildtypes (Miko, Nakamura, Henkemeyer, & Cramer, 2007). Taken together, Eph/ephrin signaling plays multiple roles in axon guidance, tonotopic map formation, and assembly of the ILD circuit (reviews: Cramer, 2005; Cramer & Gabriele, 2014).

Slit-robo and netrin-DCC interactions are also involved in axon guidance during ILD circuitry assembly (DCC = Deleted in Colorectal Cancer). Deletion of *Robo3* from r3 and r5 disrupts midline crossing of AVCN axons and results in an ectopic innervation of the ipsilateral MNTB (Figure 13.9E; Michalski et al., 2013; Renier et al., 2010). Mice lacking *Netrin-1* display a similar phenotype like *Robo3*-KOs, whereas KOs of the netrin-1 receptor *DCC* display almost no axonal outgrowth from the AVCN (Howell et al., 2007).

Development and Plasticity before Hearing Onset (P0–P12)

The auditory system of many altricial rodents, such as mice and rats, does not respond to airborne sound before ~P12 (Echteler, Arjmand, & Dallos, 1989; Ehret, 1976; Woolf & Ryan, 1984), as their ear canals are still closed (an exception are precocial guinea pigs). The altricial animals are therefore useful model organisms for developmental studies of the auditory system. At birth, ILD circuit assembly and initial topographic alignment by guidance molecules are largely complete (Friauf & Kandler, 1993; Kandler & Friauf, 1993; Kil et al., 1995; Sanes & Siverls, 1991). However, the LSO is still immature in many terms, namely inputs, dendritic morphology, biophysical properties, ion channels, synaptic kinetics, and transmitter phenotypes. Until hearing onset, enormous structural and functional changes lead to further maturation of the ILD circuitry. In this section, we highlight the most important changes required to yield a functional ILD circuit at the onset of hearing.

Before hearing onset, that is, in the absence of sensory input, spontaneous AP firing activity is present in the auditory system (Lippe, 1994; Sonntag, Englitz, Kopp-Scheinpflug, & Rübsamen, 2009; Sonntag, Englitz, Typlt, & Rübsamen, 2011; Tritsch, Yi, Gale, Glowatzki, & Bergles, 2007). The spontaneous activity is triggered by supporting cells, which periodically excite inner hair cells (IHCs) and induce Ca^{2+} APs (Tritsch et al., 2007; Wang et al., 2015). This results in activity propagation to central auditory targets, such as the SOC, with a conserved temporal AP pattern (Tritsch et al., 2010). Spontaneous AP activity can be recorded in vivo in the prehearing MNTB as early as P1 (Tritsch et al., 2010). However, synapses are generally weak in immature auditory circuits (Kandler & Friauf, 1995b; Marrs & Spirou, 2012). This raises the following question: What mechanisms ensure that the patterned AP firing of IHCs is efficiently conveyed synaptically to downstream nuclei like the LSO?

Biophysical Adaptations

A strategy to ensure faithful AP generation in response to weak excitation is a high R_{in} (Mongiat, Esposito, Lombardi, & Schinder, 2009). Indeed, biophysical properties of neurons in the developing ILD circuit (VCN, MNTB, LSO) differ drastically from properties in the mature circuit (Figure 13.10). At birth, the R_{in} amounts to ~1 GΩ in VCN neurons (Marrs & Spirou, 2012), ~600 MΩ in MNTB neurons (Hoffpauir, Kolson, Mathers, & Spirou, 2010; Rusu & Borst, 2011), and ~200 MΩ in LSO neurons (Kandler & Friauf, 1995a). Consequently, weak excitatory input currents are sufficient to generate APs. Between P1–6, R_{in} stays constant in LSO neurons but declines thereafter (Kandler & Friauf, 1995a; Walcher, Hassfurth, Grothe, & Koch, 2011), which is coincident with a shortening of the membrane time constant (τ_{mem}; Figures 13.10; 13.11). Neurons decrease their R_{in} by adding ion channels into their plasma membrane that are active close to the resting membrane potential (V_{rest}). Candidates for such conductances are HCN channels and I_{LT} channels. Indeed, both are highly abundant in the auditory brainstem (Barnes-Davies et al., 2004; Kopp-Scheinpflug, Pigott, & Forsythe, 2015).

Developmental changes of HCN conductances have not been demonstrated directly for LSO neurons before hearing onset. However, 92% of LSO neurons show a linear I-V relationship at hyperpolarizing potentials before P6 (Figure 13.10; Kandler & Friauf, 1995a), which argues against the expression of HCN conductances at this age. At P11, robust conductances mediated via the fast HCN1 isoform are present (Hassfurth, Magnusson, Grothe, & Koch, 2009; Leao et al., 2006), suggesting a developmental increase between P6–10. This is a likely scenario as the adjacent MSO shows a 13-fold increase in HCN conductance from P6-20, with a similar developmental decrease of the R_{in} and τ_{mem} as observed in the LSO (Khurana et al., 2012).

Similarly to HCN channels, I_L channels (like $K_v1.1$ and $K_v1.2$) are activated close to V_{rest} (Barnes-Davies et al., 2004; Hassfurth et al., 2009), and they are involved in the typical single-firing behavior found in auditory brainstem neurons (Brew & Forsythe, 1995). At P4, I_L gene expression is low in the SOC and upregulated during postnatal week 2 (Ehmann et al., 2013), consistent with a robust and topographically aligned I_L staining of the LSO at P9 (Barnes-Davies et al., 2004). The combination of a high R_{in} and low I_L abundance during postnatal week 1 predicts that at this age, LSO neurons have sustained firing properties, but a developmental switch in AP firing pattern needs to be shown. At P11, the majority of LSO neurons (~60–80%) fire a single AP upon prolonged current injection (Barnes-Davies et al., 2004; Ebbers et al., 2015; Hirtz et al., 2011).

Decreased R_{in} by addition of channel conductances and acceleration of τ_{mem} yields fast repolarization of the membrane. Consequently, kinetics of inhibitory and excitatory LSO inputs also show a developmental acceleration from P6 onwards (Figure 13.10; Figure 13.11B; Kandler & Friauf, 1995b). Synaptic kinetics are further accelerated by reorganization of the GlyR and AMPA receptor (AMPAR) subunit composition (Pilati et al., 2016). Between P8 and P11, the transcript levels of the GlyRα1 subunit increase ~5-fold, while the GluA4 subunit of the AMPAR is upregulated by ~25% (Pilati et al., 2016). Both

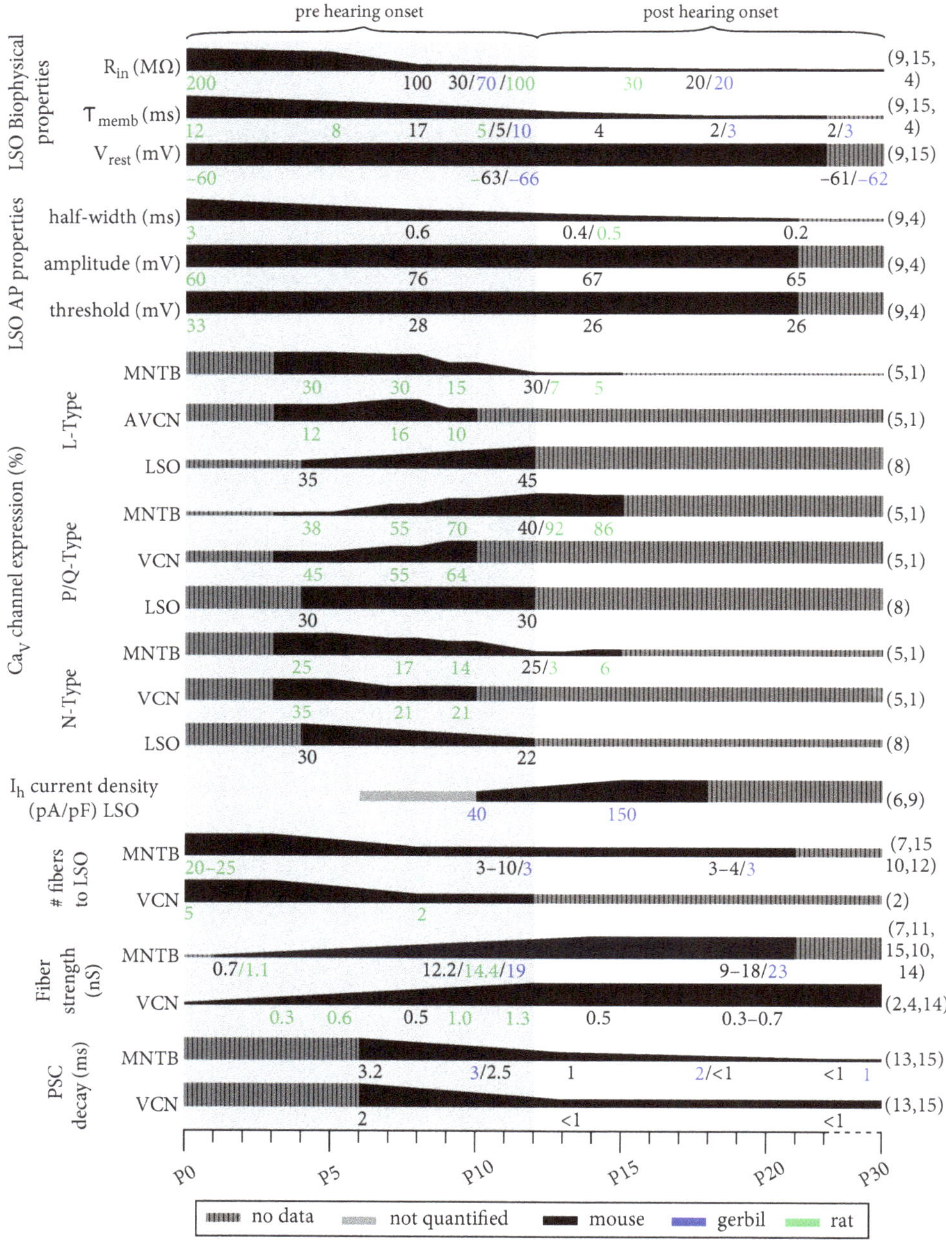

FIGURE 13.10. Prehearing and posthearing development of characteristics in the ILD pathway. Development of several presynaptic and postsynaptic parameters that influence synaptic transmission at MNTB-LSO and VCN-LSO synapses. Numbers below each timeline are exemplary values for the respective parameters. Numbers in parentheses refer to (1) Alamilla & Gillespie (2013); (2) Case, Zhao, & Gillespie (2011); (3) Ehmann et al. (2013); (4) Garcia-Pino, Gessele, & Koch (2017); (5) Giugovaz-Tropper et al. (2011); (6) Hassfurth, Magnusson, Grothe, & Koch (2009); (7) Hirtz et al. (2012); (8) Jurkovicova-Tarabova et al. (2012); (9) Kandler & Friauf (1995a); (10) Kim & Kandler (2003); (11) Kim & Kandler (2010); (12) Noh, Seal, Garver, Edwards, & Kandler (2010); (13) Pilati et al. (2016); (14) Gjoni, Zenke, Bouhours, & Schneggenburger (2018); (15) Walcher, Hassfurth, Grothe, & Koch (2011).

α1 subunits and GluA4 subunits are associated with fast kinetics (Takahashi et al., 1992; Yang et al., 2011).

Spike kinetics in LSO neurons speed up drastically during development (Figure 13.10; Figure 13.11; Kandler & Friauf, 1995a; own unpublished observations). In neonatal rodents, APs are broad with a half-width of ~3 ms but shorten ~5-fold until hearing onset (Ebbers et al., 2015; Hirtz et al., 2011; Kandler & Friauf, 1995a). Fast AP repolarization is mainly associated to high-threshold potassium channels (I_{HT} channels; Johnston, Forsythe, & Kopp-Scheinpflug, 2010). We know virtually nothing about I_{HT} function in the LSO before hearing onset. In the whole brain, I_{HT} channel transcripts increase over the first two postnatal weeks (Perney, Marshall, Martin, Hockfield, & Kaczmarek, 1992), and this may also hold for the LSO per se.

Do the normal development of biophysical parameters and the increase in channel conductance depend on spontaneous prehearing activity? Mice systemically lacking voltage-gated calcium channels 1.3 ($Ca_v1.3$ KOs), VGluT3 KO mice, and *dn/dn* mice show flat auditory brainstem responses (ABRs), thus implying a lack of correlated auditory activity (Bock, Frank, & Steel, 1982; Durham, Rubel, & Steel, 1989; Platzer et al., 2000; Seal et al., 2008). The deafness of these KOs is suggestive of impaired spontaneous activity. In VGluT3 KOs, however, this is not the case (Babola et al., 2018; Sun et al., 2018). Although in VGluT3 KOs, glutamate release from IHCs is abolished (Seal et al., 2008), spontaneous activity persists in spiral ganglion neurons (SGNs) and propagates to the IC, albeit with a changed temporal pattern. This is the case because hyperexcitable SGNs are activated directly by supporting cells (Babola et al., 2018), a scenario which could generate spontaneous pre-hearing activity in other KO models as well (Sun et al., 2018).

LSO neurons in systemic $Ca_v1.3$ KOs display increased R_{in} values, reflecting an immature state (Hirtz et al., 2011). Moreover, I_{LT} channel labeling in the LSO of systemic $Ca_v1.3$ KOs is sparse, whereas age-matched wildtype mice show strong somatic labeling. Consequently, 80% of LSO neurons in P11 systemic $Ca_v1.3$ KOs fire multiple APs upon current injection. Furthermore, the AP half width is increased due to altered expression of I_{LT} channels and, probably, I_{HT} channels as well. In contrast to systemic $Ca_v1.3$ KOs, systemic VGluT3 KOs have normal membrane properties (Noh, Seal, Garver, Edwards, & Kandler, 2010). In *dn/dn* mice, the percentage of single and multiple firing LSO neurons is shifted towards more single firing neurons (Couchman et al., 2011). Whereas the R_{in} of multiple-firing *dn/dn* LSO neurons does not differ from that of multiple firing wildtype neurons, it is increased in single-firing neurons. Interestingly, HCN channel conductances are upregulated in *dn/dn* mice. In general, deficits in biophysical properties are most severe in systemic $Ca_v1.3$ KOs, milder in *dn/dn* mice, and absent in systemic VGluT3 KOs. A potential explanation is the difference in spontaneous activity propagation and the on-site expression of $Ca_v1.3$ in LSO neurons (Hirtz et al., 2011). Ca^{2+} influx through L-type calcium channels, for example $Ca_v1.3$, is involved in triggering genetic cascades (Greer & Greenberg, 2008), potentially necessary for normal development of LSO neurons. Indeed, brainstem-specific $Ca_v1.3$ KO reproduces the sparse labeling pattern of I_{LT} channels seen in systemic $Ca_v1.3$ KOs (Satheesh et al., 2012). Therefore, a combination of peripheral (missing spontaneous activity) and central effects (missing $Ca_v1.3$ in the SOC) may explain the more severe deficits seen in systemic $Ca_v1.3$ KOs. Further studies in brainstem-specific KOs should resolve this open issue.

Taken together, biophysical properties change drastically in ILD nuclei between P0–12 and adapt to the developmental needs of the system (Figure 13.10; Figure 13.11). At P0, a high R_{in} ensures high excitability from weak inputs to promote activity propagation through the immature system, likely enabling activity-dependent maturation processes. From ~P5 until hearing onset, the channel conductance increases in LSO neurons. This results in a gradual decrease in R_{in} and τ_{mem} and, consequently, increases the temporal precision, an attribute crucial for ILD computation.

Neurotransmitter Phenotype of LSO Input and D/H Shift

During postnatal week 1, MNTB-LSO synapses are special toward their transmitter phenotype, as they release (at least) three types of transmitter, namely GABA (Kotak et al., 1998), glycine (Nabekura et al., 2004), and glutamate (Figure 13.11A; Gillespie et al., 2005). Glycine and GABA appear to be released from the same synaptic vesicles (Nabekura et al., 2004), yet glutamate release likely occurs from other vesicles (Case & Gillespie, 2011; Cooper & Gillespie, 2011). GABA release is most prominent at P3–5 (reportedly ~75% of the total inhibitory current), after which the GABAergic proportion gradually drops until hearing onset (~10%; Kotak et al., 1998). At hearing onset, the main inhibitory neurotransmitter is glycine (90%; Figure 13.11A). The developmental neurotransmitter switch is disturbed in systemic $Ca_v1.3$ KOs, as shown by an increased number of GABAergic and a decreased number of glycinergic MNTB boutons, paralleled by a higher incidence of GABAergic miniature IPSCs (Hirtz et al., 2012). Between P0–8, virtually every LSO neuron shows glutamate responses from MNTB inputs (Gillespie et al., 2005). After P8, glutamate release diminishes, such that at hearing onset glutamate responses occur in only ~25% of LSO neurons. In deaf cir/cir mice, glutamate release from MNTB terminals persists and contributes largely to the total MNTB-mediated transmission, even after P8 (Hong, Kim, & Ahn, 2008). A similar pattern of results occurs after kanamycin-induced cochlea damage or unilateral cochlea ablation. Both manipulations lead to an increased glutamatergic component in MNTB-LSO transmission and higher VGluT3 immunoreactivity in MNTB terminals (Lee et al., 2011).

Interestingly, immature LSO neurons show a high internal Cl^- concentration ($[Cl]_i$) during postnatal week 1 (Balakrishnan et al., 2003; Ehrlich, Löhrke, & Friauf, 1999; Löhrke et al., 2005). The high $[Cl]_i$ is due to low activity of the Cl^--extruding potassium-chloride cotransporter 2 (KCC2; Balakrishnan et al., 2003; Friauf, Rust, Schulenborg, & Hirtz, 2011). It results in a Cl^- reversal potential more positive than V_{rest} (Balakrishnan et al., 2003; Ehrlich et al., 1999). Consequently, the "inhibitory" neurotransmitters GABA and glycine are depolarizing in the LSO during postnatal week 1 (Kandler & Friauf, 1995b), whereas they become "classically" hyperpolarizing during postnatal

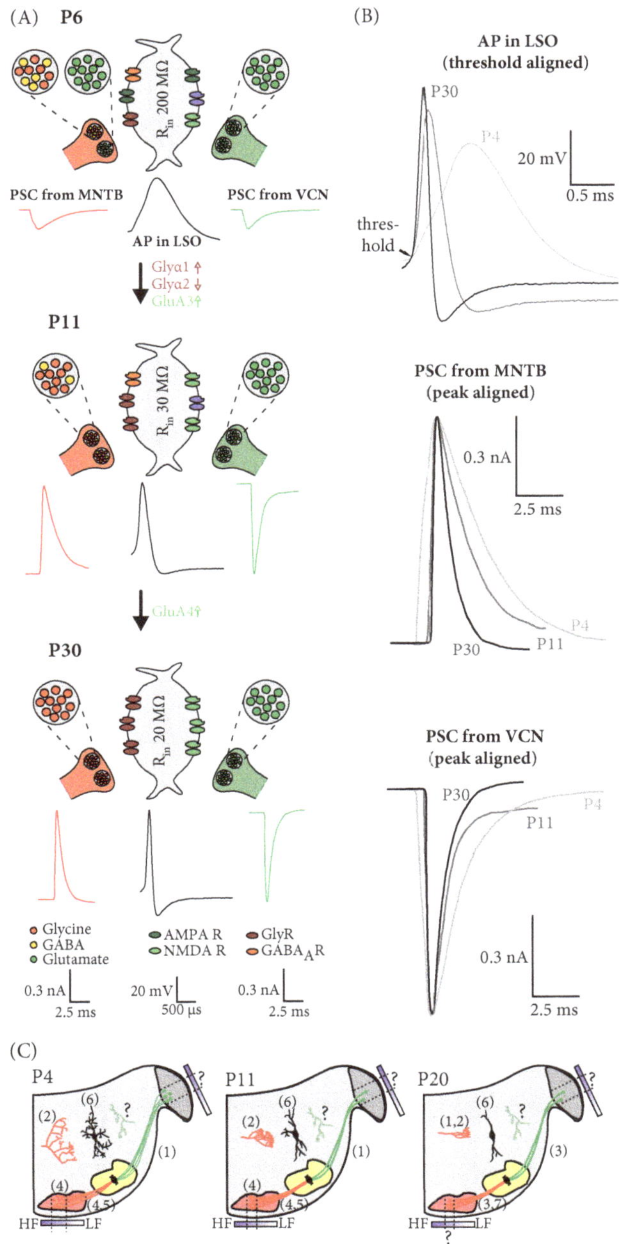

FIGURE 13.11. Postnatal development of synaptic input and output parameters in rodent LSO. **A.** Principal neuron (grey) and its synaptic inputs from MNTB (left, red) and VCN (right, green) before, around, and after hearing onset (P6, P11, P30). Presynaptic transmitter type, postsynaptic receptors, and input resistance (R_{in}) provided for each age. Evoked inhibitory postsynaptic current (eIPSCs; red) and eIPSCs (green) and APs (black) are shown as well. PSCs are modified from Pilati et al. (2016); APs are based on own unpublished data. Green and red arrows depict upregulation and downregulation in neurotransmitter receptors. **B.** Overlay of APs and PSCs from various ages (cf. panel A). **C.** Semi-schematic drawings depicting changes in fiber convergence and strength, tonotopic organization of the ILD circuit, as well as dendrite morphology of LSO neurons and architecture of MNTB (red) and CN (green) terminals (insets). Color gradients reflect the tonotopy in CN and MNTB. Open issues are highlighted with question marks. Numbers in parentheses refer to (1) Case et al. (2011); (2) Clause et al. (2014); (3) Garcia-Pino et al. (2017); (4) Kim & Kandler (2003); (5) Kim & Kandler (2010); (6) Rietzel & Friauf (1998); (7) Walcher et al. (2011).

week 2 (Figure 13.11; Kandler & Friauf, 1995b; Kullmann, Ene, & Kandler, 2002), a process named D/H shift. The early depolarizing period does not cause shunting inhibition (Friauf et al., 2011). It is indeed excitatory, because MNTB fiber stimulation in neonates can elicit APs in LSO perforated-patch recordings, a technique which maintains the native $[Cl^-]_i$ (Kullmann & Kandler, 2001; Löhrke et al., 2005). Furthermore, MNTB-mediated APs and application of GABA and glycine increase $[Ca^{2+}]_i$ of LSO neurons (Kullmann, Ene, & Kandler, 2002), possibly inducing genetic cascades. Taken together, the immature MNTB-LSO projection shows several transient features during postnatal week 1, such as GABA release, GABA/glycine-mediated depolarization, and glutamate corelease (Figure 13.11A). These features coincide temporally with the structural and functional reorganization in the immature ILD circuit. A potential involvement of glutamate corelease and glycinergic/GABAergic depolarization in these processes will be discussed in the section, "Structural and Functional Circuit Refinement."

Short-Term Plasticity

Upon repetitive activation, LSO inputs undergo STP (Friauf, Fischer, & Fuhr, 2015), that is, they dynamically adapt the strength of synaptic transmission (Zucker & Regehr, 2002). All LSO inputs respond to repetitive activation with STD. Thereby, the level of depression can depend on the activation frequency and the maturation state. In general, STD level decrease between birth and hearing onset and synaptic transmission becomes more robust (Case & Gillespie, 2011; Case, Zhao, & Gillespie, 2011; Krächan et al., 2017; Kramer et al., 2014). Developmental adaptions are coincident with a transition of presynaptic Ca^{2+} channels. During postnatal week 1, synaptic MNTB-LSO transmission in rats relies on L-type, N-type and P/Q-type Ca^{2+} channels to a similar extent, while P/Q type channels predominantly (> 90%) mediate transmission at hearing onset (Figure 13.10; Alamilla & Gillespie, 2013). Forty percent P/Q type channels are present at hearing onset in mice (Giugovaz-Tropper et al., 2011), potentially showing species-dependent differences. In contrast, the CN-LSO transmission employs mainly P/Q type (45%) and N-type channels (35%) in the first postnatal week, only increasing the percentage of P/Q type channels slightly (55%) until hearing onset (Alamilla & Gillespie, 2013).

Structural and Functional Circuit Refinement

As stated in section "Circuit Formation", the ILD circuit shows topographic features at birth. Nevertheless, the initial topography of MTNB-LSO inputs is coarse and further sharpened between P4–8 (Clause, Kim, et al., 2014; Hirtz et al., 2012; Kandler, Clause, & Noh, 2009; Kim & Kandler, 2003). Sharpening is ~2-fold and achieved by functional elimination of synaptic inputs, resulting in reduced MNTB-LSO input areas (Figure 13.11C; Kim & Kandler, 2003, 2010). At P3, fibers of 20–25 MNTB neurons converge on a single LSO neuron, while only 3–10 remain by P11 (Hirtz et al., 2012; Kim & Kandler,

2003, 2010; Noh et al., 2010; Walcher et al., 2011). In parallel to functional elimination, there is a 10–12-fold strengthening of the remaining MNTB fibers (Figure 13.10; Figure 13.11C; Hirtz et al., 2012; Kim & Kandler, 2003; Noh et al., 2010). The strengthening comprises a 2-fold increase in quantal size (i.e., postsynaptic current elicited by fusion of a single vesicle), but the main contribution is the increase in quantal content, very likely due to the addition of release sites to MNTB fibers (Kim & Kandler, 2010). Addition of release sites is supported by structural data from MNTB terminals, which show a 3-fold increase in bouton number of single MNTB fibers between P4 and P13 (Figure 13.10; Figure 13.11C; Clause, Kim, et al., 2014). In accordance with the topographical sharpening of MNTB inputs during postnatal week 1, dendrites of LSO neurons undergo pruning during the same period (Figure 13.11C; Rietzel & Friauf, 1998).

We know little about the molecular mechanisms of synaptic refinement. Ca^{2+}-dependent signaling may be involved in refinement, and LSO neurons possess several candidate molecules, such as NMDARs (Figure 13.11A; Case & Gillespie, 2011; Gillespie et al., 2005; Hirtz et al., 2011; Kalmbach, Kullmann, & Kandler, 2010) and functional L-type voltage-gated Ca^{2+} channels (Figure 13.10; Hirtz et al., 2011; Jurkovicova-Tarabova et al., 2012; Kullmann et al., 2002). Both molecules are involved in synaptic plasticity and genetic cascades (Citri & Malenka, 2008). NMDAR conductance peaks between P4–8, coincident with synaptic refinement. A causal link between synaptic elimination and long-term depression (LTD) and synaptic strengthening and long-term potentiation (LTP) is discussed (Kandler, 2004) and causality is likely when considering the visual system and the hippocampus (Lee et al., 2014; Wiegert & Oertner, 2013). Such causality remains to be shown for the ILD circuit. Both LTP and LTD have been demonstrated in the MNTB-LSO projection (Chang, Kotak, & Sanes, 2003; Kotak & Sanes, 2014; Pradhan, Maskey, & Ahn, 2012).

Compared with MNTB-LSO, we know less about CN-LSO synaptic refinement, mainly because the projection is difficult to preserve in slice preparations (Kronander, Michalski, Lebrand, Hornung, & Schneggenburger, 2017; Lohmann, Ilic, & Friauf, 1998). The CN-LSO projection refines roughly during the same period as the MNTB-LSO projection (Figure 13.10; Figure 13.11C; Case et al., 2011). At P3, ~5 fibers from CN neurons converge on a single LSO neuron, while ~3 fibers remain at P12 (Figure 13.10; Figure 13.11C; Case et al., 2011). Remaining CN-LSO fibers are also developmentally strengthened (~6-fold) within postnatal week 1–2. In contrast to the MNTB-LSO projections, CN-LSO fibers undergo further strengthening after the period of functional elimination (> P8; Case et al., 2011). Strengthening mechanisms for the CN-LSO projection are less clear. Quantal and structural analysis of CN-LSO terminals could clarify this open topic.

Are the temporally coincident features of the developing ILD circuit, such as prehearing spontaneous activity (CN-LSO; MNTB-LSO), glutamate corelease (MNTB-LSO), GABAergic transmission, and glycine and GABA mediated depolarization (MNTB-LSO) involved in ILD circuit refinement? To address this question, several studies have employed genetic approaches. They thus overcome invasive procedures such as surgical cochlea ablation, which often have severe side effects. VGluT3 KO mice are deaf (Seal et al., 2008), but spontaneous activity persists with a slightly changed temporal pattern (Babola et al., 2018; Sun et al., 2018). Furthermore, glutamate corelease from glycinergic MNTB terminals is abolished (Noh et al., 2010). VGluT3 KOs also show an impaired synaptic elimination and strengthening of the MNTB-LSO pathway (2-fold broader MNTB input width, 3-fold weaker MNTB fiber strength). Interestingly, the CN-LSO projection shows normal refinement (Noh et al., 2010), indicating a specific role of glutamate corelease for tonotopic refinement and strengthening of inhibitory (MNTB) synapses. Both synaptic elimination and strengthening of the MNTB-LSO projection are similarly impaired in systemic $Ca_V1.3$ KOs, which display a ~2-fold broader MNTB input width and a ~2-fold higher MNTB-LSO convergence (Hirtz et al., 2012). Single MNTB fiber strength is ~5-fold weaker, resulting from a reduced quantal size and a lower bouton number (Hirtz et al., 2012). A potential caveat of systemic $Ca_V1.3$ KOs is the on-site presence of $Ca_V1.3$ in the wildtype LSO, which makes it impossible to pinpoint the origin of the impairments to spontaneous peripheral activity, on-site effects or a combination of both. Cochlea—and brainstem-specific $Ca_V1.3$ KOs should clarify the respective role of $Ca_V1.3$ in the peripheral and the central auditory system.

In contrast to the harsh reduction of spontaneous peripheral activity in systemic $Ca_V1.3$ KOs, a genetic deletion of the α9 subunit of the acetylcholine receptor causes only modest activity alterations. Prehearing α9 KOs display a normal overall frequency of spontaneous activity, but shorter spike bursts and increased spiking between bursts, leading to a changed temporal fine structure. This subtle manipulation is sufficient to impair synaptic elimination and strengthening at the MNTB-LSO projection (Clause, Kim, et al., 2014). The results imply that spontaneous prehearing activity carries information that is crucial for normal synaptic refinement. The impact of glycine and GABA-mediated depolarization on synaptic refinement is not well known. First steps to disentangle the importance of the D/H shift (cf. section "Neurotransmitter Phenotype of LSO Input and D/H Shift") were performed by using KCC2 knockdown mice in which GABA and glycine neurotransmission remains depolarizing (Lee, Bach, Noh, Delpire, & Kandler, 2016). Synaptic elimination and strengthening of the MNTB-LSO pathway was normal in these animals. This result underlines that the D/H shift itself is not required for synaptic refinement, but it still leaves the impact of the transient GABAergic and glycinergic depolarizing period unclear.

As mentioned previously, we know relatively little about CN-LSO refinement. During early development, LSO neurons are innervated by noradrenergic afferents which originate from the locus coeruleus (Mulders & Robertson, 2001). Pharmacological blockade of adrenoceptors between P2–8 strongly impairs functional synaptic elimination and strengthening of the CN-LSO connection, thus arguing for a crucial role of noradrenergic signaling (Hirao et al., 2015). It is very likely that molecules other than noradrenaline also play a modulatory role during CN-LSO refinement. For example, somatostatin is heavily present in the CN-LSO connection of rats, yet only between P1–11 (Kungel & Friauf, 1995). Somatostatin depletion during this period results in less complex dendritic trees (Kungel, Piechotta, Rietzel, & Friauf, 1997), providing evidence for a trophic role during CN-LSO refinement.

Taken together, prehearing development yields an ILD circuit in the auditory brainstem with a plethora of structural and functional hallmarks that are uncommon to many other brain areas. The hallmarks include topographically aligned projections and fast output and input kinetics, the latter with a high temporal precision and resistance to synaptic fatigue. Spontaneous activity is necessary for several maturation processes before hearing onset. Future research should aim at revealing the role of several transient features, for example high $[Cl]_i$, GABA release, and high NMDA conductance. In addition, research needs to identify the molecular pathways controlling circuit maturation and to disentangle the impact of peripheral versus central activity.

Development and Plasticity after Hearing Onset

Hearing thresholds drop drastically around P12 in altricial rodents, coincident with hearing onset (Echteler et al., 1989; Woolf & Ryan, 1984, 1985). By this age, characteristic features of auditory brainstem circuits, such as temporal and topographical precision, synaptic reliability, and fast input and output kinetics are present in the ILD circuit (Trussell, 1999; von Gersdorff & Borst, 2002). Nevertheless, further developmental steps after hearing onset improve the aforementioned features. In this chapter, we will highlight the most important steps at the biophysical, structural, and functional level and discuss the impact of auditory experience on the maturation process.

Biophysical Adaptations

Several biophysical parameters of LSO neurons continue to maturate after hearing onset (Figure 13.10). First, R_{in} declines from ~70 MΩ to 20 MΩ until P20 in gerbils (Walcher et al., 2011). Second, τ_{mem} accelerates ~4-fold in gerbils and ~2-fold in mice, reaching ~2 ms in both species (Garcia-Pino, Gessele, & Koch, 2017; Walcher et al., 2011). Third, HCN conductance increases ~3-fold in gerbils (Hassfurth et al., 2009). The HCN half-activation voltage decreases from ~-90 mV to -70–80 mV between P10–17 (Garcia-Pino et al., 2017; Hassfurth et al., 2009), yielding HCN-mediated conductances close to V_{rest}. A low R_{in} and large HCN channel conductance are characteristics of temporally precise circuits (Khurana et al., 2012). Functionally, an HCN conductance reduces τ_{mem}, resulting in local acceleration of EPSP kinetics, thus minimizing temporal summation of LSO inputs (Leao, Leao, & Walmsley, 2011). Pharmacological blockade of HCN channels hyperpolarize LSO neurons, increase the R_{in} and τ_{mem} (Hassfurth et al., 2009). This highlights the functional importance of the HCN channel conductance in the LSO as a basis of temporally precise processing and ILD computation.

Another key conductance for temporally precise computation is provided by I_{LT} (Golding & Oertel, 2012). I_{LT} is highly abundant in the LSO of P30 rats, increasing from medial to lateral (Barnes-Davies et al., 2004), suggesting different firing properties at different isofrequency bands. Indeed, single-firing LSO neurons are more abundant in the lateral limb (Barnes-Davies et al., 2004). Similar to the situation before hearing onset, little is known about I_{HT} in the LSO after hearing onset. Robust staining for $K_v3.3$, but not $K_v3.1$, suggests a more prominent role of $K_v3.3$ (Grigg, Brew, & Tempel, 2000; Li, Kaczmarek, & Perney, 2001). AP kinetics of LSO neurons speed up drastically after hearing onset, characterized by a fast rising phase and a similarly fast repolarization, which results in a half width of ~200 μs at P21 (Figure 13.11B; Garcia-Pino et al., 2017).

Synaptic kinetics also accelerate further after hearing onset. The decay time of MNTB-mediated IPSCs is ~0.8 ms for young adults (Pilati et al., 2016), which is among the fastest glycinergic kinetics in the brain. Other studies report similar values (Kramer et al., 2014; Walcher et al., 2011). CN-mediated EPSCs accelerate after hearing onset to 0.9 ms in young adults (Pilati et al., 2016). Consequently, they match IPSC kinetics (Figure 13.10; Figure 13.11). This contrasts with many other brain regions, in which kinetics of EPSCs are usually several-fold faster than IPSC kinetics (Xie & Manis, 2013). The fast, sub-ms kinetics are likely due a low R_{in}, which becomes manifested after hearing onset. Another contribution is the developmental reorganization of glycine and AMPAR subunits. The abundance of the fast GluA4 AMPAR subunit increases > 2-fold (Pilati et al., 2016).

The developmental EPSC acceleration in the LSO very likely depends on normal auditory experience. Acoustic trauma results in increased ABR thresholds and prolonged EPSCs in the LSO due to reorganization in the AMPAR subunit composition (Pilati et al., 2016). Because IPSC kinetics are unchanged, subunit composition of GlyRs is likely less plastic than that of AMPARs. Due to the prolonged EPSC kinetics, ILD functions are shifted toward the contralateral side after acoustic trauma. The effect is fully reversible after ~2 months, after which EPSC kinetics have returned to normal (Pilati et al., 2016). Taken together, biophysical parameters of LSO neurons maturate further after hearing onset. In combination, decrease of the R_{in} and acceleration of τ_{mem}, APs, and GlyR and AMPAR kinetics to an adult-like state are all crucial for temporally precise processing in the ILD circuit (Golding & Oertel, 2012).

Short-Term Plasticity

Synapses in the auditory brainstem are active at a high rate. Spontaneous MNTB spike activity at P28 is ~30 Hz, reaching ~350 Hz upon sound stimulation (Sonntag et al., 2009). Synapses of the ILD circuit must be able to transmit such high frequencies in order to function properly. Indeed, MNTB-LSO and CN-LSO synapses show little synaptic failures upon repetitive high-frequency stimulation. At P21, the CN-LSO projection shows steady-state depression levels of 20–30% even at 200 Hz after 20 pulses (Garcia-Pino et al., 2017; Walcher et al., 2011). MNTB-LSO synapses depress to a steady-state level of ~15% at this frequency. Extending the stimulus duration to 60 s, steady-state depression is ~10% (Kramer et al., 2014). Thus, the MNTB-LSO and CN-LSO synapses can cope with high activation rates despite profound synaptic depression, and they are resistant to synaptic fatigue over prolonged periods. Highly efficient replenishment mechanisms are most likely at both MNTB-LSO and CN-LSO synapses, but the issue needs further investigation. Potential developmental specializations after hearing onset, such as nanodomain coupling, maturation of the readily releasable pool, or replenishment mechanisms are yet to be resolved.

Structural and Functional Refinement of the ILD Circuit

MNTB axon terminals in the LSO become pruned between P13–20, and the number of boutons per MNTB fiber is reduced by ~50%, accompanied by a ~50% reduction of the bouton area (Figure 13.11C; Clause, Kim, et al., 2014). As a result, the bouton spread along the tonotopic axis is reduced, further sharpening the topographic map (Clause, Kim, et al., 2014; Sanes & Siverls, 1991). The topographic sharpening is disrupted in gerbils upon unilateral cochlea ablation; these animals show a larger spread of boutons within the LSO (Sanes & Takacs, 1993). In parallel with bouton pruning during normal development, dendrites of LSO neurons undergo pruning after hearing onset as well (Figure 13.11C). For example, the number of primary dendrites is reduced from 6 to 4 between P11–36, and the number of dendritic endpoints is reduced even 5-fold, from ~150 to ~25 (Rietzel & Friauf, 1998).

Effects of deafferentation on the structural refinement in the ILD circuit have often been studied in deafened rodents. Early deafferentation by means of surgical ablation of the cochlea or treatment with ototoxins causes a variety of abnormalities, including neuronal loss (Moore, 1990, 1992; Moore, Rogers, & O'Leary, 1998), changed synaptic strength (Kotak & Sanes, 1996, 1997), and changed morphology (Sanes & Takacs, 1993). Unilateral cochlea ablation at P7 weakens excitatory VCN-LSO transmission on the ablated side and inhibitory MNTB-LSO transmission on the unablated side (Kotak & Sanes, 1996, 1997). Furthermore, ectopic VCN-MNTB projections form as VCN neurons of the non-ablated side project to previously inappropriate targets, including the ipsilateral MNTB and the contralateral LSO (Kitzes, Kageyama, Semple, & Kil, 1995; Russell & Moore, 1995). Another common denominator of such studies is a reduced topographic precision due to broader spread of axon terminals or LSO dendrites. For example, unilateral cochlea ablation at P7 results in more dendritic branch points in the LSO of the ablated side by P21 (Sanes & Chokshi, 1992; Sanes, Markowitz, Bernstein, & Wardlow, 1992). As a cautionary note, several early cochlea ablation studies (≤ P7) have a big drawback: if structural pruning is analyzed 1–2 weeks later, spontaneous prehearing as well as acoustically evoked activity is affected and, therefore, a clear causal conclusion toward the lacking activity cannot be drawn. Consequently, an important field of study will be to determine the impact of acoustic experience in isolation.

Little is known about critical periods during development of the ILD circuit. Sprouting of MNTB terminals is likely to be restricted to the time before hearing onset and hence does not depend on auditory experience, as cochlea ablation at P10, very shortly before hearing onset, does not yield *de novo* sprouting of AVCN-LSO projections (Russell & Moore, 1995). Nevertheless, even in adult rats, unilateral cochlea lesions or acoustic traumata induce several anatomical, cellular, and molecular changes in the brainstem, for example, a long-lasting (> 1 year) reappearance of the growth-associated protein 43 (GAP-43) in the LSO, as well as the CN and IC, the input and target nuclei of the LSO (Illing et al., 2000; Michler & Illing, 2002). The results corroborate earlier findings of a higher density of GlyRs in the contralateral LSO five months after unilateral cochleotopy (Suneja, Benson, & Potashner, 1998). They provide evidence for substantial adult auditory brainstem plasticity, possibly lasting throughout life, and can be interpreted toward reweighting synaptic inputs and readjusting neuronal tuning to prevent the ILD network from delivering false signals to higher auditory centers.

Does auditory experience yield further functional elimination or strengthening of inputs to the LSO? At P18, fibers of 3–4 MNTB neurons innervate a single LSO neuron in mice and gerbils, similar to P10. The data suggest no further functional elimination after hearing onset (Walcher et al., 2011). MNTB fiber strength also stays constant after hearing onset (Figure 13.10, Figure 13.11C). This contrasts with two reports of a developmental decline of the MNTB fiber conductance from prehearing until after hearing onset (Kramer et al., 2014; Pilati et al., 2016). The latter reports have not determined single fiber strength, which potentially explains the discrepancies. CN-LSO single fiber strength remains unchanged after hearing onset, but maximal CN-LSO strength increases. An unchanged quantal size after hearing onset suggests a developmental addition of release sites (Garcia-Pino et al., 2017). Interestingly, in a mouse model for Fragile X syndrome (fragile X mental retardation protein [FRMP] KOs), the maximal strength of CN-LSO synapses is abnormally high after hearing onset, whereas the MNTB-LSO strength develops normally. Increased excitation, combined with normal inhibition, results in shifted binaural sensitivity and increased firing rates in the LSO of FRMP KOs (Garcia-Pino et al., 2017). The changes potentially underlie the auditory hypersensitivity and processing deficits described in Fragile X patients.

As further functional refinement after hearing onset is not observed in the MNTB-LSO projection until P20, structural refinement appears to be temporally segregated from functional refinement (Clause, Kim, et al., 2014). Interestingly, disruption of the temporal pattern of spontaneous prehearing activity in α9 KOs affects not only the functional refinement before hearing onset, but also the structural refinement thereafter (Clause, Kim, et al., 2014). This is surprising because α9 KOs lack obvious hearing deficits (May, Prosen, Weiss, & Vetter, 2002; Vetter et al., 1999) besides a disturbed frequency discrimination (Clause, Lauer, & Kandler, 2017), consistent with a disturbed MNTB-LSO circuit refinement (Clause, Kim, et al., 2014). Axonal end branches of MNTB neurons stay unpruned after hearing onset in α9 KOs and thus remain in an immature state, exhibiting a higher bouton number and a larger topographic spread than normally. These results suggest that structural refinement after hearing onset is predefined by the functional elimination before hearing onset, even though both processes are temporally segregated.

Very little is known about structural and functional refinement after hearing onset in KO models. While several studies have investigated systemic $Ca_V1.3$, VGluT3, and α9 KOs during prehearing age, these models are thus far rarely employed after P20. This leaves a multitude of open questions about ILD circuit development in these models (Figure 13.11). Taken together, the ILD circuit further matures after hearing onset mainly by structural refinement, finally yielding an astonishing degree of topographic alignment.

Conclusion

In this monumental book chapter on the LSO, we aimed to provide an overview of our current knowledge about this fascinating nucleus in the auditory brainstem, in terms of organization, development, and plasticity—unlike previous reviews, which have tried to combine several seemingly diverse aspects of the 'ILD detector' in a single article. To our knowledge, this is the first attempt to do so. Our motto has been 'All in one go what one ought to know about the LSO.' Thus far, no review has put the LSO in the center of its work. It is our hope that the reader will find the insights provided by the chapters helpful in better understanding a major station of the central auditory system. For further reading and to the die-hard LSO aficionados, we recommend the following reviews published over the past 20 years or so. Structure and function of central auditory system: Altschuler & Shore, 2010; Malmierca & Hackett, 2010; Schofield, 2010. SOC: Schwartz, 1992. Binaural sound localization cues: Grothe, Pecka, & McAlpine, 2010; Middlebrooks, 2015; Tollin, 2003; Yin, 2013; Yin, 2002; Yin & Kuwada, 2010. Development of central auditory system: Cant, 1998; Sanes & Walsh, 1998. Development and plasticity of the SOC: Friauf, 2004; Moore & King, 2004. Development of sound localization circuits: Clause, Sturm, Altien, Maricich, & Kandler, 2014; Kandler & Gillespie, 2005.

Several structural and functional specializations in the ILD circuit place LSO neurons into the position to process binaural information with high speed, precision, and fidelity, even during sustained activity. The acquisition of these features is set via genetic programs and shaped by processes comprising activity-dependent remodeling. The latter make the LSO circuit crucially dependent on proper cochlea function. Although the mechanisms for sound localization are among the most thoroughly studied of central auditory information processing, many open issues remain and request future research. For example, there is compelling and growing evidence that LSO neurons have more diverse attributes than previously thought. It is therefore important to determine whether various cell types mediate complementary functions in binaural processing. Methods that combine morphology, physiology, and genetics will shed light on these issues. Likewise, it is mandatory to bring in vivo and in vitro data together. Finally, aging, with its various functional and behavioral changes, involves not only deterioration of the auditory periphery, but also deficits in central auditory processing. It will be interesting to investigate how much an impaired performance of the LSO contributes to this important issue.

Acknowledgments

This work was supported by the Priority Program 1608 "Ultrafast and temporally precise information processing: normal and dysfunctional hearing" of the Deutsche Forschungsgemeinschaft (grant Fr1784/17-1 to EF). Special thanks to Drs. Jan Hirtz and Karl Kandler for valuable comments on the manuscript and to Ulrike Eschbach for providing expert secretarial help.

References

Abdul-Latif, M. L., Salazar, J. A., Marshak, S., Dinh, M. L., & Cramer, K. S. (2015). Ephrin-A2 and ephrin-A5 guide contralateral targeting but not topographic mapping of ventral cochlear nucleus axons. *Neural Development, 10*, 27. doi:10.1186/s13064-015-0054-6

Adam, T. J., Finlayson, P. G., & Schwarz, D. W. (2001). Membrane properties of principal neurons of the lateral superior olive. *Journal of Neurophysiology, 86*(2), 922–934. doi:10.1152/jn.2001.86.2.922

Adam, T. J., Schwarz, D. W. F., & Finlayson, P. G. (1999). Firing properties of chopper and delay neurons in the lateral superior olive of the rat. *Experimental Brain Research, 124*(4), 489–502.

Akazawa, C., Ishibashi, M., Shimizu, C., Nakanishi, S., & Kageyama, R. (1995). A mammalian helix-loop-helix factor structurally related to the product of Drosophila proneural gene atonal is a positive transcriptional regulator expressed in the developing nervous system. *Journal of Biological Chemistry, 270*(15), 8730–8738.

Alamilla, J., & Gillespie, D. C. (2013). Maturation of calcium-dependent GABA, glycine, and glutamate release in the glycinergic MNTB-LSO pathway. *PLoS One, 8*(9), e75688. doi:10.1371/journal.pone.0075688

Alexander, S. P., Peters, J. A., Kelly, E., Marrion, N. V., Faccenda, E., Harding, S. D., . . . Davies, J. A.; CGTP Collaborators. (2017). The concise guide to pharmacology 2017/18: Ligand-gated ion channels. *British Journal of Pharmacology, 174 Suppl. 1*, S130–S159. doi:10.1111/bph.13879

Altieri, S. C., Jalabi, W., Zhao, T., Romito-DiGiacomo, R. R., & Maricich, S. M. (2015). En1 directs superior olivary complex neuron positioning, survival, and expression of FoxP1. *Developmental Biology, 408*(1), 99–108. doi:10.1016/j.ydbio.2015.10.008

Altman, J., & Bayer, S. A. (1980). Development of the brain stem in the rat. III. Thymidine-radiographic study of the time of origin of neurons of the vestibular and auditory nuclei of the upper medulla. *Journal of Comparative Neurology, 194*(4), 877–904. doi:10.1002/cne.901940410

Altschuler, R. A., & Shore, S. E. (2010). Central auditory neurotransmitters. In A. Rees & A. R. Palmer (Eds.), *Oxford handbook of auditory science: The auditory brain* (Vol. 2, pp. 965–989). Oxford, New York: Oxford University Press.

Aschoff, A., & Ostwald, J. (1987). Different origins of cochlear efferents in some bat species, rats, and guinea pigs. *Journal of Comparative Neurology, 264*(1), 56–72. doi:10.1002/cne.902640106

Azeredo, W. J., Kliment, M. L., Morley, B. J., Relkin, E., Slepecky, N. B., Sterns, A., . . . Woods, C. I. (1999). Olivocochlear neurons in the chinchilla: a retrograde fluorescent labelling study. *Hearing Research, 134*(1–2), 57–70. doi:10.1016/s0378-5955(99)00069-6

Babola, T. A., Li, S., Gribizis, A., Lee, B. J., Issa, J. B., Wang, H. C., . . . Bergles, D. E. (2018). Homeostatic control of spontaneous activity in the developing auditory system. *Neuron, 99*(3), 511–524. e515. doi:10.1016/j.neuron.2018.07.004

Balakrishnan, V., Becker, M., Löhrke, S., Nothwang, H. G., Güresir, E., & Friauf, E. (2003). Expression and function of chloride transporters during development of inhibitory neurotransmission in the auditory brainstem. *Journal of Neuroscience, 23*(10), 4134–4145.

Barnes-Davies, M., Barker, M. C., Osmani, F., & Forsythe, I. D. (2004). Kv1 currents mediate a gradient of principal neuron excitability across the tonotopic axis in the rat lateral superior olive. *European Journal of Neuroscience, 19*(2), 325–333.

Batra, R., Kuwada, S., & Fitzpatrick, D. C. (1997a). Sensitivity to interaural temporal disparities of low—and high-frequency neurons in the superior olivary complex. I. Heterogeneity of responses. *Journal of Neurophysiology, 78*(3), 1222–1236. doi:10.1152/jn.1997.78.3.1222

Batra, R., Kuwada, S., & Fitzpatrick, D. C. (1997b). Sensitivity to interaural temporal disparities of low—and high-frequency neurons in the superior olivary complex. II. Coincidence detection. *Journal of Neurophysiology, 78*(3), 1237–1247. doi:10.1152/jn.1997.78.3.1237

Bazwinsky, I., Bidmon, H. J., Zilles, K., & Hilbig, H. (2005). Characterization of the rhesus monkey superior olivary complex by calcium binding proteins and synaptophysin. *Journal of Anatomy, 207*(6), 745–761. doi:10.1111/j.1469-7580.2005.00491.x

Bazwinsky-Wutschke, I., Härtig, W., Kretzschmar, R., & Rübsamen, R. (2016). Differential morphology of the superior olivary complex of *Meriones unguiculatus* and *Monodelphis domestica* revealed by calcium-binding proteins. *Brain Structure and Function, 221*(9), 4505–4523. doi:10.1007/s00429-015-1181-x

Beiderbeck, B., Myoga, M. H., Müller, N. I. C., Callan, A. R., Friauf, E., Grothe, B., & Pecka, M. (2018). Precisely timed inhibition facilitates action potential firing for spatial coding in the auditory brainstem. *Nature Communications, 9*(1), 1771. doi:10.1038/s41467-018-04210-y

Ben-Arie, N., McCall, A. E., Berkman, S., Eichele, G., Bellen, H. J., & Zoghbi, H. Y. (1996). Evolutionary conservation of sequence and expression of the bHLH protein Atonal suggests a conserved role in neurogenesis. *Human Molecular Genetics, 5*(9), 1207–1216.

Bernstein, E., Caudy, A. A., Hammond, S. M., & Hannon, G. J. (2001). Role for a bidentate ribonuclease in the initiation step of RNA interference. *Nature, 409*(6818), 363–366. doi:10.1038/35053110

Bledsoe, S. C., Snead, C. R., Helfert, R. H., Prasad, V., Wenthold, R. J., & Altschuler, R. A. (1990). Immunocytochemical and lesion studies support the hypothesis that the projection from the medial nucleus of the trapezoid body to the lateral superior olive Is glycinergic. *Brain Research, 517*(1–2), 189–194. doi:10.1016/0006-8993(90)91025-C

Bock, G. R., Frank, M. P., & Steel, K. P. (1982). Preservation of central auditory function in the deafness mouse. *Brain Research, 239*(2), 608–612.

Borst, J. G., & Soria van Hoeve, J. (2012). The calyx of Held synapse: From model synapse to auditory relay. *Annual Review of Physiology, 74*, 199–224. doi:10.1146/annurev-physiol-020911-153236

Boudreau, J. C., & Tsuchitani, C. (1968). Binaural interaction in the cat superior olive S segment. *Journal of Neurophysiology, 31*(3), 442–454. doi:10.1152/jn.1968.31.3.442

Bouhours, B., Gjoni, E., Kochubey, O., & Schneggenburger, R. (2017). Synaptotagmin2 (Syt2) drives fast release redundantly with Syt1 at the output synapses of parvalbumin-expressing inhibitory neurons. *Journal of Neuroscience*, *37*(17), 4604–4617. doi:10.1523/jneurosci.3736-16.2017

Brew, H. M., & Forsythe, I. D. (1995). Two voltage-dependent K+ conductances with complementary functions in postsynaptic integration at a central auditory synapse. *Journal of Neuroscience*, *15*(12), 8011–8022.

Brownell, W. E., Manis, P. B., & Ritz, L. A. (1979). Ipsilateral inhibitory responses in the cat lateral superior olive. *Brain Research*, *177*(1), 189–193.

Brunso-Bechtold, J. K., Linville, M. C., & Henkel, C. K. (1994). Terminal types on ipsilaterally and contralaterally projecting lateral superior olive cells. *Hearing Research*, *77*(1–2), 99–104.

Caicedo, A., & Eybalin, M. (1999). Glutamate receptor phenotypes in the auditory brainstem and mid-brain of the developing rat. *European Journal of Neuroscience*, *11*(1), 51–74.

Caird, D., & Klinke, R. (1983). Processing of binaural stimuli by cat superior olivary complex neurons. *Experimental Brain Research*, *52*(3), 385–399.

Cant, N. B. (1984). The fine structure of the lateral superior olivary nucleus of the cat. *Journal of Comparative Neurology*, *227*(1), 63–77. doi:10.1002/cne.902270108

Cant, N. B. (1998). Structural development of the mammalian auditory pathways. In E. W. Rubel, A. N. Popper, & R. R. Fay (Eds.), *Development of the Auditory System* (pp. 315–413). New York: Springer.

Case, D. T., & Gillespie, D. C. (2011). Pre- and postsynaptic properties of glutamatergic transmission in the immature inhibitory MNTB-LSO pathway. *Journal of Neurophysiology*, *106*(5), 2570–2579. doi:10.1152/jn.00644.2010

Case, D. T., Zhao, X., & Gillespie, D. C. (2011). Functional refinement in the projection from ventral cochlear nucleus to lateral superior olive precedes hearing onset in rat. *PLoS One*, *6*(6), e20756. doi:10.1371/journal.pone.0020756

Casey, M. A. (1990). The effects of aging on neuron number in the rat superior olivary complex. *Neurobiology of Aging*, *11*(4), 391–394.

Casey, M. A., & Feldman, M. L. (1982). Aging in the rat medial nucleus of the trapezoid body. I. Light microscopy. *Neurobiology of Aging*, *3*(3), 187–195.

Casey, M. A., & Feldman, M. L. (1985). Aging in the rat medial nucleus of the trapezoid body. II. Electron microscopy. *Journal of Comparative Neurology*, *232*(3), 401–413. doi:10.1002/cne.902320311

Caspary, D. M., & Faingold, C. L. (1989). Non-N-methyl-D-aspartate receptors may mediate ipsilateral excitation at lateral superior olivary synapses. *Brain Research*, *503*(1), 83–90. doi:10.1016/0006-8993(89)91707-1

Caspary, D. M., & Finlayson, P. G. (1991). Superior olivary complex: Functional neuropharmacology of the principal cell types. In R. A. Altschuler, R. P. Bobbin, B. M. Clopton, & D. W. Hoffman (Eds.), *Neurobiology of hearing: The central auditory system* (Vol. 1, pp. 141–161). New York: Raven Press, Ltd.

Caspary, D. M., Ling, L., Turner, J. G., & Hughes, L. F. (2008). Inhibitory neurotransmission, plasticity and aging in the mammalian central auditory system. *Journal of Experimental Biology*, *211*(Pt 11), 1781–1791. doi:10.1242/jeb.013581

Casseday, J. H., & Neff, W. D. (1973). Localization of pure tones. *Journal of the Acoustical Society of America*, *54*(2), 365–372.

Chang, E. H., Kotak, V. C., & Sanes, D. H. (2003). Long-term depression of synaptic inhibition is expressed postsynaptically in the developing auditory system. *Journal of Neurophysiology*, *90*(3), 1479–1488. doi:10.1152/jn.00386.2003

Chavrier, P., Vesque, C., Galliot, B., Vigneron, M., Dolle, P., Duboule, D., & Charnay, P. (1990). The segment-specific gene Krox-20 encodes a transcription factor with binding sites in the promoter region of the Hox-1.4 gene. *EMBO Journal*, *9*(4), 1209–1218.

Chen, C., Arai, I., Satterfield, R., Young, S. M., Jr., & Jonas, P. (2017). Synaptotagmin 2 is the fast Ca^{2+} sensor at a central inhibitory synapse. *Cell Reports*, *18*(3), 723–736. doi:10.1016/j.celrep.2016.12.067

Chen, Q. C., Cain, D., & Jen, P. H. (1995). Sound pressure transformation at the Pinna of *Mus deopmesticus*. *Journal of Experimental Biology*, *198*(9), 2007–2023.

Citri, A., & Malenka, R. C. (2008). Synaptic plasticity: Multiple forms, functions, and mechanisms. *Neuropsychopharmacology*, *33*(1), 18–41. doi:10.1038/sj.npp.1301559

Clause, A., Kim, G., Sonntag, M., Weisz, C. J., Vetter, D. E., Rübsamen, R., & Kandler, K. (2014). The precise temporal pattern of prehearing spontaneous activity is necessary for tonotopic map refinement. *Neuron*, *82*(4), 822–835. doi:10.1016/j.neuron.2014.04.001

Clause, A., Lauer, A. M., & Kandler, K. (2017). Mice lacking the alpha9 subunit of the nicotinic acetylcholine receptor exhibit deficits in frequency difference limens and sound localization. *Frontiers in Cellular Neuroscience*, *11*, 167. doi:10.3389/fncel.2017.00167

Clause, A., Sturm, J., Altien, S. C., Maricich, S. M., & Kandler, K. (2014). Development of mammalian primary sound localization circuits. In R. Romand & V.-N. I. (Eds.), *Development of auditory and vestibular systems* (4th ed., pp. 249–285). Amsterdam: Elsevier.

Coomes, D. L., & Schofield, B. R. (2004). Projections from the auditory cortex to the superior olivary complex in guinea pigs. *European Journal of Neuroscience*, *19*(8), 2188–2200. doi:10.1111/j.0953-816X.2004.03317.x

Coomes Peterson, D., & Schofield, B. R. (2007). Projections from auditory cortex contact ascending pathways that originate in the superior olive and inferior colliculus. *Hearing Research*, *232*(1–2), 67–77. doi:10.1016/j.heares.2007.06.009

Cooper, A. P., & Gillespie, D. C. (2011). Synaptotagmins I and II in the developing rat auditory brainstem: Synaptotagmin I is transiently expressed in glutamate-releasing immature inhibitory terminals. *Journal of Comparative Neurology*, *519*(12), 2417–2433. doi:10.1002/cne.22634

Cordes, S. P., & Barsh, G. S. (1994). The mouse segmentation gene kr encodes a novel basic domain-leucine zipper transcription factor. *Cell*, *79*(6), 1025–1034.

Couchman, K., Garrett, A., Deardorff, A. S., Rattay, F., Resatz, S., Fyffe, R., . . . Leao, R. N. (2011). Lateral superior olive function in congenital deafness. *Hearing Research*, *277*(1–2), 163–175. doi:10.1016/j.heares.2011.01.012

Covey, E., Jones, D. R., & Casseday, J. H. (1984). Projections from the superior olivary complex to the cochlear nucleus in the tree shrew. *Journal of Comparative Neurology*, *226*(2), 289–305. doi:10.1002/cne.902260212

Covey, E., Vater, M., & Casseday, J. H. (1991). Binaural properties of single units in the superior olivary complex of the mustached bat. *Journal of Neurophysiology*, *66*(3), 1080–1094. doi:10.1152/jn.1991.66.3.1080

Cramer, K. S. (2005). Eph proteins and the assembly of auditory circuits. *Hearing Research*, *206*(1–2), 42–51. doi:10.1016/j.heares.2004.11.024

Cramer, K. S., & Gabriele, M. L. (2014). Axon guidance in the auditory system: Multiple functions of Eph receptors. *Neuroscience*, *277*, 152–162. doi:10.1016/j.neuroscience.2014.06.068

Darrow, K. N., Benson, T. E., & Brown, M. C. (2012). Planar multipolar cells in the cochlear nucleus project to medial olivocochlear neurons in mouse. *Journal of Comparative Neurology*, *520*(7), 1365–1375. doi:10.1002/cne.22797

Darrow, K. N., Maison, S. F., & Liberman, M. C. (2006). Cochlear efferent feedback balances interaural sensitivity. *Nature Neuroscience*, *9*(12), 1474–1476. doi:10.1038/nn1807

Deol, M. S. (1964). The abnormalities of the inner ear in *kreisler* mice. *Journal of Embryology and Experimental Morphology*, *12*, 475–490.

Di Bonito, M., Narita, Y., Avallone, B., Sequino, L., Mancuso, M., Andolfi, G., . . . Studer, M. (2013). Assembly of the auditory circuitry by a Hox genetic network in the mouse brainstem. *PLoS Genetics*, *9*(2), e1003249. doi:10.1371/journal.pgen.1003249

Doucet, J. R., & Ryugo, D. K. (2003). Axonal pathways to the lateral superior olive labeled with biotinylated dextran amine injections in the dorsal cochlear nucleus of rats. *Journal of Comparative Neurology*, *461*(4), 452–465. doi:10.1002/cne.10722

Doucet, J. R., & Ryugo, D. K. (2006). Structural and functional classes of multipolar cells in the ventral cochlear nucleus. *Anatomical Record*, *288*(4), 331–344. doi:10.1002/ar.a.20294

Durham, D., Rubel, E. W., & Steel, K. P. (1989). Cochlear ablation in *deafness* mutant mice: 2-deoxyglucose analysis suggests no spontaneous activity of cochlear origin. *Hearing Research*, *43*(1), 39–46. doi:10.1016/0378-5955(89)90057-9

Ebbers, L., Satheesh, S. V., Janz, K., Rüttiger, L., Blosa, M., Hofmann, F., . . . Nothwang, H. G. (2015). L-type calcium channel $Ca_v1.2$ is required for maintenance of auditory brainstem nuclei. *Journal of Biological Chemistry*, *290*(39), 23692–23710. doi:10.1074/jbc.M115.672675

Echteler, S. M., Arjmand, E., & Dallos, P. (1989). Developmental alterations in the frequency map of the mammalian cochlea. *Nature*, *341*(6238), 147–149. doi:10.1038/341147a0

Ehmann, H., Hartwich, H., Salzig, C., Hartmann, N., Clement-Ziza, M., Ushakov, K., . . . Nothwang, H. G. (2013). Time-dependent gene expression analysis of the developing superior olivary complex. *Journal of Biological Chemistry*, *288*(36), 25865–25879. doi:10.1074/jbc.M113.490508

Ehret, G. (1976). Development of absolute auditory thresholds in the house mouse (*Mus musculus*). *Journal of the American Academy of Audiology*, *1*(5), 179–184.

Ehret, G., & Dreyer, A. (1984). Localization of tones and noise in the horizontal plane by unrestrained house mice (*Mus musculus*). *Journal of Experimental Biology*, *109*, 163–174.

Ehrlich, I., Löhrke, S., & Friauf, E. (1999). Shift from depolarizing to hyperpolarizing glycine action in rat auditory neurons is due to age-dependent Cl^- regulation. *Journal of Physiology*, *520*, 121–137. doi:10.1111/j.1469-7793.1999.00121.x

Farago, A. F., Awatramani, R. B., & Dymecki, S. (2006). Assembly of the brainstem cochlear nuclear complex is revealed by intersectional and subtractive genetic fate maps. *Neuron*, *50*(2), 205–218. doi:10.1016/j.neuron.2006.03.014

Fech, T., Calderon-Garciduenas, L., & Kulesza, R. J., Jr. (2017). Characterization of the superior olivary complex of *Canis lupus domesticus*. *Hearing Research*, *351*, 130–140. doi:10.1016/j.heares.2017.06.010

Feliciano, M., Saldaña, E., & Mugnaini, E. (1995). Direct projections from the rat primary auditory neocortex to nucleus sagulum, paralemniscal regions, superior olivary complex and cochlear nuclei. *Auditory Neuroscience*, *1*, 287–308.

Finlayson, P. G. (1995). Decreased inhibition to lateral superior olive neurons in young and aged Sprague-Dawley rats. *Hearing Research*, *87*(1–2), 84–95.

Finlayson, P. G., & Caspary, D. M. (1989). Synaptic potentials of chinchilla lateral superior olivary neurons. *Hearing Research*, *38*(3), 221–228.

Finlayson, P. G., & Caspary, D. M. (1991). Low-frequency neurons in the lateral superior olive exhibit phase-sensitive binaural inhibition. *Journal of Neurophysiology*, *65*(3), 598–605. doi:10.1152/jn.1991.65.3.598

Finlayson, P. G., & Caspary, D. M. (1993). Response properties in young and old Fischer-344 rat lateral superior olive neurons: A quantitative approach. *Neurobiology of Aging*, *14*(2), 127–139.

Fischl, M. J., Burger, R. M., Schmidt-Pauly, M., Alexandrova, O., Sinclair, J. L., Grothe, B., . . . Kopp-Scheinpflug, C. (2016). Physiology and anatomy of neurons in the medial superior olive of the mouse. *Journal of Neurophysiology*, *116*(6), 2676–2688. doi:10.1152/jn.00523.2016

Franken, T. P., Joris, P. X., & Smith, P. H. (2018). Principal cells of the brainstem's interaural sound level detector are temporal differentiators rather than integrators. *Elife*, *7*. doi:10.7554/eLife.33854

Franken, T. P., Smith, P. H., & Joris, P. X. (2016). *In vivo* whole-cell recordings combined with electron microscopy reveal unexpected morphological and physiological properties in the lateral nucleus of the trapezoid body in the auditory brainstem. *Frontiers in Neural Circuits*, *10*, 69. doi:10.3389/fncir.2016.00069

Fredrich, M., Reisch, A., & Illing, R. B. (2009). Neuronal subtype identity in the rat auditory brainstem as defined by molecular profile and axonal projection. *Experimental Brain Research*, *195*(2), 241–260. doi:10.1007/s00221-009-1776-7

Friauf, E. (2004). Developmental changes and cellular plasticity in the superior olivary complex. In T. N. Parks, E. W. Rubel, R. R. Fay, & A. N. Popper (Eds.), *Plasticity of the auditory system* (pp. 49–95). New York: Springer.

Friauf, E., Aragon, C., Löhrke, S., Westenfelder, B., & Zafra, F. (1999). Developmental expression of the glycine transporter GLYT2 in the auditory system of rats suggests involvement in synapse maturation. *Journal of Comparative Neurology*, *412*(1), 17–37.

Friauf, E., Fischer, A. U., & Fuhr, M. F. (2015). Synaptic plasticity in the auditory system: a review. *Cell and Tissue Research*, *361*(1), 177–213. doi:10.1007/s00441-015-2176-x

Friauf, E., Hammerschmidt, B., & Kirsch, J. (1997). Development of adult-type inhibitory glycine receptors in the central auditory system of rats. *Journal of Comparative Neurology*, *385*(1), 117–134.

Friauf, E., & Herbert, H. (1985). Topographic organization of facial motoneurons to individual pinna muscles in rat (*Rattus rattus*) and bat (*Rousettus aegyptiacus*). *Journal of Comparative Neurology*, *240*(2), 161–170. doi:10.1002/cne.902400206

Friauf, E., & Kandler, K. (1993). Cell birth, formation of efferent connections, and establishment of tonotopic order in the rat cochlear nucleus. In M. A. Merchán, J. M. Juiz, D. A. Godfrey, & E. Mugnaini (Eds.), *The mammalian cochlear nuclei: Organization and function* (Vol. 1, pp. 19–28). New York: Plenum.

Friauf, E., & Ostwald, J. (1988). Divergent projections of physiologically characterized rat ventral cochlear nucleus neurons as shown by intraaxonal injection of horseradish peroxidase. *Experimental Brain Research*, *73*(2), 263–284.

Friauf, E., Rust, M. B., Schulenborg, T., & Hirtz, J. J. (2011). Chloride cotransporters, chloride homeostasis, and synaptic inhibition in the developing auditory system. *Hearing Research*, *279*(1–2), 96–110. doi:10.1016/j.heares.2011.05.012

Frisina, D. R. (2010). Aging changes in the central auditory system. In A. Rees & A. R. Palmer (Eds.), *Oxford handbook of auditory science: The auditory brain* (Vol. 2, pp. 417–440). Oxford: Oxford University Press.

Fujino, K., Koyano, K., & Ohmori, H. (1997). Lateral and medial olivocochlear neurons have distinct electrophysiological properties in the rat brain slice. *Journal of Neurophysiology*, *77*(5), 2788–2804.

Fukui, H., & Raphael, Y. (2013). Gene therapy for the inner ear. *Hearing Research*, *297*, 99–105. doi:10.1016/j.heares.2012.11.017

Garcia-Pino, E., Gessele, N., & Koch, U. (2017). Enhanced excitatory connectivity and disturbed sound processing in the auditory brainstem of Fragile X mice. *Journal of Neuroscience*, *37*(31), 7403–7419. doi:10.1523/jneurosci.2310-16.2017

Gessele, N., Garcia-Pino, E., Omerbasic, D., Park, T. J., & Koch, U. (2016). Structural changes and lack of HCN1 channels in the binaural auditory brainstem of the naked mole-rat (*Heterocephalus glaber*). *PLoS One*, *11*(1), e0146428. doi:10.1371/journal.pone.0146428

Gilardi, P., Schneider-Maunoury, S., & Charnay, P. (1991). Krox-20: A candidate gene for the regulation of pattern formation in the hindbrain. *Biochimie*, *73*(1), 85–91.

Gillespie, D. C., Kim, G., & Kandler, K. (2005). Inhibitory synapses in the developing auditory system are glutamatergic. *Nature Neuroscience*, *8*(3), 332–338.

Giugovaz-Tropper, B., Gonzalez-Inchauspe, C., Di Guilmi, M. N., Urbano, F. J., Forsythe, I. D., & Uchitel, O. D. (2011). P/Q-type calcium channel ablation in a mice glycinergic synapse mediated by multiple types of Ca^{2+} channels alters transmitter release and short term plasticity. *Neuroscience*, *192*, 219–230. doi:10.1016/j.neuroscience.2011.06.021

Gjoni, E., Aguet, C., Sahlender, D. A., Knott, G., & Schneggenburger, R. (2018). Ultrastructural basis of strong unitary inhibition in a binaural neuron. *Journal of Physiology*, 596(20), 4969–4982. doi:10.1113/jp276015

Gjoni, E., Zenke, F., Bouhours, B., & Schneggenburger, R. (2018). Specific synaptic input strengths determine the computational properties of excitation-inhibition integration in a sound localization circuit. *Journal of Physiology*, 596(20), 4945–4967. doi:10.1113/jp276012

Gleich, O., Weiss, M., & Strutz, J. (2004). Age-dependent changes in the lateral superior olive of the gerbil (*Meriones unguiculatus*). *Hearing Research*, *194*(1–2), 47–59. doi:10.1016/j.heares.2004.03.016

Glendenning, K. K., & Baker, B. N. (1988). Neuroanatomical distribution of receptors for three potential inhibitory neurotransmitters in the brainstem auditory nuclei of the cat. *Journal of Comparative Neurology*, *275*(2), 288–308. doi:10.1002/cne.902750210

Glendenning, K. K., Baker, B. N., Hutson, K. A., & Masterton, R. B. (1992). Acoustic chiasm V: Inhibition and excitation in the ipsilateral and contralateral projections of LSO. *Journal of Comparative Neurology*, *319*(1), 100–122.

Glendenning, K. K., Hutson, K. A., Nudo, R. J., & Masterton, R. B. (1985). Acoustic chiasm II: Anatomical basis of binaurality in lateral superior olive of cat. *Journal of Comparative Neurology*, *232*(2), 261–285. doi:10.1002/cne.902320210

Glendenning, K. K., & Masterton, R. B. (1983). Acoustic chiasm: Efferent projections of the lateral superior olive. *Journal of Neuroscience*, *3*(8), 1521–1537.

Glendenning, K. K., & Masterton, R. B. (1998). Comparative morphometry of mammalian central auditory systems: Variation in nuclei and form of the ascending system. *Brain, Behavior and Evolution*, *51*(2), 59–89. doi:10.1159/000006530

Glendenning, K. K., Masterton, R. B., Baker, B. N., & Wenthold, R. J. (1991). Acoustic chiasm. III: Nature, distribution, and sources of afferents to the lateral superior olive in the cat. *Journal of Comparative Neurology*, *310*(3), 377–400. doi:10.1002/cne.903100308

Goldberg, J. M., & Brown, P. B. (1968). Functional organization of the dog superior olivary complex to dichotic tonal stimuli: An anatomical and electrophysiological study. *Journal of Neurophysiology*, *31*(4), 639–655.

Goldberg, J. M., & Brown, P. B. (1969). Response of binaural neurons of dog superior olivary complex to dichotic tonal stimuli: Some physiological mechanism of sound localization. *Journal of Neurophysiology*, *32*(4), 613–636.

Golding, N. L., & Oertel, D. (2012). Synaptic integration in dendrites: Exceptional need for speed. *Journal of Physiology*, *590*(22), 5563–5569. doi:10.1113/jphysiol.2012.229328

Gomez-Alvarez, M., & Saldana, E. (2016). Different tonotopic regions of the lateral superior olive receive a similar combination of afferent inputs. *Journal of Comparative Neurology*, *524*(11), 2230–2250. doi:10.1002/cne.23942

Gomez-Nieto, R., Rubio, M. E., & Lopez, D. E. (2008). Cholinergic input from the ventral nucleus of the trapezoid body to cochlear root neurons in rats. *Journal of Comparative Neurology*, *506*(3), 452–468. doi:10.1002/cne.21554

Greene, N. T., Anbuhl, K. L., Williams, W., & Tollin, D. J. (2014). The acoustical cues to sound location in the guinea pig (*Cavia porcellus*). *Hearing Research*, *316*, 1–15. doi:10.1016/j.heares.2014.07.004

Greene, N. T., Lomakin, O., & Davis, K. A. (2010). Monaural spectral processing differs between the lateral superior olive and the inferior colliculus: Physiological evidence for an acoustic chiasm. *Hearing Research*, *269*(1–2), 134–145. doi:10.1016/j.heares.2010.06.018

Greer, P. L., & Greenberg, M. E. (2008). From synapse to nucleus: Calcium-dependent gene transcription in the control of synapse development and function. *Neuron*, *59*(6), 846–860. doi:10.1016/j.neuron.2008.09.002

Grigg, J. J., Brew, H. M., & Tempel, B. L. (2000). Differential expression of voltage-grated potassium channel genes in auditory nuclei of the mouse brainstem. *Hearing Research*, *140*(1–2), 77–90. doi:10.1016/S0378-5955(99)00187-2

Grothe, B., & Park, T. J. (1995). Time can be traded for intensity in the lower auditory system. *Naturwissenschaften*, *82*(11), 521–523. doi:Doi 10.1007/Bf01134488

Grothe, B., & Park, T. J. (2000). Structure and function of the bat superior olivary complex. *Microscopy Research and Technique*, *51*(4), 382–402. doi:10.1002/1097-0029(20001115)51:4<382::AID-JEMT7>3.0.CO;2-7

Grothe, B., & Pecka, M. (2014). The natural history of sound localization in mammals: A story of neuronal inhibition. *Frontiers in Neural Circuits*, *8*, 116. doi:10.3389/fncir.2014.00116

Grothe, B., Pecka, M., & McAlpine, D. (2010). Mechanisms of sound localization in mammals. *Physiological Reviews*, *90*(3), 983–1012. doi:10.1152/physrev.00026.2009

Guinan, J. J., Norris, B. E., & Guinan, S. S. (1972). Single auditory units in the superior olivary complex. II: Locations of unit categories and tonotopic organization. *International Journal of Neuroscience*, *4*(4), 147–166. doi:10.3109/00207457209164756

Hackney, C. M. (1987). Anatomical features of the auditory pathway from cochlea to cortex. *British Medial Bulletin*, *43*(4), 780–801.

Harnischfeger, G., Neuweiler, G., & Schlegel, P. (1985). Interaural time and intensity coding in superior olivary complex and inferior colliculus of the echolocating bat molossus ater. *Journal of Neurophysiology*, *53*(1), 89–109.

Harrison, J. M., & Irving, R. (1966). Visual and nonvisual auditory systems in mammals. Anatomical evidence indicates two kinds of auditory pathways and suggests two kinds of hearing in mammals. *Science*, *154*(3750), 738–743.

Harrison, J. M., & Warr, W. B. (1962). A study of the cochlear nuclei and ascending auditory pathways of the medulla. *Journal of Comparative Neurology*, *119*, 341–380.

Hassfurth, B., Magnusson, A. K., Grothe, B., & Koch, U. (2009). Sensory deprivation regulates the development of the hyperpolarization-activated current in auditory brainstem neurons. *European Journal of Neuroscience*, *30*(7), 1227–1238. doi:10.1111/j.1460-9568.2009.06925.x

He, C., Chen, F., Li, B., & Hu, Z. (2014). Neurophysiology of HCN channels: From cellular functions to multiple regulations. *Progress in Neurobiology*, *112*, 1–23. doi:10.1016/j.pneurobio.2013.10.001

Heffner, R. S., & Heffner, H. E. (1993). Degenerate hearing and sound localization in naked mole rats (*Heterocephalus glaber*), with an overview of central auditory structures. *Journal of Comparative Neurology*, *331*(3), 418–433. doi:10.1002/cne.903310311

Heffner, R. S., & Heffner, H. E. (2010). Explaining high-frequency hearing. *Anatomical Record (Hoboken)*, *293*(12), 2080–2082. doi:10.1002/ar.21292

Heffner, R. S., Koay, G., & Heffner, H. E. (2001). Audiograms of five species of rodents: Implications for the evolution of hearing and the perception of pitch. *Hearing Research*, *157*(1–2), 138–152.

Helfert, R. H., Bonneau, J. M., Wenthold, R. J., & Altschuler, R. A. (1989). GABA and glycine immunoreactivity in the guinea pig superior olivary complex. *Brain Research*, *501*(2), 269–286.

Helfert, R. H., Juiz, J. M., Bledsoe, S. C., Bonneau, J. M., Wenthold, R. J., & Altschuler, R. A. (1992). Patterns of glutamate, glycine, and GABA immunolabeling in four synaptic terminal classes in the lateral superior olive of the guinea pig. *Journal of Comparative Neurology*, *323*(3), 305–325. doi:10.1002/cne.903230302

Helfert, R. H., & Schwartz, I. R. (1986). Morphological evidence for the existence of multiple neuronal classes in the cat lateral superior olivary nucleus. *Journal of Comparative Neurology*, *244*(4), 533–549. doi:10.1002/cne.902440409

Helfert, R. H., & Schwartz, I. R. (1987). Morphological features of five neuronal classes in the gerbil lateral superior olive. *American Journal of Anatomy*, *179*(1), 55–69. doi:10.1002/aja.1001790108

Henkel, C. K., & Gabriele, M. L. (1999). Organization of the disynaptic pathway from the anteroventral cochlear nucleus to the lateral superior olivary nucleus in the ferret. *Anatomy and Embryology*, *199*, 149–160.

Hilbig, H., Beil, B., Hilbig, H., Call, J., & Bidmon, H. J. (2009). Superior olivary complex organization and cytoarchitecture may be correlated with function and catarrhine primate phylogeny. *Brain Structure and Function*, *213*(4–5), 489–497. doi:10.1007/s00429-008-0201-5

Hirao, K., Eto, K., Nakahata, Y., Ishibashi, H., Nagai, T., & Nabekura, J. (2015). Noradrenergic refinement of glutamatergic neuronal circuits in the lateral superior olivary nucleus before hearing onset. *Journal of Neurophysiology*, *114*(3), 1974–1986. doi:10.1152/jn.00813.2014

Hirtz, J. J., Boesen, M., Braun, N., Deitmer, J. W., Kramer, F., Lohr, C., . . . Friauf, E. (2011). $Ca_V1.3$ calcium channels are required for normal development of the auditory brainstem. *Journal of Neuroscience*, *31*(22), 8280–8294. doi:10.1523/JNEUROSCI.5098-10.2011

Hirtz, J. J., Braun, N., Griesemer, D., Hannes, C., Janz, K., Löhrke, S., . . . Friauf, E. (2012). Synaptic refinement of an inhibitory topographic map in the auditory brainstem requires functional $Ca_V1.3$ calcium channels. *Journal of Neuroscience*, *32*(42), 14602–14616. doi:10.1523/JNEUROSCI.0765-12.2012

Hoffpauir, B. K., Kolson, D. R., Mathers, P. H., & Spirou, G. A. (2010). Maturation of synaptic partners: functional phenotype and synaptic organization tuned in synchrony. *Journal of Physiology*, *588*(Pt 22), 4365–4385. doi:10.1113/jphysiol.2010.198564

Hong, S. H., Kim, M. J., & Ahn, S. C. (2008). Glutamatergic transmission is sustained at a later period of development of medial nucleus of the trapezoid body-lateral superior olive synapses in circling mice. *Journal of Neuroscience, 28*(48), 13003–13007. doi:10.1523/Jneurosci.3002-08.2008

Hossain, W. A., D'Sa, C., & Morest, D. K. (2006). Site-specific interactions of neurotrophin-3 and fibroblast growth factor (FGF2) in the embryonic development of the mouse cochlear nucleus. *Journal of Neurobiology, 66*(9), 897–915. doi:10.1002/neu.20264

Howell, D. M., Morgan, W. J., Jarjour, A. A., Spirou, G. A., Berrebi, A. S., Kennedy, T. E., & Mathers, P. H. (2007). Molecular guidance cues necessary for axon pathfinding from the ventral cochlear nucleus. *Journal of Comparative Neurology, 504*(5), 533–549. doi:10.1002/cne.21443

Hsieh, C. Y., Nakamura, P. A., Luk, S. O., Miko, I. J., Henkemeyer, M., & Cramer, K. S. (2010). Ephrin-B reverse signaling is required for formation of strictly contralateral auditory brainstem pathways. *Journal of Neuroscience, 30*(29), 9840–9849. doi:10.1523/Jneurosci.0386-10.2010

Illing, R. B., Kraus, K. S., & Michler, S. A. (2000). Plasticity of the superior olivary complex. *Microscopy Research and Technique, 51*(4), 364–381. doi:10.1002/1097-0029(20001115)51:4<364::AID-JEMT6>3.0.CO;2-E

Irvine, D. R. F. (1992). Physiology of the auditory brainstem. In A. N. Popper & R. R. Fay (Eds.), *The mammalian auditory pathway: Neurophysiology* (pp. 153–231). New York: Springer.

Irving, R., & Harrison, J. M. (1967). The superior olivary complex and audition: A comparative study. *Journal of Comparative Neurology, 130*(1), 77–86. doi:10.1002/cne.901300105

Ito, T., & Oliver, D. L. (2010). Origins of glutamatergic terminals in the inferior colliculus identified by retrograde transport and expression of VGLUT1 and VGLUT2 genes. *Frontiers in Neuroanatomy, 4*, 135. doi:10.3389/fnana.2010.00135

Jalabi, W., Kopp-Scheinpflug, C., Allen, P. D., Schiavon, E., DiGiacomo, R. R., Forsythe, I. D., & Maricich, S. M. (2013). Sound localization ability and glycinergic innervation of the superior olivary complex persist after genetic deletion of the medial nucleus of the trapezoid body. *Journal of Neuroscience, 33*(38), 15044–15049. doi:10.1523/JNEUROSCI.2604-13.2013

Jenkins, S. A., & Simmons, D. D. (2006). GABAergic neurons in the lateral superior olive of the hamster are distinguished by differential expression of gad isoforms during development. *Brain Research, 1111*(1), 12–25. doi:10.1016/j.brainres.2006.06.067

Johnston, J., Forsythe, I. D., & Kopp-Scheinpflug, C. (2010). Going native: Voltage-gated potassium channels controlling neuronal excitability. *Journal of Physiology, 588*(Pt 17), 3187–3200. doi:10.1113/jphysiol.2010.191973

Joris, P. X. (1996). Envelope coding in the lateral superior olive. II. Characteristic delays and comparison with responses in the medial superior olive. *Journal of Neurophysiology, 76*(4), 2137–2156. doi:10.1152/jn.1996.76.4.2137

Joris, P. X., & Yin, T. C. (1995). Envelope coding in the lateral superior olive. I. Sensitivity to interaural time differences. *Journal of Neurophysiology, 73*(3), 1043–1062. doi:10.1152/jn.1995.73.3.1043

Joris, P. X., & Yin, T. C. (1998). Envelope coding in the lateral superior olive. III. Comparison with afferent pathways. *Journal of Neurophysiology, 79*(1), 253–269. doi:10.1152/jn.1998.79.1.253

Jurkovicova-Tarabova, B., Griesemer, D., Pirone, A., Sinnegger-Brauns, M. J., Striessnig, J., & Friauf, E. (2012). Repertoire of high voltage-activated Ca^{2+} channels in the lateral superior olive: Functional analysis in wild-type, $Ca_v1.3^{-/-}$, and $Ca_v1.2DHP^{-/-}$ mice. *Journal of Neurophysiology, 108*(2), 365–379. doi:10.1152/jn.00948.2011

Kalmbach, A., Kullmann, P. H., & Kandler, K. (2010). NMDAR-mediated calcium transients elicited by glutamate co-release at developing inhibitory synapses. *Frontiers in Synaptic Neuroscience, 2*, 27. doi:10.3389/fnsyn.2010.00027

Kandler, K. (2004). Activity-dependent organization of inhibitory circuits: lessons from the auditory system. *Current Opinion in Neurobiology, 14*(1), 96–104. doi:10.1016/j.conb.2004.01.017

Kandler, K., Clause, A., & Noh, J. (2009). Tonotopic reorganization of developing auditory brainstem circuits. *Nature Neuroscience, 12*(6), 711–717. doi:10.1038/nn.2332

Kandler, K., & Friauf, E. (1993). Pre- and postnatal development of efferent connections of the cochlear nucleus in the rat. *Journal of Comparative Neurology, 328*(2), 161–184. doi:10.1002/cne.903280202

Kandler, K., & Friauf, E. (1995a). Development of electrical membrane properties and discharge characteristics of superior olivary complex neurons in fetal and postnatal rats. *European Journal of Neuroscience, 7*(8), 1773–1790.

Kandler, K., & Friauf, E. (1995b). Development of glycinergic and glutamatergic synaptic transmission in the auditory brainstem of perinatal rats. *Journal of Neuroscience, 15*(10), 6890–6904.

Kandler, K., & Gillespie, D. C. (2005). Developmental refinement of inhibitory sound-localization circuits. *Trends in Neurosciences, 28*(6), 290–296. doi:10.1016/j.tins.2005.04.007

Karcz, A., Hennig, M. H., Robbins, C. A., Tempel, B. L., Rübsamen, R., & Kopp-Scheinpflug, C. (2011). Low-voltage activated Kv1.1 subunits are crucial for the processing of sound source location in the lateral superior olive in mice. *Journal of Physiology, 589*(Pt 5), 1143–1157. doi:10.1113/jphysiol.2010.203331

Karis, A., Pata, I., van Doorninck, J. H., Grosveld, F., De Zeeuw, C. I., de Caprona, D., & Fritzsch, B. (2001). Transcription factor GATA-3 alters pathway selection of olivocochlear neurons and affectrs morphogenesis of the ear. *Journal of Comparative Neurology, 429*(4), 615–630.

Kelly, J. B., Liscum, A., van Adel, B., & Ito, M. (1998). Projections from the superior olive and lateral lemniscus to tonotopic regions of the rat's inferior colliculus. *Hearing Research, 116*(1–2), 43–54.

Kelly, J. B., van Adel, B. A., & Ito, M. (2009). Anatomical projections of the nuclei of the lateral lemniscus in the albino rat (*Rattus norvegicus*). *Journal of Comparative Neurology, 512*(4), 573–593. doi:10.1002/cne.21929

Khurana, S., Liu, Z., Lewis, A. S., Rosa, K., Chetkovich, D., & Golding, N. L. (2012). An essential role for modulation of hyperpolarization-activated current in the development of binaural temporal precision. *Journal of Neuroscience, 32*(8), 2814–2823. doi:10.1523/JNEUROSCI.3882-11.2012

Kiecker, C., & Lumsden, A. (2005). Compartments and their boundaries in vertebrate brain development. *Nature Reviews. Neuroscience, 6*(7), 553–564. doi:10.1038/nrn1702

Kil, J., Kageyama, G. H., Semple, M. N., & Kitzes, L. M. (1995). Development of ventral cochlear nucleus projections to the superior olivary complex in gerbil. *Journal of Comparative Neurology, 353*(3), 317–340. doi:10.1002/cne.903530302

Kim, G., & Kandler, K. (2003). Elimination and strengthening of glycinergic/GABAergic connections during tonotopic map formation. *Nature Neuroscience, 6*(3), 282–290. doi:10.1038/nn1015

Kim, G., & Kandler, K. (2010). Synaptic changes underlying the strengthening of GABA/glycinergic connections in the developing lateral superior olive. *Neuroscience, 171*(3), 924–933. doi:10.1016/j.neuroscience.2010.09.054

Kim, K. X., & Rutherford, M. A. (2016). Maturation of NaV and KV channel topographies in the auditory nerve spike initiator before and after developmental onset of hearing function. *Journal of Neuroscience, 36*(7), 2111–2118. doi:10.1523/jneurosci.3437-15.2016

Kitzes, L. M., Kageyama, G. H., Semple, M. N., & Kil, J. (1995). Development of ectopic projections from the ventral cochlear nucleus to the superior olivary complex induced by neonatal ablation of the contralateral cochlea. *Journal of Comparative Neurology, 353*(3), 341–363. doi:10.1002/cne.903530303

Koay, G., Heffner, R. S., & Heffner, H. E. (1998). Hearing in a megachiropteran fruit bat (*Rousettus aegyptiacus*). *Journal of Comparative Psychology, 112*(4), 371–382.

Kochubey, O., Babai, N., & Schneggenburger, R. (2016). A synaptotagmin isoform switch during the development of an identified CNS synapse. *Neuron, 90*(5), 984–999. doi:10.1016/j.neuron.2016.04.038

Koka, K., Read, H. L., & Tollin, D. J. (2008). The acoustical cues to sound location in the rat: Measurements of directional transfer functions. *Journal of the Acoustical Society of America, 123*(6), 4297–4309. doi:10.1121/1.2916587

Kole, M. H., Letzkus, J. J., & Stuart, G. J. (2007). Axon initial segment Kv1 channels control axonal action potential waveform and synaptic efficacy. *Neuron, 55*(4), 633–647. doi:10.1016/j.neuron.2007.07.031

Kopp-Scheinpflug, C., Fuchs, K., Lippe, W. R., Tempel, B. L., & Rübsamen, R. (2003). Decreased temporal precision of auditory signaling in *Kcna1*-null mice: An electrophysiological study *in vivo*. *Journal of Neuroscience, 23*(27), 9199–9207.

Kopp-Scheinpflug, C., Pigott, B. M., & Forsythe, I. D. (2015). Nitric oxide selectively suppresses IH currents mediated by HCN1-containing channels. *Journal of Physiology, 593*(7), 1685–1700. doi:10.1113/jphysiol.2014.282194

Korada, S., & Schwartz, I. R. (1999). Development of GABA, glycine, and their receptors in the auditory brainstem of gerbil: A light and electron microscopic study. *Journal of Comparative Neurology, 409*(4), 664–681. doi:10.1002/(Sici)1096-9861(19990712)409:4<664::Aid-Cne10>3.0.Co;2-S

Kotak, V. C., Korada, S., Schwartz, I. R., & Sanes, D. H. (1998). A developmental shift from GABAergic to glycinergic transmission in the central auditory system. *Journal of Neuroscience, 18*(12), 4646–4655.

Kotak, V. C., & Sanes, D. H. (1996). Developmental influence of glycinergic transmission: regulation of NMDA receptor-mediated EPSPs. *Journal of Neuroscience, 16*(5), 1836–1843.

Kotak, V. C., & Sanes, D. H. (1997). Deafferentation weakens excitatory synapses in the developing central auditory system. *European Journal of Neuroscience, 9*(11), 2340–2347.

Kotak, V. C., & Sanes, D. H. (2014). Developmental expression of inhibitory synaptic long-term potentiation in the lateral superior olive. *Frontiers in Neural Circuits, 8*, 67. doi:10.3389/fncir.2014.00067

Krächan, E. G., Fischer, A. U., Franke, J., & Friauf, E. (2017). Synaptic reliability and temporal precision are achieved via high quantal content and effective replenishment: Auditory brainstem versus hippocampus. *Journal of Physiology, 595*(3), 839–864. doi:10.1113/JP272799

Kramer, F., Griesemer, D., Bakker, D., Brill, S., Franke, J., Frotscher, E., & Friauf, E. (2014). Inhibitory glycinergic neurotransmission in the mammalian auditory brainstem upon prolonged stimulation: Short-term plasticity and synaptic reliability. *Frontiers in Neural Circuits, 8*, 14. doi:10.3389/fncir.2014.00014

Kraus, K. S., & Illing, R. B. (2004). Superior olivary contributions to auditory system plasticity: Medial but not lateral olivocochlear neurons are the source of cochleotomy-induced GAP-43 expression in the ventral cochlear nucleus. *Journal of Comparative Neurology, 475*(3), 374–390. doi:10.1002/cne.20180

Kronander, E., Michalski, N., Lebrand, C., Hornung, J. P., & Schneggenburger, R. (2017). An organotypic slice culture to study the formation of calyx of Held synapses *in-vitro*. *PLoS One, 12*(4), e0175964. doi:10.1371/journal.pone.0175964

Kudo, M., Kitao, Y., Okoyama, S., Moriya, M., & Kawano, J. (1996). Crossed projection neurons are generated prior to uncrossed projection neurons in the lateral superior olive of the rat. *Brain Research. Developmental Brain Research, 95*(1), 72–78.

Kudo, M., Sakurai, H., Kurokawa, K., & Yamada, H. (2000). Neurogenesis in the superior olivary complex in the rat. *Hearing Research, 139*(1–2), 144–152.

Kulesza, R. J., Jr. (2007). Cytoarchitecture of the human superior olivary complex: Medial and lateral superior olive. *Hearing Research, 225*(1–2), 80–90. doi:10.1016/j.heares.2006.12.006

Kulesza, R. J., Jr. (2008). Cytoarchitecture of the human superior olivary complex: Nuclei of the trapezoid body and posterior tier. *Hearing Research, 241*(1–2), 52–63.

Kullmann, P. H., Ene, F. A., & Kandler, K. (2002). Glycinergic and GABAergic calcium responses in the developing lateral superior olive. *European Journal of Neuroscience, 15*(7), 1093–1104.

Kullmann, P. H., & Kandler, K. (2001). Glycinergic/GABAergic synapses in the lateral superior olive are excitatory in neonatal C57Bl/6J mice. *Brain Research. Developmental Brain Research, 131*(1–2), 143–147.

Kungel, M., & Friauf, E. (1995). Somatostatin and leu-enkephalin in the rat auditory brainstem during fetal and postnatal development. *Anatomy and Embryology, 191*(5), 425–443. doi:10.1007/BF00304428

Kungel, M., Piechotta, K., Rietzel, H. J., & Friauf, E. (1997). Influence of the neuropeptide somatostatin on the development of dendritic morphology: A cysteamine-depletion study in the rat auditory brainstem. *Brain Research. Developmental Brain Research, 101*(1–2), 107–114. doi:10.1016/S0165-3806(97)00053-9

Kuwabara, N., & Zook, J. M. (1991). Classification of the principal cells of the medial nucleus of the trapezoid body. *Journal of Comparative Neurology, 314*(4), 707–720. doi:10.1002/cne.903140406

Kuwabara, N., & Zook, J. M. (1992). Projections to the medial superior olive from the medial and lateral nuclei of the trapezoid body in rodents and bats. *Journal of Comparative Neurology, 324*(4), 522–538. doi:10.1002/cne.903240406

Leao, K. E., Leao, R. N., Sun, H., Fyffe, R. E., & Walmsley, B. (2006). Hyperpolarization-activated currents are differentially expressed in mice brainstem auditory nuclei. *Journal of Physiology, 576*(Pt 3), 849–864. doi:10.1113/jphysiol.2006.114702

Leao, K. E., Leao, R. N., & Walmsley, B. (2011). Modulation of dendritic synaptic processing in the lateral superior olive by hyperpolarization-activated currents. *European Journal of Neuroscience, 33*(8), 1462–1470. doi:10.1111/j.1460-9568.2011.07627.x

Lee, H., Bach, E., Noh, J., Delpire, E., & Kandler, K. (2016). Hyperpolarization-independent maturation and refinement of GABA/glycinergic connections in the auditory brain stem. *Journal of Neurophysiology, 115*(3), 1170–1182. doi:10.1152/jn.00926.2015

Lee, H., Brott, B. K., Kirkby, L. A., Adelson, J. D., Cheng, S., Feller, M. B., . . . Shatz, C. J. (2014). Synapse elimination and learning rules co-regulated by MHC class I H2-Db. *Nature*, *509*(7499), 195–200. doi:10.1038/nature13154

Lee, J. H., Pradhan, J., Maskey, D., Park, K. S., Hong, S. H., Suh, M. W., . . . Ahn, S. C. (2011). Glutamate co-transmission from developing medial nucleus of the trapezoid body: Lateral superior olive synapses is cochlear dependent in kanamycin-treated rats. *Biochemical and Biophysical Research Communications*, *405*(2), 162–167. doi:10.1016/j.bbrc.2010.12.129

Li, W., Kaczmarek, L. K., & Perney, T. M. (2001). Localization of two high-threshold potassium channel subunits in the rat central auditory system. *Journal of Comparative Neurology*, *437*(2), 196–218.

Lippe, W. R. (1994). Rhythmic spontaneous activity in the developing avian auditory system. *Journal of Neuroscience*, *14*(3 Pt 2), 1486–1495. doi:10.1523/JNEUROSCI.14-03-01486.1994

Lohmann, C., Ilic, V., & Friauf, E. (1998). Development of a topographically organized auditory network in slice culture is calcium dependent. *Journal of Neurobiology*, *34*(2), 97–112. doi:10.1002/(Sici)1097-4695(19980205)34:2<97::Aid-Neu1>3.0.Co;2-6

Löhrke, S., Srinivasan, G., Oberhofer, M., Doncheva, E., & Friauf, E. (2005). Shift from depolarizing to hyperpolarizing glycine action occurs at different perinatal ages in superior olivary complex nuclei. *The European Journal of Neuroscience*, *22*(11), 2708–2722. doi:10.1111/j.1460-9568.2005.04465.x

Lumsden, A., & Krumlauf, R. (1996). Patterning the vertebrate neuraxis. *Science*, *274*(5290), 1109–1115.

Magnusson, A. K., Park, T. J., Pecka, M., Grothe, B., & Koch, U. (2008). Retrograde GABA signaling adjusts sound localization by balancing excitation and inhibition in the brainstem. *Neuron*, *59*(1), 125–137. doi:10.1016/j.neuron.2008.05.011

Majorossy, K., & Kiss, A. (1990). Types of neurons and synaptic relations in the lateral superior olive of the cat: Normal structure and experimental observations. *Acta Morphologica Hungarica*, *38*(3–4), 207–215.

Maki, K., & Furukawa, S. (2005). Acoustical cues for sound localization by the Mongolian gerbil, *Meriones unguiculatus*. *Journal of the Acoustical Society of America*, *118*(2), 872–886.

Malmierca, M. S., & Hackett, T. A. (2010). Structural organization of the ascending auditory pathway. In A. Rees & A. R. Palmer (Eds.), *Oxford handbook of auditory science: The auditory brain* (Vol. 2, pp. 9–42). Oxford: Oxford University Press.

Malmierca, M. S., & Ryugo, D. (2012). Auditory system. In C. Watson, G. Paxinos, & L. Puelles (Eds.), *The mouse nervous system* (pp. 607–645). Amsterdam: Elsevier.

Manis, P. B. (2008). Biophysical specializations of neurons that encode timing. In P. Dallos & D. Oertel (Eds.), *The senses: A comprehensive reference. Audition* (Vol. 3, pp. 565–586). San Diego, Academic Press.

Maricich, S. M., Xia, A., Mathes, E. L., Wang, V. Y., Oghalai, J. S., Fritzsch, B., & Zoghbi, H. Y. (2009). Atoh1-lineal neurons are required for hearing and for the survival of neurons in the spiral ganglion and brainstem accessory auditory nuclei. *Journal of Neuroscience*, *29*(36), 11123–11133. doi:10.1523/JNEUROSCI.2232-09.2009

Marrs, G. S., Morgan, W. J., Howell, D. M., Spirou, G. A., & Mathers, P. H. (2013). Embryonic origins of the mouse superior olivary complex. *Developmental Neurobiology*, *73*(5), 384–398. doi:10.1002/dneu.22069

Marrs, G. S., & Spirou, G. A. (2012). Embryonic assembly of auditory circuits: Spiral ganglion and brainstem. *Journal of Physiology*, *590*(10), 2391–2408. doi:10.1113/jphysiol.2011.226886

Masterton, B., Jane, J. A., & Diamond, I. T. (1967). Role of brainstem auditory structures in sound localization. I. Trapezoid body, superior olive, and lateral lemniscus. *Journal of Neurophysiology*, *30*(2), 341–359. doi:10.1152/jn.1967.30.2.341

May, B. J., Prosen, C. A., Weiss, D., & Vetter, D. (2002). Behavioral investigation of some possible effects of the central olivocochlear pathways in transgenic mice. *Hearing Research*, *171*(1–2), 142–157. doi:10.1016/S0378-5955(02)00495-1

McCullagh, E. A., Salcedo, E., Huntsman, M. M., & Klug, A. (2017). Tonotopic alterations in inhibitory input to the medial nucleus of the trapezoid body in a mouse model of Fragile X syndrome. *Journal of Comparative Neurology*, *525*(16), 3543–3562. doi:10.1002/cne.24290

McKay, I. J., Mucharmore, I., Krumlauf, R., Maden, M., Lumsden, A., & Lewis, J. (1994). The *kreisler* mouse: A hindbrain segmentation mutant that lacks two rhombomeres. *Development*, *120*(8), 2199–2211.

Michalski, N., Babai, N., Renier, N., Perkel, D. J., Chedotal, A., & Schneggenburger, R. (2013). Robo3-driven axon midline crossing conditions functional maturation of a large commissural synapse. *Neuron*, *78*(5), 855–868. doi:10.1016/j.neuron.2013.04.006

Michler, S. A., & Illing, R. B. (2002). Acoustic trauma induces reemergence of the growth- and plasticity-associated protein GAP-43 in the rat auditory brainstem. *Journal of Comparative Neurology*, *451*(3), 250–266. doi:10.1002/cne.10348

Middlebrooks, J. C. (2015). Sound localization. *Handbook of Clinical Neurology*, *129*, 99–116. doi:10.1016/b978-0-444-62630-1.00006-8

Middlebrooks, J. C., & Green, D. M. (1991). Sound localization by human listeners. *Annual Review of Psychology*, *42*, 135–159. doi:10.1146/annurev.ps.42.020191.001031

Middlebrooks, J. C., Makous, J. C., & Green, D. M. (1989). Directional sensitivity of sound-pressure levels in the human ear canal. *Journal of the Acoustical Society of America*, *86*(1), 89–108.

Miko, I. J., Nakamura, P. A., Henkemeyer, M., & Cramer, K. S. (2007). Auditory brainstem neural activation patterns are altered in EphA4-and ephrin-B2-deficient mice. *Journal of Comparative Neurology*, *505*(6), 669–681. doi:10.1002/cne.21530

Mongiat, L. A., Esposito, M. S., Lombardi, G., & Schinder, A. F. (2009). Reliable activation of immature neurons in the adult hippocampus. *PLoS One*, *4*(4), e5320. doi:10.1371/journal.pone.0005320

Moore, D. R. (1990). Auditory brainstem of the ferret: early cessation of developmental sensitivity of neurons in the cochlear nucleus to removal of the cochlea. *Journal of Comparative Neurology*, *302*(4), 810–823. doi:10.1002/cne.903020412

Moore, D. R. (1992). Trophic influences of excitatory and inhibitory synapses on neurones in the auditory brain stem. *Neuroreport*, *3*(3), 269–272.

Moore, D. R., & King, A. J. (2004). Plasticity of binaural systems. In T. N. Parks (Ed.), *Plasticity of the Auditory System* (pp. 98–172). New York: Springer.

Moore, D. R., Rogers, N. J., & O'Leary, S. J. (1998). Loss of cochlear nucleus neurons following aminoglycoside antibiotics or cochlear removal. *Annals of Otology, Rhinology, and Laryngology*, *107*(4), 337–343. doi:10.1177/000348949810700413

Moore, D. R., Russell, F. A., & Cathcart, N. C. (1995). Lateral superior olive projections to the inferior colliculus in normal and unilaterally deafened ferrets. *Journal of Comparative Neurology*, *357*(2), 204–216. doi:10.1002/cne.903570203

Moore, J. K. (2000). Organization of the human superior olivary complex. *Microscopy Research and Technique*, *51*(4), 403–412. doi:10.1002/1097-0029(20001115)51:4<403::AID-JEMT8>3.0.CO;2-Q

Moore, M. J., & Caspary, D. M. (1983). Strychnine blocks binaural inhibition in lateral superior olivary neurons. *Journal of Neuroscience*, *3*(1), 237–242.

Moritz, C. P., Eckstein, E., Tenzer, S., & Friauf, E. (2015). Neuroproteomics in the auditory brainstem: Candidate proteins for ultrafast and precise information processing. *Molecular and Cellular Neurosciences*, *64*, 9–23. doi:10.1016/j.mcn.2014.08.006

Mulders, W. H., & Robertson, D. (2001). Origin of the noradrenergic innervation of the superior olivary complex in the rat. *Journal of Chemical Neuroanatomy*, *21*(4), 313–322.

Munemoto, Y., Kuriyama, H., Doi, T., Sato, K., Matsumoto, A., Sugatani, J., . . . Yamashita, T. (1998). Auditory pathway and auditory brainstem response in mice lacking NMDA receptor epsilon 1 and epsilon 4 subunits. *Neuroscience Letters*, *251*(2), 101–104.

Musicant, A. D., Chan, J. C., & Hind, J. E. (1990). Direction-dependent spectral properties of cat external ear: New data and cross-species comparisons. *Journal of the Acoustical Society of America*, *87*(2), 757–781.

Nabekura, J., Katsurabayashi, S., Kakazu, Y., Shibata, S., Matsubara, A., Jinno, S., . . . Ishibashi, H. (2004). Developmental switch from GABA to glycine release in single central synaptic terminals. *Nature Neuroscience*, *7*(1), 17–23. doi:10.1038/nn1170

Nakagawa, H., Sato, K., Shiraishi, Y., Kuriyama, H., & Altschuler, R. A. (2000). NMDAR1 isoforms in the rat superior olivary complex and changes after unilateral cochlear ablation. *Brain Research. Molecular Brain Research*, *77*(2), 246–257.

Nakamura, P. A., Hsieh, C. Y., & Cramer, K. S. (2012). EphB signaling regulates target innervation in the developing and deafferented auditory brainstem. *Developmental Neurobiology*, *72*(9), 1243–1255. doi:10.1002/dneu.20990

Niblock, M. M., Brunso-Bechtold, J. K., & Henkel, C. K. (1995). Fiber outgrowth and pathfinding in the developing auditory brainstem. *Brain Research. Developmental Brain Research*, *85*(2), 288–292.

Noh, J., Seal, R. P., Garver, J. A., Edwards, R. H., & Kandler, K. (2010). Glutamate co-release at GABA/glycinergic synapses is crucial for the refinement of an inhibitory map. *Nature Neuroscience*, *13*(2), 232–238. doi:10.1038/nn.2478

Nordeen, K. W., Killackey, H. P., & Kitzes, L. M. (1983). Ascending auditory projections to the inferior colliculus in the adult gerbil, *Meriones unguiculatus*. *Journal of Comparative Neurology*, *214*(2), 131–143. doi:10.1002/cne.902140203

Nothwang, H. G. (2016). Evolution of mammalian sound localization circuits: A developmental perspective. *Progress in Neurobiology*, *141*, 1–24. doi:10.1016/j.pneurobio.2016.02.003

Oertel, D., Wright, S., Cao, X. J., Ferragamo, M., & Bal, R. (2011). The multiple functions of T stellate/multipolar/chopper cells in the ventral cochlear nucleus. *Hearing Research*, *276*(1–2), 61–69. doi:10.1016/j.heares.2010.10.018

Oliver, D. L. (2000). Ascending efferent projections of the superior olivary complex. *Microscopy Research and Technique*, *51*(4), 355–363. doi:10.1002/1097-0029(20001115)51:4<355::AID-JEMT5>3.0.CO;2-J

Ollo, C., & Schwartz, I. R. (1979). The superior olivary complex in C57BL/6 mice. *American Journal of Anatomy*, *155*(3), 349–374. doi:10.1002/aja.1001550306

O'Neill, W. E., Zettel, M. L., Whittemore, K. R., & Frisina, R. D. (1997). Calbindin D-28k immunoreactivity in the medial nucleus of the trapezoid body declines with age in C57BL/6, but not CBA/CaJ, mice. *Hearing Research*, *112*(1–2), 158–166. doi:10.1016/S0378-5955(97)00116-0

Osmanski, M. S., & Wang, X. (2011). Measurement of absolute auditory thresholds in the common marmoset (*Callithrix jacchus*). *Hearing Research*, *277*(1–2), 127–133. doi:10.1016/j.heares.2011.02.001

Paoletti, P., Bellone, C., & Zhou, Q. (2013). NMDA receptor subunit diversity: Impact on receptor properties, synaptic plasticity and disease. *Nature Reviews. Neuroscience*, *14*(6), 383–400. doi:10.1038/nrn3504

Park, T. J., Grothe, B., Pollak, G. D., Schuller, G., & Koch, U. (1996). Neural delays shape selectivity to interaural intensity differences in the lateral superior olive. *Journal of Neuroscience*, *16*(20), 6554–6566.

Park, T. J., Monsivais, P., & Pollak, G. D. (1997). Processing of interaural intensity differences in the LSO: role of interaural threshold differences. *Journal of Neurophysiology*, *77*(6), 2863–2878. doi:10.1152/jn.1997.77.6.2863

Perney, T. M., Marshall, J., Martin, K. A., Hockfield, S., & Kaczmarek, L. K. (1992). Expression of the mRNAs for the Kv3.1 potassium channel gene in the adult and developing rat brain. *Journal of Neurophysiology*, *68*(3), 756–766. doi:10.1152/jn.1992.68.3.756

Pickles, J. O. (1982). *An introduction to the physiology of hearing*. London, New York, Paris, San Diego, San Francisco, Sao Paulo, Sydney, Tokyo, Toronto: Academic Press.

Pierce, E. T. (1967). Histogenesis of the dorsal and ventral cochlear nuclei in the mouse. An autoradiographic study. *Journal of Comparative Neurology*, *131*(1), 27–54. doi:10.1002/cne.901310104

Pilati, N., Linley, D. M., Selvaskandan, H., Uchitel, O., Hennig, M. H., Kopp-Scheinpflug, C., & Forsythe, I. D. (2016). Acoustic trauma slows AMPA receptor-mediated EPSCs in the auditory brainstem, reducing GluA4 subunit expression as a mechanism to rescue binaural function. *Journal of Physiology*, *594*(13), 3683–3703. doi:10.1113/JP271929

Platzer, J., Engel, J., Schrott-Fischer, A., Stephan, K., Bova, S., Chen, H., . . . Striessnig, J. (2000). Congenital deafness and sinoatrial node dysfunction in mice lacking class D L-type Ca^{2+} channels. *Cell*, *102*(1), 89–97.

Populin, L. C., & Yin, T. C. (1998). Behavioral studies of sound localization in the cat. *Journal of Neuroscience*, *18*(6), 2147–2160.

Pradhan, J., Maskey, D., & Ahn, S. C. (2012). Long term depression of MNTB-LSO synapses is expressed postsynaptically in developing circling mice. *Neuroscience Letters*, *531*(1), 30–34. doi:10.1016/j.neulet.2012.09.049

Radtke-Schuller, S., Seeler, S., & Grothe, B. (2015). Restricted loss of olivocochlear but not vestibular efferent neurons in the senescent gerbil (*Meriones unguiculatus*). *Frontiers in Aging Neuroscience*, *7*, 4. doi:10.3389/fnagi.2015.00004

Raman, I. M., Zhang, S., & Trussell, L. O. (1994). Pathway-specific variants of AMPA receptors and their contribution to neuronal signaling. *Journal of Neuroscience*, *14*(8), 4998–5010.

Rayleigh, L. (1907). XII. On our perception of sound direction. *The London, Edinburgh, and Dublin Philosophical Magazine and Journal of Science*, *13*(74), 214–232. doi:10.1080/14786440709463595

Renier, N., Schonewille, M., Giraudet, F., Badura, A., Tessier-Lavigne, M., Avan, P., . . . Chedotal, A. (2010). Genetic dissection of the function of hindbrain axonal commissures. *PLoS Biology*, *8*(3), e1000325. doi:10.1371/journal.pbio.1000325

Reuss, S., Disque-Kaiser, U., Antoniou-Lipfert, P., Gholi, M. N., Riemann, E., & Riemann, R. (2009). Neurochemistry of olivocochlear neurons in the hamster. *Anatomical Record (Hoboken)*, *292*(4), 461–471. doi:10.1002/ar.20881

Rietzel, H. J., & Friauf, E. (1998). Neuron types in the rat lateral superior olive and developmental changes in the complexity of their dendritic arbors. *Journal of Comparative Neurology*, *390*(1), 20–40.
Rooney, B. J., Kavanagh, G. L., & Kelly, J. B. (1991). Kainic acid lesions of the superior olivary complex: A horseradish peroxidase study of surviving brain-stem projections. *Journal of Neuroscience Methods*, *39*(1), 65–75.
Rose, M. F., Ahmad, K. A., Thaller, C., & Zoghbi, H. Y. (2009). Excitatory neurons of the proprioceptive, interoceptive, and arousal hindbrain networks share a developmental requirement for Math1. *Proceedings of the National Academy of Sciences of the United States of America*, *106*(52), 22462–22467. doi:10.1073/pnas.0911579106
Rosengauer, E., Hartwich, H., Hartmann, A. M., Rudnicki, A., Satheesh, S. V., Avraham, K. B., & Nothwang, H. G. (2012). Egr2::cre mediated conditional ablation of dicer disrupts histogenesis of mammalian central auditory nuclei. *PLoS One*, *7*(11), e49503. doi:10.1371/journal.pone.0049503
Rothman, J. S., & Manis, P. B. (2003). The roles potassium currents play in regulating the electrical activity of ventral cochlear nucleus neurons. *Journal of Neurophysiology*, *89*(6), 3097–3113. doi:10.1152/jn.00127.2002
Rudy, B. (1988). Diversity and ubiquity of K channels. *Neuroscience*, *25*(3), 729–749.
Ruhland, J. L., Jones, A. E., & Yin, T. C. (2015). Dynamic sound localization in cats. *Journal of Neurophysiology*, *114*(2), 958–968. doi:10.1152/jn.00105.2015
Russell, F. A., & Moore, D. R. (1995). Afferent reorganisation within the superior olivary complex of the gerbil: Development and induction by neonatal, unilateral cochlear removal. *Journal of Comparative Neurology*, *352*(4), 607–625. doi:10.1002/cne.903520409
Rusu, S. I., & Borst, J. G. (2011). Developmental changes in intrinsic excitability of principal neurons in the rat medial nucleus of the trapezoid body. *Developmental Neurobiology*, *71*(4), 284–295. doi:10.1002/dneu.20856
Ryugo, D. K., & Fekete, D. M. (1982). Morphology of primary axosomatic endings in the anteroventral cochlear nucleus of the cat: a study of the endbulbs of Held. *Journal of Comparative Neurology*, *210*(3), 239–257. doi:10.1002/cne.902100304
Saint Marie, R. L., & Baker, R. A. (1990). Neurotransmitter-specific uptake and retrograde transport of [3H]glycine from the inferior colliculus by ipsilateral projections of the superior olivary complex and nuclei of the lateral lemniscus. *Brain Research*, *524*(2), 244–253.
Saint Marie, R. L., Ostapoff, E. M., Morest, D. K., & Wenthold, R. J. (1989). Glycine-immunoreactive projection of the cat lateral superior olive: possible role in midbrain ear dominance. *Journal of Comparative Neurology*, *279*(3), 382–396. doi:10.1002/cne.902790305
Saldana, E., & Berrebi, A. S. (2000). Anisotropic organization of the rat superior paraolivary nucleus. *Anatomy and Embryology*, *202*(4), 265–279. doi:10.1007/s004290002020265.429
Sanes, D. H. (1990). An *in vitro* analysis of sound localization mechanisms in the gerbil lateral superior olive. *Journal of Neuroscience*, *10*(11), 3494–3506.
Sanes, D. H., & Chokshi, P. (1992). Glycinergic transmission influences the development of dendrite shape. *Neuroreport*, *3*(4), 323–326.
Sanes, D. H., Geary, W. A., Wooten, G. F., & Rubel, E. W. (1987). Quantitative distribution of the glycine receptor in the auditory brain stem of the gerbil. *Journal of Neuroscience*, *7*(11), 3793–3802.
Sanes, D. H., Markowitz, S., Bernstein, J., & Wardlow, J. (1992). The influence of inhibitory afferents on the development of postsynaptic dendritic arbors. *Journal of Comparative Neurology*, *321*(4), 637–644. doi:10.1002/cne.903210410

Sanes, D. H., Merickel, M., & Rubel, E. W. (1989). Evidence for an alteration of the tonotopic map in the gerbil cochlea during development. *Journal of Comparative Neurology, 279*(3), 436–444. doi:10.1002/cne.902790308

Sanes, D. H., & Rubel, E. W. (1988). The ontogeny of inhibition and excitation in the gerbil lateral superior olive. *Journal of Neuroscience, 8*(2), 682–700.

Sanes, D. H., & Siverls, V. (1991). Development and specificity of inhibitory terminal arborizations in the central nervous system. *Journal of Neurobiology, 22*(8), 837–854. doi:10.1002/neu.480220805

Sanes, D. H., Song, J., & Tyson, J. (1992). Refinement of dendritic arbors along the tonotopic axis of the gerbil lateral superior olive. *Brain Research. Developmental Brain Research, 67*(1), 47–55.

Sanes, D. H., & Takacs, C. (1993). Activity-dependent refinement of inhibitory connections. *European Journal of Neuroscience, 5*(6), 570–574.

Sanes, D. H., & Walsh, E. J. (1998). The development of central auditory processing. In E. W. Rubel, A. N. Popper, & R. R. Fay (Eds.), *Development of the auditory system* (pp. 271–314). New York: Springer.

Satheesh, S. V., Kunert, K., Rüttiger, L., Zuccotti, A., Schönig, K., Friauf, E., . . . Nothwang, H. G. (2012). Retrocochlear function of the peripheral deafness gene Cacna1d. *Human Molecular Genetics, 21*(17), 3896–3909. doi:10.1093/hmg/dds217

Sato, K., Nakagawa, H., Kuriyama, H., & Altschuler, R. A. (1999). Differential distribution of N-methyl-D-aspartate receptor-2 subunit messenger RNA in the rat superior olivary complex. *Neuroscience, 89*(3), 839–853.

Sato, K., Shiraishi, S., Nakagawa, H., Kuriyama, H., & Altschuler, R. A. (2000). Diversity and plasticity in amino acid receptor subunits in the rat auditory brain stem. *Hearing Research, 147*(1–2), 137–144.

Scheibel, M. E., & Scheibel, A. B. (1974). Neuropil organization in the superior olive of the cat. *Experimental Neurology, 43*(2), 339–348.

Schlüter, T., Berger, C., Rosengauer, E., Fieth, P., Krohs, C., Ushakov, K., . . . Nothwang, H. G. (2018). miR-96 is required for normal development of the auditory hindbrain. *Human Molecular Genetics, 27*(5), 860–874. doi:10.1093/hmg/ddy007

Schmid, S., Guthmann, A., Ruppersberg, J. P., & Herbert, H. (2001). Expression of AMPA receptor subunit flip/flop splice variants in the rat auditory brainstem and inferior colliculus. *Journal of Comparative Neurology, 430*(2), 160–171.

Schneggenburger, R., & Forsythe, I. D. (2006). The calyx of Held. *Cell and Tissue Research, 326*(2), 311–337.

Schneider-Maunoury, S., Gilardi-Hebenstreit, P., & Charnay, P. (1998). How to build a vertebrate hindbrain. Lessons from genetics. *Comptes Rendus de l'Academie des Sciences Serie III-Sciences de la Vie-Life Sciences, 321*(10), 819–834. doi:10.1016/S0764-4469(99)80022-5

Schneider-Maunoury, S., Topilko, P., Seitandou, T., Levi, G., Cohen-Tannoudji, M., Pournin, S., . . . Charnay, P. (1993). Disruption of Krox-20 results in alteration of rhombomeres 3 and 5 in the developing hindbrain. *Cell, 75*(6), 1199–1214.

Schofield, B. R. (2010). Structural organization of the descending auditory pathway. In A. Rees & A. R. Palmer (Eds.), *Oxford handbook of auditory science: The auditory brain* (Vol. 2, pp. 43–64). Oxford: Oxford University Press.

Schofield, B. R., & Cant, N. B. (1991). Organization of the superior olivary complex in the guinea pig. I. Cytoarchitecture, cytochrome oxidase histochemistry, and dendritic morphology. *Journal of Comparative Neurology, 314*(4), 645–670. doi:10.1002/cne.903140403

Schwartz, I. R. (1992). The superior olivary complex and lateral lemniscal nuclei. In D. B. Webster, A. N. Popper, & R. R. Fay (Eds.), *The mammalian auditory pathway: Neuroanatomy* (pp. 117–167). New York: Springer.

Seal, R. P., Akil, O., Yi, E., Weber, C. M., Grant, L., Yoo, J., . . . Edwards, R. H. (2008). Sensorineural deafness and seizures in mice lacking vesicular glutamate transporter 3. *Neuron*, *57*(2), 263–275. doi:10.1016/j.neuron.2007.11.032

Shaw, E. A., & Vaillancourt, M. M. (1985). Transformation of sound-pressure level from the free field to the eardrum presented in numerical form. *Journal of the Acoustical Society of America*, *78*(3), 1120–1123.

Shneiderman, A., Stanforth, D. A., Henkel, C. K., & Saint Marie, R. L. (1999). Input-output relationships of the dorsal nucleus of the lateral lemniscus: Possible substrate for the processing of dynamic spatial cues. *Journal of Comparative Neurology*, *410*(2), 265–276.

Smith, P. H., Joris, P. X., Carney, L. H., & Yin, T. C. (1991). Projections of physiologically characterized globular bushy cell axons from the cochlear nucleus of the cat. *Journal of Comparative Neurology*, *304*(3), 387–407. doi:10.1002/cne.903040305

Sommer, I., Lingenhöhl, K., & Friauf, E. (1993). Principal cells of the rat medial nucleus of the trapezoid body: An intracellular in vivo study of their physiology and morphology. *Experimental Brain Research*, *95*(2), 223–239.

Song, M. S., & Rossi, J. J. (2017). Molecular mechanisms of Dicer: Endonuclease and enzymatic activity. *Biochemical Journal*, *474*(10), 1603–1618. doi:10.1042/BCJ20160759

Sonntag, M., Englitz, B., Kopp-Scheinpflug, C., & Rübsamen, R. (2009). Early postnatal development of spontaneous and acoustically evoked discharge activity of principal cells of the medial nucleus of the trapezoid body: An *in vivo* study in mice. *Journal of Neuroscience*, *29*(30), 9510–9520. doi:10.1523/JNEUROSCI.1377-09.2009

Sonntag, M., Englitz, B., Typlt, M., & Rübsamen, R. (2011). The calyx of Held develops adult-like dynamics and reliability by hearing onset in the mouse *in vivo*. *Journal of Neuroscience*, *31*(18), 6699–6709. doi:10.1523/JNEUROSCI.0575-11.2011

Spangler, K. M., Warr, W. B., & Henkel, C. K. (1985). The projections of principal cells of the medial nucleus of the trapezoid body in the cat. *Journal of Comparative Neurology*, *238*(3), 249–262. doi:10.1002/cne.902380302

Spirou, G. A., & Berrebi, A. S. (1997). Glycine immunoreactivity in the lateral nucleus of the trapezoid body of the cat. *Journal of Comparative Neurology*, *383*(4), 473–488.

Srinivasan, G., Friauf, E., & Löhrke, S. (2004). Functional glutamatergic and glycinergic inputs to several superior olivary nuclei of the rat revealed by optical imaging. *Neuroscience*, *128*(3), 617–634.

Sterenborg, J. C., Pilati, N., Sheridan, C. J., Uchitel, O. D., Forsythe, I. D., & Barnes-Davies, M. (2010). Lateral olivocochlear (LOC) neurons of the mouse LSO receive excitatory and inhibitory synaptic inputs with slower kinetics than LSO principal neurons. *Hearing Research*, *270*(1–2), 119–126. doi:10.1016/j.heares.2010.08.013

Sun, S., Babola, T., Pregernig, G., So, K. S., Nguyen, M., Su, S. M., . . . Müller, U. (2018). Hair cell mechanotransduction regulates spontaneous activity and spiral ganglion subtype specification in the auditory system. *Cell*, *174*, 1247–1263 e15. doi:10.1016/j.cell.2018.07.008

Suneja, S. K., Benson, C. G., & Potashner, S. J. (1998). Glycine receptors in adult guinea pig brain stem auditory nuclei: Regulation after unilateral cochlear ablation. *Experimental Neurology*, *154*(2), 473–488. doi:10.1006/exnr.1998.6946

Takahashi, T., Momiyama, A., Hirai, K., Hishinuma, F., & Akagi, H. (1992). Functional correlation of fetal and adult forms of glycine receptors with developmental changes in inhibitory synaptic receptor channels. *Neuron*, *9*(6), 1155–1161.

Thompson, A. M., & Thompson, G. C. (1987). Efferent projections from posteroventral cochlear nucleus to lateral superior olive in guinea pig. *Brain Research*, *421*(1–2), 382–386.

Tollin, D. J. (2003). The lateral superior olive: a functional role in sound source localization. *Neuroscientist*, *9*(2), 127–143. doi:10.1177/1073858403252228

Tollin, D. J., & Yin, T. C. (2002). The coding of spatial location by single units in the lateral superior olive of the cat. II. The determinants of spatial receptive fields in azimuth. *Journal of Neuroscience*, *22*(4), 1468–1479.

Tollin, D. J., & Yin, T. C. (2005). Interaural phase and level difference sensitivity in low-frequency neurons in the lateral superior olive. *Journal of Neuroscience*, *25*(46), 10648–10657. doi:10.1523/JNEUROSCI.1609-05.2005

Tollin, D. J., & Yin, T. C. T. (2002). The coding of spatial location by single units in the lateral superior olive of the cat. I. Spatial receptive fields in azimuth. *Journal of Neuroscience*, *22*(4), 1454–1467. doi:Doi 10.1523/Jneurosci.22-04-01454.2002

Triplett, J. W., & Feldheim, D. A. (2012). Eph and ephrin signaling in the formation of topographic maps. *Seminars in Cell & Developmental Biology*, *23*(1), 7–15. doi:10.1016/j.semcdb.2011.10.026

Tritsch, N. X., Rodriguez-Contreras, A., Crins, T. T. H., Wang, H. C., Borst, J. G. G., & Bergles, D. E. (2010). Calcium action potentials in hair cells pattern auditory neuron activity before hearing onset. *Nature Neuroscience*, *13*(9), 1050–1052. doi:10.1038/nn.2604

Tritsch, N. X., Yi, E., Gale, J. E., Glowatzki, E., & Bergles, D. E. (2007). The origin of spontaneous activity in the developing auditory system. *Nature*, *450*(7166), 50–55. doi:10.1038/nature06233

Trussell, L. O. (1999). Synaptic mechanisms for coding timing in auditory neurons. *Annual Review of Physiology*, *61*, 477–496. doi:10.1146/annurev.physiol.61.1.477

Tsuchitani, C. (1977). Functional organization of lateral cell groups of cat superior olivary complex. *Journal of Neurophysiology*, *40*(2), 296–318. doi:10.1152/jn.1977.40.2.296

Tsuchitani, C. (1988a). The inhibition of cat lateral superior olive unit excitatory responses to binaural tone bursts. I. The transient chopper response. *Journal of Neurophysiology*, *59*(1), 164–183. doi:10.1152/jn.1988.59.1.164

Tsuchitani, C. (1988b). The inhibition of cat lateral superior olive unit excitatory responses to binaural tone bursts. II. The sustained discharges. *Journal of Neurophysiology*, *59*(1), 184–211. doi:10.1152/jn.1988.59.1.184

Tsuchitani, C., & Boudreau, J. C. (1966). Single unit analysis of cat superior olive S segment with tonal stimuli. *Journal of Neurophysiology*, *29*(4), 684–697. doi:10.1152/jn.1966.29.4.684

Tsuchitani, C., & Boudreau, J. C. (1967). Encoding of stimulus frequency and intensity by cat superior olive S-segment cells. *Journal of the Acoustical Society of America*, *42*(4), 794–805.

Tsuchitani, C., & Johnson, D. H. (1991). Binaural cues and signal processing in the superior olivary complex. In R. A. Altschuler, R. P. Bobbin, B. M. Clopton, & D. W. Hoffman (Eds.), *Neurobiology of hearing: The central auditory system* (Vol. 1, pp. 163–193). New York: Raven Press.

van Adel, B. A., & Kelly, J. B. (1998). Kainic acid lesions of the superior olivary complex: Effects on sound localization by the albino rat. *Behavioral Neuroscience*, *112*(2), 432–446.

Vetter, D. E., Adams, J. C., & Mugnaini, E. (1991). Chemically distinct rat olivocochlear neurons. *Synapse*, *7*(1), 21–43. doi:10.1002/syn.890070104

Vetter, D. E., Liberman, M. C., Mann, J., Barhanin, J., Boulter, J., Brown, M. C., . . . Elgoyhen, A. B. (1999). Role of a9 nicotinic ACh receptor subunits in the development and function of cochlear efferent innervation. *Neuron*, *23*(1), 93–103.

Vetter, D. E., & Mugnaini, E. (1992). Distribution and dendritic features of three groups of rat olivocochlear neurons. A study with two retrograde cholera toxin tracers. *Anatomy and Embryology*, *185*(1), 1–16.

Vitten, H., Reusch, M., Friauf, E., & Löhrke, S. (2004). Expression of functional kainate and AMPA receptors in developing lateral superior olive neurons of the rat. *Journal of Neurobiology*, *59*(3), 272–288. doi:10.1002/neu.10326

von Gersdorff, H., & Borst, J. G. (2002). Short-term plasticity at the calyx of Held. *Nature Reviews. Neuroscience*, *3*(1), 53–64. doi:10.1038/nrn705

Walcher, J., Hassfurth, B., Grothe, B., & Koch, U. (2011). Comparative posthearing development of inhibitory inputs to the lateral superior olive in gerbils and mice. *Journal of Neurophysiology*, *106*(3), 1443–1453. doi:10.1152/jn.01087.2010

Walker, V. A., Peremans, H., & Hallam, J. C. T. (1998). One tone, two ears, three dimensions: A robotic investigation of pinnae movements used by rhinolophid and hipposiderid bats. *Journal of the Acoustical Society of America*, *104*(1), 569–579. doi:10.1121/1.423256

Wallace, M. M., Harris, J. A., Brubaker, D. Q., Klotz, C. A., & Gabriele, M. L. (2016). Graded and discontinuous EphA-ephrinB expression patterns in the developing auditory brainstem. *Hearing Research*, *335*, 64–75. doi:10.1016/j.heares.2016.02.013

Wang, H. C., Lin, C. C., Cheung, R., Zhang-Hooks, Y., Agarwal, A., Ellis-Davies, G., . . . Bergles, D. E. (2015). Spontaneous activity of cochlear hair cells triggered by fluid secretion mechanism in adjacent support cells. *Cell*, *163*(6), 1348–1359. doi:10.1016/j.cell.2015.10.070

Wang, V. Y., Rose, M. F., & Zoghbi, H. Y. (2005). Math1 expression redefines the rhombic lip derivatives and reveals novel lineages within the brainstem and cerebellum. *Neuron*, *48*(1), 31–43. doi:10.1016/j.neuron.2005.08.024

Warr, W. B. (1992). Organization of olivocochlear efferent systems in mammals. In D. B. Webster, A. N. Popper, & R. R. Fay (Eds.), *The mammalian auditory pathway: Neuroanatomy* (Vol. 1, pp. 410–448). New York: Springer Verlag.

Warr, W. B., Beck Boche, J. E., Ye, Y., & Kim, D. O. (2002). Organization of olivocochlear neurons in the cat studied with the retrograde tracer cholera toxin-B. *Journal of the Association for Research in Otolaryngology*, *3*(4), 457–478.

Warr, W. B., & Beck, J. E. (1996). Multiple projections from the ventral nucleus of the trapezoid body in the rat. *Hearing Research*, *93*(1–2), 83–101.

Warr, W. B., & Boche, J. E. (2003). Diversity of axonal ramifications belonging to single lateral and medial olivocochlear neurons. *Experimental Brain Research*, *153*(4), 499–513. doi:10.1007/s00221-003-1682-3

Weinrich, L., Sonntag, M., Arendt, T., & Morawski, M. (2018). Neuroanatomical characterization of perineuronal net components in the human cochlear nucleus and superior olivary complex. *Hearing Research*, *367*, 32–47. doi:10.1016/j.heares.2018.07.005

Wenthold, R. J., Huie, D., Altschuler, R. A., & Reeks, K. A. (1987). Glycine immunoreactivity localized in the cochlear nucleus and superior olivary complex. *Neuroscience*, *22*(3), 897–912.

Wiegert, J. S., & Oertner, T. G. (2013). Long-term depression triggers the selective elimination of weakly integrated synapses. *Proceedings of the National Academy of Sciences of the United States of America*, *110*(47), E4510–4519. doi:10.1073/pnas.1315926110

Wilkinson, D. G., Bhatt, S., Chavrier, P., Bravo, R., & Charnay, P. (1989). Segment-specific expression of a zinc-finger gene in the developing nervous system of the mouse. *Nature*, *337*(6206), 461–464. doi:10.1038/337461a0

Willard, F. H., & Martin, G. F. (1983). The auditory brainstem nuclei and some of their projections to the inferior colliculus in the North American opossum. *Neuroscience, 10*(4), 1203–1232.

Willaredt, M. A., Schluter, T., & Nothwang, H. G. (2015). The gene regulatory networks underlying formation of the auditory hindbrain. *Cellular and Molecular Life Sciences, 72*(3), 519–535. doi:10.1007/s00018-014-1759-0

Willott, J. F. (1997). *Pathology of the aging mouse*. Washington, DC: ILSI Press.

Winter, I. M., Robertson, D., & Cole, K. S. (1989). Descending projections from auditory brainstem nuclei to the cochlea and cochlear nucleus of the guinea pig. *Journal of Comparative Neurology, 280*(1), 143–157. doi:10.1002/cne.902800110

Woolf, N. K., & Ryan, A. F. (1984). The development of auditory function in the cochlea of the mongolian gerbil. *Hearing Research, 13*(3), 277–283.

Woolf, N. K., & Ryan, A. F. (1985). Ontogeny of neural discharge patterns in the ventral cochlear nucleus of the mongolian gerbil. *Brain Research, 349*(1–2), 131–147.

Wu, S. H., & Kelly, J. B. (1991). Physiological properties of neurons in the mouse superior olive: Membrane characteristics and postsynaptic responses studied in vitro. *Journal of Neurophysiology, 65*(2), 230–246. doi:10.1152/jn.1991.65.2.230

Wu, S. H., & Kelly, J. B. (1992a). Binaural interaction in the lateral superior olive: Time difference sensitivity studied in mouse brain slice. *Journal of Neurophysiology, 68*(4), 1151–1159. doi:10.1152/jn.1992.68.4.1151

Wu, S. H., & Kelly, J. B. (1992b). Synaptic pharmacology of the superior olivary complex studied in mouse brain slice. *Journal of Neuroscience, 12*(8), 3084–3097.

Wu, S. H., & Kelly, J. B. (1993). Response of neurons in the lateral superior olive and medial nucleus of the trapezoid body to repetitive stimulation: Intracellular and extracellular recordings from mouse brain slice. *Hearing Research, 68*(2), 189–201.

Wu, S. H., & Kelly, J. B. (1995). Inhibition in the superior olivary complex: pharmacological evidence from mouse brain slice. *Journal of Neurophysiology, 73*(1), 256–269. doi:10.1152/jn.1995.73.1.256

Wullimann, M. F., Mueller, T., Distel, M., Babaryka, A., Grothe, B., & Koster, R. W. (2011). The long adventurous journey of rhombic lip cells in jawed vertebrates: a comparative developmental analysis. *Frontiers in Neuroanatomy, 5*, 27. doi:10.3389/fnana.2011.00027

Xie, R., & Manis, P. B. (2013). Target-specific IPSC kinetics promote temporal processing in auditory parallel pathways. *Journal of Neuroscience, 33*(4), 1598–1614. doi:10.1523/JNEUROSCI.2541-12.2013

Xue, C., & Liu, F. (2014). Structured synaptic inhibition has a critical role in multiple-choice motion-discrimination tasks. *Journal of Neuroscience, 34*(40), 13444–13457. doi:10.1523/JNEUROSCI.0001-14.2014

Yang, Y. M., Aitoubah, J., Lauer, A. M., Nuriya, M., Takamiya, K., Jia, Z., . . . Wang, L. Y. (2011). GluA4 is indispensable for driving fast neurotransmission across a high-fidelity central synapse. *Journal of Physiology, 589*(17), 4209–4227. doi:10.1113/jphysiol.2011.208066

Yin, T. C. (2013). Physiological and behavioral studies of sound localization. *Journal of the Acoustical Society of America, 133*, 050050–050050. doi:10.1121/1.4799510

Yin, T. C. T. (2002). Neural mechanisms of encoding binaural localization cues in the auditory brainstem. In D. Oertel, R. R. Fay, & A. N. Popper (Eds.), *Integrative functions in the mammalian auditory pathway* (pp. 99–159). New York: Springer.

Yin, T. C. T., & Kuwada, S. (1983). Binaural interaction in low-frequency neurons in inferior colliculus of the cat. III. Effects of changing frequency. *Journal of Neurophysiology*, *50*(4), 1020–1042. doi:10.1152/jn.1983.50.4.1020

Yin, T. C. T., & Kuwada, S. (2010). Binaural localization cues. In A. Rees & A. R. Palmer (Eds.), *Oxford handbook of auditory science: The auditory brain.* (Vol. 2, pp. 271–302). Oxford: Oxford University Press.

Young, E. D., Rice, J. J., & Tong, S. C. (1996). Effects of pinna position on head-related transfer functions in the cat. *Journal of the Acoustical Society of America*, *99*(5), 3064–3076.

Zucker, R. S., & Regehr, W. G. (2002). Short-term synaptic plasticity. *Annual Review of Physiology*, *64*, 355–405. doi:10.1146/annurev.physiol.64.092501.114547

CHAPTER 14

THE SUPERIOR PARAOLIVARY NUCLEUS

ANNA K. MAGNUSSON AND
MARCELO GÓMEZ-ÁLVAREZ

Abstract

This chapter summarizes the current concepts of the superior paraolivary nucleus (SPON)—a structure embedded in the superior olivary complex in the mammalian auditory brainstem. SPON is driven by input pathways from two of the most temporally secure neurons in the brain: the octopus cells in the cochlear nucleus and the neurons of the medial nucleus of the trapezoid body. These inputs activate spiking activity that marks the onset and offset of sound, the latter based on a rebound depolarization mechanism. This makes the SPON an excellent detector of transient sound energy. Robust detection of the coarse sound pattern over time further gives SPON the capacity to track the temporal envelope of complex sounds with supreme precision. Since the SPON circuitry is constant in mammals and resilient to sensory perturbation, it indicates its high survival value. A possible neuroevolutionary role of SPON in the processing of vocalizations is discussed.

Keywords: brainstem, auditory pathways, temporal processing, rebound spiking, feature detection, segmentation, prosodic stress pattern

The SPON Is Present in All Mammals

The superior olivary complex (SOC) comprises a group of morphologically-defined nuclei in the ventral brainstem. Within the SOC, the superior paraolivary nucleus (SPON) is a prominent GABAergic nucleus (González-Hernández, Mantolán-Sarmiento, González-González, & Pérez-González, 1996; Kulesza & Berrebi, 2000), which has been implicated in processing rhythmic sound cues of importance for the perception of vocalized communication (Felix et al., 2011; Kadner & Berrebi, 2008; Kopp-Scheinpflug et al., 2011). Perceiving sound rhythms is especially important in humans, who rely on the ability to identify distinct speech units for language perception (Rosen, 1992) and speech production (Lieberman, 2002). Compared to other SOC nuclei, which are well-known for their role in deriving sound localization cues (McAlpine, 2005; Tollin, 2003) or as a model for studying the developmental organization of the auditory pathways (Kandler et al., 2009; Sanes & Friauf, 2000), the SPON has received relatively little attention. This chapter summarizes recent progress in understanding the role of the SPON for hearing, and its implications for interspecies communication.

Based on cytoarchitecture, the SPON (sometimes also referred to as the SPN) is a well-defined auditory brainstem nucleus in lower mammals, such as mice (Felix et al., 2011; Kopp-Scheinpflug et al., 2011; Leijon et al., 2016), rats (Caminos et al., 2007; Kulesza & Berrebi, 2000), gerbils (Behrend et al., 2002; Dehmel et al., 2002; Stange et al., 2013), and guinea-pigs (Schofield, 1991; Schofield & Cant, 1991, 1992). In other species, cells located dorsomedially of the medial superior olive (MSO), referred to as the dorsomedial periolivary nucleus (DMPO), are commonly speculated to be the SPON homologue in, for example, bats (Grothe, 1994; Zook & Casseday, 1985;), cats (Adams, 1983; Spirou et al., 1990), chinchillas (Azeredo et al., 1999; Kelley et al., 1992), and primates (Bazwinsky et al., 2005; Moore & Moore, 1971; Strominger et al., 1977), including humans (Bazwinsky et al., 2003; Moore et al., 1998; Moore, 2000). Although studies to systematically characterize the physiological properties of DMPO in vivo are largely missing in the mustached bat, the medial SOC exhibit SPON-like properties in response to monaural sound stimulation (Grothe, 1994; Kulesza et al., 2003), thus showing it as being homologous to the rodent SPON (Grothe, 2000). Recently, the nomenclature in humans has shifted from the DMPO to the SPON (Kulesza, 2008, 2014; Kulesza & Grothe, 2015; Schmidt et al., 2010).

Numerous anatomical investigations of the SOC reveal that the SPON/DMPO is present in all mammals investigated thus far (see Figure 14.1). An inspection of the nuclear morphology in SOC brain sections containing the MSO, SPON/DMPO and medial nucleus of the trapezoid body (MNTB; Figure 14.1) demonstrate that these areas expand proportionally in line with the increase in brainstem size from small rodents to

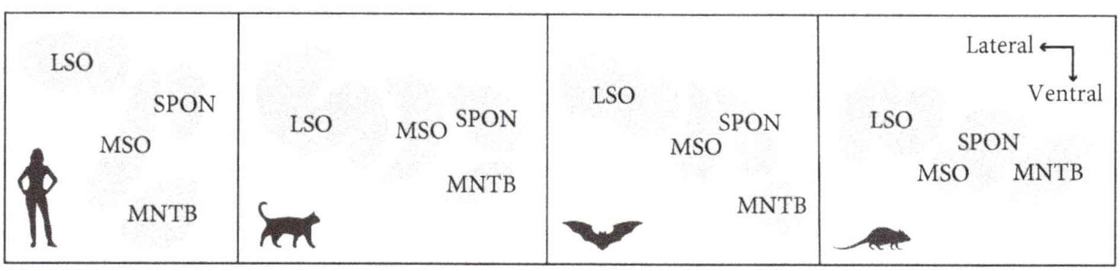

FIGURE 14.1 Schematic representation of the superior olivary complex in humans, cats, bats, and rats. The lateral (LSO) and the medial superior olivary nuclei (MSO) vary in size depending on the animal's natural acoustic niche (Heffner, 2004), whereas the superior paraolivary nucleus (SPON) and the medial nucleus of the trapezoid body (MNTB) are more uniformly represented throughout the animal chain. The nuclear structures are based on transverse brainstem sections and are inspired from, for example, Moore (2000); Zook & Casseday (1985).

primates, including humans (Figure 14.1; Kulesza, 2008, 2014; Moore, 1987, 2000; Moore et al., 1998). The size of the SPON/DMPO (Moore & Moore, 1971), however, does not depend on the animals hearing range (Heffner, 2004). Thus, the SPON is a major part of the SOC in animals in which high-frequency hearing dominates, such as mice and rats (Kulesza et al., 2002), as well as those in which low-frequency hearing is more prominent, such as gerbils (Behrend et al., 2002; Dehmel et al., 2002; Stange et al., 2013) and guinea-pigs (Schofield, 1991; Schofield & Cant, 1991, 1992). Accordingly, species that capitalize on both high and low sound frequency cues, such as the cat (Heffner, 2004), exhibit a balanced ratio between the LSO, MSO and DMPO (Figure 14.1; Moore, 2000). The naked mole rat is a special case since it is most sensitive to very low-frequency sounds (<1 kHz; Lange et al., 2007), which may lead to an expansion of the SPON at the expense of the high frequency-sensitive LSO, a hypothesis that needs to be verified by identifying the SPON neurons using, for example, GABA markers.

The SPON Receives Monaural Temporal Information

In rodents, one set of afferents to the SPON come from a mixed population of octopus and multipolar stellate cells in the contralateral posteroventral cochlear nucleus (PVCN; Friauf & Ostwald, 1988; Saldaña et al., 2009; Schofield, 1995; Thompson & Thompson, 1991; Zook & Casseday, 1985). The multipolar stellate cell type has also been described as forming an ipsilateral projection from the PVCN to the SPON (Friauf & Ostwald, 1988). Recently, this view was challenged by Felix et al. (2017), who demonstrated that a focal injection of a retrograde tracer in the SPON of mice only labeled the octopus cells in the contralateral PVCN (see Figure 14.2), whereas virtually no multipolar stellate cells were labeled in either the ipsilateral or contralateral PVCN. No tracer was observed in the ventral acoustic stria or in the anteroventral cochlear nucleus (Felix et al., 2017). The latter result confirms previous studies in SPON of rodents (Friauf & Ostwald, 1988; Kuwabara et al., 1991), whereas in the cat there is conflicting evidence for a globular bushy cell projection from the contralateral anterior ventral cochlear nucleus (AVCN). to the DMPO (Smith et al., 1991; Spirou et al., 1990). However, the slightest spread of tracer into adjacent areas of the SOC targets globular bushy cells and multipolar stellate cells in, respectively, AVCN and PVCN on both sides of the brainstem (Felix et al., 2017). Therefore, the most parsimonious interpretation is that SPON receives a single input from the octopus cells located in the contralateral PVCN (Figure 14.2; Felix et al., 2017). A statistical analysis of miniature excitatory currents (mEPSCs) recorded and pharmacologically isolated in the SPON and LSO neurons lends further support to the concept of a single input to the principal neurons of these nuclei. In contrast, the lateral olivocochlear neurons, also residing in the LSO (Aschoff & Ostwald, 1987; Motts et al., 2008), but with distinct morphological and physiological properties from the principal

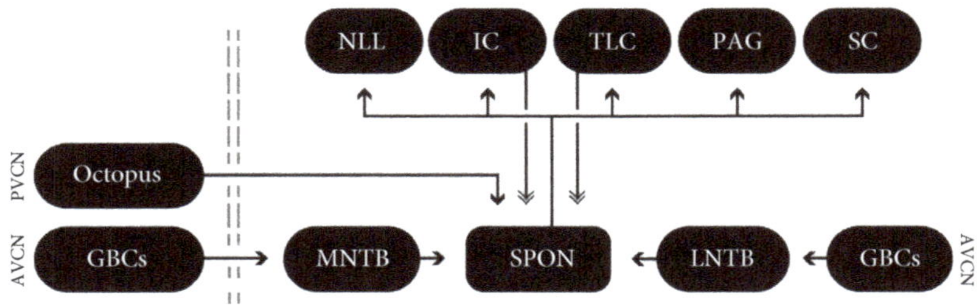

FIGURE 14.2 The superior paraolivary nucleus (SPON) connectome. The SPON receives direct excitatory input from the octopus cells in the contralateral posteroventral cochlear nucleus (PVCN), via the intermediate acoustic stria (Felix et al., 2017), and an indirect inhibitory glycinergic input from the medial nucleus of the trapezoid body (MNTB) via the globular bushy cells (GBCs) in the contralateral anteroventral cochlear nucleus (AVCN). The ipsilateral lateral nucleus of the trapezoid body (LNTB) provides an additional source of glycinergic inhibition of unknown function via GBCs in the ipsilateral AVCN. The SPON projects tonotopically to the ipsilateral inferior colliculus (IC) via the nuclei of the lateral lemniscus (NLL) (Saldaña et al., 2009; Viñuela et al., 2011). The SPON also projects to the ipsilateral and, to a lesser degree, to the contralateral tectal longitudinal column (TLC), the periaqueductal gray substance (PAG), and the deep layers of the contralateral superior colliculus (SC) in the midbrain tectum (Viñuela et al., 2011).

neurons (Adam et al., 1999; Fujino et al., 1997; Leijon & Magnusson, 2014; Sterenborg et al., 2010), displayed evidence for two or more inputs (Felix et al., 2017; Gómez-Álvarez & Saldaña, 2016). Recordings from the SPON in vivo show that sound primarily actives the SPON from the contralateral ear (bat: Grothe, 1994; rabbit: Kuwada & Batra, 1999; gerbil: Behrend et al., 2002; Dehmel et al., 2002; rat: Kadner & Berrebi, 2008; Kulesza et al., 2003, 2007; mouse: Felix et al., 2011; Kopp-Scheinpflug et al., 2011), although there have been reports of some responses, putatively from SPON neurons, that are binaural (Behrend et al., 2002; Dehmel et al., 2002). A monaural activation of the SPON, driven by octopus cells, is consistent with the hypothesis that the SPON extracts temporal information induced by broadband sounds (Felix et al., 2013, 2017; Gómez-Álvarez et al., 2018; Oertel et al., 2000; Rhode, 1998).

Another documented major projection to the SPON is from the ipsilateral principal neurons in the medial nucleus of the trapezoid body (MNTB; Figure 14.2; Banks & Smith, 1992; Bledsoe et al., 1990; Ford et al., 2009; Kuwabara & Zook, 1991, 1992; Sommer et al., 1993; Spangler et al., 1985; Warr, 1966). The MNTB neurons receive input from the globular bushy cells in the contralateral AVCN, the axons of which travel in the ventral acoustic stria and terminate with the calyx-of-Held endings onto the MNTB principal neurons (Kuwabara et al., 1991; Smith et al., 1991; Spirou et al., 1990). The MNTB-projection to the SPON gives rise to a powerful feed-forward glycinergic inhibition that quenches SPON activity during contralateral sound stimulation but, paradoxically, drives the neurons to spike at the sound offset (Kadner et al., 2006; Kulesza et al., 2007). Interestingly, a single afferent from the MNTB can branch and innervate several nuclei within the SOC (Kuwabara & Zook, 1991, 1992; Gómez-Álvarez & Saldaña, 2016; Sommer et al., 1993). It is not clear how these afferent collaterals from the MNTB contribute to sound processing in areas fulfilling vastly different roles for acoustic processing. Presumably, neuron-specific properties, such as voltage-operated mechanisms (Felix et al., 2011, 2013; Kopp-Scheinpflug et al., 2011, 2015; Yassin et al., 2014), enable the SPON, perhaps in combination with the termination pattern in relation to the cellular geometry (Felix et al., 2013; Ollo & Schwartz, 1979), to decode specific aspects of the incoming signals. In addition, the SPON receives projections from the ipsilateral lateral nucleus of the trapezoid body (LNTB; Figure 14.2; Felix et al., 2017; Saldaña et al., 2009; Viñuela et al., 2011). The LNTB is innervated by ipsilateral collateral branches of the globular bushy cell axons, (Kuwabara et al., 1991; Spirou et al., 1990), thus providing the SPON with an ipsilateral inhibitory glycinergic (Magnusson et al., 2005; Roberts et al., 2014) projection of hitherto unknown function.

The SPON Relays Temporally Precise Inhibition

The main output from the SPON is a tonotopically organized inhibitory, GABAergic projection to the ipsilateral inferior colliculus (IC) via the nuclei of the lateral lemniscus (NLL; see Figure 14.2; Saldaña et al., 2009; Viñuela et al., 2011). The function of such tonotopic GABA-ergic drive from the SPON was recently tested by performing paired recordings from the SPON and the IC, which demonstrated that the selective blockade of SPON-derived inhibition decreased IC spiking precision in response to the envelope of amplitude-modulated sounds (Felix et al., 2015). This fit well with the envelope-synchronized spiking response to amplitude-modulated sounds recorded in SPON (Behrend et al., 2002; Felix et al., 2011; Grothe, et al., 1994; Kadner & Berrebi, 2008; Kulesza et al., 2003; Kuwada & Batra, 1999). The inhibitory output from the SPON would, therefore, be suitable to tune the IC neurons to sound envelope cues (Barsz, et al., 1998; Krishna & Semple, 2000; Zheng & Escabí, 2008) and periodicity patterns, that is, how often these coarse fluctuations occur (Langner, 1992; Rees & Palmer, 1989; Schreiner & Langner, 1988). It is tempting to speculate that the topographical representation of sound periodicity, visualized by functional magnetic resonance imaging (fMRI) on the IC level (Baumann et al., 2011), may depend on inhibition from lower brainstem areas, such as the input from SPON. A shift in sensitivity from high to low modulation-frequencies in the ascending auditory pathways, from the cochlear nucleus to the IC (Frisina, 2001; Joris et al., 2004; Nelson & Carney, 2004), suggests that the auditory brainstem would be a suitable locus to perform the conversion needed to give rise to the IC periodicity map. The SPON is a suitable candidate for changing the coding strategy. Because rebound spiking in SPON neurons depends on the activation of slowly activating h-currents (Felix et al., 2011; Kopp-Scheinpflug et al.,

2011), offset spiking to sound depends on relatively long-lasting MNTB activity, which results in temporal summation of the hyperpolarizing inputs (Felix et al., 2011). By acting as a low-pass filter, Ih-dependent rebound spiking in SPON would be well suited to encode slow changes in sound energy over time as it typically occurs in periodic natural sounds, such as speech (Rosen, 1992; Shannon et al., 1995). By providing robust inhibition, synchronized to the negative edge of sound segments, SPON may not only help to enhance the "peaks" of the envelope signal by unmasking excitation (Grothe, 1994; Yang & Pollak, 1997) or phasic disinhibition of inhibitory interneurons in the IC (Malmierca et al., 2009; Oliver & Morest, 1984), but could also trigger rebound spiking in the IC (Koch & Grothe, 2003; Nagtegaal & Borst, 2010; Sun & Wu, 2008; Tan et al., 2007). The slightly delayed SPON input could, therefore, contribute to further lowering the preferred modulation frequency of the neurons in the IC (Langner, 1992; Rees & Palmer, 1989; Schreiner & Langner, 1988), while inverting the sign of the auditory signal from excitation to inhibition in SPON would enhance the modulation depth of the IC envelope-response at both the "peaks" and the "troughs" (Felix et al., 2015). The "troughs" could, according to de Cheveigné's cancellation model for pitch perception (1998), equally well serve as a periodicity cue as the "peaks." Another suggested role for SPON-derived inhibition is related to post-stimulus inhibition, which produces a forward masking effect in the IC (Nelson et al., 2009; Salimi et al., 2017). This mechanism could further enhance the contrast between sound units and aid perception of communication sounds.

Ascending SPON axons continue from the ipsilateral IC and travel through the commissure of the IC (CoIC) before terminating in the tectal longitudinal column (TLC). The newly discovered TLC is a distinct group of reticular neurons spanning the midbrain tectum longitudinally, very close to the midline and immediately above the periaqueductal gray (PAG; Figure 14.2; Aparicio et al., 2010; Aparicio & Saldaña, 2014; Marshall et al., 2008; Saldaña et al., 2007, 2009; Viñuela et al., 2011). The SPON projects densely to the ipsilateral TLC, and sparsely to the contralateral TLC (Saldaña et al., 2009; Viñuela et al., 2011). A small fraction of the ascending SPON axons circumvent the IC and cross to innervate the deep layers of the contralateral superior colliculus (SC) and the PAG (Figure 14.2; Viñuela et al., 2011), which are multimodal areas expected to trigger automated motor actions in response to external and internal signals of importance for the organism's survival (Holstege, 1998; Sparks & Hartwich-Young, 1989). Notably, injections of pseudorabies virus in the rabbit eyelid has recently demonstrated tentative evidence for a projection from the SPON to the superior salivatory nucleus (SSN; Wang et al., 2017). The SSN is a group of parasympathetic neurons that innervate the lacrimal, sublingual and submandibular glands (Tóth et al., 1999). Although a connection between the SPON and areas involved in autonomic regulation still has to be confirmed, it is tempting to speculate that the SPON, with its high sensitivity to the sound envelope (Behrend et al., 2002; Felix et al., 2011; Kadner & Berrebi, 2008; Kulesza et al., 2003; Kuwada & Batra, 1999), may be part of an old gateway mediating innate reactions to sounds, for instance, in response to the affective qualities of the voice (Pihan et al., 2008).

The SPON Receives Descending Projections but Is Most Likely Not a Major Part of the Medial Olivocochlear Efferent System

The SPON has long been considered to be a subdivision of the medial olivocochlear efferent system projecting from the brainstem to the cochlear nucleus and the cochlea. This concept builds mostly on anatomical studies performed in cats (Adams & Warr, 1976; Smith et al., 1991; Warr, 1975; Warr et al., 2002), but also studies in chinchillas (Azeredo et al., 1999), guinea-pig (Winter et al., 1989), mice (Ollo & Schwartz, 1979), and bats and rats (Aschoff & Ostwald, 1987). A close, specific, examination of the periolivary cells in the cat demonstrated that the ventromedial part of the SOC, including the SPON, the MNTB and the ventral nucleus of the trapezoid body (VNTB), are indeed targeted by the retrograde transporter HRP injected in the cochlea (Adams, 1983). However, the SPON was also targeted by HRP-injections into the ipsilateral IC. These IC retrogradely labeled neurons far outnumbered those that projected back to the cochlear nucleus or cochlea and importantly, were other neurons than the efferent ones (Adams, 1983; Adams & Warr, 1976). Instead, the majority of the cochlear-projecting neurons were confined to the VNTB (Adams, 1983). This result is consistent with other species that demonstrate that cholinergic neurons, known to be the main neurotransmitter of the olivocochlear system (Simmons, 2002), are predominantly located within the LSO and the VNTB (human: Moore et al., 1999; monkey: Thompson & Thompson, 1986; guinea-pig: Motts et al., 2008; gerbil: Kaiser et al., 2011; hamster: Simmons et al., 1999; rat; Yao & Godfrey, 1998; mouse: Brown & Levine, 2008; Leijon & Magnusson, 2014). In a rat study that traced the inputs from the SOC to the cochlea, only neurons in the LSO and the VNTB were highlighted; thus, White & Warr (1983) concluded that the VNTB is the only periolivary nucleus that has been invariably targeted by anatomical tract tracing of the olivocochlear efferent system in all species studied thus far.

Corticofugal projections primarily target the VNTB (Coomes Peterson, & Schofield, 2007; Coomes & Schofield, 2004; Feliciano et al., 1995; Mulders & Robertson, 2000), and more rarely the SPON/DMPO (Coomes & Schofield, 2004; Coomes Peterson & Schofield, 2007; Feliciano et al., 1995); however, more extensive descending cortical input to the SPON has been described in the gerbil (Budinger et al., 2000; 2013). A study combining tracer injections into the cortex and the IC revealed that corticofugal fibers predominantly connect to the ipsilateral SPON neurons projecting to the ipsilateral IC, and to a lesser degree the contralateral SPON neurons that project to the ipsilateral IC (Coomes Peterson & Schofield, 2007). The ipsilateral IC is, in itself, a source of descending input to the SPON (see Figure 14.2; Caicedo & Herbert, 1993; Vetter et al., 1993), indicating that there is reciprocal contact between the SPON and its ascending targets. In analogy with this notion, the SPON is reciprocally connected to the ipsilateral TLC (Figure 14.2; Aparicio & Saldaña, 2014; Viñuela et al., 2011). It is also worth mentioning that there is a thalamic input to the SPON, consisting of a bilateral projection from the subparafascicular nucleus (SPF) with an ipsilateral dominance (Yasui et al., 1992). The SPF is, as the auditory cortex, also reciprocally connected with the external layers of the IC (LeDoux et al., 1985). The external IC region (shell region) is involved in adaptive processes that participate in the alignment of the external representation of the environment (Gutfreund & Knudsen, 2006; Knudsen & Konishi, 1978) based on its multiple sensory inputs (Jain & Shore, 2006). Strong feedback arising from such extralemniscal pathways, via the SPF to the SPON, implies that the ascending relay of auditory information routed via the SPON may be modulated in a "top-down" manner.

Rebound Spiking Enables a High Fidelity Response to Sound Rhythms in SPON Neurons

SPON activity is characteristically triggered at the cessation of contralateral sound stimulation, resulting in an offset response (see Figure 14.3A), which has been documented in vivo in all mammals studied so far (bat: Grothe et al., 1994; rabbit: Kuwada & Batra, 1999; gerbil: Behrend et al., 2002; Dehmel et al., 2002; rat: Kadner & Berrebi, 2008; Kulesza et al., 2003; 2007; mouse: Felix et al., 2011; 2013; Kopp-Scheinpflug et al., 2011). In addition, the SPON exhibits well-timed transient spiking at the sound onset (Figure 14.3A; Behrend et al., 2002; Dehmel et al., 2002; Felix et al., 2013, 2015; Grothe, 1994; Kulesza et al., 2003; Kuwada & Batra, 1999). This typical on-off spiking behavior is driven by, respectively, the temporally specialized octopus cells (Golding et al., 1999) and the MNTB neurons (Klug & Trussell, 2006) has been speculated to convey information about the coarse temporal sound structure. Periodicity patterns, such as abrupt changes in sound energy (Kadner & Berrebi, 2008; Kulesza et al., 2003), silent gaps in ongoing sounds (Kopp-Scheinpflug et al., 2011), or the temporal envelope of sounds (Felix et al., 2011; 2013; Grothe, 1994; Kuwada & Batra, 1999), are examples of cues that would be compatible with the response properties of the SPON. In line with the notion that the SPON is suited to faithfully transmission sound rhythms, the SPON neurons fire with high precision in synchrony with more temporally complex stimuli than tones (see Figure 14.3B). For instance, the SPON phase-locks extremely well to the envelope of sinusoidally amplitude-modulated sounds (Figure 14.3B; Behrend et al., 2002; Felix et al., 2011, 2013; Kadner & Berrebi, 2008; Kulesza et al., 2003; Kuwada & Batra, 1999), implying that the on-off-spiking (Figure 14.3A) is acting in tandem to ensure precise spiking with the upstroke of the signal (Figure 14.3B).

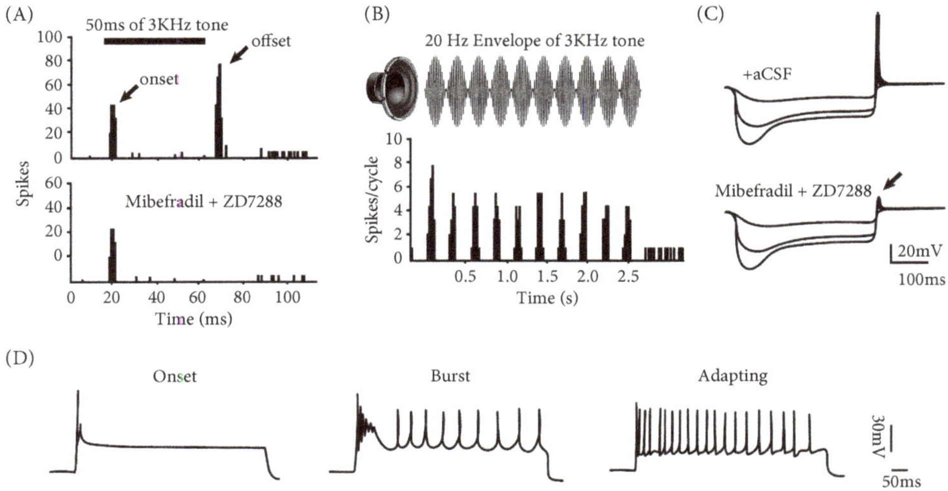

FIGURE 14.3 Electrophysiological responses of superior paraolivary nucleus (SPON) neurons. (A) The typical SPON neuron response recorded in an anesthetized animal, elicited by a pure tone at the neuron's best frequency, that is, at 3 kHz, and presented at the contralateral ear, characteristically triggers spiking at the onset and at the offset of the sound. Note that there is no spiking during the actual tone presentation since the SPON is inhibited by its medial nucleus of the trapezoid body (MNTB) input. The preceding onset response is elicited by excitation from the octopus cells. (B) Presentation of a sinusoidal amplitude modulation of the 3 kHz pure tone produces spiking activity, which phase-locks to the envelope of the modulated tone. (C) The underlying cellular mechanism for the sound-evoked offset response in the SPON neuron (A) builds upon the membrane potential rebounding to more depolarized levels at the cessation of a hyperpolarization. When the rebound depolarization reaches the spike threshold, action potentials are elicited. Rebound spiking is abolished by applying the T-type calcium channel blocker Mibefradil and the HCN-channel blocker ZD7288, verifying that these two voltage-operated cation channels act in tandem to cause the rebound depolarization. (D) Three SPON response types are found based on the firing pattern triggered by depolarizing intracellular current steps in vitro. Onset neurons typically only fire one or a few spikes, while adapting and burst neurons fire multiple spikes, the latter with an initial burst of spikelets.

Figures are adapted from Felix et al. (2011, 2013).

The SPON's spiking response is suppressed during the sound presentation (Figure 14.3A; Kulesza et al., 2003), due to the fact that the SPON is subjected to powerful glycinergic inhibition when activated by tone stimulation at the contralateral ear (Kulesza et al., 2007; Kuwabara et al., 1991). Pharmacological blockade of glycine receptors in the SPON has confirmed that the inhibitory drive from the MNTB is essential for generating the transient offset spiking response (Kulesza et al., 2007). The cellular mechanism underlying the offset response in vivo has been causally linked to rebound spiking by studying SPON neurons in vitro (Felix et al., 2011; Kopp-Scheinpflug et al., 2011). Rebound spiking occurs when the membrane potential depolarizes abruptly after hyperpolarization (Aizenman & Linden, 1999) for instance, caused by glycine receptor activation (Kopp-Scheinpflug et al., 2011). In SPON neurons, the rebound depolarization builds upon activation of two voltage-dependent currents: the non-selective cation h-current (Ih) and the low voltage-activated calcium current of T-type (see Figure 14.3D; Felix et al., 2011; Kopp-Scheinpflug et al., 2011). The Ih is partially activated at the resting membrane potential, but activates fully at more negative voltages with a $V_{1/2}$ around −90 mV in SPON (Felix et al., 2011; Kopp-Scheinpflug et al., 2011). The depolarizing effect of the Ih on the membrane potential is manifested as a "voltage-sag" when a hyperpolarizing current is injected into the neurons (see Figure 14.3C; Felix et al., 2011; Kopp-Scheinpflug et al., 2011), as previously demonstrated in auditory brainstem neurons (Koch & Grothe, 2003; Nagtegaal & Borst, 2010; Sun & Wu, 2008; Tan et al., 2007). The non-inactivating property of the Ih (Robinson & Siegelbaum, 2003) rapidly depolarizes the neuron upon release from hyperpolarization, which can exceed action potential threshold, leading to a Na^+-spike (Figure 14.3D; Felix et al., 2011; Kopp-Scheinpflug et al., 2011). This rebound spiking mechanism depends on both the duration and strength of the preceding hyperpolarization (inhibition) in SPON neurons (Felix et al., 2011; Kopp-Scheinpflug et al., 2011). Inhibition-driven hyperpolarization in the SPON neuron is enhanced by an extraordinarily low (~ −100 mV) chloride reversal potential (Kopp-Scheinpflug et al., 2011; Löhrke et al., 2005). Another mechanism that enables the rebound depolarization to reach spike threshold is the T-type calcium current (Figure 14.3C; Felix et al., 2011; Kopp-Scheinpflug et al., 2011). Due to its activation properties (Pérez-Reyes, 2003), the T-type calcium current operates in a limited voltage range and depends on intermittent hyperpolarizations for its deinactivation (McCormick & Huguenard, 1992). Periodic influx of calcium through T-type channels may underlie network-related theta oscillations (Dickson et al., 2000; Fisahn et al., 2002; Pape & McCormick, 1989; Strohmann et al., 1994) or rhythmic pacemaker activity (Park et al., 2010; Steriade et al., 1993) in neurons. A subclass of SPON neurons located in its dorsolateral quadrant show complex rebound spiking driven by T-type currents (Felix et al., 2011, 2013; Kopp-Scheinpflug et al., 2011; Leijon et al., 2016). SPON neurons responding in vitro with single versus complex spiking at the rebound are likely to relate to the offset-response types: *offset transient* and *offset-chopper*, documented in vivo (Kulesza et al., 2003). The functional significance of a calcium-dependent, robust, but temporally less defined offset spiking response in a subset of SPON neurons remains to be explored. Importantly, rebound spiking has been unequivocally linked to SPON's physiological response to sounds in living animals. Blocking the Ih and the T- type calcium current with specific antagonists ZD7288 and Mibefradil, while simultaneously presenting a tone at the contra-ear, invariably abolishes offset spiking in SPON in a reversible manner (Figure 14.3A, C; Felix et al., 2011).

The SPON Develops Properties Compatible with Precise Spiking

The developmental plasticity of SOC neurons and their inputs are well investigated (reviewed elsewhere: e.g., Hoffpauir et al., 2009; Kandler et al., 2009). Although earlier studies have demonstrated that SPON neurons are subjected to early postnatal developmental plasticity (Caicedo et al., 1998; Friauf, 2000; Friauf et al., 1999; Kandler & Friauf, 1995; Löhrke et al., 2005), it is only recently that we have begun to understand the development of the SPON's cellular properties, mostly as a result of intracellular patch-clamp recordings in acute brain slices in mice. The period of hearing onset, which occurs at P10–P12 in mice (Mikaelian & Ruben 1965), is commonly used to demark the period around which developmental plasticity occurs in the SPON (Felix et al., 2011; Felix & Magnusson, 2016; Leijon et al., 2016). The most important finding is that the membrane time constant of SPON neurons decreases to a value of around ~3ms during the weeks surrounding hearing onset (Felix et al., 2013). This intrinsic membrane property is related to a strong up-regulation of the Ih in SPON neurons (Leijon et al., 2016). Since the Ih is constitutively active in SPON neurons at the resting membrane potential, it lowers the membrane time constant which supports fast processing of the synaptic inputs (Felix & Magnusson, 2016). SPON neurons share the fast integrative property with other SOC neurons (Chirila et al., 2007; Hassfurth et al., 2009; Kandler & Friauf 1995; Magnusson et al., 2005; Sanes 1993; Scott et al., 2005, thus emphasizing the importance of the SOC for preserving temporal information. A fast membrane time constant also promotes brief action potentials (~1ms) in the SPON (Felix et al., 2013), providing further support for the idea that the SPON is specialized for extracting and relaying information about transient events by integrating synaptic input from temporally specialized pathways, that is, the octopus cell (Felix et al., 2017) and the MNTB pathway (Kuwabara et al., 1991).

The developmental aspects of the excitatory input to SPON were recently explored by stimulating the fibers of the intermediate acoustic stria around hearing onset in brainstem slices from mice (Felix & Magnusson, 2016). By comparing the ratio of minimal and maximal stimulation of the input fibers, it was shown that the SPON receives few excitatory input fibers, albeit with high release probability, throughout the postnatal maturation of the auditory brainstem (Felix & Magnusson, 2016). A strong, all-or-nothing excitation in SPON neurons is consistent with one type of excitatory input (Felix & Magnusson, 2016), giving rise to a well-defined onset response to sounds in vivo (Behrend et al., 2002; Dehmel et al., 2002; Felix et al., 2013; Grothe, 1994; Kulesza et al., 2003; Kuwada & Batra, 1999). It is worth mentioning here that when the SPON is subjected to depolarizing steps, equivalent to strong supra-threshold excitation, the corresponding firing pattern clearly reveals three response groups: *onset* spiking neurons that respond with a single spike, *burst* spiking neurons, and *adapting* neurons responding with sustained spiking that is adaptive (see Figure 14.3D; Felix et al., 2013). Since the ratio between response groups does not change with auditory development (Felix et al., 2013), this subunit classification probably reflects the postsynaptic properties of the SPON neurons (Felix et al., 2011, 2013) rather than differential connectivity (Felix et al., 2017). In line with this notion, the dendritic morphology (Ollo & Schwartz, 1979) correlates with the response groups in the SPON neurons independently of their developmental stage (Felix et al., 2013).

The SPON Is Resilient to Sensory Deprivation

Despite a consensus regarding the importance of preserving rhythmical sound information for an optimal outcome of auditory prostheses in the deaf condition (Rauschecker & Shannon, 2002; Wilson et al., 1991), the SPON has not been investigated thoroughly in the deaf or sensory deprived condition. Recently, the influence of congenital deafness on the postnatal development of SPON was investigated (Leijon et al., 2016) in mice lacking activity in the auditory nerve due to genetic deletion of the voltage-gated L-type Ca^{2+} channel isoform (Platzer et al., 2000). A sequence of cellular plasticity compensated for the sensory deprivation and rescued the rebound spiking in the deaf SPON. At an early postnatal age, corresponding to pre-hearing onset in the sensory activity-deprived SPON neurons, calcium currents compensate for low Ih levels and rescue the rebound depolarization. Later, at an equivalent post-hearing onset age, hyperpolarization-activated cyclic nucleotide-gated ion (HCN)2-channels are more strongly expressed than HCN1-channels, which upregulate the Ih to normal levels comparable to the hearing SPON (Leijon et al., 2016). Presumably, the HCN2 channel subtype, being less voltage sensitive, makes the SPON neurons more excitable (Kopp-Scheinpflug et al., 2015). The stereotyped timeline of compensatory mechanisms allowing for near normal development of rebound spiking even in absence of sensory inputs to SPON implies that the final set point of excitability may be under genetic control in these neurons. The robustness of the SPON circuitry to sensory perturbation is further illustrated by genetic ablation of its main inhibitory input from the MNTB, which surprisingly results in still normal inhibitory responses in the SPON (Altieri et al., 2014; Jalabi et al., 2013). The inhibitory input from the ipsilateral LNTB (Felix et al., 2017; Viñuela et al., 2011), could possibly be a vestigial pathway, which can serve as a replacement for inhibition in such conditions. The fact that the pathways and cellular mechanisms underlying the processing of the coarse temporal sound cues are preserved in the sensory deprived SPON could be a key aspect in the success of cochlear implants. These devices, which provide means of hearing to deaf individuals by conveying temporal envelope cues (Bacon & Viemeister, 1985) directly to the brain by electrical train stimulation of the auditory nerve—that is, providing speech rhythm cues (Rauschecker & Shannon, 2002; Wilson et al., 1991) —could hypothetically be dependent on an intact SPON circuitry.

The SPON: Early-Level Processing of Prosodic Information?

The serial nature of communicating sounds demands that the auditory system can perceive the vocalizations as single elements, preserve their temporal sequence, and simultaneously segregate them from other sounds, that is, sustained background noise (Shamma & Micheyl, 2010). Accordingly, detection of intervals in between the communicative sound elements or steep amplitude fluctuations is crucial for speech perception (Bertoncini et al., 2009; Drullman et al., 1994; Shannon et al., 1995; Smith et al., 2002). The frequency analysis performed by the cochlea is an important tool for analyzing complex sounds (Bidelman & Bhagat, 2017; Licklider, 1951), but how temporal patterns carried by the voice are singled out and preserved by neural activity in the brain is less well understood.

Mouse vocalizations are characterized by a rich repertoire of social calls (Arriaga et al., 2012; Ehret & Bernecker, 1986; Gaub & Ehret, 2005; Grimsley et al., 2011, 2016; Liu et al., 2006, Portfors, 2007), including mouse courtship song (Holy & Guo, 2005; reviewed by Egnor & Seagraves, 2016). There are theories that the perception of communication sounds specifically builds on the mammalian auditory system's inherent sensitivities to detect small differences or discontinuities in sound, giving rise to auditory contrasts (Kuhl, 1986). Indeed, the sensitivity to auditory contrasts in harmonically structured vocalizations coincides in humans and mice (Ehret, 2005; Ehret & Riecke, 2002; Geissler & Ehret, 2002). If such common basic-biological rules exist for the auditory processing of temporal and tonal information embedded in vocalizations, it establishes an important evolutionary connection between animal communication and human speech and language perception (Kuhl, 1986). Given that the production of innate vocalizations, such as laughter, are conserved on a midbrain level in both rats and humans (Holstege & Subramanian, 2016; Panksepp, 2007; Panksepp & Burgdorf, 2003), it is tempting to suggest that the neural substrate for auditory processing of non-syntactic communication cues, such as voice prosody recognized and used by infants to communicate with a parent (Gervain & Werker, 2013; Mampe et al., 2009; Sambeth et al., 2008), critically builds on subcortical processes that extract the sound envelope rhythm. We hypothesize that rhythmic voice modulations, a capacity rooted in the concept of proto-musicality (Bannan, 2012; Bryant, 2013; Falk, 2004; Fitch, 2006; Panksepp & Trevarthen, 2009), is at least partially extracted in the evolutionarily hardwired SPON circuitry (Jalabi et al., 2013; Leijon et al., 2016; Löhrke et al., 2005). We further suggested that such tonal patterns extracted on a brainstem level (Musacchia et al., 2007) may be of importance for driving the development of language and other social communication skills in a bottom-up brain-mind maturation process (Aitken & Trevarthen, 1997; Panksepp, 2015; Panksepp & Trevarthen, 2009). Interestingly, the SPON is malformed in autistic subjects (Kulesza & Mangunay, 2008), as well as in animal models of autism (Lukose et al., 2011). Studying the SPON in autistic animal models may help us to better understand human conditions that are related to difficulties in processing rhythmic information in socially-relevant communication sounds, including centrally rooted auditory processing disorders (Bamiou et al., 2001), developmental dyslexia (Goswami, 2015) and autistic spectrum disorders (Trevarthen & Delafield-Butt, 2013).

Summary

This chapter highlights the current concepts regarding the SPON from phylogenetic, developmental, mechanistic, and functional points of view. It is speculated that the SPON, being a highly conserved nucleus across mammals, plays a role in processing vocalizations and other natural sounds by decoding sound rhythms and other temporal patterns. To better understand the hierarchically structured abilities to use sound rhythms for interspecies communication, including human speech, it is important to reveal the basic biological processes in animal models, which reduce the level of communicative complexity. Knowledge gained from studying how the brain analyzes the acoustic aspects of voiced communication in animal models will eventually help us to understand various human communication disorders that are rooted in temporal processing deficits or affective-emotional communicative dysfunctions, such as autism. The genetic basis underlying variations in sensory processing is only in its infancy. More nuanced animal models of communication disorders, for instance, taking into account the level of speaking fluency, or mice with communication learning disabilities, applied together with behavioral perception tasks, provide a tantalizing prospect of shedding light on the biology of spoken language in all its forms.

Dedicated to the late Jaak Panksepp—a great scholar and friend

Acknowledgments

This chapter was written during a scholarship from The Consejo Nacional de Ciencia y Tecnología—CONACYT (M. Gómez-Álvarez; grant 665699).

References

Adam, T. J., Schwartz, D. W., & Finlayson, P. G. (1999). Firing properties of chopper and delay neurons in the lateral superior olive of the rat. *Experimental Brain Research 124*(4), 489–502.

Adams, J. C. (1983). Cytology of periolivary cells and the organization of their projections in the cat. *Journal of Comparative Neurology 215*(3), 275–289.

Adams, J. C., & Warr, W. B. (1976). Origins of axons in the cat's acoustic striae determined by injection of horseradish peroxidase into severed tracts. *Journal of Comparative Neurology 170*(1), 107–121.

Aitken, K. J., & Trevarthen, C. (1997). Self/other organization in human psychological development. *Development and Psychopathology 9*(4), 653–677.

Aizenman, C. D., & Linden, D. J. (1999). Regulation of the rebound depolarization and spontaneous firing patterns of deep nuclear neurons in slices of rat cerebellum. *Journal of Neurophysiology 82*(4), 1697–1709.

Altieri, S. C., Zhao, T., Jalabi, W., & Maricich, S. M. (2014). Development of glycinergic innervation to the murine LSO and SPN in the presence and absence of the MNTB. *Frontiers in Neural Circuits 8*, 109.

Aparicio, M. A., & Saldaña, E. (2014). The dorsal tectal longitudinal column (TLCd): A second longitudinal column in the paramedian region of the midbrain tectum. *Brain Structure and Function 219*(2), 607–630.

Aparicio, M. A., Viñuela, A., & Saldaña, E. (2010). Projections from the inferior colliculus to the tectal longitudinal column in the rat. *Neuroscience 166*(2), 653–664.

Arriaga, G., Zhou, E. P., & Jarvis, E. D. (2012). Of mice, birds, and men: The mouse ultrasonic song system has some features similar to humans and song-learning birds. *PloS One 264*(1), 56–72.

Aschoff, A., & Ostwald, J. (1987). Different origins of cochlear efferents in some bat species, rats, and guinea pigs. *Journal of Comparative Neurology 264*(1), 56–72.

Azeredo, W. J., Kliment, M. L., Morley, B. J., Relkinn, E., Slepecky, N. B., Sterns, A., . . . Woods, C. I. (1999). Olivocochlear neurons in the chinchilla: A retrograde fluorescent labelling study. *Hearing Research 134*(1–2), 57–70

Bacon, S. P., & Viemeister, N. F. (1985). Temporal modulation transfer functions in normal-hearing and hearing-impaired listeners. *Audiology: Official Organ of the International Society of Audiology 24*(2), 117–134.

Bamiou, D. E., Musiek, F. E., & Luxon, L. M. (2001). Aetiology and clinical presentations of auditory processing disorders—a review. *Archives of Disease in Childhood 85*(5), 361–365.

Banks, M. I., & Smith, P. H. (1992). Intracellular recordings from neurobiotin-labeled cells in brain slices of the rat medial nucleus of the trapezoid body. *Journal of Neuroscience 12*(7), 2819–2837.

Bannan, N. (2012). Harmony and its role in human evolution. In N. Bannan (Ed.), *Music, Language, and Human Evolution* (pp. 288–339). Oxford, England: Oxford University Press.

Barsz, K., Benson, P. K., & Walton, J. P. (1998). Gap encoding by inferior collicular neurons is altered by minimal changes in signal envelope. *Hearing Research 115*(1–2), 13–26.

Baumann, S., Griffiths, T. D., Sun, L., Petkov, C. I., Thiele, A., & Rees, A. (2011). Orthogonal representation of sound dimensions in the primate midbrain. *Nature Neuroscience 14*(4), 423–425.

Bazwinsky, I., Bidmon, H. J., Zilles, K., & Hilbig, H. (2005). Characterization of the rhesus monkey superior olivary complex by calcium binding proteins and synaptophysin. *Journal of Anatomy 207*(6), 745–761.

Bazwinsky, I., Hilbig, H., Bidmon, H. J., & Rübsamen, R. (2003). Characterization of the human superior olivary complex by calcium binding proteins and neurofilament H (SMI-32). *Journal of Comparative Neurology 456*(3), 292–303.

Behrend, O., Brand, A., Kapfer, C., & Grothe, B. (2002). Auditory response properties in the superior paraolivary nucleus of the gerbil. *Journal of Neurophysiology 87*(6), 2915–2928.

Bertoncini, J., Serniclaes, W., & Lorenzi, C. (2009). Discrimination of speech sounds based upon temporal envelope versus fine structure cues in 5- to 7-year-old children. *Journal of Speech, Language, and Hearing Research* 52(3), 682–695.

Bidelman, G. M., & Bhagat, S. P. (2017). Cochlear, brainstem, and psychophysical responses show spectrotemporal tradeoff in human auditory processing. *Neuroreport* 28(1), 17–22.

Bledsoe, S. C., Snead, C. R., Helfert, R. H., Prasad, V., Wenthold, R. J., & Altschuler, R. A. (1990). Immunocytochemical and lesion studies support the hypothesis that the projection from the medial nucleus of the trapezoid body to the lateral superior olive is glycinergic. *Brain Research* 517(1–2), 189–194.

Brown, M. C., & Levine, J. L. (2008). Dendrites of medial olivocochlear neurons in mouse. *Neuroscience* 154(1), 147–159.

Bryant, G.A. (2013). Animal signals and emotion in music: Coordinating affect across groups. *Frontiers in Psychology* 4, 990.

Budinger, E., Brosch, M., Scheich, H., & Mylius, J. (2013). The subcortical auditory structures in the Mongolian gerbil: II. Frequency-related topography of the connections with cortical field AI. *Journal of Comparative Neurology* 521(12), 2772–2797.

Budinger, E., Heil, P., & Scheich, H. (2000). Functional organization of auditory cortex in the Mongolian gerbil (Meriones unguiculatus). IV. Connections with anatomically characterized subcortical structures. *European Journal of Neuroscience* 12(7), 2452–2474.

Caicedo, A., & Herbert, H. (1993). Topography of descending projections from the inferior colliculus to auditory brainstem nuclei in the rat. *Journal of Comparative Neurology* 328(3), 377–392.

Caicedo, A., Kungel, M., Pujol, R., & Friauf, E. (1998). Glutamate-induced Co^{2+} uptake in rat auditory brainstem neurons reveals developmental changes in Ca^{2+} permeability of glutamate receptors. *European Journal of Neuroscience* 10(3), 941–954.

Caminos, E., García-Pino, E., Martínez-Galán, J. R., & Juiz, J. M. (2007). The potassium channel KCNQ5/Kv7.5 is localized in synaptic endings of auditory brainstem nuclei of the rat. *The Journal of Comparative Neurology* 505(4), 363–378.

Chirila, F. V., Rowland, K. C., Thompson, J. M., & Spirou, G. A. (2007). Development of gerbil medial superior olive: Integration of temporally delayed excitation and inhibition at physiological temperature. *Journal of Physiology* 584(Pt 1), 167–190.

Coomes, D. L., & Schofield, B. R. (2004). Projections from the auditory cortex to the superior olivary complex in guinea pigs. *European Journal of Neuroscience* 19(8), 2188–2200.

Coomes Peterson, D., & Schofield, B. R. (2007). Projections from auditory cortex contact ascending pathways that originate in the superior olive and inferior colliculus. *Hearing Research* 232(1–2), 67–77.

de Cheveigné, A. (1998). Cancellation model of pitch perception. *Journal of the Acoustical Society of America* 103(3), 1261–1271.

Dehmel, S., Kopp-Scheinpflug, C., Dörrscheidt, G. J., & Rübsamen, R. (2002). Electrophysiological characterization of the superior paraolivary nucleus in the Mongolian gerbil. *Hearing Research* 172(1–2), 18–36.

Dickson, C. T., Magistretti, J., Shalinsky, M. H., Fransén, E., Hasselmo, M. E., & Alonso, A. (2000). Properties and role of I(h) in the pacing of subthreshold oscillations in entorhinal cortex layer II neurons. *Journal of Neurophysiology* 83(5), 2562–2579.

Drullman, R., Festen, J. M., & Plomp, R. (1994). Effect of temporal envelope smearing on speech reception. *Journal of the Acoustical Society of America* 95(2), 1053–1064.

Egnor, S. R., & Seagraves, K. M. (2016). The contribution of ultrasonic vocalizations to mouse courtship. *Current Opinion in Neurobiology 38*, 1–5.

Ehret, G. (2005). Infant rodent ultrasounds—a gate to the understanding of sound communication. *Behavior Genetics 35*(1), 19–29.

Ehret, G., & Bernecker, C. (1986). Low-frequency sound communication by mouse pups (Mus musculus): Wriggling calls release maternal behaviour. *Animal Behaviour 34*(3), 821–830.

Ehret, G., & Riecke, S. (2002). Mice and humans perceive multiharmonic communication sounds in the same way. *Proceedings of the National Academy of Sciences of the United States of America 99*(1), 479–482.

Falk, D. (2004). Prelinguistic evolution in early hominins: Whence motherese? *The Behavioral and Brain Sciences 27*(4), 491–503.

Feliciano, M., Saldaña, E., & Mugnaini, E. (1995). Direct projection from the rat primary auditory neocortex to the nucleus sagulum, paralemniscal regions, superior olivary complex and cochlear nuclei. *Auditory Neuroscience 1*(1), 287–308.

Felix, R. A., Fridberger, A., Leijon, S., Berrebi, A. S., & Magnusson, A. K. (2011). Sound rhythms are encoded by postinhibitory rebound spiking in the superior paraolivary nucleus. *Journal of Neuroscience 31*(35), 12566–12578.

Felix, R. A., Gourévitch, B., Gómez-Álvarez, M., Leijon, S. C. M., Saldaña, E., & Magnusson, A. K. (2017). Octopus cells in the posteroventral cochlear nucleus provide the main excitatory input to the superior paraolivary nucleus. *Frontiers in Neural Circuits 11*, 37.

Felix, R. A., & Magnusson, A. K. (2016). Development of excitatory synaptic transmission to the superior paraolivary and lateral superior olivary nuclei optimizes differential decoding strategies. *Neuroscience 334*(1), 1–12.

Felix, R. A., Magnusson, A. K., & Berrebi, A. S. (2015). The superior paraolivary nucleus shapes temporal response properties of neurons in the inferior colliculus. *Brain Structure & Function 220*(5), 2639–2652.

Felix, R. A., Vonderschen, K., Berrebi, A. S., & Magnusson, A. K. (2013). Development of on-off spiking in superior paraolivary nucleus neurons of the mouse. *Journal of Neurophysiology 109*(11), 2691–2704.

Fisahn, A., Yamada, M., Duttaroy, A., Gan, J.-W., Deng, C.-X., McBain, C. J., & Wess, J. (2002). Muscarinic induction of hippocampal gamma oscillations requires coupling of the M1 receptor to two mixed cation currents. *Neuron 33*(4), 615–624.

Fitch, T. W. (2006). The biology and evolution of music: A comparative perspective. *Cognition 100*(1), 173–215.

Ford, M. C., Grothe, B., & Klug, A. (2009). Fenestration of the calyx of Held occurs sequentially along the tonotopic axis, is influenced by afferent activity, and facilitates glutamate clearance. *Journal of Comparative Neurology 514*(1), 92–106.

Friauf, E. (2000). Development of chondroitin sulfate proteoglycans in the central auditory system of rats correlates with acquisition of mature properties. *Audiology & Neuro-Otology 5*(5) 251–262.

Friauf, E., Aragón, C., Löhrke, S., Westenfelder, B., & Zafra, F. (1999). Developmental expression of the glycine transporter GLYT2 in the auditory system of rats suggests involvement in synapse maturation. *The Journal of Comparative Neurology 412*(1), 17–37.

Friauf, E., & Ostwald, J. (1988). Divergent projections of physiologically characterized rat ventral cochlear nucleus neurons as shown by intra-axonal injection of horseradish peroxidase. *Experimental Brain Research 73*(2), 263–284.

Frisina, R. D. (2001). Subcortical neural coding mechanisms for auditory temporal processing. *Hearing Research 158*(1–2), 1–27.

Fujino, K., Koyano, K., & Ohmori, H. (1997). Lateral and medial olivocochlear neurons have distinct electrophysiological properties in the rat brain slice. *Journal of Neurophysiology 77*(5), 2788–2804.

Gaub, S., & Ehret, G. (2005). Grouping in auditory temporal perception and vocal production is mutually adapted: The case of wriggling calls of mice. *Journal of Comparative Physiology A: Neuroethology, Sensory, Neural, and Behavioral Physiology 191*(12), 1131–1135.

Geissler, D. B., & Ehret, G. (2002). Time-critical integration of formants for perception of communication calls in mice. *Proceedings of the National Academy of Sciences of the United States of America 99*(13), 9021–9025.

Gervain, J., & Werker, J. F. (2013). Prosody cues word order in 7-month-old bilingual infants. *Nature Communications 4*, 1490.

Golding, N. L., Ferragamo, M. J., & Oertel, D. (1999). Role of intrinsic conductances underlying responses to transients in octopus cells of the cochlear nucleus. The Journal of Neuroscience *19*(8), 2897–2905.

Gómez-Álvarez, M., & Saldaña, E. (2016). Different tonotopic regions of the lateral superior olive receive a similar combination of afferent inputs. *Journal of Comparative Neurology 524*(11), 2230–2250.

Gómez-Álvarez, M., Gourévitch, B., Felix, R. A., Nyberg, T., Hernández-Montiel, H. L., & Magnusson, A. K. (2018). Temporal information in tones, broadband noise and natural vocalizations is conveyed by differential spiking responses in the superior paraolivary nucleus. *European Journal of Neuroscience 8*(4), 2030–2049

González-Hernández, T., Mantolán-Sarmiento, B., González-González, B., & Pérez-González, H. (1996). Sources of GABAergic input to the inferior colliculus of the rat. *Journal of Comparative Neurology 372*(2), 309–326.

Goswami, U. (2015). Sensory theories of developmental dyslexia: three challenges for research. *Nature Reviews: Neuroscience 16*(1), 43–54.

Grimsley, J. M. S., Monaghan, J. J. M., & Wenstrup, J. J. (2011). Development of social vocalizations in mice. *PloS One 6*(3), e17460.

Grimsley, J. M. S., Sheth, S., Vallabh, N., Grimsley, C. A., Bhattal, J., Latsko, M., & Wenstrup, J. J. (2016). Contextual modulation of vocal behavior in mouse: Newly identified 12 khz “mid-frequency” vocalization emitted during restraint. *Frontiers in Behavioral Neuroscience 10*, 38.

Grothe, B. (1994). Interaction of excitation and inhibition in processing of pure tone and amplitude-modulated stimuli in the medial superior olive of the mustached bat. *Journal of Neurophysiology 71*(2), 706–721.

Grothe, B. (2000). The evolution of temporal processing in the medial superior olive, an auditory brainstem structure. *Progress in Neurobiology 61*(6), 581–610.

Gutfreund, Y., & Knudsen, E. I. (2006). Adaptation in the auditory space map of the barn owl. *Journal of Neurophysiology 96*(2), 813–825.

Hassfurth, B., Magnusson, A. K., Grothe, B., & Koch, U. (2009). Sensory deprivation regulates the development of the hyperpolarization-activated current in auditory brainstem neurons. *European Journal of Neuroscience 30*(7), 1227–1238.

Heffner, R.S. (2004). Primate hearing from a mammalian perspective. Anatomical Record. *Part A, Discoveries in Molecular, Cellular, and Evolutionary Biology 281*(1), 1111–1122.

Hoffpauir, B. K., Marrs, G. S., Mathers, P. H., & Spirou, G. A. (2009). Does the brain connect before the periphery can direct? A comparison of three sensory systems in mice. *Brain Research 1277*, 115–129.

Holstege, G. (1998). The emotional motor system in relation to the supraspinal control of micturition and mating behavior. *Behavioural Brain Research 92*(2), 103–109.

Holstege, G., & Subramanian, H. H. (2016). Two different motor systems are needed to generate human speech. *The Journal of Comparative Neurology 524*(8), 1558–1577.

Holy, T. E., & Guo, Z. (2005). Ultrasonic songs of male mice. *PloS Biology 3*(12), e386.

Jain, R., & Shore, S. (2006). External inferior colliculus integrates trigeminal and acoustic information: Unit responses to trigeminal nucleus and acoustic stimulation in the guinea pig. *Neuroscience Letters 395*(1), 71–75

Jalabi, W., Kopp-Scheinpflug, C., Allen, P. D., Schiavon, E., DiGiacomo, R. R., Forsythe, I. D., & Maricich, S. M. (2013). Sound localization ability and glycinergic innervation of the superior olivary complex persist after genetic deletion of the medial nucleus of the trapezoid body. *Journal of Neuroscience 33*(38), 15044–15049.

Joris, P. X., Schreiner, C. E., & Rees, A. (2004). Neural processing of amplitude-modulated sounds. *Physiological Reviews 84*(2), 541–577.

Kadner, A., & Berrebi, A.S. (2008). Encoding of temporal features of auditory stimuli in the medial nucleus of the trapezoid body and superior paraolivary nucleus of the rat. *Neuroscience, 151*(3) 868–887

Kadner, A., Kulesza, R. J., & Berrebi, A. S. (2006). Neurons in the medial nucleus of the trapezoid body and superior paraolivary nucleus of the rat may play a role in sound duration coding. *Journal of Neurophysiology 95*(3), 1499–1508.

Kaiser, A., Alexandrova, O., & Grothe, B. (2011). Urocortin-expressing olivocochlear neurons exhibit tonotopic and developmental changes in the auditory brainstem and in the innervation of the cochlea. *The Journal of Comparative Neurology 519*(14), 2758–2778.

Kandler, K., Clause, A., & Noh, J. (2009). Tonotopic reorganization of developing auditory brainstem circuits. *Nature Neuroscience 12*(6), 711–717.

Kandler, K., & Friauf, E. (1995). Development of electrical membrane properties and discharge characteristics of superior olivary complex neurons in fetal and postnatal rats. *European Journal of Neuroscience 7*(8), 1773–1790.

Kelley, P. E., Frisina, R. D., Zettel, M. L., & Walton, J. P. (1992). Differential calbindin-like immunoreactivity in the brain stem auditory system of the chinchilla. *Journal of Comparative Neurology 320*(2), 196–212.

Klug, A., & Trussell, L. O. (2006). Activation and deactivation of voltage-dependent K^+ channels during synaptically driven action potentials in the MNTB. *Journal of Neurophysiology 96*(3), 1547–1555.

Knudsen, E. I., & Konishi, M. (1978). A neural map of auditory space in the owl. *Science 200*(4343), 795–797.

Koch, U., & Grothe, B. (2003). Hyperpolarization-activated current (Ih) in the inferior colliculus: Distribution and contribution to temporal processing. *Journal of Neurophysiology 90*(6), 3679–3687.

Kopp-Scheinpflug, C., Pigott, B. M., & Forsythe, I. D. (2015). Nitric oxide selectively suppresses IH currents mediated by HCN1-containing channels. *Journal of Physiology 593*(7), 1685–1700.

Kopp-Scheinpflug, C., Tozer, A. J. B., Robinson, S. W., Tempel, B. L., Hennig, M. H., & Forsythe, I. D. (2011). The sound of silence: Ionic mechanisms encoding sound termination. *Neuron 71*(5), 911–925.

Krishna, B. S., & Semple, M. N. (2000). Auditory temporal processing: responses to sinusoidally amplitude-modulated tones in the inferior colliculus. *Journal of Neurophysiology 84*(1), 255–273.

Kuhl, P. K. (1986). Theoretical contributions of tests on animals to the special-mechanisms debate in speech. *Experimental Biology 45*(3), 233–265.

Kulesza, R. J. (2008). Cytoarchitecture of the human superior olivary complex: Nuclei of the trapezoid body and posterior tier. *Hearing Research 241*(1–2), 52–63.

Kulesza, R. J. (2014). Characterization of human auditory brainstem circuits by calcium-binding protein immunohistochemistry. *Neuroscience 258*, 318–331.

Kulesza, R. J., & Berrebi, A. S. (2000). Superior paraolivary nucleus of the rat is a GABAergic nucleus. *Journal of the Association for Research in Otolaryngology 1*(4), 255–269.

Kulesza, R. J., & Grothe, B. (2015). Yes, there is a medial nucleus of the trapezoid body in humans. *Frontiers in Neuroanatomy 9*, 35.

Kulesza, R. J., Kadner, A., & Berrebi, A. S. (2007). Distinct roles for glycine and GABA in shaping the response properties of neurons in the superior paraolivary nucleus of the rat. *Journal of Neurophysiology 97*(2), 1610–1620.

Kulesza, R. J., & Mangunay, K. (2008). Morphological features of the medial superior olive in autism. *Brain Research 1200*, 132–137.

Kulesza, R. J., Spirou, G. A., & Berrebi, A. S. (2003). Physiological response properties of neurons in the superior paraolivary nucleus of the rat. *Journal of Neurophysiology 89*(4), 2299–2312.

Kulesza, R. J., Viñuela, A., Saldaña, E., & Berrebi, A. S. (2002). Unbiased stereological estimates of neuron number in subcortical auditory nuclei of the rat. *Hearing Research 168*(1–2), 12–24.

Kuwabara, N., DiCaprio, R. A., & Zook, J. M. (1991). Afferents to the medial nucleus of the trapezoid body and their collateral projections. *The Journal of Comparative Neurology 314*(4), 684–706.

Kuwabara, N., & Zook, J. M. (1991). Classification of the principal cells of the medial nucleus of the trapezoid body. *Journal of Comparative Neurology 314*(4), 707–720.

Kuwabara, N., & Zook, J. M. (1992). Projections to the medial superior olive from the medial and lateral nuclei of the trapezoid body in rodents and bats. *Journal of Comparative Neurology 324*(4), 522–538.

Kuwada, S., & Batra, R. (1999). Coding of sound envelopes by inhibitory rebound in neurons of the superior olivary complex in the unanesthetized rabbit. *Journal of Neuroscience 19*(6), 2273–2287.

Lange, S., Burda, H., Wegner, R. E., Dammann, P., Begall, S., & Kawalika, M. (2007). Living in a "stethoscope": Burrow-acoustics promote auditory specializations in subterranean rodents. *Die Naturwissenschafte 94*(2), 134–138.

Langner, G. (1992). Periodicity coding in the auditory system. *Hearing Research 60*(2), 115–142.

LeDoux, J. E., Ruggiero, D. A., & Reis, D. J. (1985). Projections to the subcortical forebrain from anatomically defined regions of the medial geniculate body in the rat. *Journal of Comparative Neurology 242*(2), 182–213.

Leijon, S., & Magnusson, A. K. (2014). Physiological characterization of vestibular efferent brainstem neurons using a transgenic mouse model. *PloS One 9*(5), e98277.

Leijon, S. C. M., Peyda, S., & Magnusson, A. K. (2016). Temporal processing capacity in auditory-deprived superior paraolivary neurons is rescued by sequential plasticity during early development. *Neuroscience 337*, 315–330.

Licklider, J. C. R. (1951). A duplex theory of pitch perception. *Experientia 7*(4), 128–133.

Lieberman, P. (2002). On the nature and evolution of the neural bases of human language. *American Journal of Physical Anthropology 35*, 36–62.

Liu, R. C., Linden, J. F., & Schreiner, C. E. (2006). Improved cortical entrainment to infant communication calls in mothers compared with virgin mice. *European Journal of Neuroscience 23*(11), 3087–3097.

Löhrke, S., Srinivasan, G., Oberhofer, M., Doncheva, E., & Friauf, E. (2005). Shift from depolarizing to hyperpolarizing glycine action occurs at different perinatal ages in superior olivary complex nuclei. *The European Journal of Neuroscience 22*(11), 2708–2722.

Lukose, R., Schmidt, E., Wolski, T. P., Murawski, N. J., & Kulesza, R. J. (2011). Malformation of the superior olivary complex in an animal model of autism. *Brain Research 1398*, 102–112.

Magnusson, A. K., Kapfer, C., Grothe, B., & Koch, U. (2005). Maturation of glycinergic inhibition in the gerbil medial superior olive after hearing onset. *Journal of Physiology 568*(Pt 2), 497–512.

Malmierca, M. S., Cristaudo, S., Pérez-González, D., & Covey, E. (2009). Stimulus-specific adaptation in the inferior colliculus of the anesthetized rat. *Journal of Neuroscience 29*(17), 5483–5493.

Mampe, B., Friederici, A. D., Christophe, A., & Wermke, K. (2009). Newborns' cry melody is shaped by their native language. *Current Biology 19*(23), 1994–1997.

Marshall, A. F., Pearson, J. M., Falk, S. E., Skaggs, J. D., Crocker, W. D., Saldaña, E., & Fitzpatrick, D. C. (2008). Auditory response properties of neurons in the tectal longitudinal column of the rat. *Hearing Research 244*(1–2), 35–44.

McAlpine, D. (2005). Creating a sense of auditory space. *Journal of Physiology 566*, 21–28.

McCormick, D. A., & Huguenard, J. R. (1992). A model of the electrophysiological properties of thalamocortical relay neurons. *Journal of Neurophysiology 566*(Pt 1), 21–28.

Mikaelian, D. & Ruben, R.J. (1965) Development of Hearing in the Normal Cba-J Mouse: Correlation of Physiological Observations with Behavioral Responses and with Cochlear Anatomy. *Acta oto-laryngologica*, *59*(2–6), 451–461.

Moore, J. K. (1987). The human auditory brain stem as a generator of auditory evoked potentials. *Hearing Research 29*(1), 33–43

Moore, J. K. (2000). Organization of the human superior olivary complex. *Microscopy Research and Technique 51*(4), 403–412.

Moore, J. K., Guan, Y. L., & Shi, S. R. (1998). MAP2 expression in developing dendrites of human brainstem auditory neurons. *Journal of Chemical Neuroanatomy 16*(1), 1–15.

Moore, J. K., & Moore, R. Y. (1971). A comparative study of the superior olivary complex in the primate brain. *Folia Primatologica: International Journal of Primatology 16*(1), 35–51.

Moore, J. K., Simmons, D. D., & Guan, Y. (1999). The human olivocochlear system: Organization and development. *Audiology & Neuro-Otology 4*(6), 311–325.

Motts, S. D., Slusarczyk, A. S., Sowick, C. S., & Schofield, B. R. (2008). Distribution of cholinergic cells in guinea pig brainstem. *Neuroscience 154*(1), 186–195.

Mulders, W.H., & Robertson, D. (2000). Evidence for direct cortical innervation of medial olivocochlear neurones in rats. *Hearing Research 144*(1–2), 65–72.

Musacchia, G., Sams, M., Skoe, E., & Kraus, N. (2007). Musicians have enhanced subcortical auditory and audiovisual processing of speech and music. *Proceedings of the National Academy of Sciences of the United States of America 104*(40), 15894–15898.

Nagtegaal, A. P., & Borst, J. G. G. (2010). *In vivo* dynamic clamp study of I(h) in the mouse inferior colliculus. *Journal of Neurophysiology 104*(2), 940–948.

Nelson, P. C., & Carney, L. H. (2004). A phenomenological model of peripheral and central neural responses to amplitude-modulated tones. *The Journal of the Acoustical Society of America 116*(4 Pt 1), 2173–2186.

Nelson, P. C., Smith, Z. M., & Young, E. D. (2009). Wide-dynamic-range forward suppression in marmoset inferior colliculus neurons is generated centrally and accounts for perceptual masking. *Journal of Neuroscience 29*(8), 2553–2562.

Oertel, D., Bal, R., Gardner, S. M., Smith, P. H., & Joris, P. X. (2000). Detection of synchrony in the activity of auditory nerve fibers by octopus cells of the mammalian cochlear nucleus. *Proceedings of the National Academy of Sciences of the United States of America 97*(22), 11773–11779.

Oliver, D. L., & Morest, D. K. (1984). The central nucleus of the inferior colliculus of the cat. *Journal of Comparative Neurology 222*, 237–264.

Ollo, C., & Schwartz, I. R. (1979). The superior olivary complex in C57BL/6 mice. *American Journal of Anatomy 155*(3), 349–373.

Panksepp, J. (2007). Neuroevolutionary sources of laughter and social joy: Modeling primal human laughter in laboratory rats. *Behavioural Brain Research 182*(2), 231–244.

Panksepp, J. (2015). Primal emotions and cultural evolution of language: Primal affects empower words. In U. M. Lüdtke (Ed.), *Emotion in Language: Theory—research—application* (pp. 27–48). Amsterdam, Netherlands: John Benjamins Publishing.

Panksepp, J., & Burgdorf, J. (2003). "Laughing" rats and the evolutionary antecedents of human joy? *Physiology and Behavior 79*(3), 533–547.

Panksepp, J., & Trevarthen, C. (2009). The neuroscience of emotion in music. In S. Malloch & C. Trevarthen (Eds.), *Communicative musicality: Exploring the basis of human companionship* (pp. 105–146). New York, NY: Oxford University Press.

Pape, H. C., & McCormick, D. A. (1989). Noradrenaline and serotonin selectively modulate thalamic burst firing by enhancing a hyperpolarization-activated cation current. *Nature 340*(6236), 715–718.

Park, Y.G., Park, H.Y., Lee, C. J., Choi, S., Jo, S., Choi, H., . . . Kim, D. (2010). Ca(V)3.1 is a tremor rhythm pacemaker in the inferior olive. *Proceedings of the National Academy of Sciences of the United States of America, 107*(23), 10731–10736.

Pérez-Reyes, E. (2003). Molecular physiology of low-voltage-activated t-type calcium channels. *Physiological Reviews 83*(1), 117–161.

Pihan, H., Tabert, M., Assuras, S., & Borod, J. (2008). Unattended emotional intonations modulate linguistic prosody processing. *Brain and Language 105*(2), 141–147.

Platzer, J., Engel, J., Schrott-Fischer, A., Stephan, K., Bova, S., Chen, H., Zheng, H, & Striessnig, J. (2000). Congenital deafness and sinoatrial node dysfunction in mice lacking class D L-type Ca^{2+} channels. *Cell 102*(1), 89–97.

Portfors, C. V. (2007). Types and functions of ultrasonic vocalizations in laboratory rats and mice. *Journal of the American Association for Laboratory Animal Science 46*(1), 28–34.

Rauschecker, J. P., & Shannon, R. V. (2002). Sending sound to the brain. *Science 295*(5557), 1025–1029.

Rees, A., & Palmer, A.R. (1989). Neuronal responses to amplitude-modulated and pure-tone stimuli in the guinea pig inferior colliculus, and their modification by broadband noise. *Journal of the Acoustical Society of America 85*(5), 1978–1994.

Rhode, W. S. (1998). Neural encoding of single-formant stimuli in the ventral cochlear nucleus of the chinchilla. *Hearing Research 117*(1–2), 39–56.

Roberts, M. T., Seeman, S. C., & Golding, N. L. (2014). The relative contributions of MNTB and LNTB neurons to inhibition in the medial superior olive assessed through single and paired recordings. *Frontiers in Neural Circuits* 8, 49.

Robinson, R. B., & Siegelbaum, S. A. (2003). Hyperpolarization-activated cation currents: From molecules to physiological function. *Annual Review of Physiology* 65, 453–480.

Rosen, S. (1992). Temporal information in speech: Acoustic, auditory and linguistic aspects. *Philosophical Transactions of the Royal Society of London. Series B, Biological Sciences*, *336*(1278) 367–373.

Saldaña, E., Aparicio, M. A., Fuentes-Santamaría, V., & Berrebi, A. S. (2009). Connections of the superior paraolivary nucleus of the rat: Projections to the inferior colliculus. *Neuroscience 163*(1), 372–387.

Saldaña, E., Viñuela, A., Marshall, A. F., Fitzpatrick, D. C., & Aparicio, M. A. (2007). The TLC: A novel auditory nucleus of the mammalian brain. *Journal of Neuroscience 27*(48), 13108–13116.

Salimi, N., Zilany, M. S. A., & Carney, L. H. (2017). Modeling responses in the superior paraolivary nucleus: Implications for forward masking in the inferior colliculus. *Journal of the Association for Research in Otolaryngology 18*(3), 441–456

Sambeth, A., Ruohio, K., Alku, P., Fellman, V., & Huotilainen, M. (2008). Sleeping newborns extract prosody from continuous speech. *Clinical Neurophysiology: Official Journal of the International Federation of Clinical Neurophysiology 119*(2), 332–341.

Sanes, D. H. (1993). The development of synaptic function and integration in the central auditory system. *Journal of Neuroscience 13*(6), 2627–2637.

Sanes, D. H., & Friauf, E. (2000). Review: Development and influence of inhibition in the lateral superior olivary nucleus. *Hearing Research 147*(1–2), 46–58.

Schmidt, E., Wolski, T. P., & Kulesza, R. J. (2010). Distribution of perineuronal nets in the human superior olivary complex. *Hearing Research 265*(1–2), 15–24.

Schofield, B. R. (1991). Superior paraolivary nucleus in the pigmented guinea pig: Separate classes of neurons project to the inferior colliculus and the cochlear nucleus. *Journal of Comparative Neurology 312*(1), 68–76.

Schofield, B. R. (1995). Projections from the cochlear nucleus to the superior paraolivary nucleus in guinea pigs. *Journal of Comparative Neurology 360*(1), 135–149.

Schofield, B. R., & Cant, N. B. (1991). Organization of the superior olivary complex in the guinea pig. I. Cytoarchitecture, cytochrome oxidase histochemistry, and dendritic morphology. *Journal of Comparative Neurology 314*(4), 645–670.

Schofield, B. R., & Cant, N. B. (1992). Organization of the superior olivary complex in the guinea pig: II. Patterns of projection from the periolivary nuclei to the inferior colliculus. *Journal of Comparative Neurology 317*(4), 438–455.

Schreiner, C. E., & Langner, G. (1988). Periodicity coding in the inferior colliculus of the cat. II. Topographical organization. *Journal of Neurophysiology 60*(6), 1823–1840.

Scott, L. L., Mathews, P. J., & Golding, N. L. (2005). Posthearing developmental refinement of temporal processing in principal neurons of the medial superior olive. *Journal of Neuroscience 25*(35), 7887–7895.

Shamma, S. A., & Micheyl, C. (2010). Behind the scenes of auditory perception. *Current Opinion in Neurobiology 20*(3), 361–366.

Shannon, R. V., Zeng, F. G., Kamath, V., Wygonski, J., & Ekelid, M. (1995). Speech recognition with primarily temporal cues. *Science 270*(5234), 303–304.

Simmons, D.D. (2002). Development of the inner ear efferent system across vertebrate species. *Journal of Neurobiology 53*(2), 228–250.

Simmons, D. D., Bertolotto, C., Typpo, K., Clay, A., & Wu, M. (1999). Differential development of cholinergic-like neurons in the superior olive: a light microscopic study. *Anatomy and Embryology 200*(6), 585–595.

Smith, P. H., Joris, P. X., Carney, L. H., & Yin, T. C. (1991). Projections of physiologically characterized globular bushy cell axons from the cochlear nucleus of the cat. *Journal of Comparative Neurology 304*(3), 387–407.

Smith, Z. M., Delgutte, B., & Oxenham, A. J. (2002). Chimaeric sounds reveal dichotomies in auditory perception. *Nature 416*(6876), 87–90.

Sommer, I., Lingenhöhl, K., & Friauf, E. (1993). Principal cells of the rat medial nucleus of the trapezoid body: an intracellular *in vivo* study of their physiology and morphology. *Experimental Brain Research 95*(2), 223–239.

Spangler, K. M., Warr, W. B., & Henkel, C. K. (1985). The projections of principal cells of the medial nucleus of the trapezoid body in the cat. *The Journal of Comparative Neurology 238*(3), 249–262.

Sparks, D. L., & Hartwich-Young, R. (1989). The deep layers of the superior colliculus. *Reviews of Oculomotor Research 3*, 213–255.

Spirou, G. A., Brownell, W. E., & Zidanic, M. (1990). Recordings from cat trapezoid body and HRP labeling of globular bushy cell axons. *Journal of Neurophysiology 63*(5), 1169–1190.

Stange, A., Myoga, M. H., Lingner, A., Ford, M. C., Alexandrova, O., Felmy, F., & Grothe, B. (2013). Adaptation in sound localization: from GABA (B) receptor-mediated synaptic modulation to perception. *Nature Neuroscience 16*(12), 1840–1847.

Sterenborg, J. C., Pilati, N., Sheridan, C. J., Uchitel, O. D., Forsythe, I. D., & Barnes-Davies, M. (2010). Lateral olivocochlear (LOC) neurons of the mouse LSO receive excitatory and inhibitory synaptic inputs with slower kinetics than LSO principal neurons. *Hearing Research 270*(1–2), 119–126.

Steriade, M., McCormick, D. A., & Sejnowski, T. J. (1993). Thalamocortical oscillations in the sleeping and aroused brain. *Science 262*(5134), 679–685.

Ströhmann, B., Schwarz, D. W., & Puil, E. (1994). Subthreshold frequency selectivity in avian auditory thalamus. *Journal of Neurophysiology 71*(4), 1361–1372.

Strominger, N. L., Nelson, L. R., & Dougherty, W. J. (1977). Second order auditory pathways in the chimpanzee. *Journal of Comparative Neurology 172*(2), 349–365.

Sun, H., & Wu, S. H. (2008). Modification of membrane excitability of neurons in the rat's dorsal cortex of the inferior colliculus by preceding hyperpolarization. *Neuroscience 154*(1), 257–272.

Tan, M. L., Theeuwes, H. P., Feenstra, L., & Borst, J. G. G. (2007). Membrane properties and firing patterns of inferior colliculus neurons: An *in vivo* patch-clamp study in rodents. *Journal of Neurophysiology 98*(1), 443–453.

Thompson, A. M., & Thompson, G. C. (1991). Posteroventral cochlear nucleus projections to olivocochlear neurons. *Journal of Comparative Neurology 303*(2), 267–285.

Thompson, G. C., & Thompson, A. M. (1986). Olivocochlear neurons in the squirrel monkey brainstem. *Journal of Comparative Neurology 254*(2), 246–258.

Tollin, D. J. (2003). The lateral superior olive: A functional role in sound source localization. *The Neuroscientist: A Review Journal Bringing Neurobiology, Neurology and Psychiatry 9*(2), 127–143.

Tóth, I. E., Boldogkoi, Z., Medveczky, I., & Palkovits, M. (1999). Lacrimal preganglionic neurons form a subdivision of the superior salivatory nucleus of rat: Transneuronal labelling by pseudorabies virus. *Journal of the Autonomic Nervous System 77*(1), 45–54.

Trevarthen, C., & Delafield-Butt, J. T. (2013). Autism as a developmental disorder in intentional movement and affective engagement. *Frontiers in Integrative Neuroscience 7*, 49.
Vetter, D. E., Saldaña, E., & Mugnaini, E. (1993). Input from the inferior colliculus to medial olivocochlear neurons in the rat: a double label study with PHA-L and cholera toxin. *Hearing Research 70*(2), 173–186.
Viñuela, A., Aparicio, M. A., Berrebi, A. S., & Saldaña, E. (2011). Connections of the Superior Paraolivary Nucleus of the Rat: II. Reciprocal Connections with the Tectal Longitudinal Column. *Frontiers in Neuroanatomy 5*, 1.
Wang, J., Zhou, R., & Gao, W. (2017). The neural pathway for lacrimal gland tear secretion in New Zealand White rabbits. *Neuroscience Letters 649*, 14–19.
Warr, W. B. (1966). Fiber degeneration following lesions in the anterior ventral cochlear nucleus of the cat. *Experimental Neurology 14*(4), 453–474.
Warr, W. B. (1975). Olivocochlear and vestibular efferent neurons of the feline brain stem: Their location, morphology and number determined by retrograde axonal transport and acetylcholinesterase histochemistry. *Journal of Comparative Neurology 161*(2), 159–181.
Warr, W. B., Beck Boche, J. E., Ye, Y., & Kim, D. O. (2002). Organization of olivocochlear neurons in the cat studied with the retrograde tracer cholera toxin-B. *Journal of the Association for Research in Otolaryngology 3*(4), 457–478.
White, J. S., & Warr, W. B. (1983). The dual origins of the olivocochlear bundle in the albino rat. *Journal of Comparative Neurology 219*(2), 203–214.
Wilson, B. S., Finley, C. C., Lawson, D. T., Wolford, R. D., Eddington, D. K., & Rabinowitz, W. M. (1991). Better speech recognition with cochlear implants. *Nature 352*(6332), 236–238.
Winter, I. M., Robertson, D., & Cole, K. S. (1989). Descending projections from auditory brainstem nuclei to the cochlea and cochlear nucleus of the guinea pig. *Journal of Comparative Neurology 280*(1), 143–157.
Yang, L. C., & Pollak, G. D. (1997). Differential response properties to amplitude modulated signals in the dorsal nucleus of the lateral lemniscus of the mustache batand the roles of GABAergic inhibition. *Journal of Neurophysiology* (1), 324–340.
Yao, W., & Godfrey, D. A. (1998). Immunohistochemical evaluation of cholinergic neurons in the rat superior olivary complex. *Microscopy Research and Technique 41*(3), 270–283.
Yassin, L., Radtke-Schuller, S., Asraf, H., Grothe, B., Hershfinkel, M., Forsythe, I. D., & Kopp-Scheinpflug, C. (2014). Nitric oxide signaling modulates synaptic inhibition in the superior paraolivary nucleus (SPN) via cGMP-dependent suppression of KCC2. *Frontiers in Neural Circuits 8*, 65.
Yasui, Y., Nakano, K., & Mizuno, N. (1992). Descending projections from the subparafascicular thalamic nucleus to the lower brain stem in the rat. *Experimental Brain Research 90*(3), 508–518.
Zheng, Y., & Escabí, M. A. (2008). Distinct roles for onset and sustained activity in the neuronal code for temporal periodicity and acoustic envelope shape. *Journal of Neuroscience 28*(52), 14230–14244.
Zook, J. M., & Casseday, J. H. (1985). Projections from the cochlear nuclei in the mustache bat, Pteronotus parnellii. *Journal of Comparative Neurology 237*(3), 307–324.

CHAPTER 15

PERINEURONAL NETS IN THE SUPERIOR OLIVARY COMPLEX

Development, Function, and Plasticity

MARKUS MORAWSKI AND MANDY SONNTAG

Abstract

This chapter addresses perineuronal nets in the superior olivary complex, a collection of nuclei in the auditory brainstem that are involved in the processing of sound source location. Perineuronal nets, a specific form of extracellular matrix, are believed to control synaptic plasticity. They surround neuronal somata and dendrites of specific types of neurons, among which are many neurons of the superior olivary complex. The chapter describes the distribution of perineuronal nets in the superior olivary complex, focusing on controversial results and discussing underlying reasons. In addition, it considers the development of perineuronal nets and highlights differences between the main components of perineuronal nets, including the proteoglycans aggrecan, brevican, and neurocan. Finally, it introduces current concepts on the function of perineuronal nets that are specifically based on experimental data collected in the superior olivary complex and point to a contribution of perineuronal nets to synaptic transmission and neuronal excitability.

Keywords: superior olivary complex, auditory brainstem, perineuronal nets, extracellular matrix, development, aggrecan, brevican, neurocan, synaptic transmission

Introduction

The central nervous system (CNS) has nowadays to be considered as a functional network of neurons, glia, and extracellular matrix (ECM) molecules. Compared to neurons and glia, the ECM has received less attention despite the fact that the ECM constitutes up to 20% of brain volume (Bignami, Hosley, & Dahl, 1993; Lau, Cua, Keough, Haylock-Jacobs, & Yong, 2013). Perhaps the most interesting and complex functions of the CNS are the ability to encode new information (learning) and to store this information (memory). During learning a high degree of plasticity is required, while the storage of memory requires a high degree of stability (Alberini, 2011). The identification of molecules and mechanisms that modulate these processes are therefore key to the understanding of CNS function. Recent studies suggest that the neural ECM and especially the perineuronal nets (PNs) are important regulators of this plasticity (for review see Takesian & Hensch, 2013; Wang & Fawcett, 2012).

PNs are composed of different ECM molecules that form a lattice-like sheath that surrounds the somata and proximal dendrites of particular neurons. Different chondroitin sulfate proteoglycans (CSPGs) of the lectican family (e.g., aggrecan, brevican, and neurocan) bind via their G1 domains to hyaluronan, which is constantly secreted by the neuronal membrane- anchored hyaluronan synthase. This hyaluronan–CSPG bond is stabilized via hyaluronan and proteoglycan link proteins (HAPLN 1–4). Finally tenascin-R is bound to the CSPGs, cross-linking the complexes of hyaluronan, HAPLN, and CSPGs and stabilizing PNs into a quaternary complex (Chiquet-Ehrismann & Tucker, 2011; Morawski, Bruckner, Arendt, & Matthews, 2012; Yamaguchi, 2000). A special feature of the CSPGs is the numerous attached glycosaminoglycan chains (GAGs), creating the chondroitin sulfate (CS) rich region which is responsible for the specific hydrodynamic properties of strongly hydrated polyanionic ECM (Morawski et al., 2015). Each glycosaminoglycan chain consists of repeated pairs of glucuronic acid and N-acetylgalactosamine. The latter can be sulfated in position 6, 4, or even be unsulfated leading to hundreds of potential glycan combinations (Cummings, 2009); for review see (Caterson, 2012).

The systematic investigation of PNs in the CNS of different species under physiological and pathological conditions has revealed possible functions of PNs in brain development, neuronal signal processing, synaptic plasticity and neuroprotection (Bruckner et al., 2000; Matthews et al., 2002; Morawski, Bruckner, Jager et al., 2012; Morawski, Bruckner, Riederer, Bruckner, & Arendt, 2004; for reviews see Takesian & Hensch, 2013; Wang & Fawcett, 2012; Zimmermann & Dours-Zimmermann, 2008). It was even hypothesized that PNs are part of the cortical long-term memory storage system (Tsien, 2013). Still, to date a specific function of the PN remains elusive. However, there is increasing evidence that the different CSPGs may serve distinct functions in the PN as a structural entity (Avram, Shaposhnikov, Buiu, & Mernea, 2014; Balmer, 2016; Blosa et al., 2015; Favuzzi et al., 2017; Suttkus et al., 2014).

PNs are neither evenly distributed in the CNS nor generally present on most types of neurons. They only appear on specialized subsets of neurons. In the cortex, around 60–80% of these neurons belong to the group of parvalbumin-positive GABAergic interneurons, which are characterized by high-frequency action potential activity (i.e., fast-spiking neurons") and the expression of the high-voltage gated potassium channel subunit $K_v3.1$ (Hartig et al., 1999; Suttkus et al., 2014). While in most cortical areas only a minor proportion of neurons are surrounded by PNs (Bruckner et al., 2000; Morawski, Pavlica et al., 2010; Seeger, Brauer, Hartig, & Bruckner, 1994; Suttkus et al., 2014), the nuclei of the central auditory system, especially those of the superior olivary complex

(SOC), have exceptionally high proportions of PN-bearing neurons. As the functional role of PNs might best be studied in brain areas rich in these ECM components, the SOC has gained increasing attention in the last years and has become a model system to study the cellular and systemic function of PNs and their subcomponents in the brain (Sonntag, Blosa, Schmidt, Rubsamen, & Morawski, 2015).

This chapter addresses the cell-specific distribution of PNs in the nuclei of the SOC, considering species-specific differences and discussing controversial results based on the application of distinct markers and antibodies used for the detection of PNs. It further describes the development of PNs in the SOC, pointing out differences in the developmental profile and expression pattern of the PN subcomponents. The chapter concludes with current concepts on the function of PNs within the SOC, focusing on the impact of PNs on synaptic transmission, synaptic plasticity, and neuronal excitability.

Distribution of Perineuronal Nets in the Superior Olivary Complex

The SOC is composed of several nuclei that contribute to the processing of sound source location. Among those are the medial, lateral, and ventral nucleus of the trapezoid body (MNTB, LNTB, and VNTB), the lateral and medial superior olive (LSO and MSO), and the superior paraolivary nucleus (SPN). The distribution of PNs within these nuclei is well described across many mammalian species.

Medial Nucleus of the Trapezoid Body

Within the SOC, the MNTB stands out because virtually all of its principal neurons are surrounded by a PN. The high prevalence of PNs in the MNTB is consistent across many different species (gerbil: Lurie, Pasic, Hockfield, & Rubel, 1997; Sonntag, Blosa, Schmidt, Rubsamen, & Morawski, 2015; rat: Friauf, 2000; Hartig et al., 2001; Myers, Ray, & Kulesza, 2012; Seeger, Brauer, Hartig, & Bruckner, 1994; mouse: Balmer, 2016; Blosa et al., 2013; Blosa et al., 2015; Kolson et al., 2016; tenrec: Morawski, Bruckner, Jager, Seeger, Kunzle et al., 2010; dog: Fech, Calderon-Garciduenas, & Kulesza, 2017; rhesus monkey: Hilbig, Nowack, Boeckler, Bidmon, & Zilles, 2007). PNs in the MNTB densely cover the principal neurons' cell bodies but rarely extend into proximal dendrites (Blosa et al., 2013; Hartig et al., 2001; Lurie, Pasic, Hockfield, & Rubel, 1997). They form cotton wool-like structures (Blosa et al., 2013; Hartig et al., 2001; Kolson et al., 2016; Lurie, Pasic, Hockfield, & Rubel, 1997) that deviate from the typical lattice-like appearance of PNs around cortical neurons (Blosa et al., 2013; Celio & Blumcke, 1994; Celio, Spreafico, Biasi, & Vitellaro-Zuccarello, 1998; Deepa et al., 2006; Hockfield & McKay, 1983; Zaremba, Guimaraes, Kalb, & Hockfield, 1989). The shape of PNs around MNTB principal cells is most likely an adaptation to its specialized synaptic input (Blosa et al., 2013), a single giant synapse, the calyx of Held, which is formed by the axons of the globular bushy cells in the ventral cochlear nucleus and covers ~50% of the MNTB neuron's cell body (Morest, 1968; Satzler et al., 2002; see also chapter by Spirou in this book).

Various markers have been applied to identify PNs in the MNTB. While labeling of aggrecan and brevican yielded the highest number of PN positive MNTB neurons in all investigated species (gerbil: Lurie et al., 1997; rats: Myers et al., 2012; mice: Blosa et al., 2013; Kolson et al., 2016), results obtained using Wisteria floribunda agglutinin (WFA), which binds to N-acetylgalactosamine residues on the CS-GAG-chains of aggrecan (Giamanco, Morawski, & Matthews, 2010; Morawski, Bruckner, Arendt, & Matthews, 2012), were controversial, perhaps reflecting species differences. In dogs, the majority of MNTB principal cells (80%) showed WFA-labeled PNs (Fech et al., 2017). Similar observations were made in rats, where ~90% of neurons in the MNTB revealed WFA binding sites (Myers et al., 2012). However, in mice >90% of MNTB neurons were found to reveal aggrecan- and brevican positive PNs, while only ~25% of the neurons in the same nucleus were additionally reactive to WFA (Blosa et al., 2013). In the MNTB of rhesus monkeys, WFA labeling was found to follow a medio-lateral gradient with the number of WFA-reactive neurons in the medial MNTB being higher compared to the lateral MNTB (Hilbig et al., 2007). Further, MNTB neurons with WFA binding sites were shown to express the potassium channel subunit Kv3.1β which is supposed to facilitate high-frequency activity (Rudy & McBain, 2001) and which also exhibits a mediolateral gradient in the MNTB (Gazula et al., 2010; Hilbig, Nowack, Boeckler, Bidmon, & Zilles, 2007; Leao et al., 2006).

Lateral Superior Olive

In contrast to the MNTB, PNs in the LSO enclose neuronal somata as well as proximal dendrites of mainly fusiform cells (Friauf, 2000), thereby exhibiting the characteristic net-like shape (Friauf, 2000; Lurie, Pasic, Hockfield, & Rubel, 1997). PNs in the LSO were identified in various species, including gerbil (Lurie et al., 1997), rat (Friauf, 2000; Myers, Ray, & Kulesza, 2012; Seeger, Brauer, Hartig, & Bruckner, 1994), dog (Atoji & Suzuki, 1992; Atoji, Yamamoto, Suzuki, Matsui, & Oohira, 1997; Fech, Calderon-Garciduenas, & Kulesza, 2017), tenrec (Morawski, Bruckner, Jager, Seeger, Kunzle et al., 2010) and rhesus monkey (Hilbig et al., 2007), though species-specific differences have been documented. While in dogs, medial LSO neurons were less frequently enclosed by WFA positive PNs (68%) than lateral LSO neurons (83%; Fech et al., 2017), the opposite was found in the rhesus monkey, where especially the medial LSO neurons exhibited strongly labeled WFA -positive PNs (Hilbig et al., 2007).

Discrepancies in the estimated number of PN-bearing LSO neurons have also been emerged with respect to the utilized PN marker. While more than 85% of LSO neurons in rats are surrounded by PNs when using WFA, only about 53% of the LSO neurons exhibit PNs when using the glycosylation-dependent anti-CSPG antibody Cat-315 (Myers et al., 2012). These results point to chemical variations in the subcomponents of PNs, such as glycosylation state (Dino, Harroch, Hockfield, & Matthews, 2006; Matthews et al., 2002) which might affect the suitability of PN markers and further lead to repeated misinterpretations in the literature (Morawski, Bruckner, Jager et al., 2012).

Medial Superior Olive

PNs have been found around principal neurons of the MSO in rats (Friauf, 2000; Myers, Ray, & Kulesza, 2012; Seeger, Brauer, Hartig, & Bruckner, 1994), gerbils (Lurie et al., 1997), and dogs (Atoji & Suzuki, 1992; Atoji, Yamamoto, Suzuki, Matsui, & Oohira, 1997; Fech, Calderon-Garciduenas, & Kulesza, 2017). PNs in the MSO are associated with bipolar shaped cell bodies and with medially and laterally oriented dendritic processes, remarkably at larger extent than dendrites of other nuclei in the SOC (Lurie et al., 1997).

Gradients in PN expression along the tonotopic axis have been reported for dogs. In the dorsal, high-frequency part of the MSO only 35% of the neurons are enclosed by WFA-positive PNs, while in the ventral, low-frequency portion of the MSO 78% of the neurons reveal WFA-positive PNs (Fech et al., 2017).

Other Nuclei of the Superior Olivary Complex

The remaining nuclei of the SOC, including the LNTB, VNTB, and SPN, are not well examined regarding the distribution of PNs. The little information that is available was collected in rats and dogs. In adult rats, about 70–80% of SPN neurons were found to be surrounded by PNs labeled with either WFA or anti-Cat-315 (Myers et al., 2012). In dogs, more than half of the LNTB (59%) and VNTB neurons (65%) revealed WFA-positive PNs.

Perineuronal Nets in the Superior Olivary Complex of Humans

Perineuronal nets have been detected in SOC nuclei of many species, ranging from rodents, such as gerbils, mice and rats, to dogs and rhesus monkey. However, PNs have also been found in the human SOC, but the investigations are mainly restricted to older individuals (>70 years old).

Although the neuroanatomy of the human SOC was described to be largely comparable to what has been reported for other species (Kulesza, 2007, 2008; Schmidt, Wolski,

& Kulesza, 2010), the distribution of PNs was found to differ in some respects. In the MNTB, only about 25% of the neurons were associated with PNs, using either WFA or an anti-CSPG antibody. PNs were primarily associated with round-shaped neurons (59%) but were also found around stellate (39%) and fusiform cells (2%) within this nucleus. Similar results were found in the LNTB, VNTB, and SPN, where the number of neurons surrounded by PNs varied between 10 and 32% and were also distributed among fusiform, stellate, and round or oval-shaped neurons (Schmidt et al., 2010). Thus, the number of neurons surrounded by PNs is remarkably reduced compared to other mammalian species. Surprisingly, the labeling of PNs in the MSO and LSO by WFA or an anti-CSPG antibody did only rarely reveal net-like structure in the LSO (<1% of the neurons) and virtually never in the MSO (Schmidt et al., 2010). These data are to some extent conflicting with results documented in most of the other species tested so far where labeling of the LSO and MSO presented a clear, net-like structure surrounding the cell bodies and dendrites.

The interpretation of these results needs to be done with caution. The absence of WFA binding sites and the negative immunosignal in response to the used anti-CSPG antibody does not necessarily mean that MSO and LSO neurons in the human SOC do not express PNs. The suitability of some PN markers, including WFA, as well as PN-specific antibodies, has been increasingly doubted in the last years (Sonntag et al., 2015). WFA detects N-acetylgalactosamine residues on CS-GAG chains of aggrecan (Table 15.1, Figure 15.1; Giamanco et al., 2010). Still, studies conducted in the hippocampus and neocortex clearly demonstrated that many neurons that are surrounded by aggrecan do not reveal WFA binding sites (Ajmo, Eakin, Hamel, & Gottschall, 2008; Morawski, Bruckner, Jager, Seeger, & Arendt, 2010; Suttkus et al., 2014). Further, the glycosylation state of aggrecan may vary among neurons, which affects the binding properties of some glycosylation-dependent anti-CSPG antibodies, such as Cat-315 and Cat-316 (Table 15.1, Figure 15.1; Dino, Harroch, Hockfield, & Matthews, 2006; Matthews et al., 2002). It might thus be possible that the biochemical properties of aggrecan around LSO and MSO neurons in the human SOC deviate from that of other species, where WFA and various glycosylation-independent, anti-aggrecan, and anti-CSPG antibodies (Table 15.1, Figure 15.1) yielded clear PNs around MSO and LSO neurons (Fech, Calderon-Garciduenas, & Kulesza, 2017; Friauf, 2000; Lurie, Pasic, Hockfield, & Rubel, 1997; Morawski, Bruckner, Jager, Seeger, Kunzle et al., 2010; Myers, Ray, & Kulesza, 2012). Surprisingly, most of the currently recommended PN-specific antibodies that mainly detect the core proteins of various PN subcomponents (such as aggrecan, brevican, neurocan, and HAPLN 1 and 4), and which were demonstrated to specifically label PNs around neurons in the auditory brainstem of mice and gerbils (Blosa et al., 2013; Blosa et al., 2015; Kolson et al., 2016; Sonntag, Blosa, Schmidt, Rubsamen, & Morawski, 2015), have not been applied to the human auditory brainstem yet. It most likely can be assumed that these antibodies will prove to be the better choice to clarify whether neurons in the human MSO and LSO are surrounded by or devoid of PNs (Morawski, Bruckner, Jager et al., 2012).

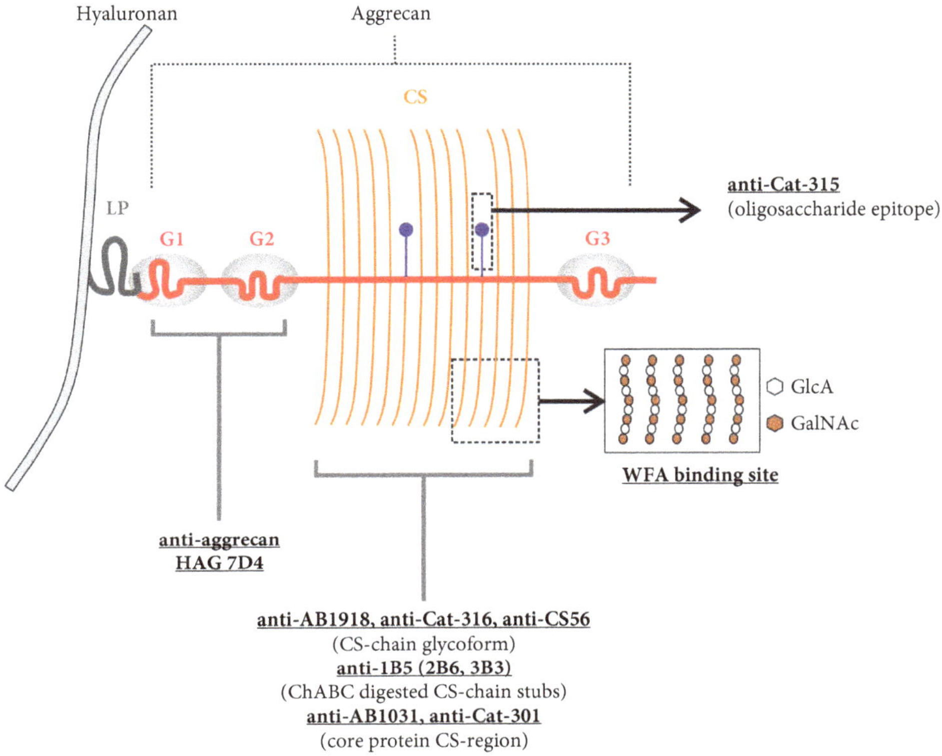

FIGURE 15.1. Antibodies detecting the core protein and chondroitin sulfate glycosaminoglycan side chains of aggrecan. Schematic illustration of the aggrecan protein (including the three globular domains G1–G3 of the core protein and attached CS side chains) and respective antibodies direct against different components of aggrecan. CS—chondroitin sulfate; G—globular domain; GalNAc—N-acetylgalactosamine; GlcA—glucuronic acid; LP—link protein

Development of Perineuronal Nets in the Superior Olivary Complex

PNs gradually mature during late stages of postnatal development, being established first in brainstem areas and last in cortical areas (Bruckner et al., 2000; Friauf, 2000). The formation of PNs coincides with the end of critical periods, which indicate developmental epochs with heightened plasticity (Kalb & Hockfield, 1988; Pizzorusso et al., 2002; for review see Zimmermann & Dours-Zimmermann, 2008).

The development of PNs in the superior olivary complex is well described in rodents (gerbil, mice and rats) and is characterized by profound changes between the end of the first postnatal week and the end of the first postnatal month (Bruckner et al., 2000;

Table 15.1. Commonly used antibodies/markers for the detection of aggrecan in perineuronal nets.

Marker	Detected Region	Detected Component	Specific for Aggrecan	Reference	Source
	Core protein				
MAB anti-human aggrecan (clone HAG 7D4)		Aggrecan core protein at G1-G2 domain	Yes	(Bruckner, Morawski, & Arendt, 2008); (Virgintino et al., 2009)	Bio-Rad (AbD Serotec)
MAB 5284 anti-Cat-301		Aggrecan core protein at CS-region	Yes	Matthews et al. 2002	Merck (Millipore)
AB1031 anti-aggrecan		Aggrecan core protein at CS-region	Yes	Blosa et al. 2013	Merck (Millipore)
	CS-Chain (glycoform)				
AB1918 anti-CSPG		Unspecified CS-chain potentially on aggrecan	Unclear	Bruckner et al. 2000; Friauf 2000	Chemicon dis-continued
ab11570 anti-pan CS56		Unspecified CS-chain on PGs	No	(Balmer, Carels, Frisch, & Nick, 2009; Miyata, Komatsu, Yoshimura, Taya, & Kitagawa, 2012)	Merck, Abcam, LSBio, Bio-Rad
MAB 15812 anti-Cat-316		Unspecified CS-chain potentially on aggrecan	Unclear	Matthews et al. 2002	Merck (Millipore)
	CS-Chain (digested)				
Anti-CS Delta Di-OS (clone 1B5)		OS CS-stub after ChABC digestion	Unclear	Caterson 2012	AMSBio
anti-CS Delta Di-4S (clone 2B6)		4S CS-stub after ChABC digestion	Unclear	Caterson 2012	AMSBio
anti-CS Delta Di-6S (clone 3B3)		6S CS-stub after ChABC digestion	Unclear	Caterson 2012	AMSBio

Table 15.1. **Continued**

Marker	Detected Region	Detected Component	Specific for Aggrecan	Reference	Source
	Oligosaccharide on PGs				
MAB 1581 anti-Cat-315		In development: RPTPζ/phosphacan In adult: oligo-epitope on aggrecan	Unclear	Matthews et al. 2002; Dino et al. 2006	Merck (Millipore)
	N-acetyl-galactosamine				
Wisteria Floribunda agglutinin (WFA)		N-acetyl-Galactosamine on CS-chain of aggrecan	Yes	(Bruckner et al., 1993); Giamanco et al. 2010	Merck (Sigma-Aldrich), Vector Labs

Antibodies and markers commonly used for the detection of aggrecan can be directed against the core protein, chondroitin sulfate (CS) chains, oligosaccharides, or N-acetylgalactosamines.

Friauf, 2000; Kolson et al., 2016; Lurie, Pasic, Hockfield, & Rubel, 1997; Myers, Ray, & Kulesza, 2012). These changes include an increase in the number of PN-positive neurons in the MNTB, LSO, and MSO (Myers et al., 2012), an increase in gene expression of PN components, demonstrated in the MNTB (Kolson et al., 2016), and an increase in staining intensity of PN components, indicating an increase in protein expression levels in the MNTB, LSO, and MSO (Bruckner et al., 2000; Friauf, 2000; Kolson et al., 2016; Lurie, Pasic, Hockfield, & Rubel, 1997).

In detail, aggrecan and brevican first appear around P6-P7 in the MNTB and are mainly diffusely distributed in the neuropil (Figure 15.2), although occasional punctate accumulations of aggrecan were observed at the surface of principal neurons at this age (Friauf, 2000; Kolson et al., 2016; Lurie, Pasic, Hockfield, & Rubel, 1997). In contrast to this, HAPLN 1 already shows ring-like patterns around the principal neurons at this age and thus seems to develop much faster than brevican and aggrecan (Kolson et al., 2016). Similar observations were made for neurocan, which also clearly encircles MNTB principal cells already at P4–7 in mice (Figure 15.2; Bruckner et al., 2000). The early presence of HAPLN 1 might be directly linked to the development of neurocan, since HAPLN 1 interacts with neurocan and stabilizes the connection between this proteoglycan and hyaluronan (Zimmermann & Dours-Zimmermann, 2008). Around hearing onset (P12–P14), labeling of aggrecan, brevican, and HAPLN 1 is significantly increased in intensity and appears as a ring clearly delineating neuronal cell bodies (Bruckner et al., 2000; Friauf, 2000; Kolson et al., 2016; Lurie, Pasic, Hockfield, & Rubel, 1997). Between P21 and P28 intensity of PN labeling further increases and adult-like shape is reached (Figure 15.2; Friauf, 2000; Lurie, Pasic, Hockfield, & Rubel, 1997).

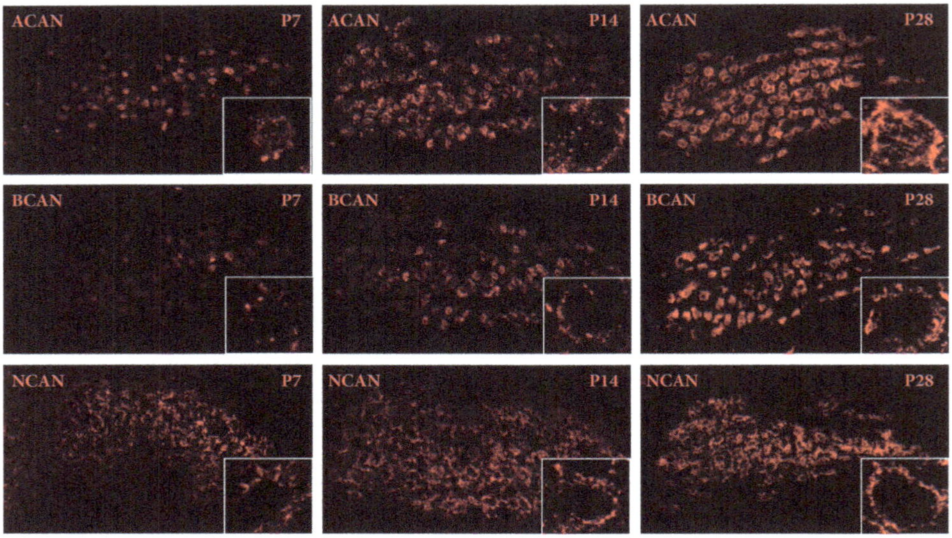

FIGURE 15.2. Development of chondroitin-sulfate proteoglycans in the medial nucleus of the trapezoid body of the mouse. Immunohistochemical labeling of the chondroitin-sulfated proteoglycans aggrecan (ACAN, top row), brevican (BCAN, middle row) and neurocan (NCAN, bottom row) at the ages P7, P14, and P28 indicates differences in the developmental expression patterns between ACAN and BCAN versus NCAN. ACAN and BCAN show weak, mainly intracellular immunolabeling at P7, consistent with incomplete transportation into the extracellular space. ACAN and BCAN immunoreactivity strongly increases during further development, finally forming the typical ring-like structures at P28. NCAN is characterized by early high-expression levels and is accumulated extracellularly around neurons already at P7, with only minor changes up to P28.

The developmental profiles of PNs in the LSO and MSO were largely comparable to what has been described in the MNTB. At the end of the first postnatal week, aggrecan exhibits a faint and diffuse labeling. Neuron-specific labeling of aggrecan is first detected around P11–P12, surrounding dendrites and cell bodies of the principal neurons in the LSO and MSO. During the next two postnatal weeks, intensity of aggrecan labeling heavily increases, exhibiting an adult-like appearance at P28 (Friauf, 2000; Lurie, Pasic, Hockfield, & Rubel, 1997).

In rodents, the expression and maturation of PNs in the SOC coincides with critical morphological and physiological developmental processes and the onset of response to airborne sound (Sonntag et al., 2009). In the MNTB, these changes encompass the (1) transition from multiple inputs to mono-innervation by the large calyx of Held during the first postnatal week (Bergsman, Camilli, & McCormick, 2004; Holcomb et al., 2013; Rodriguez-Contreras, van Hoeve, John Silvio Soria, Habets, Locher, & Borst, 2008; for review see Yu & Goodrich, 2014); (2) the growth and fenestration of the calyx of Held up to the age of P14 (Ford, Grothe, & Klug, 2009; Hoffpauir, Grimes, Mathers, & Spirou, 2006; Kandler & Friauf, 1993; Morest, 1968; for review see Yu & Goodrich, 2014); and (3) the acceleration of synaptic transmission speed, shortening of action potential duration, and increase in synaptic fidelity along with changes in the composition and expression of receptors and channels during the second postnatal week (Sonntag,

Englitz, Typlt, & Rubsamen, 2011; Taschenberger & Gersdorff, 2000; for review see Gersdorff & Borst, 2002; Schneggenburger & Forsythe, 2006). Likewise, developmental changes with respect to refinement, pruning, and strengthening of synaptic contacts occur in the MSO and LSO during the second postnatal week, resulting in functional networks around hearing onset (Kandler, Clause, & Noh, 2009).

The strong temporal correlation between PN development and maturation of morphological and physiological features of SOC neurons suggests that PNs are involved in processes involved in closing the critical period in hearing system development. This was also suggested for the visual system where the appearance of PNs is likewise linked to the onset of sensory information processing (Hockfield & Sur, 1990; Kalb & Hockfield, 1988; Pizzorusso et al., 2002). The underlying mechanisms are not clarified up to now, but previous reports indicate that PNs stabilize synaptic contacts and functional networks by restricting synaptic plasticity. This was experimentally demonstrated in the visual cortex, where synaptic plasticity remained at juvenile levels after enzymatic digestion of the CS-GAG side chains of proteoglycans of PNs (Carulli et al., 2010; Pizzorusso et al., 2002; Wang & Fawcett, 2012).

In addition, it was shown that the expression and maturation of PNs does not only correlate with the onset of sensory information processing but might also directly be dependent on sensory information. Visual deprivation was found to be linked to reduced levels of aggrecan in the visual cortex (Hockfield & Sur, 1990). The effects of auditory deprivation on PN expression has also been investigated in neurons of the SOC in rats, yielding reduced numbers of PN bearing neurons in the MNTB and MSO compared to normal hearing controls (Myers et al., 2012).

In contrast to the early development, the effect of aging on the expression of PNs in the auditory brainstem is not well understood. Comparative analysis of PN expression in the SOC in 4-week old and 1-year old gerbils did not yield any differences (Lurie et al., 1997). Investigations in other brain regions yielded similar results. In the auditory cortex of CBA mice, no differences in the intensity of PN staining were found between young (1–3 months) and old (14–24 months) animals (Brewton, Kokash, Jimenez, Pena, & Razak, 2016). Likewise, the number of PN-bearing neurons in the human amygdala was not related to the age of the individuals (Pantazopoulos, Murray, & Berretta, 2008). Interestingly, the sulfation pattern of GAG side chains of PNs in the auditory, visual, and motor cortex of rats was demonstrated to change with increasing age (Foscarin, Raha-Chowdhury, Fawcett, & Kwok, 2017), indicating functional modifications in the aging brain.

Structure and Molecular Composition of Perineuronal Nets in the Medial Nucleus of the Trapezoid Body

The characterization of the PNs in the SOC is currently mainly constrained to a qualitative and (less frequently) quantitative estimation of the distribution of PNs in the individual SOC nuclei. Structural details, such as molecular composition of PNs as well as interaction of PNs with neurons and synapses, have only been investigated in the MNTB so far (Blosa et al., 2013).

Elaborate immunohistochemical analyses confirmed the presence of all major PN constituents around MNTB principal cells, including hyaluronan, the CSPGs aggrecan, brevican, and neurocan, different oligosaccharide epitopes, HAPLN 1 and tenascin-R (Blosa et al., 2013; Blosa et al., 2015; Kolson et al., 2016). The typical, strong interaction of PNs and synapses terminating on the neuronal surface and on dendrites was also demonstrated in the MNTB, since both glutamatergic and GABAergic synaptic boutons, as well as the huge glutamatergic calyx of Held, were tightly enwrapped by aggrecan immunoreactivity. These data indicate that PNs in the MNTB enclose synapses irrespective of the prevalent neurotransmitter (Blosa et al., 2013).

Interestingly, the CSPGs seemed to differ in their extension and distribution around the neuronal surface. While aggrecan revealed a prominent, cotton wool-like appearance surrounding the entire neuron as well as the outer surface of the calyx of Held, brevican, and neurocan were found to be more delicate forming thinner rings around the neuronal cell bodies (Blosa et al., 2013; Kolson et al., 2016). In addition, electron microscopical analyses yielded that brevican is especially located in the perisynaptic space, around unmyelinated parts of presynaptic axons, and even in the calyceal, subsynaptic space, but it is sparsely present in the soma-free neuropil within the MNTB (Blosa et al., 2013; Blosa et al., 2015). Thus, PNs around MNTB principal neurons appear to be composed of an inner brevican/neurocan ring and an outer aggrecan ring (Blosa et al., 2013; Kolson et al., 2016). Remarkably, the extracellular space filled with perineuronal extracellular matrix revealed an extension of up to 2 μm in the MNTB (Blosa et al., 2013), which matches the bulky appearance of PNs around MNTB principal neurons and is significantly larger than what has been generally found around other neurons (20–70 nm (Sykova & Nicholson, 2008; van Harreveld, 1965). This 100-times bigger ECM coat around neurons in the SOC, especially in the MNTB, might point to an outstanding role of PNs for the physiology of these neurons (Morawski et al., 2015).

Function of Perineuronal Nets in the Superior Olivary Complex

The heterogeneous distribution and the different developmental periods of appearance of aggrecan, brevican and neurocan in the PN gives rise to the assumption that these CSPGS may occupy different functions within the PN. Depending on the brain region of interest and the considered PN subcomponent, PNs contribute to synaptic stabilization and plasticity, to synaptic transmission and to neuroprotection. However, the specific function of PNs or their subcomponents in the SOC remains largely elusive. Given the high density of PNs in the SOC, it is surprising that so far only two very recent studies considered the MNTB as a model system to estimate the PNs' role in synaptic transmission and neuronal activity (Balmer, 2016; Blosa et al., 2015).

Chondroitin Sulfate Side Chains and Their Impact on Neuronal Excitability and Synaptic Plasticity

Injection of chondroitinase ABC in the visual cortex and amygdala yielded reactivation of juvenile states of synaptic plasticity in these systems (Gogolla, Caroni, Luthi, & Herry, 2009; Pizzorusso et al., 2002), thus indicating that PNs restrict synaptic plasticity after the closure of the critical window (Dityatev & Fellin, 2008; Gundelfinger, Frischknecht, Choquet, & Heine, 2010; Wang & Fawcett, 2012). This is supposed to be based on the PNs' contribution to the stabilization of neuron-synapse and synapse-dendrite interactions (Hockfield & Sur, 1990; Vivo et al., 2013; Wang & Fawcett, 2012) and potentially also on the PNs' control of neuronal activity. The latter theory mainly relies on the fact that PNs provide a strong polyanionic charge determined by the high number of negatively charged chondroitin sulfate side chains bound to aggrecan (Giamanco, Morawski, & Matthews, 2010; Morawski et al., 2015; Morawski, Bruckner, Arendt, & Matthews, 2012). Thus, PNs, especially aggrecan, are believed to act as a diffusion barrier or spatial buffer for positively charged ions and proteins, a function thatwas found to be important for the protection of neurons against toxic accumulations of cations or other positively charged molecules (Morawski, Bruckner, Arendt, & Matthews, 2012; Morawski, Bruckner, Jager, Seeger, & Arendt, 2010; Morawski, Bruckner, Riederer, Bruckner, & Arendt, 2004; Suttkus et al., 2014; Suttkus, Morawski, & Arendt, 2016; Suttkus, Rohn, Jager, Arendt, & Morawski, 2012) but might further be essential for high-frequency neuronal activity by controlling ion availability and homeostasis (Hartig et al., 1999; Hrabetova, Masri, Tao, Xiao, & Nicholson, 2009; Morawski et al., 2015). This idea is supported by an elaborate electrophysiological work, recently published by (Balmer, 2016), who demonstrated the impact of PNs on neuronal activity in the MNTB. After enzymatic digestion of chondroitin sulfate side chains by chondroitinase ABC, MNTB principal cells revealed greatly reduced excitability in response to white noise currents, and thus needed more current for spiking compared to untreated MNTB neurons (Figure 15.3). This change was not based on alterations in passive membrane properties, since resting membrane potential and input resistance were comparable between enzyme-treated and control cells. Instead, the spike thresholds of the enzyme-treated neurons were elevated. The underlying mechanisms are still unclear, but given the fact that chondroitinase ABC cuts off negatively charged side chains, loss of the polyanionic character is a likely reason for the observed physiological changes. In cortical and hippocampal slices, the diffusion of calcium is increased after chondroitinase ABC- digestion of PNs (Hrabetova et al., 2009), supporting the hypothesis that PNs bind cations (Morawski et al., 2015). Sodium and potassium ions might likewise be controlled by PNs, though not yet verified experimentally (Hartig et al., 1999; Morawski et al., 2015). It is also assumed that the voltage-dependency of ion channels is regulated by the PNs anionic side chains. By increasing the negative charge of the membrane and shifting the activation of voltage-dependent currents toward more hyperpolarized potentials, the excitability of neurons might be increased (Balmer, 2016; Morawski et al., 2015).

The elevated neuronal excitability was suggested to be one principle underlying the PN-mediated restriction of synaptic plasticity (Balmer, 2016). However, only little is known about the influence of PNs on synaptic plasticity in the auditory system. A recent study published by (Happel et al., 2014) demonstrated that the enzymatic digestion of PNs in the auditory cortex of gerbils considerably affects the reversal learning behavior which is known to be based on plastic modifications of neuronal interactions. Whether PNs also control synaptic plasticity in the SOC is virtually elusive and needs to be investigated in future studies. Previous findings demonstrate that MNTB principal cells reveal heterogeneous properties with respect to short-term plasticity (Grande & Wang, 2011). Likewise, it was shown that not all PN-bearing MNTB principal cells reveal binding sites for the lectin WFA which detects the negatively charged side chains bound to proteoglycans (Blosa et al., 2013). In this regard, it might be of importance to figure out whether PNs are heterogeneous with respect to their negative charge (Morawski et al., 2015) and whether they differ in their potential to control synaptic plasticity in the MNTB.

Brevican and Its Role in Synaptic Transmission and Organization of Subsynaptic Space

The primarily perisynaptic location of brevican was assumed to be connected to the contribution to physiological processes at synapses. Electrophysiological in vivo investigations of MNTB principal neurons of brevican-deficient mice supported this theory by showing that the duration of synaptic transmission as well as of pre- and postsynaptic action potentials were significantly prolonged in comparison to wildtype mice (Figure 15.3; Blosa et al., 2015). These data point to an essential role of brevican for high-speed synaptic transmission, which in turn is a precondition for high-frequency activity. These physiological changes were accompanied by a reduction of the amount of the presynaptic vesicular glutamate transporter 1, which controls the amount of glutamate in each vesicle as well as the amount of glutamate released by each vesicle. In addition, striking ultrastructural alterations at the calyx of Held were found in brevican-deficient mice. Brevican is expressed in the extracellular space underneath the calyx of Held forming subsynaptic cavities which were found to separate adjacent postsynaptic densities from each other (Blosa et al., 2013; Blosa et al., 2015). These cavities were significantly reduced in size in brevican-deficient mice (Blosa et al., 2015), indicating that brevican might contribute to the compartmentalization of this huge synapse. The calyx

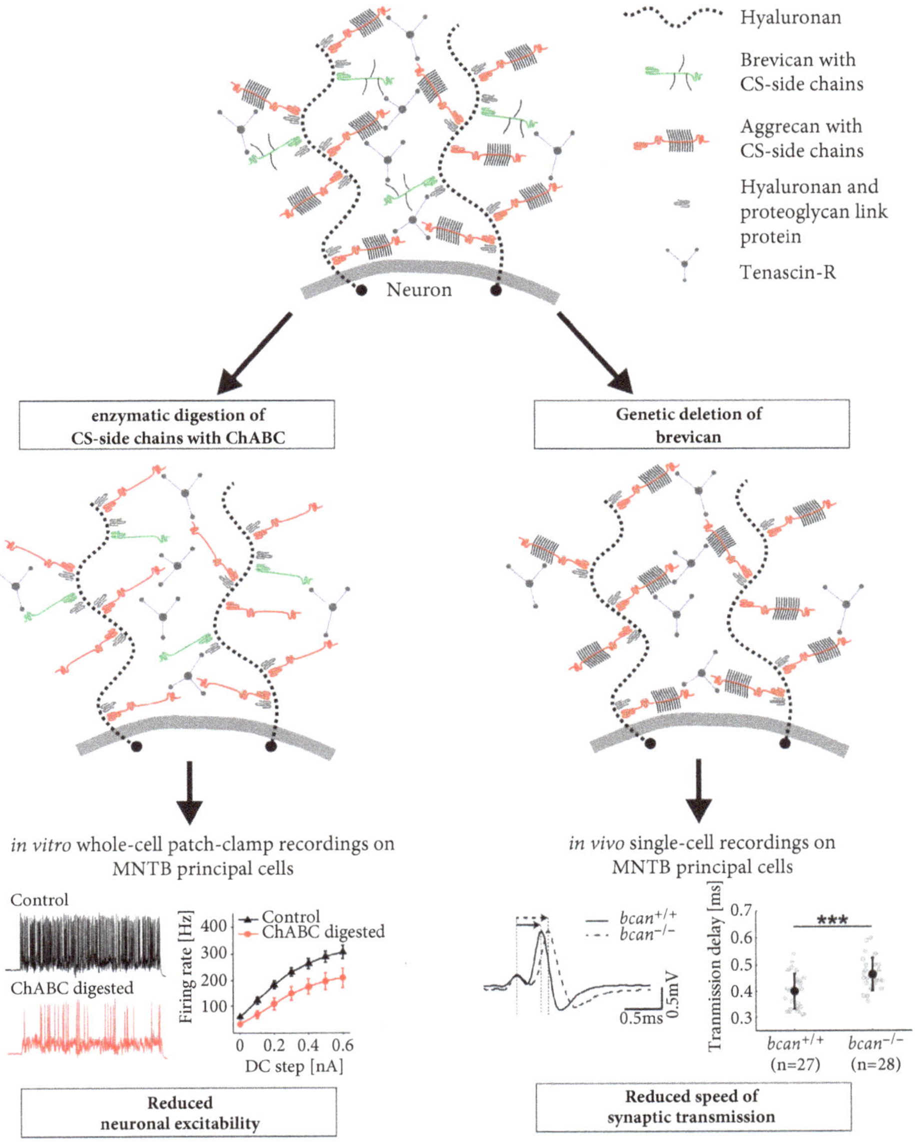

FIGURE 15.3. Impact of perineuronal nets on synaptic transmission and neuronal excitability in the medial nucleus of the trapezoid body. Electrophysiological measurements in the medial nucleus of the trapezoid body (MNTB) after targeted manipulation of perineuronal net (PN) subcomponents indicate that brevican and chondroitin sulfate (CS) side chains, mainly bound to aggrecan, serve different functions. After genetic deletion of brevican (*bcan*$^{-/-}$) in the mouse, a significant reduction in speed of synaptic transmission at the calyx of Held is observed (left, figures were modified from Blosa et al., 2015). After enzymatic digestion of CS side chains with chondroitinase ABC (ChABC) whole-cell patch-clamp recordings indicate a reduced excitability of MNTB principal neurons (right, figures were modified from Balmer, 2016). *** $p < 0.001$

of Held is a morphologically specialized synapse exhibiting several hundreds of active zones (Gersdorff & Borst, 2002; Taschenberger, Leao, Rowland, Spirou, & Gersdorff, 2002). The brevican-filled subsynaptic cavities are believed to be important for the spatial and functional organization of synaptic release sites which is indispensable for fast and high-frequency transmission. In this regard, brevican is assumed to restrict transmitter spillover and to control the reuptake of glutamate into the presynaptic terminal (Blosa et al., 2013; Yamada et al., 1997). Altogether, these findings indicate that brevican acts presynaptically by controlling transmitter recycling and vesicular release (Blosa et al., 2013). However, postsynaptic actions of brevican were also suggested since in hippocampal neurons brevican physically interacts with AMPA receptor subunits GluR1, GluR2/3 and GluR4 (Favuzzi et al., 2017; Saroja et al., 2014), perhaps controlling the mobility of AMPA receptors (Frischknecht et al., 2009). Further investigations are needed to elucidate the molecular mechanisms behind the action of brevican underlying its impact on glutamatergic signaling in the MNTB.

Brevican and Its Impact on Hearing

Fast, temporally precise, reliable, and high-frequency synaptic transmission are important preconditions for the proper processing of auditory information within the SOC. Disruptions of one of these critical features are supposed to result in the impairment of hearing function. Since brevican was shown to be essential for achieving the very high speed of synaptic transmission in the MNTB, it is not surprising at all that auditory signal processing in the MNTB in brevican-deficient mice was also deteriorated. In detail, in vivo single-cell recordings in brevican-deficient mice yielded reduced hearing thresholds and sound-evoked discharge rates in the MNTB (Blosa et al., 2015). Interestingly, the MNTB could be excluded as the origin of these effects since the reliability of synaptic transmission at the calyx of Held—MNTB synapse was not changed in brevican-deficient mice (Blosa et al., 2015). Since these brevican-deficient mice are a systemic knockout line, it is to be expected that brevican controls synaptic transmission throughout the entire brain, and thus the cochlear nucleus, which precedes the MNTB, might be a potential source of the demonstrated alterations in sensitivity and firing rates (Blosa et al., 2015), a possibility that remains to be examined. In addition, the questions remain whether the positive influence of brevican on synaptic transmission speed is a general phenomenon, valid for all synapses along the auditory pathway (or even in the whole CNS), and whether the absence of brevican affects the localization of sound sources, a function that strongly depends on temporally precise and fast synaptic transmission in the CN and SOC.

Conclusion

PNs are a specialized form of ECM that surround specific types of neurons in the central nervous system. In most regions of the CNS, especially in the cortex, PNs are only associated with about 1–10% of the neurons, strongly depending on the area investigated (Morawski, Pavlica et al., 2010; Suttkus et al., 2014). A remarkably high density of PNs was found in the nuclei of the auditory brainstem, especially of the SOC, which seems to be consistent across many mammalian species, including humans. Thus, the PNs might serve as a suitable marker for the identification of the SOC and its subnuclei in species where the neuroanatomy is not yet well described.

Structural details and functional aspects of PNs so far have been mainly studied in cortical and hippocampal interneurons, the preferred model system for investigation of PN function (Brakebusch et al., 2002; Favuzzi et al., 2017; Geissler et al., 2013; Pizzorusso et al., 2002). The nuclei of the SOC have only been addressed in a few studies, which is surprising given the high prevalence of PNs around the neurons within this complex. One reason might be that the neurons within the SOC form a group of very active neurons partly characterized by morphologically specialized synapses, and therefore greatly differ from most of the other PN-bearing neurons, such as interneurons in the cortex and hippocampus (Sonntag et al., 2015). This might foster doubts whether the results obtained in the SOC can be generalized for other brain regions. However, in a recent comparative study it was shown that enzymatic digestion of PNs around neurons in the MNTB and around cortical interneurons results in a similar reduction of excitability in both types of neurons, thus indicating that the function of PNs might be the same irrespective of the type of neuron or transmitter (Balmer, 2016). In addition, especially the huge calyx of Held in the MNTB, which is a unique model synapse for the investigation of glutamatergic synaptic transmission (Gersdorff & Borst, 2002; Schneggenburger & Forsythe, 2006), might greatly help to study the influence of PNs on synaptic transmission. It is currently not possible to elucidate this in the same extent in the cortex and hippocampus as the direct access to the synapses is hampered due to their small sizes.

Despite of the remaining uncertainty of whether the contribution of PNs to neuronal activity and synaptic transmission observed in the MNTB can be assumed as a general PN function, these findings strongly support the previously introduced concept of the tetrapartite synapse (Dityatev & Rusakov, 2011), where the pre- and postsynapse, glia cells, and PNs conjointly control the physiology of the synapses and neurons.

References

Ajmo, J. M., Eakin, A. K., Hamel, M. G., & Gottschall, P. E. (2008). Discordant localization of WFA reactivity and brevican/ADAMTS-derived fragment in rodent brain. *BMC Neuroscience*, *9*, 14. https://doi.org/10.1186/1471-2202-9-14

Alberini, C. M. (2011). The role of reconsolidation and the dynamic process of long-term memory formation and storage. *Frontiers in Behavioral Neuroscience*, *5*, 12. https://doi.org/10.3389/fnbeh.2011.00012

Atoji, Y., & Suzuki, Y. (1992). Chondroitin sulfate in the extracellular matrix of the medial and lateral superior olivary nuclei in the dog. *Brain Research*, *585*(1–2), 287–290.

Atoji, Y., Yamamoto, Y., Suzuki, Y., Matsui, F., & Oohira, A. (1997). Immunohistochemical localization of neurocan in the lower auditory nuclei of the dog. *Hearing Research*, *110*(1–2), 200–208.

Avram, S., Shaposhnikov, S., Buiu, C., & Mernea, M. (2014). Chondroitin sulfate proteoglycans: Structure-function relationship with implication in neural development and brain disorders. *BioMed Research International*, *2014*, 642798. https://doi.org/10.1155/2014/642798

Balmer, T. S. (2016). Perineuronal nets enhance the excitability of fast-spiking neurons. *eNeuro*, *3*(4). https://doi.org/10.1523/ENEURO.0112-16.2016

Balmer, T. S., Carels, V. M., Frisch, J. L., & Nick, T. A. (2009). Modulation of perineuronal nets and parvalbumin with developmental song learning. *The Journal of Neuroscience*, *29*(41), 12878–12885. https://doi.org/10.1523/JNEUROSCI.2974-09.2009

Bergsman, J. B., Camilli, P. de, & McCormick, D. A. (2004). Multiple large inputs to principal cells in the mouse medial nucleus of the trapezoid body. *Journal of Neurophysiology*, *92*(1), 545–552. https://doi.org/10.1152/jn.00927.2003

Bignami, A., Hosley, M., & Dahl, D. (1993). Hyaluronic acid and hyaluronic acid-binding proteins in brain extracellular matrix. *Anatomy and Embryology*, *188*(5), 419–433.

Blosa, M., Sonntag, M., Bruckner, G., Jager, C., Seeger, G., Matthews, R. T., . . . Morawski, M. (2013). Unique features of extracellular matrix in the mouse medial nucleus of trapezoid body: Implications for physiological functions. *Neuroscience*, *228*, 215–234. https://doi.org/10.1016/j.neuroscience.2012.10.003

Blosa, M., Sonntag, M., Jager, C., Weigel, S., Seeger, J., Frischknecht, R., . . . Morawski, M. (2015). The extracellular matrix molecule brevican is an integral component of the machinery mediating fast synaptic transmission at the calyx of Held. *The Journal of Physiology*, *593*(19), 4341–4360. https://doi.org/10.1113/JP270849

Brakebusch, C., Seidenbecher, C. I., Asztely, F., Rauch, U., Matthies, H., Meyer, H., . . . Fassler, R. (2002). Brevican-deficient mice display impaired hippocampal CA1 long-term potentiation but show no obvious deficits in learning and memory. *Molecular and Cellular Biology*, *22*(21), 7417–7427.

Brewton, D. H., Kokash, J., Jimenez, O., Pena, E. R., & Razak, K. A. (2016). Age-related deterioration of perineuronal nets in the primary auditory cortex of mice. *Frontiers in Aging Neuroscience*, *8*, 270. https://doi.org/10.3389/fnagi.2016.00270

Bruckner, G., Brauer, K., Hartig, W., Wolff, J. R., Rickmann, M. J., Derouiche, A., . . . Reichenbach, A. (1993). Perineuronal nets provide a polyanionic, glia-associated form of microenvironment around certain neurons in many parts of the rat brain. *Glia*, *8*(3), 183–200. https://doi.org/10.1002/glia.440080306

Bruckner, G., Grosche, J., Schmidt, S., Hartig, W., Margolis, R. U., Delpech, B., . . . Schachner, M. (2000). Postnatal development of perineuronal nets in wild-type mice and in a mutant deficient in tenascin-R. *Journal of Comparative Neurology*, *428*(4), 616–629.

Bruckner, G., Morawski, M., & Arendt, T. (2008). Aggrecan-based extracellular matrix is an integral part of the human basal ganglia circuit. *Neuroscience*, *151*(2), 489–504. https://doi.org/10.1016/j.neuroscience.2007.10.033

Carulli, D., Pizzorusso, T., Kwok, J. C. F., Putignano, E., Poli, A., Forostyak, S., . . . Fawcett, J. W. (2010). Animals lacking link protein have attenuated perineuronal nets and persistent plasticity. *Brain: A Journal of Neurology*, *133*(Pt 8), 2331–2347. https://doi.org/10.1093/brain/awq145

Caterson, B. (2012). Fell-Muir Lecture: Chondroitin sulphate glycosaminoglycans: Fun for some and confusion for others. *International Journal of Experimental Pathology*, *93*(1), 1–10. https://doi.org/10.1111/j.1365-2613.2011.00807.x

Celio, M. R., & Blümcke, I. (1994). Perineuronal nets: A specialized form of extracellular matrix in the adult nervous system. *Brain Research Reviews*, *19*(1), 128–145.

Celio, M. R., Spreafico, R., Biasi, S. de, & Vitellaro-Zuccarello, L. (1998). Perineuronal nets: Past and present. *Trends in Neurosciences*, *21*(12), 510–515.

Chiquet-Ehrismann, R., & Tucker, R. P. (2011). Tenascins and the importance of adhesion modulation. *Cold Spring Harbor Perspectives in Biology*, *3*(5). https://doi.org/10.1101/cshperspect.a004960

Cummings, R. D. (2009). The repertoire of glycan determinants in the human glycome. *Molecular bioSystems*, *5*(10), 1087–1104. https://doi.org/10.1039/b907931a

Deepa, S. S., Carulli, D., Galtrey, C., Rhodes, K., Fukuda, J., Mikami, T., . . . Fawcett, J. W. (2006). Composition of perineuronal net extracellular matrix in rat brain: A different disaccharide composition for the net-associated proteoglycans. *The Journal of Biological Chemistry*, *281*(26), 17789–17800. https://doi.org/10.1074/jbc.M600544200

Dino, M. R., Harroch, S., Hockfield, S., & Matthews, R. T. (2006). Monoclonal antibody Cat-315 detects a glycoform of receptor protein tyrosine phosphatase beta/phosphacan early in CNS development that localizes to extrasynaptic sites prior to synapse formation. *Neuroscience*, *142*(4), 1055–1069. https://doi.org/10.1016/j.neuroscience.2006.07.054

Dityatev, A., & Fellin, T. (2008). Extracellular matrix in plasticity and epileptogenesis. *Neuron Glia Biology*, *4*(3), 235–247. https://doi.org/10.1017/S1740925X09000118

Dityatev, A., & Rusakov, D. A. (2011). Molecular signals of plasticity at the tetrapartite synapse. *Current Opinion in Neurobiology*, *21*(2), 353–359. https://doi.org/10.1016/j.conb.2010.12.006

Favuzzi, E., Marques-Smith, A., Deogracias, R., Winterflood, C. M., Sanchez-Aguilera, A., Mantoan, L., . . . Rico, B. (2017). Activity-dependent gating of parvalbumin interneuron function by the perineuronal net protein brevican. *Neuron*, *95*(3), 639–655.e10. https://doi.org/10.1016/j.neuron.2017.06.028

Fech, T., Calderon-Garciduenas, L., & Kulesza, R. J., JR. (2017). Characterization of the superior olivary complex of Canis lupus domesticus. *Hearing Research*, *351*, 130–140. https://doi.org/10.1016/j.heares.2017.06.010

Ford, M. C., Grothe, B., & Klug, A. (2009). Fenestration of the calyx of Held occurs sequentially along the tonotopic axis, is influenced by afferent activity, and facilitates glutamate clearance. *Journal of Comparative Neurology*, *514*(1), 92–106. https://doi.org/10.1002/cne.21998

Foscarin, S., Raha-Chowdhury, R., Fawcett, J. W., & Kwok, J. C. F. (2017). Brain ageing changes proteoglycan sulfation, rendering perineuronal nets more inhibitory. *Aging*, *9*(6), 1607–1622. https://doi.org/10.18632/aging.101256

Friauf, E. (2000). Development of chondroitin sulfate proteoglycans in the central auditory system of rats correlates with acquisition of mature properties. *Audiology & Neuro-otology*, *5*(5), 251–262. https://doi.org/10.1159/000013889

Frischknecht, R., Heine, M., Perrais, D., Seidenbecher, C. I., Choquet, D., & Gundelfinger, E. D. (2009). Brain extracellular matrix affects AMPA receptor lateral mobility and short-term synaptic plasticity. *Nature Neuroscience*, *12*(7), 897–904. https://doi.org/10.1038/nn.2338

Gazula, V.-R., Strumbos, J. G., Mei, X., Chen, H., Rahner, C., & Kaczmarek, L. K. (2010). Localization of Kv1.3 channels in presynaptic terminals of brainstem auditory neurons. *The Journal of Comparative Neurology*, *518*(16), 3205–3220. https://doi.org/10.1002/cne.22393

Geissler, M., Gottschling, C., Aguado, A., Rauch, U., Wetzel, C. H., Hatt, H., & Faissner, A. (2013). Primary hippocampal neurons, which lack four crucial extracellular matrix molecules, display abnormalities of synaptic structure and function and severe deficits in perineuronal net formation. *Journal of Neuroscience*, *33*(18), 7742–7755. https://doi.org/10.1523/JNEUROSCI.3275-12.2013

Gersdorff, H. von, & Borst, J. G. G. (2002). Short-term plasticity at the calyx of Held. *Nature Reviews. Neuroscience*, *3*(1), 53–64. https://doi.org/10.1038/nrn705

Giamanco, K. A., Morawski, M., & Matthews, R. T. (2010). Perineuronal net formation and structure in aggrecan knockout mice. *Neuroscience*, *170*(4), 1314–1327. https://doi.org/10.1016/j.neuroscience.2010.08.032

Gogolla, N., Caroni, P., Luthi, A., & Herry, C. (2009). Perineuronal nets protect fear memories from erasure. *Science*, *325*(5945), 1258–1261. https://doi.org/10.1126/science.1174146

Grande, G., & Wang, L.-Y. (2011). Morphological and functional continuum underlying heterogeneity in the spiking fidelity at the calyx of Held synapse in vitro. *Journal of Neuroscience*, *31*(38), 13386–13399. https://doi.org/10.1523/JNEUROSCI.0400-11.2011

Gundelfinger, E. D., Frischknecht, R., Choquet, D., & Heine, M. (2010). Converting juvenile into adult plasticity: a role for the brain's extracellular matrix. *European Journal of Neuroscience*, *31*(12), 2156–2165. https://doi.org/10.1111/j.1460-9568.2010.07253.x

Happel, M. F. K., Niekisch, H., Castiblanco Rivera, L. L., Ohl, F. W., Deliano, M., & Frischknecht, R. (2014). Enhanced cognitive flexibility in reversal learning induced by removal of the extracellular matrix in auditory cortex. *Proceedings of the National Academy of Sciences of the United States of America*, *111*(7), 2800–2805. https://doi.org/10.1073/pnas.1310272111

Hartig, W., Derouiche, A., Welt, K., Brauer, K., Grosche, J., Mader, M., . . . Bruckner, G. (1999). Cortical neurons immunoreactive for the potassium channel Kv3.1b subunit are predominantly surrounded by perineuronal nets presumed as a buffering system for cations. *Brain Research*, *842*(1), 15–29.

Hartig, W., Singer, A., Grosche, J., Brauer, K., Ottersen, O. P., & Bruckner, G. (2001). Perineuronal nets in the rat medial nucleus of the trapezoid body surround neurons immunoreactive for various amino acids, calcium-binding proteins and the potassium channel subunit Kv3.1b. *Brain Research*, *899*(1–2), 123–133.

Hilbig, H., Nowack, S., Boeckler, K., Bidmon, H.-J., & Zilles, K. (2007). Characterization of neuronal subsets surrounded by perineuronal nets in the rhesus auditory brainstem. *Journal of Anatomy*, *210*(5), 507–517. https://doi.org/10.1111/j.1469-7580.2007.00713.x

Hockfield, S., & McKay, R. D. (1983). A surface antigen expressed by a subset of neurons in the vertebrate central nervous system. *Proceedings of the National Academy of Sciences of the United States of America*, *80*(18), 5758–5761.

Hockfield, S., & Sur, M. (1990). Monoclonal antibody Cat-301 identifies Y-cells in the dorsal lateral geniculate nucleus of the cat. *Journal of Comparative Neurology, 300*(3), 320–330. https://doi.org/10.1002/cne.903000305

Hoffpauir, B. K., Grimes, J. L., Mathers, P. H., & Spirou, G. A. (2006). Synaptogenesis of the calyx of Held: Rapid onset of function and one-to-one morphological innervation. *Journal of Neuroscience, 26*(20), 5511–5523. https://doi.org/10.1523/JNEUROSCI.5525-05.2006

Holcomb, P. S., Hoffpauir, B. K., Hoyson, M. C., Jackson, D. R., Deerinck, T. J., Marrs, G. S., . . . Spirou, G. A. (2013). Synaptic inputs compete during rapid formation of the calyx of Held: A new model system for neural development. *Journal of Neuroscience, 33*(32), 12954–12969. https://doi.org/10.1523/JNEUROSCI.1087-13.2013

Hrabetova, S., Masri, D., Tao, L., Xiao, F., & Nicholson, C. (2009). Calcium diffusion enhanced after cleavage of negatively charged components of brain extracellular matrix by chondroitinase ABC. *Journal of Physiology, 587*(Pt 16), 4029–4049. https://doi.org/10.1113/jphysiol.2009.170092

Kalb, R. G., & Hockfield, S. (1988). Molecular evidence for early activity-dependent development of hamster motor neurons. *Journal of Neuroscience, 8*(7), 2350–2360.

Kandler, K., Clause, A., & Noh, J. (2009). Tonotopic reorganization of developing auditory brainstem circuits. *Nature Neuroscience, 12*(6), 711–717. https://doi.org/10.1038/nn.2332

Kandler, K., & Friauf, E. (1993). Pre- and postnatal development of efferent connections of the cochlear nucleus in the rat. *Journal of Comparative Neurology, 328*(2), 161–184. https://doi.org/10.1002/cne.903280202

Kolson, D. R., Wan, J., Wu, J., Dehoff, M., Brandebura, A. N., Qian, J., . . . Spirou, G. A. (2016). Temporal patterns of gene expression during calyx of held development. *Developmental Neurobiology, 76*(2), 166–189. https://doi.org/10.1002/dneu.22306

Kulesza, R. J., Jr. (2007). Cytoarchitecture of the human superior olivary complex: Medial and lateral superior olive. *Hearing Research, 225*(1–2), 80–90. https://doi.org/10.1016/j.heares.2006.12.006

Kulesza, R. J., Jr. (2008). Cytoarchitecture of the human superior olivary complex: nuclei of the trapezoid body and posterior tier. *Hearing research, 241*(1–2), 52–63. https://doi.org/10.1016/j.heares.2008.04.010

Lau, L. W., Cua, R., Keough, M. B., Haylock-Jacobs, S., & Yong, V. W. (2013). Pathophysiology of the brain extracellular matrix: a new target for remyelination. *Nature reviews. Neuroscience, 14*(10), 722–729. https://doi.org/10.1038/nrn3550

Leao, R. N., Sun, H., Svahn, K., Berntson, A., Youssoufian, M., Paolini, A. G., . . . Walmsley, B. (2006). Topographic organization in the auditory brainstem of juvenile mice is disrupted in congenital deafness. *Journal of Physiology, 571*(Pt 3), 563–578. https://doi.org/10.1113/jphysiol.2005.098780

Lurie, D. I., Pasic, T. R., Hockfield, S. J., & Rubel, E. W. (1997). Development of Cat-301 immunoreactivity in auditory brainstem nuclei of the gerbil. *Journal of Comparative Neurology, 380*(3), 319–334.

Matthews, R. T., Kelly, G. M., Zerillo, C. A., Gray, G., Tiemeyer, M., & Hockfield, S. (2002). Aggrecan glycoforms contribute to the molecular heterogeneity of perineuronal nets. *Journal of Neuroscience, 22*(17), 7536–7547.

Miyata, S., Komatsu, Y., Yoshimura, Y., Taya, C., & Kitagawa, H. (2012). Persistent cortical plasticity by upregulation of chondroitin 6-sulfation. *Nature Neuroscience, 15*(3), 414–422, S1–S2. https://doi.org/10.1038/nn.3023

Morawski, M., Bruckner, G., Arendt, T., & Matthews, R. T. (2012). Aggrecan: Beyond cartilage and into the brain. *International Journal of Biochemistry & Cell Biology*, *44*(5), 690–693. https://doi.org/10.1016/j.biocel.2012.01.010

Morawski, M., Bruckner, G., Jager, C., Seeger, G., & Arendt, T. (2010). Neurons associated with aggrecan-based perineuronal nets are protected against tau pathology in subcortical regions in Alzheimer's disease. *Neuroscience*, *169*(3), 1347–1363. https://doi.org/10.1016/j.neuroscience.2010.05.022

Morawski, M., Bruckner, G., Jager, C., Seeger, G., Kunzle, H., & Arendt, T. (2010). Aggrecan-based extracellular matrix shows unique cortical features and conserved subcortical principles of mammalian brain organization in the Madagascan lesser hedgehog tenrec (Echinops telfairi Martin, 1838). *Neuroscience*, *165*(3), 831–849. https://doi.org/10.1016/j.neuroscience.2009.08.018

Morawski, M., Bruckner, G., Jager, C., Seeger, G., Matthews, R. T., & Arendt, T. (2012). Involvement of perineuronal and perisynaptic extracellular matrix in Alzheimer's disease neuropathology. *Brain Pathology*, *22*(4), 547–561. https://doi.org/10.1111/j.1750-3639.2011.00557.x

Morawski, M., Bruckner, M. K., Riederer, P., Bruckner, G., & Arendt, T. (2004). Perineuronal nets potentially protect against oxidative stress. *Experimental Neurology*, *188*(2), 309–315. https://doi.org/10.1016/j.expneurol.2004.04.017

Morawski, M., Pavlica, S., Seeger, G., Grosche, J., Kouznetsova, E., Schliebs, R., . . . Arendt, T. (2010). Perineuronal nets are largely unaffected in Alzheimer model Tg2576 mice. *Neurobiology of Aging*, *31*(7), 1254–1256. https://doi.org/10.1016/j.neurobiolaging.2008.07.023

Morawski, M., Reinert, T., Meyer-Klaucke, W., Wagner, F. E., Troger, W., Reinert, A., . . . Arendt, T. (2015). Ion exchanger in the brain: Quantitative analysis of perineuronally fixed anionic binding sites suggests diffusion barriers with ion sorting properties. *Scientific Reports*, *5*, 16471. https://doi.org/10.1038/srep16471

Morest, D. K. (1968). The growth of synaptic endings in the mammalian brain: A study of the calyces of the trapezoid body. *Zeitschrift fur Anatomie und Entwicklungsgeschichte*, *127*(3), 201–220.

Myers, A. K., Ray, J., & Kulesza, R. J., Jr. (2012). Neonatal conductive hearing loss disrupts the development of the Cat-315 epitope on perineuronal nets in the rat superior olivary complex. *Brain Research*, *1465*, 34–47. https://doi.org/10.1016/j.brainres.2012.05.024

Pantazopoulos, H., Murray, E. A., & Berretta, S. (2008). Total number, distribution, and phenotype of cells expressing chondroitin sulfate proteoglycans in the normal human amygdala. *Brain Research*, *1207*, 84–95. https://doi.org/10.1016/j.brainres.2008.02.036

Pizzorusso, T., Medini, P., Berardi, N., Chierzi, S., Fawcett, J. W., & Maffei, L. (2002). Reactivation of ocular dominance plasticity in the adult visual cortex. *Science*, *298*(5596), 1248–1251. https://doi.org/10.1126/science.1072699

Rodriguez-Contreras, A., van Hoeve, John Silvio Soria, Habets, R. L. P., Locher, H., & Borst, J. G. G. (2008). Dynamic development of the calyx of Held synapse. *Proceedings of the National Academy of Sciences USA*, *105*(14), 5603–5608. https://doi.org/10.1073/pnas.0801395105

Rudy, B., & McBain, C. J. (2001). Kv3 channels: voltage-gated K+ channels designed for high-frequency repetitive firing. *Trends in Neurosciences*, *24*(9), 517–526.

Saroja, S. R., Sase, A., Kircher, S. G., Wan, J., Berger, J., Hoger, H., . . . Lubec, G. (2014). Hippocampal proteoglycans brevican and versican are linked to spatial memory of Sprague-Dawley rats in the Morris water maze. *Journal of Neurochemistry*, *130*(6), 797–804. https://doi.org/10.1111/jnc.12783

Satzler, K., Sohl, L. F., Bollmann, J. H., Borst, J. G. G., Frotscher, M., Sakmann, B., & Lubke, J. H. R. (2002). Three-dimensional reconstruction of a calyx of Held and its postsynaptic principal neuron in the medial nucleus of the trapezoid body. *Journal of Neuroscience*, *22*(24), 10567–10579.

Schmidt, E., Wolski, T. P., Jr., & Kulesza, R. J., Jr. (2010). Distribution of perineuronal nets in the human superior olivary complex. *Hearing research*, *265*(1–2), 15–24. https://doi.org/10.1016/j.heares.2010.03.077

Schneggenburger, R., & Forsythe, I. D. (2006). The calyx of Held. *Cell and Tissue Research*, *326*(2), 311–337. https://doi.org/10.1007/s00441-006-0272-7

Seeger, G., Brauer, K., Hartig, W., & Bruckner, G. (1994). Mapping of perineuronal nets in the rat brain stained by colloidal iron hydroxide histochemistry and lectin cytochemistry. *Neuroscience*, *58*(2), 371–388.

Sonntag, M., Blosa, M., Schmidt, S., Rubsamen, R., & Morawski, M. (2015). Perineuronal nets in the auditory system. *Hearing Research*, *329*, 21–32. https://doi.org/10.1016/j.heares.2014.12.012

Sonntag, M., Englitz, B., Typlt, M., & Rubsamen, R. (2011). The calyx of Held develops adult-like dynamics and reliability by hearing onset in the mouse in vivo. *Journal of Neuroscience*, *31*(18), 6699–6709. https://doi.org/10.1523/JNEUROSCI.0575-11.2011

Suttkus, A., Morawski, M., & Arendt, T. (2016). Protective properties of neural extracellular matrix. *Molecular Neurobiology*, *53*(1), 73–82. https://doi.org/10.1007/s12035-014-8990-4

Suttkus, A., Rohn, S., Jager, C., Arendt, T., & Morawski, M. (2012). Neuroprotection against iron-induced cell death by perineuronal nets: An in vivo analysis of oxidative stress. *American Journal of Neurodegenerative Disease*, *1*(2), 122–129.

Suttkus, A., Rohn, S., Weigel, S., Glockner, P., Arendt, T., & Morawski, M. (2014). Aggrecan, link protein and tenascin-R are essential components of the perineuronal net to protect neurons against iron-induced oxidative stress. *Cell Death & Disease*, *5*, e1119. https://doi.org/10.1038/cddis.2014.25

Sykova, E., & Nicholson, C. (2008). Diffusion in brain extracellular space. *Physiological Reviews*, *88*(4), 1277–1340. https://doi.org/10.1152/physrev.00027.2007

Takesian, A. E., & Hensch, T. K. (2013). Balancing plasticity/stability across brain development. *Progress in Brain Research*, *207*, 3–34. https://doi.org/10.1016/B978-0-444-63327-9.00001-1

Taschenberger, H., & Gersdorff, H. von. (2000). Fine-tuning an auditory synapse for speed and fidelity: Developmental changes in presynaptic waveform, EPSC kinetics, and synaptic plasticity. *The Journal of Neuroscience*, *20*(24), 9162–9173.

Taschenberger, H., Leao, R. M., Rowland, K. C., Spirou, G. A., & Gersdorff, H. von. (2002). Optimizing synaptic architecture and efficiency for high-frequency transmission. *Neuron*, *36*(6), 1127–1143.

Tsien, R. Y. (2013). Very long-term memories may be stored in the pattern of holes in the perineuronal net. *Proceedings of the National Academy of Sciences USA*, *110*(30), 12456–12461. https://doi.org/10.1073/pnas.1310158110

van Harreveld, A. (1965). Effect of cerebral asphyxiation on a well-established conditioned reflex. *Journal of Comparative and Physiological Psychology*, *60*(2), 299–302.

Virgintino, D., Perissinotto, D., Girolamo, F., Mucignat, M. T., Montanini, L., Errede, M., . . . Perris, R. (2009). Differential distribution of aggrecan isoforms in perineuronal nets of the human cerebral cortex. *Journal of Cellular and Molecular Medicine*, *13*(9B), 3151–3173. https://doi.org/10.1111/j.1582-4934.2009.00694.x

Vivo, L. de, Landi, S., Panniello, M., Baroncelli, L., Chierzi, S., Mariotti, L., . . . Ratto, G. M. (2013). Extracellular matrix inhibits structural and functional plasticity of dendritic spines in the adult visual cortex. *Nature communications*, *4*, 1484. https://doi.org/10.1038/ncomms2491

Wang, D., & Fawcett, J. (2012). The perineuronal net and the control of CNS plasticity. *Cell and Tissue Research*, *349*(1), 147–160. https://doi.org/10.1007/s00441-012-1375-y

Yamada, H., Fredette, B., Shitara, K., Hagihara, K., Miura, R., Ranscht, B., . . . Yamaguchi, Y. (1997). The brain chondroitin sulfate proteoglycan brevican associates with astrocytes ensheathing cerebellar glomeruli and inhibits neurite outgrowth from granule neurons. *Journal of Neuroscience*, *17*(20), 7784–7795.

Yamaguchi, Y. (2000). Lecticans: Organizers of the brain extracellular matrix. *Cellular and Molecular Life Sciences*, *57*(2), 276–289. https://doi.org/10.1007/PL00000690

Yu, W.-M., & Goodrich, L. V. (2014). Morphological and physiological development of auditory synapses. *Hearing Research*, *311*, 3–16. https://doi.org/10.1016/j.heares.2014.01.007

Zaremba, S., Guimaraes, A., Kalb, R. G., & Hockfield, S. (1989). Characterization of an activity-dependent, neuronal surface proteoglycan identified with monoclonal antibody Cat-301. *Neuron*, *2*(3), 1207–1219.

Zimmermann, D. R., & Dours-Zimmermann, M. T. (2008). Extracellular matrix of the central nervous system: From neglect to challenge. *Histochemistry and Cell Biology*, *130*(4), 635–653. https://doi.org/10.1007/s00418-008-0485-9

CHAPTER 16

THE NUCLEI OF THE LATERAL LEMNISCUS

FELIX FELMY

Abstract

Parallel processing streams guide ascending auditory information through the processing hierarchy of the auditory brainstem. Many of these processing streams converge in the lateral lemnisucus, the fiber bundle that connects the cochlear nuclei and superior olivary complex with the inferior colliculus. The neuronal populations within the lateral lemniscus can be segregated according to their gross structure-function relationships into three distinct nuclei. These nuclei are termed ventral, intermedial, and dorsal nucleus, according to their position within the lemniscal fiber bundle. The complexity of their input pattern increases in an ascending fashion. The three nuclei employ different neurotransmitters and exhibit distinct synaptic and biophysical features. Yet they all share a large heterogeneity. Functionally, the ventral nucleus of the lateral lemniscus has been hypothesized to reduce spectral splatter by generating a rapid, temporally precise feedforward onset inhibition in the inferior colliculus. In the intermedial nucleus of the lateral lemniscus a cross-frequency integration has been observed. The hallmark of the dorsal nucleus of the lateral lemniscus is the generation of a long-lasting inhibition in its contralateral counterpart and the inferior colliculus. This inhibition is proposed to generate a suppression of sound sources during reverberations and could act as a temporal filter capable of removing spurious interaural time differences. While great advances have been made in understanding the role that these nuclei play in auditory processing, the functional diversity of the individual neuronal responsiveness within each nucleus remains largely unsolved.

Keywords: nuclei of the lateral lemniscus, auditory brainstem, structure-function relationship, tonotopy, synaptic integration, supra-threshold spike pattern, spectral filter, temporal filter

In this chapter, we summarize and discuss the current literature concerning the auditory brainstem nuclei located in the lateral lemniscus (LL). In line with classical neuroscience research, we relate structure to function in order to elucidate the processing mechanisms of these auditory brainstem nuclei. We first look at the structure of the auditory nuclei, which are embedded within this fiber bundle. We summarize the different types of transmitters, specific expression patterns, specialized morphologies, and how the tonotopy is arranged. We continue to review the biophysical properties of the different cell types within the LL. These properties include action potential generation and firing behavior, as well as synaptic input properties. Furthermore, we discuss functional data showing how sound information is integrated in the nuclei of the LL. These considerations will guide us to form a hypothesis regarding their functional significance. Finally, by bringing these different aspects together, we seek to obtain a glimpse of the processing power of the auditory nuclei that are immersed in the fiber bundle of the LL.

The Structure and Connectivity of the Auditory Nuclei within the Lateral Lemniscus

The LL is formed by a thick fiber bundle, which connects the auditory brainstem with the auditory midbrain (Figure 16.1). Auditory information travels from the cochlear nucleus, the superior olivary complex (SOC), and the neurons within the LL to the inferior colliculus (IC). Within this thick axonal bundle, several nuclei are intermingled, the nuclei of the LL.

Separation into Nuclei

The neuronal populations in the LL can be separated. The most distinct part of the LL is the dorsal part that makes up the dorsal nucleus of the lateral lemniscus (DNLL). This structure is well defined as a roundish nucleus at the junction of the LL and commissure of Probst, ventral to the border of the IC. DNLL neurons are separated by those that follow ventrally in the LL. In bats, a region of the intermedial nucleus of the lateral lemniscus (INLL) is well defined. In rodents, this region merges more continuously into the elongated ventral nucleus of the lateral lemniscus (VNLL). Thus, the border between INLL/VNLL is difficult to define in some species. The boarders of the VNLL are best defined at lateral and ventral edge.

Ventral nucleus of the lateral lemniscus.

The overall organization of the VNLL seems complex and is species dependent. In general, the VNLL consists of a heterogeneous group of various cell types. This heterogeneity is obvious in the echolocating bat *Eptesicus fuscus*, where a subset of globular cells is aggregated to form the columnar region (Covey & Casseday, 1986), while the

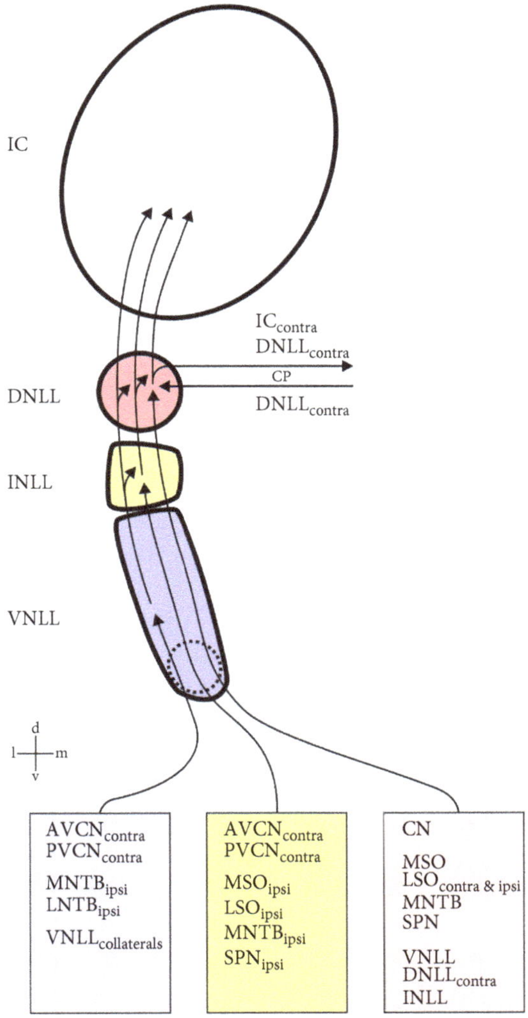

FIGURE 16.1. Simplified input output pattern of the nuclei of the lateral lemniscus (NLL). The ventral nucleus receives inputs from the anterior and posterior ventral cochlear nucleus (AVCN and PVCN) and the medial and lateral nucleus of the trapezoid body (MNTB and LNTB) from the superior olivary complex (SOC). In addition, ventral nucleus of the lateral lemniscus (VNLL) neurons themselves are indicated to generate collaterals within the VNLL while their ascending projections target the intermedial nucleus of the lateral lemniscus (INLL), dorsal nucleus of the lateral lemniscus (DNLL), and inferior colliculus (IC). The INLL receives also input from the ventral cochlear nuclei (CN) and the SOC. Input from the SOC is derived from medial and lateral superior olive neurons (MSO and LSO) the MNTB, and the superior paraolivary nucleus (SPN). INLL input projects the DNLL and IC. DNLL neurons receive inputs from the CN, SOC, and the LL nuclei. The output structures of the DNLL are the ipsilateral IC and the contralateral IC and DNLL via the commissure of Probst (CP). All nuclei of the LL receive cholinergic modulator inputs. Descending inputs from cortical structure appear in all LL nuclei, in the DNLL with a tonotopic arrangement.

rest of the VNLL contains other cell types. These other cell types are dominated by multipolar neurons (Covey & Casseday, 1986). In rodents, this organization is absent, but the ventral and dorsal VNLL parts still hold differences in the neuronal population. In the gerbil VNLL globular cells are more prominent in the ventral aspect compared to the dorsal part (Mylius, Brosch, Scheich, & Budinger, 2013). In the same species multipolar and elongated cells are present in the entire VNLL with a bias toward the dorsal part (Mylius et al., 2013). This distribution of neuronal morphologies appears to match with that of guinea pig (Schofield & Cant, 1997), rat (Merchan & Berbel, 1996; Zhao & Wu, 2001), cat (Adams, 1979), and humans (Adams, 1997). Thus, as a general emerging picture, the VNLL is composed of a morphologically heterogeneous cell population, with biased localizations for most mammals: globular cells being located in the ventral region, while elongated and multipolar cells are more frequent in the dorsal part.

A morphological specialty of ventral, globular VNLL neurons is their large glutamatergic input that is targeted toward their soma. This endbulb type synapse was found in cats (Adams, 1997; Smith, Massie, & Joris, 2005; Stotler, 1953), guinea pig (Schofield & Cant, 1997), mice (Caspari, Baumann, Garcia-Pino, & Koch, 2015), gerbils (Berger, Meyer, Ammer, & Felmy, 2014), rats (Friauf & Ostwald, 1988), bats (Covey & Casseday, 1986; Vater, Covey, & Casseday, 1997), and humans (Adams, 1997). Globular VNLL neurons therefore form a similar synaptic input-output structure as has been found in the MNTB (calyx of Held) and the anterior ventral cochlear nucleus (endbulb of Held).

The heterogeneity of VNLL cells is also given in the expression of the diverse transmitter types. In the VNLL, glycinergic and GABergic cells are present (Moore & Trussell, 2017; Riquelme, Saldana, Osen, Ottersen, & Merchan, 2001; Saint Marie, Shneiderman, & Stanforth, 1997; Ueyama et al., 1999; Vater, Kossl, & Horn, 1992). The lack of glutamatergic neurons in the VNLL is further documented by in-situ hybridizations that showed only expression of vesicular inhibitory amino acid transporter (T. Ito, Bishop, & Oliver, 2011). Interestingly, it was recently demonstrated that glycine and γ-aminobutyric acid (GABA) are co-released simultaneously from a subset of VNLL neurons in the IC (Moore & Trussell, 2017). Besides GABAergic and glycinergic cells, a population of neurons in the VNLL stains for neither (Riquelme et al., 2001; Saint Marie et al., 1997), indicating a small portion of neurons with an unresolved transmitter type. With respect to calcium binding proteins, VNLL neurons have been shown to be parvalbuminergic (Caicedo, d'Aldin, Puel, & Eybalin, 1996; Lohmann & Friauf, 1996). In guinea pigs, VNLL neurons are also positive for calbindin (Caicedo et al., 1996), while in bats and in rats calretinin positive staining is observed (Lohmann & Friauf, 1996; Vater & Braun, 1994). Ion channel labelling showed that VNLL neurons in bats express Kv1.1. This labelling was most prominent in the columnar region (Rosenberger, Fremouw, Casseday, & Covey, 2003). In rodents, HCN1 staining is more prominent in the dorsal part, while HCN2 staining is present throughout the VNLL (Caspari et al.,

2015; Koch, Braun, Kapfer, & Grothe, 2004). $GABA_B$ receptors have been described in the VNLL with a stronger density in the dorsal aspect (Jamal, Zhang, Finlayson, Porter, & Zhang, 2011). $GABA_A$ receptors appear to differ in subunit composition between the dorsal and the ventral VNLL (Campos, de Cabo, Wisden, Juiz, & Merlo, 2001). Finally, nicotinic acetylcholine (ACH) receptors have been detected throughout the VNLL (Happe & Morley, 2004). Taken together, neurons in the VNLL form a heterogeneous population based on morphology and protein expression patterns. Since globular cells receive a specific type of synaptic input and are located mainly in the ventral aspect of the VNLL, they constitute a rather distinct population of specialized neurons. It is expected that overall the VNNL cell populations show different biophysical adaptations as indicated by the antibody staining for membrane channels.

The tonotopic organization of the VNLL is less clear cut compared to other auditory brainstem nuclei. In vivo recordings and tracing studies suggest that the tonotopic organization is complex in the VNLL (Covey & Casseday, 1986, 1991; Kelly, Liscum, van Adel, & Ito, 1998; Malmierca, Leergaard, Bajo, Bjaalie, & Merchan, 1998; Merchan & Berbel, 1996). In rats, it has been shown that the most lateral neurons of the VNLL represent largely low frequencies and more central neurons high frequencies (Kelly, Liscum, et al., 1998; Merchan & Berbel, 1996). In the cat, frequency domains are originally reported to be organized in a dorso-ventral order (Aitkin, Anderson, & Brugge, 1970), but have since been shown to be organized in a patchy way (Malmierca et al., 1998). Only in the bat columnar region, the tonotopy is well defined and follows a high- to low-frequency gradient along the ventro-dorsal axis (Covey & Casseday, 1986, 1991).

VNLL neurons receive inputs mainly from the cochlear nuclei and the medial nucleus of the trapezoid body (Glendenning, Brunso-Bechtold, Thompson, & Masterton, 1981; Huffman & Covey, 1995; Kelly, van Adel, & Ito, 2009; Spangler, Warr, & Henkel, 1985; Zook & Casseday, 1987). In bats, evidence for a small projection from the lateral nucleus of the trapezoid body was presented (Huffman & Covey, 1995). The large somatic endbulb synapses on globular VNLL neurons originates from neurons in the posterior ventral cochlear nuclei most likely from octopus cells (Adams, 1997; Friauf & Ostwald, 1988; Schofield & Cant, 1997; Smith et al., 2005). In addition bushy cells innervate the region of the VNLL (Friauf & Ostwald, 1988; Huffman & Covey, 1995; Smith, Joris, Carney, & Yin, 1991; Smith, Joris, & Yin, 1993), most likely without the restriction towards globular VNLL neurons. Also axons originating in the core of the posterior cochlear nucleus innervate the overall VNLL (Thompson, 1998; Warr, 1969). Inhibitory inputs to the VNLL originate from the medial nucleus of the trapezoid body or stem from internal collaterals. Thus, both excitatory and inhibitory inputs to VNLL neurons are fast and precisely timed. The main projection of VNLL neurons is to the IC (Kelly et al., 2009; Moore & Trussell, 2017; Tanaka, Otani, Tokunaga, & Sugita, 1985; Willard & Martin, 1983; Zook & Casseday, 1982, 1987). Besides these direct projections, axons of VNLL neurons are thought to terminate on INLL and the DNLL neurons (Kelly et al., 2009) and within the VNLL itself, where globular neurons might feedforward inhibition to other VNLL neurons (Nayagam, Clarey, & Paolini, 2005). In addition, VNLL neurons receive cholinergic inputs, most likely in form of volume transmission. This follows from the presence of nicotinic (Happe & Morley, 2004) and metabotropic (Franzen et al., 2015) ACH receptors. Where these cholinergic fibers might originate from is so far not fully clarified.

Intermedial nucleus of the lateral lemniscus

As some authors define a short segment of the lateral lemniscus dorsal to the VNLL and ventral to the DNLL as INLL, we will discuss the anatomical and morphological properties of these neurons. This region appears morphologically better defined in bats compared to other mammals.

Elongated cells sending their dendrites orthogonal to the ascending fibers are the hallmark of the INLL, as described in bats (Covey & Casseday, 1986) and gerbils (Mylius et al., 2013). In addition, the presence of globular cells and multipolar cells has been described in bats (Covey & Casseday, 1986) and gerbils respectively (Mylius et al., 2013). In cats, elongated and multipolar neurons are also located in this region (Adams, 1979; Glendenning et al., 1981). Thus, the common denominator of neuron types in the INLL across species appears to be elongated, bipolar morphologies.

The neuronal population assigned to the INLL expresses predominantly parvalbumin (Caicedo et al., 1996; Lohmann & Friauf, 1996; Vater & Braun, 1994). Some of these neurons are GABAergic in bats (Vater et al., 1992), but in cats, rats and mice most neurons are non-GABAergic and non-glycinergic (T. Ito et al., 2011; Riquelme et al., 2001; Saint Marie et al., 1997; Ueyama et al., 1999). Using in-situ hybridizations T. Ito et al. (2011) observed only vesicular glutamate expressing cells in the INLL of rats and mice. Thus, the interface between the VNLL and the DNLL is generated by a population of glutamatergic, excitatory neurons. As in the VNLL, the INLL region expresses nicotinic ACH receptors (Happe & Morley, 2004). In INLL Kv1.1 was only expressed in a third of all INLL neurons (Rosenberger et al., 2003).

For the tonotopy of the INLL, the best frequencies of neurons decrease along a ventro-dorso axis, along the ascending fibers in bats (Covey & Casseday, 1991; Yavuzoglu, Schofield, & Wenstrup, 2010). In rats, however, a specific tonotopic organization of this INLL region seems not apparent at a first glance (Kelly, Buckthought, & Kidd, 1998). Neurons of the INLL receive inputs from the major nuclei of the superior olivary complex and the cochlear nuclei (Kelly et al., 2009; Thompson, 1998) and send their axons to the inferior colliculus (Kelly et al., 2009; Zook & Casseday, 1982).

Dorsal nucleus of the lateral lemniscus

The crossing of two fiber bundles is an excellent landmark of the DNLL. Here, the fibers of the lateral lemniscus and the commissure of Probst generate a T-junction. The commissure of Probst is a fiber bundle that connects the DNLL hemispheres with each other. The neurons at this fiber crossing represent the first cluster of neurons ventral to the IC border. Thus, the DNLL is one of the "simplest to spot" nuclei in the LL. However, lateral to the DNLL, a small cell population resides that has been attributed to a different nucleus called the sagulum nucleus, a neuronal population that will not be addressed here further.

Neurons in the DNLL come in different shapes. In one study, the axial diameters of the soma were quantified and subsequently separated based on their shape. Nine types of neurons could be identified (Kane & Barone, 1980), categorized into round ovoid and elongated, each with three different sizes. Other studies defined multipolar, bipolar, round and elongated cell types (Adams, 1979; Bajo, Merchan, Lopez, & Rouiller, 1993; Iwahori, 1986; Mylius et al., 2013; Wu & Kelly, 1995). Importantly, all of the different morphological cell types exhibited the same action potential firing properties (Wu & Kelly, 1995). Therefore, the morphological differentiation seems not to segregate DNLL neurons into biophysically distinct neurons. The dendrites of DNLL neurons have received little attention regarding their extent and orientation. Morphologically, these dendrites are relatively thin and without spiny protrusions. Overall, the heterogeneity of DNLL neurons might rather reflect a large continuum of morphological variability than clearly defined subsets of neurons. Whether such a large morphological variability supports a specific function remains unresolved.

Despite this morphological heterogeneity at least 80% of DNLL neurons were shown to be GABAergic (Riquelme et al., 2001; Saint Marie et al., 1997; Ueyama et al., 1999; Vater et al., 1992). The remaining 20% of neurons were also negative for glycine (Saint Marie et al., 1997). It remains unclear whether this cell population contains glutamatergic or neuro-modulatory transmitters and how it is inter-connected within the auditory brainstem pathways. Expression patterns have been determined by immunohistochemistry showing that DNLL neurons preferentially express the slow calcium buffer parvalbumin (Ammer, Grothe, & Felmy, 2012; Caicedo et al., 1996; Lohmann & Friauf, 1996; Seto-Ohshima, Aoki, Semba, Emson, & Heizmann, 1990; Vater & Braun, 1994). Interestingly, 20% of DNLL neurons are calbindinergic (Ammer et al., 2012; Caicedo et al., 1996; Lohmann & Friauf, 1996). Whether this calbindinergic subset matches with the non-GABAergic neurons is not known. Other functional markers whose expression has been demonstrated are Kv1.1 (Rosenberger et al., 2003), HCN2 but not HCN1 (Koch et al., 2004), $GABA_A$ receptors (Campos et al., 2001), low amounts of $GABA_{B2}$ receptors (Jamal et al., 2011), and VGlut2 (Di Bonito et al., 2013).

Like many other auditory brainstem nuclei, the DNLL is tonotopically organized. The tonotopic organization has been evaluated either by activity markers or by synaptic connectivity with respect to other well-known topographic maps. In gerbils, early studies suggested that low frequencies are represented in the dorso-medial portion, while high frequencies are present in the ventro-medial part (Ryan, Woolf,

& Sharp, 1982). This dorso-medial tonotopical arrangement was also described by retrograde labeling of the IC (Bajo, Merchan, Malmierca, Nodal, & Bjaalie, 1999; Shneiderman, Stanforth, Henkel, & Saint Marie, 1999) and anterograde labeling of the SOC (Shneiderman, Oliver, & Henkel, 1988; Shneiderman et al., 1999). Moreover, the dorso-ventral tonotopic axis is in agreement with in vivo studies performed in bats (Covey, 1993; Markovitz & Pollak, 1994). In rats, however, two studies indicated that the tonotopy follows a concentric arrangement. Here, low frequencies are represented in the center, while high frequencies are present in the outer shell of the DNLL (Kelly, Liscum, et al., 1998; Merchan, Saldana, & Plaza, 1994).

Ascending projections arrive at the DNLL from the nuclei of the SOC, and information is then forwarded from the DNLL to the IC. Inputs arise mainly from the medial and lateral superior olive (Glendenning et al., 1981; Henkel, 1997; Huffman & Covey, 1995; Kelly et al., 2009; Shneiderman et al., 1999; Siveke, Pecka, Seidl, Baudoux, & Grothe, 2006). Besides these inputs, it has been indicated that some axons originate in the superior para-olivary nuclei (Kelly et al., 2009) and the medial nucleus of the trapezoid body (Siveke et al., 2006; Spangler et al., 1985). For rats (Kelly et al., 2009) and bats (Covey & Casseday, 1986; Huffman & Covey, 1995; Yang, Liu, & Pollak, 1996; Zook & Casseday, 1985) connections from the VNLL and INLL and in cats (Glendenning et al., 1981) also minor collaterals from the cochlear nucleus to DNLL neurons have been described. Also inputs from the cochlear nucleus to the DNLL have been observed (Thompson, 1998; Warr, 1969). Besides this ascending input, a small number of descending inputs from higher brain areas enter and likely terminate in the DNLL in a tonotopic fashion (Budinger, Brosch, Scheich, & Mylius, 2013). Thus, feedback from cortical structures might be able to influence auditory processing at the stage of the DNLL. The DNLL in turn projects only to two nuclei. One nucleus is the contralateral DNLL; the other nuclei are the both IC hemispheres. Retrograde labeling from the IC stains the DNLL (Gonzalez-Hernandez, Mantolan-Sarmiento, Gonzalez-Gonzalez, & Perez-Gonzalez, 1996; Kelly et al., 2009; Shneiderman et al., 1999; Tanaka et al., 1985; Willard & Martin, 1983; Zook & Casseday, 1982). Retrograde tracing of the DNLL labels its contralateral counterpart (Glendenning et al., 1981; Huffman & Covey, 1995; Oliver & Shneiderman, 1989), and anterograde labeling of the DNLL output yields staining in the contralateral DNLL and the IC (Bajo et al., 1993).

Taken together, the DNLL receives tonotopically organized excitatory inputs from the medial superior olive, the lateral superior olive and, to a smaller extent, from the cochlear nucleus. Glycinergic inhibitory inputs are provided by the VNLL, the medial nucleus of the trapezoid body, and the lateral superior olive, while GABAergic inputs originate predominantly from the contralateral DNLL and from the superior para-olivary nuclei. The tonotopically organized output of the DNLL is GABAergic and projects to the contralateral DNLL and both IC hemispheres. Thus, the DNLL integrates information from a large number of lower auditory brainstem areas. This connectivity suggests that the DNLL functions as an inhibitory gate for the IC by using highly processed auditory information from various sources.

Cellular Features of Neurons in the Auditory Nuclei of the Lateral Lemniscus

In the following section the synaptic and biophysical properties of neurons in the LL are discussed. The data for this section is largely based on single cell recordings in vitro obtained from rodents.

Ventral Nucleus of the Lateral Lemniscus

Similar to their morphological heterogeneity, VNLL neurons show a wide range of firing behaviors when recorded in vitro (Zhao & Wu, 2001). Neurons located in the dorsal part exhibit sustained firing with very rapid onset and strong hyperpolarizing current (I_h) (Caspari et al., 2015). In the ventral region, firing patterns are characterized by a single rapid onset action potential (Caspari et al., 2015; Franzen et al., 2015). For globular cells in the ventral part of the VNLL, the onset firing pattern emerges during development (Franzen et al., 2015). Interestingly, during late postnatal refinement, the input resistance and membrane time constant decrease (Franzen et al., 2015), resulting in a decreased cell capacitance (Baumann & Koch, 2017; Franzen et al., 2015). Thus, smaller and leakier neurons with large somatic excitation are generated during late postnatal development. This process generates neurons suited for rapid voltage signaling with very short latencies (Franzen et al., 2015). Furthermore, globular VNLL neurons display membrane resonance properties. These intrinsic membrane dynamics are thought to facilitate action potential generation at a certain input frequency. For globular VNLL neurons, the resonance frequencies are low compared to neurons of the medial and lateral superior olive, despite exhibiting similar onset firing patterns in vitro (Fischer, Leibold, & Felmy, 2018). This difference is due to a larger input resistance compared to the extremely leaky neurons in the SOC (Fischer et al., 2018). The resonance frequency in the VNLL ranges between 10 and 100 Hz and therefore promotes matching input rates. Thus, based on their intrinsic biophysical properties, VNLL neurons are ideally suited to respond rapidly and with high precision to sounds whose amplitude is modulated at 10 to 100 Hz.

VNLL neurons receive inhibitory and excitatory inputs (Baumann & Koch, 2017; Irfan, Zhang, & Wu, 2005; Zhao & Wu, 2001). Individual neurons receive inhibitory input via $GABA_A$ receptors only or via both $GABA_A$ and glycine-receptors, while excitation is mediated by non-NMDA and NMDA-receptors (Irfan et al., 2005). Where the GABAergic input originates is not fully understood. It may originate from a possible GABA-positive subpopulation of neurons of the lateral nucleus of the trapezoid body, which in bats is connected to the VNLL (Huffman & Covey, 1995). Excitatory inputs appear to be distributed through the VNLL in a size-dependent manner—the excitatory post-synaptic current (EPSC) of a single fiber being the fastest and largest in the ventral aspect of the VNLL (Caspari et al., 2015). This distinct distribution of input size appears not be present for the inhibitory inputs (Caspari et al., 2015). The strong excitation delivered by a single somatic fiber in juvenile gerbil ventral VNLL neurons is unable to drive supra-threshold output reliably (Berger et al., 2014), thus indicating that integration is required. During late postnatal development, these large inputs increase even more in size (Baumann & Koch, 2017); F. Felmy, unpublished results). This increase in synaptic current and an increase in excitability are probably sufficient to generate a faithful one-to-one transmission in fully matured VNLL neurons. This is consistent with in vivo on-cell recordings that show a pre-potential followed by the large postsynaptic spike (Adams, 1997). Contrary, however to the situation in the medial nucleus of the trapezoid body, it seems that more than one large somatic synapse targets a single globular VNLL neuron (Berger et al., 2014), possibly generating additional safety-factors for synaptic transmission during periods of high activity.

The development of large synaptic inputs to globular, ventral VNLL neurons is modulated by acetylcholine. Treating mice with nicotine during development leads to smaller excitatory inputs (Baumann & Koch, 2017). This treatment appears selective for the synaptic inputs as membrane properties were unchanged. The effect was driven by nicotinic ACH-Rs, some of which are calcium permeable and thereby able to modulate gene expression. Besides this influence of nACH-Rs on development, mACH-Rs can be activated on globular VNLL neurons (Franzen et al., 2015). These receptors reduce the action potential current threshold, which leads to changes in firing behavior in juvenile neurons. Thus, acetylcholine influences VNLL neurons on various levels at least during late postnatal development.

Intermedial Nucleus of the Lateral Lemniscus

The cellular features of the INLL have not been quantified. Since it is difficult to distinguish between the dorsal part of the VNLL and the INLL in rodents and both nuclei contain elongated cells, it is likely that INLL cell properties match those reported for dorsal VNLL neurons.

Dorsal Nucleus of the Lateral Lemniscus

The biophysical properties of DNLL neurons have been studied in various species and age groups. The membrane properties of DNLL neurons change during late postnatal development (Ahuja & Wu, 2000; Ammer et al., 2012). As in many other brainstem nuclei, input resistance and time constant become smaller during development, while the resting potential remains stable. Overall, the variability of membrane properties at rest is high for DNLL neurons. In mature neurons, for example, the membrane resistance can vary by a factor of 10, ranging from 20 to 200 MOhm. Despite their strong heterogeneity, it is difficult to assign firing properties to specific neuronal morphologies (Wu & Kelly, 1995). Neurons in the DNLL generate large action potentials when challenged with current injections or synaptic stimulations. During long-lasting current injections, these neurons fire sustained action potentials with little adaptation (Ahuja & Wu, 2000; Ammer et al., 2012; Porres, Meyer, Grothe, & Felmy, 2011; Wu & Kelly, 1995). In general, DNLL neurons appear highly excitable and the high-input resistance allows incoming EPSCs to have a strong impact on voltage signaling. During late postnatal development, the somatic action potential size increases and the half-width decreases (Ahuja & Wu, 2000; Ammer et al., 2012). Mature DNLL neurons exhibit a small I_h that activates at low membrane potentials (Fu, Brezden, & Wu, 1997). In gerbils this I_h current hardly becomes activated upon strong inhibition (Ammer, Siveke, & Felmy, 2015). Whether activation kinetics of this channel change during heavy synaptic inputs in an NO dependent manner, like in the MNTB (Steinert et al., 2008), and thereby increase its impact on voltage signaling, remains unknown. The presence of high-voltage-gated and A-type potassium currents has been described (Fu, Wu, Brezden, & Kelly, 1996). It should be noted that DNLL neurons express hardly any low–voltage-gated potassium currents (Fu et al., 1996), consistent with the expression analysis in bats (Rosenberger et al., 2003). In addition, somatic action potentials were shown to activate calcium influx through voltage-gated calcium channels (Porres et al., 2011).

Neurons in the DNLL receive all three major synaptic inputs: GABA, glycine, and glutamate. Inhibitory inputs are hyperpolarizing, since the chloride reversal is negative in respect to the resting potential (Ammer et al., 2015). GABAergic inputs are driven by ionotropic $GABA_A$ receptors (Pecka et al., 2007). These inputs show a frequency-dependent buildup (Ammer et al., 2015). In addition, spillover and asynchronous release prolong the decay of the synaptic GABAergic conductance in a frequency-dependent manner (Ammer et al., 2015). Since little I_h or low-voltage-activated potassium current (K_{LT}) are activated between maximal hyperpolarization and action potential threshold, the GABAergic inhibition is integrated passively. Passive integration enhances the time course of the GABAergic IPSP (Ammer et al., 2015). Thus, strong activity in the GABAergic inputs prolongs the time courses of IPSPs and generates long-lasting inhibitory action. The pattern and synaptic parameters of the glycinergic inhibition remain unclear. Some of our initial recordings indicate that glycinergic inputs show asynchronous release during and after high-frequency stimulation similar to GABAergic inputs.

Postsynaptic glutamatergic currents are mediated by α-amino-3-hydroxy-5-methyl-4-isoxazolepropionic acid (AMPA) and *N*-methyl-D-aspartate acid (NMDA) receptors (Ammer et al., 2012; Fu, Brezden, Kelly, & Wu, 1997; Kelly & Kidd, 2000; Porres et al., 2011; Siveke et al., 2018; Wu & Kelly, 1996). Consistent with the strong heterogeneity of morphological, passive, and active membrane parameters, glutamatergic inputs to the DNLL show a large variability. This variability applies to the time constants, the size, the short-term plasticity, and the NMDA/AMPA ratio of glutamatergic inputs (Ammer et al., 2012; Porres et al., 2011). Importantly, action potential generation is supported by NMDA receptors even under normal extracellular Mg^{2+} concentrations (Ammer et al., 2012; Fu, Brezden, Kelly et al., 1997; Kelly & Kidd, 2000; Porres et al., 2011; Siveke et al.,

2018). Thus, NMDA currents enhance the output firing rate and thereby the information content of DNLL neurons (Ammer et al., 2012; Porres et al., 2011; Siveke et al., 2018). This NMDA action is also interesting because, first, the NMDA dependent increase in sensory information content in the DNLL might be a blueprint for other auditory brainstem nuclei. NMDA receptor activation and electrogenic signaling has also been documented in the IC (Sanchez, Gans, & Wenstrup, 2007; Sivaramakrishnan & Oliver, 2006; Wu, Ma, & Kelly, 2004), the AVCN (Pliss, Yang, & Xu-Friedman, 2009), and in the VNLL. This NMDA receptor-mediated increased information content matches the increase in sensory information that has been described along the ascending auditory brainstem pathways before (Kuwada, Fitzpatrick, Batra, & Ostapoff, 2006; Pecka, Siveke, Grothe, & Lesica, 2010). Second, the addition of NMDA conductances will help overcome the strong GABAergic long-lasting inhibition generated by contralateral DNLL neurons. At the same time, NMDA receptor amplified excitation will lead to an even greater inhibition on the contralateral counterpart. Thus, the push-pull mechanism between the DNLL hemispheres is strongly dependent on NMDA currents.

DNLL neurons exhibit basic similarities, yet with a large parameter range. The function of this variability is obscure and might simply reflect the nuclear organization or adaptations to the various input nuclei. Alternatively, the variability might indicate that DNLL neurons can use a large set of cellular features to adjust their function to the specific sound-processing tasks.

Functional Aspects of the Auditory Nuclei in the Lateral Lemniscus

After reviewing the cellular features of neurons of the LL we turn to discuss functional apsects of each nucleus. These considerations are largely based on in vivo recordings. In this section finally we aim to identify some functional tasks that these neurons perform during the processing of auditory information to support the generation of the wonderfull auditory space which we perceive in our everyday life.

Ventral Nucleus of the Lateral Lemniscus

VNLL neurons are predominantly driven by monaural sounds; however, binaurality has also been documented in cats, rats, and rabbits (Batra & Fitzpatrick, 1999; Guinan, Norris, & Guinan, 1972; Recio-Spinoso & Joris, 2014; Zhang & Kelly, 2006b), but little binaurality exists in bats (Covey & Casseday, 1991). Sound-evoked responses can be segregated in different classes amongst VNLL neurons. Covey and Casseday (1991) found that neurons in the columnar region of the VNLL in bats fire predominantly with a very rapid onset response. Neurons in the rest of the VNLL could be classified into the main groups of onset, onset-sustained, sustained, and chopping-response types (Covey & Casseday, 1991; Huffman, Argeles, & Covey, 1998; Metzner & Radtke-Schuller, 1987). These types of neurons were also described in other mammals. In cats, rats, mice, and rabbits, onset and onset-sustained cells with various forms of adaptations predominate in the VNLL (Adams, 1997; Batra & Fitzpatrick, 1999; Liu, Huang, & Wang, 2014; Recio-Spinoso & Joris, 2014; Zhang & Kelly, 2006b). One hallmark of the columnar neurons in the bat VNLL is that they have a very short latency and this latency is invariant to the increase in sound intensity (Covey & Casseday, 1991; Haplea, Covey, & Casseday, 1994). Such constant latency neurons are also found in cats (Recio-Spinoso & Joris, 2014), mice (Liu et al., 2014), and rats (Zhang & Kelly, 2006b). Thus, within the VNLL, a subset of neurons shows a very high temporal precision to sound transients that is barely affected by intensity. As these neurons are located in the columnar region in bats, they are known to be innervated with a large somatic synapse arising from the octopus cell area. Thus, the constant latency might arise from strong synaptic inputs integrated by small round neurons. Frequency tuning of VNLL neurons to sound is heterogeneous and, in bats, it seemed to segregate again into neurons that show a rapid temporal precise onset and neurons that fire more sustained to brief tone stimulations. In the bat's columnar neurons, broad frequency tuning is dominant (Covey & Casseday, 1991; Haplea et al., 1994). However, in mice and cats, the width of the frequency tuning seemed not to correlate with the firing pattern of sustained or onset response type (Liu et al., 2014; Recio-Spinoso & Joris, 2014). Here, tuning curves correlate with the characteristic frequency of the neuron (Liu et al., 2014; Recio-Spinoso & Joris, 2014), with wider tunings in lower frequencies. These tuning characteristics are consistent with in vivo data from the octopus cell area recorded in cats (Rhode & Smith, 1986). Thus, overall frequency tuning in the VNLL might be inherited from its input structure. Taken together, rapid onset neurons generate fast, temporally precise inhibition in the ascending pathways targeting the dorsal VNLL and, importantly, the IC. Such fast-onset inhibitions have been indeed observed in VNLL and IC neurons (Nayagam et al., 2005; Spencer et al., 2015; Xie, Gittelman, Li, & Pollak, 2008; Xie, Gittelman, & Pollak, 2007). This inhibition covers a broad frequency range, extending the frequency range that triggers excitation in the same neuron. Thus, based on the frequency range and temporal precision, the onset inhibition is considered to originate in the ventral VNLL. This inhibitory signaling can be interpreted as a "shut up and listen" input. Such an onset inhibition might enhance the contrast of excitatory inputs and may generate ideal spike triggers due to the relief of sodium channel inactivation. Functionally, fast-onset inhibition was shown to reduce spectral splatter (Spencer et al., 2015). Spectral splatter emerges during sharp onset activation and consists of the resultant noise generated in the frequency domain. This function arises from its ability to suppress onset information over a broad frequency range. A spectral filter is thereby generated that suppresses spurious sound frequencies when integrated in the IC.

Furthermore, the modulation transfer-functions of VNLL neurons show that these neurons do not follow very high-input frequencies (Zhang & Kelly, 2006a). This finding is consistent with their intrinsic resonance (Fischer et al., 2018), which is tuned to low frequencies. Therefore, one might argue that VNLL neurons are designed to transmit especially loud low-frequency-modulated sounds. As low-frequency modulation of sound is one feature of salient sounds, including natural alarm sounds (Arnal, Flinker, Kleinschmidt, Giraud, & Poeppel, 2015), the octopus-VNLL circuit might be designed to process such auditory features initially. The rapid feedforward inhibition from VNLL to IC might furthermore enhance contrast and modulate gain for the processing of such salient-sounds features. Interestingly, contrast enhancement is supposed to be one possible mechanism mediating saliency (Huang & Elhilali, 2017; Itti & Koch, 2001). Thus, this circuit holds the requirements for early processing of the salient-sounds feature.

Intermedial Nucleus of the Lateral Lemniscus

In vivo recordings selectively performed in the INLL are sparse, with most data being collected in bats and rats. As in the VNLL, the response characteristics in the INLL are fairly heterogeneous. INLL neurons responded to sounds with sustained, onset, or onset-sustained patterns in some cases with chopping behavior (Huffman et al., 1998; Kelly, Buckthought, et al., 1998; Xie, Meitzen, & Pollak, 2005). All frequencies an animal can hear are represented in the INLL (Covey & Casseday, 1991; Kelly, Buckthought, et al., 1998). Another response feature that received attention in INLL neurons is spike latency. This feature is particular interesting, as it might segregate VNLL from INLL neurons. INLL first-spike latencies were longer compared to columnar neurons but not to other VNLL neurons (Covey & Casseday, 1991). Overall, VNLL and INLL latencies were shown to present a continuum, with the shortest being in the columnar VNLL and the longest in INLL neurons (Covey & Casseday, 1991). Compared to DNLL neurons, INLL neurons showed shorter latencies in rats (Kelly, Buckthought, et al., 1998).

The sharpness of frequency tuning in the INLL is very variable, covering a large range of Q_{dB} values (Covey & Casseday, 1991; Xie et al., 2005). There is evidence that for some cells, tuning is acuminated by side band inhibition (Xie et al., 2005). This side band inhibition is mediated by either GABAergic or both GABAergic and glycinergic inputs. The mixed input is intriguing, as VNLL neurons were shown to release both GABA and glycine simultaneously (Moore & Trussell, 2017). Thus, ascending VNLL axons might be sending of collaterals into the INLL on their way to the IC, thereby sharpening the tuning of INLL neurons.

The physiological features of INLL neurons described so far are based on monaural activation. However, some INLL neurons were shown to receive binaural inputs. Despite the fact that most INLL neurons respond similarly to monaural and binaural sounds, a fraction showed increased responsiveness to stimulation of both ears, while others showed lower responsiveness when stimulated binaurally (Covey & Casseday, 1991; Kelly, Buckthought, et al., 1998; Xie et al., 2005). Thus, for both the VNLL and the INLL a fraction of neurons integrate binaural information.

A physiological hallmark that was recently assigned to INLL neurons, and possibly to some VNLL neurons, is their ability to integrate information across different sound frequencies. Thus, these neurons pool information between different frequency channels. In some neurons, low-frequency sounds can suppress the response rate to higher-frequency tones even at best frequency (Peterson, Nataraj, & Wenstrup, 2009). In other neurons facilitation of neuronal response rates was observed upon cross-frequency integration (Mittmann & Wenstrup, 1995). This integration was sensitive to glycine but not GABA antagonists. The glycinergic inputs mediating this response were traced to originate mainly in the medial and lateral nucleus of the trapezoid body and to a minor extend in the VNLL (Yavuzoglu et al., 2010; Yavuzoglu, Schofield, & Wenstrup, 2011). Thus, ascending inhibition sharpens well-defined cross-frequency integration in the INLL.

Dorsal Nucleus of the Lateral Lemniscus

In the DNLL the frequency tuning is narrower compared to the VNLL (Bajo, Villa, de Ribaupierre, & Rouiller, 1998; Covey, 1993; Kelly, Buckthought, et al., 1998; Markovitz & Pollak, 1994) and is directly inherited from the ascending pathways, as no side band glycinergic or GABAergic inhibition was observed (Xie et al., 2005). Sound-evoked response patterns recorded at best frequency can be categorized into onset, sustained, on-off, and off responses (Bajo et al., 1998; Covey, 1993; Kelly, Buckthought, et al., 1998; Kuwada et al., 2006; Markovitz & Pollak, 1994; Metzner & Radtke-Schuller, 1987). On-neurons encode time more faithfully as they follow higher modulation frequencies in sinusoidal amplitude modulated paradigms, compared to sustained firing cells (Yang & Pollak, 1997). Overall, specific sound-evoked response patterns vary significantly. It has not fully been elucidated whether these variations are related to tonotopy, location, or input structures within the DNLL. Nevertheless, this functional heterogeneity matches well with the heterogeneity of the membrane and synaptic parameters described in the DNLL part of the section about the cellular features. Functionally, these diverse responses do not underlie a detection of distinct con-specific calls, as in bats DNLL neurons were not selective for a specific call, but responded to any call well (Bauer, Klug, & Pollak, 2002). In addition, sound-evoked response latencies vary considerably in the DNLL (Covey, 1993; Markovitz & Pollak, 1994) and clearly depend on sound intensity (Markovitz & Pollak, 1994). Spontaneous activity recorded in the DNLL was subdivided into modes of bursting or regular spiking (Bajo et al., 1998), again implicating different cellular categories. The presence of spontaneous activity matches the notion that DNLL neurons appear highly excitable in in vitro recordings. Moreover, in vivo recordings additionally demonstrated that DNLL neurons are sensitive to excitatory non-NMDA- and NMDA-receptor antagonists (Kelly & Kidd, 2000; Siveke et al., 2018). Inhibitory inputs to DNLL neurons can be blocked by antagonists of GABA and glycine receptors (Yang & Pollak, 1994a, 1994b).

It follows from the inputs of the binaural coincidence detectors located in the SOC that DNLL neurons are sensitive to interaural time differences (ITDs) and interaural level differences (ILDs) (Covey, 1993; Kelly, Buckthought, et al., 1998; Kuwada et al., 2006;

Siveke et al., 2006). That ITD and ILD coding is inherited from the SOC is also indicated by the observed peak and trough type ITDs (Kuwada et al., 2006; Siveke et al., 2006). The binaural accuracy or the information content of ITDs is higher in the DNLL compared to the SOC (Kuwada et al., 2006; Pecka et al., 2010). Such an enhancement could be mediated on the circuit level by integrating over a large range of inputs. Alternatively, the increase could be mediated by postsynaptic amplification mechanisms. Porres et al. (2011) have shown that NMDA receptors are ideally suited to amplify the output rates of DNLL neurons. That the sensory information content is indeed enhanced in an NMDA-dependent manner was recently demonstrated in vivo (Siveke et al., 2018). This NMDA-dependent mechanism might be a blueprint for increasing the information contents in the ascending auditory pathways as glutamatergic synapses drive NMDA-receptors at least in DNLL and IC neurons (Sanchez et al., 2007; Sivaramakrishnan & Oliver, 2006; Wu et al., 2004). Furthermore, as will be described, the NMDA-receptor dependent amplification of DNLL outputs might be crucial to adjust long-lasting GABAergic inhibition in both the DNLL and the IC (Bauer, Klug, & Pollak, 2000; Porres et al., 2011; Yang & Pollak, 1994b).

Besides the processing of binaural information that is inherited from the SOC, DNLL neurons have the potential to interact via the commissure of Probst with their contralateral counterparts to generate additional binaural interactions. In agreement with the GABAergic nature of DNLL neurons, this hemispherical interaction is dominated by GABA. GABAergic, but not glycinergic, blockers reduce the long-lasting inhibition generated in the DNLL from its contralateral counterpart (Yang & Pollak, 1994b). The GABAergic action is mediated by ionotropic GABA receptors. This contralaterally initiated inhibition can outlast sound presentations by tens of milliseconds (Burger & Pollak, 2001; Pecka et al., 2007; Siveke et al., 2018; Yang & Pollak, 1994b, 1998). The time course of this GABAergic inhibition depends first on the firing rate of the presynaptic DNLL neuron (Ammer et al., 2015). Higher output rates lead to a frequency-dependent buildup of GABAergic transmitter in the synaptic cleft and to asynchronous release from presynaptic terminals, thereby prolonging activation of postsynaptic GABA receptors. Second, passive postsynaptic integration of hyperpolarizing inhibition prolongs the GABAergic action (Ammer et al., 2015). These mechanisms together are suitable and sufficient to explain the long-lasting suppression of activity in the DNLL (Ammer et al., 2015). Whether similar biophysical properties on the pre- and postsynaptic site are the basis of the long-lasting inhibition observed in the IC (Bauer et al., 2000) has not been elucidated.

The importance of the DNLL in binaural processing has been demonstrated by a series of behavioral and elegant in vivo pharmacological experiments. By cutting the commissure of Probst, M. Ito, van Adel, and Kelly (1996) demonstrated that the minimal audible angle increased dramatically. Along the same lines, Kelly, Li, and van Adel (1996) used unilateral and bilateral kainic acid induced lesions of the DNLL to show that its loss led to an increase in minimal audible angle. To demonstrate binaural processing in vivo, the approach was to change the activity in one DNLL and recorded in the contralateral counterpart or the IC. Li and Kelly (1992) demonstrated that by silencing the DNLL, the

ILD functions of contralateral IC neurons lost tuning, a finding corroborated by Burger and Pollak (2001). Additionally, these authors could link the long-lasting GABAergic effect toward the change in ILD function in the IC. Silencing DNLL neurons either by GABA agonists or non-NMDA-receptor and NMDA-receptor antagonists shows the suppressive effect of DNLL neurons in the IC (Faingold, Anderson, & Randall, 1993; Kelly & Kidd, 2000). These authors thereby demonstrate that the GABAergic reciprocal inhibition between the DNLL hemispheres is crucial for binaural responsiveness in the IC. Conversely, electrically evoked activity of the DNLL was able to suppress IC activity to contralateral sound stimulation in a manner that matched binaural activation (Faingold et al., 1993). Together these data demonstrate that based on synaptic integration of AMPA, NMDA, and GABA receptors, binaural activity in the DNLL shapes ITD and ILD coding, and hence the space representation, in the IC.

The function of long-lasting GABAergic inhibition in the DNLL was proposed to generate suppression of location information of sound source during reverberations (Pecka et al., 2007). Mechanistically, rapid alterations in the location of sound sources could generate relief of GABAergic suppression (disinhibition) in one IC hemisphere. In this model (Pecka et al., 2007), a preceding sound blocks the activity of the sound source ipsilateral DNLL via the commissure of Probst. Therefore, the suppression of this DNLL leads to a disinhibition of the IC that is contralateral to the sound. Since the inhibition of the DNLL is supposed to be longer-lasting than the sound itself, the suppression of the ipsilateral DNLL by the preceding sound will persist into the activity generated by a rapidly occurring second sound. When the second sound comes from the opposite direction while the disinhibition in the IC is still present, the second sound will be represented in both IC hemispheres. Thus, for the time of the long-lasting inhibition an ambiguous representation of the second sound is generated that might suppress the accurate detection of its localization. Such an ambiguous sound representation might suppress the localization without quenching the sensory evoked activation. Since the IC is activated on both hemispheres during the second sound we can speculate that this second sound can be detected but not accurately localized. That a second sound can be detected but not localized is observed in human listeners during an echo, or lead lag detection paradigm (Litovsky, Colburn, Yost, & Guzman, 1999; Pecka et al., 2007). A key element for this GABAergic dis-inhibition is thereby the reciprocal inhibition between the DNLL/IC hemispheres. Such reciprocal inhibitory connections were indicated to be ideally suited to underlie context-dependent sensory processing (Mysore & Knudsen, 2012). A more overarching scenario for DNLL function could be a possible role as a selective filter. As we have seen, the long-lasting inhibition creates a time window that quenches unambiguous localizations. Evidence was presented that during rapid sound fluctuations, the DNLL circuit might suppress the presence of acoustically generated spurious sound information (Meffin & Grothe, 2009). The properties of the DNLL circuit were shown to match the temporal structure of a filter that suppresses a frequency of spuriously generated ITDs larger than 100 Hz. Thus, ITDs and ILDs that are stable and do not fluctuate between the different locations in space rapidly will be allowed to be processed further. This selective filtering is consistent with the idea of a long-lasting

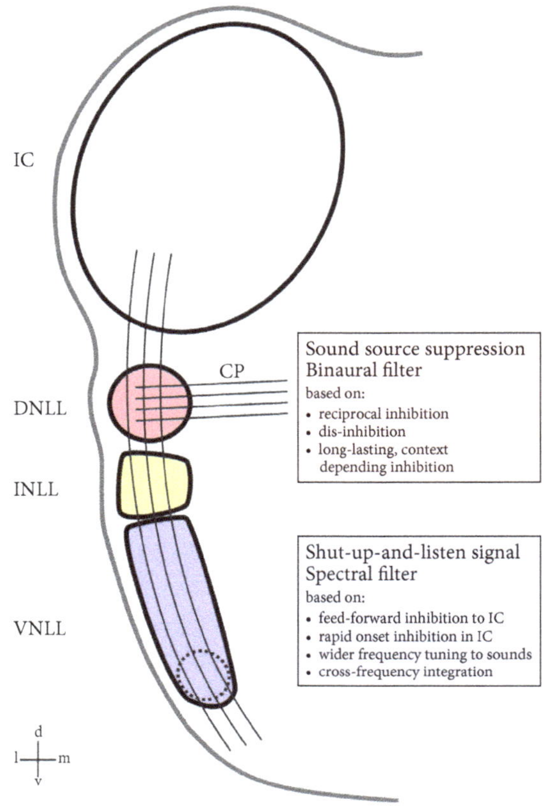

FIGURE 16.2. Three main nuclei can be delineated in the fiber bundle of the lateral lemniscus (LL) that connects lower auditory brainstem nuclei with the inferior colliculus (IC). The glycinergic/GABAergic ventral nucleus of the lateral lemniscus (VNLL) is considered temporally precise and generates a rapid feed-forward inhibition. One functional feature might be the suppression of spectral splatter, spurious frequencies that are generated by the onset of a rapid sound transient. A subregion (dotted circle) is temporally most precise and receives a large glutamatergic somatic input. The glutamatergic neurons of the intermediate nuclei of the lateral lemniscus (INLL) are likely to be involved in cross-frequency integration. The GABAergic dorsal nucleus of the lateral lemniscus (DNLL) is reciprocally connected via the commissure of Probst (CP). It acts as a binaural filter suppressing spurious interaural information and is implicated in the suppression of sound source localization during reverberations.

suppression that might be involved in the suppression of space information during reverberations, and with the finding that DNLL neurons process con-specific sounds irrespective of the call type (Bauer et al., 2002). Thus, the DNLL might represent a filter specifically tuned for slower temporal aspects that acts in a context dependent manner. Data from our group indeed supports this idea of a context-dependent filter, as the time course of the long-lasting suppression evoked in the contralateral DNLL depends on the overall sound intensity. Thus, the temporal properties of this filter are dynamically adjusted to sound intensities.

We can put together a scenario in which the VNLL and DNLL act as specific filters (Figure 16.2). The function of the VNLL and the DNLL might be to filter out spurious frequencies and space information, respectively. We put forward that these nuclei cut out perturbing material and enhance the remaining information. In doing so, the LL enhances sound representation in the IC by increasing signal to noise. Based on their filter properties, sound processing in the IC becomes focused. In light of these properties, the LL might be regarded as a gate keeper for the IC.

Acknowledgments

I grateful to Dr. Elisabeth M.M. Meyer who for her comments and help with the manuscript. I thank Sönke von den Berg for help with the figure. Our current work on the LL is supported by DFG789/6-1 and DFG789/7-1

References

Adams, J. C. (1979). Ascending projections to the inferior colliculus. *Journal of Comparative Neurology, 183*(3), 519–538. doi: 10.1002/cne.901830305

Adams, J. C. (1997). Projections from octopus cells of the posteroventral cochlear Nucleus to the ventral nucleus of the lateral lemniscus in cat and human. *Auditory Neuroscience, 3*(4), 335–350.

Ahuja, T. K., & Wu, S. H. (2000). Developmental changes in physiological properties in the rat's dorsal nucleus of the lateral lemniscus. *Hearing Research, 149*(1–2), 33–45.

Aitkin, L. M., Anderson, D. J., & Brugge, J. F. (1970). Tonotopic organization and discharge characteristics of single neurons in nuclei of the lateral lemniscus of the cat. *Journal of Neurophysiology, 33*(3), 421–440.

Ammer, J. J., Grothe, B., & Felmy, F. (2012). Late postnatal development of intrinsic and synaptic properties promotes fast and precise signaling in the dorsal nucleus of the lateral lemniscus. *Journal of Neurophysiology, 107*(4), 1172–1185. doi: 10.1152/jn.00585.2011

Ammer, J. J., Siveke, I., & Felmy, F. (2015). Activity-dependent transmission and integration control the timescales of auditory processing at an inhibitory synapse. *Current Biology, 25*(12), 1562–1572. doi: 10.1016/j.cub.2015.04.026

Arnal, L. H., Flinker, A., Kleinschmidt, A., Giraud, A. L., & Poeppel, D. (2015). Human screams occupy a privileged niche in the communication soundscape. *Current Biology, 25*(15), 2051–2056. doi: 10.1016/j.cub.2015.06.043

Bajo, V. M., Merchan, M. A., Lopez, D. E., & Rouiller, E. M. (1993). Neuronal morphology and efferent projections of the dorsal nucleus of the lateral lemniscus in the rat. *Journal of Comparative Neurology, 334*(2), 241–262. doi: 10.1002/cne.903340207

Bajo, V. M., Merchan, M. A., Malmierca, M. S., Nodal, F. R., & Bjaalie, J. G. (1999). Topographic organization of the dorsal nucleus of the lateral lemniscus in the cat. *Journal of Comparative Neurology, 407*(3), 349–366.

Bajo, V. M., Villa, A. E., de Ribaupierre, F., & Rouiller, E. M. (1998). Discharge properties of single neurons in the dorsal nucleus of the lateral lemniscus of the rat. *Brain Research Bulletin*, *47*(6), 595–610. doi: S0361-9230(98)00127-0 [pii]

Batra, R., & Fitzpatrick, D. C. (1999). Discharge patterns of neurons in the ventral nucleus of the lateral lemniscus of the unanesthetized rabbit. *Journal of Neurophysiology*, *82*(3), 1097–1113. doi: 10.1152/jn.1999.82.3.1097

Bauer, E. E., Klug, A., & Pollak, G. D. (2000). Features of contralaterally evoked inhibition in the inferior colliculus. *Hearing Research*, *141*(1–2), 80–96.

Bauer, E. E., Klug, A., & Pollak, G. D. (2002). Spectral determination of responses to species-specific calls in the dorsal nucleus of the lateral lemniscus. *Journal of Neurophysiology*, *88*(4), 1955–1967. doi: 10.1152/jn.2002.88.4.1955

Baumann, V. J., & Koch, U. (2017). Perinatal nicotine exposure impairs the maturation of glutamatergic inputs in the auditory brainstem. *Journal of Physiology*, *595*(11), 3573–3590. doi: 10.1113/JP274059

Berger, C., Meyer, E. M., Ammer, J. J., & Felmy, F. (2014). Large somatic synapses on neurons in the ventral lateral lemniscus work in pairs. *Journal of Neuroscience*, *34*(9), 3237–3246. doi: 10.1523/JNEUROSCI.3664-13.2014

Budinger, E., Brosch, M., Scheich, H., & Mylius, J. (2013). The subcortical auditory structures in the Mongolian gerbil: II. Frequency-related topography of the connections with cortical field AI. *Journal of Comparative Neurology*, *521*(12), 2772–2797. doi: 10.1002/cne.23314

Burger, R. M., & Pollak, G. D. (2001). Reversible inactivation of the dorsal nucleus of the lateral lemniscus reveals its role in the processing of multiple sound sources in the inferior colliculus of bats. *Journal of Neuroscience*, *21*(13), 4830–4843.

Caicedo, A., d'Aldin, C., Puel, J. L., & Eybalin, M. (1996). Distribution of calcium-binding protein immunoreactivities in the guinea pig auditory brainstem. *Anatomy of Embryology (Berlin)*, *194*(5), 465–487.

Campos, M. L., de Cabo, C., Wisden, W., Juiz, J. M., & Merlo, D. (2001). Expression of GABA(A) receptor subunits in rat brainstem auditory pathways: Cochlear nuclei, superior olivary complex and nucleus of the lateral lemniscus. *Neuroscience*, *102*(3), 625–638.

Caspari, F., Baumann, V. J., Garcia-Pino, E., & Koch, U. (2015). Heterogeneity of intrinsic and synaptic properties of neurons in the ventral and dorsal parts of the ventral nucleus of the lateral lemniscus. *Frontiers in Neural Circuits*, *9*, 74. doi: 10.3389/fncir.2015.00074

Covey, E. (1993). Response properties of single units in the dorsal nucleus of the lateral lemniscus and paralemniscal zone of an echolocating bat. *Journal of Neurophysiology*, *69*(3), 842–859. doi: 10.1152/jn.1993.69.3.842

Covey, E., & Casseday, J. H. (1986). Connectional basis for frequency representation in the nuclei of the lateral lemniscus of the bat Eptesicus fuscus. *Journal of Neuroscience*, *6*(10), 2926–2940.

Covey, E., & Casseday, J. H. (1991). The monaural nuclei of the lateral lemniscus in an echolocating bat: Parallel pathways for analyzing temporal features of sound. *Journal of Neuroscience*, *11*(11), 3456–3470.

Di Bonito, M., Narita, Y., Avallone, B., Sequino, L., Mancuso, M., Andolfi, G., . . . Studer, M. (2013). Assembly of the auditory circuitry by a Hox genetic network in the mouse brainstem. *PLoS Genetics*, *9*(2), e1003249. doi: 10.1371/journal.pgen.1003249

Faingold, C. L., Anderson, C. A., & Randall, M. E. (1993). Stimulation or blockade of the dorsal nucleus of the lateral lemniscus alters binaural and tonic inhibition in contralateral inferior colliculus neurons. *Hearing Research*, *69*(1–2), 98–106.

Fischer, L., Leibold, C., & Felmy, F. (2018). Resonance properties in auditory brainstem neurons. *Frontiers in Cellular Neuroscience, 12*, 8. doi: 10.3389/fncel.2018.00008

Franzen, D. L., Gleiss, S. A., Berger, C., Kumpfbeck, F. S., Ammer, J. J., & Felmy, F. (2015). Development and modulation of intrinsic membrane properties control the temporal precision of auditory brain stem neurons. *Journal of Neurophysiology, 113*(2), 524–536. doi: 10.1152/jn.00601.2014

Friauf, E., & Ostwald, J. (1988). Divergent projections of physiologically characterized rat ventral cochlear nucleus neurons as shown by intra-axonal injection of horseradish peroxidase. *Experimental Brain Research, 73*(2), 263–284.

Fu, X. W., Brezden, B. L., Kelly, J. B., & Wu, S. H. (1997). Synaptic excitation in the dorsal nucleus of the lateral lemniscus: Whole-cell patch-clamp recordings from rat brain slice. *Neuroscience, 78*(3), 815–827.

Fu, X. W., Brezden, B. L., & Wu, S. H. (1997). Hyperpolarization-activated inward current in neurons of the rat's dorsal nucleus of the lateral lemniscus in vitro. *Journal of Neurophysiology, 78*(5), 2235–2245. doi: 10.1152/jn.1997.78.5.2235

Fu, X. W., Wu, S. H., Brezden, B. L., & Kelly, J. B. (1996). Potassium currents and membrane excitability of neurons in the rat's dorsal nucleus of the lateral lemniscus. *Journal Neurophysiology, 76*(2), 1121–1132. doi: 10.1152/jn.1996.76.2.1121

Glendenning, K. K., Brunso-Bechtold, J. K., Thompson, G. C., & Masterton, R. B. (1981). Ascending auditory afferents to the nuclei of the lateral lemniscus. *Journal of Compative Neurology, 197*(4), 673–703.

Gonzalez-Hernandez, T., Mantolan-Sarmiento, B., Gonzalez-Gonzalez, B., & Perez-Gonzalez, H. (1996). Sources of GABAergic input to the inferior colliculus of the rat. *Journal of Comparative Neurology, 372*(2), 309–326. doi: 10.1002/(SICI)1096-9861(19960819)372:2<309::AID-CNE11>3.0.CO;2-E [pii] 10.1002/(SICI)1096-9861(19960819)372:2<309::AID-CNE11>3.0.CO;2-E

Guinan, J. J., Jr., Norris, B. E., & Guinan, S. S. (1972). Single auditory units in the superior olivary complex: II: Locations of unit categories and tonotopic organization. *International Journal of Neuroscience, 4*, 147–166. doi: 10.3109/00207457209164756

Haplea, S., Covey, E., & Casseday, J. H. (1994). Frequency tuning and response latencies at three levels in the brainstem of the echolocating bat, *Eptesicus fuscus. Journal of Comparative Physiology A, 174*(6), 671–683.

Happe, H. K., & Morley, B. J. (2004). Distribution and postnatal development of alpha 7 nicotinic acetylcholine receptors in the rodent lower auditory brainstem. *Brain Research Developmental Brain Research, 153*(1), 29–37. doi: 10.1016/j.devbrainres.2004.07.004

Henkel, C. K. (1997). Axonal morphology in fibrodendritic laminae of the dorsal nucleus of the lateral lemniscus: Afferent projections from the medial superior olivary nucleus. *Journal of Comparative Neurology, 380*(1), 136–144.

Huang, N., & Elhilali, M. (2017). Auditory salience using natural soundscapes. *Journal of the Acoustical Society of America, 141*(3), 2163. doi: 10.1121/1.4979055

Huffman, R. F., Argeles, P. C., & Covey, E. (1998). Processing of sinusoidally amplitude modulated signals in the nuclei of the lateral lemniscus of the big brown bat, Eptesicus fuscus. *Hearing Research, 126*(1–2), 181–200.

Huffman, R. F., & Covey, E. (1995). Origin of ascending projections to the nuclei of the lateral lemniscus in the big brown bat, Eptesicus fuscus. *Journal of Comparative Neurology, 357*(4), 532–545.

Irfan, N., Zhang, H., & Wu, S. H. (2005). Synaptic transmission mediated by ionotropic glutamate, glycine and GABA receptors in the rat's ventral nucleus of the lateral lemniscus. *Hearing Research*, *203*(1–2), 159–171. doi: 10.1016/j.heares.2004.11.021

Ito, M., van Adel, B., & Kelly, J. B. (1996). Sound localization after transection of the commissure of Probst in the albino rat. *Journal of Neurophysiology*, *76*(5), 3493–3502. doi: 10.1152/jn.1996.76.5.3493

Ito, T., Bishop, D. C., & Oliver, D. L. (2011). Expression of glutamate and inhibitory amino acid vesicular transporters in the rodent auditory brainstem. *Journal of Comparative Neurology*, *519*(2), 316–340. doi: 10.1002/cne.22521

Itti, L., & Koch, C. (2001). Computational modelling of visual attention. *Nature Reviews Neuroscience*, *2*(3), 194–203. doi: 10.1038/35058500

Iwahori, N. (1986). A Golgi study on the dorsal nucleus of the lateral lemniscus in the mouse. *Neuroscience Research*, *3*(3), 196–212.

Jamal, L., Zhang, H., Finlayson, P. G., Porter, L. A., & Zhang, H. (2011). The level and distribution of the GABA(B)R2 receptor subunit in the rat's central auditory system. *Neuroscience*, *181*, 243–256. doi: 10.1016/j.neuroscience.2011.02.050

Kane, E. S., & Barone, L. M. (1980). The dorsal nucleus of the lateral lemniscus in the cat: Neuronal types and their distributions. *Journal of Comparative Neurology*, *192*(4), 797–826. doi: 10.1002/cne.901920412

Kelly, J. B., Buckthought, A. D., & Kidd, S. A. (1998). Monaural and binaural response properties of single neurons in the rat's dorsal nucleus of the lateral lemniscus. *Hearing Research*, *122*(1–2), 25–40.

Kelly, J. B., & Kidd, S. A. (2000). NMDA and AMPA receptors in the dorsal nucleus of the lateral lemniscus shape binaural responses in rat inferior colliculus. *Journal of Neurophysiology*, *83*(3), 1403–1414.

Kelly, J. B., Li, L., & van Adel, B. (1996). Sound localization after kainic acid lesions of the dorsal nucleus of the lateral lemniscus in the albino rat. *Behavioral Neuroscience*, *110*(6), 1445–1455.

Kelly, J. B., Liscum, A., van Adel, B., & Ito, M. (1998). Projections from the superior olive and lateral lemniscus to tonotopic regions of the rat's inferior colliculus. *Hearing Research*, *116*(1–2), 43–54.

Kelly, J. B., van Adel, B. A., & Ito, M. (2009). Anatomical projections of the nuclei of the lateral lemniscus in the albino rat (*Rattus norvegicus*). *Journal of Comparative Neurology*, *512*(4), 573–593. doi: 10.1002/cne.21929

Koch, U., Braun, M., Kapfer, C., & Grothe, B. (2004). Distribution of HCN1 and HCN2 in rat auditory brainstem nuclei. *European Journal of Neuroscience*, *20*(1), 79–91. doi: 10.1111/j.0953-816X.2004.03456.x

Kuwada, S., Fitzpatrick, D. C., Batra, R., & Ostapoff, E. M. (2006). Sensitivity to interaural time differences in the dorsal nucleus of the lateral lemniscus of the unanesthetized rabbit: comparison with other structures. *Journal of Neurophysiology*, *95*(3), 1309–1322. doi: 10.1152/jn.00901.2005

Li, L., & Kelly, J. B. (1992). Inhibitory influence of the dorsal nucleus of the lateral lemniscus on binaural responses in the rat's inferior colliculus. *Journal of Neuroscience*, *12*(11), 4530–4539.

Litovsky, R. Y., Colburn, H. S., Yost, W. A., & Guzman, S. J. (1999). The precedence effect. *Journal of the Acoustical Society of America*, *106*(4 Pt 1), 1633–1654.

Liu, H. H., Huang, C. F., & Wang, X. (2014). Acoustic signal characteristic detection by neurons in ventral nucleus of the lateral lemniscus in mice. *Dongwuxue Yanjiu*, *35*(6), 500–509. doi: 10.13918/j.issn.2095-8137.2014.6.500

Lohmann, C., & Friauf, E. (1996). Distribution of the calcium-binding proteins parvalbumin and calretinin in the auditory brainstem of adult and developing rats. *Journal of Comparative Neurology*, *367*(1), 90–109. doi: 10.1002/(SICI)1096-9861(19960325)367:1<90::AID-CNE7>3.0.CO;2-E

Malmierca, M. S., Leergaard, T. B., Bajo, V. M., Bjaalie, J. G., & Merchan, M. A. (1998). Anatomic evidence of a three-dimensional mosaic pattern of tonotopic organization in the ventral complex of the lateral lemniscus in cat. *Journal of Neuroscience*, *18*(24), 10603–10618.

Markovitz, N. S., & Pollak, G. D. (1994). Binaural processing in the dorsal nucleus of the lateral lemniscus. *Hearing Research*, *73*(1), 121–140.

Meffin, H., & Grothe, B. (2009). Selective filtering to spurious localization cues in the mammalian auditory brainstem. *Journal of the Acoustical Society of Amerika*, *126*(5), 2437–2454. doi: 10.1121/1.3238239

Merchan, M. A., & Berbel, P. (1996). Anatomy of the ventral nucleus of the lateral lemniscus in rats: A nucleus with a concentric laminar organization. *Journal of Comparative Neurology*, *372*(2), 245–263. doi: 10.1002/(SICI)1096-9861(19960819)372:2<245::AID-CNE7>3.0.CO;2-3

Merchan, M. A., Saldana, E., & Plaza, I. (1994). Dorsal nucleus of the lateral lemniscus in the rat: Concentric organization and tonotopic projection to the inferior colliculus. *Journal of Comparative Neurology*, *342*(2), 259–278. doi: 10.1002/cne.903420209

Metzner, W., & Radtke-Schuller, S. (1987). The nuclei of the lateral lemniscus in the rufous horseshoe bat, *Rhinolophus rouxi*. A neurophysiological approach. *Journal of Comparative Physiology A*, *160*(3), 395–411.

Mittmann, D. H., & Wenstrup, J. J. (1995). Combination-sensitive neurons in the inferior colliculus. *Hearing Research*, *90*(1–2), 185–191.

Moore, L. A., & Trussell, L. O. (2017). Corelease of inhibitory neurotransmitters in the mouse auditory midbrain. *Journal of Neuroscience*, *37*(39), 9453–9464. doi: 10.1523/JNEUROSCI.1125-17.2017

Mylius, J., Brosch, M., Scheich, H., & Budinger, E. (2013). Subcortical auditory structures in the Mongolian gerbil: I. Golgi architecture. *Journal of Comparative Neurology*, *521*(6), 1289–1321. doi: 10.1002/cne.23232

Mysore, S. P., & Knudsen, E. I. (2012). Reciprocal inhibition of inhibition: A circuit motif for flexible categorization in stimulus selection. *Neuron*, *73*(1), 193–205. doi: 10.1016/j.neuron.2011.10.037

Nayagam, D. A., Clarey, J. C., & Paolini, A. G. (2005). Powerful, onset inhibition in the ventral nucleus of the lateral lemniscus. *Journal of Neurophysiology*, *94*(2), 1651–1654. doi: 10.1152/jn.00167.2005

Oliver, D. L., & Shneiderman, A. (1989). An EM study of the dorsal nucleus of the lateral lemniscus: Inhibitory, commissural, synaptic connections between ascending auditory pathways. *Journal of Neuroscience*, *9*(3), 967–982.

Pecka, M., Siveke, I., Grothe, B., & Lesica, N. A. (2010). Enhancement of ITD coding within the initial stages of the auditory pathway. *Journal of Neurophysiology*, *103*(1), 38–46. doi: 00628.2009 [pii] 10.1152/jn.00628.2009

Pecka, M., Zahn, T. P., Saunier-Rebori, B., Siveke, I., Felmy, F., Wiegrebe, L., . . . Grothe, B. (2007). Inhibiting the inhibition: A neuronal network for sound localization in reverberant environments. *Journal of Neuroscience*, *27*(7), 1782–1790. doi: 27/7/1782 [pii] 10.1523/JNEUROSCI.5335-06.2007

Peterson, D. C., Nataraj, K., & Wenstrup, J. (2009). Glycinergic inhibition creates a form of auditory spectral integration in nuclei of the lateral lemniscus. *Journal Neurophysiology*, *102*(2), 1004–1016. doi: 10.1152/jn.00040.2009

Pliss, L., Yang, H., & Xu-Friedman, M. A. (2009). Context-dependent effects of NMDA receptors on precise timing information at the endbulb of Held in the cochlear nucleus. *Journal of Neurophysiology*, *102*(5), 2627–2637. doi: 10.1152/jn.00111.2009

Porres, C. P., Meyer, E. M., Grothe, B., & Felmy, F. (2011). NMDA currents modulate the synaptic input-output functions of neurons in the dorsal nucleus of the lateral lemniscus in Mongolian gerbils. *Journal of Neuroscience*, *31*(12), 4511–4523. doi: 10.1523/JNEUROSCI.6054-10.2011

Recio-Spinoso, A., & Joris, P. X. (2014). Temporal properties of responses to sound in the ventral nucleus of the lateral lemniscus. *Journal of Neurophysiology*, *111*(4), 817–835. doi: 10.1152/jn.00971.2011

Rhode, W. S., & Smith, P. H. (1986). Encoding timing and intensity in the ventral cochlear nucleus of the cat. *Journal of Neurophysiology*, *56*(2), 261–286. doi: 10.1152/jn.1986.56.2.261

Riquelme, R., Saldana, E., Osen, K. K., Ottersen, O. P., & Merchan, M. A. (2001). Colocalization of GABA and glycine in the ventral nucleus of the lateral lemniscus in rat: An in situ hybridization and semiquantitative immunocytochemical study. *Journal of Comparative Neurology*, *432*(4), 409–424.

Rosenberger, M. H., Fremouw, T., Casseday, J. H., & Covey, E. (2003). Expression of the Kv1.1 ion channel subunit in the auditory brainstem of the big brown bat, *Eptesicus fuscus*. *Journal of Comparative Neurology*, *462*(1), 101–120. doi: 10.1002/cne.10713

Ryan, A. F., Woolf, N. K., & Sharp, F. R. (1982). Tonotopic organization in the central auditory pathway of the Mongolian gerbil: A 2-deoxyglucose study. *Journal of Comparative Neurology*, *207*(4), 369–380. doi: 10.1002/cne.902070408

Saint Marie, R. L., Shneiderman, A., & Stanforth, D. A. (1997). Patterns of gamma-aminobutyric acid and glycine immunoreactivities reflect structural and functional differences of the cat lateral lemniscal nuclei. *Journal of Comparative Neurology*, *389*(2), 264–276.

Sanchez, J. T., Gans, D., & Wenstrup, J. J. (2007). Contribution of NMDA and AMPA receptors to temporal patterning of auditory responses in the inferior colliculus. *Journal of Neuroscience*, *27*(8), 1954–1963. doi: 10.1523/JNEUROSCI.2894-06.2007

Schofield, B. R., & Cant, N. B. (1997). Ventral nucleus of the lateral lemniscus in guinea pigs: Cytoarchitecture and inputs from the cochlear nucleus. *Journal of Comparative Neurology*, *379*(3), 363–385.

Seto-Ohshima, A., Aoki, E., Semba, R., Emson, P. C., & Heizmann, C. W. (1990). Parvalbumin immunoreactivity in the central auditory system of the gerbil: A developmental study. *Neuroscience Letters*, *119*(1), 60–63.

Shneiderman, A., Oliver, D. L., & Henkel, C. K. (1988). Connections of the dorsal nucleus of the lateral lemniscus: An inhibitory parallel pathway in the ascending auditory system? *Journal of Comparative Neurology*, *276*(2), 188–208. doi: 10.1002/cne.902760204

Shneiderman, A., Stanforth, D. A., Henkel, C. K., & Saint Marie, R. L. (1999). Input-output relationships of the dorsal nucleus of the lateral lemniscus: Possible substrate for the processing of dynamic spatial cues. *Journal of Comparative Neurology*, *410*(2), 265–276.

Sivaramakrishnan, S., & Oliver, D. L. (2006). Neuronal responses to lemniscal stimulation in laminar brain slices of the inferior colliculus. *Journal of the Association of Research Otolaryngology*, *7*(1), 1–14. doi: 10.1007/s10162-005-0017-4

Siveke, I., Ammer, J. J., Gleiss, S. A., Grothe, B., Leibold, C., & Felmy, F. (2018). Electrogenic N-methyl-D-aspartate receptor signaling enhances binaural responses in the adult brainstem. *European Journal of Neuroscience*, *47*(7), 858–865. doi: 10.1111/ejn.13859

Siveke, I., Pecka, M., Seidl, A. H., Baudoux, S., & Grothe, B. (2006). Binaural response properties of low-frequency neurons in the gerbil dorsal nucleus of the lateral lemniscus. *Journal of Neurophysiology*, *96*(3), 1425–1440. doi: 10.1152/jn.00713.2005

Smith, P. H., Joris, P. X., Carney, L. H., & Yin, T. C. (1991). Projections of physiologically characterized globular bushy cell axons from the cochlear nucleus of the cat. *Journal of Comparative Neurology*, *304*(3), 387–407. doi: 10.1002/cne.903040305

Smith, P. H., Joris, P. X., & Yin, T. C. (1993). Projections of physiologically characterized spherical bushy cell axons from the cochlear nucleus of the cat: Evidence for delay lines to the medial superior olive. *Journal of Comparative Neurology*, *331*(2), 245–260. doi: 10.1002/cne.903310208

Smith, P. H., Massie, A., & Joris, P. X. (2005). Acoustic stria: Anatomy of physiologically characterized cells and their axonal projection patterns. *Journal of Comparative Neurology*, *482*(4), 349–371. doi: 10.1002/cne.20407

Spangler, K. M., Warr, W. B., & Henkel, C. K. (1985). The projections of principal cells of the medial nucleus of the trapezoid body in the cat. *Journal of Comparative Neurology*, *238*(3), 249–262. doi: 10.1002/cne.902380302

Spencer, M. J., Nayagam, D. A., Clarey, J. C., Paolini, A. G., Meffin, H., Burkitt, A. N., & Grayden, D. B. (2015). Broadband onset inhibition can suppress spectral splatter in the auditory brainstem. *PLoS One*, *10*(5), e0126500. doi: 10.1371/journal.pone.0126500

Steinert, J. R., Kopp-Scheinpflug, C., Baker, C., Challiss, R. A., Mistry, R., Haustein, M. D., . . . Forsythe, I. D. (2008). Nitric oxide is a volume transmitter regulating postsynaptic excitability at a glutamatergic synapse. *Neuron*, *60*(4), 642–656. doi: 10.1016/j.neuron.2008.08.025

Stotler, W. A. (1953). An experimental study of the cells and connections of the superior olivary complex of the cat. *Journal of Comparative Neurology*, *98*(3), 401–431.

Tanaka, K., Otani, K., Tokunaga, A., & Sugita, S. (1985). The organization of neurons in the nucleus of the lateral lemniscus projecting to the superior and inferior colliculi in the rat. *Brain Research*, *341*(2), 252–260.

Thompson, A. M. (1998). Heterogeneous projections of the cat posteroventral cochlear nucleus. *Journal of Comparative Neurology*, *390*(3), 439–453.

Ueyama, T., Sato, K., Kakimoto, S., Houtani, T., Sakuma, S., Ohishi, H., . . . Sugimoto, T. (1999). Comparative distribution of GABAergic and peptide-containing neurons in the lateral lemniscal nuclei of the rat. *Brain Research*, *849*(1–2), 220–225.

Vater, M., & Braun, K. (1994). Parvalbumin, calbindin D-28k, and calretinin immunoreactivity in the ascending auditory pathway of horseshoe bats. *Journal of Comparative Neurology*, *341*(4), 534–558. doi: 10.1002/cne.903410409

Vater, M., Covey, E., & Casseday, J. H. (1997). The columnar region of the ventral nucleus of the lateral lemniscus in the big brown bat (*Eptesicus fuscus*): Synaptic arrangements and structural correlates of feedforward inhibitory function. *Cell Tissue Res*, *289*(2), 223–233.

Vater, M., Kossl, M., & Horn, A. K. (1992). GAD- and GABA-immunoreactivity in the ascending auditory pathway of horseshoe and mustached bats. *Journal of Comparative Neurology*, *325*(2), 183–206. doi: 10.1002/cne.903250205

Warr, W. B. (1969). Fiber degeneration following lesions in the posteroventral cochlear nucleus of the cat. *Experimental Neurology*, *23*(1), 140–155.

Willard, F. H., & Martin, G. F. (1983). The auditory brainstem nuclei and some of their projections to the inferior colliculus in the North American opossum. *Neuroscience, 10*(4), 1203–1232.

Wu, S. H., & Kelly, J. B. (1995). In vitro brain slice studies of the rat's dorsal nucleus of the lateral lemniscus. II. Physiological properties of biocytin-labeled neurons. *Journal of Neurophysiology, 73*(2), 794–809.

Wu, S. H., & Kelly, J. B. (1996). In vitro brain slice studies of the rat's dorsal nucleus of the lateral lemniscus. III. synaptic pharmacology. *Journal of Neurophysiology, 75*(3), 1271–1282.

Wu, S. H., Ma, C. L., & Kelly, J. B. (2004). Contribution of AMPA, NMDA, and GABA(A) receptors to temporal pattern of postsynaptic responses in the inferior colliculus of the rat. *Journal of Neuroscience, 24*(19), 4625–4634. doi: 10.1523/JNEUROSCI.0318-04.2004

Xie, R., Gittelman, J. X., Li, N., & Pollak, G. D. (2008). Whole cell recordings of intrinsic properties and sound-evoked responses from the inferior colliculus. *Neuroscience, 154*(1), 245–256. doi: 10.1016/j.neuroscience.2008.02.039

Xie, R., Gittelman, J. X., & Pollak, G. D. (2007). Rethinking tuning: in vivo whole-cell recordings of the inferior colliculus in awake bats. *Journal of Neuroscience, 27*(35), 9469–9481. doi: 10.1523/JNEUROSCI.2865-07.2007

Xie, R., Meitzen, J., & Pollak, G. D. (2005). Differing roles of inhibition in hierarchical processing of species-specific calls in auditory brainstem nuclei. *Journal of Neurophysiology, 94*(6), 4019–4037. doi: 10.1152/jn.00688.2005

Yang, L., Liu, Q., & Pollak, G. D. (1996). Afferent connections to the dorsal nucleus of the lateral lemniscus of the mustache bat: Evidence for two functional subdivisions. *Journal of Comparative Neurology, 373*(4), 575–592. doi: 10.1002/(SICI)1096-9861(19960930)373:4<575::AID-CNE7>3.0.CO;2-Z

Yang, L., & Pollak, G. D. (1994a). GABA and glycine have different effects on monaural response properties in the dorsal nucleus of the lateral lemniscus of the mustache bat. *Journal of Neurophysiology, 71*(6), 2014–2024.

Yang, L., & Pollak, G. D. (1994b). The roles of GABAergic and glycinergic inhibition on binaural processing in the dorsal nucleus of the lateral lemniscus of the mustache bat. *Journal of Neurophysiology, 71*(6), 1999–2013.

Yang, L., & Pollak, G. D. (1997). Differential response properties to amplitude modulated signals in the dorsal nucleus of the lateral lemniscus of the mustache bat and the roles of GABAergic inhibition. *Journal of Neurophysiology, 77*(1), 324–340. doi: 10.1152/jn.1997.77.1.324

Yang, L., & Pollak, G. D. (1998). Features of ipsilaterally evoked inhibition in the dorsal nucleus of the lateral lemniscus. *Hearing Research, 122*(1–2), 125–141. doi: S0378-5955(98)00088-4 [pii]

Yavuzoglu, A., Schofield, B. R., & Wenstrup, J. J. (2010). Substrates of auditory frequency integration in a nucleus of the lateral lemniscus. *Neuroscience, 169*(2), 906–919. doi: 10.1016/j.neuroscience.2010.04.073

Yavuzoglu, A., Schofield, B. R., & Wenstrup, J. J. (2011). Circuitry underlying spectrotemporal integration in the auditory midbrain. *Journal of Neuroscience, 31*(40), 14424–14435. doi: 10.1523/JNEUROSCI.3529-11.2011

Zhang, H., & Kelly, J. B. (2006a). Responses of neurons in the rat's ventral nucleus of the lateral lemniscus to amplitude-modulated tones. *Journal of Neurophysiology, 96*(6), 2905–2914. doi: 10.1152/jn.00481.2006

Zhang, H., & Kelly, J. B. (2006b). Responses of neurons in the rat's ventral nucleus of the lateral lemniscus to monaural and binaural tone bursts. *Journal of Neurophysiology, 95*(4), 2501–2512. doi: 10.1152/jn.01215.2005

Zhao, M., & Wu, S. H. (2001). Morphology and physiology of neurons in the ventral nucleus of the lateral lemniscus in rat brain slices. *Journal of Comparative Neurology*, *433*(2), 255–271.
Zook, J. M., & Casseday, J. H. (1982). Origin of ascending projections to inferior colliculus in the mustache bat, *Pteronotus parnellii*. *Journal of Comparative Neurology*, *207*(1), 14–28. doi: 10.1002/cne.902070103
Zook, J. M., & Casseday, J. H. (1985). Projections from the cochlear nuclei in the mustache bat, *Pteronotus parnellii*. *Journal of Comparative Neurology*, *237*(3), 307–324. doi: 10.1002/cne.902370303
Zook, J. M., & Casseday, J. H. (1987). Convergence of ascending pathways at the inferior colliculus of the mustache bat, Pteronotus parnellii. *Journal of Comparative Neurology*, *261*(3), 347–361. doi: 10.1002/cne.902610303

CHAPTER 17

AXON TRAJECTORIES IN THE AUDITORY BRAINSTEM

NELL BEATTY CANT

Abstract

This chapter summarizes what is known about the organization of the axons that make up the white matter of the auditory brainstem. The sources of the axons in each of the major fiber bundles (the dorsal and intermediate acoustic striae, the ventral acoustic stria or trapezoid body, and the lateral lemniscus) are reviewed, and, where information is available, the organization of specific groups of axons within the fiber bundles is described. The chapter collects the extensive but scattered information about axon trajectories into one place, both to provide a summary of what is known and also to indicate important gaps in our knowledge. The emphasis is almost entirely on the routes followed by groups of axons over the relatively long distances between structures and on the organization of specific types of axons within the fiber bundles; information about the termination patterns of the axons can be obtained from the references cited and throughout the chapter. Because knowledge about axon trajectories has considerable practical value (as, for example, in designing and interpreting both anatomical and physiological studies), the most useful information is species specific. Fortunately, at least at our current level of understanding, the components and relative positions of the major fiber bundles are remarkably similar across species (undoubtedly reflecting a common mammalian developmental plan).

Keywords: dorsal acoustic stria, intermediate acoustic stria, ventral acoustic stria, trapezoid body, lateral lemniscus, white matter, auditory brainstem

THE auditory brainstem is made up of many types of neurons grouped into a number of complex structures. Understanding the interconnections among these structures has been a major focus of neuroanatomical studies for over a century. An important goal of the studies has been the construction of detailed maps of the connections with respect to the origins and termination patterns of the numerous neuronal populations that constitute the basic units of the system. Such maps form a logical foundation for interpretation of physiological and functional studies, often lead to the development of new hypotheses, and can provide inspiration for computational models.

The auditory system is one of the more complicated sensory systems in terms of the number of brainstem structures that form its parts, and many reviews of the connections among these structures are available (e.g., Rouiller, 1997; Thompson & Schofield, 2000; Oertel & Wickesberg, 2002; Smith & Spirou, 2002; Malmierca, 2003; Cant, 2005; Schofield, 2005; Malmierca & Hackett, 2010; Schofield, 2011; Cant & Oliver, 2018). In broad outline, inputs from the cochlea are distributed to the dorsal and ventral cochlear nuclei in the caudal brainstem. Specific neuronal populations in the cochlear nuclei project to nuclei in the superior olivary complex, the nuclei of the lateral lemniscus, and/or the inferior colliculus. The inferior colliculus additionally receives inputs from neurons in the superior olive and nuclei of the lateral lemniscus, which are also interconnected with each other. The inferior colliculus, in turn, provides most (although not quite all) ascending auditory input to the forebrain. Some auditory structures are interconnected by commissural projections, and descending projections arise and terminate at all levels from the forebrain to the lower brainstem.

Summary information about the interconnections among auditory nuclei and the constituent neuronal populations is generally presented in the form of schematic representations known as "wiring diagrams." Although such diagrams are often quite detailed, they almost never provide realistic information about the routes followed by the axons as they pass between structures. In this sense, the wiring diagrams might be compared to the commonly used maps of underground train systems in large cities, in which spatial information is ignored in order to emphasize links between origins and terminations.[1] Just as the subway maps do not accurately depict geographical relationships, neuronal wiring diagrams are almost always distorted topologically with respect to the complex three-dimensional arrangements of the axons that provide the links. Obviously, the rationale for both types of maps is that the nodes or connection points are the sites of functional significance and the routes travelled are of lesser interest. Nevertheless, information about the trajectories followed by particular axon bundles is important, and sometimes essential, for the implementation and interpretation of experiments designed to investigate both structure and function.

Although detailed information about the three-dimensional organization of the white matter is generally omitted from reviews of auditory neuroanatomy, a considerable amount is known about the trajectories taken by specific groups of axons through the brainstem. The period from the late 1800s through the 1960s was a time of intense neuroanatomical study of the brains of many species, both mammalian and nonmammalian. The major fiber bundles that carry auditory information were described by investigators who used degeneration and myelin staining techniques to study auditory connectivity (history reviewed by Papez, 1930; Rasmussen, 1946). Since these methods were better suited to establishing fiber trajectories and general patterns of connectivity than to establishing details of synaptic organization, the early papers often went into great detail about the organization of the white matter. By the 1970s, the main structures in both the gray and white matter were known, and as better methods became available for the study of nuclear and synaptic organization, less emphasis was devoted to the details of fiber trajectories. However, a number of assiduous authors have taken care to describe the routes followed by projection neurons, and new information about the organization of the tracts is still being gathered.

In this review, I have attempted to collect the extensive but scattered information about axon trajectories into one place, both to provide a summary of what is known and also to indicate important gaps in our knowledge. The emphasis is almost entirely on the routes followed by groups of axons over the relatively long distances between structures and on the organization of specific types of axons within the fiber bundles; information about the termination patterns of the axons can be obtained from the references cited throughout the chapter. Because knowledge about axon trajectories has considerable practical value (as, for example, in designing and interpreting both anatomical and physiological studies), the most useful information is species specific. Fortunately, at least at our current level of understanding, the components and relative positions of the major fiber bundles are remarkably similar across species (undoubtedly reflecting a common mammalian developmental plan; cf. Cant, 1998). The most detailed descriptions are available for the cat, but information is also available for species as diverse as commonly used laboratory rodents, opossum, various species of bats, various species of monkeys, baboon, chimpanzee, and human (cited where appropriate).

Routes Followed by Ascending Auditory Axons

The principal cell axons that connect the cochlear nuclei with other parts of the brainstem travel in one of three major fiber tracts, named according to their relative location along the dorsal to ventral dimension of the neuraxis: the dorsal acoustic stria (DAS; stria of Monakow), the intermediate acoustic stria (IAS; stria of Held), and the ventral acoustic stria (commonly referred to as the trapezoid body [TB]). The striae may contain axons from sources other than the cochlear nuclei as well. A fourth major brainstem auditory fiber bundle, the lateral lemniscus (LL), includes the rostral extension of axons in the three acoustic striae and also contains ascending axons that arise in the superior olivary complex and the nuclei of the lateral lemniscus. All of the major tracts may further contain descending projections, as well as commissural fibers. The components (and/or the organization) of a tract usually vary along its extent as axons join and leave it. (For this reason, a tract should not generally be equated with one particular set of axons.) Some of the components of the major auditory tracts that are described in this chapter are illustrated in Figures 17.1–3, and information about known components of the tracts is summarized in Figure 17.4.

Dorsal Acoustic Stria

The DAS extends from the medial border of the dorsal cochlear nucleus, forming a cap of axons on the dorsal aspect of the inferior cerebellar peduncle,[2] to the ventral pole of the lateral lemniscus, which many of its axons join. The axons of both types of principal cells in the dorsal cochlear nucleus, the fusiform and giant cells, form the main components of the DAS as they leave the cochlear nucleus (cat: Fernandez & Karapas, 1967; van Noort, 1969; Osen, 1972; Adams & Warr, 1976; Smith et al., 2005; opossum: Willard & Martin, 1983; horseshoe bat: Vater & Feng, 1990; Rhesus monkey: Barnes et al., 1943; Strominger, 1973; human: Moore & Osen, 1979). These axons form major components of the DAS throughout its course and so define the trajectory of the entire tract. The stria travels rostrally and medially away from the dorsal cochlear nucleus while also dipping ventrally as it spreads out through the middle of the pontine tegmentum, where it crosses the midline (Figure 17.2, panels 4 and 5). The tract then dips further ventrally toward the rostral and dorsal aspect of the superior olivary complex, where many of its axons turn to join the lateral lemniscus. Fernandez and Karapas (1967, their Figure 4) illustrate the course of the DAS in the cat at eight transverse levels through the brainstem, providing a good appreciation of its three-dimensional extent (see also Adams & Warr, 1976, their figure 1; Smith et al., 2005).[3] As they enter the tegmentum, the axons from the dorsal cochlear nucleus appear to split into two or more separate bundles (cat: Papez, 1930; Adams & Warr, 1976); the significance of the split is not clear.

In the pontine tegmentum, the axons from the dorsal cochlear nucleus are joined in the DAS by axons from the principal cells of the lateral superior olivary nucleus that innervate the contralateral inferior colliculus. These axons leave the olivary complex dorsally and then turn medially to join the DAS (cat: van Noort, 1969; Elverland, 1978; Glendenning & Masterton, 1983; ferret: Henkel et al., 2007, see their figure 1C for an illustration of the convergence of the axons from the dorsal cochlear nucleus and the lateral superior olivary nucleus in the pontine tegmentum; mustache bat: Vater et al., 1995). After crossing the midline, the axons from the dorsal cochlear nucleus and those from the lateral superior olivary nucleus turn ventrally before then turning rostrally and dorsally to enter the lateral lemniscus.

Intermediate Acoustic Stria

The IAS is the smallest of the three acoustic striae (cat: Fernandez & Karapas, 1967; Adams & Warr, 1976; Smith et al., 1993a, 2005; Adams, 1997; rat: Harrison & Feldman, 1970; horseshoe bat: Vater & Feng, 1990; Rhesus monkey: Barnes et al., 1943; Strominger, 1973; chimpanzee: Strominger et al., 1977; human: Moore & Osen, 1979). Earlier literature contains some confusion about the cells of origin but it seems now generally agreed that most, if not all, of the ascending fibers in the IAS are the axons of octopus cells, which travel dorsally from the posteroventral cochlear nucleus, forming a bundle caudal to the DAS (cat: Warr, 1969, 1982; Osen, 1972; Adams, 1997; Smith et al., 2005; rat: Harrison & Feldman, 1970; Friauf & Ostwald, 1988; mouse: Felix et al., 2017). Like those of the DAS, the axons of the IAS loop over the inferior cerebellar peduncle as they leave the cochlear nucleus, but they then make a sharp turn ventrally to course along the medial border of the spinal trigeminal nucleus. As they reach the level of the caudal superior olivary complex, they turn medially and course parallel to the dorsal surface of that complex to cross the midline. On the contralateral side, the bundle of axons splits into several fascicles, some of which pass through olivary regions before rejoining the others to enter the lateral lemniscus (cat: Warr, 1982; rat: Friauf & Ostwald, 1988). The octopus cell axons in the IAS terminate in elaborate calyx-like terminations in the ventral portion of the contralateral ventral nucleus of the lateral lemniscus (cat: Stotler, 1953; Adams, 1997; Smith et al., 2005; rat: Friauf & Oswald, 1988; mouse: Felix et al., 2017; guinea pig: Schofield & Cant, 1997; human: Adams, 1997).

Ventral Acoustic Stria

The largest and most complex of the three acoustic striae, the ventral acoustic stria, is more commonly referred to as the trapezoid body (TB) in reference to the shape of the fiber bundle at the midline. The tract spans the width of the ventral brainstem at the level of the superior olivary complex; axons in the tract pass through and around the olivary nuclei. At the midline, it lies dorsal to the medullary pyramids. The TB contains almost all of the ascending axons of principle cells in the ventral cochlear nucleus (cat: Warr, 1966, 1969, 1972, 1982; van Noort, 1969; rat: Harrison & Warr, 1962; Harrison & Irving, 1966a, b; Harrison & Feldman, 1970; gerbil: Russell & Moore, 1995; guinea pig: Thompson & Thompson, 1991; dog (beagle): Goldberg & Brown, 1968; several species of bats: Zook & Casseday, 1985; Vater & Feng, 1990; Rhesus monkey: Strominger & Strominger, 1971; chimpanzee: Strominger et al., 1977; human: Moore & Osen, 1979). The tract is highly organized across its three dimensions (cat: van Noort, 1969; Brownell, 1975; Warr, 1982; rat: Harrison & Feldman, 1970). As axons leave the ventral cochlear nucleus, those from rostral regions are located rostrally and those from caudal parts are located caudally. The fibers travel in parallel as they course to the midline so the same rostral-to-caudal organization is evident there. The axons are further organized with respect to axon diameter and at least some of them are organized topographically with respect to frequency (cat: Brownell, 1975; Warr, 1982; Spirou et al., 1990). The differences in axon diameter give the TB a layered appearance. The dorsal-most layer contains medium-sized axons; the middle layer, which does not extend all the way to the rostral pole of the TB, contains large axons. The ventral, superficial layer, which is enlarged at the rostral pole of the TB, contains mainly thin axons. Some mixing of axon diameters occurs between the dorsal and middle axon layers (cat: Brownell, 1975). The axons of most of the cell populations in the cochlear nuclei and other neurons that send axons into the TB have been associated with one of these layers.

The medium-diameter axons of the spherical bushy cells in the anteroventral cochlear nucleus project through the dorsal half of the TB (cat: Warr, 1966, 1982; Brownell, 1975; Smith et al., 1993b; gerbil: N. B. Cant, unpublished observations; Figure 17.1) and occupy approximately the rostral two-thirds at the midline, where they are organized according to frequency (cat: Brownell, 1975; Spirou et al., 1990). The spherical bushy cell axons pass through or around the lateral and medial superior olivary nuclei on the ipsilateral side (forming terminations), traverse the medial nucleus of the trapezoid body (without terminating), cross the midline (forming terminations in the contralateral medial superior olivary nucleus), and turn rostrally to join the lateral lemniscus, where they terminate in the ventral nucleus (cat: Warr, 1966; Smith et al., 1993b; Beckius et al., 1999; rat: Harrison & Irving, 1966a). (The path followed by these axons is "dorsal" relative to the position of other axons in the TB; as they pass through the superior olivary complex itself, many of the axons may run ventral to the main nuclei [Warr, 1966; Smith et al., 1993b; Harrison & Irving, 1966a]).

The large-diameter axons of the globular bushy cells in the ventral cochlear nucleus project into the middle layer of the TB. These axons are among the largest in the auditory system and are the source of calyces in the contralateral medial nucleus of the trapezoid body (cat: Warr, 1969, 1972, 1982; Tolbert et al., 1982; Spirou et al., 1990; Smith et al., 1991; rat: Harrison & Warr, 1962; Harrison & Irving, 1966a, b; Friauf & Ostwald, 1988; mouse, gerbil, and several species of bat: Kuwabara et al., 1991). The very large, heavily myelinated axons course ventral to the nuclei of the superior olivary complex along most of its caudal-to-rostral dimension, although they are not present at the rostral pole (Brownell, 1975; Warr, 1982). They give off collateral branches to several periolivary nuclei on the ipsilateral side, cross the midline in the ventral half of the TB, send thick branches into the contralateral medial nucleus of the trapezoid body, and continue laterally and rostrally to join the lateral lemniscus. The axons terminate in the ventral nucleus of the lateral lemniscus. Unlike the fibers in the dorsal half of the TB at the midline, the ventral fibers do not appear to be organized topographically with respect to frequency (Brownell, 1975; Spirou et al., 1990). In the rat, a small number of equally thick axons arise from cells of the cochlear nerve root but travel in the most ventral part of the TB (rat: Lee et al., 1996; López et al., 1999).

Many of the multipolar neurons in the ventral cochlear nucleus project directly to the inferior colliculus. These neurons are referred to by a number of different names (cf. Oertel et al., 2011), but it is generally agreed that those that project to the IC have thin axons and leave the cochlear nucleus via the TB (cat: Warr, 1969, 1972, 1982; van Noort, 1969; Brownell, 1975; Smith & Rhode, 1989; Spirou et al., 1990; Smith et al., 1993a; Thompson, 1998; guinea pig: Thompson & Thompson, 1991; gerbil and chinchilla: Ostapoff et al., 1994; mouse: Oertel et al., 1990). Many of the multipolar cell axons enter the most ventral fiber layer in the TB, but axons of multipolar cells may be found throughout the dorsal-to-ventral dimension of the tract (cat: Warr, 1969; Smith et al., 1993a; rat: Doucet & Ryugo, 2003; mouse: Darrow et al., 2012; guinea pig: Thompson & Thompson, 1991). The trajectory pattern of the multipolar cell axons from the rostral

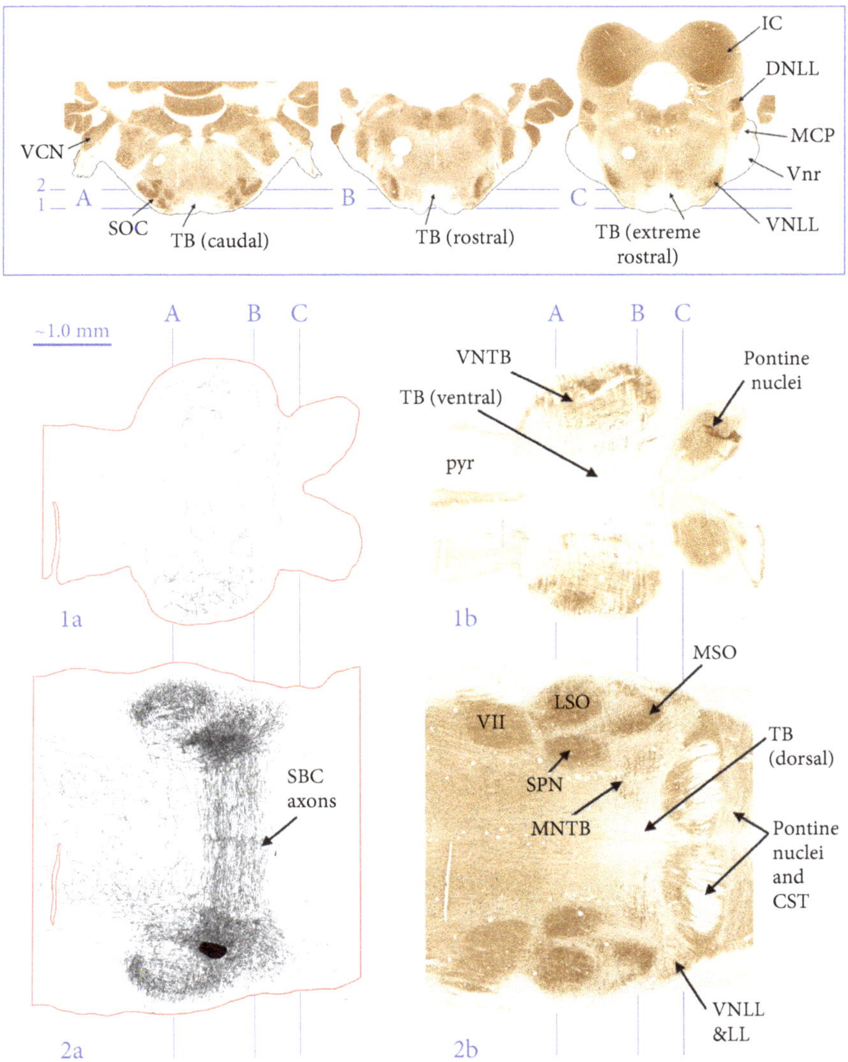

FIGURE 17.1. Drawings to illustrate the path followed by spherical bushy cell (SBC) axons through the dorsal and rostral part of the trapezoid body. Panels 1a and 2a: Horizontal sections through the superior olivary complex of a gerbil in which biotinylated dextran amine (BDA) was injected into the medial superior olivary nucleus (MSO; injection site indicated by the black spot), filling SBC axons from the anteroventral cochlear nuclei on both sides of the brain. (These sections are from Case 644, described in Cant, 2013.) Panels 1b and 2b: Cytochrome oxidase-reacted sections adjacent to the BDA-reacted sections in panels 1a and 2a, respectively. Rostral is to the right for all horizontal sections. Inset: For purposes of orientation, the approximate levels of the horizontal sections are cross-referenced to the levels of three transverse sections from another gerbil. Dorsal is to the top for the transverse sections. Abbreviations for all figures: AVCN, anteroventral cochlear nucleus; BDA, biotinylated dextran amine (a tracer that is transported

pole of the ventral cochlear nucleus differs in detail from that of those that arise more caudally. The most rostral axons take an "obliquely anterior [rostral]" course and cross the midline at the rostral extreme of the TB (rostral to the nuclei themselves, sometimes straying into the area of the pontine nuclei; cat: Warr, 1966; gerbil: N. B. Cant, unpublished observations; Figure 17.2, panels 1–3). These axons do not appear to innervate the olivary nuclei; on the contralateral side they enter the LL at its ventral pole (Figure 17.2, panel 3).

In contrast, the axons that arise from the multipolar cells in the "multipolar cell area" of the ventral cochlear nucleus (Osen, 1969) travel in the caudal half of the TB and cross the midline in parallel with the other groups of TB axons (cat: Warr, 1972). Just after they pass ventral to the contralateral medial nucleus of the trapezoid body, these axons make an almost right-angle turn and course rostrally so that they are now oriented perpendicular to the crossing TB axons (cat: Warr, 1972, 1982; Smith et al., 1993b; gerbil: N. B. Cant, unpublished observations, Figure 17.2, panels 1 and 2). Therefore, whereas the TB contains axons arranged in parallel order at the midline, in the region of the superior olivary complex, it also contains axons that course longitudinally with respect to the long axis of the brainstem. Along their caudal-to-rostral course, the multipolar cell axons give rise to terminals in the ventral nucleus of the trapezoid body (cat: Warr, 1972; Smith et al., 1993a).

A small contingent of axons that project from the caudal cochlear nucleus to the midbrain do not enter the TB directly but rather course rostrally along the medial margin of the anteroventral cochlear nucleus to enter the TB at its rostral extreme (cat: Warr, 1972, 1982; Thompson, 1998). This small bundle of axons was called the "lateral trapezoid body tract" by Warr (1972), who traced it as far as the ventral part of the LL. It may arise from small cells in the region of the granule cell layer (Thompson, 1998).

Lateral Lemniscus and Paralemniscal Fibers

The LL (Figure 17.3) contains ascending inputs to the IC from the cochlear nuclei, superior olivary complex, and nuclei of the lateral lemniscus, and it is also the route of

---

both anterogradely and retrogradely through axons); CST, corticospinal tract; DAS, dorsal acoustic stria; DCN, dorsal cochlear nucleus; DNLL, dorsal nucleus of the lateral lemniscus; IC, inferior colliculus; IPF, interpeduncular fossa; LL, lateral lemniscus; LNTB, lateral nucleus of the trapezoid body; LSO, lateral superior olivary nucleus; MCP, middle cerebellar peduncle; MG, medial geniculate nucleus; MNTB, medial nucleus of the trapezoid body; MSO, medial superior olivary nucleus; PVCN, posteroventral cochlear nucleus; pyr, medullary pyramid; SBC, spherical bushy cell; SOC, superior olivary complex; SPN, superior paraolivary nucleus; TB, trapezoid body; VCN, ventral cochlear nucleus; VII, motor nucleus of the seventh nerve; VNLL, ventral nucleus of the lateral lemniscus; VNTB, ventral nucleus of the trapezoid body; Vnr, trigeminal nerve root.

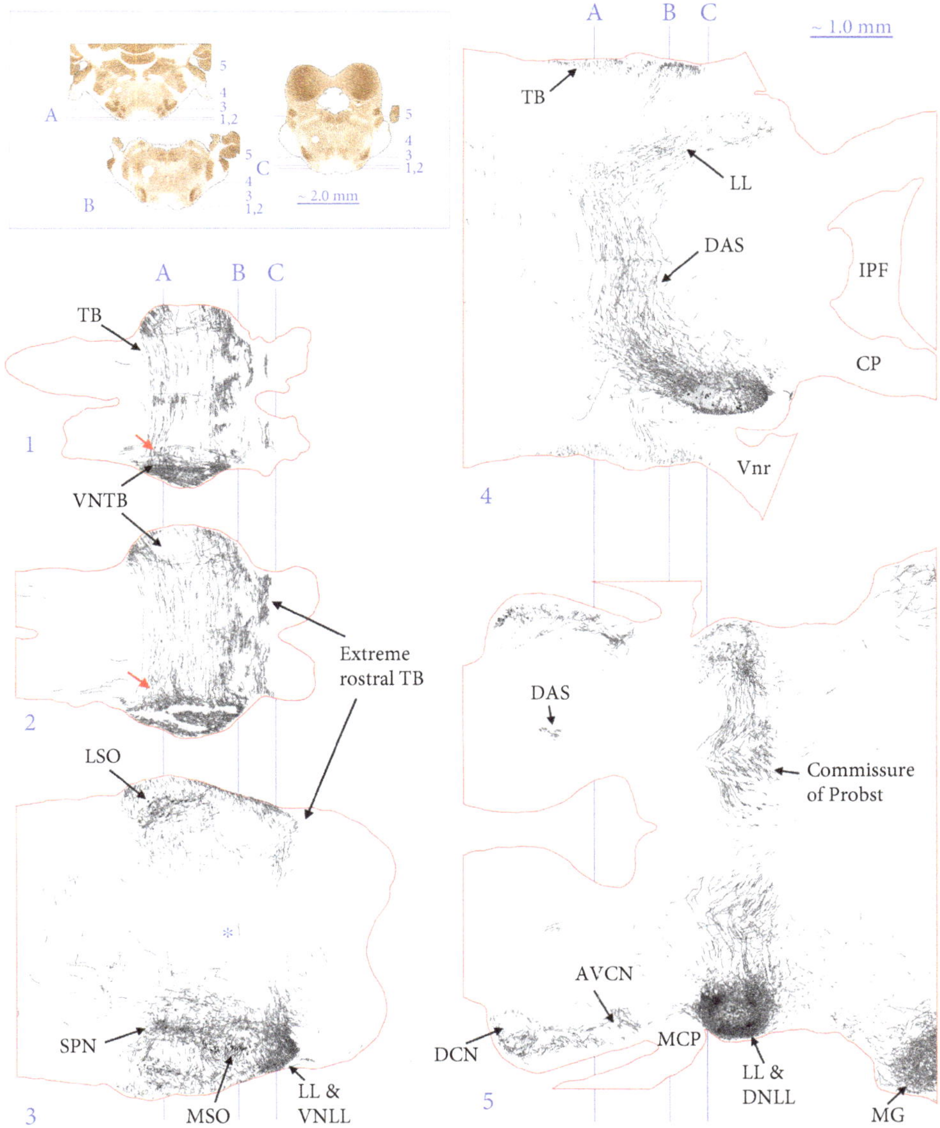

FIGURE 17.2. Drawings to illustrate the paths followed by axons that project into and out of the inferior colliculus (IC). Panels 1–5: Horizontal sections through the brainstem of a gerbil in which BDA was injected into the right IC. The rostral direction is to the right of the figure. (These sections are from Case 419, described in Cant and Benson, 2006.) The approximate levels of the horizontal sections are indicated at three transverse levels in the inset (the same transverse sections shown in Figure 17.1). In this case, many axons are labeled in the ventral TB (both ascending and descending axons) but almost no axons are labeled in the dorsal TB (asterisk on panel 3; the spherical bushy cells do not project to the IC and so are not labeled in this case). Multipolar cells of the AVCN travel in the extreme rostral part of the TB (panels 1–3). Multipolar cells of the PVCN cross the midline more caudally and then turn rostrally to run parallel to the VNTB. The red arrows on panels 1 and 2 indicate the area in which the axons make the turn. Descending fibers from the inferior colliculus also run parallel to the VNTB and may be intermingled with those from the cochlear nucleus. Gray fill on the drawings indicates places where terminal branching of the axons was so dense that it was impossible to mark individual axons. Abbreviations as in legend for Figure 17.1.

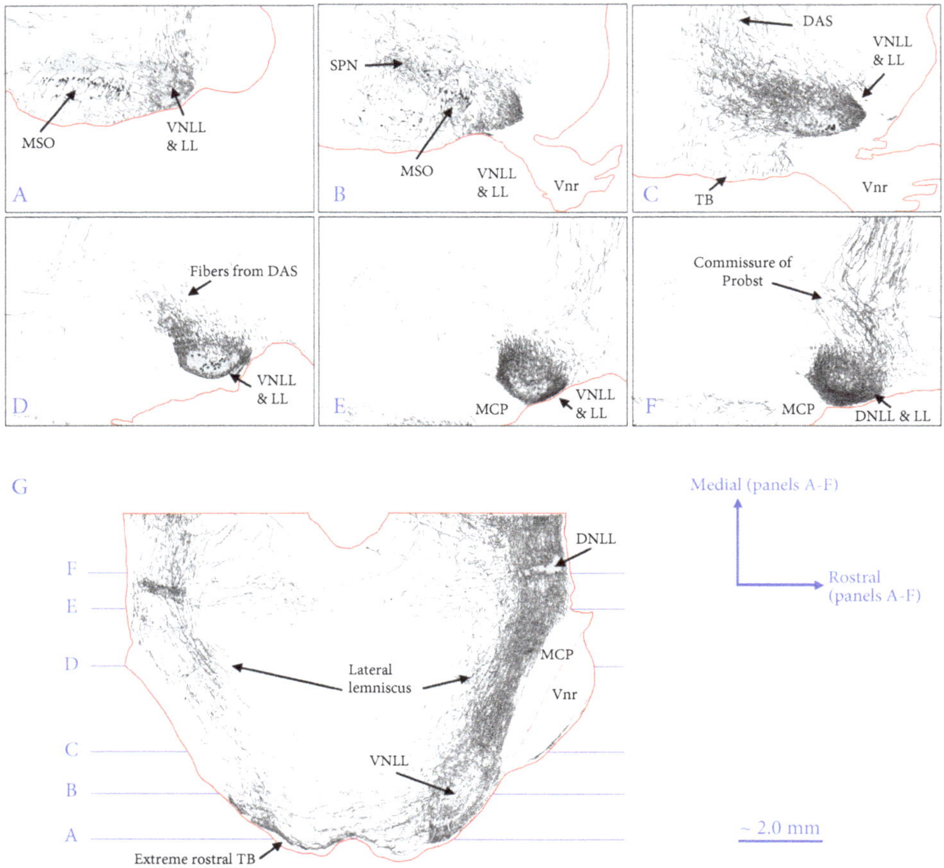

FIGURE 17.3. Panels A–F: Drawings to illustrate axons in the LL in the same case shown in Figure 17.2. Panel G: Transverse section from a gerbil in which BDA was injected into the inferior colliculus (Case 430, described in Cant & Benson, 2006). The approximate levels for the top six panels are indicated by the blue lines on the transverse section. (The sections lie near those shown in Figure 17.2 but are at slightly different dorsal-to-ventral levels. The top edge of each box indicates the same distance from the midline for each section, and the right edge indicates the same distance from the front of the brain.) Abbreviations as in Figure 17.1.

some descending systems. It is the most complex of the major auditory fiber tracts and is also the least well-understood in terms of the organization of its components. Detailed studies, such as those described for the TB (e.g., Warr, 1966, 1982; van Noort, 1969; Brownell, 1975; Spirou et al., 1990), have not been reported. The LL lies near the lateral surface of the brainstem and spans the distance between the ventral pons (immediately rostral to the superior olivary complex) and the dorsal midbrain, where its ascending fibers enter the inferior colliculus. The LL surrounds the dorsal and ventral nuclei of the lateral lemniscus, and the nuclei themselves are penetrated by bundles of fasciculated axons.

The rostral, caudal, and lateral boundaries of the LL are fairly well defined, but the medial boundary is less distinct, fading into the adjacent lateral tegmentum in an area known as the paralemniscal region (also referred to as Monakow's area in the older literature; see Varga et al., 2008, for a detailed discussion of this complex tegmental region). Rasmussen (1946) called the fibers surrounding the rostral, lateral, and caudal aspects of the nuclei the LL proper and the region medial to the nuclei the paralemniscal zone. In contrast to the more restricted sources of axons in the LL proper, the paralemniscal zone is traversed by a large variety of fibers from both auditory and non-auditory areas (e.g., Herbert et al., 1997). Axons in this region from nuclei in the lower brainstem that project directly to the medial geniculate nucleus, bypassing the inferior colliculus (e.g., Henkel, 1983), have been referred to as the central acoustic tract (discussed in, e.g., Casseday et al., 1989).

The LL, like the TB, is organized such that axons of some cell types are segregated from one another while others appear to be intermingled. The topography is complex. Axons of different cell types occupy specific zones within the medial-to-lateral and rostral-to-caudal dimensions. Further, because some axons join the tract along its ventral-to-dorsal axis, others terminate in the nuclei of the lateral lemniscus, and a few appear to change position as they course through the tract, there is also a dorsal-to-ventral organization. As noted in the following sections, many authors have noted whether axons from specific sources run in lateral or medial "bands" of the LL (i.e., lateral or medial with respect to the nuclear groups), but only a few comment on the rostral-to-caudal organization of the component axons. This an important omission because the white matter surrounding the nuclei of the lateral lemniscus appears thicker in the rostral-to-caudal dimension than in the lateral-to-medial dimension (Figure 17.3), and it is highly likely that axons that are described as having a lateral or medial location are distributed differentially in the rostral-to-caudal dimension as well.

Axons from the Cochlear Nuclei that Enter the Lateral Lemniscus

Most, if not all of the axons that arise in the cochlear nuclei and travel in one of the three acoustic striae described previously continue into the LL. Axons in the TB, IAS, and DAS join the LL near the rostral boundary of the superior olivary complex or along its ventral-to-dorsal extent. Some of these axons terminate in the nuclei of the lateral lemniscus, while others continue to the midbrain to terminate in the inferior colliculus. Axons from different parts of the cochlear nuclear complex travel in different parts of the LL.

After the fibers of the DAS that originate from the contralateral dorsal cochlear nucleus cross the midline, they dip ventrally toward the superior olivary complex and then turn dorsally and rostrally to ascend to the midbrain in the paralemniscal tegmentum (cat: Rasmussen, 1946; Warr, 1966; Fernandez & Karapas, 1967; van Noort, 1969; Osen, 1972; Glendenning et al., 1981; Smith et al., 2005; rabbit: Borg, 1973; horseshoe bat: Vater & Feng, 1990; Rhesus monkey: Barnes et al., 1943). As they course dorsally, they also move laterally so that they appear to enter the inferior colliculus with the other fibers of the LL proper (the white matter). Observations by Osen (1972) in kittens suggested that the axons of the giant cells and fusiform cells may be separate as they enter the inferior colliculus; lesions of the rostral part of the LL, near its entrance to the inferior colliculus, led to degeneration of fusiform cells but not of giant cells in the dorsal cochlear nucleus. In contrast to the route followed by the contralateral axons from the dorsal cochlear nucleus, the axons that arise in the *ipsilateral* dorsal cochlear nucleus (a relatively small number) travel in the lateral band of the LL (Warr, 1966).

The multipolar cell axons that project from both the contralateral and ipsilateral ventral cochlear nuclei to the inferior colliculus travel in the lateral band of the LL (cat: Warr, 1966, Osen, 1972; Glendenning et al., 1981; Oliver, 1987; rat: Harrison & Warr, 1962; gerbil: Benson & Cant, 2008; opossum: Willard & Martin, 1983; horseshoe bat: Vater & Feng, 1990). Some of them may also be located in the white matter rostral to the nuclei (cat: Osen, 1972; Warr, 1972, 1982; gerbil: Benson & Cant, 2008), a point that is better appreciated in horizontal and sagittal planes of section than in the more commonly used transverse plane. Some authors also report that axons from the ventral cochlear nucleus may travel through the nuclei rather than in the white matter surrounding them (cat: Osen, 1972; rat: Saldaña et al., 2009; horseshoe bat: Vater & Feng, 1990); these may be the axons of cells other than the multipolar cells.

The axons of globular and spherical bushy cells and octopus cells also send branches into the LL (cat: Warr, 1982; Smith et al., 1991, 1993b, 2005; rat: Friauf & Ostwald, 1988; guinea pig: Schofield & Cant, 1997). These axons terminate in the nuclei of the lateral lemniscus and do not reach the inferior colliculus. The octopus cell axons terminate in the ventral part of the ventral nucleus, but the bushy cell axons probably terminate throughout the ventral nuclei (reviewed by Oertel & Wickesberg, 2002). Whether the projection from the ventral cochlear nucleus to the dorsal nucleus of the lateral lemniscus (Glendenning et al., 1981; Shneiderman et al., 1988) is solely from multipolar cells on their way to the inferior colliculus or whether the axons of other cell types project so far dorsally is not known. Some or all of these axons may travel in fascicles interspersed among the cells of the nuclei of the lateral lemniscus rather than in the surrounding tract itself (cat: Glendenning & Masterton 1983; horseshoe bat: Vater & Feng, 1990). In the rat, the large axons that arise from cochlear root neurons ascend for some distance in the rostral band of the LL before leaving the tract to innervate multiple tegmental areas (rat: López et al., 1999; Nodal & Lopéz, 2003).

Axons from the Nuclei of the Superior Olivary Complex that Enter the LL

Most projections from the superior olivary complex to the inferior colliculus arise from principal cells in the medial and lateral superior olivary nuclei (MSO and LSO, respectively), but there are also projections from other olivary nuclei (reviewed by Schofield, 2005). Axons that arise from the ipsilateral MSO course dorsally through that nucleus (guinea pig: Smith, 1995; gerbil: Kuwabara & Zook, 1999) and then turn rostrally and laterally to join the LL, where most, if not all of them, travel in the medial band close to the nuclei of the lateral lemniscus (cat: Rasmussen, 1946; van Noort, 1969; Elverland, 1978; Henkel & Spangler, 1983, their Figure 5; Henkel, 1997; mustache bat: Zook & Casseday, 1987; Vater et al. 1995). Some of the MSO axons may course in the LL rostral to the nuclei (Henkel & Spangler 1983). Axons from principal cells in the LSO that project to the ipsilateral inferior colliculus (mainly glycinergic, Saint Marie et al., 1989 [cat]) also exit the nucleus dorsally and join those from the MSO to travel to the inferior colliculus in the medial band or paralemniscal region (cat: Rasmussen, 1946; van Noort, 1969; Elverland, 1978; Glendenning et al., 1981; mustache bat: Vater et al., 1995). Like those from the MSO, some of the axons from the LSO may also run in the rostral LL (Glendenning et al., 1981, their Figure 10). Some authors report that a few axons from the MSO and LSO run in the lateral band of the LL, but Henkel & Spangler (1983) argue that the axons in question probably arise from other olivary sources.

Axons from the LSO that project to the contralateral inferior colliculus cross the midline in the DAS (see previous discussion) and appear to remain together with the axons from the dorsal cochlear nucleus as they travel to the inferior colliculus in the medial (paralemniscal) band of the LL (suggested by figures in Elverland, 1978 [cat]; Glendenning et al., 1981 [cat]; Casseday et al., 1988 [horseshoe bat]). The organization of these fibers in the medial band with respect to those from the ipsilateral LSO and MSO is not known. If the axons from the two sides do remain segregated in the LL, the organization prefigures that in the central nucleus of the inferior colliculus, where the terminations from the ipsilateral and contralateral LSOs are non-overlapping, terminations from the contralateral dorsal cochlear nucleus overlap those from the contralateral LSO, and those from the ipsilateral MSO overlap those from the ipsilateral LSO (cat: Shneiderman & Henkel, 1987; Oliver et al., 1997; Loftus et al., 2004).

Axons from several additional populations of olivary cells appear to be located in specific parts of the LL. Thick axons of GABAergic cells in the superior paraolivary nucleus travel to the inferior colliculus in the paralemniscal zone, passing through the paralemniscal nucleus (rat: Saldaña et al., 2009). Axons from the medial and ventral nuclei of the trapezoid body, on the other hand, ascend through the nuclei or are located in the lateral and/or rostral bands of the LL (cat: Glendenning & Masterton, 1983; Henkel & Spangler, 1983; Spangler et al., 1985; Smith et al., 1998; rat: Sommer et al., 1993; Warr & Beck, 1996; horseshoe bat: Casseday et al., 1988). Many of these projections, like the ipsilateral projections from the lateral superior olivary nucleus, are glycinergic (chinchilla and guinea pig: Saint Marie & Baker, 1990).

Projections to the inferior colliculus from the nuclei of the lateral lemniscus themselves appear to course dorsally through the nuclei rather than in the surrounding fiber tract (cat: Kudo, 1981; Whitley & Henkel, 1984; rat: Merchán et al., 1994).

Routes Followed by Descending Auditory Axons

Almost all auditory structures contain populations of neurons that send axons to nuclei at lower levels of the neuraxis. Collectively, these projections make up the descending auditory pathways (reviewed by Saldaña, 1993; Thompson, 2005; Schofield, 2011). Routes taken by the descending axons have not been documented as completely as those of the ascending systems, but some authors have taken care to illustrate and discuss the routes taken by specific systems. Like the fibers of the ascending pathways, those of the descending pathways appear to follow defined, stereotypic routes (e.g., Feliciano et al., 1995).

Descending Pathways from the Auditory Cortex

Axons arising from pyramidal cells in most, if not all, fields of auditory cortex travel with other corticobulbar and corticospinal fibers through the internal capsule and cerebral peduncles, where they occupy its most lateral part (cat: Rasmussen, 1964; rat: Feliciano et al. 1995; Saldaña et al., 1996; reviewed by Saldaña, 2015). Descending axons follow at least three routes into the ipsilateral inferior colliculus (rat: Feliciano et al., 1995). Two bundles of thick axons leave the peduncle at the level of the midbrain. One of these runs directly into the inferior colliculus through its rostral pole. The second runs more laterally to enter via the brachium of the inferior colliculus. A third group of axons leaves the descending cortical tract at the pontine level and then courses dorsally in the paralemniscal region and rostral band of the LL. Some of these fibers reach the inferior colliculus but others appear to terminate in tegmental areas (rat: Feliciano et al., 1995; Saldaña et al., 1996). Within the inferior colliculus, terminations from the three groups appear to intermingle. Whether the three groups of fibers arise from separate sources and/or have different targets within the inferior colliculus is not known. A few of the cortical fibers cross to the contralateral inferior colliculus via the collicular commissure.

For the most part, the cortical projections to the superior olivary complex and cochlear nuclei arise from different populations of neurons (rat: Doucet et al., 2002) and follow different routes through the brainstem (rat: Feliciano et al. 1995; guinea pig: Coomes and Schofield 2004). The cortical fibers that innervate the superior olivary complex travel with the corticospinal tract as far as the medullary pyramids, where they turn to enter the superior olivary complex and split into two bundles, a small bundle that spreads over the dorsal aspect of the complex and a larger bundle that courses caudally, giving rise to terminals along the rostral-to-caudal extent of the ventral nucleus of the trapezoid body (perpendicular to the crossing fibers of the TB).

On the other hand, most of the cortical fibers that innervate the cochlear nuclei follow a route unrelated to the major auditory fiber bundles (rat: Feliciano et al., 1995). These axons leave the cerebral peduncles in the midbrain and run in a dorsal and caudal direction to reach the level of the middle cerebellar peduncle. They course next to the peduncle until they reach the dorsal aspect of the anteroventral cochlear nucleus, which they enter through the dorsal region known as the subpeduncular area (cat, rat and mouse: Mugnaini et al., 1980; Osen et al., 1984; Weedman et al., 1996). The few cortical fibers that innervate the contralateral superior olivary complex and/or cochlear nucleus cross the midline in the TB and those that innervate the cochlear nucleus may then follow a circuitous route into the subpeduncular corner that mimics that of the ipsilateral projection (rat: Feliciano et al., 1995; guinea pig: Coomes & Schofield, 2004).

Descending Pathways from the Inferior Colliculus to the Superior Olivary Complex and the Cochlear Nuclei

Projections to the superior olivary complex and cochlear nuclei appear to arise from largely separate populations of neurons in the inferior colliculus (rat: Okoyama et al., 2006; guinea pig: Coomes & Schofield, 2004). Both projections reach their targets via the LL, but whether they travel in the same or separate parts of the tract is not clear. Most authors report that descending collicular fibers travel through the nuclei or in the lateral band of the LL (cat: van Noort, 1969; rat: Faye-Lund, 1986; Caicedo & Herbert, 1993; Saldaña, 1993; Malmierca et al., 1996; rabbit: Borg, 1973; Rhesus monkey: Moore & Goldberg, 1966). However, Rasmussen (1960) states that the axons destined for the cochlear nucleus travel in "Monakow's bundle" (i.e., the medial band of the LL).

At the rostral pole of the superior olive, collicular fibers that innervate olivary nuclei leave the LL to run along the rostral-to-caudal axis of the ventral nucleus of the trapezoid body, forming terminations along its length (rat: Vetter et al., 1993; guinea pig: Thompson & Thompson, 1993). Thus, these axons course perpendicular to the crossing fibers of the trapezoid body and parallel to the cortical axons that also innervate the ventral nucleus.

The collicular axons that innervate the cochlear nucleus also travel from rostral to caudal through the TB. In the caudal part of the tract, they turn laterally or medially to travel to the ipsilateral or contralateral cochlear nuclei, respectively (cat: Conlee & Kane, 1982). At the border of the cochlear nucleus, they turn dorsally to pass between the medial border of the posteroventral cochlear nucleus and the lateral boundary of the inferior cerebellar peduncle as the "centrifugal bundle of Lorente de Nó" (cat: Rasmussen,

1960; van Noort, 1969; Adams & Warr, 1976; rat: Caicedo & Herbert, 1993; Malmierca et al., 1996; mouse: Lorente de Nó, 1981, his figure 6-4). The major target of the recurrent bundle is the granule cell layer associated with the dorsal cochlear nucleus (Malmierca et al., 1996). As already noted, this is also the major target of projections from the auditory cortex. Thus, the terminations of the cortical and collicular projections ultimately appear to overlap, although the axons reach the nucleus via quite different routes.

Descending Pathways from the Superior Olivary Complex to the Cochlear Nucleus and Cochlea

Nuclei of the superior olivary complex send bilateral projections to the cochlear nuclei via all three acoustic striae (cat: van Noort, 1969; Elverland, 1977; Adams & Warr, 1976; Spangler et al. 1987; rat: Warr & Beck, 1996; rabbit: Borg, 1973). These projections include the only descending inputs to the cochlear nucleus that have been identified as inhibitory (guinea pig: Benson & Potashner, 1990; Ostapoff et al., 1997). Most of the contralateral projections are GABAergic, whereas the ipsilateral projections are mainly glycinergic.

At the midline, crossing axons from the ventral nucleus of the trapezoid body (the main source of contralateral projections to the cochlear nucleus) travel in rostral and dorsal portions of the trapezoid body (cat: Spangler et al., 1987; rat: Warr & Beck, 1996; Gómez-Nieto et al., 2008). Whether they are segregated from the axons of the spherical bushy cells or interspersed among them is not known, but as descending axons approach the medial boundary of the cochlear nucleus, both glycinergic (large) axons and GABAergic (small) axons are gathered into distinct fascicles, separated from the ascending fibers of the TB (guinea pig: Kolston et al., 1992; but not present in baboon: Moore et al., 1996).

Cholinergic axons of the olivocochlear bundle (to be discussed further) send branches into the cochlear nucleus as they pass by it in the vestibular nerve root; the branches enter the ventral cochlear nucleus all along its medial border (cat: Osen & Roth, 1969; Brown et al., 1988; rat: White & Warr, 1983; Osen et al., 1984; mouse: Brown et al., 1988, 1991; Brown, 1993; guinea pig: Winter et al., 1989; gerbil: Ryan et al., 1990; Brown et al., 1988; but apparently not present in human: Moore & Osen, 1979). In rodents, another group of cholinergic axons that arise in the ventral nucleus of the trapezoid body travel to the ventral cochlear nucleus in the TB and innervate the large neurons in the cochlear nerve root (rat: Sherriff & Henderson, 1994; Gómez-Nieto et al., 2008).

The best-characterized descending auditory projections are those from neurons in the superior olivary complex that travel in the olivocochlear bundle to the cochlea (reviewed by Warr, 1992). The discovery of this projection was a consequence of keen interest in the so-called olivary peduncle, a bundle of axons present in a variety of species that extends almost vertically between the superior olivary complex and the floor of the fourth ventricle (Papez, 1930; Rasmussen, 1946; see Rasmussen for a concise history of the long interest in this bundle of axons). Rasmussen (1946) discovered the source of these fibers in the superior olivary complex and demonstrated that they crossed the midline in the floor of the fourth ventricle and travelled with the vestibular nerve root out of the brain. He gave the bundle the name used today, the olivocochlear bundle (OCB; see White & Warr, 1983, their figures 2 and 3, for detailed illustrations of the course of the OCB fibers in the brainstem [rat]). At the level of the cochlea, the OCB fibers form the vestibular anastomosis of Oort, leaving the vestibular nerve root and entering the cochlear modiolus (e.g., cat: Arnesen & Osen, 1984).

Not all OCB fibers cross the midline (see e.g., Warr, 1992); those that do not cross course parallel and lateral to the crossing fibers in the olivary peduncle (Rasmussen, 1960). Brown (1993) followed individually labeled axons of these lateral OCB fibers and demonstrated that many of them turn medially (with the crossing fibers) before looping back to project out of the brain on the same side (see his figure 17.1 for illustrations of the course taken by both medial and lateral OCB fibers [mouse]). The anatomical detail is significant for interpretation of lesion studies because it suggests that large lesions, even if placed near the midline, could damage both crossed and uncrossed axons (Brown, 1993). Although it is sometimes suggested that axons that project out of the medial and lateral superior olivary nuclei join the olivary peduncle before entering the LL, this was explicitly denied by Papez (1930) and Rasmussen (1946). Rather, for a short distance, these axons run lateral and parallel to the fibers of the olivary peduncle.

Brainstem Commissures

In addition to the decussating axons that connect auditory nuclei with those at different levels of the brainstem, commissural projections interconnect the right and left cochlear nuclei and inferior colliculi. In both cases, these projections are made up of both excitatory and inhibitory axons.

Connections between the Cochlear Nuclei on the Two Sides of the Brain

Commissural connections between the cochlear nuclei (cat: Adams & Warr, 1976; Cant & Gaston, 1982; guinea pig: Shore et al., 1992; Schofield & Cant, 1996) consist of both excitatory and inhibitory components (guinea pig: Wenthold, 1987; rat: Alibardi, 1998, 2006). Large inhibitory (glycinergic) axons arise from multipolar neurons in the ventral cochlear nucleus and leave via the "commissural stria," a loose bundle of glycine-positive axons adjacent and rostral to the DAS (cat: Smith et al., 2005; guinea pig: Kolston et al., 1992; mouse: Brown et al., 2013; baboon: Moore et al., 1996). The commissural fibers cross the midline in the DAS (mouse: Brown et al., 2013), where they spread out in the dorsal-to-ventral dimension and so appear to be intermingled with the crossing axons from the dorsal cochlear nucleus and the lateral superior olivary nucleus. Near the point where the DAS joins the LL, some of the commissural axons peel off ventrally to enter the TB. Others course dorsally to enter the dorsal cochlear nucleus via the DAS (or perhaps the adjacent commissural stria). Some of the commissural axons do not turn but rather course straight toward the cochlear nucleus (passing through the trigeminal nucleus and tract) to enter the ventral cochlear nucleus along its medial border (cat: Cant & Gaston, 1982; Smith et al., 2005; guinea pig: Schofield & Cant, 1996; mouse: Brown, et al., 2013, their figures 2 and 3; baboon: Moore et al., 1996). Whether the excitatory component of the commissure follows the same or different routes is not known.

Midbrain Commissures

Thick axons arising from the GABAergic cells of one dorsal nucleus of the lateral lemniscus project across the midline to the nucleus on the opposite side via the prominent commissure of Probst (cat: Adams & Mugnaini, 1984; Henkel & Shneiderman, 1988; Hutson et al., 1991; squirrel monkey: Goldberg & Moore, 1967; gerbil: N. B. Cant, unpublished observations; Figure 17.1, panel 5). The commissure takes an almost straight path across the midline ventral to the periaqueductal gray nuclei, and the large axons enter the opposite dorsal nucleus from its rostral aspect (cat: Kudo, 1981; Figure 17.3, panel F). The only other known components of this commissure are axons that project from the dorsal nucleus of the lateral lemniscus to the contralateral inferior colliculus and axons that project from the nucleus sagulum on one side to that on the other (cat: Henkel & Shneiderman, 1988; Hutson et al., 1991).

Projections from one inferior colliculus to that on the opposite side travel via the prominent collicular commissure that lies dorsal to the cerebral aqueduct (reviewed by Saldaña and Merchán, 2005). Other axons that travel in this commissure include projections from the inferior colliculus to the contralateral medial geniculate nucleus and axons from lower brainstem nuclei that first enter the ipsilateral colliculus and then cross to the opposite side (cat: Hutson et al., 1991; rat: Viñuela et al., 2011).

Routes Followed by Non-auditory Inputs to Auditory Nuclei

Several somatosensory nuclei, including the dorsal column nuclei and spinal nuclei of the trigeminal nerve provide input to the auditory system (e.g., tree shrew: Schroeder & Jane, 1971; rat: Massopust et al., 1985). Like other axons leaving the dorsal column nuclei, the axons that innervate auditory structures course ventrally and medially as internal arcuate fibers, cross the midline, and join the contralateral medial lemniscus to run rostrally. At the level of the pontine nuclei, axons destined for the inferior colliculus move into the nearby LL and travel in its most lateral part to reach the dorsal midbrain (Schroeder & Jane, 1971). Presumably, axons destined for the cochlear nuclei (e.g., rat: Weinburg & Rustioni, 1987) leave the medial lemniscus at the level of the superior olivary complex to join the trapezoid body, but this has not been explicitly demonstrated.

Axons from the spinal nucleus of the trigeminal nerve that project to the inferior colliculus cross to the contralateral side and course ventrally to join the trigeminothalamic tract adjacent to the medial lemniscus. At the pontine level, the axons peel away from this tract to enter the LL and ascend to the inferior colliculus (Zhou & Shore, 2006). The location of the axons within the lateral lemniscus was not specified. Axons that project from the spinal nucleus of the trigeminal nerve to the cochlear nuclei course along the spinal trigeminal tract and enter the cochlear nucleus via either the IAS or the DAS (Zhou & Shore, 2004). Routes taken by other non-auditory inputs to the brainstem auditory structures (reviewed by Cant & Oliver, 2018; Schofield & Hurley, 2018) have not been described in detail.

Some axons that initially travel in the medial lemniscus and the trigeminothalamic tract enter the LL before again peeling off to innervate portions of the midbrain reticular formation and the deep layers of the superior colliculus (rat: Massopust et al., 1985; Macaque monkey: Wiberg et al., 1987). Thus, a few axons that travel in the ventral LL may not be part of the auditory system.

Conclusion

Information about the trajectories followed by specific groups of axons (summarized in Figure 17.4) has been used by experimental psychologists, neurophysiologists, molecular and cellular biologists, developmental neurobiologists, and neuroanatomists to design and interpret experiments that have furthered our knowledge of auditory function. However, there are important gaps in our knowledge concerning the organization of the white matter of the auditory system, and it is logical to suggest that filling the gaps could lead to improved experimental protocols and more informed interpretation of a wide variety of studies. Descriptions of the organization of axons in the lateral lemniscus and the associated nuclei of the lateral lemniscus are especially incomplete. It is possible that axons from specific sources are bundled together in that tract and segregated from axons from other sources (as is the case to a large extent in the trapezoid body), but the descriptions of the trajectories are insufficient to allow even tentative conclusions about many of the axons that travel in this tract. Even relatively simple analyses of axons in cross section at several dorsal-to-ventral levels of the lateral lemniscus (as was done for

(A) Components of the acoustic striae

Stria	Border of cochlear nucleus	Midline
DAS & commissural stria	DCN fusiform cell axons (i) DCN giant cell axons (i) VCN commissural cell axons from both sides Descending axons from SOC (i) Axons from somatosensory nuclei	DCN fusiform cell axons from both sides DCN giant cell axons from both sides VCN commissural cell axons from both sides LSO principal cell axons from both sides
IAS	VCN octopus cell axons (i) Descending axons from SOC (i)	VCN octopus cell axons from both sides
TB	VCN spherical cell axons (i) VCN globular cell axons (i) AVCN multipolar cell axons (i) PVCN multipolar cell axons (i) Descending axons from SOC (i & c) Descending axons from IC (i & c)	Spherical cell axons from both sides (dorsal and rostral) Globular cell axons from both sides (middle and caudal) AVCN multipolar cell axons from both sides (extreme rostral) PVCN multipolar cell axons from both sides (ventral and caudal) Descending axons from SOC and IC to contralateral VCN

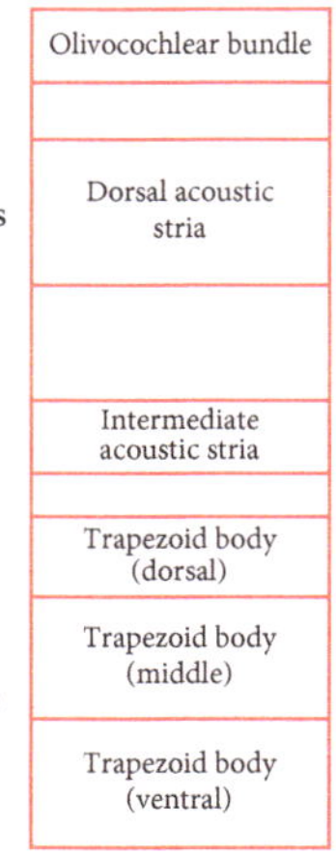

(B) Components of the lateral lemniscus

Sources of axons in the lateral LL	Sources of axons in the medial LL (and paralemniscal area)
Contralateral ventral cochlear nucleus Ipsilateral ventral cochlear nucleus Ipsilateral dorsal cochlear nucleus Descending axons from IC to SOC and DCN Dorsal column nuclei and spinal nucleus of the trigeminal nerve Ipsilateral LNTB, VNTB, and MNTB (may travel through VNLL rather than in white matter)	Contralateral dorsal cochlear nucleus Contralateral lateral superior olivary nucleus Ipsilateral superior paraolivary nucleus Ipsilateral medial superior olivary nucleus Ipsilateral lateral superior olivary nucleus Ipsilateral auditory cortical axons to IC (few)

FIGURE 17.4. Summary of the components of the three acoustic striae (A) and of the lateral lemniscus (B), as described in the text. The red box indicates the relative locations (from dorsal to ventral) of auditory fiber bundles in the pons at the midline. (i, ipsilateral; c, contralateral; other abbreviations as in Figure 17.1.)

the trapezoid body at the midline) could lead to new insights into the organization of that tract. Studies in which glycinergic and/or GABAergic axons are specifically labeled could add further information about the organization of axons of specific cell types. As noted at the beginning of this chapter, some of the earliest studies of the auditory pathways emphasized descriptions of the major tracts. With the continuing improvement of non-invasive methods of imaging fiber tracts in the brain, methods that can be used in both humans and experimental animals, there is reason for renewed interest in the specific details of the organization of those tracts (e.g., Schmahmann et al., 2007; Calabrese et al., 2015; Tarabichi et al., 2018). These new methods are becoming available at a time when there is also increasing recognition that abnormalities in the brainstem may contribute significantly to hearing disorders (e.g., Felix et al., 2018; Palmer & Berger, 2018). Neuroanatomical studies of the tracts will continue to be important for validating and interpreting new methods that have potential for improved understanding of human disease.

Notes

1. The fascinating history of the development of topological subway maps begins in the 1930s with Harry Beck, who developed the first such map for users of the London Underground (e.g., Toor, 2013). Similar maps are now used in most major cities of the world, with the interesting exception of New York City (Rawsthorn, 2012). Nowadays, we take such maps for granted, but we know better than to rely on them when navigating above ground.
2. In marsupials, the dorsal cochlear nucleus is located medial to the peduncle so that the DAS does not pass over it (e.g., Aitkin, 1996).
3. Although Fernandez and Karapas (1967) appear to equate the DAS with the axons from the dorsal cochlear nucleus, here it is considered (in conformity with most authors) that the DAS extends only as far as the rostral aspect of the superior olivary complex, where many of its axons enter the lateral lemniscus.

References

Adams, J. C. (1997). Projections from octopus cells of the posteroventral cochlear nucleus to the ventral nucleus of the lateral lemniscus in cat and human. *Auditory Neuroscience 3*(4), 335–350.

Adams, J. C., & Mugnaini, E. (1984). Dorsal nucleus of the lateral lemniscus: A nucleus of GABAergic projection neurons. *Brain Research Bulletin 13*(4), 585–590.

Adams, J. C., & Warr, W. B. (1976). Origins of axons in the cat's acoustic striae determined by injection of horseradish peroxidase into severed tracts. *Journal of Comparative Neurology 170*(1), 107–122.

Aitkin, L. (1996). The anatomy of the cochlear nuclei and superior olivary complex of arboreal Australian marsupials. *Brain, Behavior and Evolution 48*(1), 103–114.

Alibardi, L. (1998). Ultrastructural and immunocytochemical characterization of commissural neurons in the ventral cochlear nucleus of the rat. *Annals of Anatomy 180*(5), 427–438.

Alibardi, L. (2006). Review: Cytological characteristics of commissural and tuberculo-ventral neurons in the rat dorsal cochlear nucleus. *Hearing Research 216–217*(June-July), 73–80.

Arnesen, A. R., & Osen, K. K. (1984). Fibre population of the vestibulocochlear anastomosis in the cat. *Acta Otolaryngologica (Stockholm) 98*(3–4), 255–269.

Barnes, W. T., Magoun, H. W., & Ranson, S. W. (1943). The ascending auditory pathway in the brain stem of the monkey. *Journal of Comparative Neurology 79*(1), 129–152.

Beckius, G. E., Batra, R., & Oliver, D. L. (1999). Axons from anteroventral cochlear nucleus that terminate in medial superior olive of cat: observations related to delay lines. *Journal of Neuroscience 19*(8), 3146–3161.

Benson, C. G., & Cant, N. B. (2008). The ventral nucleus of the lateral lemniscus of the gerbil (*Meriones unguiculatus*): organization of connections with the cochlear nucleus and the inferior colliculus. *Journal of Comparative Neurology 510*(6), 673–690.

Benson, C. G., & Potashner, S. J. (1990). Retrograde transport of [3H]glycine from the cochlear nucleus to the superior olive in the guinea pig. *Journal of Comparative Neurology 296*(3), 415–426.

Borg, E. (1973). A neuroanatomical study of the brainstem auditory system of the rabbit. Part II. Descending connections. *Acta Morphologica Neerlando-Scandinavica 11*(1), 49–62.

Brown, M. C. (1993). Fiber pathways and branching patterns of biocytin-labeled olivocochlear neurons in the mouse brainstem. *Journal of Comparative Neurology 337*(4), 600–613.

Brown, M. C., Drottar, M., Benson, T. E., & Darrow, K. (2013). Commissural axons of the mouse cochlear nucleus. *Journal of Comparative Neurology 521*(7), 1683–1696.

Brown, M. C., Liberman, M. C., Benson, T. E., & Ryugo, D. K. (1988). Brainstem branches from olivocochlear axons in cats and rodents. *Journal of Comparative Neurology 278*(4), 591–603.

Brown, M. C., Pierce, S., & Berglund, A. M. (1991). Cochlear-nucleus branches of thick (medial) olivocochlear fibers in the mouse: a cochleotopic projection. *Journal of Comparative Neurology 303*(2), 300–315.

Brownell, W. E. (1975). Organization of the cat trapezoid body and the discharge characteristics of its fibers. *Brain Research 94*(3), 413–433.

Caicedo, A., & Herbert, H. (1993). Topography of descending projections from the inferior colliculus to auditory brainstem nuclei in the rat. *Journal of Comparative Neurology 328*(3), 377–392.

Calabrese, E., Badea, A., Cofer, G., Qi, Y., & Johnson, G. A. (2015). A diffusion MRI tractography connectome of the mouse brain and comparison with neuronal tracer data. *Cerebral Cortex 25*(11), 4628–4637.

Cant, N. B. (1998). Structural development of the mammalian auditory pathways. In E. W. Rubel, A. N. Popper, & R. R. Fay (eds.), *Development of the auditory system* (pp. 315–413). New York, NY: Springer-Verlag.

Cant, N. B. (2005). Projections from the cochlear nuclear complex to the inferior colliculus. In J. A. Winer & C. E. Schreiner (eds.), *The inferior colliculus* (pp. 115–131). New York, NY: Springer.

Cant, N. B. (2013). Patterns of convergence in the central nucleus of the inferior colliculus of the Mongolian gerbil: organization of inputs from the superior olivary complex in the low frequency representation. *Frontiers in Neural Circuits 7*, 29. doi: 10.3389/fncir.2013.00029.

Cant, N. B., & Benson, C. G. (2006). Organization of the inferior colliculus of the gerbil (*Meriones unguiculatus*): differences in distribution of projections from the cochlear nuclei and the superior olivary complex. *Journal of Comparative Neurology 495*(5), 511–528.

Cant, N. B., & Gaston, K. C. (1982). Pathways connecting the right and left cochlear nuclei. *Journal of Comparative Neurology 212*(3), 313–326.

Cant, N. B., & Oliver, D. L. (2018). Overview of auditory projection pathways and intrinsic microcircuits. In D. L. Oliver, N. B. Cant, R. R. Fay, & A. N. Popper (eds.), *The mammalian auditory pathways. Synaptic organization and microcircuits* (pp. 7–39). New York, NY: Springer.

Casseday, J. H., Covey, E., & Vater, M. (1988). Connections of the superior olivary complex in the rufous horseshoe bat *Rhinolophus rouxi*. *Journal of Comparative Neurology 278*(3), 313–329.

Casseday, J. H., Kobler, J. B., Isbey, S. F., & Covey, E. (1989). Central acoustic tract in an echolocating bat: an extralemniscal auditory pathway to the thalamus. *Journal of Comparative Neurology 287*(2), 247–259.

Conlee, J. W., & Kane, E. S. (1982). Descending projections from the inferior colliculus to the dorsal cochlear nucleus in the cat: an autoradiographic study. *Neuroscience 7*(1), 161–178.

Coomes, D. L., & Schofield, B. R. (2004). Projections from the auditory cortex to the superior olivary complex in guinea pigs. *European Journal of Neuroscience 19*(8), 2188–2200.

Darrow, K. N., Benson, T. E., & Brown, M. C. (2012). Planar multipolar cells in the cochlear nucleus project to medial olivocochlear neurons in mouse. *Journal of Comparative Neurology* 520(7), 1365–1375.

Doucet, J. R., Rose, L., & Ryugo, D. K. (2002). The cellular origin of corticofugal projections to the superior olivary complex in the rat. *Brain Research* 925(1), 28–41.

Doucet, J. R., & Ryugo, D. K. (2003). Axonal pathways to the lateral superior olive labeled with biotinylated dextran amine injections in the dorsal cochlear nucleus of rats. *Journal of Comparative Neurology* 461(4), 452–464.

Elverland, H. H. (1977). Descending connections between the superior olivary and cochlear nuclear complexes in the cat studied by autoradiographic and horseradish peroxidase methods. *Experimental Brain Research* 27(3–4), 397–412.

Elverland, H. H. (1978). Ascending and intrinsic projections of the superior olivary complex in the cat. *Experimental Brain Research* 32(1), 117–134.

Faye-Lund, H. (1986). Projection from the inferior colliculus to the superior olivary complex in the albino rat. *Anatomy and Embryology* 175(1), 35–52.

Feliciano, M., Saldaña, E., & Mugnaini, E. (1995). Direct projections from the rat primary auditory neocortex to nucleus sagulum, paralemniscal regions, superior olivary complex and cochlear nuclei. *Auditory Neuroscience* 1(1), 287–308.

Felix, R. A., II, Gourévitch, B., Gómez-Álvarez, M., Leijon, S. C. M., Saldaña, E., & Magnusson, A. K. (2017). Octopus cells in the posteroventral cochlear nucleus provide the main excitatory input to the superior paraolivary nucleus. *Frontiers in Neural Circuits* 11, 37. doi.org/10.3389/fncir.2017.00037.

Felix, R. A., II, Gourévitch, B., & Portfors, C. V. (2018). Subcortical pathways: towards a better understanding of auditory disorders. *Hearing Research* 362(May), 48–60.

Fernandez, C., & Karapas, F. (1967). The course and termination of the striae of Monakow and Held in the cat. *Journal of Comparative Neurology* 131(3), 371–386.

Friauf, E., & Ostwald, J. (1988). Divergent projections of physiologically characterized rat ventral cochlear nucleus neurons as shown by intra-axonal injection of horseradish peroxidase. *Experimental Brain Research* 73(2), 263–284.

Glendenning, K. K., Brunso-Bechtold, J. K., Thompson, G. C., & Masterton, R. B. (1981). Ascending auditory afferents to the nuclei of the lateral lemniscus. *Journal of Comparative Neurology* 197(4), 673–703.

Glendenning, K. K., & Masterton, R. B. (1983). Acoustic chiasm: efferent projections of the lateral superior olive. *Journal of Neuroscience* 3(8), 1521–1537.

Goldberg, J. M., & Brown, P. B. (1968). Functional organization of the dog superior olivary complex: an anatomical and elecrophysiological study. *Journal of Neurophysiology* 31(4), 639–656.

Goldberg, J. M., & Moore, R. Y. (1967). Ascending projections of the lateral lemniscus in the cat and monkey. *Journal of Comparative Neurology* 129(2), 143–156.

Goméz-Nieto, R., Rubio, M. E., & López, D. E. (2008). Cholinergic input from the ventral nucleus of the trapezoid body to cochlear root neurons in rats. *Journal of Comparative Neurology* 506(3), 452–468.

Harrison, J. M., & Feldman, M. L. (1970). Anatomical aspects of the cochlear nucleus and superior olivary complex. In W. D. Neff (ed.), *Contributions to sensory physiology* (Vol. 49, pp. 95–142). New York, NY: Academic Press.

Harrison, J. M., & Irving, R. (1966a). Ascending connections of the anterior ventral cochlear nucleus in the rat. *Journal of Comparative Neurology* 126(1), 51–64.

Harrison, J. M., & Irving, R. (1966b). The organization of the posterior ventral cochlear nucleus in the rat. *Journal of Comparative Neurology 126*(3), 391–402.

Harrison, J. M., & Warr, W. B. (1962) A study of the cochlear nuclei and ascending auditory pathways of the medulla. *Journal of Comparative Neurology 119*(3), 341–352.

Henkel, C. K. (1983). Evidence of sub-collicular auditory projections to the medial geniculate nucleus in the cat: an autoradiographic and horseradish peroxidase study. *Brain Research 259*(1), 21–30.

Henkel, C. K. (1997). Axonal morphology in fibrodendritic laminae of the dorsal nucleus of the lateral lemniscus: afferent projections from the medial superior olivary nucleus. *Journal of Comparative Neurology 380*(1), 136–144.

Henkel, C. K., Keiger, C. J., Franklin, S. R., & Brunso-Bechtold, J. K. (2007). Development of banded afferent compartments in the inferior colliculus before onset of hearing in ferrets. *Neuroscience 146*(1), 225–235.

Henkel, C. K., & Shneiderman, A. (1988). Nucleus sagulum: projections of a lateral tegmental area to the inferior colliculus in the cat. *Journal of Comparative Neurology 271*(4), 577–588.

Henkel, C. K., & Spangler, K. M. (1983). Organization of the efferent projections of the medial superior olivary nucleus in the cat as revealed by HRP and autoradiographic tracing methods. *Journal of Comparative Neurology 221*(4), 416–428.

Herbert, H., Klepper, A., & Ostwald, J. (1997). Afferent and efferent connections of the ventrolateral tegmental area in the rat. *Anatomy and Embryology 196*(3), 235–259.

Hutson, K. A., Glendenning, K. K., & Masterton, R. B. (1991). Acoustic chiasm IV: Eight midbrain decussations of the auditory system in the cat. *Journal of Comparative Neurology 312*(1), 105–131.

Kolston, J., Osen, K. K., Hackney, C. M., Ottersen, O. P., & Storm-Mathisen, J. (1992). An atlas of glycine—and GABA-like immunoreactivity and colocalization in the cochlear nuclear complex of the guinea pig. *Anatomy and Embryology 186*(5), 443–465.

Kudo, M. (1981). Projections of the nuclei of the lateral lemniscus in the cat: an autoradiographic study. *Brain Research 221*(1), 57–69.

Kuwabara, N., DiCaprio, R. A., & Zook, J. M. (1991). Afferents to the medial nucleus of the trapezoid body and their collateral projections. *Journal of Comparative Neurology 314*(4), 684–706.

Kuwabara, N. & Zook, J. M. (1999). Local collateral projections from the medial superior olive to the superior paraolivary nucleus in the gerbil. *Brain Research 846*(1), 59–71.

Lee, Y., López, D. E., Meloni, E. G., & Davis, M. (1996). A primary acoustic startle pathway: Obligatory role of cochlear root neurons and the nucleus reticularis pontis caudalis. *Journal of Neuroscience 16*(11), 3775–3789.

Loftus, W. C., Bishop, D. C., Saint Marie, R. L., & Oliver, D. L. (2004). Organization of binaural excitatory and inhibitory inputs to the inferior colliculus from the superior olive. *Journal of Comparative Neurology 472*(3), 330–344.

López, D. E., Saldaña, E., Nodal, F. R., Merchán, M., & Warr, W. B. (1999). Projections of cochlear root neurons, sentinels of the rat auditory pathway. *Journal of Comparative Neurology 415*(2), 160–174.

Lorente de Nó, R. (1981). *The primary acoustic nuclei*. New York, NY: Raven Press.

Malmierca, M. S. (2003). The structure and physiology of the rat auditory system: an overview. *International Reviews of Neurobiology 56*, 147–211.

Malmierca, M. S., & Hackett, T. A. (2010). Structural organization of the ascending auditory pathway. In A. R. Palmer & A. Rees (eds.), *The Oxford handbook of auditory science: the auditory brain* (pp. 9–42). Oxford, England: Oxford University Press.

Malmierca, M. S., Le Beau, F. E. N., & Rees, A. (1996). The topographical organization of descending projections from the central nucleus of the inferior colliculus in guinea pig. *Hearing Research 93*(1–2), 167–180.

Massopust, L. C., Hauge, D. H., Ferneding, J. C., Doubek, W. G., & Taylor, J. J. (1985). Projection systems and terminal localization of dorsal column afferents: an autoradiographic and horseradish peroxidase study in the rat. *Journal of Comparative Neurology 237*(4), 533–544.

Merchán, M. A., Saldaña, E., & Plaza, I. (1994). Dorsal nucleus of the lateral lemniscus in the rat: concentric organization and tonotopic projection to the inferior colliculus. *Journal of Comparative Neurology 342*(2), 259–278.

Moore, J. K., & Osen, K. K. (1979). The cochlear nuclei in man. *American Journal of Anatomy 154*(3), 393–418.

Moore, J. K., Osen, K. K., Storm-Mathisen, J., & Otttersen, O. P. (1996). γ-Aminobutyric acid and glycine in the baboon cochlear nuclei: an immunocytochemical colocalization study with reference to interspecies differences in inhibitory systems. *Journal of Comparative Neurology 369*(4), 497–519.

Moore, R. Y., & Goldberg, J. M. (1966). Projections of the inferior colliculus in the monkey. *Experimental Neurology 14*(4), 429–438.

Mugnaini, E., Warr, W. B., & Osen, K. K. (1980). Distribution and light microscopic features of granule cells in the cochlear nuclei of cat, rat, and mouse. *Journal of Comparative Neurology 191*(4), 581–606.

Nodal, F. R., & López, D. E. (2003). Direct input from cochlear root neurons to pontine reticulospinal neurons in albino rat. *Journal of Comparative Neurology 460*(1), 80–93.

Oertel, D., & Wickesberg, R. E. (2002). Ascending pathways through ventral nuclei of the lateral lemniscus and their possible role in pattern recognition in natural sounds. In D. Oertel, R. R. Fay, & A. N. Popper (eds.), *Integrative functions in the mammalian auditory pathway* (pp. 207–237). New York, NY: Springer.

Oertel, D., Wright, S., Cao, X.-J., Ferragamo, M., & Bal, R. (2011). The multiple functions of T stellate/multipolar/chopper cells in the ventral cochlear nucleus. *Hearing Research 276*(1), 61–69.

Oertel, D., Wu, S. H., Garb, M. W., & Dizack, C. (1990). Morphology and physiology of cells in slice preparations of the posteroventral cochlear nucleus of mice. *Journal of Comparative Neurology 295*(1), 136–154.

Okoyama, S., Ohbayashi, M., Ito, M., & Harada, S. (2006). Neuronal organization of the rat inferior colliculus participating in four major auditory pathways. *Hearing Research 218*(1–2), 72–80.

Oliver, D. L. (1987). Projections to the inferior colliculus from the anteroventral cochlear nucleus in the cat: possible substrates for binaural interaction. *Journal of Comparative Neurology 264*(1), 24–46.

Oliver, D. L., Beckius, G. E., Bishop, D. C., & Kuwada, S. (1997). Simultaneous anterograde labeling of axonal layers from lateral superior olive and dorsal cochlear nucleus in the inferior colliculus of cat. *Journal of Comparative Neurology 382*(2), 215–229.

Osen, K. K. (1969). Cytoarchitecture of the cochlear nuclei in the cat. *Journal of Comparative Neurology 136*(4), 453–484.

Osen, K. K. (1972). Projections of the cochlear nuclei on the inferior colliculus in the cat. *Journal of Comparative Neurology 144*(3), 355–372.

Osen, K. K., Mugnaini, E., Dahl, A.-L., & Christiansen, A. H. (1984). Histochemical localization of acetylcholinesterase in the cochlear and superior olivary nuclei. A reappraisal with emphasis on the cochlear granule cell system. *Archives Italiennes de Biologie 122*(3), 169–212.

Osen, K. K., & Roth, K. (1969). Histochemical localization of cholinesterases in the cochlear nuclei of the cat, with notes on the origin of acetylcholinesterase-positive afferents and the superior olive. *Brain Research 16*(1), 165–185.

Ostapoff, E.-M., Benson, C. G., & Saint Marie, R. L. (1997). GABA- and glycine-immunoreactive projections from the superior olivary complex to the cochlear nucleus in guinea pig. *Journal of Comparative Neurology 381*(4), 500–512.

Ostapoff, E.-M., Feng, J. J., & Morest, D. K. (1994). A physiological and structural study of neuron types in the cochlear nucleus. II. Neuron types and their structural correlates with response properties. *Journal of Comparative Neurology 346*(1), 19–42.

Palmer, A. R., & Berger, J. I. (2018). Changes in the inferior colliculus associated with hearing loss: noise-induced hearing loss, age-related hearing loss, tinnitus and hyperacusis. In K. Kandler (ed.), *The Oxford handbook of the auditory brainstem* (pp. 1–26). doi: 10.1093/oxfordhb/9780190849061.

Papez, J. W. (1930). Superior olivary nucleus. Its fiber connections. *Archives of Neurology and Psychiatry 24*(1), 1–20.

Rasmussen G. L. (1960). Efferent fibers of the cochlear nerve and cochlear nucleus. In G. L. Rasmussen & W. Windle (eds.), *Neural mechanisms of the auditory and vestibular system* (pp. 105–115). Springfield, IL: Charles C Thomas.

Rasmussen, G. L. (1946). The olivary peduncle and other fiber projections of the superior olivary complex. *Journal of Comparative Neurology 84*(2), 141–219.

Rasmussen, G. L. (1964). Anatomic relationships of the ascending and descending auditory systems. In W. S. Fields & B. R. Alford (eds.) *Neurological aspects of auditory & vestibular disorders* (pp. 1–19). Springfield, IL: Charles C. Thomas.

Rawsthorn, A. (2012). The subway map that rattled New Yorkers. *New York Times*. http://nytimes.com/2012/08/06/arts/design.

Rouiller, E. M. (1997). Functional organization of the auditory pathways. In G. Ehret & R. Romand (eds.), *The central auditory system* (pp. 3–96). New York, NY: Oxford University Press.

Russell, F. A., & Moore, D. R. (1995). Afferent reorganization within the superior olivary complex of the gerbil: Development and induction by neonatal, unilateral cochlear removal. *Journal of Comparative Neurology 352*(4), 607–625.

Ryan, A. F., Keithley, E. M., Wang, Z.-X., & Schwartz, I. R. (1990). Collaterals from lateral and medial olivocochlear efferent neurons innervate different regions of the cochlear nucleus and adjacent brainstem. *Journal of Comparative Neurology 300*(4), 572–582.

Saint Marie, R. L., & Baker, R. A. (1990). Neurotransmitter-specific uptake and retrograde transport of [H3]glycine from the inferior colliculus by ipsilateral projections of the superior olivary complex and nuclei of the lateral lemniscus. *Brain Research 524*(2), 244–253.

Saint Marie, R. L., Ostapoff, E.-M., Morest, D. K., & Wenthold, R. J. (1989). Glycine-immunoreactive projection of the cat lateral superior olive: possible role in midbrain ear dominance. *Journal of Comparative Neurology 279*(3), 382–396.

Saldaña, E. (1993). Descending projections from the inferior colliculus to the cochlear nuclei in mammals. In M. A. Merchán, J. M. Juiz, D. A. Godfrey, & E. Mugnaini (eds.), *The mammalian cochlear nuclei. Organization and function* (pp. 153–165). New York, NY: Plenum Press.

Saldaña, E. (2015). All the way from the cortex: a review of auditory corticosubcollicular pathways. *Cerebellum 14*(5), 584–596.

Saldaña, E., & Merchán, M. A. (2005). Intrinsic and commissural connections of the inferior colliculus. In J. A. Winer & C. E. Schreiner (eds.), *The inferior colliculus* (pp. 155–181). New York, NY: Springer,.

Saldaña, E., Aparicio, M.-A., Fuentes-Santamaría, V., & Berrebi, A. S. (2009). Connections of the superior paraolivary nucleus of the rat: Projections to the inferior colliculus. *Neuroscience 163*(1), 372–387.

Saldaña, E., Feliciano, M., & Mugnaini, E. (1996). Distribution of descending projections from primary auditory neocortex to inferior colliculus mimics the topography of intracollicular projections. *Journal of Comparative Neurology 371*(1), 15–40.

Schmahmann, J. D., Pandya, D. N., Wang, R., Dai, G., D'Arceuil, H. E., de Crespigny, A. J., & Wedeen, V. J. (2007). Association fibre pathways of the brain: parallel observations from diffusion spectrum imaging and autoradiography. *Brain 130*(3), 630–653.

Schofield, B. R. (2005). Superior olivary complex and lateral lemniscal connections of the auditory midbrain. In J. A. Winer & C. E. Schreiner (eds.), *The inferior colliculus* (pp. 115–131). New York: Springer.

Schofield, B. R. (2011). Central descending auditory pathways. In D. Ryugo & R. R. Fay (eds.), *Auditory and vestibular efferents* (pp. 261–290). New York, NY: Springer.

Schofield, B. R., & Cant, N. B. (1996). Origins and targets of commissural connections between the cochlear nuclei in guinea pigs. *Journal of Comparative Neurology 375*(1), 128–146.

Schofield, B. R., & Cant, N. B. (1997). Ventral nucleus of the lateral lemniscus in guinea pigs: cytoarchitecture and inputs from the cochlear nucleus. *Journal of Comparative Neurology 379*(3), 363–385.

Schofield, B. R., & Hurley, L. (2018). Circuits for modulation of auditory function. In D. L. Oliver, N. B. Cant, R. R. Fay, & A. N. Popper (eds.), *The mammalian auditory pathways. Synaptic organization and microcircuits* (pp. 235–267). New York, NY: Springer.

Schroeder, D. M., & Jane, J. A. (1971). Projection of dorsal column nuclei and spinal cord in the brainstem and thalamus in the tree shrew, *Tupaia glis*. *Journal of Comparative Neurology 142*(3), 309–350.

Sherriff, F. E., & Henderson, Z. (1994). Cholinergic neurons in the ventral trapezoid nucleus project to the cochlear nuclei in the rat. *Neuroscience 58*(3), 627–633.

Shneiderman, A., & Henkel, C. K. (1987). Banding of lateral superior olivary nucleus afferents in the inferior colliculus: a possible substrate for sensory integration. *Journal of Comparative Neurology 266*(4), 519–534.

Shneiderman, A., Oliver, D. L., & Henkel, C. K. (1988). Connections of the dorsal nucleus of the lateral lemniscus: an inhibitory parallel pathway in the ascending auditory system? *Journal of Comparative Neurology 276*(2), 188–208.

Shore, S. E., Godfrey, D. A., Helfert, R. H., Altschuler, R. A., & Bledsoe, S. C. (1992). Connections between the cochlear nuclei in guinea pig. *Hearing Research 62*(1), 16–26.

Smith, P. H. (1995). Structural and functional differences distinguish principal from nonprincipal cells in the guinea pig MSO slice. *Journal of Neurophysiology 73*(4), 1653–1667.

Smith, P. H., Joris, P. X., Banks, M. I., & Yin, T. C. T. (1993a). Responses of cochlear nucleus cells and projections of their axons. In M. A. Merchán, J. M. Juiz, D. A. Godfrey, & E. Mugnaini (eds.), *The mammalian cochlear nuclei. Organization and function* (pp. 349–371). New York, NY: Plenum Press.

Smith, P. H., Joris, P. X., & Yin, T. C. T. (1993b). Projections of physiologically characterized spherical bushy cell axons from the cochlear nucleus of the cat: evidence for delay lines to the medial superior olive. *Journal of Comparative Neurology 331*(2), 245–260.

Smith, P. H., Joris, P. X., & Yin, T. C. T. (1998). Anatomy and physiology of principal cells of the medial nucleus of the trapezoid body (MNTB) of the cat. *Journal of Neurophysiology 79*(6), 3127–3142.

Smith, P. H., Massie, A., & Joris, P. X. (2005). Acoustic stria: anatomy of physiologically characterized cells and their axonal patterns. *Journal of Comparative Neurology 482*(4), 349–371.

Smith, P. H., & Rhode, W. S. (1989). Structural and functional properties distinguish two types of multipolar cells in the ventral cochlear nucleus. *Journal of Comparative Neurology 282*(4), 595–616.

Smith, P. H., & Spirou, G. A. (2002). From the cochlea to the cortex and back. In D. Oertel, R. R. Fay, & A. N. Popper (eds.), *Integrative functions in the mammalian auditory pathway* (pp. 6–71). New York: Springer.

Sommer, I., Lingenhöhl, K., & Friauf, E. (1993). Principal cells of the rat medial nucleus of the trapezoid body: an intracellular in vivo study of their physiology and morphology. *Experimental Brain Research 95*(2), 223–239.

Spangler, K. M., Cant, N. B., Henkel, C. K., Farley, G. R., & Warr, W. B. (1987). Descending projections from the superior olivary complex to the cochlear nucleus of the cat. *Journal of Comparative Neurology 259*(3), 452–465.

Spangler, K. M., Warr, W. B., & Henkel, C. K. (1985). The projections of principal cells of the medial nucleus of the trapezoid body in the cat. *Journal of Comparative Neurology 238*(3), 249–262.

Spirou, G. A., Brownell, W. E., & Zidanic, M. (1990). Recordings from cat trapezoid body and HRP labeling of globular bushy cell axons. *Journal of Neurophysiology 63*(5), 1169–1189.

Stotler, W. A. (1953). An experimental study of the cells and connections of the superior olivary complex of the cat. *Journal of Comparative Neurology 98*(3), 401–431.

Strominger, N. L. (1973). The origins, course and distribution of the dorsal and intermediate acoustic striae in the Rhesus monkey. *Journal of Comparative Neurology 147*(2), 209–234.

Strominger, N. L., Nelson, L. R., & Dougherty, W. J. (1977). Second order auditory pathways in the chimpanzee. *Journal of Comparative Neurology 172*(2), 349–366.

Strominger, N. L., & Strominger, A. I. (1971). Ascending brain stem projections of the anteroventral cochlear nucleus in the Rhesus monkey. *Journal of Comparative Neurology 143*(2), 217–242.

Tarabichi, O., Kozin, E. D., Kanumuri, V. V., Barber, S., Ghosh, S., Sitek, K. R., . . . Lee, D. J. (2018). Diffusion tensor imaging of central auditory pathways in patients with sensorineuronal hearing loss: a systematic review. *Otolaryngology Head and Neck Surgery 158*(3), 432–442.

Thompson, A. M. (1998). Heterogeneous projections of the cat posteroventral cochlear nucleus. *Journal of Comparative Neurology 390*(3), 439–453.

Thompson, A. M. (2005). Descending connections of the auditory midbrain. In J. A. Winer & C. E. Schreiner (eds.), *The inferior colliculus* (pp. 182–199). New York: Springer.

Thompson, A. M., & Schofield, B. R. (2000). Afferent projections of the superior olivary complex. *Microscopy Research and Technique 51*(4), 330–354.

Thompson, A. M., & Thompson, G. C. (1991). Projections from the posteroventral cochlear nucleus to the superior olivary complex in guinea pig: light and EM observations with the PHA-L method. *Journal of Comparative Neurology 311*(4), 495–508.

Thompson, A. M., & Thompson, G. C. (1993). Relationship of descending inferior colliculus projections to olivocochlear neurons. *Journal of Comparative Neurology 33*(3), 402–412.

Tolbert, L. P., Morest D. K., & Yurgelun-Todd, D. A. (1982). The neuronal architecture of the anteroventral cochlear nucleus of the cat in the region of the cochlear nerve root: horseradish peroxidase labelling of identified cell types. *Neuroscience 7*(22), 3031–3052.

Toor, A. (2013). Meet Harry Beck, the genius behind London's iconic subway map. *The Verge* http://www.theverge.com/2013/3/29/4160028.

Van Noort, J. (1969). *The structure and connections of the inferior colliculus: an investigation of the lower auditory system*. Leiden, Netherlands: Assen, Van Gorcum.

Varga, T., Palkovits, M., Usdin, T. B., & Dobolyi, A. (2008). The medial paralemniscal nucleus and its afferent neuronal connections in rat. *Journal of Comparative Neurology 511*(2), 221–237.

Vater, M., Casseday, J. H., & Covey, E. (1995). Convergence and divergence of ascending binaural and monaural pathways from the superior olives of the mustached bat. *Journal of Comparative Neurology 351*(4), 632–646.

Vater, M., & Feng, A. S. (1990). Functional organization of ascending and descending connections of the cochlear nucleus of horseshoe bats. *Journal of Comparative Neurology 292*(3), 373–395.

Vetter, D. E., Saldaña, E., & Mugnaini, E. (1993). Input from the inferior colliculus to medial olivocochlear neurons in the rat: a double label study with PHA-L and cholera toxin. *Hearing Research 70*(2), 173–186.

Viñuela, A., Aparicio, M.-A., Berrebi, A. S., & Saldaña, E. (2011). Connections of the superior paraolivary nucleus of the rat: II. Reciprocal connections with the tectal longitudinal column. *Frontiers in Neuroanatomy 5*, 1. doi:10.3389/fnana.2011.00001.

Warr, W. B. (1966). Fiber degeneration following lesions in the anterior ventral cochlear nucleus of the cat. *Experimental Neurology 14*(4), 453–474.

Warr, W. B. (1969). Fiber degeneration following lesions in the posteroventral cochlear nucleus of the cat. *Experimental Neurology 23*(1), 140–155.

Warr, W. B. (1972). Fiber degeneration following lesions in the multipolar and globular cell areas in the ventral cochlear nucleus of the cat. *Brain Research 40*(2), 247–270.

Warr, W. B. (1982). Parallel ascending pathways from the cochlear nucleus: Neuroanatomical evidence of functional specialization. In: D. Neff (ed.), *Contributions to sensory physiology*, (Vol. 7, pp. 1–38). New York, NY: Academic Press.

Warr, W. B. (1992). Organization of olivocochlear efferent systems in mammals. In D. B. Webster, A. N. Popper, & R. R. Fay (eds.), *The mammalian auditory pathways: neuroanatomy* (pp. 410–448). New York, NY: Springer-Verlag.

Warr, W. B., & Beck, J. E. (1996). Multiple projections from the ventral nucleus of the trapezoid body in the rat. *Hearing Research 93*(1–2), 83–101.

Weedman, D. L., Pongstaporn, T., & Ryugo, D. K. (1996). Ultrastructural study of the granule cell domain of the cochlear nucleus in rats: mossy fiber endings and their targets. *Journal of Comparative Neurology 369*(3), 345–360.

Weinburg, R. J., & Rustioni, A. (1987). A cuneocochlear pathway in the rat. *Neuroscience 20*(1), 209–219.

Wenthold, R. J. (1987). Evidence for a glycinergic pathway connecting the two cochlear nuclei: an immunocytochemical and retrograde transport study. *Brain Research 415*(1), 183–187.

White, J. S., & Warr, W. B. (1983). The dual origins of the olivocochlear bundle in the albino rat. *Journal of Comparative Neurology 219*(2), 203–214.

Whitley, J. M., & Henkel, C. K. (1984). Topographical organization of the inferior collicular projection and other connections of the ventral nucleus of the lateral lemniscus in the cat. *Journal of Comparative Neurology 229*(2), 257–270.

Wiberg, M., Westman, J., & Blomqvist, A. (1987). Somatosensory projection to the mesencephalon: an anatomical study in the monkey. *Journal of Comparative Neurology 264*(1), 92–117.

Willard, F. H., & Martin, G. F. (1983). The auditory brainstem nuclei and some of their projections to the inferior colliculus in the North American opossum. *Neuroscience 10*(4), 1203–1232.

Winter, I. M., Robertson, D., & Cole, K. S. (1989). Descending projections from auditory brainstem nuclei to the cochlea and cochlear nucleus of the guinea pig. *Journal of Comparative Neurology 280*(1), 143–157.

Zhou, J., & Shore, S. (2004). Projections from the trigeminal nuclear complex to the cochlear nuclei: a retrograde and anterograde tracing study in the guinea pig. *Journal of Neuroscience Research 78*(6), 901–907.

Zhou, J., & Shore, S. (2006). Convergence of spinal trigeminal and cochlear nucleus projections in the inferior colliculus of the guinea pig. *Journal of Comparative Neurology 495*(1), 100–112.

Zook, J. M., & Casseday, J. H. (1985). Projections from the cochlear nuclei in the mustache bat, *Pteronotus parnellii*. *Journal of Comparative Neurology 237*(3), 307–324.

Zook, J. M., & Casseday, J. H. (1987). Convergence of ascending pathways at the inferior colliculus of the mustache bat, *Pteronotus parnellii*. *Journal of Comparative Neurology 261*(3), 347–361.

CHAPTER 18

NEURON TYPES, INTRINSIC CIRCUITS, AND PLASTICITY IN THE INFERIOR COLLICULUS

TETSUFUMI ITO, MUNENORI ONO, AND DOUGLAS L. OLIVER

Abstract

The inferior colliculus is a critical auditory center in the midbrain which virtually acts as a hub of all ascending and descending auditory information flows. Wide variety of neuronal responses to sound is found in the IC, and this variety emerges not only from the wide range of extrinsic afferent inputs, but also from the complex features of the local circuits in the IC, for example, the mosaic pattern of extrinsic fiber termination, the various neuronal types each of which compose different patterns of local connection, and the unique forms of synaptic plasticity *de novo*. This chapter reviews the recent progress in understanding these features, and identifies the key issues for future research.

Keywords: glutamatergic neurons, GABAergic neurons, dendritic morphology, axonal arborization, synaptic domain, stimulus specific adaptation, long-lasting sound-evoked after-discharge

Neurons, intrinsic circuits and plasticity in the inferior colliculus (IC) are best discussed within the framework of the overall structure of the auditory midbrain. The IC contains a central nucleus (ICc) that is surrounded by a cortex. The ICc is the primary terminus and integration center for the lateral lemniscus and the dorsal acoustic stria, the ascending inputs from the lower auditory brainstem (see chapter by Cant in this volume), and it is easily identified by prominent cytochrome oxidase staining. The ICc contains subregions where some inputs are more prevalent than others. ICc is the primary source of ascending projections to the portions of the medial geniculate body that supply the core auditory cortex.

In contrast, the cortex of the IC differs in its structure, which consists of layers that parallel the surface of the IC laterally, dorsally, caudally, and in some species rostrally. In general, the cortex has prominent staining with nicotinamide adenine dinucleotide phosphate (NADPH) diaphorase. The lateral cortex of IC is the main structure through which the tectothalamic and corticotectal pathways exit and enter the IC. However, its neuronal structure indicates that it is more than just a gateway, and the inputs and outputs of these lateral cortex neurons are distinct from those in the ICc. The dorsal cortex of the IC contains layers that parallel the dorsal surface of the IC. These layers are typically thicker than the lateral cortex layers, and their size is correlated with the size of the auditory cortex that provides its major input. The neuronal types, local, afferent, and efferent connections also differ from that of ICc. The caudal cortex is thin and superficial, while the rostral cortex is complex and merges with the intercollicular tegmentum.

Neuron Types

IC neurons are subdivided into several categories according to criteria such as dendritic morphology, molecular profiles, synaptic organization, intrinsic membrane properties, or response types to sound. Unfortunately, with some exceptions, no definite agreement of correspondence of categories defined by different criteria.

Morphology

Neurons in the IC exhibit various morphology. Even with simple Nissl staining, neuronal types can be distinguished by the size and shape of the neuron bodies. Dendritic morphology was described by Golgi-impregnation (Malmierca, Blackstad, Osen, Karagulle, & Molowny, 1993; Oliver & Morest, 1984), intra- or juxtacellular staining (Oliver, Kuwada, Yin, Haberly, & Henkel, 1991; Wallace, Shackleton, & Palmer, 2012), or virally introduced labeling (Ito & Oliver, 2014) methods. Neurons also show variety in cytoplasmic features that can be studied with electron microscopy and correlate with dendritic morphology (Paloff, Usunoff, & Hinova-Palova, 1992).

In the ICc, Golgi impregnated materials revealed that several distinctive neuron types can be identified based on the arborization of the dendritic tree. Neuron types in the ICc are well-studied. In the cat, disc-shaped neurons and stellate neurons were identified based on the orientation of the dendritic trees (Oliver & Morest, 1984). Disc-shaped neurons have flat dendritic trees roughly 70 μm wide that are parallel to each other and the major lemniscal afferent fibers and form the characteristic fibrodendritic laminae of the ICc. Stellate neurons have dendritic trees that are either un-oriented or oriented orthogonal to the fibrodendritic laminae. In Nissl stained sections, disc-shaped neurons are seen as flattened neuron bodies that align with the fibrodendritic laminae. In rats, two neuron types, flat and less-flat, were identified by 3D reconstruction and quantitative analyses (Malmierca et al., 1993). Flat neurons are likely to correspond with disc-shaped neurons, and the thickness of dendritic arbor is 50–70 μm. Unlike stellate neurons, dendritic trees of less-flat neurons in the rat are "oriented" to the axis of fibrodendritic laminae, although the dendritic trees are thicker than those of flat neurons and the thickness is about 100 μm. When recordings of the characteristic frequency (CF) of ICc neurons are made in an orientation orthogonal to the fibrodendritic laminae, every 150–180 microns there is a step in the CF of about 0.24 to 0.33 octave (Malmierca et al., 2008; Schreiner & Langner, 1997). This is roughly the same size as the diameter of an axonal lamina and suggests that two or three flat, disc-shaped neurons, side by side, form the functional unit of the fibrodendritic lamina in ICc (Malmierca et al., 2008).

In the lateral cortex of IC, there are three layers (Faye-Lund & Osen, 1985; Loftus, Malmierca, Bishop, & Oliver, 2008). Layer 1 contains small, flattened neurons that extend dendrites parallel to the surface of the IC (T. Ito, unpublished observation). Layer 2 is densely packed with small and medium-sized neurons. Many of layer 2 neurons are GABAergic (Ono, Yanagawa, & Koyano, 2005) and likely to extend the dendritic trees within the layer. Layer 2 GABAergic neurons make distinct dense clusters (Chernock, Larue, & Winer, 2004; Lesicko, Hristova, Maigler, & Llano, 2016) that are called GABA modules. Some of layer 2 neurons are densely covered with dendritic spines (Malmierca, Blackstad, & Osen, 2011). Layer 1 and 2 of the lateral cortex continue medially to the same layers in the dorsal cortex, and rostrally to brachium and brachial nucleus of the IC, respectively. Layer 3 of the lateral cortex receives banded lemniscal axons which are orthogonal to the fibrodendritic laminae in the ICc (Saldana & Merchan, 1992). In layer 3, several neuron types are identified and their dendritic arbor is related to the layering of the ascending axons as well as layered structure of the cortex (Malmierca et al., 2011). Pyramidal-like neurons (Figure 18.1D) are spiny neurons and resemble pyramidal neurons in neocortex, as they have thick tufted apical dendrites that extend to layer 1, as well as basal dendrites. The basal dendrites may receive inputs from layered lemniscal axons in layer 3, while the tips of basal dendrites intermingle with the lateral-most fibrodendritic laminae of the ICc. Bitufted neurons have a spindle-shaped, middle to large soma with two or three dendritic trees that extend in opposite directions, parallel to apical dendrites of pyramidal-like neurons. Chandelier neurons have 3 or more dendrites that are sharply branched and oriented toward the surface of the IC. The different layers of lateral cortex receive inputs from different sources, that is, visual inputs to layer 1 (Paloff, Usunoff, Hinova-Palova, & Ivanov, 1985), somatosensory inputs to layer 2 (Lesicko et al., 2016), and auditory inputs to layer 3 (Loftus et al., 2008), and differential neuromodulatory inputs to layers (Henderson & Sherriff, 1991; Klepper & Herbert, 1991). Since all three neuron types have dendrites directed to the surface to the lateral cortex, it suggests these neurons participate in multimodal integration. As these neurons have dendritic spines, they may control synaptic strength independently, and this may contribute to plasticity in this region.

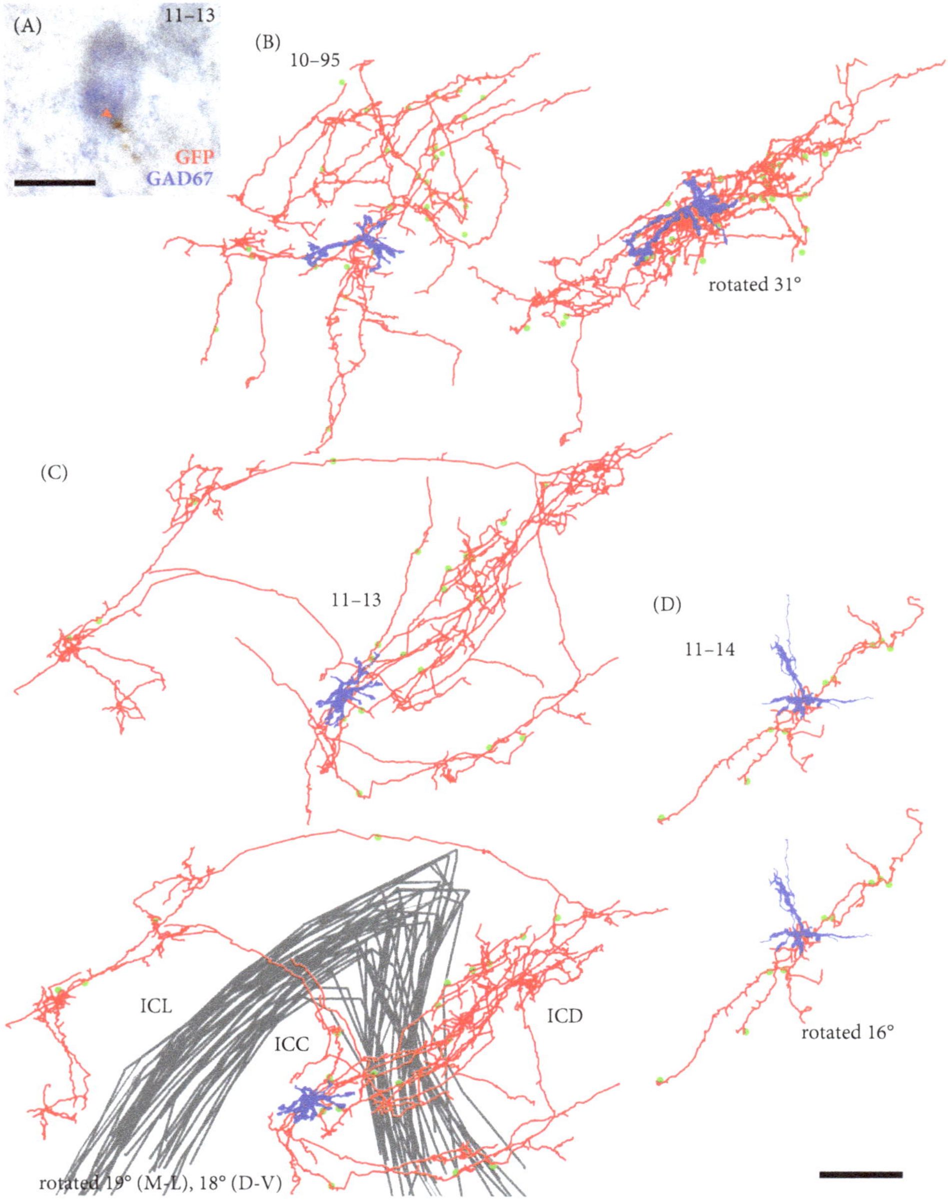

FIGURE 18.1. Spatial distribution of GAD67-positive (+) neuron bodies receiving axosomatic contact from axons of a single glutamatergic neuron. (A) An example of GAD67+ neuron (blue) that received axosomatic contact (a red arrow) with a GFP+ axon (brown). Case 11–13. (B–D) Reconstructed dendrites (blue) and axons (red) of GFP– neurons. Dots indicate neuron bodies of GAD67+ neurons that receive one or more axosomatic contacts. In case 10–95 (B), the axonal plexus became flatter when the neuron was rotated 31 degrees around the mediolateral axis. In the case 11–13 (C), axon collaterals made two planar plexuses in the ICC and dorsal cortex, and one plexus in the lateral cortex. The GAD67+ neurons receiving the axosomatic contacts were located in the dorsal and lateral cortices as well as in the ICC. Gray lines indicate the border of the ICC. In case 11–14 (D), the neuron had a poorly arborized axon, and the GAD67+ neurons aligned well after a rotation of –16 degree around the mediolateral axis. Scale bars = 20 μm in A; 250 μm in B–D.

From Ito and Oliver (2014) with permission from Wiley.

The dorsal cortex contains three to four layers depending on the species (Faye-Lund & Osen, 1985; Morest & Oliver, 1984). Layer 1 is mostly free of neurons except for small cells whose dendrites parallel the surface of IC. Layers 2 and 3 have successively larger neurons in the rat. Dorsal cortex is more extensive in the cat and other species that exhibit a more elaborately developed cerebral cortex. The largest cells are in layer 4 (Morest & Oliver, 1984). In the deep layers of dorsal cortex, ascending axons are found that are the continuum of fibers that compose the fibrodendritic lamina of the ICc (Saldana & Merchan, 1992). Some neurons have dendritic trees that parallel the fibrodendritic laminae like flat neurons in the ICc (Malmierca et al., 2011; Oliver et al., 1991). In the same region, many large multipolar neurons are present whose dendrites extend orthogonal to the orientation of the lamina in ICc (Morest & Oliver, 1984; Oliver & Morest, 1984).

In the rostral cortex, there is no sign of lamination, and most neurons are classified as multipolar that do not have dendritic trees with a specific orientation (Malmierca et al., 2011; Morest & Oliver, 1984). Small multipolar neurons tend to have medium number of spines, while larger neurons tend to have fewer spines. Although inputs to the rostral cortex have not been well described, it is likely the region receives converged inputs from cerebral cortex, brainstem somatosensory nuclei, and ICc (Lesicko, Hristova, Maigler, & Llano, 2016).

Neurotransmitter Type or Other Molecular Markers

Inferior colliculus expresses wide variety of neurotransmitters or other molecular markers, which can be examined on a database (http://mouse.brain-map.org/). It appears that almost all IC neurons contain either glutamate or GABA as a neurotransmitter (Fujimoto, Konno, Watanabe, & Jinno, 2017), that is, excitatory or inhibitory, respectively. IC neurons are unlikely to use glycine as a neurotransmitter because GLYT2, a key molecule for a glycinergic phenotype (Aubrey et al., 2007), is not expressed by neurons in the IC (Tanaka & Ezure, 2004). GLYT2 is found in lemniscal axons from the auditory brainstem that terminate in ICc (Choy Buentello, Bishop, & Oliver, 2015). GABAergic neurons express glutamic acid decarboxylase 65 and 67 (GAD65 and GAD67). IC glutamatergic neurons express vesicular glutamate transporter 2 (VGLUT2) but not VGLUT1 or VGLUT3 (Ito, Bishop, & Oliver, 2009).

Approximately 20–30% of IC neurons are GABAergic (Merchan, Aguilar, Lopez-Poveda, & Malmierca, 2005; Oliver, Winer, Beckius, & Saint Marie, 1994). In the central nucleus, the density of GABAergic neurons is higher than in the dorsal, caudal, and rostral cortical areas. GABAergic neurons within the GABA modules in lateral cortex also are densely clustered. GABAergic neurons are subdivided into at least 2 populations, large and small GABAergic (LG and SG) neurons (Ito et al., 2009; Ito & Oliver, 2012): LG neurons receive dense VGLUT2-positive axosomatic synapses while SG or glutamatergic neurons not. The somatic size of SG and glutamatergic neurons are similar, and LG neurons have the largest cell bodies in the IC. The LG and SG neurons have a different synaptic organization and different projection targets (described in

Synaptic Organization and Morphology of Local Circuit). The functional classification of IC GABAergic neurons is further subdivided into 4 categories by the presence of axosomatic VGLUT2-positive excitatory terminals and an extracellular matrix structure, the perineuronal net (Beebe, Young, Mellott, & Schofield, 2016; Foster, Mellott, & Schofield, 2014). The perineuronal nets are found mainly around large neurons and are on most but not all LG neurons. Since perineuronal nets may stabilize synapses on dendrites and inhibit structural plasticity (Corvetti & Rossi, 2005), the GABAergic LG neurons with perineuronal nets may have reduced plasticity relative to other IC neurons.

Many IC neurons appear to co-release neuromodulators together with classical neurotransmitters such as glutamate and GABA. Neuromodulators, such as nitric oxide, enkephalin, neuropeptide-Y, somatostatin, substance P, and cholecystokinin are prevalent in the IC cortex but not in the ICc (Coote & Rees, 2008; Nakagawa et al., 1995; Tongjaroenbuangam et al., 2006; Wynne, Harvey, Robertson, & Sirinathsinghji, 1995; Wynne & Robertson, 1997). In the lateral cortex, the labeling density of neuromodulators appeared to be layer-specific, suggesting that they control the gain of multimodal inputs. Since GABAergic neurons of all sizes may or may not express nitric oxide synthase (Fujimoto et al., 2017), the expression of nitric oxide is not likely related to the LG/SG classification.

In addition to neuromodulators, IC neurons express other molecular markers. For example, calcium binding proteins like parvalbumin (PV), calretinin, and calbindin are expressed in the IC (Friauf, 1994; Lohmann & Friauf, 1996). The expression of calcium binding protein is also layer- and subdivision-specific. PV is strongly expressed in the ICc and in the GABA modules of layer 2 lateral cortex (Chernock et al., 2004). Calretinin and calbindin is rich in layer 1 of the IC cortex and appears to be almost absent in GABA modules (Friauf, 1994; Lohmann & Friauf, 1996). In many brain regions, PV is used as a marker of GABAergic neurons, and in the IC, almost all GABAergic neurons are positive for PV (Fujimoto et al., 2017). However, a substantial number of GAD67-negative neurons also express PV (Fujimoto et al., 2017), so PV cannot be used as a marker of GABAergic neurons in the IC. Expression patterns of calcium binding proteins change during development (Friauf, 1994; Fujimoto et al., 2017; Lohmann & Friauf, 1996).

Synaptic Organization

IC receives ascending inputs from all auditory brainstem nuclei (Adams, 1979), descending inputs from the auditory cortex (Winer, 2005) and several non-lemniscal thalamic nuclei (Winer, Chernock, Larue, & Cheung, 2002), as well as neuromodulatory inputs from dopaminergic (Nevue, Elde, Perkel, & Portfors, 2015), noradrenergic, serotoninergic (Klepper & Herbert, 1991), and cholinergic (Motts & Schofield, 2009) neurons, and multisensory inputs (Lesicko et al., 2016). Axons from each input source tend to terminate in specific subregions in the IC, some of which are smaller than the obvious anatomical subdivisions (Oliver, 2005). One example is layer 2 of the lateral cortex where somatosensory inputs terminate within the GABA modules and auditory cortex inputs terminate outside the modules (Lesicko et al., 2016). Even within the ICc, there are subregions which differ in terms of the specific combination of inputs from extrinsic sources (Cant & Benson, 2007; Loftus, Bishop, & Oliver, 2010). This "synaptic domain" organization limits the variety of synaptic inputs available to neurons in different parts of the IC (Oliver, 2005). Within the ICc, this concept extends down to the level of the fibrodendritic laminae where adjacent laminae may contain axons from different sources (Loftus, Bishop, Saint Marie, & Oliver, 2004; Shneiderman & Henkel, 1987). A flat, disc-shaped neuron may have both its cell body and dendritic tree confined to one fibrodendritic lamina and receive only one set of synaptic inputs. In contrast, an adjacent large stellate neuron may have dendrites that extend into two or three adjacent laminae and receive inputs from several sets of inputs. Thus, adjacent neurons in the ICc may have very different patterns of synaptic input and receive excitatory or inhibitory synaptic inputs from different sources.

Since the patterns of synaptic distribution on LG, SG, and glutamatergic neurons are very different (Ito et al., 2009), studies about the synaptic organization should account for the type of postsynaptic neuron. The identification of inputs to the dendrites of identified neurons is technically challenging, thus our current knowledge is limited (Oliver, Ostapoff, & Beckius, 1999), and future studies must generate the details about axodendritic synapses on identified neuron types. In the following, the patterns of axosomatic synapses are described.

Both excitatory and inhibitory axosomatic synapses are present in the IC. In an electron microscopic study (Paloff, Usunoff, Hinova-Palova, & Ivanov, 1989), inhibitory axosomatic synapses were common for most neuron types, while excitatory axosomatic synapses were found mainly on large neurons. The large neurons in that study appear to be the GABAergic LG neurons as they share the same ultrastructural features (Ito et al., 2009; Ito & Oliver, 2014). The number of excitatory axosomatic terminals is positively correlated with the somatic size of the LG but not SG neurons (Ito et al., 2009), and this suggests that the density of the axosomatic terminals is kept constant on LG neurons to maintain excitability. The sources of fibers that make VGLUT2-positive excitatory axosomatic contacts on LG neurons include the IC itself, dorsal cochlear nucleus, superior olivary complex, and intermediate nucleus of the lateral lemniscus. Auditory cortex and ventral cochlear nuclei are not likely sources because projection neurons in these regions express VGLUT1 (Ito, Bishop, & Oliver, 2011; Ito & Oliver, 2010), which is not expressed in axosomatic terminals on LG neurons (Ito et al., 2009). Quantitative analysis of the axosomatic contacts from single VGLUT2-expressing axons revealed that a single excitatory axon makes 1–7 axosomatic contacts, so this suggests that an LG neuron receives axosomatic inputs from hundreds of excitatory neurons (Ito et al.,

2015; Ito & Oliver, 2014). Furthermore, a single LG neuron receives inputs from both lemniscal fibers and local neurons which indicates a convergence of inputs from many sources (Ito et al., 2015). Since each lower brainstem auditory nucleus encodes different auditory information, LG neurons are likely to integrate auditory information analyzed in parallel in lower brainstem nuclei.

The spatial origins of excitatory and inhibitory local inputs to single IC neurons were revealed in experiments that combined whole-neuron recording with the uncaging of glutamate (Sturm, Zhang-Hooks, Roos, Nguyen, & Kandler, 2017; Sturm, Nguyen, & Kandler, 2014). Because synaptic responses caused by focal glutamate uncaging indicate the presence of presynaptic neurons in the stimulation sites, maps of regions with neurons which make inputs on recorded neurons can be revealed. Inhibitory and excitatory inputs were isolated by holding membrane voltage at the reversal potentials of glutamate receptors and chloride, respectively. Furthermore, the inputs specific to glutamatergic and GABAergic neurons were identified in recordings from VGLUT2-Cre-dT-loxP and VGAT-Cre-dT-loxP mice, respectively. In glutamatergic neurons in the normal condition, the map of inputs from GABAergic neurons was larger than the map of inputs from glutamatergic neurons (Figure 18.2A). This suggests that excitatory inputs originate in a spatially restricted region, fibrodendritic lamina, while the origin of inhibitory inputs was not restricted in the same lamina. In contrast, the GABAergic neurons were subdivided into 2 groups based on the shape of the map. Type 1 GABAergic neurons received an inhibitory input area from a larger area than the excitatory one. Type 2 neurons received predominantly excitatory inputs with very few or no inhibitory inputs. The amplitude of the excitatory inputs was larger in type 2 neurons than in type 1. The authors suggested that type 1 and type 2 GABAergic neurons correspond to the SG and LG neurons, respectively. Interestingly, noise trauma altered the input maps and synaptic electrical charges to glutamatergic and type 1 GABAergic neurons, but not to type 2 GABAergic neurons. The lack of plasticity in type 2 GABAergic, presumably LG neurons, is also suggested by the fact that most of LG neurons possess perineuronal nets, which may inhibit structural plastic changes (see Neurotransmitter Type or Other Molecular Markers).

Intrinsic Properties

The IC consists of the neurons with diverse intrinsic membrane properties, and this results in different firing patterns in response to depolarization (Geis & Borst, 2013; Moore & Trussell, 2017; Ono et al., 2005; Peruzzi, Sivaramakrishnan, & Oliver, 2000; Sivaramakrishnan & Oliver, 2001; Tan & Borst, 2007). The majority of the IC neurons showed the repetitive firing during the depolarization evoked by square current injection, while the others showed transient firing only at the onset of the depolarization (Moore & Trussell, 2017; Peruzzi et al., 2000; Sivaramakrishnan &

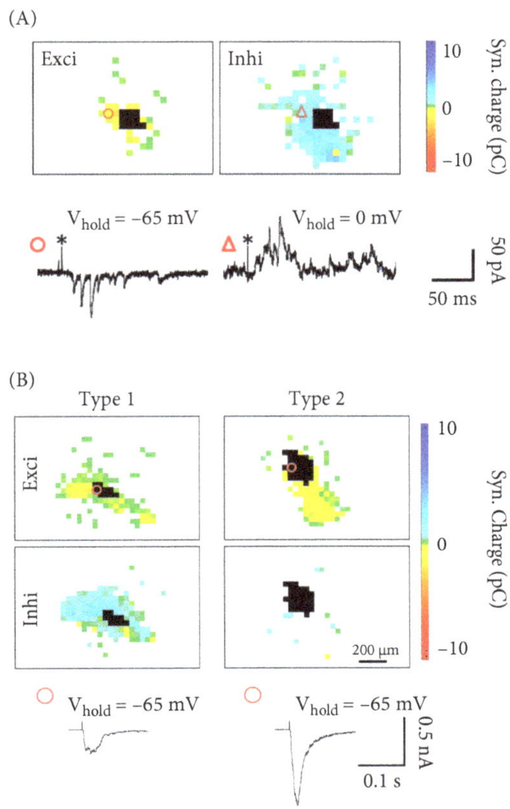

FIGURE 18.2 Spatial distribution of synaptic input sources on single ICC neurons. (A) Maps of excitatory and inhibitory inputs on a glutamatergic neuron. Excitatory and inhibitory maps are obtained at a membrane holding voltage of −65 mV and 0 mV, respectively. Traces illustrate excitatory (circle) and inhibitory (triangle) synaptic responses to glutamate uncaging (*) at the locations indicated by symbols. Uncaging sites that elicited direct responses in the recorded neuron are marked as black. Example maps and recording traces are from single stimulation iterations. (B) Input maps of a type 1 and type 2 GABAergic neuron. Type 1 neurons receive both excitatory and inhibitory inputs while type 2 neurons receive predominantly excitatory inputs.

Modified from Sturm et al. (2017) with permission.

Oliver, 2001; Tan & Borst, 2007). The neurons with repetitive firing were subdivided by the temporal pattern of the firing: regular sustained, adapting, build-up, pauser, and so forth. The diversity in the firing is shaped by the different potassium currents (Sivaramakrishnan & Oliver, 2001). In addition to the firing pattern to depolarization, IC neurons were subdivided based on the presence of rebound firing to hyperpolarization. This rebound firing was shown to involve the T-type calcium current and the hyperpolarization-activated current (I_h) (Koch & Grothe, 2003;

Ono et al., 2005), but the I_h does not determine the firing properties by itself (Koch & Grothe, 2003).

The IC neurons with different firing patterns were not related to specific morphological types (Peruzzi et al., 2000). Moreover, they were not spatially organized in the IC, but it is possible that the neurons with different firing properties are distributed in a mosaic pattern. Both glutamatergic and GABAergic neurons were heterogeneous in terms of their firing patterns, although the patterns in glutamatergic neurons were more diverse than GABAergic neurons (Ono et al., 2005). Consequently, to date, the different firing patterns have not been related to other characteristics of cell types in the IC with a few exceptions. One exception is the GABAergic neurons in the GABA module in the lateral cortex region (Ono et al., 2005). These neurons are a homogenous group with transient firing to depolarization and rebound firing to hyperpolarization. In the dorsal cortex, all the large GABAergic neurons had lower membrane resistance than other types of neurons (Geis & Borst, 2013) despite not being a single firing type. In the future, additional neuronal classifiers will be necessary to associate the firing properties with specific neuron types, and this will help dissect the design of the neural circuits in the IC.

Response Properties to Sound

It is well known that IC neurons have diverse responses to sound. In the response to pure tones, they vary in their frequency response areas (Palmer, Shackleton, Sumner, Zobay, & Rees, 2013), post-stimulus time histograms (PSTH) patterns (Rees, Sarbaz, Malmierca, & Le Beau, 1997), and the degree of temporal adaptation (Perez-Gonzalez & Malmierca, 2014). They also have diverse responses to binaural, amplitude-modulated (AM) (Joris, Schreiner, & Rees, 2004), and frequency-modulated (FM) sounds (Williams & Fuzessery, 2012). This diversity in the IC partly reflects the processing in the neural circuits of the brainstem. In many cases, the responses of the IC neurons reflect their inputs from the neurons in the brainstem. This diversity of inputs was demonstrated directly in recent in vivo whole-cell studies that revealed the synaptic currents evoked by sound in IC neurons (Ono & Oliver, 2014a, 2014b). However, the IC is not merely a relay station. It can integrate information from multiple sources in the brainstem. An anatomical study combined with electrophysiological recordings showed that IC neurons that differed in their responses to binaural stimuli received inputs from different combinations of nuclei in the brainstem (Loftus et al., 2010). In that case, inputs from the different sources were related to neural circuits with distinct roles in binaural processing (or the absence of binaural processing). In some cases, neurons in the IC have complex responses to binaural sound that are likely due to convergence of inputs from at least two of the binaural circuits (Batra, Kuwada, & Stanford, 1993; Li, Gittelman, & Pollak, 2010; McAlpine, Jiang, Shackleton, & Palmer, 1998). The results of these studies strongly suggest that the convergence of afferent inputs generates de novo responses to sound in the IC.

Consistent with these observations, virtually all IC neurons were shown to receive both excitatory and inhibitory synaptic inputs, and this is critical in shaping the response properties of IC neurons. Among the properties shaped by the interaction of the excitatory and inhibitory inputs are: threshold (Ono & Oliver, 2014a), frequency tuning (Xie, Gittelman, & Pollak, 2007), PSTH pattern (Ono & Oliver, 2014a), binaural responses (Li et al., 2010; Ono & Oliver, 2014b; Xiong et al., 2013), FM direction selectivity (Gittelman, Li, & Pollak, 2009; Kuo & Wu, 2012) and others. While all the excitatory synaptic inputs are glutamatergic in the IC, the inhibitory inputs are both GABAergic and glycinergic, and this may lead to a diversity of function. The GABAergic and glycinergic inhibitory currents are known to have distinct kinetics (Moore & Trussell, 2017). Since GABAergic and glycinergic terminals are distributed differentially in the IC (Choy Buentello et al., 2015), it raises the possibility of a segregation of function related to different inputs using these two inhibitory transmitters.

Interestingly, combination-sensitive neurons in the bat appear to depend exclusively on glycinergic inputs and are independent of GABAergic inputs (Nataraj & Wenstrup, 2005; Sanchez, Gans, & Wenstrup, 2008; Wenstrup, Nataraj, & Sanchez, 2012). In addition, FM-rate selectivity in the bat was reported to depend exclusively on glycinergic inputs (Williams & Fuzessery, 2011). Thus, in some cases, the GABAergic and glycinergic inputs are likely to have different functions and terminate on different neurons. However, in other IC neurons, GABAergic and glycinergic inputs may work cooperatively instead of having distinct roles in processing. Previous pharmacological studies have shown that sound-evoked responses of many IC neurons were modulated by blocking either GABAergic or glycinergic inputs. In support of this view, a recent in vitro study showed that some ascending fibers from ventral nucleus of the lateral lemniscus co-released GABA and glycine (Moore & Trussell, 2017). This may be the ultimate form of cooperation between GABAergic and glycinergic in the IC.

In IC neurons, it was reported that there was no one-to-one correspondence between the sound-evoked responses and morphology (Wallace et al., 2012) or intrinsic firing properties (Tan, Theeuwes, Feenstra, & Borst, 2007). The morphology of a neuron is often an important factor in the neuronal response. Morphology largely affects the spread of passive currents within the neuron and constrains the spatial distribution of the synaptic terminals. It is likely that the orientation and length of the dendritic tree affect the combination of the synaptic inputs on the IC neuron since the IC has a tonotopic structure as well as synaptic domains which are created by the different termination zones of different subcortical nuclei. One would expect that neurons with the largest dendritic fields would have the most diverse responses. However, a study using the juxtacellular labeling technique failed to find an explicit relationship between the dendritic morphology and the responses to sound (Wallace et al., 2012). In addition to the morphology, the intrinsic firing properties are expected to influence the neural responses strongly. Again, a study using in vivo whole-cell recording showed that the temporal pattern of the responses of IC neurons to sound did not always match that of firing during the depolarization evoked by square current injection (Tan et al., 2007). In both the case of morphology and intrinsic properties, the lack of correspondence between response pattern and cell morphology is likely due to the diversity in the afferent inputs. Neurons with the same morphology and intrinsic membrane properties may have different responses to sound if the sources of the afferents are different. Further studies will be required to understand the contribution of these cellular properties to sound processing in the IC.

As described in Neurotransmitter Type or Other Molecular Markers, the IC contains both glutamatergic and GABAergic neurons. A recent study elucidated the response properties of glutamatergic and GABAergic IC neurons to sound using transgenic mice that express channelrhodopsin-2 (ChR2) exclusively in the inhibitory neurons. The glutamatergic and GABAergic neurons could not be distinguished in vivo by their spike shapes (Ono, Bishop, & Oliver, 2017) unlike in the neocortex or the hippocampus. Overall, the sound-evoked responses in both classes of neurons were similar, although glutamatergic neurons responded better to amplitude modulations at high rate. However, the responses of both classes were affected by their locations (Ono et al., 2017). These results suggest that the location of the neuron in a specific synaptic domain (described in Synaptic Organization) might be the dominant influence on the response to sound regardless of the cell types. However, the caveat here is that both glutamatergic and GABAergic neurons have subtypes (see Morphology, and Neurotransmitter Type or Other Molecular Markers). It is possible that one subtype might have distinct sound-evoked responses. Today, the development of optogenetics will allow specific cell types in IC to be identified and studied in vivo and in vitro. With this approach, it will be possible to characterize the function of all the neuronal types in the IC and investigate their role in the circuitry of the auditory midbrain.

Intrinsic Circuits

IC neurons receive inputs not only from extrinsic fibers but also from other IC neurons, making complex local circuitry. The complex local circuitry produces variety and similarity of response patterns among nearby neurons and emerges various forms of plasticity.

Morphology of Local Circuits

The IC has a complex local circuitry. Most neurons with axons that project out of the IC also have a local axonal plexus (Oliver et al., 1991). Single neuron labeling studies showed with intracellular or juxtacellular dye injection or recombinant viral tracers that most IC neurons possessed axons with local collaterals (Ito & Oliver, 2014; Oliver et al., 1991; Wallace et al., 2012). Although the presence of true interneurons is under debate, neurons with well-developed local axons without collaterals entering the brachium of the IC have been observed (Ito & Oliver, 2014; Wallace et al., 2012).

The morphology of the local circuit in the ICc is best viewed in relationship to the fibrodendritic laminae. In cats, disc-shaped neurons have flattened local collaterals that are parallel to the dendritic field of the neuron and extend within the same fibrodendritic laminae as the dendritic field. In contrast, stellate neurons with dendritic trees that are unoriented or orthogonal to the laminae have axonal collaterals that enter multiple fibrodendritic laminae (Oliver et al., 1991). The former circuit may enhance or suppress many neurons within a lamina that share similar tuning, while the latter pattern suggests a circuitry with broad spectral sensitivity used to connect many neurons with different frequency tuning. In rodents, neurons with a laminar axonal plexus can originate from both flat neurons and moderately-oriented, less-flat neurons (Ito & Oliver, 2014; Wallace et al., 2012). Although, most neurons had single local plexuses in the same laminae as the dendritic trees, a few neurons had plexuses in different laminae. These results suggest that the local axons can influence the IC circuitry in various ways. Mapping of local connections with uncaging glutamate in slices showed that IC neurons receive local excitatory as well as inhibitory inputs along the fibrodendritic laminae in which they reside (J. J. Sturm, Nguyen, & Kandler, 2016). This is in line with the anatomical studies (Ito & Oliver, 2014; Wallace et al., 2012) and further shows that the organization of local excitatory and inhibitory circuits is similarity organized. Some ICc neurons also send their local axons into the cortex of the IC, and these neurons are likely to convey auditory information to the multimodal regions of IC.

Since the local IC circuit contains subtypes of both excitatory and inhibitory neurons, identifying the circuitry between specific neuron types is important. Little is known about this topic except for a recent study where three GAD67-negative, putative glutamatergic neurons without visible projection axons were reconstructed, and the apposition of axonal terminals on GABAergic neuron bodies was examined (Ito & Oliver, 2014) (Figure 18.1). Two ICc neurons had well-developed local axonal plexuses, and the axons made contact on 20 and 30 LG somata. The LG somata receiving contacts were well-aligned on a plane, and this suggested that local glutamatergic neurons innervate many LG neurons in the same fibrodendritic laminae. In the lateral cortex, one pyramidal-like neuron had a poorly developed axon within layer 3, but this axon made contacts with 9 LG somata.

Physiological Properties of Nearby Neurons

It is likely that the local circuit of the IC contains subtypes of neurons with different intrinsic membrane properties, but these neurons receive similar synaptic inputs, as synaptic domain hypothesis suggests. As described in Intrinsic Properties, a spatial organization in the IC has not been reported that could segregate neurons with different firing properties, except for the neurons in the GABA modules. Consistent with this, the expression of voltage sensitive ion channels also appears to lack any specific spatial distribution in IC.

How then are the responses properties to sound organized in the local circuits of the IC? Although few, several studies have reported the relationship of the nearby neurons in the IC, using different recording techniques [single microelectrode; (Ono et al., 2017; Syka, Radionova, & Popelar, 1981), tetrode; (Chen, Rodriguez, Read, & Escabi, 2012; Seshagiri & Delgutte, 2007), multichannel silicon probe; (Atencio, Shen, & Schreiner, 2016)]. In all the studies, the characteristic (CF) or best frequency (BF) were the parameters of the sound-evoked responses that were most highly correlated among the nearby neurons. In three studies, the bandwidths of the frequency response area were also well correlated in the nearby neurons although less so than CF and BF (Atencio et al., 2016; Chen et al., 2012; Ono et al., 2017). However, in another study (Seshagiri & Delgutte, 2007), the bandwidths of the frequency response areas were not significantly correlated. When pairs of identified GABAergic and glutamatergic neurons or pairs of glutamatergic neurons were compared, the pairs shared similar frequency tuning (Ono et al., 2017). This suggests that within a lamina both classes of neurons share inputs with similar frequency tuning, but adjacent laminae could have differences in spectral sensitivity depending on whether the same inputs are present in the adjacent laminae.

The temporal properties of neurons within a local circuit may be less well correlated. The PSTH to pure tones may be highly variable among the nearby neurons (Atencio et al., 2016; Ono et al., 2017; Seshagiri & Delgutte, 2007). This may be true for both GABAergic-glutamatergic and glutamatergic-glutamatergic neuronal pairs (Ono et al., 2017). This could be a function of local neurons with similar inputs but different intrinsic membrane properties. When an array of tetrodes is used, the neurons near one tetrode recording site had spectro-temporal response patterns that were more similar to each other than the neurons at other recording sites (Chen et al., 2012). However, the temporal response patterns to a dynamic moving ripple sound were less well correlated at different sites than the spectral responses. The nature of temporal processing within the local IC circuit and the mechanisms that create the response diversity in the local IC circuit remain unresolved.

Plasticity

Plasticity is ubiquitous and plays a critical role in the organization of functional neural circuits in the CNS. In the IC, it is well known that the corticofugal projection to IC can induce plastic changes in the responses of IC neurons to sound. This top-down plasticity is likely to be critical in the learning of the auditory tasks (Bajo, Nodal, Moore, & King, 2010; Slee & David, 2015). A series of studies by Suga's group (Suga, 2012; Xiao & Suga, 2005; Zhang & Suga, 1997) showed that the activation or inactivation of the primary auditory cortex changes the response properties of the IC neurons to sound. The plasticity induced by the cortex affects the response properties in the frequency, temporal and intensity domains (reviewed in Suga, 2012). Acoustic fear conditioning induced dramatic frequency changes in the IC via corticofugal projection (Gao & Suga, 1998).

The plastic changes in the IC may not be solely due to changes in the IC local circuit. Corticofugal activity is known to affect multiple levels in the auditory pathway: medial geniculate body, IC, superior olivary nuclei, cochlear nuclei, and cochlea. However, local changes in the IC are likely since because local application of atropine, an acetylcholine blocker, can block the BF changes in IC induced by the acoustic fear conditioning (Ji, Gao, & Suga, 2001). The cholinergic inputs driven by corticofugal projection is likely from pontomesencephalic tegmentum (Schofield, Motts, & Mellott, 2011), but the relationships of these cholinergic inputs to the auditory corticofugal system remains unclear.

In addition to the top-down plasticity, some forms of bottom-up plasticity have been reported in the IC. Stimulus specific adaptation (SSA) is a plastic neuronal processing that is not found caudal to the IC (Ayala, Perez-Gonzalez, Duque, Nelken, & Malmierca, 2013; Carbajal & Malmierca, 2018; Perez-Gonzalez & Malmierca, 2014) (see also chapter by Malmierca et al., in this volume). Given a series of repetitive tones, the neurons with SSA show reduced responses to a common sound, while they respond well to a tone that is rarely presented. SSA was considered to be relevant to novelty detection in the acoustic environment and was first discovered in the auditory cortex (Ulanovsky, Las, & Nelken, 2003). The neurons with SSA are located in the cortices of the IC (Ayala et al., 2015; Carbajal & Malmierca, 2018; Malmierca, Cristaudo, Perez-Gonzalez, & Covey, 2009) that are heavily innervated by the corticofugal projections from auditory cortex. In line with this observation, it was shown that the deactivation of the auditory cortex modified the responses of the neurons with SSA in the IC (Anderson & Malmierca, 2013). However, cortical deactivation did not affect half of the neurons with SSA and did not completely eliminate the SSA in the majority of neurons with decreased SSA after cortical deactivation. Thus, local processing in the IC must contribute to the SSA in the IC neurons. Synaptic depression is likely the major determinant of SSA. Indeed, some IC neurons showed synaptic depression in sound evoked EPSCs when the sound interval was longer than 1 s (Ono & Oliver, 2014a), which is much longer than the 2–8 Hz repetition rate used in SSA experiments suggesting that synaptic depression is even more likely during stimulus presentations in SSA. The highly depressive synaptic inputs might be from IC intrinsic connections because the SSA neuron were shown to receive minimal inputs from brainstem in comparison to non-SSA neurons (Ayala et al., 2015). Further, pharmacological studies have shown that inhibition (Ayala & Malmierca, 2018) and neuromodulators (Ayala & Malmierca, 2015; Valdes-Baizabal, Parras, Ayala, & Malmierca, 2017) modified the SSA in the IC, and this suggests that the SSA in the IC is likely to be shaped by complex neuronal processing.

Another example of bottom-up plasticity is long-lasting sound-evoked afterdischarge (Ono, Bishop, & Oliver, 2016). Most neurons in the auditory pathway as well as IC neurons usually respond to sound during its presentation and cease spike discharges at the sound termination. However, when presented a long duration sound (more than 30 s) or repetitive sequential sounds over a long duration, a subpopulation of IC neurons continued to fire for several tens of seconds to a few minutes after the sound termination (after-discharge). Both glutamatergic and GABAergic neurons could exhibit the long-duration sound-evoked after-discharge (LSA). The neurons with LSA were distributed broadly in the ICc, however most were located in the ventral ICc, the area tuned to high sound frequencies (Ono et al., 2016). Although the cellular mechanism that generates LSA remains unknown, it is likely to be shaped in the IC because most neurons in lower brainstem nuclei show a suppression of activity after long-lasting sound stimuli. The functional significance of LSA is also unknown, but it might be a neuronal gain control mechanism dependent on the input strength, and it might be relevant to tinnitus as an abnormal gain enhancement in the auditory pathway (Auerbach, Rodrigues, & Salvi, 2014).

To elucidate the mechanism of these plastic changes in vivo, it is necessary to learn the cellular properties of the neural circuit. In vitro brain slice preparations are helpful in this regard. Most IC neurons show long-term potentiation or long-term depression with tetanic stimulation in the brain slice (Wu, Ma, Sivaramakrishnan, & Oliver, 2002; Zhang & Wu, 2000). Moreover, a plateau potential is seen in the IC in response to electrical stimulation of axons in the lateral lemniscus (Sivaramakrishnan & Oliver, 2006). A sustained depolarization might be relevant to potentiation, depression or LSA. However, studies using IC slice preparations are still limited, and further in vitro investigations of the neural circuits of the IC would promote our understanding of the plastic responses in response to sound.

Finally, the responses of IC neurons can be altered by auditory experiences (Irvine, 2017), for example, partial hearing loss (Chambers et al., 2016; Popescu & Polley, 2010) or specific sound-rearing (Yu, Sanes, Aristizabal, Wadghiri, & Turnbull, 2007). In vitro slice recordings have also shown that hearing loss can modify synaptic strength in the IC neural circuit (J. J. Sturm et al., 2017; Vale, Juiz, Moore, & Sanes, 2004; Vale & Sanes, 2000, 2002). These changes may be a product of a large-scale reorganization within the auditory pathway and interactions between the different structures including the IC. Examples include the application of atropine to the IC of fear-conditioned animals which abolishes the plastic changes in the IC and also reduces the changes in the auditory cortex (Ji et al., 2001). Thus, it might be possible to reduce the symptoms induced by maladaptive plasticity in the auditory pathway (leading to tinnitus) by manipulating the neural activity in the IC.

Key Issues to Address in the Future

To better understand the functional organization of the IC, we need to identify and manipulate specific cell types which are involved in a particular functional unit inside the IC local circuit. Followings are our proposal for the future research direction.

Molecular Markers for Specific Neuronal Types

At this point, we do not have molecular markers that identify subtypes of glutamatergic or GABAergic neurons. For example, it is likely that subtypes of GABAergic neurons (LG, SG, or neurons with perineuronal nets) have different projection patterns and serve different functions. With single molecular markers to define neuronal subtypes, one may create transgenic mice that target specific types of IC neurons to label or modify specific components of the neural circuitry.

Identification of Functional Circuits through the IC and Specific Microcircuits within the IC

Since the IC consists of neuron subtypes, which have different patterns of circuit connectivity, their roles in auditory processing are likely to be different. On the other hand, synaptic domains in the IC suggest the wiring of microcircuit is different between regions. The former implies neuron-type-specific functional organization, while latter implies microdomain-based or map-based functional organization in the IC. Future study may determine which is the case in the IC. It is also possible that dual modes of coding, that is, both neuron-type-based and map-based, are present in the IC. Neuron type identification using molecular markers and recording from large number of neurons will help to clarify this issue. Neighboring neurons with different dendritic arborizations may receive different combination of inputs even their neuron bodies are in the same synaptic domain. Therefore, in future studies of the synaptic organization, the composition of inputs should be related to the neuron type as well as the location of the cell body.

References

Adams, J. C. (1979). Ascending projections to the inferior colliculus. *Journal of Comparative Neurology*, *183*(3), 519–538.

Anderson, L. A., & Malmierca, M. S. (2013). The effect of auditory cortex deactivation on stimulus-specific adaptation in the inferior colliculus of the rat. *European Journal of Neuroscience*, *37*(1), 52–62. doi: 10.1111/ejn.12018

Atencio, C. A., Shen, V., & Schreiner, C. E. (2016). Synchrony, connectivity, and functional similarity in auditory midbrain local circuits. *Neuroscience*, *335*, 30–53. doi: 10.1016/j.neuroscience.2016.08.024

Aubrey, K. R., Rossi, F. M., Ruivo, R., Alboni, S., Bellenchi, G. C., Le Goff, A., . . . Supplisson, S. (2007). The transporters GlyT2 and VIAAT cooperate to determine the vesicular glycinergic phenotype. *Journal of Neuroscience*, *27*(23), 6273–6281. doi: 27/23/6273 [pii] 10.1523/JNEUROSCI.1024-07.2007

Auerbach, B. D., Rodrigues, P. V., & Salvi, R. J. (2014). Central gain control in tinnitus and hyperacusis. *Frontiers in Neurology*, *5*, 206. doi: 10.3389/fneur.2014.00206

Ayala, Y. A., & Malmierca, M. S. (2015). Cholinergic modulation of stimulus-specific adaptation in the inferior colliculus. *Journal of Neuroscience*, *35*(35), 12261–12272. doi: 10.1523/Jneurosci.0909-15.2015

Ayala, Y. A., & Malmierca, M. S. (2018). The effect of inhibition on stimulus-specific adaptation in the inferior colliculus. *Brain Structure and Function*, *223*(3), 1391–1407. doi: 10.1007/s00429-017-1546-4

Ayala, Y. A., Perez-Gonzalez, D., Duque, D., Nelken, I., & Malmierca, M. S. (2013). Frequency discrimination and stimulus deviance in the inferior colliculus and cochlear nucleus. *Frontiers in Neural Circuits*, *6*. doi: Artn 119 10.3389/Fncir.2012.00119

Ayala, Y. A., Udeh, A., Dutta, K., Bishop, D., Malmierca, M. S., & Oliver, D. L. (2015). Differences in the strength of cortical and brainstem inputs to SSA and non-SSA neurons in the inferior colliculus. *Scientific Reports*, *5:10383*. doi: Artn 10383 10.1038/Srep10383

Bajo, V. M., Nodal, F. R., Moore, D. R., & King, A. J. (2010). The descending corticocollicular pathway mediates learning-induced auditory plasticity. *Nature Neuroscience*, *13*(2), 253–260. doi: 10.1038/nn.2466

Batra, R., Kuwada, S., & Stanford, T. R. (1993). High-frequency neurons in the inferior colliculus that are sensitive to interaural delays of amplitude-modulated tones: Evidence for dual binaural influences. *Journal of Neurophysiology*, *70*(1), 64–80. doi: 10.1152/jn.1993.70.1.64

Beebe, N. L., Young, J. W., Mellott, J. G., & Schofield, B. R. (2016). Extracellular molecular markers and soma size of inhibitory neurons: Evidence for four subtypes of GABAergic cells in the inferior colliculus. *Journal of Neuroscience*, *36*(14), 3988–3999.

Cant, N. B., & Benson, C. G. (2007). Multiple topographically organized projections connect the central nucleus of the inferior colliculus to the ventral division of the medial geniculate nucleus in the gerbil, Meriones unguiculatus. *Journal of Comparative Neurology*, *503*(3), 432–453.

Carbajal, Guillermo V., & Malmierca, Manuel S. (2018). The neuronal basis of predictive coding along the auditory pathway: From the subcortical roots to cortical deviance detection. *Trends in Hearing*, *22*: 1–33. doi: 10.1177/2331216518784822

Chambers, A. R., Resnik, J., Yuan, Y., Whitton, J. P., Edge, A. S., Liberman, M. C., & Polley, D. B. (2016). Central gain restores auditory processing following near-complete cochlear denervation. *Neuron*, *89*(4), 867–879. doi: 10.1016/j.neuron.2015.12.041

Chen, C., Rodriguez, F. C., Read, H. L., & Escabi, M. A. (2012). Spectrotemporal sound preferences of neighboring inferior colliculus neurons: Implications for local circuitry and processing. *Frontiers in Neural Circuits*, *6*, 62. doi: 10.3389/fncir.2012.00062

Chernock, M. L., Larue, D. T., & Winer, J. A. (2004). A periodic network of neurochemical modules in the inferior colliculus. *Hearing Research*, *188*(1–2), 12–20.

Choy Buentello, D., Bishop, D. C., & Oliver, D. L. (2015). Differential distribution of GABA and glycine terminals in the inferior colliculus of rat and mouse. *Journal of Comparative Neurology*, *523*(18), 2683–2697. doi: 10.1002/cne.23810

Coote, E. J., & Rees, A. (2008). The distribution of nitric oxide synthase in the inferior colliculus of guinea pig. *Neuroscience*, *154*(1), 218–225.

Corvetti, L., & Rossi, F. (2005). Degradation of chondroitin sulfate proteoglycans induces sprouting of intact purkinje axons in the cerebellum of the adult rat. *Journal of Neuroscience*, *25*(31), 7150–7158. doi: 10.1523/JNEUROSCI.0683-05.2005

Faye-Lund, H., & Osen, K. K. (1985). Anatomy of the inferior colliculus in rat. *Anatomy of Embryology (Berlin)*, *171*(1), 1–20.

Foster, N. L., Mellott, J. G., & Schofield, B. R. (2014). Perineuronal nets and GABAergic cells in the inferior colliculus of guinea pigs. *Frontiers in Neuroanatomy*, *7*, 53.

Friauf, E. (1994). Distribution of calcium-binding protein calbindin-D28k in the auditory system of adult and developing rats. *Journal of Comparative Neurology*, *349*(2), 193–211.

Fujimoto, H., Konno, K., Watanabe, M., & Jinno, S. (2017). Late postnatal shifts of parvalbumin and nitric oxide synthase expression within the GABAergic and glutamatergic phenotypes of inferior colliculus neurons. *Journal of Comparative Neurology*, *525*(4), 868–884. doi: 10.1002/cne.24104

Gao, E., & Suga, N. (1998). Experience-dependent corticofugal adjustment of midbrain frequency map in bat auditory system. *Proceedings of the National Academy of Sciences of the United States of America*, *95*(21), 12663–12670.

Geis, H. R., & Borst, J. G. (2013). Large GABAergic neurons form a distinct subclass within the mouse dorsal cortex of the inferior colliculus with respect to intrinsic properties, synaptic inputs, sound responses, and projections. *Journal of Comparative Neurology*, *521*(1), 189–202. doi: 10.1002/cne.23170

Gittelman, J. X., Li, N., & Pollak, G. D. (2009). Mechanisms underlying directional selectivity for frequency-modulated sweeps in the inferior colliculus revealed by in vivo whole-cell recordings. *Journal of Neuroscience*, *29*(41), 13030–13041. doi: 10.1523/JNEUROSCI.2477-09.2009

Henderson, Z., & Sherriff, F. E. (1991). Distribution of choline acetyltransferase immunoreactive axons and terminals in the rat and ferret brainstem. *Journal of Comparative Neurology*, *314*(1), 147–163.

Irvine, D. R. F. (2017). Plasticity in the auditory system. *Hearing Research* doi: 10.1016/j.heares.2017.10.011

Ito, T., Bishop, D. C., & Oliver, D. L. (2009). Two classes of GABAergic neurons in the inferior colliculus. *Journal of Neuroscience*, *29*(44), 13860–13869.

Ito, T., Bishop, D. C., & Oliver, D. L. (2011). Expression of glutamate and inhibitory amino acid vesicular transporters in the rodent auditory brainstem. *Journal of Comparative Neurology*, *519*(2), 316–340. doi: 10.1002/cne.22521

Ito, T., Hioki, H., Sohn, J., Okamoto, S., Kaneko, T., Iino, S., & Oliver, D. L. (2015). Convergence of lemniscal and local excitatory inputs on large GABAergic tectothalamic neurons. *Journal of Comparative Neurology*, *523*, 2277–2296.

Ito, T., & Oliver, D. L. (2010). Origins of glutamatergic terminals in the inferior colliculus identified by retrograde transport and expression of VGLUT1 and VGLUT2 Genes. *Frontiers in Neuroanatomy*, *4*, 135. doi: 10.3389/fnana.2010.00135

Ito, T., & Oliver, D. L. (2012). The basic circuit of the IC: Tectothalamic neurons with different patterns of synaptic organization send different messages to the thalamus. *Frontiers in Neural Circuits*, *6*, 48. doi: 10.3389/fncir.2012.00048

Ito, T., & Oliver, D. L. (2014). Local and commissural IC neurons make axosomatic inputs on large GABAergic tectothalamic neurons. *Journal of Comparative Neurology*, *522*(15), 3539–3554.

Ji, W., Gao, E., & Suga, N. (2001). Effects of acetylcholine and atropine on plasticity of central auditory neurons caused by conditioning in bats. *Journal of Neurophysiology*, *86*(1), 211–225. doi: 10.1152/jn.2001.86.1.211

Joris, P. X., Schreiner, C. E., & Rees, A. (2004). Neural processing of amplitude-modulated sounds. *Physiology Review*, *84*(2), 541–577. doi: 10.1152/physrev.00029.2003

Klepper, A., & Herbert, H. (1991). Distribution and origin of noradrenergic and serotonergic fibers in the cochlear nucleus and inferior colliculus of the rat. *Brain Research*, *557*(1–2), 190–201.

Koch, U., & Grothe, B. (2003). Hyperpolarization-activated current (Ih) in the inferior colliculus: Distribution and contribution to temporal processing. *Journal of Neurophysiology*, *90*(6), 3679–3687. doi: 10.1152/jn.00375.2003

Kuo, R. I., & Wu, G. K. (2012). The generation of direction selectivity in the auditory system. *Neuron*, *73*(5), 1016–1027. doi: 10.1016/j.neuron.2011.11.035

Lesicko, A. M., Hristova, T. S., Maigler, K. C., & Llano, D. A. (2016). Connectional modularity of top-down and bottom-up multimodal inputs to the lateral cortex of the mouse inferior colliculus. *Journal of Neuroscience*, *36*(43), 11037–11050.

Li, N., Gittelman, J. X., & Pollak, G. D. (2010). Intracellular recordings reveal novel features of neurons that code interaural intensity disparities in the inferior colliculus. *Journal of Neuroscience*, *30*(43), 14573–14584. doi: 10.1523/JNEUROSCI.2228-10.2010

Loftus, W. C., Bishop, D. C., & Oliver, D. L. (2010). Differential patterns of inputs create functional zones in central nucleus of inferior colliculus. *Journal of Neuroscience*, *30*(40), 13396–13408. doi: 30/40/13396 [pii] 10.1523/JNEUROSCI.0338-10.2010

Loftus, W. C., Bishop, D. C., Saint Marie, R. L., & Oliver, D. L. (2004). Organization of binaural excitatory and inhibitory inputs to the inferior colliculus from the superior olive. *Journal of Comparative Neurology*, *472*(3), 330–344. doi: 10.1002/cne.20070

Loftus, W. C., Malmierca, M. S., Bishop, D. C., & Oliver, D. L. (2008). The cytoarchitecture of the inferior colliculus revisited: A common organization of the lateral cortex in rat and cat. *Neuroscience*, *154*(1), 196–205.

Lohmann, C., & Friauf, E. (1996). Distribution of the calcium-binding proteins parvalbumin and calretinin in the auditory brainstem of adult and developing rats. *Journal of Comparative Neurology*, *367*(1), 90–109.

Malmierca, M. S., Blackstad, T. W., & Osen, K. K. (2011). Computer-assisted 3-D reconstructions of Golgi-impregnated neurons in the cortical regions of the inferior colliculus of rat. *Hearing Research*. 274(1–2):13–26. doi: S0378-5955(10)00316-3 [pii] 10.1016/j.heares.2010.06.011

Malmierca, M. S., Blackstad, T. W., Osen, K. K., Karagulle, T., & Molowny, R. L. (1993). The central nucleus of the inferior colliculus in rat: A Golgi and computer reconstruction study of neuronal and laminar structure. *Journal of Comparative Neurology*, *333*(1), 1–27.

Malmierca, M. S., Cristaudo, S., Perez-Gonzalez, D., & Covey, E. (2009). Stimulus-specific adaptation in the inferior colliculus of the anesthetized rat. *Journal of Neuroscience*, *29*(17), 5483–5493. doi: 10.1523/JNEUROSCI.4153-08.2009

Malmierca, M. S., Izquierdo, M. A., Cristaudo, S., Hernandez, O., Perez-Gonzalez, D., Covey, E., & Oliver, D. L. (2008). A discontinuous tonotopic organization in the inferior colliculus of the rat. *Journal of Neuroscience*, *28*(18), 4767–4776.

McAlpine, D., Jiang, D., Shackleton, T. M., & Palmer, A. R. (1998). Convergent input from brainstem coincidence detectors onto delay-sensitive neurons in the inferior colliculus. *Journal of Neuroscience*, *18*(15), 6026–6039.

Merchan, M., Aguilar, L. A., Lopez-Poveda, E. A., & Malmierca, M. S. (2005). The inferior colliculus of the rat: Quantitative immunocytochemical study of GABA and glycine. *Neuroscience*, *136*(3), 907–925.

Moore, L. A., & Trussell, L. O. (2017). Corelease of inhibitory neurotransmitters in the mouse auditory midbrain. *Journal of Neuroscience*, *37*(39), 9453–9464. doi: 10.1523/JNEUROSCI.1125-17.2017

Morest, D. K., & Oliver, D. L. (1984). The neuronal architecture of the inferior colliculus in the cat: Defining the functional anatomy of the auditory midbrain. *Journal of Comparative Neurology*, *222*(2), 209–236.

Motts, S. D., & Schofield, B. R. (2009). Sources of cholinergic input to the inferior colliculus. *Neuroscience*, *160*(1), 103–114.

Nakagawa, H., Ikeda, M., Houtani, T., Ueyama, T., Baba, K., Kondoh, A., . . . Sugimoto, T. (1995). Immunohistochemical evidence for enkephalin and neuropeptide Y in rat inferior colliculus neurons that provide ascending or commissural fibers. *Brain Research*, *690*(2), 236–240.

Nataraj, K., & Wenstrup, J. J. (2005). Roles of inhibition in creating complex auditory responses in the inferior colliculus: Facilitated combination-sensitive neurons. *Journal of Neurophysiology*, *93*(6), 3294–3312. doi: 10.1152/jn.01152.2004

Nevue, A. A., Elde, C. J., Perkel, D. J., & Portfors, C. V. (2015). Dopaminergic input to the inferior colliculus in mice. *Frontiers in Neuroanatomy*, *9*, 168. doi: 10.3389/fnana.2015.00168

Oliver, D. L. (2005). Neuronal organization in the inferior colliculus. Chapter 2. In J. A. Winer & C. E. Schreiner (Eds.), *The Inferior Colliculus* (pp. 69–114). New York: Springer.

Oliver, D. L., Kuwada, S., Yin, T. C., Haberly, L. B., & Henkel, C. K. (1991). Dendritic and axonal morphology of HRP-injected neurons in the inferior colliculus of the cat. *Journal of Comparative Neurology*, *303*(1), 75–100.

Oliver, D. L., & Morest, D. K. (1984). The central nucleus of the inferior colliculus in the cat. *Journal of Comparative Neurology*, *222*(2), 237–264.

Oliver, D. L., Ostapoff, E. M., & Beckius, G. E. (1999). Direct innervation of identified tectothalamic neurons in the inferior colliculus by axons from the cochlear nucleus. *Neuroscience*, *93*(2), 643–658.

Oliver, D. L., Winer, J. A., Beckius, G. E., & Saint Marie, R. L. (1994). Morphology of GABAergic neurons in the inferior colliculus of the cat. *Journal of Comparative Neurology*, *340*(1), 27–42.

Ono, M., Bishop, D. C., & Oliver, D. L. (2016). Long-lasting sound-evoked afterdischarge in the auditory midbrain. *Science Reports*, *6*, 20757. doi: 10.1038/srep20757

Ono, M., Bishop, D. C., & Oliver, D. L. (2017). Identified GABAergic and glutamatergic neurons in the mouse inferior colliculus share similar response properties. *Journal of Neuroscience*, *37*(37), 8952–8964. doi: 10.1523/JNEUROSCI.0745-17.2017

Ono, M., & Oliver, D. L. (2014a). Asymmetric temporal interactions of sound-evoked excitatory and inhibitory inputs in the mouse auditory midbrain. *Journal of Physiology*, *592*(16), 3647–3669. doi: 10.1113/jphysiol.2014.275446

Ono, M., & Oliver, D. L. (2014b). The balance of excitatory and inhibitory synaptic inputs for coding sound location. *Journal of Neuroscience*, *34*(10), 3779–3792. doi: 10.1523/JNEUROSCI.2954-13.2014

Ono, M., Yanagawa, Y., & Koyano, K. (2005). GABAergic neurons in inferior colliculus of the GAD67-GFP knock-in mouse: electrophysiological and morphological properties. *Neuroscience Research*, *51*(4), 475–492.

Palmer, A. R., Shackleton, T. M., Sumner, C. J., Zobay, O., & Rees, A. (2013). Classification of frequency response areas in the inferior colliculus reveals continua not discrete classes. *Journal of Physiology*, *591*(16), 4003–4025. doi: 10.1113/jphysiol.2013.255943

Paloff, A. M., Usunoff, K. G., & Hinova-Palova, D. V. (1992). Ultrastructure of Golgi-impregnated and gold-toned neurons in the central nucleus of the inferior colliculus in the cat. *Journal für Hirnforschung*, *33*(4–5), 361–407.

Paloff, A. M., Usunoff, K. G., Hinova-Palova, D. V., & Ivanov, D. P. (1985). Retinal innervation of the inferior colliculus in adult cats: Electron microscopic observations. *Neuroscience Letters*, *54*(2–3), 339–344.

Paloff, A. M., Usunoff, K. G., Hinova-Palova, D. V., & Ivanov, D. P. (1989). The fine structure of the inferior colliculus in the cat. I. Neuronal perikarya in the central nucleus. *Journal für Hirnforschung*, *30*(1), 69–90.

Perez-Gonzalez, D., & Malmierca, M. S. (2014). Adaptation in the auditory system: An overview. *Frontiers in Integrative Neuroscience*, *8*, 19. doi: 10.3389/fnint.2014.00019

Peruzzi, D., Sivaramakrishnan, S., & Oliver, D. L. (2000). Identification of cell types in brain slices of the inferior colliculus. *Neuroscience*, *101*(2), 403–416.

Popescu, M. V., & Polley, D. B. (2010). Monaural deprivation disrupts development of binaural selectivity in auditory midbrain and cortex. *Neuron*, *65*(5), 718–731. doi: 10.1016/j.neuron.2010.02.019

Rees, A., Sarbaz, A., Malmierca, M. S., & Le Beau, F. E. (1997). Regularity of firing of neurons in the inferior colliculus. *Journal of Neurophysiology*, *77*(6), 2945–2965. doi: 10.1152/jn.1997.77.6.2945

Saldana, E., & Merchan, M. A. (1992). Intrinsic and commissural connections of the rat inferior colliculus. *Journal of Comparative Neurology*, *319*(3), 417–437.

Sanchez, J. T., Gans, D., & Wenstrup, J. J. (2008). Glycinergic "inhibition" mediates selective excitatory responses to combinations of sounds. *Journal of Neuroscience*, *28*(1), 80–90. doi: 10.1523/JNEUROSCI.3572-07.2008

Schofield, B. R., Motts, S. D., & Mellott, J. G. (2011). Cholinergic cells of the pontomesencephalic tegmentum: Connections with auditory structures from cochlear nucleus to cortex. *Hearing Research*, *279*(1–2), 85–95. doi: 10.1016/j.heares.2010.12.019

Schreiner, C. E., & Langner, G. (1997). Laminar fine structure of frequency organization in auditory midbrain. *Nature*, *388*(6640), 383–386.

Seshagiri, C. V., & Delgutte, B. (2007). Response properties of neighboring neurons in the auditory midbrain for pure-tone stimulation: A tetrode study. *Journal of Neurophysiology*, *98*(4), 2058–2073. doi: 10.1152/jn.01317.2006

Shneiderman, A., & Henkel, C. K. (1987). Banding of lateral superior olivary nucleus afferents in the inferior colliculus: A possible substrate for sensory integration. *Journal of Comparative Neurology*, *266*(4), 519–534.

Sivaramakrishnan, S., & Oliver, D. L. (2001). Distinct K currents result in physiologically distinct cell types in the inferior colliculus of the rat. *Journal of Neuroscience*, *21*(8), 2861–2877.

Sivaramakrishnan, S., & Oliver, D. L. (2006). Neuronal responses to lemniscal stimulation in laminar brain slices of the inferior colliculus. *Journal of the Association of Research Otolaryngology*, *7*(1), 1–14. doi: 10.1007/s10162-005-0017-4

Slee, S. J., & David, S. V. (2015). Rapid task-related plasticity of spectrotemporal receptive fields in the auditory midbrain. *Journal of Neuroscience*, *35*(38), 13090–13102. doi: 10.1523/Jneurosci.1671-15.2015

Sturm, J. J., Nguyen, T., & Kandler, K. (2016). Mapping auditory synaptic circuits with photostimulation of caged glutamate. *Methods in Molecular Biology*, *1427*, 525–537. doi: 10.1007/978-1-4939-3615-1_30

Sturm, J. J., Zhang-Hooks, Y. X., Roos, H., Nguyen, T., & Kandler, K. (2017). Noise trauma-induced behavioral gap detection deficits correlate with reorganization of excitatory and inhibitory local circuits in the inferior colliculus and are prevented by acoustic enrichment. *Journal of Neuroscience*, *37*(26), 6314–6330. doi: 10.1523/JNEUROSCI.0602-17.2017

Sturm, J., Nguyen, T., & Kandler, K. (2014). Development of intrinsic connectivity in the central nucleus of the mouse inferior colliculus. *Journal of Neuroscience*, *34*(45), 15032–15046.

Suga, N. (2012). Tuning shifts of the auditory system by corticocortical and corticofugal projections and conditioning. *Neuroscience & Biobehavioral Reviews*, *36*(2), 969–988. doi: 10.1016/j.neubiorev.2011.11.006

Syka, J., Radionova, E. A., & Popelar, J. (1981). Discharge characteristics of neuronal pairs in the rabbit inferior colliculus. *Experimental Brain Research*, *44*(1), 11–18.

Tan, M. L., & Borst, J. G. (2007). Comparison of responses of neurons in the mouse inferior colliculus to current injections, tones of different durations, and sinusoidal amplitude-modulated tones. *Journal of Neurophysiology*, *98*(1), 454–466. doi: 10.1152/jn.00174.2007

Tan, M. L., Theeuwes, H. P., Feenstra, L., & Borst, J. G. (2007). Membrane properties and firing patterns of inferior colliculus neurons: an in vivo patch-clamp study in rodents. *Journal of Neurophysiology*, *98*(1), 443–453. doi: 10.1152/jn.01273.2006

Tanaka, I., & Ezure, K. (2004). Overall distribution of GLYT2 mRNA-containing versus GAD67 mRNA-containing neurons and colocalization of both mRNAs in midbrain, pons, and cerebellum in rats. *Neuroscience Research*, *49*(2), 165–178.

Tongjaroenbuangam, W., Jongkamonwiwat, N., Phansuwan-Pujito, P., Casalotti, S. O., Forge, A., Dodson, H., & Govitrapong, P. (2006). Relationship of opioid receptors with GABAergic neurons in the rat inferior colliculus. *European Journal of Neuroscience*, *24*(7), 1987–1994.

Ulanovsky, N., Las, L., & Nelken, I. (2003). Processing of low-probability sounds by cortical neurons. *Nature Neuroscience*, *6*(4), 391–398. doi: 10.1038/nn1032

Valdes-Baizabal, C., Parras, G. G., Ayala, Y. A., & Malmierca, M. S. (2017). Endocannabinoid modulation of stimulus-specific adaptation in inferior colliculus neurons of the rat. *Scientific Reports*, *7*. doi: Artn 6997 10.1038/S41598-017-07460-W

Vale, C., Juiz, J. M., Moore, D. R., & Sanes, D. H. (2004). Unilateral cochlear ablation produces greater loss of inhibition in the contralateral inferior colliculus. *European Journal of Neuroscience*, *20*(8), 2133–2140. doi: 10.1111/j.1460-9568.2004.03679.x

Vale, C., & Sanes, D. H. (2000). Afferent regulation of inhibitory synaptic transmission in the developing auditory midbrain. *Journal of Neuroscience*, *20*(5), 1912–1921.

Vale, C., & Sanes, D. H. (2002). The effect of bilateral deafness on excitatory and inhibitory synaptic strength in the inferior colliculus. *European Journal of Neuroscience*, *16*(12), 2394–2404.

Wallace, M. N., Shackleton, T. M., & Palmer, A. R. (2012). Morphological and physiological characteristics of laminar cells in the central nucleus of the inferior colliculus. *Frontiers in Neural Circuits*, *6*, 55. doi: 10.3389/fncir.2012.00055

Wenstrup, J. J., Nataraj, K., & Sanchez, J. T. (2012). Mechanisms of spectral and temporal integration in the mustached bat inferior colliculus. *Frontiers in Neural Circuits*, *6*, 75. doi: 10.3389/fncir.2012.00075

Williams, A. J., & Fuzessery, Z. M. (2011). Differential roles of GABAergic and glycinergic input on FM selectivity in the inferior colliculus of the pallid bat. *Journal of Neurophysiology*, *106*(5), 2523–2535. doi: 10.1152/jn.00569.2011

Williams, A. J., & Fuzessery, Z. M. (2012). Multiple mechanisms shape FM sweep rate selectivity: Complementary or redundant? *Frontiers in Neural Circuits*, *6*, 54. doi: 10.3389/fncir.2012.00054

Winer, J. A. (2005). Three systems of descending projections to the inferior colliculus. In J. A. Winer & C. E. Schreiner (Eds.), *The inferior colliculus* (pp. 231–247). New York, NY: Springer.

Winer, J. A., Chernock, M. L., Larue, D. T., & Cheung, S. W. (2002). Descending projections to the inferior colliculus from the posterior thalamus and the auditory cortex in rat, cat, and monkey. *Hearing Research*, *168*(1–2), 181–195.

Wu, S. H., Ma, C. L., Sivaramakrishnan, S., & Oliver, D. L. (2002). Synaptic modification in neurons of the central nucleus of the inferior colliculus. *Hearing Research*, *168*(1–2), 43–54.

Wynne, B., Harvey, A. R., Robertson, D., & Sirinathsinghji, D. J. (1995). Neurotransmitter and neuromodulator systems of the rat inferior colliculus and auditory brainstem studied by in situ hybridization. *Journal of Chemical Neuroanatomy*, *9*(4), 289–300.

Wynne, B., & Robertson, D. (1997). Somatostatin and substance P-like immunoreactivity in the auditory brainstem of the adult rat. *Journal of Chemical Neuroanatomy*, *12*(4), 259–266.

Xiao, Z., & Suga, N. (2005). Asymmetry in corticofugal modulation of frequency-tuning in mustached bat auditory system. *Proceedings of the National Academy of Sciences of the United States of America*, *102*(52), 19162–19167. doi: 10.1073/pnas.0509761102

Xie, R., Gittelman, J. X., & Pollak, G. D. (2007). Rethinking tuning: In vivo whole-cell recordings of the inferior colliculus in awake bats. *Journal of Neuroscience*, *27*(35), 9469–9481. doi: 10.1523/JNEUROSCI.2865-07.2007

Xiong, X. R., Liang, F., Li, H., Mesik, L., Zhang, K. K., Polley, D. B., . . . Zhang, L. I. (2013). Interaural level difference-dependent gain control and synaptic scaling underlying binaural computation. *Neuron*, *79*(4), 738–753. doi: 10.1016/j.neuron.2013.06.012

Yu, X., Sanes, D. H., Aristizabal, O., Wadghiri, Y. Z., & Turnbull, D. H. (2007). Large-scale reorganization of the tonotopic map in mouse auditory midbrain revealed by MRI. *Proceedings of the National Academy of Sciences of the United States of America*, *104*(29), 12193–12198. doi: 10.1073/pnas.0700960104

Zhang, Y., & Suga, N. (1997). Corticofugal amplification of subcortical responses to single tone stimuli in the mustached bat. *Journal of Neurophysiology*, *78*(6), 3489–3492. doi: 10.1152/jn.1997.78.6.3489

Zhang, Y., & Wu, S. H. (2000). Long-term potentiation in the inferior colliculus studied in rat brain slice. *Hearing Research*, *147*(1–2), 92–103.

CHAPTER 19

CHANGES IN THE INFERIOR COLLICULUS ASSOCIATED WITH HEARING LOSS

Noise-Induced Hearing Loss, Age-Related Hearing Loss, Tinnitus and Hyperacusis

ALAN R. PALMER AND JOEL I. BERGER

Abstract

The inferior colliculus is an important auditory relay center that undergoes fundamental changes following hearing loss, whether noise induced (NIHL) or age related (ARHL). These changes may contribute to the induction or maintenance of phenomena such as tinnitus (phantom auditory sensations) and hyperacusis (increased sensitivity to sound). Here, we outline changes that can occur in the inferior colliculus following damage to the periphery and/or as a result of the ageing process, both immediate and long-term, and attempt to disentangle which changes relate to either tinnitus or hyperacusis, as opposed to solely hearing loss. Understanding these changes is ultimately important to reversing the underlying pathology and treating these conditions.

Keywords: inferior colliculus, noise-induced hearing loss, age-related hearing loss, presbycusis, tinnitus, hyperacusis

Introduction

Trauma to the ear, either by ototoxic drugs or acoustic over-exposure (AOE) or simply as a result of ageing, can result in hearing loss. Age-related hearing loss (ARHL) or presbycusis is the major cause of hearing problems in elderly people. It is usually, but not always, associated with a progressive elevation in hearing thresholds and its prevalence increases with age so that it affects almost two-thirds of adults in their mid-70s (Gopinath et al., 2009). With or without elevation of thresholds, with ageing there can be a deterioration in speech intelligibility, temporal processing, and sound localization (Lee, 2013; Strouse, Ashmead, Ohde, & Grantham, 1998). Many factors may trigger or exacerbate ARHL, including lifetime exposure to environmental noise; exposure to ototoxic agents; or dietary, metabolic, hormonal or vascular changes (Masoro, 1991). There is, however, a considerable genetic component at least of ARHL of cochlear origin, with many genes that either contribute to noise-induced hearing loss (NIHL), promote ARHL, or promote both NIHL and ARHL (e.g., Ohlemiller, 2006). In humans, Schuknecht defined three forms of presbycusis (based on the analysis of human temporal bones) that affect different elements of the transduction process: sensory, neural, and metabolic (Schuknecht, 1955, 1964). A variety of aetiologies of ARHL has been described for different rodent models in the auditory periphery (Fetoni, Picciotti, Paludetti, & Troiani, 2011). In addition, ageing results in other widespread changes in morphology and neurochemistry of the whole brain (e.g., Banay-Schwartz, Lajtha, & Palkovits, 1989; McGeer & McGeer, 1975), and age-related changes have been documented at all stations of auditory processing within the central nervous system from cochlear nucleus to auditory cortex (Caspary, Ling, Turner, & Hughes, 2008).

Hearing loss (as a result of ageing or AOE) is considered the most common trigger for chronic tinnitus, a phantom auditory sensation in the absence of an external stimulus (Eggermont & Roberts, 2004). Tinnitus is extremely widespread, affecting 8–15% of the adult population (Shargorodsky, Curhan, & Farwell, 2010). Historically, the causes of tinnitus were assumed to be within the inner ear, although studies demonstrating its persistence following severance of the auditory nerve or ablation of the cochlea indicated that central auditory system changes must contribute to the phantom percept (House & Brackmann, 1981; Zacharek, Kaltenbach, Mathog, & Zhang, 2002). As an important center for binaural integration from the two ears, as well as a near-obligatory relay for ascending auditory information, the inferior colliculus (IC) has been proposed as a key structure in the generation and maintenance of subjective tinnitus (Robertson, Bester, Vogler, & Mulders, 2012).

Concurrently with the presence of tinnitus, hyperacusis—an oversensitivity to loud sounds—can also occur following cochlear trauma, and tinnitus is comorbid in up to 86% of patients with hyperacusis (Anari, Axelsson, Eliasson, & Magnusson, 1999), findings that suggest common underlying aetiologies. Here, we discuss immediate and early changes in the IC following different types of cochlear trauma and examine pathophysiology in the IC that could underlie hyperacusis. We then examine long-term changes and consider evidence linking these to tinnitus, attempting to identify alterations solely related to hearing loss wherever possible. We also assess how the IC changes as a result of age-related hearing loss (presbycusis). Finally, we discuss how pathological IC activity may be modulated by various interventions.

Noise-Induced Hearing Loss and Its Sequelae

Immediate and Short-Term Changes Following Cochlear Trauma

Here we describe immediate and short-term changes (defined as ≤ 30 days after the insult) that occur in the IC following damage to the cochlea. Spontaneous firing rates (neural activity during silence) appear either unchanged immediately after an acoustic trauma (Dong, Mulders, Rodger, Woo, & Robertson, 2010; Groschel, Ryll, Gotze, Ernst, & Basta, 2014; Wang, Salvi, & Powers, 1996) or even decreased (Niu, Kumaraguru, Wang, & Sun, 2013), but significant increases are usually evident within 12 hours (Mulders & Robertson, 2013). This increase in spontaneous firing is persistent and evident between 1 to 4 weeks later (Hesse et al., 2016; Manzoor, Gao, Licari, & Kaltenbach, 2013; Mulders & Robertson, 2013; Vogler, Robertson, & Mulders, 2014; Wang et al., 2013). Initially, increased spontaneous activity appears to occur over a broad range of frequencies and later narrows to frequencies corresponding to the region of hearing loss (Manzoor et al., 2013; Mulders & Robertson, 2013; Vogler et al., 2014). Such increased spontaneous activity may be caused by a shift in the balance of excitatory and inhibitory inputs to GABAergic and glutamatergic IC neurons observed after noise exposure (Sturm, Zhang-Hooks, Roos, Nguyen, & Kandler, 2017). Similar changes in spontaneous activity are found in recordings from mouse brain slices, but over different time courses—either no change or a reduction in IC spontaneous firing after 1 week, with hyperactivity only apparent 2 weeks after noise exposure (Basta & Ernst, 2005; Groschel et al., 2014). However, it is possible that these differences are a result of the type of recording (*in vivo* vs. *in vitro*), as *in vivo* neural responses may be affected by input from other auditory regions. Certainly, there is evidence that ablation or lesioning of the cochlea or dorsal cochlear nucleus (DCN) can reduce or prevent IC hyperactivity in the early stages of changes following noise exposure (Brozoski, Wisner, Sybert, & Bauer, 2012; Manzoor et al., 2012; Mulders & Robertson, 2009), thereby suggesting a dependence on ascending input.

A number of studies have examined evoked activity following an acoustic insult. Recently, Sheppard et al. (2017) demonstrated that long-term exposure to low-level noise produced enhanced evoked responses immediately after the exposure, despite a reduction in suprathreshold compound action potential (CAP) amplitudes. One week later, IC local field potential amplitudes were enhanced at frequencies corresponding to the noise exposure but suppressed at frequencies above, while CAP amplitudes were also enhanced at this time point. Wang et al. (2002) also demonstrated enhancements in IC responses within 24 hours after noise exposure, at frequencies below the hearing loss, possibly reflecting a decrease in inhibition at these frequencies (as observed in Heeringa

& van Dijk, 2016). However, changes in IC-evoked firing rates following noise trauma, as with other changes, may depend on the specific subregion recorded from the central nucleus (CNIC), external nucleus (ICx), or dorsal cortex (ICD). Szczepaniak and Moller (1996b) demonstrated that during exposure to loud tones, generally considered non-traumatic (either 95 dB or 104 dB SPL), click-evoked responses recorded from neurons in the ICx in rats were reduced compared to pre-exposure. However, 15 minutes after exposure, the same responses were significantly larger than baseline recordings, possibly reflecting some degree of hypersensitivity. All such changes could indicate evidence of a neural basis for hyperacusis.

Contrary to these studies, both Popelar et al. (1987) and Sun et al. (2012) demonstrated decreases in IC sound-evoked activity 1 hour following acoustic trauma. Recordings were made from the CNIC in Popelar et al. (1987), while the precise recording location was not specified in Sun et al. (2012), although it is possible that these responses could be restricted to the CNIC. Therefore, extra-lemniscal IC regions, such as the ICx, are likely to exhibit responses different to those from the CNIC following noise exposure. This is perhaps unsurprising, as there are fundamental differences in input between the subregions: the CNIC receives much of its afferent input from the cochlear nucleus, superior olivary complex, and lateral lemniscus, while ICx has many multisensory connections and ICD primarily receives descending input (see Huffman & Henson, 1990).

Corresponding to and probably underlying such functional alterations, there are clear changes in neurotransmission in the short term following cochlear trauma. Extensive evidence indicates that GABAergic inhibition is altered rapidly following noise exposure, which could underlie changes in spontaneous firing rates, although the time courses over which these changes take place vary between studies. Levels of the glutamic acid decarboxylase (GAD) isoform GAD_{67}, the primary enzyme in producing gamma-aminobutyric acid (GABA), were elevated immediately after noise exposure (Abbott, Hughes, Bauer, Salvi, & Caspary, 1999). Two to 30 days later, levels of GAD_{67} and another isoform, GAD_{65}, were decreased compared to controls. Similarly, Argence et al. (2006) demonstrated that unilateral cochleotomy resulted in a decrease of GAD_{67} and glycine receptor α1 subunits in contralateral CNIC, starting one day after the procedure and continuing until 8 days later, at which point both measures remained low. Furthermore, Dong et al. (2010) observed that two weeks after noise exposure $GABA_A$α1 subunit expression, which is related to fast inhibitory neurotransmission, decreased in areas of the IC corresponding to frequencies close to the exposure frequency. Complete destruction of the organ of Corti also downregulated GAD_{67} and GABAtp (another gene associated with inhibitory transmission), although downregulation was also apparent for VGLUT2, which is associated with excitatory neurotransmission (Fyk-Kolodziej et al., 2015). However, there are likely to be significant differences between changes induced by widespread mechanical trauma compared with noise exposure (which is more focused).

All of these studies indicate a net decrease in inhibition following trauma to the periphery. Although Suneja et al. (1998) actually found an increase in GABA release following both cochlear ablation and ossicle removal, this was combined with a decrease in GABA uptake, again suggesting that inhibition was pathologically altered. By contrast, Tan et al. (2007) found an increase in GABA-positive neurons, in conjunction with an elevation in brain-derived neurotrophic factor (BDNF) 6 days after noise exposure, which may be an indication of synaptic plasticity induced by the trauma. Shorter-term increases in BDNF activation were also evident 30 minutes following noise exposure (Meltser & Canlon, 2010), which coincides with an increase in c-fos expression (Saint Marie, Luo, & Ryan, 1999), although here increases in BDNF were no longer significant 24 hours later. Milbrandt et al. (2000) also demonstrated that GAD_{65} in IC was decreased following noise exposure, both immediately after and 48 hours later, but this completely recovered 30 days post-exposure. However, [3H]muscimol binding was increased at this time point, which is indicative of an increase in $GABA_A$ binding sites. Interestingly, Holt et al. (2010) demonstrated that the ICD was the only auditory area with an increase in manganese uptake two days after noise exposure, which is suggestive of increased glutamatergic activity (Takeda, 2003). Therefore, although there is a general consensus that IC neurotransmission is altered following cochlear trauma, there is clearly complexity in how these changes take place.

Long-Term Changes Following Cochlear Trauma

Spontaneous firing rates in the IC remain increased in the long term (> 30 days) following trauma to the cochlea (Berger, Coomber, Wells, Wallace, & Palmer, 2014; Coomber et al., 2014; Longenecker & Galazyuk, 2016; Mulders & Robertson, 2011; Ropp, Tiedemann, Young, & May, 2014; Vogler, Robertson, & Mulders, 2016). Given that evidence of chronic tinnitus-like behavior can take up to 5–8 weeks to emerge (e.g., Turner, Larsen, Hughes, Moechars, & Shore, 2012), this is a time at which it becomes important to differentiate between changes underlying tinnitus compared to those that are simply a result of the noise exposure. Although increases in spontaneous firing rate have classically been considered an underlying contributor to the perception of tinnitus, recent studies, demonstrating no differences between animals with behavioral evidence of tinnitus and those without, raise the possibility that these increases may simply be a product of the hearing loss but not necessarily associated with tinnitus (Coomber et al., 2014; Longenecker & Galazyuk, 2016; Ropp et al., 2014). Furthermore, one recent study demonstrated that repetitive transcranial magnetic stimulation in guinea pigs successfully eliminated behavioral evidence of tinnitus, although IC hyperactivity (increased spontaneous activity) remained unchanged (Mulders, Vooys, Makowiecki, Tang, & Rodger, 2016).

It appears that there is a time-dependent change in the way that increased spontaneous activity is maintained within the IC following noise exposure. Cochlear ablation within 6 weeks can reverse noise-induced hyperactivity (Mulders & Robertson, 2009) but is ineffective beyond this time (Mulders & Robertson, 2011). Furthermore, DCN ablation in the first few weeks following an acoustic insult significantly reduced noise-induced IC hyperactivity (Manzoor et al., 2012). This is supported by evidence indicating that bilateral DCN lesions prior to noise exposure prevented tinnitus-like behavior from emerging (Brozoski et al., 2012), although DCN ablation 3–5 months after acoustic trauma did not reverse preexisting tinnitus-like behavior (Brozoski & Bauer, 2005). However, it is possible that there may still be some dependence on peripheral input at this later stage, as Ropp et al. (2014) demonstrated that IC neurons receiving VCN input were hyperactive 1–4 months following noise exposure, whereas those receiving DCN input were not. Further research is required to determine whether the VCN modulates noise-induced changes in IC activity in the long term. In summary, the evidence just described suggests that IC hyperactivity is generally dependent on ascending input in the short term following noise exposure, but it may later become intrinsic.

There are distinct changes in the firing patterns of IC neurons following long-term recovery from noise exposure. Several weeks after noise exposure, patterns of burst firing emerge, which are associated with increased neural synchrony (Bauer, Turner, Caspary, Myers, & Brozoski, 2008; Coomber et al., 2014). These bursting patterns occur at the same time as a shift in the balance of response profiles, whereby the proportion of IC onset-type responses increases, along with a decrease in sustained responses (Berger et al., 2014), although these were evident regardless of the the presence of behavioral evidence of tinnitus. Furthermore, noise exposure in juvenile rats can impair sound processing (frequency selectivity) in adulthood: the dynamic range of IC neurons is reduced, inhibitory sidebands are reduced, and excitatory areas are expanded (Bures, Grecova, Popelar, & Syka, 2010; Grecova, Bures, Popelar, Suta, & Syka, 2009).

There is limited evidence for some form of tonotopic reorganization of the IC 1–10 months following noise exposure (Izquierdo, Gutierrez-Conde, Merchan, & Malmierca, 2008), although this reorganization does not occur in the same manner or to the same extent as in the auditory cortex and may simply be a passive process. There is also evidence of changes in IC neurotransmitters which persist following long-term recovery. Three to sixteen weeks following noise trauma, decreases in the density of serotonergic fibers in the CNIC are evident, an effect that is exacerbated in aging mice (Papesh & Hurley, 2012). Given that the neuromodulatory serotonergic system appears to be involved in regulating plasticity, this could reflect plastic changes, underlying alterations in neuronal firing rates, caused by the noise exposure.

Browne et al. (2012) demonstrated that although GAD_{67} levels were decreased in contralateral IC 4 days after noise exposure, these were at near-normal levels 32 days after. Expression of *N*-methyl-D-aspartate receptor subunit 2A in the IC, related to excitatory neurotransmission, was decreased at this later time point. Although this seems surprising, given the wealth of evidence showing that firing rates are increased, the authors suggested that reduced excitatory transmission might be to compensate for the hyperactivity. Five months after noise exposure, glutamate and aspartate (related to glutamate synthesis) levels were increased. At that time there was also an unexpected increase in GABA and decreased taurine production, possibly linked to GABA or glycine function (Godfrey et al., 2012). Therefore, while levels of GABA were increased, it is possible that inhibitory function in the IC may have decreased.

Age-Related Changes in the Inferior Colliculus

The standard paradigm for investigating ARHL has been to compare young and old individuals of the same strain. This has been facilitated by using rodent models with shorter lifespans and further by using strains that have accelerated ARHL (see Hazzard & Soban, 1988 for early examples). Most of these models exhibit a progressive hearing loss and this is particularly pronounced in the C57BL/6 strain investigated at the inferior colliculus level by Willott (1986). In this strain, the progressive hearing loss of cochlear origin starts at high-frequency and leads to broader frequency tuning and an enhancement of mid-frequency hearing in the IC, before almost total hearing loss at only 14 months of age. The hearing loss is of cochlear origin in these mice, but there are significant changes in the inferior colliculus of C57BL/6 mice that accompany the hearing loss, which include decrease in the size of principal neurons, reduced numbers of synapses on principal neurons, and a reduction in the area of the soma covered by synapses (Kazee et al., 1995). This very rapid and profound progression of hearing loss is a little extreme compared to other strains (Willott, 1986), and in subsequent work investigators have tended to use other models such as CBA mice or Fischer 344 rats, which do eventually show high-frequency hearing loss but not as early or as profoundly, more in keeping with most human presbycusis. Indeed, the changes in principal cells and synapses, found with ageing in C57BL/6 mice, appear not to occur in CBA mice (Kazee & West, 1999). This suggests that synaptic changes may be a result of the reduced afferent inflow rather than ageing per se. In rats, at least, it is unlikely that presbycusis is mainly associated with changes in the total number of neurons in the IC (Burianova, Ouda, & Syka, 2015).

Despite progressive hearing loss (reaching profound levels) with ageing, the projections from the ventral cochlear nucleus and superior olive to the IC remain stable (Byrd, Frisina, Lynch-Armour, & Walton, 1995; Willott, Pankow, Hunter, & Kordyban, 1985), although one report suggests that inputs from all divisions of the cochlear nucleus to the inferior colliculus decline with age (Lynch-Armour, Frisina, McReynolds, Byrd, & Walton, 1995). Clearly, any ARHL effects that are described at the level of the inferior colliculus can have several elements, some of which may be inherited from lower levels or result from descending influences from higher levels.

Changes to Neurotransmitter Systems with Ageing

As we described earlier, reduced afferent inflow to the inferior colliculus as a result of a variety of causes, including noise overexposure, manifests as significant changes, particularly in the inhibitory (GABAergic) neurotransmission systems. It is not yet known whether changes in the IC with ageing are occurring at this level for the first time or whether they are a consequence of the gradual loss of afferent input as result of age-related changes in the cochlea. However, there are age-related changes in the neurotransmitter systems that occur at the level of the inferior colliculus that may not necessarily reflect peripheral hearing loss, nor appear to simply mirror changes taking place in the rest of the brain. Some morphological changes occur with ageing such as a reorganization of the synaptic endings on the soma and dendrites (Helfert, Sommer, Meeks, Hofstetter, & Hughes, 1999). The exact functional significance of such alterations is unknown, but more obviously functional are a range of different indicators of GABAergic synaptic transmission that have all been shown to change with age. Presynaptically these include a reduction in the number of GABA immunostained neurons (Caspary et al., 1990); reductions in the levels of GABA (Banay-Schwartz et al., 1989; Caspary, Raza, Lawhorn Armour, Pippin, & Arneric, 1990) and in GABA receptor subunits (Gutierrez, Khan, Morris, & De Blas, 1994); reduction in GAD activity (Burianova, Ouda, Profant, & Syka, 2009; Gutierrez et al., 1994); and reduced $GABA_A$ and $GABA_B$ receptor binding (Milbrandt, Albin, & Caspary, 1994; Milbrandt, Albin, Turgeon & Caspary 1996).

There are also (possibly as a consequence of the presynaptic changes already described) age-related alterations in the postsynaptic GABA receptor. The GABA receptor consists of pentameric subunit complexes, and with ageing there is a significant downregulation of the α1 subunit and an upregulation of the α3 and γ1 subunits (Caspary et al., 1999; Gutierrez et al., 1994; Milbrandt, Hunter, & Caspary, 1997). Co-expression of various subunits with the γ1 produces an increase in the GABA affinity (Caspary et al., 1999; Milbrandt et al., 1997), which is confirmed by oocyte expression studies and microsac/synapsosome preparations (Caspary et al., 1999; Ducic, Caruncho, Zhu, Vicini, & Costa, 1995). Aquaporin expression changes transiently with ageing in the IC, which may also have an effect on neurotransmitter cycling (Christensen, D'Souza, Zhu, & Frisina, 2009). A combination of all of these factors suggests an age-related reduction in inhibitory function in the inferior colliculus (Caspary, Milbrandt, & Helfert, 1995).

Excitatory neurotransmission in the IC is also altered in ageing. Subunits of the *N*-methyl-D-aspartate receptor are downregulated and nitric oxide signaling is reduced (Jung, Na, & Huh, 2012; Osumi et al., 2012; Sanchez-Zuriaga, Marti-Gutierrez, De La Cruz, & Peris-Sanchis, 2007). Glutamate related genes are also altered in expression with ageing and hearing loss, leading on the one hand to increased glutamate availability (and possibly toxicity) and, on the other, to an upregulation of a high affinity glutamate transporter that may be compensatory (Tadros et al., 2007).

While the relationship of various calcium-binding proteins to neurotransmission is not fully understood, these proteins are still useful markers of distinct neuronal types and have been shown to change in the ageing IC. Calbindin is present only in the nucleus of the commissure of the inferior colliculus but declines by up to 25% in ageing mice, whereas Calretinin is absent in the central nucleus of the IC but high in the pericentral regions (dorsal cortex and external nucleus), where there was a 40–60% increase in immunoreactivity for calretinin with ageing in CBA mice but not C57 mice (Zettel, Frisina, Haider, & O'Neill, 1997). Parvalbumin (co-expressed in GABAergic neurons) immunoreactivity changes in ageing, but in a strain-dependent manner such that an increase was found in Long Evans rat IC but a decrease in Fischer 344 rat cortex (Ouda, Druga, & Syka, 2008). Parvalbumin is also upregulated in the IC of ageing macaques (Engle, Gray, Turner, Udell, & Recanzone, 2014).

Age-Related Changes in Inferior Colliculus Physiological Responses

Mentioned earlier (Willott, 1986), are changes in responses in the IC in C57BL/6 mice that are consequent on threshold elevations due to peripheral pathology (Fetoni et al., 2011). These changes in frequency responsiveness and tuning affect the tonotopic arrangement in the IC, as also documented using 2-deoxyglucose labelling in rats (Keithley, Lo, & Ryan, 1994). In C57BL/6 mice there was an increase with age in the numbers of spontaneously active neurons, an increase in poorly responsive neurons and pronounced changes in frequency tuning (Willott, Parham, & Hunter, 1988). However, the effect of ageing is, perhaps not surprisingly, species and strain specific (given the different pathologies). In ageing CBA mice, major threshold elevation and changes in tonotopic organization do not occur, with mostly normal activity retained (Walton, Frisina, & O'Neill, 1994; Willott, 1986), although changes in spontaneous rates and the proportion of poorly responsive neurons have been reported (Willott et al., 1988). However, a detailed study of ageing CBA frequency response areas (FRAs; Leong, Barsz, Allen, & Walton, 2011) indicated broader and more symmetric FRAs in middle-aged and old mice, with fewer closed response areas and consequently an increase in monotonic rate level functions. Many of the usual response characteristics can be unchanged in ageing animals: for example in the inferior colliculus of Fischer 344 rats, with only modest threshold elevations of about 30 dB, spontaneous rate, first-spike latency, dynamic range, the proportion of non-monotonic rate level functions, and sensitivity to tone presentation rate show no differences with ageing (Palombi & Caspary, 1996). There were, however, somewhat more subtle changes with ageing in these rats: more units were unresponsive, the maximum discharge rate was lower (by 12%), 12% more units were onset responders, and the iso-intensity functions were 18% wider. Overall, however, neurons in these rats responded to most simple auditory stimuli like those in young animals.

Across a range of studies in different animal models, a consistent finding is that temporal coding measured by a variety of metrics is worse in the ageing inferior colliculus. Fine temporal coding is important for speech recognition and localization, both of which are poorer in elderly individuals (e.g., Gordon-Salant & Fitzgibbons, 1993; Strouse et al., 1998). In particular, the ability to identify gaps in sound is important and this has been the focus of several studies of neural responses in ageing mice. Interestingly, there are neurons in aged CBA mice that have minimal gap detection thresholds of only 1–2 ms, which matches the behaviorally measured ability (Walton, Frisina, Ison, & O'Neill, 1997, Walton, Frisina & Meierhans, 1995). The main difference is, however, that such neurons (which have onset or phasic responses to tone bursts) are much less common in the aged animals (Walton, Frisina, & O'Neill, 1998). In addition, the recovery of the response after the silent gap was generally slower and less complete in neurons from aged animals. A similar increased recovery time has been found using gross potentials such as the auditory brainstem response (Allen, Burkard, Ison, & Walton, 2003) and paired tones (Finlayson, 2002).

Equally important for the discrimination of species-specific vocalizations are fluctuations in amplitude and frequency. Sensitivity to such fluctuations has been studied with sinusoidal amplitude modulated signals and with frequency sweeps. Somewhat surprisingly, although there is a deterioration in sensitivity to the speed of frequency- modulated sweeps in the auditory cortex, this is not evident at the level of the inferior colliculus (Lee, Wallani, & Mendelson, 2002; Mendelson & Lui, 2004). Sensitivity to amplitude modulation in IC is, however, affected by the ageing process. Responses to amplitude modulation are usually quantified using modulation transfer functions (MTFs). These plot either the discharge rate (the rate MTF or rMTF) or the activity locked to the modulation envelope (the temporal MTF or tMTF) as a function of the modulation rate. In young Fischer 344 rats the tMTFs were more commonly band-pass in shape, whereas in older rats the tMTFs were more commonly low-pass in shape, while the proportions of rMTF shapes were similar across the ages, as was the response gain and median maximum discharge rate (Shaddock Palombi, Backoff, & Caspary, 2001).

In aged CBA mice, by using noise carriers the overall response rate to amplitude modulated stimuli was increased by a factor about two and the median upper cut-off frequency of the rMTFs was reduced to about half that in young mice (Walton, Simon, & Frisina, 2002).

In the ageing gerbil there is a decrease in the selectivity to temporally variable pulse trains leading to an increase in signal correlations such that the population response as a whole becomes more homogeneous and less efficient in coding complex sounds (Khouri, Lesica, & Grothe, 2011). A similar result has recently been shown in the auditory cortex of ageing Macaques (Chi-Wing & Recanzone, 2017).

Finally, middle-aged mice C57BL/6J are less able to benefit from spatial separation of signal and masker (McFadden & Willott, 1994) presumably again as a result of the loss of fine temporal coding.

Modulation of Pathological IC Activity

Despite the fact that there is no uniformly effective treatment for either tinnitus or hyperacusis, a number of studies have demonstrated modulation of noise-induced pathological activity related to these conditions in the IC. On the basis that inhibition is suppressed following cochlear trauma, Szczepaniak and Moller (1996a) successfully attenuated noise-induced sound-evoked hyperactivity by systemically administering a $GABA_B$ agonist, L-baclofen, to rats. Although L-baclofen, administered at a high dose, also diminished behavioral evidence of tinnitus in rats (Zheng, Vagal, McNamara, Darlington, & Smith, 2012), its efficacy as a treatment in humans is highly variable (Smith, Zheng, & Darlington, 2012), and in some cases it may actually induce tinnitus (Auffret et al., 2014). In a similar scenario, noise-induced hyperactivity in the IC and behavioral evidence of tinnitus have both been suppressed in guinea pigs by acute and chronic administration of the diuretic furosemide (Mulders, Barry, & Robertson, 2014; Mulders, McMahen, & Robertson, 2014). However, once again, although in some patients intravenous administration of furosemide reduced their symptoms of tinnitus (Risey, Guth, & Amedee, 1995), in high doses it may actually cause tinnitus (see Salvi, Lobarinas, & Sun, 2009 for a review).

A phenomenon known as residual inhibition, whereby tinnitus can be temporarily suppressed or eliminated following presentation of a particular auditory stimulus, is evident to some degree in approximately 70% of patients (Roberts, Moffat, & Bosnyak, 2006). Voytenko and Galazyuk (2011) proposed a possible underlying mechanism for residual inhibition, demonstrating that the spontaneous firing of single IC neurons may be suppressed following the presentation of a short stimulus, an effect that was mediated by metabotropic glutamate receptors. Furthermore, Galazyuk et al. (2017) recently demonstrated that this effect is present in approximately 40% of spontaneously active IC neurons, and is similarly evident in animals with behavioral evidence of noise-induced tinnitus, wherein IC neurons were hyperactive. While this method only provides temporary cessation of the phantom percept, it offers a promising tool for examining neuronal states with and without the presence of tinnitus, and further implies a possible role for the IC in the modulation of tinnitus.

A number of studies have examined electrical stimulation of the inferior colliculus as a potential basis for development of an auditory midbrain implant. Offutt et al. (2014) demonstrated that direct electrical stimulation of the ICD resulted in modulation of CNIC firing that persisted after stimulation had ceased, which they proposed as a possible methodology for treating tinnitus. In a follow-up to this study, Smit et al. (2016) found that stimulation of ICx in rats suppressed noise-induced deficits in behavioral gap detection, consistent with the reduction of tinnitus-like behavior. Furthermore, a recent study showed that electrical IC stimulation can result in frequency percepts that correlate with the frequency tuning of the IC (Pages et al., 2016), thus suggesting that this may also be an effective treatment for hearing loss in humans who would not be suitable candidates for cochlear implants. It has also been demonstrated that stimulation of the round window of the cochlea within two-to-three weeks after noise exposure can suppress hyperactivity in IC neurons (Mulders, Spencer, & Robertson, 2016; Norena, Mulders, & Robertson, 2015).

One consideration when examining modulation of noise-induced IC pathology is the time after noise exposure at which interventions are employed. As described earlier, there may be a particular temporal window following a traumatic event, during which time the dependence of the IC on peripheral activity allows treatments that target the cochlea, auditory nerve, or cochlear nucleus to also affect IC activity. However, if IC pathology underlies or contributes to tinnitus or hyperacusis, any treatments targeting the periphery at a later time may not be successful. Clearly, the complexity in the development of tinnitus over time, as well as the uncertainty in differentiating between noise-induced pathology and tinnitus-specific pathology, complicates this process.

Conclusions and Discussion

A finding common to NIHL and ARHL is that there are changes to the machinery of neurotransmitter release in the inferior colliculus. This has been extensively studied for the inhibitory neurotransmitter GABA, and it has been shown that several factors combine to make GABA less available in both NIHL and ARHL. It is somewhat surprising therefore that many studies of ARHL fail to reveal large changes in the physiological response profiles, although other detailed analyses do indeed reveal somewhat subtle changes. Such findings have prompted several authors to suggest that there are compensatory changes occurring in both excitatory and inhibitory neurotransmission (Caspary et al., 1999; Helfert, Sommer, Hughes, Jeffery, & Caspary, 1994; Mendelson & Lui, 2004). In the case of GABA, the presynaptic downregulation and other changes that make GABA less available are offset by a change in the subunit structure, which increases the efficacy of the GABA receptors in transporting chloride ions. In ageing there is also a downregulation in excitatory amino acids such that the balance of excitation and inhibition is less disrupted by the changes in GABA. It is unclear whether changes in neurotransmission due to NIHL and those due to ARHL are both initiated by reduction in afferent activity, since the changes in ARHL appear to occur in some instances without large threshold elevations. A consistent finding, at least in ARHL, is that the temporal coding in the IC is somewhat disrupted, which could provide some basis for the poorer discrimination and speech intelligibility shown by subjects with ARHL.

Hearing loss of cochlear origin that generates a profound high-frequency loss with a sharp frequency transition (beyond an "edge-frequency") can result in long-term plastic changes in the tonotopic mapping in the auditory cortex (Eggermont & Komiya, 2000; Robertson & Irvine, 1989). This takes the form of a spread of the sensitivity to the edge-frequency across the deafferented cortex. This active reorganization of tonotopy has not been reported in the IC, despite experiments specifically designed to reveal such changes, although some degree of passive reorganization may occur (Irvine, Rajan, & Smith, 2003; Izquierdo et al., 2008).

NIHL has been reported to result in increased spontaneous discharge rates at a variety of levels in the auditory pathway, not least in the inferior colliculus (e.g., Coomber et al., 2014; Mulders & Robertson, 2009; Ropp et al., 2014). This increase has been linked to the changes in neurotransmission suggesting increased "gain" in the processing circuitry (Schaette & McAlpine, 2011). The higher spontaneous rates have been cited as a possible correlate of tinnitus. However, several studies have now shown that such changes in spontaneous rate can be found in all animals that have been subject to damaging levels of noise whether or not there is any behavioral evidence of tinnitus (Coomber et al., 2014; Longenecker & Galazyuk, 2016; Ropp et al., 2014).

Future Directions

Although changes in the IC after NIHL and ARHL seem to correlate in some instances with conditions such as tinnitus, hyperacusis, and presbycusis, it is unclear whether this is merely a correlation or causal. Are other changes taking place (for example, at the auditory cortex) more appropriate mechanisms of tinnitus and hyperacusis and therefore more appropriate targets for intervention? What is it in the ascending input to the IC that is initiating or driving the changes in neurotransmission that eventually become more permanent and independent of peripheral input?

It is known that an enriched auditory environment can alleviate reorganization of auditory cortex caused by severe high-frequency hearing loss (Norena & Eggermont, 2005). It is also clear that enrichment following noise trauma can prevent reorganization of the IC with concomitant alleviation of behavioral indices of pathology (Sturm et al., 2017). It is yet to be determined, however, whether any practical therapy involving acoustic enrichment immediately following acoustic insults will be effective in humans.

Further research is also required to determine whether the VCN modulates noise-induced changes in IC activity in the long term.

References

Abbott, S. D., Hughes, L. F., Bauer, C. A., Salvi, R., & Caspary, D. M. (1999). Detection of glutamate decarboxylase isoforms in rat inferior colliculus following acoustic exposure. *Neuroscience*, *93*(4), 1375–1381. doi:S0306-4522(99)00300-0 [pii]

Allen, P. D., Burkard, R. F., Ison, J. R., & Walton, J. P. (2003). Impaired gap encoding in aged mouse inferior colliculus at moderate but not high stimulus levels. *Hearing Research*, *186*(1–2), 17–29. doi:S0378595503003009 [pii]

Anari, M., Axelsson, A., Eliasson, A., & Magnusson, L. (1999). Hypersensitivity to sound—questionnaire data, audiometry and classification. *Scandinavian Audiology*, *28*(4), 219–230.

Argence, M., Saez, I., Sassu, R., Vassias, I., Vidal, P. P., & de Waele, C. (2006). Modulation of inhibitory and excitatory synaptic transmission in rat inferior colliculus after unilateral cochleectomy: an in situ and immunofluorescence study. *Neuroscience*, *141*(3), 1193–1207. doi:10.1016/j.neuroscience.2006.04.058

Auffret, M., Rolland, B., Deheul, S., Loche, V., Hennaux, C., Cottencin, O., . . . Team, C. (2014). Severe tinnitus induced by off-label baclofen. *Annals of Pharmacotherapy*, *48*(5), 656–659. doi:10.1177/1060028014525594

Banay-Schwartz, M., Lajtha, A., & Palkovits, M. (1989). Changes with aging in the levels of amino acids in rat CNS structural elements. II. Taurine and small neutral amino acids. *Neurochemical Research*, *14*(6), 563–570.

Basta, D., & Ernst, A. (2005). Erratum to "Noise-induced changes of neuronal spontaneous activity in mice inferior colliculus brain slices." *Neuroscience Letters*, *374*(1), 74–79.

Bauer, C. A., Turner, J. G., Caspary, D. M., Myers, K. S., & Brozoski, T. J. (2008). Tinnitus and inferior colliculus activity in chinchillas related to three distinct patterns of cochlear trauma. *Journal of Neuroscience Research*, *86*(11), 2564–2578. doi:10.1002/jnr.21699

Berger, J. I., Coomber, B., Wells, T. T., Wallace, M. N., & Palmer, A. R. (2014). Changes in the response properties of inferior colliculus neurons relating to tinnitus. *Frontiers of Neurology*, *5*, 203. doi:10.3389/fneur.2014.00203

Browne, C. J., Morley, J. W., & Parsons, C. H. (2012). Tracking the expression of excitatory and inhibitory neurotransmission-related proteins and neuroplasticity markers after noise induced hearing loss. *PLOS One*, *7*(3). doi:10.1371/journal.pone.0033272

Brozoski, T. J., & Bauer, C. A. (2005). The effect of dorsal cochlear nucleus ablation on tinnitus in rats. *Hearing Research*, *206*(1–2), 227–236. doi:10.1016/j.heares.2004.12.013

Brozoski, T. J., Wisner, K. W., Sybert, L. T., & Bauer, C. A. (2012). Bilateral dorsal cochlear nucleus lesions prevent acoustic-trauma induced tinnitus in an animal model. *Journal of the Association for Research in Otolaryngology*, *13*(1), 55–66. doi:10.1007/s10162-011-0290-3

Bures, Z., Grecova, J., Popelar, J., & Syka, J. (2010). Noise exposure during early development impairs the processing of sound intensity in adult rats. *European Journal of Neuroscience*, *32*(1), 155–164. doi:10.1111/j.1460-9568.2010.07280.x

Burianova, J., Ouda, L., Profant, O., & Syka, J. (2009). Age-related changes in GAD levels in the central auditory system of the rat. *Experimental Gerontology*, *44*(3), 161–169. doi:10.1016/j.exger.2008.09.012

Burianova, J., Ouda, L., & Syka, J. (2015). The influence of aging on the number of neurons and levels of non-phosphorylated neurofilament proteins in the central auditory system of rats. *Frontiers in Aging Neuroscience*, *7*, 27. doi:10.3389/fnagi.2015.00027

Byrd, J., Frisina, R. D., Lynch-Armour, M. A., & Walton, J. P. (1995). Superior olivary complex inputs to the dorsomedial inferior colliculus of the CBA mouse model of presbycusis remain stable with age. *Journal of the Association for Research in Otolaryngology, Abstr. 18*, 174.

Caspary, D. M., Holder, T. M., Hughes, L. F., Milbrandt, J. C., McKernan, R. M., & Naritoku, D. K. (1999). Age-related changes in GABA(A) receptor subunit composition and function in rat auditory system. *Neuroscience*, *93*(1), 307–312. doi:S0306-4522(99)00121-9 [pii]

Caspary, D. M., Ling, L., Turner, J. G., & Hughes, L. F. (2008). Inhibitory neurotransmission, plasticity and aging in the mammalian central auditory system. *Journal of Experimental Biology*, *211*(Pt 11), 1781–1791. doi:10.1242/jeb.013581

Caspary, D. M., Milbrandt, J. C., & Helfert, R. H. (1995). Central auditory aging: GABA changes in the inferior colliculus. *Experimental Gerontology*, *30*(3–4), 349–360.

Caspary, D. M., Raza, A., Lawhorn Armour, B. A., Pippin, J., & Arneric, S. P. (1990). Immunocytochemical and neurochemical evidence for age-related loss of GABA in the inferior colliculus: Implications for neural presbycusis. *Journal of Neuroscience*, *10*(7), 2363–2372.

Chi-Wing, N., & Recanzone, G. H. (2017). Age-related changes in temporal processing of rapidly-presented sound sequences in the Macaque auditory cortex. *Cerebral Cortex*, *13*, 1–22.

Christensen, N., D'Souza, M., Zhu, X., & Frisina, R. D. (2009). Age-related hearing loss: Aquaporin 4 gene expression changes in the mouse cochlea and auditory midbrain. *Brain Research, 1253*, 27–34. doi:10.1016/j.brainres.2008.11.070

Coomber, B., Berger, J. I., Kowalkowski, V. L., Shackleton, T. M., Palmer, A. R., & Wallace, M. N. (2014). Neural changes accompanying tinnitus following unilateral acoustic trauma in the guinea pig. *European Journal of Neuroscience, 40*(2), 2427–2441. doi:10.1111/ejn.12580

Dong, S., Mulders, W. H., Rodger, J., Woo, S., & Robertson, D. (2010). Acoustic trauma evokes hyperactivity and changes in gene expression in guinea-pig auditory brainstem. *European Journal of Neuroscience, 31*(9), 1616–1628. doi:10.1111/j.1460-9568.2010.07183.x

Dong, S., Rodger, J., Mulders, W. H., & Robertson, D. (2010). Tonotopic changes in GABA receptor expression in guinea pig inferior colliculus after partial unilateral hearing loss. *Brain Research, 1342*, 24–32. doi:10.1016/j.brainres.2010.04.067

Ducic, I., Caruncho, H. J., Zhu, W. J., Vicini, S., & Costa, E. (1995). gamma-Aminobutyric acid gating of Cl- channels in recombinant GABAA receptors. *Journal of Pharmacology and Experimental Therapeutics, 272*(1), 438–445.

Eggermont, J. J., & Komiya, H. (2000). Moderate noise trauma in juvenile cats results in profound cortical topographic map changes in adulthood. *Hearing Research, 142*, 89–101.

Eggermont, J. J., & Roberts, L. E. (2004). The neuroscience of tinnitus. *Trends in Neuroscience, 27*(11), 676–682. doi:10.1016/j.tins.2004.08.010

Engle, J. R., Gray, D. T., Turner, H., Udell, J. B., & Recanzone, G. H. (2014). Age-related neurochemical changes in the rhesus macaque inferior colliculus. *Frontiers in Aging Neuroscience, 6*, 73. doi:10.3389/fnagi.2014.00073

Fetoni, A. R., Picciotti, P. M., Paludetti, G., & Troiani, D. (2011). Pathogenesis of presbycusis in animal models: A review. *Experimental Gerontology, 46*(6), 413–425. doi:10.1016/j.exger.2010.12.003

Finlayson, P. G. (2002). Paired-tone stimuli reveal reductions and alterations in temporal processing in inferior colliculus neurons of aged animals. *Journal of the Association for Research in Otolaryngology, 3*(3), 321–331. doi:10.1007/s101620020038

Fyk-Kolodziej, B. E., Shimano, T., Gafoor, D., Mirza, N., Griffith, R. D., Gong, T.-W., & Holt, A. G. (2015). Dopamine in the auditory brainstem and midbrain: Co-localization with amino acid neurotransmitters and gene expression following cochlear trauma. *Frontiers in Neuroanatomy, 9*, 88.

Galazyuk, A. V., Voytenko, S. V., & Longenecker, R. J. (2017). Long-lasting forward suppression of spontaneous firing in auditory neurons: Implication to the residual inhibition of tinnitus. *Journal of the Association for Research in Otolaryngology, 18*(2), 343–353. doi:10.1007/s10162-016-0601-9

Godfrey, D. A., Kaltenbach, J. A., Chen, K., Ilyas, O., Liu, X., Licari, F., . . . McKnight, D. (2012). Amino acid concentrations in the hamster central auditory system and long-term effects of intense tone exposure. *Journal of Neuroscience Research, 90*(11), 2214–2224. doi:10.1002/jnr.23095

Gopinath, B., Rochtchina, E., Wang, J. J., Schneider, J., Leeder, S. R., & Mitchell, P. (2009). Prevalence of age-related hearing loss in older adults: Blue Mountains Study. *Archives of Internal Medicine, 169*(4), 415–416. doi:10.1001/archinternmed.2008.597

Gordon-Salant, S., & Fitzgibbons, P. J. (1993). Temporal factors and speech recognition performance in young and elderly listeners. *Journal of Speech and Hearing Research, 36*(6), 1276–1285.

Grecova, J., Bures, Z., Popelar, J., Suta, D., & Syka, J. (2009). Brief exposure of juvenile rats to noise impairs the development of the response properties of inferior colliculus neurons. *European Journal of Neuroscience*, *29*(9), 1921–1930. doi:10.1111/j.1460-9568.2009.06739.x

Groschel, M., Ryll, J., Gotze, R., Ernst, A., & Basta, D. (2014). Acute and long-term effects of noise exposure on the neuronal spontaneous activity in cochlear nucleus and inferior colliculus brain slices. *Biomedical Research International*, *2014*, 909260. doi:10.1155/2014/909260

Gutierrez, A., Khan, Z. U., Morris, S. J., & De Blas, A. L. (1994). Age-related decrease of GABAA receptor subunits and glutamic acid decarboxylase in the rat inferior colliculus. *Journal of Neuroscience*, *14*(12), 7469–7477.

Hazzard, D. G., & Soban, J. (1988). Studies of aging using genetically defined rodents: A bibliography. *Experimental Aging Research*, *14*(2–3), 59–81. doi:10.1080/03610738808259727

Heeringa, A. N., & van Dijk, P. (2016). The immediate effects of acoustic trauma on excitation and inhibition in the inferior colliculus: A Wiener-kernel analysis. *Hearing Research*, *331*, 47–56.

Helfert, R. H., Sommer, T. J., Hughes, L. F., Jeffery, C. M., & Caspary, D. M. (1994). Age-related changes in the organization of the central nucleus of the inferior colliculus of the Fischer 344 rat. *Journal of the Association for Research in Otolaryngology*, *Abstr. 17*, 11.

Helfert, R. H., Sommer, T. J., Meeks, J., Hofstetter, P., & Hughes, L. F. (1999). Age-related synaptic changes in the central nucleus of the inferior colliculus of Fischer-344 rats. *Journal of Comparative Neurology*, *406*(3), 285–298. doi:10.1002/(SICI)1096-9861(19990412)406:3<285::AID-CNE1>3.0.CO;2-P [pii]

Hesse, L. L., Bakay, W., Ong, H.-C., Anderson, L., Ashmore, J., McAlpine, D., . . . Schaette, R. (2016). Non-monotonic relation between noise exposure severity and neuronal hyperactivity in the auditory midbrain. *Frontiers in Neurology*, *7*, 133.

Holt, A. G., Bissig, D., Mirza, N., Rajah, G., & Berkowitz, B. (2010). Evidence of key tinnitus-related brain regions documented by a unique combination of manganese-enhanced MRI and acoustic startle reflex testing. *PLOS One*, *5*(12). doi:ARTN e14260 10.1371/journal.pone.0014260

House, J. W., & Brackmann, D. E. (1981). Tinnitus: Surgical treatment. *CIBA Foundation Symposium*, *85*, 204–216.

Huffman, R. F., & Henson, O. W. (1990). The descending auditory pathway and acousticomotor systems: Connections with the inferior colliculus. *Brain Research Reviews*, *15*(3), 295–323.

Irvine, D. R. F., Rajan, R., & Smith, S. (2003). Effects of restricted cochlear lesions in adult cats on the frequency organization of the inferior colliculus *Journal of Comparative Neurology*, *467*, 354–374.

Izquierdo, M. A., Gutierrez-Conde, P. M., Merchan, M. A., & Malmierca, M. S. (2008). Non-plastic reorganization of frequency coding in the inferior colliculus of the rat following noise-induced hearing loss. *Neuroscience*, *154*(1), 355–369. doi:10.1016/j.neuroscience.2008.01.057

Jung, J., Na, C., & Huh, Y. (2012). Alterations in nitric oxide synthase in the aged CNS. *Oxidative Medicine and Cellular Longevity*, *2012*, 718976. doi:10.1155/2012/718976

Kazee, A. M., Han, L. Y., Spongr, V. P., Walton, J. P., Salvi, R. J., & Flood, D. G. (1995). Synaptic loss in the central nucleus of the inferior colliculus correlates with sensorineural hearing loss in the C57BL/6 mouse model of presbycusis. *Hearing Research*, *89*(1–2), 109–120.

Kazee, A. M., & West, N. R. (1999). Preservation of synapses on principal cells of the central nucleus of the inferior colliculus with aging in the CBA mouse. *Hearing Research*, *133*(1–2), 98–106. doi:S0378-5955(99)00058-1 [pii]

Keithley, E. M., Lo, J., & Ryan, A. F. (1994). 2-Deoxyglucose uptake patterns in response to pure tone stimuli in the aged rat inferior colliculus. *Hearing Research*, *80*(1), 79–85.

Khouri, L., Lesica, N. A., & Grothe, B. (2011). Impaired auditory temporal selectivity in the inferior colliculus of aged Mongolian gerbils. *Journal of Neuroscience*, *31*(27), 9958–9970. doi:10.1523/JNEUROSCI.4509-10.2011

Lee, H. J., Wallani, T., & Mendelson, J. R. (2002). Temporal processing speed in the inferior colliculus of young and aged rats. *Hearing Research*, *174*(1–2), 64–74. doi:S0378595502006391 [pii]

Lee, K. Y. (2013). Pathophysiology of age-related hearing loss (peripheral and central). *Korean Journal of Audiology*, *17*(2), 45–49. doi:10.7874/kja.2013.17.2.45

Leong, U. C., Barsz, K., Allen, P. D., & Walton, J. P. (2011). Neural correlates of age-related declines in frequency selectivity in the auditory midbrain. *Neurobiology of Aging*, *32*(1), 168–178. doi:10.1016/j.neurobiolaging.2009.01.006

Longenecker, R. J., & Galazyuk, A. V. (2016). Variable effects of acoustic trauma on behavioral and neural correlates of tinnitus in individual animals. *Frontiers in Behavioral Neuroscience*, *10*, 207. doi:10.3389/fnbeh.2016.00207

Lynch-Armour, M. A., Frisina, R. D., McReynolds, E. E., Byrd, J., & Walton, J. P. (1995). Cochlear nucleus inputs to a functionally-characterized region of the inferior colliculus decline with age for the CBA mouse model of presbycusis. *Journal of the Association for Research in Otolaryngology, Abstr. 18*, 71.

Manzoor, N. F., Gao, Y., Licari, F., & Kaltenbach, J. A. (2013). Comparison and contrast of noise-induced hyperactivity in the dorsal cochlear nucleus and inferior colliculus. *Hearing Research*, *295*, 114–123. doi:10.1016/j.heares.2012.04.003

Manzoor, N. F., Licari, F. G., Klapchar, M., Elkin, R. L., Gao, Y., Chen, G., & Kaltenbach, J. A. (2012). Noise-induced hyperactivity in the inferior colliculus: Its relationship with hyperactivity in the dorsal cochlear nucleus. *Journal of Neurophysiology*, *108*(4), 976–988. doi:10.1152/jn.00833.2011

Masoro, E. J. (1991). Use of rodents as models for the study of "normal aging": conceptual and practical issues. *Neurobiology of Aging*, *12*(6), 639–643.

McFadden, S. L., & Willott, J. F. (1994). Responses of inferior colliculus neurons in C57BL/6J mice with and without sensorineural hearing loss: Effects of changing the azimuthal location of a continuous noise masker on responses to contralateral tones. *Hearing Research*, *78*(2), 132–148.

McGeer, E. G., & McGeer, P. L. (1975). Age changes in the human for some enzymes associated with metabolism of catecholamines, GABA and ace- tylcholine. In J. M. Ordy. & K. R. Brizzee. (Eds.), *Neurobiology of Aging* (pp. 287–305). New York, NY: Plenum.

Meltser, I., & Canlon, B. (2010). The expression of mitogen-activated protein kinases and brain-derived neurotrophic factor in inferior colliculi after acoustic trauma. *Neurobiology of Disease*, *40*(1), 325–330. doi:10.1016/j.nbd.2010.06.006

Mendelson, J. R., & Lui, B. (2004). The effects of aging in the medial geniculate nucleus: A comparison with the inferior colliculus and auditory cortex. *Hearing Research*, *191*(1–2), 21–33. doi:10.1016/j.heares.2004.01.010

Milbrandt, J. C., Albin, R. L., & Caspary, D. M. (1994). Age-related decrease in GABAB receptor binding in the Fischer 344 rat inferior colliculus. *Neurobiology of Aging*, *15*(6), 699–703.

Milbrandt, J. C., Albin, R. L., Turgeon, S. M., & Caspary, D. M. (1996). GABAA receptor binding in the aging rat inferior colliculus. *Neuroscience*, *73*(2), 449–458. doi:0306-4522(96)00050-4 [pii]

Milbrandt, J. C., Holder, T. M., Wilson, M. C., Salvi, R. J., & Caspary, D. M. (2000). GAD levels and muscimol binding in rat inferior colliculus following acoustic trauma. *Hearing Research*, *147*(1–2), 251–260.

Milbrandt, J. C., Hunter, C., & Caspary, D. M. (1997). Alterations of GABAA receptor subunit mRNA levels in the aging Fischer 344 rat inferior colliculus. *Journal of Comparative Neurology*, *379*(3), 455–465. doi:10.1002/(SICI)1096-9861(19970317)379:3 <455::AID-CNE10>3.0.CO;2-F [pii]

Mulders, W. H., Barry, K. M., & Robertson, D. (2014). Effects of furosemide on cochlear neural activity, central hyperactivity and behavioural tinnitus after cochlear trauma in guinea pig. *PLOS One*, *9*(5), e97948. doi:10.1371/journal.pone.0097948

Mulders, W. H., McMahen, C., & Robertson, D. (2014). Effects of chronic furosemide on central neural hyperactivity and cochlear thresholds after cochlear trauma in Guinea pig. *Frontiers of Neurology*, *5*, 146. doi:10.3389/fneur.2014.00146

Mulders, W. H., & Robertson, D. (2009). Hyperactivity in the auditory midbrain after acoustic trauma: Dependence on cochlear activity. *Neuroscience*, *164*(2), 733–746. doi:10.1016/j.neuroscience.2009.08.036

Mulders, W. H., & Robertson, D. (2011). Progressive centralization of midbrain hyperactivity after acoustic trauma. *Neuroscience*, *192*, 753–760. doi:10.1016/j.neuroscience.2011.06.046

Mulders, W. H., & Robertson, D. (2013). Development of hyperactivity after acoustic trauma in the guinea pig inferior colliculus. *Hearing Research*, *298*, 104–108. doi:10.1016/j.heares.2012.12.008

Mulders, W. H., Spencer, T. C., & Robertson, D. (2016). Effects of pulsatile electrical stimulation of the round window on central hyperactivity after cochlear trauma in guinea pig. *Hearing Research*, *335*, 128–137. doi:10.1016/j.heares.2016.03.001

Mulders, W. H., Vooys, V., Makowiecki, K., Tang, A. D., & Rodger, J. (2016). The effects of repetitive transcranial magnetic stimulation in an animal model of tinnitus. *Scientific Reports*, *6*, 38234. doi:10.1038/srep38234

Niu, Y., Kumaraguru, A., Wang, R., & Sun, W. (2013). Hyperexcitability of inferior colliculus neurons caused by acute noise exposure. *Journal of Neuroscience Research*, *91*(2), 292–299.

Norena, A. J., & Eggermont, J. J. (2005). Enriched acoustic environment after noise trauma reduces hearing loss and prevents cortical map reorganization. *Journal of Neuroscience*, *25*(3), 699–705. doi:10.1523/JNEUROSCI.2226-04.2005

Norena, A. J., Mulders, W. H., & Robertson, D. (2015). Suppression of putative tinnitus-related activity by extra-cochlear electrical stimulation. *Journal of Neurophysiology*, *113*(1), 132–143. doi:10.1152/jn.00580.2014

Offutt, S. J., Ryan, K. J., Konop, A. E., & Lim, H. H. (2014). Suppression and facilitation of auditory neurons through coordinated acoustic and midbrain stimulation: Investigating a deep brain stimulator for tinnitus. *Journal of Neural Engineering*, *11*(6). doi:Artn 066001

Ohlemiller, K. K. (2006). Contributions of mouse models to understanding of age- and noise-related hearing loss. *Brain Research*, *1091*(1), 89–102. doi:10.1016/j.brainres.2006.03.017

Osumi, Y., Shibata, S. B., Kanda, S., Yagi, M., Ooka, H., Shimano, T., . . . Tomoda, K. (2012). Downregulation of N-methyl-D-aspartate receptor zeta1 subunit (GluN1) gene in inferior colliculus with aging. *Brain Research*, *1454*, 23–32. doi:10.1016/j.brainres.2012.03.018

Ouda, L., Druga, R., & Syka, J. (2008). Changes in parvalbumin immunoreactivity with aging in the central auditory system of the rat. *Experimental Gerontology*, *43*(8), 782–789. doi:10.1016/j.exger.2008.04.001

Pages, D. S., Ross, D. A., Punal, V. M., Agashe, S., Dweck, I., Mueller, J., . . . Groh, J. M. (2016). Effects of electrical stimulation in the inferior colliculus on frequency discrimination by rhesus monkeys and implications for the auditory midbrain implant. *Journal of Neuroscience, 36*(18), 5071–5083. doi:10.1523/JNEUROSCI.3540-15.2016

Palombi, P. S., & Caspary, D. M. (1996). Physiology of the aged Fischer 344 rat inferior colliculus: Responses to contralateral monaural stimuli. *Journal of Neurophysiology, 76*(5), 3114–3125.

Papesh, M. A., & Hurley, L. M. (2012). Plasticity of serotonergic innervation of the inferior colliculus in mice following acoustic trauma. *Hearing Research, 283*(1–2), 89–97. doi:10.1016/j.heares.2011.11.004

Popelar, J., Syka, J., & Berndt, H. (1987). Effect of noise on auditory evoked responses in awake guinea pigs. *Hearing Research, 26*(3), 239–247.

Risey, J. A., Guth, P. S., & Amedee, R. G. (1995). Furosemide Distinguishes Central and Peripheral Tinnitus. *The International Tinnitus Journal, 1*(2), 99–103.

Roberts, L. E., Moffat, G., & Bosnyak, D. J. (2006). Residual inhibition functions in relation to tinnitus spectra and auditory threshold shift. *Acta Oto-Laryngologica Supplementum* (556), 27–33.

Robertson, D., Bester, C., Vogler, D., & Mulders, W. H. (2012). Spontaneous hyperactivity in the auditory midbrain: Relationship to afferent input. *Hearing Research, 295*, 124–129. doi:10.1016/j.heares.2012.02.002

Robertson, D., & Irvine, D. R. F. (1989). Plasticity of frequency organization in auditory cortex of guinea pigs with partial unilateral deafness. *Journal of Comparative Neurology, 282*, 456–471.

Ropp, T. J., Tiedemann, K. L., Young, E. D., & May, B. J. (2014). Effects of unilateral acoustic trauma on tinnitus-related spontaneous activity in the inferior colliculus. *Journal of the Association for Research in Otolaryngology, 15*(6), 1007–1022. doi:10.1007/s10162-014-0488-2

Saint Marie, R. L., Luo, L., & Ryan, A. F. (1999). Effects of stimulus frequency and intensity on c-fos mRNA expression in the adult rat auditory brainstem. *Journal of Comparative Neurology, 404*(2), 258–270.

Salvi, R., Lobarinas, E., & Sun, W. (2009). Pharmacological treatments for tinnitus: New and old. *Drugs Future, 34*(5), 381–400. doi:10.1358/dof.2009.034.05.1362442

Sanchez-Zuriaga, D., Marti-Gutierrez, N., De La Cruz, M. A., & Peris-Sanchis, M. R. (2007). Age-related changes of NADPH-diaphorase-positive neurons in the rat inferior colliculus and auditory cortex. *Microscopy Research and Technique, 70*(12), 1051–1059. doi:10.1002/jemt.20512

Schaette, R., & McAlpine, D. (2011). Tinnitus with a normal audiogram: Physiological evidence for hidden hearing loss and computational model. *Journal of Neuroscience, 31*(38), 13452–13457. doi:10.1523/JNEUROSCI.2156-11.2011

Schuknecht, H. F. (1955). Presbycusis. *Laryngoscope, 65*(6), 402–419. doi:10.1288/00005537-195506000-00002

Schuknecht, H. F. (1964). Further observations on the pathology of presbycusis. *Archives of Otolaryngology, 80*, 369–382.

Shaddock Palombi, P., Backoff, P. M., & Caspary, D. M. (2001). Responses of young and aged rat inferior colliculus neurons to sinusoidally amplitude modulated stimuli. *Hearing Research, 153*(1–2), 174–180. doi:S0378595500002641 [pii]

Shargorodsky, J., Curhan, G. C., & Farwell, W. R. (2010). Prevalence and characteristics of tinnitus among US adults. *American Journal of Medicine, 123*(8), 711–718. doi:10.1016/j.amjmed.2010.02.015

Sheppard, A. M., Chen, G. D., Manohar, S., Ding, D., Hu, B. H., Sun, W., . . . Salvi, R. (2017). Prolonged low-level noise-induced plasticity in the peripheral and central auditory system of rats. *Neuroscience, 359*, 159–171. doi:10.1016/j.neuroscience.2017.07.005

Smit, J. V., Janssen, M. L., van Zwieten, G., Jahanshahi, A., Temel, Y., & Stokroos, R. J. (2016). Deep brain stimulation of the inferior colliculus in the rodent suppresses tinnitus. *Brain Research, 1650*, 118–124. doi:10.1016/j.brainres.2016.08.046

Smith, P. F., Zheng, Y., & Darlington, C. L. (2012). Revisiting baclofen for the treatment of severe chronic tinnitus. *Frontiers of Neurology, 3*, 34. doi:10.3389/fneur.2012.00034

Strouse, A., Ashmead, D. H., Ohde, R. N., & Grantham, D. W. (1998). Temporal processing in the aging auditory system. *Journal of the Acoustical Society of America, 104*(4), 2385–2399.

Sturm, J. J., Zhang-Hooks, Y. X., Roos, H., Nguyen, T., & Kandler, K. (2017). Noise trauma-induced behavioral gap detection deficits correlate with reorganization of excitatory and inhibitory local circuits in the inferior colliculus and are prevented by acoustic enrichment. *Journal of Neuroscience, 37*(26), 6314–6330. doi:10.1523/JNEUROSCI.0602-17.2017

Sun, W., Deng, A., Jayaram, A., & Gibson, B. (2012). Noise exposure enhances auditory cortex responses related to hyperacusis behavior. *Brain Research, 1485*, 108–116. doi:10.1016/j.brainres.2012.02.008

Suneja, S. K., Potashner, S. J., & Benson, C. G. (1998). Plastic changes in glycine and GABA release and uptake in adult brain stem auditory nuclei after unilateral middle ear ossicle removal and cochlear ablation. *Experimental Neurology, 151*(2), 273–288. doi:10.1006/exnr.1998.6812

Szczepaniak, W. S., & Moller, A. R. (1996a). Effects of (–)-baclofen, clonazepam, and diazepam on tone exposure-induced hyperexcitability of the inferior colliculus in the rat: Possible therapeutic implications for pharmacological management of tinnitus and hyperacusis. *Hearing Research, 97*(1–2), 46–53.

Szczepaniak, W. S., & Moller, A. R. (1996b). Evidence of neuronal plasticity within the inferior colliculus after noise exposure: A study of evoked potentials in the rat. *Electroencephalography and clinical neurophysiology, 100*(2), 158–164.

Tadros, S. F., D'Souza, M., Zettel, M. L., Zhu, X., Waxmonsky, N. C., & Frisina, R. D. (2007). Glutamate-related gene expression changes with age in the mouse auditory midbrain. *Brain Research, 1127*(1), 1–9. doi:10.1016/j.brainres.2006.09.081

Takeda, A. (2003). Manganese action in brain function. *Brain Research Reviews, 41*(1), 79–87.

Tan, J., Ruttiger, L., Panford-Walsh, R., Singer, W., Schulze, H., Kilian, S. B., . . . Knipper, M. (2007). Tinnitus behavior and hearing function correlate with the reciprocal expression patterns of BDNF and Arg3.1/arc in auditory neurons following acoustic trauma. *Neuroscience, 145*(2), 715–726. doi:10.1016/j.neuroscience.2006.11.067

Turner, J., Larsen, D., Hughes, L., Moechars, D., & Shore, S. (2012). Time course of tinnitus development following noise exposure in mice. *Journal of Neuroscience Research, 90*(7), 1480–1488. doi:10.1002/jnr.22827

Vogler, D. P., Robertson, D., & Mulders, W. H. (2014). Hyperactivity following unilateral hearing loss in characterized cells in the inferior colliculus. *Neuroscience, 265*, 28–36. doi:10.1016/j.neuroscience.2014.01.017

Vogler, D. P., Robertson, D., & Mulders, W. H. A. M. (2016). Influence of the paraflocculus on normal and abnormal spontaneous firing rates in the inferior colliculus. *Hearing Research, 333*, 1–7. doi:10.1016/j.heares.2015.12.021

Voytenko, S. V., & Galazyuk, A. V. (2011). mGluRs modulate neuronal firing in the auditory midbrain. *Neuroscience Letters, 492*(3), 145–149. doi:10.1016/j.neulet.2011.01.075

Walton, J. P., Frisina, R. D., Ison, J. R., & O'Neill, W. E. (1997). Neural correlates of behavioral gap detection in the inferior colliculus of the young CBA mouse. *Journal of Comparative Physiology A, 181*(2), 161–176.

Walton, J. P., Frisina, R. D., & Meierhans, L. R. (1995). Sensorineural hearing loss alters recovery from short-term adaptation in the C57BL/6 mouse. *Hearing Research, 88*(1–2), 19–26.

Walton, J. P., Frisina, R. D., & O'Neill, W. E. (1994). Effects of age on single-unit processing in the inferior colliculus of the CBA mouse model of presbycusis. *Journal of the Association for Research in Otolaryngology, Abstr. 17*, 83.

Walton, J. P., Frisina, R. D., & O'Neill, W. E. (1998). Age-related alteration in processing of temporal sound features in the auditory midbrain of the CBA mouse. *Journal of Neuroscience, 18*(7), 2764–2776.

Walton, J. P., Simon, H., & Frisina, R. D. (2002). Age-related alterations in the neural coding of envelope periodicities. *Journal of Neurophysiology, 88*(2), 565–578.

Wang, F., Zuo, L., Hong, B., Han, D., Range, E. M., Zhao, L., . . . Liu, L. (2013). Tonotopic reorganization and spontaneous firing in inferior colliculus during both short and long recovery periods after noise overexposure. *Journal of Biomedical Science, 20*, 91. doi:10.1186/1423-0127-20-91

Wang, J., Ding, D., & Salvi, R. J. (2002). Functional reorganization in chinchilla inferior colliculus associated with chronic and acute cochlear damage. *Hearing Research, 168*(1–2), 238–249.

Wang, J., Salvi, R. J., & Powers, N. (1996). Plasticity of response properties of inferior colliculus neurons following acute cochlear damage. *Journal of Neurophysiology, 75*(1), 171–183.

Willott, J. F. (1986). Effects of aging, hearing loss, and anatomical location on thresholds of inferior colliculus neurons in C57BL/6 and CBA mice. *Journal of Neurophysiology, 56*(2), 391–408.

Willott, J. F., Pankow, D., Hunter, K. P., & Kordyban, M. (1985). Projections from the anterior ventral cochlear nucleus to the central nucleus of the inferior colliculus in young and aging C57BL/6 mice. *Journal of Comparative Neurology, 237*(4), 545–551. doi:10.1002/cne.902370410

Willott, J. F., Parham, K., & Hunter, K. P. (1988). Response properties of inferior colliculus neurons in middle-aged C57BL/6J mice with presbycusis. *Hearing Research, 37*(1), 15–27. doi:0378-5955(88)90074-3 [pii]

Zacharek, M. A., Kaltenbach, J. A., Mathog, T. A., & Zhang, J. (2002). Effects of cochlear ablation on noise induced hyperactivity in the hamster dorsal cochlear nucleus: Implications for the origin of noise induced tinnitus. *Hearing Research, 172*(1–2), 137–143. doi:S0378595502005750 [pii]

Zettel, M. L., Frisina, R. D., Haider, S. E., & O'Neill, W. E. (1997). Age-related changes in calbindin D-28k and calretinin immunoreactivity in the inferior colliculus of CBA/CaJ and C57Bl/6 mice. *Journal of Comparative Neurology, 386*(1), 92–110. doi:10.1002/(SICI)1096-9861(19970915)386:1<92::AID-CNE9>3.0.CO;2-8 [pii]

Zheng, Y., Vagal, S., McNamara, E., Darlington, C. L., & Smith, P. F. (2012). A dose-response analysis of the effects of L-baclofen on chronic tinnitus caused by acoustic trauma in rats. *Neuropharmacology, 62*(2), 940–946. doi:10.1016/j.neuropharm.2011.09.027

CHAPTER 20

UNIFYING THE MIDBRAIN

The Commissure of the Inferior Colliculus

ADRIAN REES AND LLWYD D. ORTON

Abstract

Commissural fibres interconnecting the two sides of the brain are found at several points along the auditory pathway, thus suggesting their fundamental importance for the analysis of sound. This chapter presents an overview of what is currently known about the anatomy, physiology, and behavioral influences of the commissure of the inferior colliculus (CoIC)—the most prominent brainstem auditory commissure—that reciprocally interconnects the principal nuclei of the auditory midbrain, the inferior colliculi (IC). The primary contribution to the CoIC originates from neurons projecting from one inferior colliculus to the other, with the dorsal cortex and central nucleus providing the most extensive connections. In addition, many ascending and descending auditory centers send projections to the IC via the CoIC, together with diverse sources located outside the classically defined auditory pathway. The degree of interconnection between the two ICs suggests they function as a single entity. Recent *in vivo* evidence has established that CoIC projections modulate the neural representation of sound frequency, level, and location in the IC, thus indicating an important role for the CoIC in auditory processing. However, there is limited evidence for the influence of the CoIC on auditory behavior. This, together with the diversity of sources projecting via the CoIC, suggest unknown roles that warrant further exploration.

Keywords: auditory cortex, behavior, commissure, electrophysiology, frequency response area, GABA, hearing, inferior colliculus, neuroanatomy, sound localization

THE auditory system is unique among mammalian sensory systems in having *precortical* commissural connections that interconnect homologous structures on either side of the brain. In the somatosensory and visual systems, crossing fibers occur at the spinal cord and optic chiasm, respectively, but these are decussations where fibers travel obliquely to terminate in structures at a level above their origin. True commissural interactions in most sensory and motor systems are found in the cerebral cortex, where the two hemispheres are interconnected by the corpus callosum and the other major commissures. However, as in several aspects of its functional organization, the auditory system proves to be the maverick among sensory systems, operating according to its own distinct requirements.

The first commissural connections in the auditory pathway occur between the cochlear nuclei, the direct recipients of input from the cochlea. There are two systems: one glycinergic that originates mainly in the core of the ventral cochlear nucleus (VCN) and another, excitatory, which arises from neurons in the small cell cap of the VCN (Alibardi, 1998; Arnott, Wallace, Shackleton, & Palmer, 2004; Brown, Drottar, Benson, & Darrow, 2013; Cant & Gaston, 1982; Doucet, Lenihan, & May, 2009; Schofield & Cant, 1996; Shore, Godfrey, Helfert, Altschuler, & Bledsoe, 1992). Given their different organization, these two systems probably serve several functions, including balancing binaural interactions between the cochlear nuclei (Doucet et al., 2009; Needham & Paolini, 2006).

Commissural projections are absent between the nuclei of the superior olivary complex, and next occur near the head of the brainstem where the commissure of Probst, a primarily GABAergic pathway, interconnects the binaurally responsive neurons of the dorsal nucleus of the lateral lemniscus (Adams & Mugnaini, 1984; Chen, Kelly, & Wu, 1999; Shneiderman, Oliver, & Henkel, 1988; van Adel, Kidd, & Kelly, 1999). Interestingly, the mainly monaural neurons in the ventral nucleus of the lateral lemniscus, which receive inputs predominantly from the contralateral cochlear nucleus, are not commissurally interconnected—an observation again consistent with the idea that commissural connections are important in binaural processing.

Of all the subcortical auditory commissures, the most substantial interconnects the inferior colliculi. The significance of this reciprocal innervation is evidenced by the fact that the commissure of the inferior colliculus (CoIC) is likely the largest single external source of input the IC receives (Moore, 1988). This chapter explores what is currently known about the organisation and function of the CoIC, and speculates about its role in sound analysis.

Structure of the Review

The chapter begins by considering the anatomy of the CoIC, including the sources and connections of its fibers. These sections are followed by a discussion of experiments that have investigated the function of the CoIC, and we conclude with a consideration of the putative role of the CoIC, and identify the major gaps in our knowledge. The aim is not to be historically exhaustive, but rather to highlight the major principles of CoIC organisation.

Anatomical Organization of the CoIC

The CoIC principally interconnects neurons in the two ICs, although, as discussed later, some of its fibers originate in, or target, other structures in the auditory pathway. In appearance, the CoIC is a curvilinear tract composed of heavily myelinated fibers that interconnect the ICs dorsal to the cerebral aqueduct (Figure 20.1A; Faye Lund & Osen, 1985; Saldaña & Merchán, 2005). The number of CoIC fibers increases dorsally, medially and rostrally as they coalesce to cross the midline, forming the caudal part of the tectal commissure, a fiber bundle that also contains the commissural fibers of the superior colliculus (Faye Lund & Osen, 1985). The CoIC courses symmetrically about the midline forming a direct projection from neurons in one IC to those opposite. Intermingled between the commissural fibers are neurons that form a commissural nucleus, located between the dorsal cortex of the IC (ICD) and the periaqueductal grey in cat (Morest & Oliver, 1984) and rat (Faye Lund & Osen, 1985). This structure is now considered to be the caudal portion of a more extensive tectal longitudinal column that receives collaterals of commissural fibers (Aparicio, Viñuela, & Saldaña, 2010; Saldaña, Viñuela, Marshall, Fitzpatrick, & Aparicio, 2007). Lateral to the commissural nuclei, CoIC fibers splay across the entirety of the IC where their fascicles decrease in density as they project toward their targets.

Connectivity of Commissural Fibers Between the ICs

The overall of schema of intercollicular connectivity is highly conserved across mammalian species. The patterns of connections formed by the intercollicular fibers were first demonstrated in a variety of species using degeneration techniques (Moore & Goldberg, 1966; Powell & Hatton, 1969; van Noort, 1969; Woollard & Harpman, 1940). More recent studies using anterograde and retrograde tracers have added detail and clarity to those earlier findings, demonstrating that there are commissural neurons in IC that project contralaterally to all its subdivisions (Adams, 1980; Coleman & Clerici, 1987; Gonzalez Hernandez, Meyer, & Ferres-Torres, 1986; Malmierca, Hernández, Antunes, & Rees, 2009; Malmierca, Rees, Lebeau, & Bjaalie, 1995; Saldana & Merchan, 1992).

The first detailed study of commissural projections, using the anterograde tracer Phaseolus vulgaris-leucoagglutinin, was conducted in rat (Saldana & Merchan, 1992). Tracer deposits in the central nucleus (ICC) labelled, in the coronal plane, two bands of fibers that coursed through rostral part of the ipsilateral IC; one through the dorsal cortex (ICD) and the (ICC, the other through the lateral cortex (ICL; save for the most superficial layer). Caudally, the two bands converged to form one continuous laminar plexus. A mirror symmetric, though less extensive, distribution of axon terminal fibers was revealed in the contralateral IC. Intercollicular connections therefore follow a reciprocal topographic pattern, with terminals distributed throughout

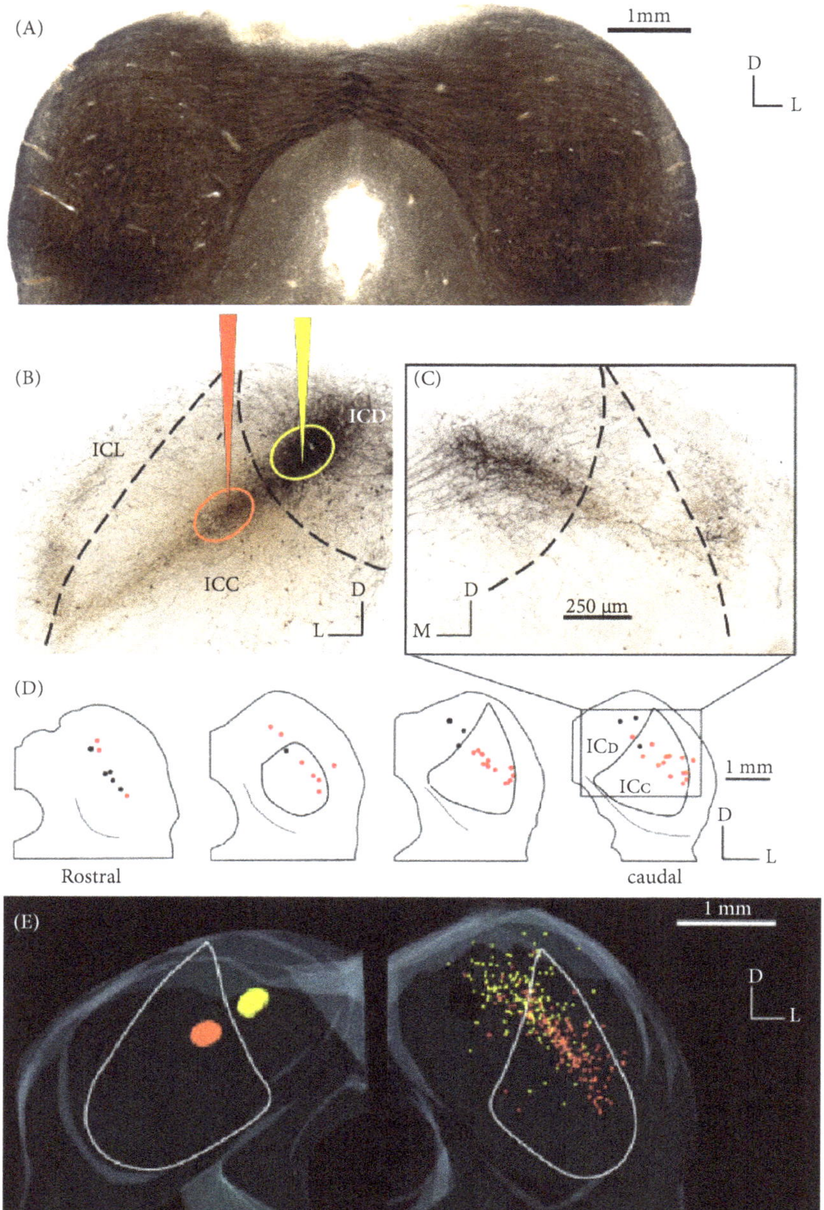

FIGURE 20.1. **A.** Coronal section (50-µm thick) of the tectal midbrain in guinea pig stained for myelin with osmium tetroxide to show the commissure of the inferior colliculus (CoIC). Commissural fibers can be seen crossing the midline and fanning out into each IC. Fibers of the lateral lemniscus can be seen entering the ICs from below. **B.** Photomicrograph showing injections of two different tracers into the same frequency band lamina in the IC of rat. The best frequency at the injection sites was determined by electrophysiological recording to sound to be 10–10.5 kHz. An injection of tetramethyl-rhodamine dextran was made in ICD (yellow circle) and

the contralateral fibrodendritic lamina in all subdivisions (Saldaña & Merchán, 2005; Saldana & Merchan, 1992).

A similar distribution of intercollicular projections was demonstrated in guinea pig using biocytin injections combined with electrophysiological recording (Malmierca et al., 1995). This approach allowed the injection sites and the resulting labelled laminae to be characterized with respect to the frequency organisation of the IC. In the IC contralateral to the tracer injection, electrolytic lesions placed at sites with the same best frequency as the tracer injection confirmed the precise symmetry of these intercollicular connections.

Thus, the consistent finding from studies using anterograde tracers was a mirror symmetric pattern of labelling in each IC defining the arc of the fibrodendritic laminae (Figure 20.1B and C; Saldana and Merchan 1992; Malmierca et al. 1995; Malmierca et al. 2009). These laminae are the structural substrate underlying the tonotopic representation of sound frequency in the IC (Merzenich & Reid, 1974; Rose, Greenwood, Goldberg, & Hind, 1963).

Although these studies show the general organisation of commissural connections between the ICs, they do not address the intricacies of the circuitry involved. Particularly pertinent is whether the ipsilateral and contralateral laminae are connected in a point-to-point fashion, or whether neurons at a single location on a lamina send divergent connections across the lamina surface? A partial answer to this question was obtained using retrograde labelling from small injections of two dextran tracers. Malmierca et al. (2009) placed tracers at different frequency locations and subdivisions in rat IC and reconstructed in 3D the locations of retrograde labelled neurons on the contralateral side. Labelled somata were distributed throughout the contralateral lamina from an injection in ICc, but the number of labelled somata in the contralateral IC was maximal at a point mirror symmetric to the injection site (Figure 20.1B–E).

The caveats of tracer studies notwithstanding, the observed pattern of labelling suggests that commissural neurons make divergent connections. Thus a single point on

---

biotinylated dextran amine into ICc (red circle). A V-shaped plexus of intrinsic axons is labelled ipsilateral to the injections with a central wing in ICc that extends into ICd, and a lateral wing that turns into ICl. **C.** In the contralateral IC, commissural fibers are labelled in mirror image distribution to those seen ipsilaterally, with retrogradely labelled neuronal somata scattered among them. **D.** Camera lucida drawings from sections at different locations along the rostro-caudal axis, showing the locations of somata labelled by the injection in ICc (red dots) and ICd (black dots), respectively. **E.** Three dimensional reconstructions in the coronal plane of the locations of the injection sites (left) and of retrogradely labelled somata (right) for the case shown in **B–D.** The injection in ICc labels somata (red points) in the contralateral ICc and ICd. Somata labelled following an injection in ICd (yellow points) are restricted to the cortical regions. (Some of the latter appear in this view to be in ICc, but viewing from other orientations shows them to be in the cortex rostral and caudal to ICc.) Neurons in ICl do not give rise to commissural projections. D, dorsal; L, lateral. (B–E adapted from Malmierca et al., 2009.)

a lamina receives convergent connections from neurons distributed over the surface of the homologous lamina in the contralateral side, but the greater weight of connections occurs between homotopic points (Figure 20.2A). Such an organisation may provide the basis for complex convergent and divergent information processing between the ICs. However, we do not know whether different classes of neurons contribute to these different projection patterns. The answer to this question awaits the detailed connectivity mapping of individual commissural neurons.

In addition to interconnecting neurons in the contralateral ICc, neurons in the ICc also receive projections from the contralateral ICd. An injection in ICc retrogradely labelled neurons in contralateral ICd whose distribution followed the axis of the lamina in ICc. In contrast, an injection in ICd resulted in a diffuse pattern of labelled somata in contralateral ICd (Malmierca et al., 2009). These distributions suggest there are two distinct populations of neurons within ICd giving rise to commissural connections: neurons in the ventral part of ICd, a region into which the frequency band laminae extend, project to the contralateral ICc and ventral ICd, whereas neurons in the dorsal part of ICd connect more widely throughout the contralateral ICd (Figure 20.2B). Neurons in ICl were rarely labelled following injections in ICc or ICd, indicating that although commissural projections terminate in this subdivision, it is not a source of commissural connections.

Together, these findings suggest that different populations of commissural neurons interconnect the two ICs in distinct ways, perhaps in a manner analogous to the functional zones identified for the multiple sources of afferent input to the IC (Cant, 2013; Cant & Benson, 2006; Loftus, Bishop, & Oliver, 2010). The search for the organizing principles of interactions within and between the fibrodendritic laminae of the IC remains an important, but unanswered, challenge.

Commissural Fibers Originating or Terminating Outside the IC

Not all fibers passing through the commissure originate in the IC. A subset of ascending lemniscal fibers cross via the commissure to the contralateral IC (Barnes, Magoun, & Ranson, 1943; Hutson, Glendenning, & Masterton, 1991). These originate from the ventral (Whitley & Henkel, 1984), intermediate (Hutson et al., 1991), and dorsal nuclei of the lateral lemniscus (Bajo, Merchan, Lopez, & Rouiller, 1993), as well as the sagulum (Henkel & Shneiderman, 1988). Some neurons in the paraolivary nucleus of the superior olivary complex similarly send collaterals to dorsal cortex of the contralateral colliculus via the commissure (Saldaña, Aparicio, Fuentes-Santamaría, & Berrebi, 2009). A recent report finds even fibers originating from a location as peripheral as the DCN can reach the ipsilateral IC by traversing the brainstem to the contralateral IC before crossing back through the CoIC to terminate in the ipsilateral ICd (Milinkeviciute, Muniak, Pongstaporn, Cho, & Ryugo, 2015). Thus, it seems projections taking this

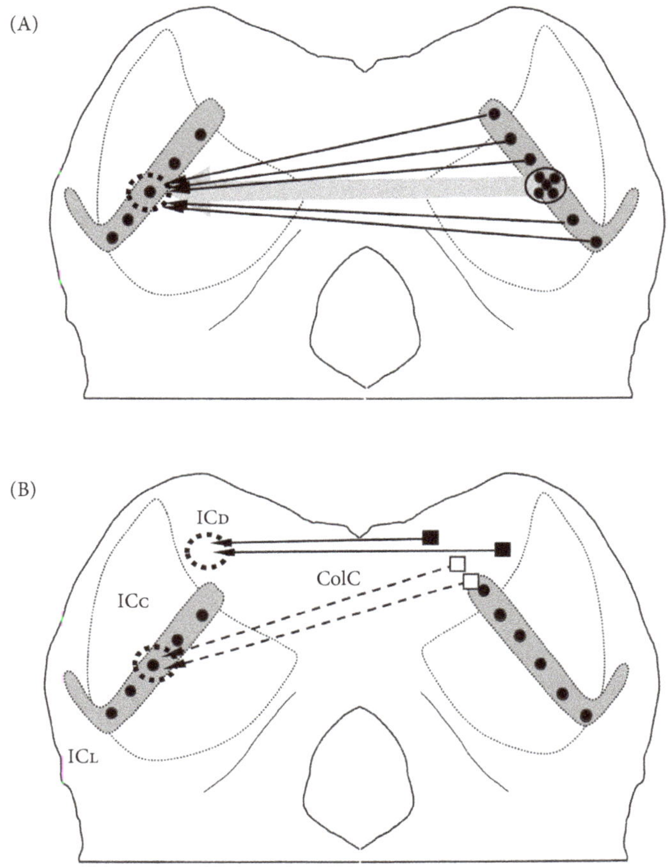

FIGURE 20.2. Schematic diagrams to illustrate the patterns of commissural connections between the different subdivisions of the IC based on retrograde labelling following tracer injections like those in Figure 20.1.

A. An injection (dotted circle) into ICc results in fibro-dendritic labelling of a V-shaped axonal plexus (grey) in both ICs (see Figure 20.1B). Retrogradely labeled somata (filled dots) are observed over the length of the lamina in the contralateral (right) IC, consistent with each of these neurons making divergent commissural projections (thin arrows) to the injection site and sites along the lamina. Cell counts show the projection is weighted (broad arrow) to a point on the lamina (solid circle) corresponding to that of the injection site. **B.** Neurons in ICd make two types of projection: an injection in ICc retrogradely labels neurons in the deeper layers of ICd (open squares) in line with the lamina, while an injection in ICd labels neurons distributed more diffusely in ICd (solid squares). (Adapted from Malmierca et al., 2009.)

circuitous route contribute to the relatively sparse input described from the ipsilateral dorsal cochlear nucleus to the IC (see Cant 2005 for review).

The CoIC also likely contains ascending projections from IC to the superior colliculus (Moore & Goldberg 1966) and to the ventral nucleus of the *contralateral* medial geniculate body (MGB; Coomes & Schofield, 2004; González-Hernández, Galindo-Mireles, Castañeyra-Perdomo, & Ferres-Torres, 1991; Kudo & Niimi, 1978; Oliver, 1984). Double labelling experiments suggest that as many as 30% of IC neurons projecting to the ipsilateral MGB also project to the contralateral MGB (González-Hernández et al., 1991). Such projections may provide a means for further bilateral integration within MGB.

In addition to conveying ascending and laterally directed fibers, the CoIC also mediates descending connections. While cortico-collicular, and thalamo-collicular connections are predominantly ipsilateral, a small proportion reach the contralateral IC directly via the commissure. Most terminals of such cortico-collicular fibers are found medially and dorsally, and in contrast to their ipsilateral counterparts, labeled terminals in the contralateral ICc only extend into its most dorsal part, and are absent in ICl (Adams & Wenthold, 1979; Rockel & Jones, 1973; Saldana, Feliciano, & Mugnaini, 1996). After tracer injections in both ICs, around 5% of cortico-collicular neurons were found to be double labelled in guinea pig and opossum (Coomes, Schofield, & Schofield, 2005; Willard & Martin, 1984). In contrast, Bajo and Moore (2005) failed to find any double-labelled cells in auditory cortex after large tracer injections in both left and right IC in gerbil. Nevertheless, it seems that, at least in some species, cortical neurons may send collateralized inputs to both ICs.

We do not know the exact proportion of commissural fibers that either originate or terminate outside the IC, but they are likely a small proportion of the total. It is also interesting, that, in contrast to the weight of intercollicular connections between the ICcs, commissural connections to the IC from extra-collicular sources are predominantly restricted to ICd.

There are a few reports of non-auditory projections *to* IC which project through the CoIC. Higher order areas such as the insula (Winer, Chernock, Larue, & Cheung, 2002) innervate IC via CoIC, while subcortical sources include the substantia nigra pars lateralis, a tonically firing GABAergic output of the basal ganglia (Afifi & Kaelber, 1965; Olazabal & Moore, 1989), the cholinergic basolateral amygdala (Marsh, Fuzessery, Grose, & Wenstrup, 2002), and bilateral projections from the hypothalamus (Adams, 1980). These little considered sources of input suggest processing in the IC goes beyond the analysis of sound per se.

The Neurochemistry of Commissural Fibers

Studies concur that the CoIC comprises both excitatory and inhibitory fibers. Saint Marie (1996) demonstrated an glutamatergic, excitatory, component based on the synaptic uptake and retrograde transport of tritiated D-aspartate. But combining retrograde labeling with immunohistochemistry for GABA or its synthesizing enzyme GAD67 reveals a substantial minority of labeled neurons are GABAergic (González-Hernández, Mantolán-Sarmiento, González-González, & Pérez-González, 1996; Nakamoto, Sowick, & Schofield, 2013). In rat, 18% of retrogradely labeled commissural neurons in the IC were

GABA positive (González-Hernández et al., 1996; Hernández, Rees, & Malmierca, 2006). Given that around 20–25% of neurons in the IC of rat are GABAergic (Merchán, Aguilar, Lopez-Poveda, & Malmierca, 2005) the percentage of inhibitory commissural projections suggests the commissural projection is representative of the population of IC GABAergic neurons. In guinea pig, co-labelling of commissurally identified neurons with GAD67 found that approximately 10% of intercollicular projections were GABAergic, but the number differed between subdivisions from only 4% in ICc, to between 12–21% in the different cortical subdivisions (Nakamoto et al., 2013). Species differences probably go some way to explain the differences between reports, but there also appears to be a dorsal to ventral gradient through ICd and ICc with respect to the number of GABAergic neurons that contribute to the commissure. In ICd up to 68% of commissural neurons are GABAergic, but there are many fewer in the more ventral parts of ICc (González-Hernández et al., 1996). Such a gradient may, therefore, explain why Zhang, Li, Kelly, & Wu (1998) failed to find any GABAergic labeled cells among commissural neurons labelled with fluorogold following injections placed ventrally in ICc. The contribution of different proportions of GABAergic neurons between different regions of IC indicates disparate roles of fibers with the CoIC, related to their afferent sources and efferent targets.

While glutamate or GABA are the principal neurotransmitters of commissural neurons, a small number of commissural neurons expressing neuropeptide Y or encephalin have been identified in the cortical subdivisions of the IC (Nakagawa et al., 1995). Further investigation into the diversity of the neurotransmitters expressed by CoIC neurons is required.

Neuronal Morphologies in IC Contributing to Commissural Connections

There is no systematic study of the neuronal types in IC that form the commissural projection. However, several reports using retrograde tracers or intracellular labeling show that IC neurons of widely differing morphologies are sources of commissural input (Adams, 1980; Coleman & Clerici, 1987; Druga & Syka, 1984; González-Hernández et al., 1996; Gonzalez Hernandez et al., 1986; Moore, 1988; Okoyama, Ohbayashi, Ito, & Harada, 2006; Saint Marie, 1996). The task of comparing these studies is somewhat hampered by the different terminologies applied to naming the neuronal types. However, it appears safe to say that the two major classes of neurons that feature in cytoarchitecture of the frequency-band laminae of the ICc (neurons with flattened disc-shaped dendritic fields and stellate neurons—also termed flat and less flat types (Malmierca, Blackstad, Osen, Karagulle, & Molowny, 1993; Malmierca & Hackett, 2010; Oliver, 2005; Oliver & Morest, 1984) are both found in the commissural population in the central nucleus, together with mainly stellate types in ICd.

In one of the few quantitative studies, Okoyama et al. (2006) report that the most frequently encountered types were small- and medium-sized disc-shaped neurons (average soma diameters 12 and 16 μm respectively) together with medium-sized stellate neurons. Neurons of both categories with large diameter somata (>20 μm) were observed, but much less frequently. These two major morphological classes are also present in studies that targeted the excitatory (Saint Marie, 1996) or inhibitory (GABAergic; González-Hernández et al., 1996; Nakamoto et al., 2013) components of the commissural projection. Following injection of tritiated aspartate to retrogradely label glutamatergic neurons, Saint Marie (1996) reported labelled neurons in ICc and ICd of the contralateral IC, including "fusiform" cells lying parallel to the orientation of the frequency band laminae, thus presumed disc-shaped neurons. Gonzalez-Hernandez et al. (1996) and Nakamoto et al. (2013) combined retrograde labelling with immunohistochemistry to identify GABAergic neurons projecting from one IC to the other. Labelling was most pronounced in ICd and the dorsal part of ICc. The labelled neurons constituted a heterogeneous population of morphologies and diameters with multipolar (stellate) and fusiform types representing somata diameters from 12 μm to over 20 μm. Comparison of these findings with the population analysis of GABAergic neuron size in the IC by Ito et al (Ito, Bishop, & Oliver, 2009), suggests that GABAergic of all sizes contribute to the commissural projection.

Intracellular and juxtacellular labelling techniques in vivo or in vitro produce smaller samples of neurons than retrograde studies, but have the advantage that labelling of dendritic arbors is more complete, and axons can often be traced along at least part of their length. Such studies have described labelled neurons with axons directed towards or into the commissure (Reetz & Ehret, 1999; Smith, 1992; Wallace, Shackleton, & Palmer, 2012). Consistent with the retrograde studies discussed previously, in ICd most of these neurons are "multipolar" (putative stellate or less flat) cells (Smith 1992), but in ICc, some have flattened dendritic arbors characteristic of neurons that aligned to form the frequency-band laminae (Reetz & Ehret, 1999; Wallace et al., 2012).

Inputs and Outputs of Commissural Neurons

Knowledge of the inputs and outputs of commissural neurons is essential to delineate their microcircuitry. Although we know relatively little about their sources of inputs, given their number and distribution in IC, it would be surprising if commissural neurons were not the recipients of extensive input from both intrinsic and external sources.

One significant source of input to commissural neurons comes from the auditory cortex. Nakamoto et al. (2013) in guinea pig used anterograde and retrograde tracers in combination to demonstrate that commissurally projecting neurons receive extensive input from the ipsilateral auditory cortex. These contacts were seen on neurons in ICd and ICc, and cortico-collicular endings were found on both presumed excitatory and identified inhibitory commissural neurons. Intriguingly, as suggested by Nakamoto et al. (2013), cortical input to commissural neurons might be the primary route whereby the IC is influenced by the *contralateral* auditory cortex.

In support of this hypothesis, spontaneous and sound-evoked firing in IC were found to be influenced by electrical stimulation of either contralateral or ipsilateral auditory cortex, but the latency of the contralateral response was longer than that for ipsilateral stimulation (11.4 vs. 7.2 ms; Torterolo, Zurita, Pedemonte, & Velluti, 1998). The longer latency of the contralateral response is consistent with the possibility that the auditory cortex influences the contralateral IC indirectly via the commissure.

With respect to the output connections of commissural neurons, studies *in vitro* show that the majority of ICc neurons activated by stimulating the commissure are also driven by stimulation of the lateral lemniscus (Moore, Kotak, & Sanes, 1998; Reetz & Ehret, 1999). In contrast, neurons in ICd receiving commissural input were not, or only weakly, driven by stimulation of the lateral lemniscus (Smith, 1992). These data support the notion of different populations of commissural neurons suggested by the anatomical findings discussed earlier (see Figure 20.2).

GABAergic neurons projecting to GABAergic neurons in the contralateral IC have been demonstrated (Lee, Yanagawa, & Imaizumi, 2015), and cell-dependent monosynaptic tracing in mouse has extended this finding. Chen, Cheng, Ito, and Song (2018) reported differences in the proportions of inhibitory neurons projecting to glutamatergic and GABAergic neurons in the other IC. About a third of GABAergic neurons projected to glutamatergic neurons, and this proportion was similar for GABAergic neurons located in either ICc or ICd. However, there was a marked, location-dependent difference in the proportion of GABAergic neurons projecting to *GABAergic* neurons, with about 60% of those in ICd projecting to GABAergic neurons compared with only 20% of those in ICc. These data suggest that commissural connections predominantly drive dis-inhibitory circuits in ICd.

Among the GABAergic neurons targeted by commissural connections are the large GABAergic neurons with diameters >16.5 μm. These neurons, characterized by the dense axosomatic contacts they receive from terminals expressing vesicular glutamate transporter 2 (VGLUT2; Altschuler, Tong, Holt, & Oliver, 2008; Ito et al., 2009), constitute the inhibitory connection from the IC to MGB (Ito et al., 2009; Winer, Saint Marie, Larue, & Oliver, 1996). These neurons receive excitatory inputs from several external and intrinsic sources, including from the contralateral IC, although these inputs are considerably sparser than from ipsilateral intrinsic neurons (Ito et al., 2015; Ito & Oliver, 2014).

Intracellular labeling demonstrates that some neurons that send axons towards the commissure also make axon collaterals that head towards the brachium or the lateral lemniscus. Although it was not possible to trace them to their terminals, this observation is consistent with commissural neurons also making ascending or descending connections external to the IC (Reetz & Ehret, 1999). More definitive double labelling tracer studies have also addressed this question. González-Hernández et al. (1991) observed that around 10% of neurons that project to MGB also project to the contralateral IC in rat, but this rose to 25–30% in regions where the two tracers showed most overlap. In contrast, Okoyama et al. (2006), also in rat, reported only about 1% of IC neurons were double labelled following injections into the contralateral IC and the ipsilateral MGB. Furthermore, the latter study showed a complete absence of neurons that contribute to both the commissural *and* the descending pathways from the IC to the cochlear nucleus or the superior olive. These conflicting findings are yet to be resolved.

Overview of Anatomical Findings

The sources and projections of commissural fibers are summarized in Figure 20.3. Together, the anatomical findings discussed emphasize several points about the organisation of the commissure. Commissural connections are responsible for extensive interaction between the two ICs. The commissure mediates excitatory and inhibitory connections roughly in proportion to the percentages in which those neuronal types are found in the IC, and cells with a wide variety of morphologies project from one side to the other. These projections, if not connecting point-to-point, are at least weighted towards the interconnection of homologous points on the fibrodendritic laminae of the ICc, while in ICd there appears to be two populations of commissural neurons with distinct patterns of connections.

Our knowledge of the micro-circuitry of the IC is rudimentary. The extent to which commissural neurons also project to the main external targets of the IC, the brainstem and the thalamus, is controversial, but within the IC their projections to output neurons converge with other inputs. It is not known if commissural neurons are directly reciprocal, though this seems likely. Commissural neurons receive feedback from the auditory cortex, providing a route for the contralateral auditory cortex to influence the IC, over and above the relatively sparse *direct* projections from the contralateral cortex.

Overall, the anatomical findings reveal the ICs to be so intimately bound to one another by the commissure, it is hard to avoid the conclusion that they function as a single entity.

Functional Properties of Commissural Projections

What is the function of these interconnections? In comparison to our knowledge of the anatomical organisation of the CoIC, our understanding of its function is far more limited. The interconnection of the left and right sides of the brain points to a commissural role in binaural interactions, including the neural representation of sounds in azimuth. However, the extent of coupling between the two ICs suggests equally extensive and wide-ranging effects on auditory processing. What knowledge we have about the functional role of commissural connections derives primarily from electrophysiological studies *in vitro*, and *in vivo*.

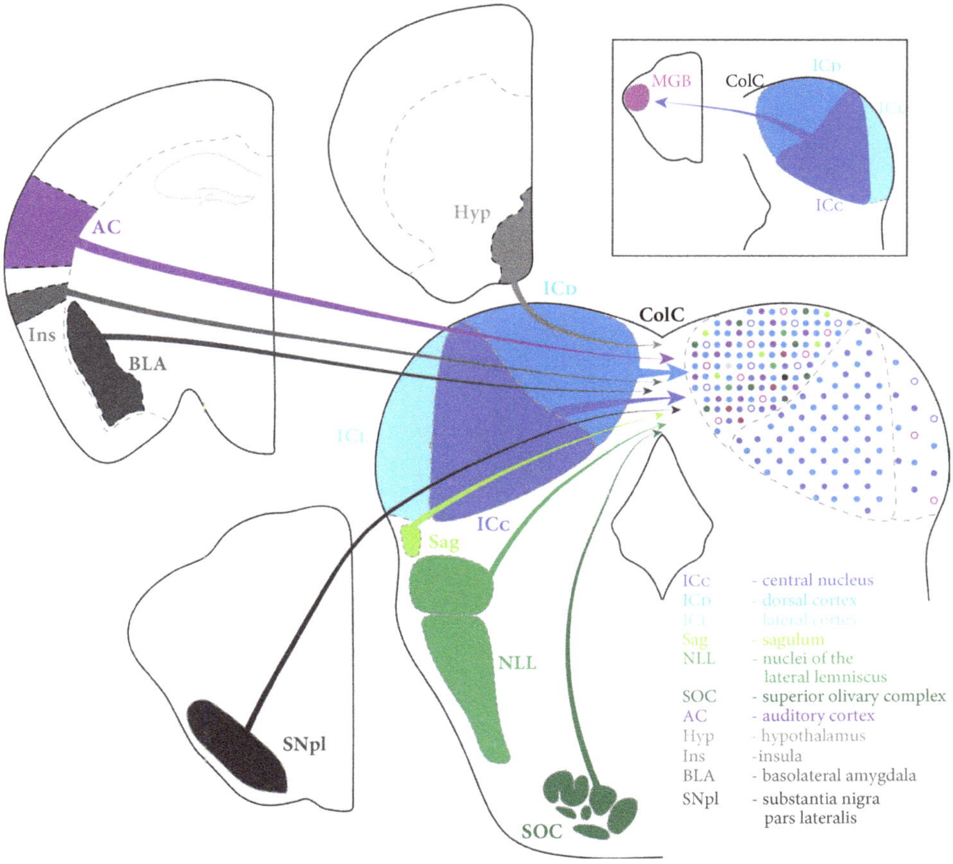

FIGURE 20.3 Summary of the sources and terminal sites of fibers projecting through the commissure of the IC. By far the largest part of the projection originates in the contralateral IC from ICc and ICd. Other centres in the brainstem, diencephalon and cerebral cortex make up smaller part of the projection and primarily terminate in the ICd. Colored stippling in the subdivisions of the IC, corresponding to the color of the incoming projections, indicates the regions where these inputs terminate. Inset top right shows that the IC also sends a minor projection to the contralateral medial geniculate body (MGB) via the CoIC (doi.org/10.6084/m9.figshare.6395990.v3)

In Vitro Studies

Electrical stimulation in brain slices, has been used to study the effects of commissural fibers on their contralateral neuronal targets. Interestingly, for neurons recorded in the central nucleus, the predominant response of stimulating the commissure was a short latency EPSP followed by a short or, more often, a long latency IPSP (Moore et al., 1998; Reetz & Ehret, 1999). In contrast, although some neurons in ICd and ICl showed only a short latency EPSP or IPSP, the dominant pattern was a short latency IPSP followed by an EPSP, often accompanied by a second, long latency, IPSP (Li, Evans, & Faingold, 1999; Smith, 1992). The short latency responses are consistent with monosynaptic excitatory and inhibitory connections, while the longer latency inhibitory effects indicate at least a di-synaptic pathway. Admittedly, the number of neurons studied in this way was relatively small, but these findings support the suggestion made earlier that there are different patterns of synaptic organisation for commissural connections between the cortices of the IC, and those of the central nucleus.

Pharmacological approaches in these studies showed that the long latency component of the inhibition was blocked by the perfusion of AMPA glutamatergic-receptor antagonists, confirming that the long-latency inhibitory component is mediated by di- or poly-synaptic pathways in which GABAergic neurons are driven by excitatory commissural fibers (Moore et al., 1998; Smith, 1992). Thus, although excitatory fibers in the commissure outnumber inhibitory fibers by around 4:1, inhibitory effects arising from commissural activation could occur more frequently than expected from this ratio. For some commissurally activated neurons in ICD, it was also possible to uncover an NMDA-receptor mediated component, suggesting that these inputs may play a role in processing that involves learning and plasticity (Li et al., 1999; Smith, 1992), as might be expected given the role of ICD in learning-induced auditory plasticity (Bajo, Nodal, Moore, & King, 2010).

In Vivo Studies

The main advantage of *in vivo* recording for auditory studies is that it can be combined with physiologically relevant sound stimulation. In the current context, such recordings have been combined with stimulating or inactivating the commissural pathway.

In principle, inactivating commissural inputs, and thus removing their normative influence, might be more informative for understanding the physiology of commissural connections. Two approaches have been used: the application of drugs, either by pressure injection (Malmierca et al., 2003; Malmierca, Hernandez, & Rees, 2005), or microdialysis (Orton, Papasavvas, & Rees, 2016; Orton & Rees, 2014) into one IC, or local cooling of one IC (Orton et al., 2016; Orton, Poon, & Rees, 2012; Orton & Rees, 2014). A limitation of pressure injection is the proximity of the recording site to the site of injection and the mechanical instability that often accompanies the injection. This is a particular problem for single-unit studies where the recording is highly sensitive to mechanical disturbance. Micro-iontophoresis avoids these issues, but the volume of drug delivered, and therefore the region of influence of the drug, is small, and, given the organisation of commissural connections, requires positioning the pipette to match the location of the recording site in the other IC. A better combination of mechanical stability and extended region of influence is obtained by delivering a drug via a microdialysis cannula (Orton et al., 2016; Orton & Rees, 2014). An alternative to blocking commissural activity is to activate the commissure via electrical stimulation of the contralateral IC (Mei, Cheng, Tang, Fu, Wang, et al., 2012). This method allows direct activation of commissural fibers with control over the pattern of stimulation. However, it may not mimic physiological activity, and could result in effects arising from the antidromic activation of neurons in the contralateral IC.

In vivo studies demonstrate that modulating commissural input has wide-ranging effects on neurons in the contralateral IC, with evidence for effects on frequency response areas, rate-level functions and the processing binaural cues.

Frequency response areas or receptive fields in the IC can be subdivided into several categories according to their shape. Many neurons have a V-shaped response area, redolent of auditory nerve fibers (LeBeau, Malmierca, & Rees, 2001; Palmer, Shackleton, Sumner, Zobay, & Rees, 2013). The other broad group, termed non-V, contains several patterns, some of which appear to have been sculpted by inhibition from a V-type shape (Alkhatib, Biebel, & Smolders, 2006; Egorova, Ehret, Vartanian, & Esser, 2001; LeBeau et al., 2001; Palmer et al., 2013). While distinct sub-types appear to occur within this group, detailed analysis of thousands of response areas suggest they do not constitute discrete classes, but lie on a continuum (Palmer et al., 2013). Experiments where recording is combined with iontophoresis of GABAergic antagonists shows differential effects on these two groups: V-shaped response areas show increased firing rate over the whole response area, with little change in receptive field area or shape. In contrast, neurons in the non-V group show changes in receptive field shape, often reverting to a more V-like appearance (LeBeau et al., 2001).

Interestingly, inactivation of the commissural connections produces changes in frequency response areas reminiscent of those seen with inhibitory blockade (LeBeau et al., 2001; Malmierca et al., 2003; Orton & Rees, 2014). V-shaped response areas typically showed an increase or reduction in firing over the whole response area, whereas in non-V type responses changes in firing rate were accompanied by an increase or decrease in receptive field area and shape (Figure 20.4; Orton & Rees, 2014). The parallels between these observations and those in which inhibitory inputs to the recorded neuron are blocked by GABAergic antagonists, suggest that commissural connections contribute to the inputs defining receptive field shape, and these can be excitatory or inhibitory in their action.

Electrical stimulation of one IC leads to changes in firing rate and broadening or narrowing of V-shaped tuning curves for neurons in the other IC, in some cases accompanied by a change in best frequency (Cheng et al., 2013; Mei, Cheng, Tang, Fu, Jen, et al., 2012). The direction of such changes depended on the difference between the frequency represented by the stimulation site in one IC and the recording site in the other. Where such a difference existed, the best frequency shifted towards that of the stimulation site (Cheng et al., 2013; Mei, Cheng, Tang, Fu, Wang, et al., 2012). These effects appear to involve plasticity, since they are sustained for 1–2 hours following 30 mins of stimulation. It is not clear to what extent these effects implicate commissural interactions between different frequency-band laminae.

As expected given changes in frequency response areas, stimulation or inactivation in the IC also influences the relationship between firing rate and sound level of neurons in the opposite side, as exemplified by rate-level functions (RLFs). Electrical stimulation

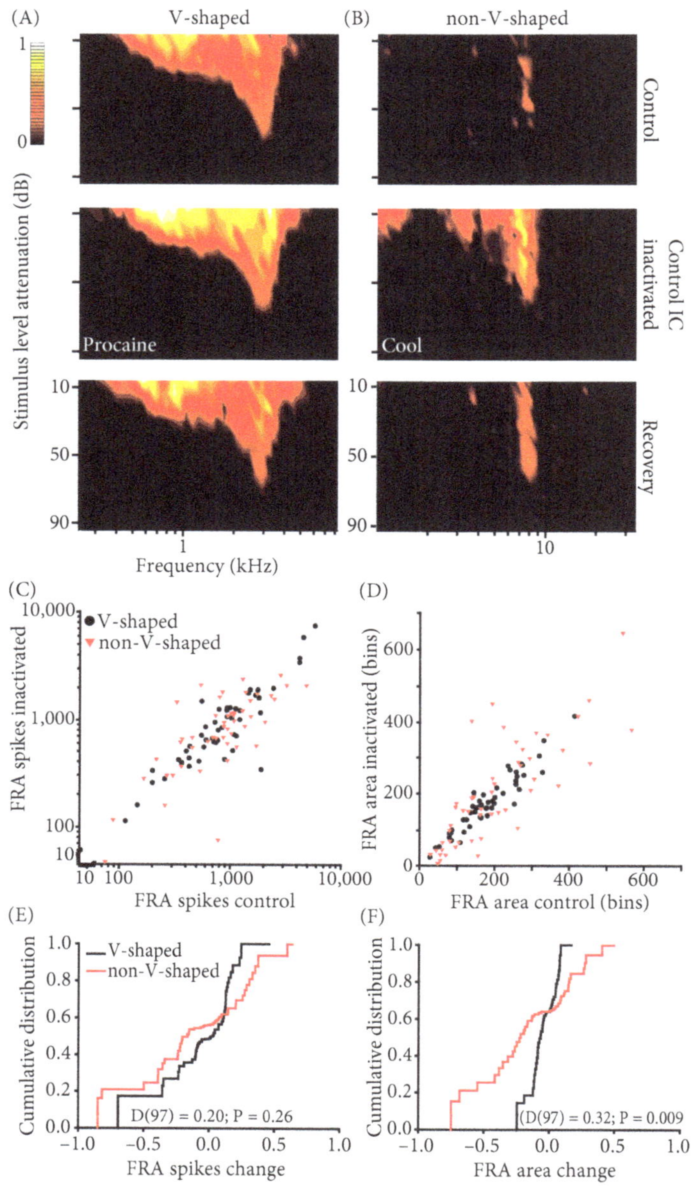

FIGURE 20.4 Influence of commissural input on frequency responses in the IC. V-shaped (**A**) and nonV-shaped (**B**) response areas for single neurons recorded in the IC of guinea pig. Control (top), during inactivation of the contralateral IC by procaine infusion or cooling (middle), and after recovery (bottom). Responses in each example normalized to the maximum value across conditions. On deactivation of the contralateral IC, the V-shaped response area showed an elevation in firing, but little change in area or shape. In contrast, the nonV-shaped response area expanded, and firing increased at frequencies to which the neuron responded in the control condition. Comparison of firing (**C**, total number of spikes) and area (**D**, above threshold bins) in the control and deactivated conditions for the populations of V-shaped (black) and nonV-shaped (red) frequency response areas (FRAs). Cumulative distributions for the change in firing (**E**) and area (**F**) of V and nonV groups. While the range over which firing changed was similar between the two groups, the nonV group showed a larger range of area change than the V group. (Adapted from Orton & Rees, 2014.)

can elicit increases or decreases in firing rate, although the majority of neurons were inhibited by stimulation of the contralateral IC (Cheng 2016; Mei 2012). Facilitation was generally only observed with small BF differences whereas inhibition occurred over a wider range of best frequency differences, again raising the possibility of interactions between within and between laminae. In general, rate level responses were suppressed by electrical stimulation with an increased slope, and a reduction in dynamic range, but no change in the degree of monotonicity. As with the effects on frequency responses, there was evidence for the involvement of short-term plasticity.

Blockade of commissural inputs, either by cooling or microdialysis of procaine, in guinea pig resulted in shifts in RLFs towards higher sound levels and reduced non-monotonicity, effects that were, in the main, due to changes in responsivity at supra-threshold sound levels (Orton & Rees, 2014). As a consequence of these changes, there was an overall reduction in the ability of neurons to discriminate sound levels, suggesting that physiologically commissural input enhances the neural representation of sound level.

Although in all these studies there was evidence for both excitatory and inhibitory commissural effects, inhibitory effects appear to occur disproportionately to the known distribution of glutamatergic and GABAergic fibers in the commissure (see *The Neurochemistry of Commissural Fibers* Malmierca et al., 2005; Mei, Cheng, & Chen, 2013; Orton & Rees, 2014). This finding concurs with the findings of *in vitro* studies (see *In Vitro Studies*) demonstrating that inhibitory effects are mediated not only monosynaptically, but also by di- or poly-synaptic circuits in which excitatory commissural fibers target local inhibitory neurons in the contralateral IC.

As we suggested earlier, it seems intuitive that commissural interactions might impact binaural processing. Physiological studies *in vivo* lend some support to this view (Malmierca et al 2005; Orton et al 2016). Orton et al (2016) addressed this issue by inactivating the IC by cooling or procaine infusion while recording neuronal responses to stimuli of varying interaural time or level difference (ITD, ILD) in the opposite IC. The dominant effect of IC inactivation was a reversible reduction or increase in firing rate at all values ITD or ILD. Across the population of recorded neurons, there was no evidence that the range of ITD or ILDs encoded changed on removal of commissural input. Nevertheless, analysis of firing rates for the control and inactivated conditions (Figure 20.5) indicated, both for ITD and ILD, that response gain was reduced following commissural inactivation. Commensurate with this reduction in gain, discriminability of these binaural cues was also reduced. Taken together, these findings suggest that in normal operation, commissural inputs enhance the ability of IC neurons to discriminate changes in the position of sounds in azimuthal space.

An important caveat that applies to all the methodologies used thus far to manipulate commissural inputs is that they might influence the contralateral IC via routes other than the commissure. These alternative pathways could go via the auditory cortex, given that both ipsilateral and contralateral cortices influence the IC, the latter, in part, via a commissural projection (Nakamoto et al., 2013). Alternatively, the descending projections from the IC to the superior olivary complex or the cochlear nucleus could

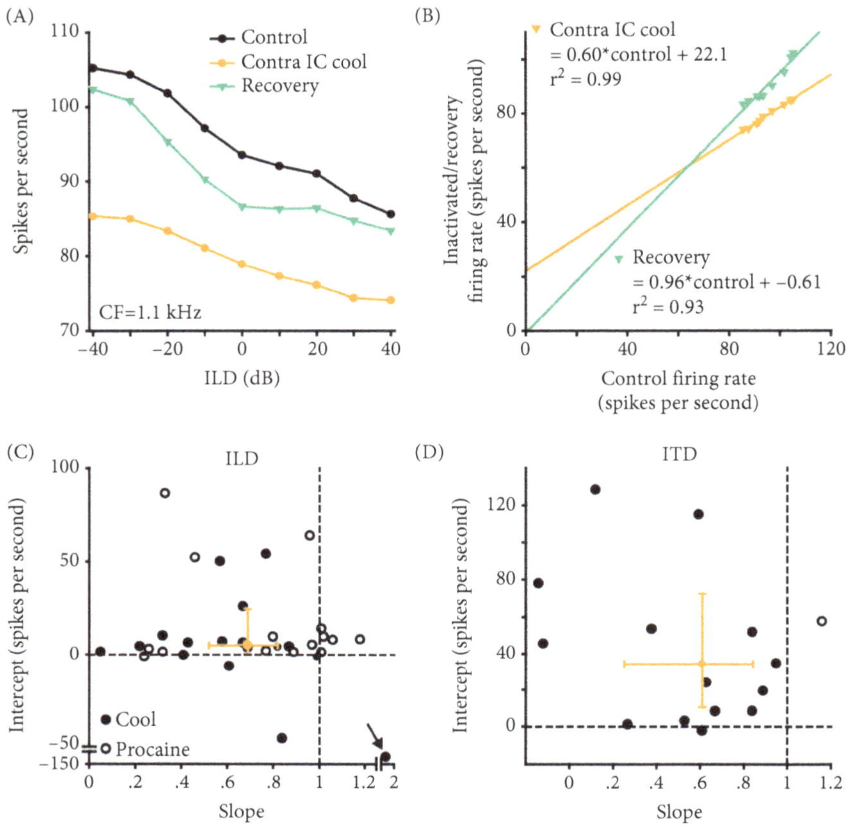

FIGURE 20.5 The influence of commissural input on response gain to interaural time and level differences in the IC. **A.** Interaural level difference (ILD, sound level in the ear ipsilateral to the recorded IC relative to that in the contralateral ear) functions for a single neuron: control (black), during deactivation of the contralateral IC (yellow) and after recovery (green). **B** Data in (**A**) replotted to show firing rate in the inactivated (yellow) or recovery conditions (green) as a function of control. The difference in slope and intercept between these two functions denotes a divisive and additive gain change in the inactivated condition. **C & D** Summary plots showing the change in slope and intercept as in (**B**) for units tested with ILD (**C**) and ITD (**D**) stimuli. Overall, for both cues of azimuthal location, removal of commissural input leads to a reduction in slope and a more positive intercept, consistent with normal commissural input enhancing response gain in a multiplicative and subtractive manner. (From Orton et al., 2016.)

also modulate the ascending input into the IC. The possibility seems less likely in view of the fact that when the IC is inactivated through cooling, the effect on sound-evoked local field potentials recorded in the opposite IC is predominantly on the later potentials rather than on the initial afferent volley (Orton et al 2012).

Some of the technical limitations of the methods used to investigate commissural function thus far could be surmounted with the application of optogenetics. This confers the possibility of targeting only those neurons that contribute to the commissural projection, a feat not possible with methods that globally modulate IC function. Furthermore, given evidence that commissural neurons may be a distinct subset of IC neurons (Okoyama et al., 2006), the ability to manipulate them in the absence of influencing IC neurons that project to upstream or downstream targets would be a distinct advantage.

Behavioral Studies

If commissural inputs are important for sound processing in the IC, then the loss of commissural input might be expected to lead to behavioral deficits in sound processing. Transecting the commissure is difficult and not reversible, and there is only one study in the literature where this has been reported (Moore, Casseday, & Neff, 1974). In this behavioral study of sound localization in cat, transection of the commissure of the IC was either performed alone, or preceded or followed by transections of the trapezoid body and/or the corpus callosum to demonstrate their cumulative effects. Only a lesion to the trapezoid body was reported to impact sound localization. Unfortunately, the study has limited utility since only two sound sources were used, situated either side of the animal's midline, thus it tested lateralization rather than localization. Subsequent studies have confirmed that following unilateral lesions within various structures in the ascending auditory pathway animals can retain the ability to lateralize sound sources, but may not be able to localize them (Jenkins & Masterton, 1982).

In the absence of studies involving commissural transection, we can look to studies in animals or humans where there is a lesion in one IC. These reports vary in the tests conducted and the effects observed, but are consistent in reporting deficits in sound localization in the spatial hemifield contralateral to the lesion (Champoux et al., 2007; Jenkins & Masterton, 1982; Kelly & Kavanagh, 1994; Litovsky, Fligor, & Traino, 2002). The extent of the lesion varied from study to study, but the most marked deficits occurred where damage extended to the nuclei of the lateral lemniscus (Kelly & Kavanagh, 1994).

For the current discussion, the question is whether such unilateral lesions had any impact on responses to stimuli presented in the hemifield ipsilateral to the lesion—the "intact hemifield". Such effects would be expected if signals to the IC, via the commissure, from the lesioned side, were ordinarily important. Although the other IC is not *necessary* for localization in the "intact hemifield," there is evidence that performance in that hemifield is affected by a lesion to the other IC. Litovsky et al.'s (2002) patient showed impaired performance, relative to controls, when localizing targets close to the midline in the "intact hemifield," and in animal studies, pre-lesion performance was consistently worse than post-lesion performance in the "intact hemifield" (Kelly & Kavanagh, 1994). Although these were small effects and could have alternative explanations, we should be cautious about ruling out the importance of the commissural pathway on the basis of these studies. Most behavioral studies tested localization using clicks or brief noise bursts, in which the main interaural cue is stimulus onset time, rather than on-going interaural time and level differences. Furthermore, tests were conducted in quiet conditions using constant intensity stimuli, and so did not fully reflect the more demanding conditions of real-world listening.

Speculations Regarding the Function of Commissural Projections

The anatomical and physiological evidence accumulated to date suggests the CoIC's extensive connections exert wide-ranging effects on sound processing that encompass at least the encoding of frequency, level, and location.

Insights into why the colliculi are interconnected may be gained by considering why is it important for one colliculus to know about the responses of its twin in response to events in the acoustic environment? One possibility is that the signal in one IC alone is insufficient to define the properties of a sound source unambiguously. For example, consider how the location of a sound source is represented in the two ICs. Signals encoding interaural time and level differences reach the ICs having been extracted in the medial and lateral nuclei, respectively, of the superior olivary complex (Grothe, Pecka, & McAlpine, 2010). The neural representation of these azimuthal cues is organized in mirror symmetric hemispheric channels. As a sound source moves from one extreme of azimuth to the other, the firing rate of neurons in one IC increases while those in the other decrease in a negatively correlated manner. However, when considering the neural activity in one IC alone, such a rate-coded representation might not code the stimulus invariantly. As represented schematically in Figure 20.6, the change in firing rate of neurons in the right IC to a sound that moves from the midline to the left side (green arrow and green dot) would be indistinguishable from that to a sound on the midline that increases in overall level (blue arrow, blue dot). These stimulus changes are distinguishable, however, if the firing rates in *both* ICs are compared. The increase in level results in an increased firing rate in both ICs, whereas the change in azimuth leads to a reduction in firing in the left IC and an increase in the right. Although such an analysis is doubtless an oversimplification of reality, it serves to demonstrate how signals sent back and forth across the commissure signalling the mutual state of the ICs could be important for resolving such ambiguities.

Other roles for the commissure are suggested by anatomical and physiological findings. One important aspect of real-world hearing is the need to adjust response properties of neurons to keep them within their operating range as overall sound levels in the acoustic environment change. Stimulus-dependent gain control in the IC has been shown to keep neurons within their operating range so maintaining their responsiveness to tones as noise levels increase (Dean, Harper, & McAlpine, 2005; Rees & Palmer, 1988; Robinson & McAlpine, 2009). It is interesting that modulation of commissural

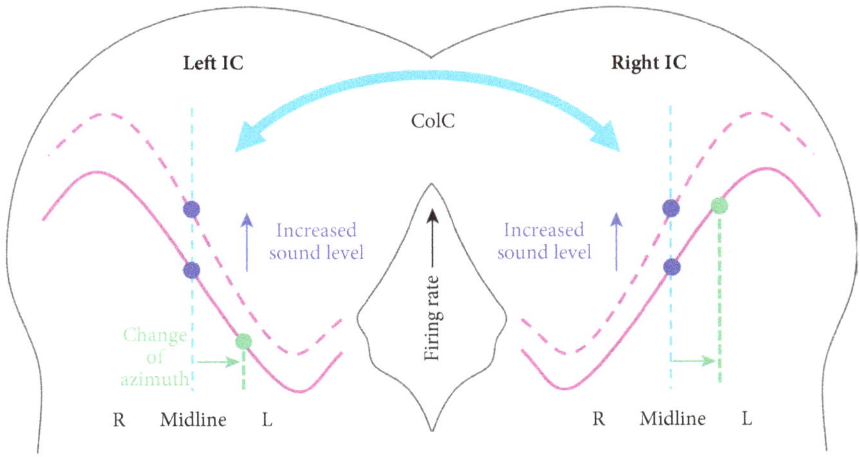

FIGURE 20.6 Schematic diagram demonstrating ambiguous stimulus representation when based on firing rates in one IC (see text for discussion). The solid magenta curves represent the response functions of IC neurons to changes in stimulus azimuth in the hemispheric channel model for sound localization. The dashed magenta curves represent the firing to similar stimuli, but at a higher sound pressure level. As a stimulus moves from the midline to the left, the firing rate in the contralateral (right) IC increases (green arrow and green dot), but the same firing rate is given by a stimulus at a higher level in the midline (blue arrow and blue dot). This ambiguity is resolved if the firing in both ICs is considered. A shift in azimuth leads to firing in the two ICs changing in opposite directions (green arrows and green dots), whereas changes in level lead to firing rates changing in the same direction (blue arrows and blue dots). Connecting the two ICs via the CoIC could provide each IC with information about the status of the other. (doi.org/10.6084/m9.figshare.6396287.v1)

activity leads to shifts in the operating ranges of rate-level functions (Mei, Cheng, Tang, Fu, Jen, et al., 2012; Mei, Tang, Fu, Cheng, & Chen, 2016; Orton & Rees, 2014).

Finally, there is increasing evidence of the important influence that corticofugal and other descending inputs have on auditory processing, including mediating various forms of plasticity (Bajo & King, 2013; Bajo et al., 2010; Suga & Ma, 2003). Such descending inputs might also mediate the types of feedback interactions postulated in predictive coding (Bastos et al., 2012). Particularly intriguing in this context is the evidence for a crossed cortical input to the contralateral IC mediated by commissural connections (Nakamoto et al., 2013).

Conclusion

This chapter has highlighted the extent to which the two inferior colliculi are tightly interconnected by commissural connections that closely integrate many aspects of their complex circuitry. The wide-ranging effects of the commissural system on the coding of fundamental parameters of sound: frequency, level and spatial location, is consistent with the possibility that responses of virtually all neurons in one IC are influenced by those in the other. Thus, functionally, the two ICs appear to operate as a single entity.

Existing studies have only scratched the surface in discovering the role of commissural connections, and it is important to avoid the fallacy of basing an understanding of commissural function on the answers to what might be the wrong questions! It is more than likely that the adequate stimulus (Sherrington, 1906) necessary to reveal the critical contribution of the CoIC has yet to be identified. Furthermore, it is increasingly evident that the inferior colliculus does much more than just integrate ascending sensory information. It receives a multitude of inputs from diverse sources, including those of corticofugal (Bajo & King, 2013) and neuromodulatory origin (Gittelman, Perkel, & Portfors, 2013; Hurley & Sullivan, 2012), that have thus far received little attention. A more complete understanding of the function of the CoIC may require experiments in an awake behaving preparation where the full impact of these diverse inputs can be assessed.

Acknowledgments

Some of our own work discussed in this chapter was supported by grants from the Wellcome Trust (066348) and BBSRC (BB/J0008680/1) to AR.

References

Adams, J. C. (1980). Crossed and descending projections to the inferior colliculus. *Neuroscience Letters*, *19*(1), 1–5.

Adams, J. C., & Mugnaini, E. (1984). Dorsal nucleus of the lateral lemniscus: A nucleus of GABAergic projection neurons. *Brain Research Bulletin*, *13*(4), 585–590.

Adams, J. C., & Wenthold, R. J. (1979). Distribution of putative amino acid transmitters, choline acetyltransferase and glutamate decarboxylase in the inferior colliculus. *Neuroscience*, *4*(12), 1947–1951.

Afifi, A., & Kaelber, W. W. (1965). Efferent connections of the substantia nigra in the cat. *Experimental Neurology*, *11*, 474–482.

Alibardi, L. (1998). Ultrastructural and immunocytochemical characterization of commissural neurons in the ventral cochlear nucleus of the rat. *Annals of Anatomy—Anatomischer Anzeiger*, *180*(5), 427–438.

Alkhatib, A., Biebel, U. W., & Smolders, J. W. T. (2006). Inhibitory and excitatory response areas of neurons in the central nucleus of the inferior colliculus in unanesthetized chinchillas. *Experimental Brain Research*, *174*(1), 124–143.

Altschuler, R. A., Tong, L., Holt, A. G., & Oliver, D. L. (2008). Immunolocalization of vesicular glutamate transporters 1 and 2 in the rat inferior colliculus. *Neuroscience*, *154*(1), 226–232.

Aparicio, M. A., Viñuela, A., & Saldaña, E. (2010). Projections from the inferior colliculus to the tectal longitudinal column in the rat. *Neuroscience*, *166*(2), 653–664.

Arnott, R. H., Wallace, M. N., Shackleton, T. M., & Palmer, A. R. (2004). Onset neurones in the anteroventral cochlear nucleus project to the dorsal cochlear nucleus. *Journal of the Association for Research in Otolaryngology*, *5*(2), 153–170.

Bajo, V. M., & King, A. J. (2013). Cortical modulation of auditory processing in the midbrain. *Frontiers in Neural Circuits*, *6*(114), 1–12. doi: 10.3389/fncir.2012.00114

Bajo, V. M., Merchan, M. A., Lopez, D. E., & Rouiller, E. M. (1993). Neuronal morphology and efferent projections of the dorsal nucleus of the lateral lemniscus in the rat. *Journal of Comparative Neurology*, *334*(2), 241–262.

Bajo, V. M., & Moore, D. R. (2005). Descending projections from the auditory cortex to the inferior colliculus in the gerbil, *Meriones unguiculatus*. *Journal of Comparative Neurology*, *486*(2), 101–116.

Bajo, V. M., Nodal, F. R., Moore, D. R., & King, A. J. (2010). The descending corticocollicular pathway mediates learning-induced auditory plasticity. *Nature Neuroscience*, *13*(2), 253–260.

Barnes, W. T., Magoun, H. W., & Ranson, S. W. (1943). The ascending auditory pathway in the brain stem of the monkey. *Journal of Comparative Neurology*, *79*(1), 129–152.

Bastos, Andre M., Usrey, W. M., Adams, Rick A., Mangun, George R., Fries, P., & Friston, Karl J. (2012). Canonical microcircuits for predictive coding. *Neuron*, *76*(4), 695–711.

Brown, M. C., Drottar, M., Benson, T. E., & Darrow, K. (2013). Commissural axons of the mouse cochlear nucleus. *Journal of Comparative Neurology*, *521*(7), 1683–1696.

Cant, N. B. (2005). Projections from the Cochlear Nuclear Complex to the Inferior Colliculus. In J. A. Winer & C. E. Schreiner (Eds.), *The Inferior Colliculus* (pp. 115–131). New York, NY: Springer.

Cant, N. B. (2013). Patterns of convergence in the central nucleus of the inferior colliculus of the Mongolian gerbil: Organization of inputs from the superior olivary complex in the low frequency representation. *Frontiers in Neural Circuits*, *7*(29), 1–22. doi: 10.3389/fncir.2013.00029

Cant, N. B., & Benson, C. G. (2006). Organization of the inferior colliculus of the gerbil (*Meriones unguiculatus*): Differences in distribution of projections from the cochlear nuclei and the superior olivary complex. *Journal of Comparative Neurology*, *495*(5), 511–528.

Cant, N. B., & Gaston, K. C. (1982). Pathways connecting the right and left cochlear nuclei. *Journal of Comparative Neurology*, *212*(3), 313–326.

Champoux, F., Paiement, P., Mercier, C., Lepore, F., Lassonde, M., & Gagné, J. P. (2007). Auditory processing in a patient with a unilateral lesion of the inferior colliculus. *European Journal of Neuroscience*, *25*(1), 291–297.

Chen, C., Cheng, M., Ito, T., & Song, S. (2018). Neuronal organization in the inferior colliculus revisited with cell-type-dependent monosynaptic tracing. *Journal of Neuroscience, 38*(13), 3318-3332.

Chen, L., Kelly, J. B., & Wu, S. H. (1999). The commissure of Probst as a source of GABAergic inhibition. *Hearing Research*, *138*(1), 106–114.

Cheng, L., Mei, H.-X., & Huang, Y. (2016). Inter-collicular suppression compresses all types of rate-amplitude functions of inferior collicular neurons in mice. *Physiological Research*, *65*, 527-536.

Cheng, L., Mei, H. X., Tang, J., Fu, Z. Y., Jen, P. H. S., & Chen, Q. C. (2013). Bilateral collicular interaction: Modulation of auditory signal processing in frequency domain. *Neuroscience*, *235*, 27–39.

Coleman, J. R., & Clerici, W. J. (1987). Sources of projections to subdivisions of the inferior colliculus in the rat. *The Journal of Comparative Neurology*, *262*(2), 215–226.

Coomes, D. L., & Schofield, B. R. (2004). Separate projections from the inferior colliculus to the cochlear nucleus and thalamus in guinea pigs. *Hearing Research, 191*(1–2), 67–78.

Coomes, D. L., Schofield, R. M., & Schofield, B. R. (2005). Unilateral and bilateral projections from cortical cells to the inferior colliculus in guinea pigs. *Brain Research, 1042*(1), 62–72.

Dean, I., Harper, N. S., & McAlpine, D. (2005). Neural population coding of sound level adapts to stimulus statistics. *Nature Neuroscience, 8*(12), 1684–1689.

Doucet, J. R., Lenihan, N. M., & May, B. J. (2009). Commissural neurons in the rat ventral cochlear nucleus. *Journal of the Association for Research in Otolaryngology, 10*(2), 269–280.

Druga, R., & Syka, J. (1984). Ascending and descending projections to the inferior colliculus in the rat *Physiologica Bohemoslovaca, 33*, 31–42.

Egorova, M., Ehret, G., Vartanian, I., & Esser, K. H. (2001). Frequency response areas of neurons in the mouse inferior colliculus. I. Threshold and tuning characteristics. *Experimental Brain Research, 140*(2), 145–161.

Faye Lund, H., & Osen, K. K. (1985). Anatomy of the inferior colliculus in rat. *Anatomy and Embryology, 171*(1), 1–20.

Gittelman, J. X., Perkel, D. J., & Portfors, C. V. (2013). Dopamine modulates auditory responses in the inferior colliculus in a heterogeneous manner. *Journal of the Association for Research in Otolaryngology, 14*(5), 719–729.

González-Hernández, T., Mantolán-Sarmiento, B., González-González, B., & Pérez-González, H. (1996). Sources of GABAergic input to the inferior colliculus of the rat. *Journal of Comparative Neurology, 372*(2), 309–326.

González-Hernández, T. H., Galindo-Mireles, D., Castañeyra-Perdomo, A., & Ferres-Torres, R. (1991). Divergent projections of projecting neurons of the inferior colliculus to the medial geniculate body and the contralateral inferior colliculus in the rat. *Hearing Research, 52*(1), 17–21.

Gonzalez Hernandez, T. H., Meyer, G., & Ferres-Torres, R. (1986). The commissural interconnections of the inferior colliculus in the albino mouse. *Brain Research, 368*(2), 268–276.

Grothe, B., Pecka, M., & McAlpine, D. (2010). Mechanisms of sound localization in mammals. *Physiological Reviews, 90*(3), 983–1012.

Henkel, C. K., & Shneiderman, A. (1988). Nucleus sagulum: Projections of a lateral tegmental area to the inferior colliculus in the cat. *Journal of Comparative Neurology, 271*(4), 577–588.

Hernández, O., Rees, A., & Malmierca, M. S. (2006). A GABAergic component in the commissure of the inferior colliculus in rat. *Neuroreport, 17*(15), 1611–1614.

Hurley, L. M., & Sullivan, M. R. (2012). From behavioral context to receptors: Serotonergic modulatory pathways in the IC. *Frontiers in Neural Circuits, 6(58), 1–17.* doi: 10.3389/fncir.2012.00058

Hutson, K. A., Glendenning, K. K., & Masterton, R. B. (1991). Acoustic chiasm. IV: Eight midbrain decussations of the auditory system in the cat. *Journal of Comparative Neurology, 312*(1), 105–131.

Ito, T., Bishop, D. C., & Oliver, D. L. (2009). Two classes of GABAergic neurons in the inferior colliculus. *Journal of Neuroscience, 29*(44), 13860–13869.

Ito, T., Hioki, H., Sohn, J., Okamoto, S., Kaneko, T., Iino, S., & Oliver, D. L. (2015). Convergence of lemniscal and local excitatory inputs on large GABAergic tectothalamic neurons. *Journal of Comparative Neurology, 523*(15), 2277–2296.

Ito, T., & Oliver, D. L. (2014). Local and commissural IC neurons make axosomatic inputs on large GABAergic tectothalamic neurons. *Journal of Comparative Neurology, 522*(15), 3539–3554.

Jenkins, W. M., & Masterton, R. B. (1982). Sound localization: effects of unilateral lesions in central auditory system. *Journal of Neurophysiology, 47*(6), 987–1016.

Kelly, J. B., & Kavanagh, G. L. (1994). Sound localization after unilateral lesions of inferior colliculus in the ferret (Mustela putorius). *Journal of Neurophysiology, 71*(3), 1078–1087.

Kudo, M., & Niimi, K. (1978). Ascending projections of the inferior colliculus onto the medial geniculate body in the cat studied by anterograde and retrograde tracing techniques. *Brain Research, 155*(1), 113–117.

LeBeau, F. E. N., Malmierca, M. S., & Rees, A. (2001). Iontophoresis in vivo demonstrates a key role for $GABA_A$ and glycinergic inhibition in shaping frequency response areas in the inferior colliculus of guinea pig. *Journal of Neuroscience, 21*(18), 7303–7312.

Lee, C. C., Yanagawa, Y., & Imaizumi, K. (2015). Commissural functional topography of the inferior colliculus assessed in vitro. *Hearing Research, 328*, 94–101.

Li, Y., Evans, M. S., & Faingold, C. L. (1999). Synaptic response patterns of neurons in the cortex of rat inferior colliculus. *Hearing Research, 137*(1–2), 15–28.

Litovsky, R. Y., Fligor, B. J., & Traino, M. J. (2002). Functional role of the human inferior colliculus in binaural hearing. *Hearing Research, 165*(1–2), 177–188.

Loftus, W. C., Bishop, D. C., & Oliver, D. L. (2010). Differential patterns of inputs create functional zones in central nucleus of inferior colliculus. *Journal of Neuroscience, 30*(40), 13396–13408.

Malmierca, M. S., Blackstad, T. W., Osen, K. K., Karagulle, T., & Molowny, R. L. (1993). The central nucleus of the inferior colliculus in rat: A Golgi and computer reconstruction study of neuronal and laminar structure. *Journal of Comparative Neurology, 333*(1), 1–27.

Malmierca, M. S., & Hackett, T. A. (2010). Structural organization of the ascending auditory pathway. In A. Rees & A. Palmer (Eds.), *The Auditory Brain* (pp. 9–41). Oxford, England: Oxford University Press.

Malmierca, M. S., Hernández, O., Antunes, F. M., & Rees, A. (2009). Divergent and point-to-point connections in the commissural pathway between the inferior colliculi. *Journal of Comparative Neurology, 514*(3), 226–239.

Malmierca, M. S., Hernandez, O., Falconi, A., Lopez-Poveda, E. A., Merchan, M., & Rees, A. (2003). The commissure of the inferior colliculus shapes frequency response areas in rat: An in vivo study using reversible blockade with microinjection of kynurenic acid. *Experimental Brain Research, 153*(4), 522–529.

Malmierca, M. S., Hernandez, O., & Rees, A. (2005). Intercollicular commissural projections modulate neuronal responses in the inferior colliculus. *European Journal of Neuroscience, 21*(10), 2701–2710.

Malmierca, M. S., Rees, A., Lebeau, F. E. N., & Bjaalie, J. G. (1995). Laminar organization of frequency-defined local axons within and between the inferior colliculi of the guinea-pig. *Journal of Comparative Neurology, 357*(1), 124–144.

Marsh, R. A., Fuzessery, Z. M., Grose, C. D., & Wenstrup, J. J. (2002). Projection to the inferior colliculus from the basal nucleus of the amygdala. *Journal of Neuroscience, 22*(23), 10449–10460.

Mei, H.-X., Cheng, L., & Chen, Q.-C. (2013). Neural interactions in unilateral colliculus and between bilateral colliculi modulate auditory signal processing. *Frontiers in Neural Circuits, 7*(68), 1–8. doi: 10.3389/fncir.2013.00068

Mei, H.-X., Cheng, L., Tang, J., Fu, Z.-Y., Jen, P. H. S., & Chen, Q.-C. (2012). Modulation of amplitude sensitivity by bilateral collicular interaction among different frequency laminae. *Neuroscience Letters*, *517*(1), 13–17.

Mei, H.-X., Cheng, L., Tang, J., Fu, Z.-Y., Wang, X., Jen, P. H. S., & Chen, Q.-C. (2012). Bilateral collicular interaction: Modulation of auditory signal processing in amplitude domain. *PLoS ONE*, *7*(7), e41311.

Mei, H.-X., Tang, J., Fu, Z.-Y., Cheng, L., & Chen, Q.-C. (2016). Plastic change in the auditory minimum threshold induced by intercollicular effects in mice. *Neural Plasticity*, *2016*, 8.

Merchán, M., Aguilar, L. A., Lopez-Poveda, E. A., & Malmierca, M. S. (2005). The inferior colliculus of the rat: Quantitative immunocytochemical study of GABA and glycine. *Neuroscience*, *136*(3), 907–925.

Merzenich, M. M., & Reid, M. D. (1974). Representation of the cochlea within the inferior colliculus of the cat. *Brain Research*, *77*(3), 397–415.

Milinkeviciute, G., Muniak, M., Pongstaporn, T., Cho, A., & Ryugo, D. (2015). Circuitry between the dorsal cochlear nucleus and the inferior colliculus in the mouse. *Journal of the Association for Research in Otolaryngology* Abs.:44

Moore, C. N., Casseday, J. H., & Neff, W. D. (1974). Sound localization: The role of the commissural pathways of the auditory system of the cat. *Brain Research*, *82*(1), 13–26.

Moore, D. R. (1988). Auditory brainstem of the ferret: Sources of projections to the inferior colliculus. *Journal of Comparative Neurology*, *269*(3), 342–354.

Moore, D. R., Kotak, V. C., & Sanes, D. H. (1998). Commissural and lemniscal synaptic input to the gerbil inferior colliculus. *Journal of Neurophysiology*, *80*(5), 2229–2236.

Moore, R. Y., & Goldberg, J. M. (1966). Projections of the inferior colliculus in the monkey. *Experimental Neurology*, *14*(4), 429–438.

Morest, D. K., & Oliver, D. L. (1984). The neuronal architecture of the inferior colliculus in the cat: defining the functional anatomy of the auditory midbrain. *Journal of Comparative Neurology*, *222*(2), 209–236.

Nakagawa, H., Ikeda, M., Houtani, T., Ueyama, T., Baba, K., Kondoh, A., . . . Sugimoto, T. (1995). Immunohistochemical evidence for enkephalin and neuropeptide Y in rat inferior colliculus neurons that provide ascending or commissural fibers. *Brain Research*, *690*(2), 236–240.

Nakamoto, K. T., Sowick, C. S., & Schofield, B. R. (2013). Auditory cortical axons contact commissural cells throughout the guinea pig inferior colliculus. *Hearing Research*, *306*(Supplement C), 131–144.

Needham, K., & Paolini, A. G. (2006). Neural timing, inhibition and the nature of stellate cell interaction in the ventral cochlear nucleus. *Hearing Research*, *216–217*, 31–42.

Okoyama, S., Ohbayashi, M., Ito, M., & Harada, S. (2006). Neuronal organization of the rat inferior colliculus participating in four major auditory pathways. *Hearing Research*, *218*(1–2), 72–80.

Olazabal, U. E., & Moore, J. K. (1989). Nigrotectal projection to the inferior colliculus: Horseradish peroxidase transport and tyrosine hydroxylase immunohistochemical studies in rats, cats, and bats. *Journal of Comparative Neurology*, *282*(1), 98–118.

Oliver, D. L. (1984). Neuron types in the central nucleus of the inferior colliculus that project to the medial geniculate-body. *Neuroscience*, *11*(2), 409–424.

Oliver, D. L. (2005). Neuronal organisation of the inferior colliculus. In J. A. Winer & C. E. Schreiner (Eds.), *The Inferior Colliculus* (pp. 69–114). New York, NY: Springer.

Oliver, D. L., & Morest, D. K. (1984). The Central Nucleus of the Inferior Colliculus in the Cat. *Journal of Comparative Neurology, 222*(2), 237–264.

Orton, L. D., Papasavvas, C. A., & Rees, A. (2016). Commissural Gain Control Enhances the Midbrain Representation of Sound Location. *Journal of Neuroscience, 36*(16), 4470–4481.

Orton, L. D., Poon, P. W. F., & Rees, A. (2012). Deactivation of the inferior colliculus by cooling demonstrates intercollicular modulation of neuronal activity. *Frontiers in Neural Circuits, 6(100),1*–15. doi: 10.3389/fncir.2012.00100

Orton, L. D., & Rees, A. (2014). Intercollicular commissural connections refine the representation of sound frequency and level in the auditory midbrain. *eLife, 3*,e03764.

Palmer, A. R., Shackleton, T. M., Sumner, C. J., Zobay, O., & Rees, A. (2013). Classification of frequency response areas in the inferior colliculus reveals continua not discrete classes. *Journal of Physiology, 591*(16), 4003–4025.

Powell, E. W., & Hatton, J. B. (1969). Projections of the inferior colliculus in cat. *Journal of Comparative Neurology, 136*(2), 183–192.

Rees, A., & Palmer, A. R. (1988). Rate-intensity functions and their modification by broadband noise for neurons in the guinea-pig inferior colliculus. *Journal of the Acoustical Society of America, 83*(4), 1488–1498.

Reetz, G., & Ehret, G. (1999). Inputs from three brainstem sources to identified neurons of the mouse inferior colliculus slice. *Brain Research, 816*(2), 527–543.

Robinson, B. L., & McAlpine, D. (2009). Gain control mechanisms in the auditory pathway. *Current Opinion in Neurobiology, 19*(4), 402–407.

Rockel, A. J., & Jones, E. G. (1973). Observations on the fine structure of the central nucleus of the inferior colliculus of the cat. *Journal of Comparative Neurology, 147*(1), 61–92.

Rose, J. E., Greenwood, D. D., Goldberg, J. M., & Hind, J. E. (1963). Some discharge characteristics of single neurons in the inferior colliculus of the cat. I. Tonotopical organization, relation of spike-counts to tone intensity, and firing patterns of single elements. *Journal of Neurophysiology, 26*, 294–320.

Saint Marie, R. L. (1996). Glutamatergic connections of the auditory midbrain: Selective uptake and axonal transport of D-[3H]aspartate. *Journal of Comparative Neurology, 373*(2), 255–270.

Saldaña, E., Aparicio, M. A., Fuentes-Santamaría, V., & Berrebi, A. S. (2009). Connections of the superior paraolivary nucleus of the rat: Projections to the inferior colliculus. *Neuroscience, 163*(1), 372–387.

Saldana, E., Feliciano, M., & Mugnaini, E. (1996). Distribution of descending projections from primary auditory neocortex to inferior colliculus mimics the topography of intracollicular projections. *Journal of Comparative Neurology, 371*(1), 15–40.

Saldaña, E., & Merchán, M. (2005). Intracollicular connections. In J. A. Winer & C. Schreiner (Eds.), *The Inferior Colliculus* (pp. 155–181). New York, NY: Springer.

Saldana, E., & Merchán, M. A. (1992). Intrinsic and commissural connections of the rat inferior colliculus. *Journal of Comparative Neurology, 319*(3), 417–437.

Saldaña, E., Viñuela, A., Marshall, A. F., Fitzpatrick, D. C., & Aparicio, M. A. (2007). The TLC: A novel auditory nucleus of the mammalian brain. *Journal of Neuroscience, 27*(48), 13108–13116.

Schofield, B. R., & Cant, N. B. (1996). Origins and targets of commissural connections between the cochlear nuclei in guinea pigs. *Journal of Comparative Neurology, 375*(1), 128–146.

Sherrington, C. S. (1906). *The integrative action of the nervous system*. New Haven, CT: Yale University Press.

Shneiderman, A., Oliver, D. L., & Henkel, C. K. (1988). Connections of the dorsal nucleus of the lateral lemniscus: An inhibitory parallel pathway in the ascending auditory-system. *Journal of Comparative Neurology*, *276*(2), 188–208.

Shore, S. E., Godfrey, D. A., Helfert, R. H., Altschuler, R. A., & Bledsoe, S. C. (1992). Connections between the cochlear nuclei in guinea pig. *Hearing Research*, *62*(1), 16–26.

Smith, P. H. (1992). Anatomy and physiology of multipolar cells in the rat inferior collicular cortex using the in vitro brain slice technique. *Journal of Neuroscience*, *12*(9), 3700–3715.

Suga, N., & Ma, X. F. (2003). Multiparametric corticofugal modulation and plasticity in the auditory system. *Nature Reviews Neuroscience*, *4*(10), 783–794.

Torterolo, P., Zurita, P., Pedemonte, M., & Velluti, R. A. (1998). Auditory cortical efferent actions upon inferior colliculus unitary activity in the guinea pig. *Neuroscience Letters*, *249*(2–3), 172–176.

van Adel, B. A., Kidd, S. A., & Kelly, J. B. (1999). Contribution of the commissure of Probst to binaural evoked responses in the rat's inferior colliculus: interaural time differences. *Hearing Research*, *130*(1–2), 115–130.

van Noort, J. (1969). *The structure and connections of the inferior colliculus. An investigation of the lower auditory system.* Assen, Netherlands: Van Gorcum.

Wallace, M. N., Shackleton, T. M., & Palmer, A. R. (2012). Morphological and physiological characteristics of laminar cells in the central nucleus of the inferior colliculus. *Frontiers in Neural Circuits*, *6*, 55.

Whitley, J. M., & Henkel, C. K. (1984). Topographical organization of the inferior collicular projection and other connections of the ventral nucleus of the lateral lemniscus in the cat. *Journal of Comparative Neurology*, *229*(2), 257–270.

Willard, F. H., & Martin, G. F. (1984). Collateral innervation of the inferior colliculus in the North American opossum: A study using fluorescent markers in a double-labeling paradigm. *Brain Research*, *303*(1), 171–182.

Winer, J. A., Chernock, M. L., Larue, D. T., & Cheung, S. W. (2002). Descending projections to the inferior colliculus from the posterior thalamus and the auditory cortex in rat, cat, and monkey. *Hearing Research*, *168*(1–2), 181–195.

Winer, J. A., Saint Marie, R. L., Larue, D. T., & Oliver, D. L. (1996). GABAergic feedforward projections from the inferior colliculus to the medial geniculate body. *Proceedings of the National Academy of Sciences of the United States of America*, *93*(15), 8005–8010.

Woollard, H. H., & Harpman, J. A. (1940). The connexions of the inferior colliculus and of the dorsal nucleus of the lateral lemniscus. *Journal of Anatomy*, *74*(4), 441–458.

Zhang, D. X., Li, L., Kelly, J. B., & Wu, S. H. (1998). GABAergic projections from the lateral lemniscus to the inferior colliculus of the rat. *Hearing Research*, *117*(1–2), 1–12.

CHAPTER 21

NEUROMODULATORY FEEDBACK TO THE INFERIOR COLLICULUS

LAURA HURLEY

Abstract

The inferior colliculus (IC) receives prominent projections from centralized neuromodulatory systems. These systems include extra-auditory clusters of cholinergic, dopaminergic, noradrenergic, and serotonergic neurons. Although these modulatory sites are not explicitly part of the auditory system, they receive projections from primary auditory regions and are responsive to acoustic stimuli. This bidirectional influence suggests the existence of auditory-modulatory feedback loops. A characteristic of neuromodulatory centers is that they integrate inputs from anatomically widespread and functionally diverse sets of brain regions. This connectivity gives neuromodulatory systems the potential to import information into the auditory system on situational variables that accompany acoustic stimuli, such as context, internal state, or experience. Once released, neuromodulators functionally reconfigure auditory circuitry through a variety of receptors expressed by auditory neurons. In addition to shaping ascending auditory information, neuromodulation within the IC influences behaviors that arise subcortically, such as prepulse inhibition of the startle response. Neuromodulatory systems therefore provide a route for integrative behavioral information to access auditory processing from its earliest levels.

Keywords: acetylcholine, dopamine, norepinephrine, serotonin, noradrenaline, auditory, midbrain

The inferior colliculus (IC) is an auditory crossroads. It receives ascending and descending inputs from auditory regions, contains functional domains defined by projections from specific auditory brainstem nuclei or by particular neurotransmitters, and responds to non-auditory events (Bajo & King, 2012; Bulkin & Groh, 2012; Choy Buentello et al., 2015; Lesicko et al., 2016; Loftus et al., 2010; Patel et al,. 2017; Zhou &

Shore 2006). Projections from these different sources converge at the level of the IC to create or refine responses to acoustic stimuli. The IC further stages ascending and descending projections to auditory as well as non-auditory targets (Bartlett, 2013; Coomes & Schofield, 2004; Ito et al., 2009; Peruzzi et al., 1997; Schofield & Cant, 1999). Because of its centrality to these converging and diverging pathways, the IC is an important site for regulatory control.

There is a growing appreciation that regulation of the excitatory-inhibitory circuitry in the IC and other auditory regions can allow auditory processing to dynamically adjust to behavioral context, internal state, or experience (Charitidi & Canlon, 2010; Hurley & Hall, 2011; Weinberger, 2015). One important mechanism underlying this type of regulation is neuromodulation (Schofield & Hurley, 2018). The process of neuromodulation has been defined in different ways. Definitions are based on the identity and source of modulatory neurochemicals, the structure of synapses releasing neuromodulators, or the action of neuromodulatory receptors through second messenger systems (Maley et al., 1990; Marder, 2012; Nadim & Bucher, 2014). A useful functional perspective is based on a longstanding view of neuromodulators as reconfiguring the neural circuitry mediated by excitatory and inhibitory amino acid neurotransmitters like glutamate, GABA, and glycine. This chapter will focus on four types of neurochemicals that can fit one or more of these definitions: acetylcholine and the monoamines serotonin, norepinephrine, and dopamine. The effects of these neuromodulators in the auditory system follow basic principles that have been intensively studied for some time in motor systems (Marder, 2012), and are becoming more widely understood as an integral component of auditory processing (see Schofield & Beebe, this volume; Schofield & Hurley, 2018).

For the most part, this chapter will deal with neuromodulation by discrete groups of neurons that are extrinsic to the auditory system. It is important to note, however, that sources of neurochemical signals like acetylcholine and dopamine are also intrinsic components of auditory circuitry in the brainstem, which underlie feedback to early stages of auditory processing (Elgoyhen & Katz, 2012; Mulders & Robertson, 2004; Sherriff & Henderson, 1994). Auditory-extrinsic neuromodulatory centers show some striking functional similarities. One of these is their broad interaction with other neural sites. Neuromodulatory centers interconnect extensively with many other brain regions, including sensory, motor, and integrative sites (Benarroch, 2013; Lee et al., 2003; Luppi et al., 1995; Pollak Dorocic et al., 2014; Reese et al., 1995b; Retson & Van Bockstaele, 2013; Wang et al., 2006). These connections place neuromodulatory centers in position to instruct the auditory system on events in nonauditory brain regions.

All of the neuromodulatory regions discussed here also receive input from the auditory system, or possess populations of neurons that respond to acoustic stimuli (Aston-Jones & Bloom, 1981; Yasui et al., 1990; Reese et al., 1995a; Rasmussen et al., 1986; Heym et al., 1982). This reciprocity suggests that neuromodulatory systems could present a type of feedback to auditory neurons. A useful parallel model consists of descending pathways from the auditory cortex and IC, which are prominent features of auditory circuitry that provide feedback to the IC and auditory brainstem (e.g., Caicedo & Herbert, 1993); Schofield & Beebe, this volume). By virtue of their extensive connectivity with integrative brain regions that "interpret" external events, neuromodulatory systems could import information into the auditory system on situational variables that accompany acoustic stimuli, such as context, state, or salience (Petersen & Hurley, 2017).

The following sections present established and recent findings on neuromodulation in the IC and brainstem auditory nuclei in the framework of a feedback model. These sections emphasize major characteristics of auditory neuromodulation that are consistent with a feedback model, starting with the sources of neuromodulatory input, which originate in a diversity of neuron groups. In many cases, modulatory neurons are sensitive to acoustic stimuli, but represent "value-added" versions of these stimuli. The topography of terminal fields of neuromodulatory projections in the IC and brainstem auditory nuclei are specific and functionally suggestive. Once released from these projections, neuromodulatory signals within auditory regions encode information on behavioral salience. These neuromodulatory signals further multiplex information on external and internal events that occur on different time scales. Finally, neuromodulators functionally reconfigure auditory circuitry and alter behavioral responses to auditory stimulation.

Sources of Neuromodulatory Input to the IC and Auditory Brainstem

Ways to Trace Neuromodulatory Sources

As prominent neuroanatomical features of the auditory system, neuromodulators in the IC and auditory brainstem have been studied for decades. Descriptions of modulatory projections to auditory brainstem nuclei based on histochemical reactions predate the use of selective labels for specific neurochemical pathways (Dahlstrom & Fuxe, 1964; Kromer & Moore, 1976; Levitt & Moore, 1979). The development of antibodies directed against specific monoamines, their synthetic enzymes, or selective transporters used in combination with tract tracing or selective neurotoxins has allowed for the sources of specific neuromodulatory inputs to the IC and many auditory brainstem nuclei to be identified (Hormigo et al., 2012; Klepper & Herbert, 1991; Motts & Schofield, 2009; Mulders & Robertson, 2005a). These studies portray a diverse set of neuromodulatory sources to the auditory system that in some cases have defied assumptions regarding their identity (Nevue et al., 2016a). This diversity is suggestive of a rich functional capability.

The extrinsic sources of neuromodulatory inputs to the IC and auditory brainstem have been extensively reviewed, for either single modulatory pathways (Schofield et al., 2011) or multiple pathways (Schofield & Hurley, 2018); this literature is therefore only briefly summarized here. Identifying modulatory sources typically involves retrograde or anterograde anatomical tracing, often accompanied by neurochemical identification of modulatory fibers or cell bodies (Klepper & Herbert, 1991; Motts & Schofield, 2009; Nevue et al., 2016a). Neurochemical identification has proven especially crucial, because most neuromodulatory nuclei house non-modulatory neurons that also project to the IC and auditory brainstem but use GABA or other neurotransmitters (Boucetta & Jones, 2009; Klepper & Herbert, 1991; Motts & Schofield, 2009; Nevue et al., 2016a; Vasudeva et al. 2011).

Where are Auditory Neuromodulators From?

There are multiple sources of cholinergic inputs to the IC and auditory brainstem nuclei. The cochlear nucleus receives inputs from cholinergic neurons in the auditory ventral nucleus of the trapezoid body, as well as tegmental cholinergic neurons in the pontomesencephalic tegmentum (Mellott et al., 2011). The IC itself receives projections from the pontomesencephalic cholinergic groups (Dautan et al., 2016; Motts & Schofield, 2009). An additional group of non-auditory cholinergic neurons projecting to the IC is found in the rostral ventrolateral medullary region (Stornetta et al., 2013). As a comparison, cholinergic innervation of the primary auditory cortex arises mainly from the basal forebrain (Bajo et al., 2014; Kamke et al., 2005). Thus, although many auditory sites receive cholinergic terminals, acetylcholine could be released under very different circumstances across auditory regions, depending on the source.

For other neuromodulatory pathways, the IC shares a dominant source with brainstem auditory nuclei. The IC and cochlear nucleus receive a majority of serotonergic projections from the dorsal raphe nucleus, with smaller although still substantial contributions from other raphe groups (Klepper & Herbert, 1991). The IC, cochlear nucleus, and superior olivary complex all receive noradrenergic input from the locus coeruleus (Klepper & Herbert, 1991; Mulders & Robertson, 2001). The understanding of dopaminergic innervation of the IC has changed with the addition of selective co-labels for the synthetic enzyme for dopamine. Although the dopaminergic substantia nigra projects to the IC (Olazábal & Moore, 1989), these projections may not be from dopaminergic neurons (Nevue et al., 2016a). Instead, some authors have suggested that the projections from substantia nigra to the IC are GABAergic (Maisonnette et al., 1996; Nobre et al., 2004). The IC and regions within the superior olivary complex receive dopaminergic projections from the subparafascicular nucleus (Nevue et al., 2016a, 2016b).

Hidden Diversity Within Neuromodulatory Sources

These findings together suggest that sources of cortical versus subcortical modulatory input are different for acetylcholine and dopamine, but similar for serotonin and norepinephrine. Even for seemingly universal modulatory sources like the dorsal raphe nucleus and locus coeruleus, however, there may be hidden variability, because these large modulatory centers are far from homogeneous (Calizo et al., 2011; Chandler et al.,

2014a; Chandler et al., 2014b). In the dorsal raphe nucleus, subgroups of serotonergic neurons are distinguished by their position along rostrocaudal, mediolateral, and dorsoventral axes. Neurons in these different groups have afferent, efferent, and intrinsic distinctions (Calizo et al., 2011; Jacobs et al., 1978; Janusonis et al., 1999; Kirifides et al., 2001; Lee et al., 2003; Peyron et al., 1998; Van Bockstaele et al., 1993). For example, overlapping but distinct groups of dorsal raphe and locus coeruleus neurons project to cortical versus subcortical sensory sites (Kirifides et al., 2001; Waterhouse et al., 1993). In the locus coeruleus, subsets of noradrenergic neurons with distinct terminal fields show differential gene expression and electrophysiological characteristics (Chandler et al., 2014a).

Subpopulations of modulatory neurons may also be defined by their receptivity to other neurochemicals and their functional projections. For example, Pet1-positive dorsal raphe neurons expressing dopamine D2 receptors are involved in regulating aggressive behavior and project to a specific set of targets, sending strong projections to the IC and other auditory regions (Niederkofler et al., 2016). In general, although there is ample evidence that neuromodulatory centers have functionally distinct subsets of neurons, and of topographic organization of projections from neuromodulatory centers (Waterhouse et al., 1993; Waterhouse et al., 1986), the functional topographies of modulatory projections to the auditory system have not yet been well characterized.

Neuromodulatory Neurons Receive Auditory and Nonauditory Inputs

Auditory Inputs

The connectivity and firing patterns of modulatory neurons provide one way of assessing the conditions that could trigger the release of neuromodulators within the auditory system. Consistent with a feedback model, all of the neuromodulatory regions relevant to this chapter either receive input from auditory regions (Figure 21.1), or respond to simple auditory stimuli like clicks and tones. Projections from different auditory regions to the pontomesencephalic tegmental nuclei or the subparafascicular nucleus have been well-documented (inferior colliculus: Wang et al., 2006; Yasui et al., 1990; medial geniculate body: LeDoux et al., 1985; auditory cortex: Schofield & Motts, 2009; Schofield, 2010; Yasui et al., 1990); some of these are described in detail in the chapter by Schofield and Beebe, in this volume. Pontomesencephalic tegmental neurons further show extremely short latency responses to clicks (< 10 ms) as well as longer-latency responses, although the auditory-responsive neurons have not been chemically identified (Reese et al., 1995a). Responses of neurons in the serotonergic dorsal raphe nucleus and noradrenergic locus coeruleus to auditory stimuli have been reported for decades (Aston-Jones & Bloom, 1981; Foote et al., 1980; Heym et al., 1982; Shima et al.,

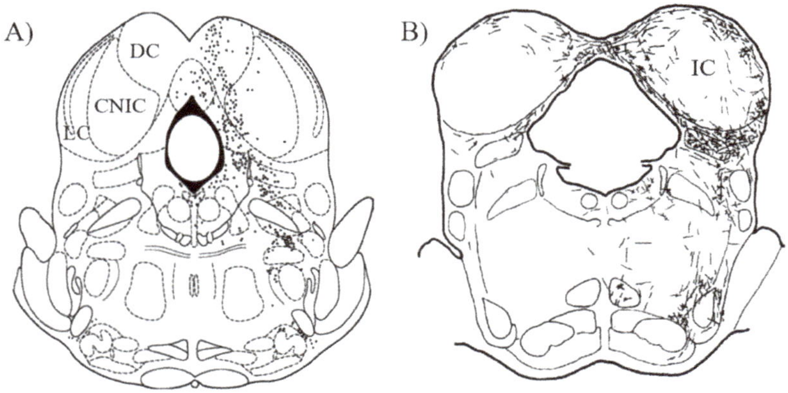

FIGURE 21.1. Evidence of anatomical connections between auditory and modulatory regions. A) Cell bodies labeled after placement of a retrograde tracer in the subparafascicular nucleus in rat. Subdivisions of the IC are labeled (LC = lateral cortex; CNIC = central nucleus of the IC; DC = dorsal cortex). (Adapted from Wang et al., 2006.) B) Fibers labeled by placement of an anterograde tracer in the magnocellular portion of the subparafascicular nucleus in rat. (Adapted from Yasui et al., 1992.) Note that projections are not neurochemically identified.

1986), and serotonergic dorsal raphe neurons receive monosynaptic inputs from the external subregion of the IC (Pollak Dorocic et al., 2014).

Nonauditory Inputs

Auditory inputs constitute only a subset of the inputs into neuromodulatory nuclei, however. These nuclei typically receive extensive projections from a wide range of brain regions. The pontomesencephalic tegmental cholinergic nuclei are notably interconnected with motor control regions, as well as with hypothalamic regions involved in sleep/wake regulation (Benarroch, 2013). The subparafascicular nucleus, which contains dopaminergic neurons, is interconnected with regions that regulate reproductive behavior (Wang et al., 2006). The dorsal raphe nucleus and locus coeruleus likewise receive afferents from a wide range of brain regions representing many different functional domains, including areas important to cognitive function, social behavior, affective state, and stress (e.g., Lee et al., 2003; Luppi et al., 1995; Pollak Dorocic et al., 2014; Retson & Van Bockstaele, 2013).

Diverse Inputs Create Integrative Responses

Corresponding to this wide range of afferents, the auditory responsiveness of neurons in modulatory areas does not simply indicate the presence of auditory stimuli, but corresponds to additional factors such as internal state. Behavioral arousal is a state often associated with neuromodulators of all types. This includes arousal associated with phases of the sleep-wake cycle. The activity patterns of modulatory neurons are frequently tied to the sleep-wake cycle (Boucetta & Jones, 2009; Foote et al., 1980; Lorincz & Adamantidis, 2017; Motts & Schofield, 2009). Higher tonic firing rates typically occur during waking states, although firing rates may vary among modulatory systems during different sleep states. Internal states other than arousal are also represented within neuromodulatory axes, in that neuromodulatory activity depends on factors like social status and reproductive state (Challis et al., 2013; Hall et al., 2012; Hanson & Hurley, 2016; Korzan & Summers, 2007; Matragrano et al., 2012a; Matragrano et al., 2012b). Neuromodulatory systems may therefore not only modulate the tone of neural activity in sensory systems according to the level of behavioral arousal, but also promote optimal processing as it relates to specific internal states.

Across internal states, it is clear that neuromodulatory neurons integrate auditory and nonauditory sources of information about specific events. Modulatory neurons are often polysensory, responding to stimuli in multiple modalities (e.g., Aston-Jones & Bloom, 1981; Heym et al., 1982). Modulatory neurons also represent the salience of acoustic stimuli, a phenomenon that is well demonstrated by the responsiveness of modulatory neurons to reward contingencies. Extrinsic reward or the natural salience associated with acoustic stimuli affect the responses of neurons in multiple modulatory centers (Fischer & Ullsperger, 2017; Maney, 2013). In the locus coeruleus, for example, pairing tones with foot shock can create frequency-selective responses to tones alone even when tones do not initially evoke responses at all (Martins & Froemke, 2015). The responses of neuromodulatory neurons to acoustic stimuli therefore often represent the behavioral significance of these stimuli.

Neuromodulatory Inputs Broadly Innervate the IC and Auditory Brainstem

What Does it Mean to Project Diffusely?

Modulatory neurons are often described as projecting diffusely. This is true in the sense that modulatory fibers take apparently nondirect pathways through neural tissue and typically have many release sites along their length (Janusonis, 2017). These release sites may contain synaptic specializations, or be asynaptic. The latter configuration has been associated with the volume release of neuromodulators. In this mode, neuromodulators may diffuse some distance from their release sites before binding to receptors or transporters (Bunin & Wightman, 1998; Eid et al., 2013; Fuxe et al., 2015;

but see Sarter et al., 2009 for a discussion of the controversy surrounding the concepts of volume versus synaptic transmission of acetylcholine). Although the synaptic configurations of neuromodulatory release sites have not been examined ultrastructurally in the IC, many serotonergic varicosities that form basket terminals around GABAergic neurons in the auditory cortex show only weak synaptic specializations (DeFelipe et al., 1991).

Neuromodulatory Fiber Patterns are Selective

At the same time, modulatory fibers selectively innervate different subregions of the IC and auditory brainstem nuclei, or even specific layers, neural subgroups, or functionally distinct domains. On the broadest scale, some auditory brainstem nuclei seem to be relatively devoid of particular types of neuromodulatory inputs. For example, in the superior olivary complex of mice, the lateral superior olive does not receive dopaminergic innervation from the subparafascicular nucleus (Nevue et al., 2016b), and the guinea pig superior olivary complex as a whole receives few dopaminergic fibers (Mulders & Robertson, 2005a). The densities of serotonergic and noradrenergic fibers are generally higher in periolivary regions than in olivary nuclei themselves, although some fibers are present within olivary nuclei (e.g., Mulders & Robertson, 2005a; Thompson & Schofield, 2000; Wynne & Robertson, 1996). The MNTB shows a species-specific pattern of innervation by serotonergic fibers, which are present in bat but very scattered in mouse and cat (Hurley & Thompson, 2001; Thompson & Hurley, 2004; Thompson & Schofield, 2000).

In some species, neuromodulatory fiber densities correspond to tonotopic organization. Serotonergic fibers are denser in the regions corresponding to low-frequency responses than to high-frequency responses in the bat lateral and medial superior olives (Hurley & Thompson, 2001). Catecholaminergic fibers similarly are denser in the low-frequency regions of bat cochlear nucleus (Kössl et al., 1988). This pattern suggests that serotonin and norepinephrine or dopamine may modulate responses of low-frequency neurons more than those of high-frequency neurons. Interestingly, although the same frequency-variable pattern of fibers is not observed in mice (Kössl et al., 1988; Thompson & Hurley, 2004), the mouse auditory brainstem response is generally more sensitive to serotonergic perturbation when stimuli consist of low-frequency tones compared to high-frequency tones, providing some functional support for frequency-selective modulatory effects (Papesh & Hurley, 2016).

Another type of pattern is for neuromodulatory inputs to be densest in integrative multimodal regions of auditory nuclei. Of the major subdivisions of the IC, serotonergic, noradrenergic, and dopaminergic fibers are denser in some pericentral subregions than in the central subdivision, although modulatory fibers are also clearly found within the central nucleus (Fyk-Kolodziej et al., 2015; Hormigo et al., 2012; Hurley & Thompson, 2001; Klepper & Herbert, 1991; Nevue et al. 2016a; Papesh and Hurley 2012; Figure 21.2). This pattern is also seen in the cochlear nucleus, in which the dorsal cochlear nucleus

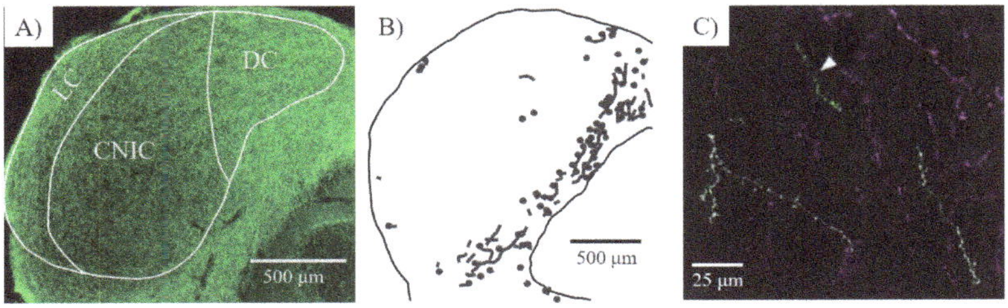

FIGURE 21.2. Projections from neuromodulatory regions to the IC. A) Dense plexus of fibers labeled with an antibody to the serotonin transporter, which labels the projections of serotonergic neurons with high specificity. (Adapted from Keesom & Morningstar et al., 2018.) B) Locations of fibers (lines) and varicosities (circles) from virally labeled cholinergic fibers originating in the rostral ventrolateral medulla in mouse. Symbols represent the locations, but not the dimensions, of fibers and varicosities. Adapted from Stornetta et al. 2013. C) Fibers in the central subdivision of the IC labeled by placement of an anterograde tracer in the subparafascicular nucleus in mouse (green) and by an antibody to tyrosine hydroxylase (purple). Co-labeled fibers appear white. Arrow indicates fiber from the subparafascicular nucleus that is not catecholaminergic. (Adapted from Nevue et al., 2016a.)

has denser serotonergic and catecholaminergic inputs than ventral subdivisions in some species (Klepper & Herbert, 1991; Kössl et al., 1988; Thompson & Thompson, 2001). These findings suggest that one role of multiple types of neuromodulators is to regulate the convergence of ascending auditory input with descending auditory input or nonauditory inputs (Hurley & Thompson, 2001; Klepper & Herbert, 1991). This hypothesis has received functional support in the case of serotonin, which alters the balance of auditory versus polysensory input at the level of fusiform neurons of the dorsal cochlear nucleus (Tang & Trussell, 2017).

Modulatory fibers even selectively innervate specific cellular layers or groups. In both the pericentral IC and the dorsal cochlear nucleus, noradrenergic fibers are sparsest in the outermost layer and denser in other layers, while serotonergic fibers show a reversed pattern; that is, are densest in the most external layer (Klepper & Herbert. 1991). These patterns are suggestive of layer-specific, complementary functions of different types of neuromodulators. Layer 2 of the lateral subregion of the IC exhibits a particularly intriguing structure of repeated neurochemical modules that co-localize acetylcholinesterase as well as cytochrome oxidase, NADPH, and glutamic acid decarboxylase (Chernock et al., 2004; Lesicko et al., 2016). Cholinergic inputs may therefore participate in a distinct neurochemical complex in these domains, which are the termination sites for somatosensory inputs (Lesicko et al., 2016). Specific neuron types also show selective anatomical targeting and functional effects of neuromodulation. In the ventral cochlear nucleus, T-stellate cells, but not D-stellate cells, are sensitive to cholinergic agonists (Fujino & Oertel, 2001). Olivocochlear neurons within the superior olivary complex are also particular targets of multiple types of neuromodulators including norepinephrine, serotonin, and peptide transmitters (Behrens et al., 2002; Mulders & Robertson, 2005a; 2000; Thompson & Schofield, 2000; Woods & Azeredo, 1999). Functionally, neurons in olivocochlear regions are responsive to application of norepinephrine and serotonin, with complementary effects on their descending targets (Mulders & Robertson, 2005b; Wang & Robertson, 1997).

All of these patterns are consistent with neuromodulatory systems targeting different kinds of anatomical domains. Although some evidence supports the functional hypotheses that arise from these patterns, these hypotheses have not been tested in many cases.

Neuromodulatory Activity in the IC and Auditory Brainstem

How is Neuromodulatory Activity in the Auditory System Measured?

The broad responsiveness of neurons within modulatory centers, combined with the prominent projections from these areas to auditory regions, creates the confusing potential for many different types of information to be imported into the auditory system. A way to resolve this ambiguity is to directly measure neuromodulatory activity under different behavioral circumstances. These types of measurements have been accomplished by microdialysis or localized tissue collection followed by HPLC measurement of neuromodulators and their major metabolites (Cransac et al., 1998; Matragrano et al., 2012b). Additionally, antibodies specific for activated forms of modulatory synthetic enzymes, or carbon fiber voltammetry, can capture neuromodulatory activity (Hall et al., 2010; Matragrano et al., 2012a). Most of the studies in this area have assessed either serotonergic or noradrenergic activity on relatively broad spatial and temporal scales rather than on the scale of synaptic events.

Acoustic and Nonacoustic Stimuli Influence Neuromodulatory Activity

Absolute changes in the levels of serotonin and norepinephrine and their major metabolites have been measured in the cochlear nucleus, IC, and auditory cortex following exposure to noise. These show activation of modulatory pathways that is specific to particular auditory nuclei and their subregions, and that varies with sound level. For example, noise alters the ratios of serotonin and norepinephrine relative to their metabolites in tissue containing both the dorsal and posteroventral cochlear nuclei, but not in the anteroventral cochlear nucleus (Cransac et al., 1998). These ratios are generally interpreted as an indication of modulatory release and subsequent metabolism, termed "turnover." Modulatory turnover is dependent on the intensity of noise; noradrenergic turnover in the cochlear nucleus and serotonergic turnover in the auditory cortex are only seen at relatively low intensities. Voltammetric measurements suggest that serotonergic activity increases modestly in the IC with moderate noise levels (Hall et al., 2010). In neither of these studies was the relationship of noise exposure to levels of systemic stress explored. However, nonauditory stressors including confinement to a small arena also increase serotonergic activity in the IC (Hall et al., 2010; Hall et al., 2012; Hanson & Hurley, 2014). Glucocorticoids do not directly evoke this release, since the systemic injection of corticosterone has no effect on serotonergic activity (Hall et al., 2012). Not all purported inducers of stress influence auditory serotonin, however. The presentation of an olfactory stressor, a chemical component of fox urine that induces strong aversive responses in mice, does not significantly alter serotonergic activity in the IC (Hall et al., 2010). Thus, increases in neuromodulatory activity in the IC in response to simple stimuli, even stimuli that share threatening qualities, are quite selective.

Neuromodulatory Activity During Social Interaction

A more complex context that increases serotonergic activity in the IC of mice is presentation of a social partner. Serotonergic increases occur across a range of different types of encounters: in males interacting males or females (Hall et al., 2011; Hurley & Hall, 2011; Keesom & Hurley, 2016) and females interacting with males (Hanson & Hurley, 2014). Within each of these types of encounters, across-individual variation in serotonergic activity corresponds to variation in behavior. In male-male interactions, for example, serotonergic activity correlates with social investigation by the experimental subjects, and with overall movement (Hall et al., 2011). Males that are more active and more socially investigative show the largest serotonergic increases. In contrast, serotonergic activity in males interacting with females correlates inversely with the rejection behaviors of the female partners, but not with behaviors of the subject males (Keesom & Hurley, 2016). Individual males that experience the most rejection, including female-produced broadband vocalizations ("squeaks"), do not show serotonergic increases. In this case, serotonin levels inversely correspond to a specific type of auditory stimulus (female-produced squeaks) and are more representative of the valence, or positive versus negative behavioral value, of the situation for individual males.

Internal State and Experience Play a Role

Serotonergic pathways within the IC are also capable of multiplexing information about behaviorally relevant events that occur on different timescales. This is accomplished through plasticity at different levels of the serotonergic system. For example, internal state is one factor that is encoded by serotonin release. Serotonergic activity in the IC increases as animals recover from anesthesia (Hall et al., 2010). This may be due to increased firing rates of neurons in the dorsal raphe nucleus (Sakai & Crochet,

2001). Reproductive cycles may also induce long-term changes in the infrastructure of serotonin in the auditory midbrain. Implanting female white-throated sparrows with estradiol, which would normally increase during their breeding season, augments the density of serotonergic fibers in an avian auditory midbrain nucleus that is a homolog of the IC (Matragrano et al., 2012b). In a parallel study in males, treatment with testosterone to mimic breeding levels results in a decrease in both serotonergic and noradrenergic fibers in the auditory midbrain (Matragrano et al., 2013). Seasonally breeding fish also experience neuromodulatory plasticity in both the auditory periphery and central auditory system (Forlano & Sisneros, 2016). Reproductively related changes in neuromodulation are not limited to seasonally reproducing animals. In female lab mice, the effects of manipulating serotonin levels on immediate early gene activity in the IC depends on the naturally cycling estrous phase (Hanson & Hurley, 2016). This result suggests change at the level of responsiveness to serotonin release, potentially in the expression of serotonin receptors by IC neurons. Neuromodulatory systems are therefore regulated at times when acoustic social signals have particular significance for reproduction.

Experience of multiple kinds also alters serotonergic infrastructure. Monaural acoustic trauma alters the bilateral balance of serotonergic fibers in the IC, decreasing fibers in the IC contralateral to trauma relative to the ipsilateral side (Papesh & Hurley, 2012). Bilateral cochlear ablation likewise decreases the density of fibers immunoreactive for tyrosine hydroxylase, a synthetic enzyme for dopamine and norepinephrine (Tong et al., 2005). Binaural acoustic trauma or ablation, as well as age-associated hearing loss, upregulate or downregulate the expression of several types of serotonin receptors in the IC relative to controls (Holt et al., 2005; Smith et al., 2014; Tadros et al., 2007). This includes at least one type of receptor that is expressed strongly in the IC as measured both immunohistochemically and by ligand binding studies, the 5-HT_{1A} receptor (Peruzzi & Dut, 2004; Smith et al., 2014; Thompson et al., 1994). This evidence suggests that serotonin receptor expression by auditory neurons is altered following hearing loss. The effects of acoustic trauma and hearing loss on modulatory systems therefore occur at levels that are both presynaptic and postsynaptic to modulatory fibers within the IC.

Postweaning social isolation is another class of experience that alters serotonergic activity in the IC (Keesom et al., 2017). Male mice housed in same-sex social groups versus in isolation for a period of weeks after the time of weaning show two key differences when acutely challenged with an unfamiliar social partner. Individually housed mice have more sluggish serotonergic responses that peak later than those of socially housed mice, although their relative amplitudes do not differ. Individually housed mice also do not exhibit the correlations between serotonergic activity and behavior that are typical for socially housed mice (Hall et al., 2011; Keesom et al., 2017). Thus, serotonin release may be dysregulated relative to variation in the social context for mice with less social experience.

Together, these types of studies illustrate that neuromodulatory activity in auditory regions does not faithfully represent acoustic stimuli, but instead may encode the value

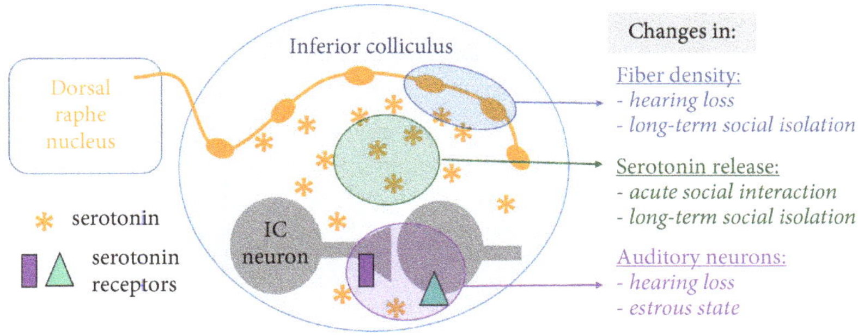

FIGURE 21.3. External events, internal state, and experience alter the serotonergic modulatory system within the IC at multiple levels. Schematic representation of serotonergic projections from the dorsal raphe nucleus to the IC. Behaviorally relevant variables alter serotonergic fiber density (orange line), serotonin availability (asterisks), and the expression of serotonin receptors (purple and green shapes) by IC neurons.

of particular situations, internal state, and different kinds of experience. These factors may be represented at multiple levels of modulatory systems, including in the level of modulatory release and responsiveness, and in neuromodulatory infrastructure including the density of fibers and receptor expression (Figure 21.3)

Neuromodulators Functionally Reconfigure Auditory Circuitry

Once released in the IC and auditory brainstem, neuromodulators have profound effects; all four neurochemicals discussed in this chapter influence the firing patterns or response properties of substantial proportions of IC neurons. These effects fit a classic model of neuromodulators as reconfiguring neural circuitry by targeting specific aspects of cellular function (Harris-Warrick & Johnson, 2010; Marder & Bucher, 2007).

Receptors Determine Modulatory Effects

The effects of neuromodulatory release on the intrinsic properties and sound-evoked responses of auditory neurons depend upon the types of receptors expressed by target neurons (Hurley & Sullivan, 2012). For example, many neuromodulators have suppressive effects on neural firing for some IC neurons, and facilitatory effects for others (e.g., acetylcholine: Habbicht & Vater, 1996; serotonin: Hurley & Pollak, 1999; dopamine: Gittelman et al., 2013). In some cases, these differences are positively attributable to the activation of different receptor types. For acetylcholine, a nicotinic antagonist increases neural activity while a broad-spectrum muscarinic antagonist generally decreases activity (Habbicht & Vater, 1996). There is further diversity even among muscarinic receptor subtypes, since m1 and m2 muscarinic acetylcholine receptor antagonists have different effects. For serotonin, selective agents for receptors in at least three of the seven receptor families have characteristic suppressive or facilitatory physiological effects on sound-evoked responses (Bohorquez & Hurley, 2009; Hurley, 2007, 2006). This general phenomenon of multiple types of effects of single neuromodulators is widespread, and is also observed in a number of auditory brainstem nuclei (e.g., Ebert, 1996; Ebert & Ostwald, 1992; Kössl & Vater, 1989; Wang & Robertson, 1997). Rather than canceling each other out, such opposing effects may result in greater selectivity for specific inputs at the level of auditory microcircuitry, may shape temporal responses, or may stabilize new circuit configurations (Harris-Warrick & Johnson, 2010; Kössl & Vater, 1989; Tang & Trussell, 2017).

Neural Phenotypes Influence Modulatory Effects

The effects of neuromodulators also depend on the identities of neurons expressing the relevant receptors. Given the importance of inhibitory inputs in the IC to the response properties of IC neurons (Pollak, 2013; Pollak et al., 2002; Pollak et al., 2011), neuromodulation of inhibition has been a particular focus for some studies. There is robust evidence for modulation of GABAergic and glycinergic inputs to IC neurons by both acetylcholine and serotonin. In slice preparations, activation of muscarinic receptors or 5-HT_2 receptors creates a dramatic increase in the frequency of spontaneous GABAergic inhibitory postsynaptic currents, and a 5-HT_2 agonist also increases their amplitude (Wang et al., 2008; Yigit et al., 2003). Serotonin also increases the frequency of glycinergic postsynaptic currents, although not as dramatically (Obara et al., 2014). Because some of these effects can be prevented by blocking action potentials with tetrodotoxin, these increases in inhibitory activity are thought to represent enhanced spontaneous firing of presynaptic inhibitory neurons. It is not clear whether these effects are limited to a specific developmental phase, as are similar effects of serotonin in the lateral superior olive (Fitzgerald & Sanes, 1999).

The 5-HT_{1B} receptor may also act through inhibitory neurons. This receptor increases sound-evoked activity of many IC neurons (Baldan Ramsey et al., 2010; Hurley, 2006; Hurley et al., 2008). In other brain regions, the 5-HT_{1B} receptor generally acts by limiting synaptic transmission, and its effects in the IC are reduced in the presence of a $GABA_A$ receptor agonist, consistent with effects of the 5-HT_{1B} receptor on presynaptic GABAergic neurons (Hurley et al., 2008; Sari, 2004). Likewise, although the D_2 receptor is the predominant dopamine receptor type in the IC, dopamine application to the IC has heterogeneous effects, potentially by influencing presynaptic GABAergic neurons (Gittelman et al., 2013). Although inhibition is clearly an important functional target of neuromodulation in the IC, neuromodulators likely influence the activity of non-GABAergic neurons too (Hurley & Sullivan, 2012; Peruzzi & Dut, 2004).

Subcellular Targets

Neuromodulators selectively target specific subcellular compartments; this type of selectivity has been most thoroughly explored in different auditory brainstem nuclei. At the Calyx of Held, both norepinephrine acting via α2 adrenergic receptors and serotonin acting via 5-HT_{1B} receptors limit calcium influx presynaptically at early developmental stages, resulting in reduced release of glutamate (Leão & Von Gersdorff, 2002; Mizutani et al., 2006). Neuromodulators can also alter intrinsic excitability by changing the membrane potential (Goyer et al., 2016; Miko & Sanes, 2009). Further, neuromodulators selectively alter neural output. For cartwheel cells in the dorsal cochlear nucleus, dopaminergic D_3 receptors shift firing patterns from a bursting to a regular-firing mode by decreasing T-type calcium current selectively in the axon initial segment (Bender et al., 2010, 2012). For MSO neurons, activation of 5-HT_{1A} receptors hyperpolarizes the membrane potential in the axon initial segment and decreases spike threshold (Ko et al., 2016). These selective effects occur partly through targeting particular types of ion currents. For example, the activation curve of the hyperpolarization-activated, cyclic nucleotide- gated cation current is shifted by norepinephrine in the MNTB and the avian nucleus laminaris (Banks et al., 1993; Yamada et al., 2005), and by serotonin in the MSO and DCN (Ko et al., 2016; Tang & Trussell, 2015).

Functional Outcomes of Targeted Effects

In the IC, this range of selective modulatory mechanisms results in the transformation of functional response properties. Neuromodulators commonly alter the spontaneous or evoked firing rates of IC neurons in response to stimuli (Curtis & Koizumi, 1961; Gittelman et al., 2013; Hurley et al., 2004; Hurley & Pollak, 1999). Neuromodulators also alter firing patterns (Gittelman et al., 2013; Habbicht & Vater, 1996), latency or latency jitter (Felix et al., 2017; Gittelman et al., 2013; Hurley, 2007; Hurley & Pollak, 2005b), or selectively alter frequency tuning (Hurley & Pollak, 2001). These types of changes can contribute to shifts in neural selectivity for spectrotemporally divergent sounds, such as tones versus FM sweeps (Hurley & Pollak, 1999), sounds of different frequency (Hurley et al., 2004; Hurley & Pollak, 2001) or different species-specific vocalizations (Hurley & Pollak, 2005a).

Responses of IC neurons to temporally complex stimuli are also altered by neuromodulation. Ionotropic 5-HT_3 receptors are responsible for a seconds-long depolarization of a few millivolts in baseline membrane potential following stimulus barrage to lemniscal inputs. This depolarization increases the gain of the neural response to a single stimulus of the input fibers (Miko & Sanes, 2009). In vivo, the same receptor type causes responses to different acoustic stimulus rates to become more similar (Bohorquez & Hurley, 2009). For neurons that show stimulus-specific adaptation, acetylcholine equalizes responses between rare and common stimuli by decreasing adaptation to the common stimulus (Ayala & Malmierca, 2015; Ayala et al., 2016). These types of effects demonstrate that neuromodulators regulate the responses to local auditory context.

A superb example of how neuromodulatory effects at the level of multiple auditory neurons within a microcircuit combine to create functionally coherent change is seen for the effects of serotonin in the dorsal cochlear nucleus. Serotonin acts through multiple receptor types and multiple cell types converging on fusiform cells to enhance multisensory responses and dampen auditory-only responses (Tang & Trussell, 2017, 2015). These types of combinatorial processes also occur in the IC. For example, 5-HT_{1A} and 5-HT_{1B} receptors both influence the responses of high proportions of neurons, but in opposite ways. Activation of 5-HT_{1A} receptors often reduces responses to acoustic stimuli and delays spikes, consistent with suppression of excitability in other brain regions by this receptor (Hurley, 2007; 2006; Ohno, 2010). In contrast, 5-HT_{1B} activation usually increases the responses of IC neurons to acoustic stimuli, consistent with a presynaptic reduction of GABAergic transmission (Hurley et al., 2008; Sari, 2004). Some IC neurons respond to activation of both of these types of receptors (Baldan Ramsey et al., 2010). For these double-responsive neurons, the effects of activating both receptor types on spike rate is linear, in that large effects of a given receptor type alone correspond to large effects when applied in combination. However, effects on spike latency are dominated by the 5-HT_{1A} receptor. Thus, different types of neuromodulatory receptor may combine in nonlinear ways to create distinct profiles of neural activity.

Neuromodulators do not Act Alone

Creating additional potential for complex regulatory effects, different neuromodulatory systems also interact with each other. In some auditory regions, neuromodulatory systems are activated during some of the same events, including associative training (dopamine and serotonin: Stark & Scheich, 1997) or exposure to noise (norepinephrine and serotonin: Cransac et al., 1998; Hall et al., 2010). In each of these cases, although multiple neuromodulators are activated in the same general stimulus paradigm, the patterns of neuromodulatory release across stimulus conditions or across auditory regions are distinct. Profiles of release across different neuromodulators could therefore be more informative than for any single neuromodulator. At the level of auditory neurons and the receptors that they express, specific neuron types in the auditory brainstem and midbrain are the targets of multiple neuromodulatory systems (e.g., cartwheel cells: (Bender et al., 2010; He et al., 2014; Kuo & Trussell, 2011), calyx of Held: (Leão & Von Gersdorff, 2002; Mizutani et al., 2006). A very few studies have also documented responsiveness of the same individual auditory neurons to multiple types of neuromodulators (Hurley et al., 2004; McCormick & Pape, 1990). Different neuromodulatory systems therefore are likely to collaborate in their influence on auditory circuitry.

Behavioral Functions of Neuromodulation in in the IC

Building and testing hypotheses for the perceptual outcomes of auditory neuromodulation requires reconciling the exceptional breadth of neuromodulatory capabilities with specific behavioral contexts and auditory circuits (Linster & Cleland, 2016). A well-explored and well-reviewed example of the influence of neuromodulators on auditory perception is plasticity in responses to the pairing of tones with aversive stimuli like shock. Multiple types of neuromodulators, including acetylcholine, dopamine, and norepinephrine, alter the representation of frequency in auditory cortex and may change behavior following associative learning in parallel (Bao et al., 2001; Martins & Froemke, 2015; Weinberger, 2015). In the auditory cortex, local modulation with a peptide neurotransmitter, oxytocin, also alters neural responses in step with maternal responses to pup calls (Marlin et al., 2015).

Neuromodulatory Regulation of Aversion

Through effects in the IC, neuromodulation influences several classes of behaviors. These include unconditioned and conditioned aversion. Electrical or chemical stimulation of the central subdivision of the IC induces a variety of unconditioned fearful or aversive behaviors, including arousal, freezing, and escape behaviors (Brandão et al., 1994; Brandão et al., 1999). IC stimulation can even serve as an unconditioned aversive stimulus in operant conditioning paradigms in which animals leave a chamber to discontinue the stimulus (Melo & Brandão, 1995). These findings have led to a model of the IC as part of a mesencephalic substrate for defensive behaviors, along with regions of the periaqueductal gray and superior colliculus (Brandão et al., 1999). Local injection of neuromodulators or their specific receptor agonists or antagonists into the IC can modify these defensive behaviors. Zimelidine, a serotonin reuptake inhibitor, reduces the number and increases the latency of conditioned aversive behaviors when it is injected into the IC (Brandão et al., 1993; Melo and Brandão 1995). Injection of 5-HT_{1A} or 5-HT_{2A} agonists have similar effects, consistent with the prevalence of each of these receptor types in the IC (Melo & Brandão, 1995; Peruzzi & Dut, 2004; Smith et al., 2014; Thompson et al., 1994; Wang et al., 2008). Injection of sulpiride, a D_2 dopaminergic receptor antagonist, into the IC increases avoidance of open arms in the elevated plus maze as well as the amplitude of the auditory evoked potential recorded locally in the IC (de Oliveira et al., 2014). Thus, multiple neuromodulatory systems dampen aversive behavioral responses to stimulation of the IC.

Neuromodulatory Regulation of Prepulse Inhibition

Auditory prepulse inhibition is another phenomenon in which the IC plays an important role (Gomez-Nieto et al., 2008; Li & Yue, 2002; Yeomans et al., 2006). The startle response to an acoustic stimulus can be reduced by a non-startling transient prepulse or by electrical stimulation of the IC, and is also disrupted by lesion of the IC (Leitner & Cohen, 1985; Li et al., 1998a; Li et al., 1998b). This suppression may protect the response to the initial sound (prepulse), and involves specific subcortical circuitry in which the IC contributes information about the prepulse (Carlson & Willott, 1998; Fendt et al., 2001; Leitner & Cohen, 1985; Li & Yue, 2002). Cholinergic pathways originating in the pontomesencephalic tegmentum are also important to this circuit (Fendt et al., 2001; Koch et al., 1993). Consistent with this model, local effects of neuromodulators in the IC alter prepulse inhibition. Unilateral injection of 2,5-Dimethoxy-4-iodoamphetamine, an agonist of 5-HT_2 receptors, reduces prepulse inhibition but does not affect the amplitude of the acoustic startle response itself (de Oliveira et al., 2017). The injection of D_2 agonists into the IC induces similar effects (Satake et al., 2012).

All together, these findings show that in addition to being a site for the modulation of ascending auditory information, the IC is involved in subcortical circuitry that modifies responses to potentially threatening stimuli. Multiple types of neuromodulators can influence these defensive behaviors through local effects within the IC.

Do Neuromodulatory Systems Really Provide Feedback to Auditory Circuits?

The previous sections illustrate that auditory and modulatory regions are anatomically interconnected. Despite this evidence, it would not be an accurate reflection of a broad body of literature to say that neuromodulatory systems simply channel instructive feedback to the auditory system. One reason for this is that modulatory systems are both downstream and upstream of integrative brain regions such as the prefrontal cortex, amygdala, hypothalamic nuclei, or bed nucleus of the stria terminalis (Benarroch, 2013; Lee et al., 2003; Luppi et al., 1995; Mena-Segovia & Bolam, 2017; Parent et al., 1981; Pollak Dorocic et al., 2014; Retson & Van Bockstaele, 2013). Modulatory systems may therefore play an important role in establishing, as well as distributing, information regarding stimulus salience.

A second way that neuromodulatory systems violate a linear model of auditory feedback circuitry is illustrated by a widely expressed anatomical feature of modulatory neurons: they often send collateral projections to divergent targets. These collaterals can potentially couple modulatory signals in different auditory regions. Dopaminergic neurons in the subparafascicular nucleus, cholinergic neurons in the pedunculopontine tegmental nucleus, and noradrenergic neurons in the locus coeruleus all send collaterals to multiple auditory targets (Klepper & Herbert, 1991; Nevue et al., 2016b; Schofield et al., 2011). As might be expected from this pattern of projections, the effects of neuromodulators at different levels interact. For example, acetylcholine applied locally to the IC influences auditory cortical plasticity, and vice versa (Ma & Suga, 2005). Many collaterals of modulatory neurons are even more divergently projecting, targeting not only sensory regions, but non-sensory regions too (e.g., Lee et al., 2009; Villar et al., 1988). This pattern could result in neuromodulatory release under the same conditions in functionally divergent brain regions. As an example, serotonin levels in both the IC and the preoptic area increase when male rodents interact with females, and depend on the females being sexually available (Fumero et al., 1994; Keesom & Hurley, 2016; Mas et al., 1995). Neuromodulatory systems are therefore capable of broadly coordinating neural activity across sensory, motor, and motivational systems.

Interactions Among the IC, Amygdala, and Modulatory Systems

The functional entanglement that arises from these types of interactions is highlighted by a series of studies illustrating the modulatory control of unconditioned aversive behavior evoked by stimulation of the IC. As described earlier, electrical stimulation of the IC evokes aversive behavior, and local injection of serotonergic and dopaminergic agents into the IC dampen some of these aversive behavioral responses. The amygdala is another site that regulates aversive behaviors and that interacts with the IC, in which neuromodulators influence behavioral output. Lesion of the central amygdala increases aversive thresholds to stimulation of the IC but lesion of the basolateral amygdala decreases them (Maisonnette et al., 1996). This finding is consistent with a model of the amygdala as downstream of the IC in the regulation of aversive behaviors. Modulatory nuclei may also act as functional intermediaries between the IC and amygdala, in that stimulation of the IC causes increased release of serotonin and dopamine within the basolateral amygdala, although less in the central amygdala (Macedo et al., 2005). The actions of serotonin and dopamine in the amygdala exert complex effects on defensive behavior. The local injection of serotonergic and dopaminergic antagonists within the basolateral amygdala dampens conditioned place aversion but enhances unconditioned aversion in response to chemical stimulation of the IC (Macedo et al., 2007). Likewise, selective neurochemical lesion of serotonergic fibers in the central amygdala increases thresholds for alertness, freezing, and escape behavior caused by IC stimulation, while neurochemical lesion within the basolateral complex decreases thresholds for these behaviors (Macedo et al., 2002). Finally, anatomical pathways from the amygdala to the IC suggest an additional route for direct amygdalo-collicular feedback (Marsh et al., 2002). Functionally, manipulation of inhibitory neurotransmission in the amygdala

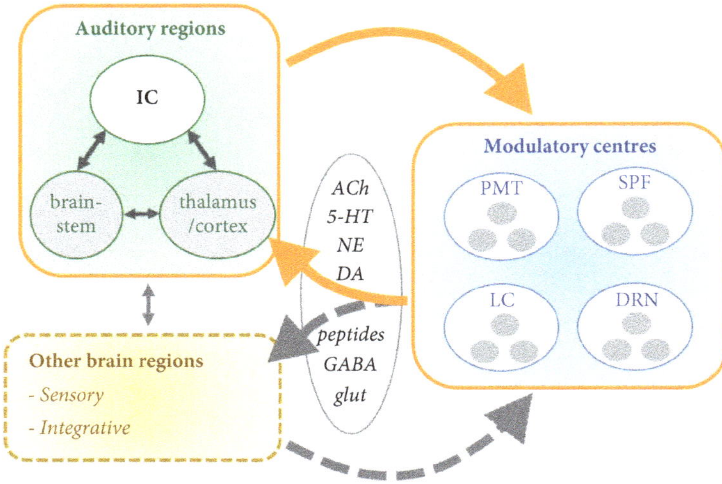

FIGURE 21.4. Schematic diagram illustrating some of the connections among auditory, modulatory, and other brain regions. Feedback loop between auditory and modulatory regions is emphasized by solid orange outlines and arrows. ACh = acetylcholine; 5-HT = serotonin; NE = norepinephrine; DA = dopamine; glut = glutamate; PMT = pontomesencephalic tegmentum; SPF = subparafascicular nucleus; LC = locus coeruleus; DRN = dorsal raphe nucleus.

alters the amplitude of locally measured auditory evoked potentials in the IC (Nobre & Brandão, 2011). Arising from these somewhat complicated results is an important general point. It is not simply the case that the auditory system and neuromodulatory systems mutually influence each another, a point made at length in this chapter. Rather, recursive connections among auditory, interpretive, and modulatory systems all interact to regulate behavior (Figure 21.4)

Conclusion: Neuromodulators Are a Substrate for Auditory and Nonauditory Integration

Understanding the actions of neuromodulatory pathways in the auditory system requires thinking about the auditory system from its earliest levels as anatomically and functionally interwoven with non-auditory regions of the brain. Neuromodulatory systems channel integrative information to the auditory system, providing the potential for auditory circuits to adjust their activity to conform to salient events, internal state, or experience. Auditory neuromodulation influences behavioral responses to sound, but the importance of modulatory pathways to behavior depends on the circuitry underlying specific behavioral tasks, the functional connectivity between modulatory subgroups and auditory regions, and the behavioral context. A circuit-based approach will therefore be crucial to better understanding auditory neuromodulation and the roles that modulatory processes play in perception and behavior.

The extensive interactions between auditory and modulatory regions also potentially give auditory neurons the power to mediate the transformation between external events and internal representations such as valence or salience (Petersen & Hurley, 2017). In part through the influence of modulatory systems, auditory neurons may be active participants in extracting information relevant to specific contexts, states, or histories of individuals, and consequently have a profound influence on behavioral output. Ultimately, mutual influence by auditory and interpretive systems may optimally shape behavior to best match the dynamics of an animal's internal and external environments.

References

Aston-Jones, G., & Bloom, F. E. (1981). Norepinephrine-containing locus coeruleus neurons in behaving rats exhibit pronounced responses to non-noxious environmental stimuli. *Journal of Neuroscience*, *1*(8), 887–900.

Ayala, Y. A., & Malmierca, M. S. (2015). Cholinergic modulation of stimulus-specific adaptation in the inferior colliculus. *Journal of Neuroscience*, *35*(35), 12261–12272. doi:10.1523/JNEUROSCI.0909-15.2015

Ayala, Y. A., Perez-Gonzalez, D., & Malmierca, M. S. (2016). Stimulus-specific adaptation in the inferior colliculus: The role of excitatory, inhibitory and modulatory inputs. *Biological Psychology*, *116*, 10–22. doi:10.1016/j.biopsycho.2015.06.016

Bajo, V. M., & King, A. J. (2012). Cortical modulation of auditory processing in the midbrain. *Frontiers in Neural Circuits*, *6*, 114. doi:10.3389/fncir.2012.00114

Bajo, V. M., Leach, N. D., Cordery, P. M., Nodal, F. R., & King, A. J. (2014). The cholinergic basal forebrain in the ferret and its inputs to the auditory cortex. *European Journal of Neuroscience*, *40*(6), 2922–2940. doi:10.1111/ejn.12653

Baldan Ramsey, L. C., Sinha, S. R., & Hurley, L. M. (2010). 5-HT1A and 5-HT1B receptors differentially modulate rate and timing of auditory responses in the mouse inferior colliculus. *European Journal of Neuroscience*, *32*(3), 368–379. doi:10.1111/j.1460-9568.2010.07299.x

Banks, M. I., Pearce, R. A., & Smith, P. H. (1993). Hyperpolarization-activated cation current (Ih) in neurons of the medial nucleus of the trapezoid body: Voltage-clamp analysis and enhancement by norepinephrine and cAMP suggest a modulatory mechanism in the auditory brain stem. *Journal of Neurophysiology*, *70*(4), 1420–1432. doi:10.1152/jn.1993.70.4.1420

Bao, S., Chan, V. T., & Merzenich, M. M. (2001). Cortical remodelling induced by activity of ventral tegmental dopamine neurons. *Nature*, *412*(6842), 79–83. doi:10.1038/35083586

Bartlett, E. L. (2013). The organization and physiology of the auditory thalamus and its role in processing acoustic features important for speech perception. *Brain and Language*, *126*(1), 29–48. doi:10.1016/j.bandl.2013.03.003

Behrens, E. G., Schofield, B. R., & Thompson, A. M. (2002). Aminergic projections to cochlear nucleus via descending auditory pathways. *Brain Research*, *955*(1–2), 34–44.

Benarroch, E. E. (2013). Pedunculopontine nucleus: Functional organization and clinical implications. *Neurology*, *80*(12), 1148–1155. doi:10.1212/WNL.0b013e3182886a76

Bender, K. J., Ford, C. P., & Trussell, L. O. (2010). Dopaminergic modulation of axon initial segment calcium channels regulates action potential initiation. *Neuron, 68*(3), 500–511. doi:10.1016/j.neuron.2010.09.026

Bender, K. J., Uebele, V. N., Renger, J. J., & Trussell, L. O. (2012). Control of firing patterns through modulation of axon initial segment T-type calcium channels. *Journal of Physiology, 590*(1), 109–118. doi:10.1113/jphysiol.2011.218768

Bohorquez, A., & Hurley, L. M. (2009). Activation of serotonin 3 receptors changes in vivo auditory responses in the mouse inferior colliculus. *Hearing Research, 251*(1–2), 29–38. doi:10.1016/j.heares.2009.02.006

Boucetta, S., & Jones, B. E. (2009). Activity profiles of cholinergic and intermingled GABAergic and putative glutamatergic neurons in the pontomesencephalic tegmentum of urethane-anesthetized rats. *Journal of Neuroscience, 29*(14), 4664–4674. doi:10.1523/JNEUROSCI.5502-08.2009

Brandão, M. L., Anseloni, V. Z., Pandóssio, J. E., De Araújo, J. E., & Castilho, V. M. (1999). Neurochemical mechanisms of the defensive behavior in the dorsal midbrain. *Neuroscience and Biobehavioral Reviews, 23*(6), 863–875.

Brandão, M. L., Cardoso, S. H., Melo, L. L., Motta, V., & Coimbra, N. C. (1994). Neural substrate of defensive behavior in the midbrain tectum. *Neuroscience and Biobehavior Reviews, 18*(3), 339–346.

Brandão, M. L., Melo, L. L., & Cardoso, S. H. (1993). Mechanisms of defense in the inferior colliculus. *Behavioural Brain Research, 58*(1–2), 49–55.

Bulkin, D. A., & Groh, J. M. (2012). Distribution of visual and saccade related information in the monkey inferior colliculus. *Frontiers in Neural Circuits, 6*, 61. doi:10.3389/fncir.2012.00061

Bunin, M. A., & Wightman, R. M. (1998). Quantitative evaluation of 5-hydroxytryptamine (serotonin) neuronal release and uptake: an investigation of extrasynaptic transmission. *Journal of Neuroscience, 18*(13), 4854–4860.

Caicedo, A., & Herbert, H. (1993). Topography of descending projections from the inferior colliculus to auditory brainstem nuclei in the rat. *Journal of Comparative Neurology, 328*(3), 377–392. doi:10.1002/cne.903280305

Calizo, L. H., Akanwa, A., Ma, X., Pan, Y. Z., Lemos, J. C., Craige, C., . . . Beck, S. G. (2011). Raphe serotonin neurons are not homogenous: electrophysiological, morphological and neurochemical evidence. *Neuropharmacology, 61*(3), 524–543. doi:10.1016/j.neuropharm.2011.04.008

Carlson, S., & Willott, J. F. (1998). Caudal pontine reticular formation of C57BL/6J mice: responses to startle stimuli, inhibition by tones, and plasticity. *Journal of Neurophysiology, 79*(5), 2603–2614. doi:10.1152/jn.1998.79.5.2603

Challis, C., Boulden, J., Veerakumar, A., Espallergues, J., Vassoler, F. M., Pierce, R. C., . . . Berton, O. (2013). Raphe GABAergic neurons mediate the acquisition of avoidance after social defeat. *Journal of Neuroscience, 33*(35), 13978–13988, 13988a. doi:10.1523/JNEUROSCI.2383-13.2013

Chandler, D. J., Gao, W. J., & Waterhouse, B. D. (2014a). Heterogeneous organization of the locus coeruleus projections to prefrontal and motor cortices. *Proceedings of the National Academy of Sciences of the United States of America, 111*(18), 6816–6821. doi:10.1073/pnas.1320827111

Chandler, D. J., Waterhouse, B. D., & Gao, W. J. (2014b). New perspectives on catecholaminergic regulation of executive circuits: evidence for independent modulation of prefrontal functions by midbrain dopaminergic and noradrenergic neurons. *Frontiers in Neural Circuits, 8*, 53. doi:10.3389/fncir.2014.00053

Charitidi, K., & Canlon, B. (2010). Estrogen receptors in the central auditory system of male and female mice. *Neuroscience, 165*(3), 923–933. doi:10.1016/j.neuroscience.2009.11.020

Chernock, M. L., Larue, D. T., & Winer, J. A. (2004). A periodic network of neurochemical modules in the inferior colliculus. *Hearing Research, 188*(1–2), 12–20. doi:10.1016/S0378-5955(03)00340-X

Choy Buentello, D., Bishop, D. C., & Oliver, D. L. (2015). Differential distribution of GABA and glycine terminals in the inferior colliculus of rat and mouse. *Journal of Comparative Neurology, 523*(18), 2683–2697. doi:10.1002/cne.23810

Coomes, D. L., & Schofield, B. R. (2004). Separate projections from the inferior colliculus to the cochlear nucleus and thalamus in guinea pigs. *Hearing Research, 191*(1–2), 67–78. doi:10.1016/j.heares.2004.01.009

Cransac, H., Cottet-Emard, J. M., Hellstrom, S., & Peyrin, L. (1998). Specific sound-induced noradrenergic and serotonergic activation in central auditory structures. *Hearing Research, 118*(1–2), 151–156.

Curtis, D. R., & Koizumi, K. (1961). Chemical transmitter substances in brain stem of cat. *Journal of Neurophysiology, 24*, 80–90. doi:10.1152/jn.1961.24.1.80

Dahlstrom, A., & Fuxe, K. (1964). Localization of monoamines in the lower brain stem. *Experientia, 20*(7), 398–399.

Dautan, D., Hacioglu Bay, H., Bolam, J. P., Gerdjikov, T. V., & Mena-Segovia, J. (2016). Extrinsic sources of cholinergic innervation of the striatal complex: A whole-brain mapping analysis. *Frontiers in Neuroanatomy, 10*, 1. doi:10.3389/fnana.2016.00001

DeFelipe, J., Hendry, S. H., Hashikawa, T., & Jones, E. G. (1991). Synaptic relationships of serotonin-immunoreactive terminal baskets on GABA neurons in the cat auditory cortex. *Cerebral Cortex, 1*(2), 117–133.

de Oliveira, A. R., Colombo, A. C., Muthuraju, S., Almada, R. C., & Brandao, M. L. (2014). Dopamine D2-like receptors modulate unconditioned fear: Role of the inferior colliculus. *PLoS One, 9*(8), e104228. doi:10.1371/journal.pone.0104228

de Oliveira, R. P., Nagaishi, K. Y., & Barbosa Silva, R. C. (2017). Atypical antipsychotic clozapine reversed deficit on prepulse inhibition of the acoustic startle reflex produced by microinjection of DOI into the inferior colliculus in rats. *Behavioural Brain Research, 325*(Pt A), 72–78. doi:10.1016/j.bbr.2017.01.053

Ebert, U. (1996). Noradrenalin enhances the activity of cochlear nucleus neurons in the rat. *European Journal of Neuroscience, 8*(6), 1306–1314.

Ebert, U., & Ostwald, J. (1992). Serotonin modulates auditory information processing in the cochlear nucleus of the rat. *Neuroscience Letters, 145*(1), 51–54.

Eid, L., Champigny, M. F., Parent, A., & Parent, M. (2013). Quantitative and ultrastructural study of serotonin innervation of the globus pallidus in squirrel monkeys. *European Journal of Neuroscience, 37*(10), 1659–1668. doi:10.1111/ejn.12164

Elgoyhen, A. B., & Katz, E. (2012). The efferent medial olivocochlear-hair cell synapse. *Journal of Physiology Paris, 106*(1–2), 47–56. doi:10.1016/j.jphysparis.2011.06.001

Felix, R. A., 2nd, Elde, C. J., Nevue, A. A., & Portfors, C. V. (2017). Serotonin modulates response properties of neurons in the dorsal cochlear nucleus of the mouse. *Hearing Research, 344*, 13–23. doi:10.1016/j.heares.2016.10.017

Fendt, M., Li, L., & Yeomans, J. S. (2001). Brain stem circuits mediating prepulse inhibition of the startle reflex. *Psychopharmacology (Berlin), 156*(2–3), 216–224.

Fischer, A. G., & Ullsperger, M. (2017). An Update on the Role of Serotonin and its Interplay with Dopamine for Reward. *Frontiers in Human Neuroscience, 11*, 484. doi:10.3389/fnhum.2017.00484

Fitzgerald, K. K., & Sanes, D. H. (1999). Serotonergic modulation of synapses in the developing gerbil lateral superior olive. *Journal of Neurophysiology, 81*(6), 2743–2752. doi:10.1152/jn.1999.81.6.2743

Foote, S. L., Aston-Jones, G., & Bloom, F. E. (1980). Impulse activity of locus coeruleus neurons in awake rats and monkeys is a function of sensory stimulation and arousal. *Proceedings of the National Academy of Sciences of the United States of America, 77*(5), 3033–3037.

Forlano, P. M., & Sisneros, J. A. (2016). Neuroanatomical evidence for catecholamines as modulators of audition and acoustic behavior in a vocal teleost. *Advances in Experimental Medical Biology, 877*, 439–475. doi:10.1007/978-3-319-21059-9_19

Fujino, K., & Oertel, D. (2001). Cholinergic modulation of stellate cells in the mammalian ventral cochlear nucleus. *Journal of Neuroscience, 21*(18), 7372–7383.

Fumero, B., Fernandez-Vera, J. R., Gonzalez-Mora, J. L., & Mas, M. (1994). Changes in monoamine turnover in forebrain areas associated with masculine sexual behavior: a microdialysis study. *Brain Research, 662*(1–2), 233–239.

Fuxe, K., Agnati, L. F., Marcoli, M., & Borroto-Escuela, D. O. (2015). Volume Transmission in Central Dopamine and Noradrenaline Neurons and Its Astroglial Targets. *Neurochemistry Research, 40*(12), 2600–2614. doi:10.1007/s11064-015-1574-5

Fyk-Kolodziej, B. E., Shimano, T., Gafoor, D., Mirza, N., Griffith, R. D., Gong, T. W., & Holt, A. G. (2015). Dopamine in the auditory brainstem and midbrain: co-localization with amino acid neurotransmitters and gene expression following cochlear trauma. *Frontiers in Neuroanatomy, 9*, 88. doi:10.3389/fnana.2015.00088

Gittelman, J. X., Perkel, D. J., & Portfors, C. V. (2013). Dopamine modulates auditory responses in the inferior colliculus in a heterogeneous manner. *Journal of the Association of Research Otolaryngology, 14*(5), 719–729. doi:10.1007/s10162-013-0405-0

Gomez-Nieto, R., Rubio, M. E., & Lopez, D. E. (2008). Cholinergic input from the ventral nucleus of the trapezoid body to cochlear root neurons in rats. *Journal of Comparative Neurology, 506*(3), 452–468. doi:10.1002/cne.21554

Goyer, D., Kurth, S., Gillet, C., Keine, C., Rubsamen, R., & Kuenzel, T. (2016). Slow cholinergic modulation of spike probability in ultra-fast time-coding sensory neurons. *eNeuro, 3*(5). doi:10.1523/ENEURO.0186-16.2016

Habbicht, H., & Vater, M. (1996). A microiontophoretic study of acetylcholine effects in the inferior colliculus of horseshoe bats: implications for a modulatory role. *Brain Research, 724*(2), 169–179.

Hall, I. C., Rebec, G. V., & Hurley, L. M. (2010). Serotonin in the inferior colliculus fluctuates with behavioral state and environmental stimuli. *Journal of Experimental Biology, 213*(Pt 7), 1009–1017. doi:10.1242/jeb.035956

Hall, I. C., Sell, G. L., Chester, E. M., & Hurley, L. M. (2012). Stress-evoked increases in serotonin in the auditory midbrain do not directly result from elevations in serum corticosterone. *Behavioural Brain Research, 226*(1), 41–49. doi:10.1016/j.bbr.2011.08.042

Hall, I. C., Sell, G. L., & Hurley, L. M. (2011). Social regulation of serotonin in the auditory midbrain. *Behavioral Neuroscience, 125*(4), 501–511. doi:10.1037/a0024426

Hanson, J. L., & Hurley, L. M. (2014). Context-dependent fluctuation of serotonin in the auditory midbrain: the influence of sex, reproductive state and experience. *Journal of Experimental Biology, 217*(Pt 4), 526–535. doi:10.1242/jeb.087627

Hanson, J. L., & Hurley, L. M. (2016). Serotonin, estrus, and social context influence c-Fos immunoreactivity in the inferior colliculus. *Behavioral Neuroscience, 130*(6), 600–613. doi:10.1037/bne0000165

Harris-Warrick, R. M., & Johnson, B. R. (2010). Checks and balances in neuromodulation. *Frontiers in Behavioral Neuroscience, 4*. doi:10.3389/fnbeh.2010.00047

He, S., Wang, Y. X., Petralia, R. S., & Brenowitz, S. D. (2014). Cholinergic modulation of large-conductance calcium-activated potassium channels regulates synaptic strength and spine calcium in cartwheel cells of the dorsal cochlear nucleus. *Journal of Neuroscience, 34*(15), 5261–5272. doi:10.1523/JNEUROSCI.3728-13.2014

Heym, J., Trulson, M. E., & Jacobs, B. L. (1982). Raphe unit activity in freely moving cats: effects of phasic auditory and visual stimuli. *Brain Research, 232*(1), 29–39.

Holt, A. G., Asako, M., Lomax, C. A., MacDonald, J. W., Tong, L., Lomax, M. I., & Altschuler, R. A. (2005). Deafness-related plasticity in the inferior colliculus: gene expression profiling following removal of peripheral activity. *Journal of Neurochemistry, 93*(5), 1069–1086. doi:10.1111/j.1471-4159.2005.03090.x

Hormigo, S., Horta Junior Jde, A., Gomez-Nieto, R., & Lopez, D. E. (2012). The selective neurotoxin DSP-4 impairs the noradrenergic projections from the locus coeruleus to the inferior colliculus in rats. *Frontiers in Neural Circuits, 6*, 41. doi:10.3389/fncir.2012.00041

Hurley, L. M. (2006). Different serotonin receptor agonists have distinct effects on sound-evoked responses in inferior colliculus. *Journal of Neurophysiology, 96*(5), 2177–2188. doi:10.1152/jn.00046.2006

Hurley, L. M. (2007). Activation of the serotonin 1A receptor alters the temporal characteristics of auditory responses in the inferior colliculus. *Brain Research, 1181*, 21–29. doi:10.1016/j.brainres.2007.08.053

Hurley, L. M., Devilbiss, D. M., & Waterhouse, B. D. (2004). A matter of focus: Monoaminergic modulation of stimulus coding in mammalian sensory networks. *Current Opinion in Neurobiology, 14*(4), 488–495. doi:10.1016/j.conb.2004.06.007

Hurley, L. M., & Hall, I. C. (2011). Context-dependent modulation of auditory processing by serotonin. *Hearing Research, 279*(1–2), 74–84. doi:10.1016/j.heares.2010.12.015

Hurley, L. M., & Pollak, G. D. (1999). Serotonin differentially modulates responses to tones and frequency-modulated sweeps in the inferior colliculus. *Journal of Neuroscience, 19*(18), 8071–8082.

Hurley, L. M., & Pollak, G. D. (2001). Serotonin effects on frequency tuning of inferior colliculus neurons. *Journal of Neurophysiology, 85*(2), 828–842. doi:10.1152/jn.2001.85.2.828

Hurley, L. M., & Pollak, G. D. (2005a). Serotonin modulates responses to species -specific vocalizations in the inferior colliculus. *Journal of Comparative Physiology, A. Neuroethology, Sensory, Neural, and Behavioral Physiology, 191*(6), 535–546. doi:10.1007/s00359-005-0623-y

Hurley, L. M., & Pollak, G. D. (2005b). Serotonin shifts first-spike latencies of inferior colliculus neurons. *Journal of Neuroscience, 25*(34), 7876–7886. doi:10.1523/JNEUROSCI.1178-05.2005

Hurley, L. M., & Sullivan, M. R. (2012). From behavioral context to receptors: serotonergic modulatory pathways in the IC. *Frontiers in Neural Circuits, 6*, 58. doi:10.3389/fncir.2012.00058

Hurley, L. M., & Thompson, A. M. (2001). Serotonergic innervation of the auditory brainstem of the Mexican free-tailed bat, *Tadarida brasiliensis*. *Journal of Comparative Neurology, 435*(1), 78–88.

Hurley, L. M., Tracy, J. A., & Bohorquez, A. (2008). Serotonin 1B receptor modulates frequency response curves and spectral integration in the inferior colliculus by reducing GABAergic inhibition. *Journal of Neurophysiology*, *100*(3), 1656–1667. doi:10.1152/jn.90536.2008

Ito, T., Bishop, D. C., & Oliver, D. L. (2009). Two classes of GABAergic neurons in the inferior colliculus. *Journal of Neuroscience*, *29*(44), 13860–13869. doi:10.1523/JNEUROSCI.3454-09.2009

Jacobs, B. L., Foote, S. L., & Bloom, F. E. (1978). Differential projections of neurons within the dorsal raphe nucleus of the rat: A horseradish peroxidase (HRP) study. *Brain Research*, *147*(1), 149–153.

Janusonis, S. (2017). Serotonin in space: Understanding single fibers. *ACS Chemical Neuroscience*, *8*(5), 893–896. doi:10.1021/acschemneuro.6b00417

Janusonis, S., Fite, K. V., & Foote, W. (1999). Topographic organization of serotonergic dorsal raphe neurons projecting to the superior colliculus in the Mongolian gerbil (Meriones unguiculatus). *Journal of Comparative Neurology*, *413*(2), 342–355.

Kamke, M. R., Brown, M., & Irvine, D. R. (2005). Origin and immunolesioning of cholinergic basal forebrain innervation of cat primary auditory cortex. *Hearing Research*, *206*(1–2), 89–106. doi:10.1016/j.heares.2004.12.014

Keesom, S. M., & Hurley, L. M. (2016). Socially induced serotonergic fluctuations in the male auditory midbrain correlate with female behavior during courtship. *Journal of Neurophysiology*, *115*(4), 1786–1796. doi:10.1152/jn.00742.2015

Keesom, S. M., Morningstar, M. D., Sandlain, R., Wise, B. M., & Hurley, L. M. (2018). Social isolation reduces serotonergic fiber density in the inferior colliculus of female, but not male, mice. *Brain Research*, *1694*, 94–103. doi:10.1016/j.brainres.2018.05.010

Keesom, S. M., Sloss, B. G., Erbowor-Becksen, Z., & Hurley, L. M. (2017). Social experience alters socially induced serotonergic fluctuations in the inferior colliculus. *Journal of Neurophysiology*, *118*(6), 3230–3241. doi:10.1152/jn.00431.2017

Kirifides, M. L., Simpson, K. L., Lin, R. C., & Waterhouse, B. D. (2001). Topographic organization and neurochemical identity of dorsal raphe neurons that project to the trigeminal somatosensory pathway in the rat. *Journal of Comparative Neurology*, *435*(3), 325–340.

Klepper, A., & Herbert, H. (1991). Distribution and origin of noradrenergic and serotonergic fibers in the cochlear nucleus and inferior colliculus of the rat. *Brain Research*, *557*(1–2), 190–201.

Ko, K. W., Rasband, M. N., Meseguer, V., Kramer, R. H., & Golding, N. L. (2016). Serotonin modulates spike probability in the axon initial segment through HCN channels. *Nature Neuroscience*, *19*(6), 826–834. doi:10.1038/nn.4293

Koch, M., Kungel, M., & Herbert, H. (1993). Cholinergic neurons in the pedunculopontine tegmental nucleus are involved in the mediation of prepulse inhibition of the acoustic startle response in the rat. *Experimental Brain Research*, *97*(1), 71–82.

Korzan, W. J., & Summers, C. H. (2007). Behavioral diversity and neurochemical plasticity: Selection of stress coping strategies that define social status. *Brain Behavior and Evolution*, *70*(4), 257–266. doi:10.1159/000105489

Kössl, M., & Vater, M. (1989). Noradrenaline enhances temporal auditory contrast and neuronal timing precision in the cochlear nucleus of the mustached bat. *Journal of Neuroscience*, *9*(12), 4169–4178.

Kössl, M., Vater, M., & Schweizer, H. (1988). Distribution of catecholamine fibers in the cochlear nucleus of horseshoe bats and mustache bats. *Journal of Comparative Neurology*, *269*(4), 523–534. doi:10.1002/cne.902690405

Kromer, L. F., & Moore, R. Y. (1976). Cochlear nucleus innervation by central norepinephrine neurons in the rat. *Brain Research, 118*(3), 531–537.

Kuo, S. P., & Trussell, L. O. (2011). Spontaneous spiking and synaptic depression underlie noradrenergic control of feed-forward inhibition. *Neuron, 71*(2), 306–318. doi:10.1016/j.neuron.2011.05.039

Leao, R. M., & Von Gersdorff, H. (2002). Noradrenaline increases high-frequency firing at the calyx of Held synapse during development by inhibiting glutamate release. *Journal of Neurophysiology, 87*(5), 2297–2306. doi:10.1152/jn.2002.87.5.2297

LeDoux, J. E., Ruggiero, D. A., & Reis, D. J. (1985). Projections to the subcortical forebrain from anatomically defined regions of the medial geniculate body in the rat. *Journal of Comparative Neurology, 242*(2), 182–213. doi:10.1002/cne.902420204

Lee, H. S., Kim, M. A., Valentino, R. J., & Waterhouse, B. D. (2003). Glutamatergic afferent projections to the dorsal raphe nucleus of the rat. *Brain Research, 963*(1–2), 57–71.

Lee, S. B., Beak, S. K., Park, S. H., Waterhouse, B. D., & Lee, H. S. (2009). Collateral projection from the locus coeruleus to whisker-related sensory and motor brain regions of the rat. *Journal of Comparative Neurology, 514*(4), 387–402. doi:10.1002/cne.22012

Leitner, D. S., & Cohen, M. E. (1985). Role of the inferior colliculus in the inhibition of acoustic startle in the rat. *Physiology and Behavior, 34*(1), 65–70.

Lesicko, A. M., Hristova, T. S., Maigler, K. C., & Llano, D. A. (2016). Connectional modularity of top-down and bottom-up multimodal inputs to the lateral cortex of the mouse inferior colliculus. *Journal of Neuroscience, 36*(43), 11037–11050. doi:10.1523/JNEUROSCI.4134-15.2016

Levitt, P., & Moore, R. Y. (1979). Origin and organization of brainstem catecholamine innervation in the rat. *Journal of Comparative Neurology, 186*(4), 505–528. doi:10.1002/cne.901860402

Li, L., Korngut, L. M., Frost, B. J., & Beninger, R. J. (1998a). Prepulse inhibition following lesions of the inferior colliculus: prepulse intensity functions. *Physiology and Behavior, 65*(1), 133–139.

Li, L., Priebe, R. P., & Yeomans, J. S. (1998b). Prepulse inhibition of acoustic or trigeminal startle of rats by unilateral electrical stimulation of the inferior colliculus. *Behavioral Neuroscience, 112*(5), 1187–1198.

Li, L., & Yue, Q. (2002). Auditory gating processes and binaural inhibition in the inferior colliculus. *Hearing Research, 168*(1–2), 98–109.

Linster, C., & Cleland, T. A. (2016). Neuromodulation of olfactory transformations. *Current Opinion in Neurobiology, 40*, 170–177. doi:10.1016/j.conb.2016.07.006

Loftus, W. C., Bishop, D. C., & Oliver, D. L. (2010). Differential patterns of inputs create functional zones in central nucleus of inferior colliculus. *Journal of Neuroscience, 30*(40), 13396–13408. doi:10.1523/JNEUROSCI.0338-10.2010

Lorincz, M. L., & Adamantidis, A. R. (2017). Monoaminergic control of brain states and sensory processing: Existing knowledge and recent insights obtained with optogenetics. *Progress in Neurobiology, 151*, 237–253. doi:10.1016/j.pneurobio.2016.09.003

Luppi, P. H., Aston-Jones, G., Akaoka, H., Chouvet, G., & Jouvet, M. (1995). Afferent projections to the rat locus coeruleus demonstrated by retrograde and anterograde tracing with cholera-toxin B subunit and Phaseolus vulgaris leucoagglutinin. *Neuroscience, 65*(1), 119–160.

Ma, X., & Suga, N. (2005). Long-term cortical plasticity evoked by electric stimulation and acetylcholine applied to the auditory cortex. *Proceedings of the National Academy of Sciences of the United States of America, 102*(26), 9335–9340. doi:10.1073/pnas.0503851102

Macedo, C. E., Castilho, V. M., de Souza e Silva, M. A., & Brandao, M. L. (2002). Dual 5-HT mechanisms in basolateral and central nuclei of amygdala in the regulation of the defensive behavior induced by electrical stimulation of the inferior colliculus. *Brain Research Bulletin*, *59*(3), 189–195.

Macedo, C. E., Martinez, R. C., Albrechet-Souza, L., Molina, V. A., & Brandao, M. L. (2007). 5-HT2- and D1-mechanisms of the basolateral nucleus of the amygdala enhance conditioned fear and impair unconditioned fear. *Behavioural Brain Research*, *177*(1), 100–108. doi:10.1016/j.bbr.2006.10.031

Macedo, C. E., Martinez, R. C., de Souza Silva, M. A., & Brandao, M. L. (2005). Increases in extracellular levels of 5-HT and dopamine in the basolateral, but not in the central, nucleus of amygdala induced by aversive stimulation of the inferior colliculus. *European Journal of Neuroscience*, *21*(4), 1131–1138. doi:10.1111/j.1460-9568.2005.03939.x

Maisonnette, S. S., Kawasaki, M. C., Coimbra, N. C., & Brandao, M. L. (1996). Effects of lesions of amygdaloid nuclei and substantia nigra on aversive responses induced by electrical stimulation of the inferior colliculus. *Brain Research Bulletin*, *40*(2), 93–98.

Maley, B. E., Engle, M. G., Humphreys, S., Vascik, D. A., Howes, K. A., Newton, B. W., & Elde, R. P. (1990). Monoamine synaptic structure and localization in the central nervous system. *Journal of Electron Microscopic Technique*, *15*(1), 20–33. doi:10.1002/jemt.1060150104

Maney, D. L. (2013). The incentive salience of courtship vocalizations: Hormone-mediated "wanting" in the auditory system. *Hearing Research*, *305*, 19–30. doi:10.1016/j.heares.2013.04.011

Marder, E. (2012). Neuromodulation of neuronal circuits: back to the future. *Neuron*, *76*(1), 1–11. doi:10.1016/j.neuron.2012.09.010

Marder, E., & Bucher, D. (2007). Understanding circuit dynamics using the stomatogastric nervous system of lobsters and crabs. *Annual Review of Physiology*, *69*, 291–316. doi:10.1146/annurev.physiol.69.031905.161516

Marlin, B. J., Mitre, M., D'Amour J. A., Chao, M. V., & Froemke, R. C. (2015). Oxytocin enables maternal behaviour by balancing cortical inhibition. *Nature*, *520*(7548), 499–504. doi:10.1038/nature14402

Marsh, R. A., Fuzessery, Z. M., Grose, C. D., & Wenstrup, J. J. (2002). Projection to the inferior colliculus from the basal nucleus of the amygdala. *Journal of Neuroscience*, *22*(23), 10449–10460.

Martins, A. R., & Froemke, R. C. (2015). Coordinated forms of noradrenergic plasticity in the locus coeruleus and primary auditory cortex. *Nature Neuroscience*, *18*(10), 1483–1492. doi:10.1038/nn.4090

Mas, M., Fumero, B., & Gonzalez-Mora, J. L. (1995). Voltammetric and microdialysis monitoring of brain monoamine neurotransmitter release during sociosexual interactions. *Behavioural Brain Research*, *71*(1–2), 69–79.

Matragrano, L. L., Beaulieu, M., Phillip, J. O., Rae, A. I., Sanford, S. E., Sockman, K. W., & Maney, D. L. (2012a). Rapid effects of hearing song on catecholaminergic activity in the songbird auditory pathway. *PLoS One*, *7*(6), e39388. doi:10.1371/journal.pone.0039388

Matragrano, L. L., LeBlanc, M. M., Chitrapu, A., Blanton, Z. E., & Maney, D. L. (2013). Testosterone alters genomic responses to song and monoaminergic innervation of auditory areas in a seasonally breeding songbird. *Developmental Neurobiology*, *73*(6), 455–468. doi:10.1002/dneu.22072

Matragrano, L. L., Sanford, S. E., Salvante, K. G., Beaulieu, M., Sockman, K. W., & Maney, D. L. (2012b). Estradiol-dependent modulation of serotonergic markers in auditory areas of a seasonally breeding songbird. *Behavioral Neuroscience, 126*(1), 110–122. doi:10.1037/a0025586

McCormick, D. A., & Pape, H. C. (1990). Noradrenergic and serotonergic modulation of a hyperpolarization-activated cation current in thalamic relay neurones. *Journal of Physiology, 431*, 319–342.

Mellott, J. G., Motts, S. D., & Schofield, B. R. (2011). Multiple origins of cholinergic innervation of the cochlear nucleus. *Neuroscience, 180*, 138–147. doi:10.1016/j.neuroscience.2011.02.010

Melo, L. L., & Brandao, M. L. (1995). Role of 5-HT1A and 5-HT2 receptors in the aversion induced by electrical stimulation of inferior colliculus. *Pharmacology, Biochemistry, and Behavior, 51*(2–3), 317–321.

Mena-Segovia, J., & Bolam, J. P. (2017). Rethinking the pedunculopontine nucleus: From cellular organization to function. *Neuron, 94*(1), 7–18. doi:10.1016/j.neuron.2017.02.027

Miko, I. J., & Sanes, D. H. (2009). Transient gain adjustment in the inferior colliculus is serotonin- and calcium-dependent. *Hearing Research, 251*(1–2), 39–50. doi:10.1016/j.heares.2009.02.003

Mizutani, H., Hori, T., & Takahashi, T. (2006). 5-HT1B receptor-mediated presynaptic inhibition at the calyx of Held of immature rats. *European Journal of Neuroscience, 24*(7), 1946–1954. doi:10.1111/j.1460-9568.2006.05063.x

Motts, S. D., & Schofield, B. R. (2009). Sources of cholinergic input to the inferior colliculus. *Neuroscience, 160*(1), 103–114. doi:10.1016/j.neuroscience.2009.02.036

Mulders, W. H., & Robertson, D. (2000). Morphological relationships of peptidergic and noradrenergic nerve terminals to olivocochlear neurones in the rat. *Hearing Research, 144*(1–2), 53–64.

Mulders, W. H., & Robertson, D. (2001). Origin of the noradrenergic innervation of the superior olivary complex in the rat. *Journal of Chemical Neuroanatomy, 21*(4), 313–322.

Mulders, W. H., & Robertson, D. (2004). Dopaminergic olivocochlear neurons originate in the high frequency region of the lateral superior olive of guinea pigs. *Hearing Research, 187*(1–2), 122–130.

Mulders, W. H., & Robertson, D. (2005a). Catecholaminergic innervation of guinea pig superior olivary complex. *Journal of Chemical Neuroanatomy, 30*(4), 230–242. doi:10.1016/j.jchemneu.2005.09.005

Mulders, W. H., & Robertson, D. (2005b). Noradrenergic modulation of brainstem nuclei alters cochlear neural output. *Hearing Research, 204*, 147–155.

Nadim, F., & Bucher, D. (2014). Neuromodulation of neurons and synapses. *Current Opinion in Neurobiology, 29*, 48–56. doi:10.1016/j.conb.2014.05.003

Nevue, A. A., Elde, C. J., Perkel, D. J., & Portfors, C. V. (2016a). Dopaminergic input to the inferior colliculus in mice. *Frontiers in Neuroanatomy, 9*, 168. doi:10.3389/fnana.2015.00168

Nevue, A. A., Felix, R. A., 2nd, & Portfors, C. V. (2016b). Dopaminergic projections of the subparafascicular thalamic nucleus to the auditory brainstem. *Hearing Research, 341*, 202–209. doi:10.1016/j.heares.2016.09.001

Niederkofler, V., Asher, T. E., Okaty, B. W., Rood, B. D., Narayan, A., Hwa, L. S., . . . Dymecki, S. M. (2016). Identification of serotonergic neuronal modules that affect aggressive behavior. *Cell Reports, 17*(8), 1934–1949. doi:10.1016/j.celrep.2016.10.063

Nobre, M. J., & Brandao, M. L. (2011). Modulation of auditory-evoked potentials recorded in the inferior colliculus by GABAergic mechanisms in the basolateral and central nuclei of the amygdala in high- and low-anxiety rats. *Brain Research, 1421*, 20–29. doi:10.1016/j.brainres.2011.09.013

Nobre, M. J., Lopes, M. G., & Brandao, M. L. (2004). Defense reaction mediated by NMDA mechanisms in the inferior colliculus is modulated by GABAergic nigro-collicular pathways. *Brain Research*, *999*(1), 124–131.

Obara, N., Kamiya, H., & Fukuda, S. (2014). Serotonergic modulation of inhibitory synaptic transmission in mouse inferior colliculus. *Biomedical Research*, *35*(1), 81–84.

Ohno, Y. (2010). New insight into the therapeutic role of 5-HT1A receptors in central nervous system disorders. *Central Nervous System Agents in Medical Chemistry*, *10*(2), 148–157.

Olazábal, U. E., & Moore, J. K. (1989). Nigrotectal projection to the inferior colliculus: Horseradish peroxidase transport and tyrosine hydroxylase immunohistochemical studies in rats, cats, and bats. *Journal of Comparative Neurology*, *282*(1), 98–118. doi:10.1002/cne.902820108

Papesh, M. A., & Hurley, L. M. (2012). Plasticity of serotonergic innervation of the inferior colliculus in mice following acoustic trauma. *Hearing Research*, *283*(1–2), 89–97. doi:10.1016/j.heares.2011.11.004

Papesh, M. A., & Hurley, L. M. (2016). Modulation of auditory brainstem responses by serotonin and specific serotonin receptors. *Hearing Research*, *332*, 121–136. doi:10.1016/j.heares.2015.11.014

Parent, A., Descarries, L., & Beaudet, A. (1981). Organization of ascending serotonin systems in the adult rat brain. A radioautographic study after intraventricular administration of [3H]5-hydroxytryptamine. *Neuroscience*, *6*(2), 115–138.

Patel, M. B., Sons, S., Yudintsev, G., Lesicko, A. M., Yang, L., Taha, G. A., . . . Llano, D. A. (2017). Anatomical characterization of subcortical descending projections to the inferior colliculus in mouse. *Journal of Comparative Neurology*, *525*(4), 885–900. doi:10.1002/cne.24106

Peruzzi, D., Bartlett, E., Smith, P. H., & Oliver, D. L. (1997). A monosynaptic GABAergic input from the inferior colliculus to the medial geniculate body in rat. *Journal of Neuroscience*, *17*(10), 3766–3777.

Peruzzi, D., & Dut, A. (2004). GABA, serotonin and serotonin receptors in the rat inferior colliculus. *Brain Research*, *998*(2), 247–250.

Petersen, C. L., & Hurley, L. M. (2017). Putting it in context: linking auditory processing with social behavior circuits in the vertebrate brain. *Integrative and Comparative Biology*, *57*(4), 865–877.

Peyron, C., Petit, J. M., Rampon, C., Jouvet, M., & Luppi, P. H. (1998). Forebrain afferents to the rat dorsal raphe nucleus demonstrated by retrograde and anterograde tracing methods. *Neuroscience*, *82*(2), 443–468.

Pollak Dorocic, I., Furth, D., Xuan, Y., Johansson, Y., Pozzi, L., Silberberg, G., . . . Meletis, K. (2014). A whole-brain atlas of inputs to serotonergic neurons of the dorsal and median raphe nuclei. *Neuron*, *83*(3), 663–678. doi:10.1016/j.neuron.2014.07.002

Pollak, G. D. (2013). The dominant role of inhibition in creating response selectivities for communication calls in the brainstem auditory system. *Hearing Research*, *305*, 86–101. doi:10.1016/j.heares.2013.03.001

Pollak, G. D., Burger, R. M., Park, T. J., Klug, A., & Bauer, E. E. (2002). Roles of inhibition for transforming binaural properties in the brainstem auditory system. *Hearing Research*, *168*(1–2), 60–78.

Pollak, G. D., Xie, R., Gittelman, J. X., Andoni, S., & Li, N. (2011). The dominance of inhibition in the inferior colliculus. *Hearing Research*, *274*(1–2), 27–39. doi:10.1016/j.heares.2010.05.010

Rasmussen, K., Strecker, R. E., & Jacobs, B. L. (1986). Single unit responses of noradrenergic, serotonergic, and dopaminergic neurons in freely moving cats to simple sensory stimuli. *Brain Research, 369*(1–2), 336–340.

Reese, N. B., Garcia-Rill, E., & Skinner, R. D. (1995a). Auditory input to the pedunculopontine nucleus: II. Unit responses. *Brain Research Bulletin, 37*(3), 265–273.

Reese, N. B., Garcia-Rill, E., & Skinner, R. D. (1995b). The pedunculopontine nucleus—auditory input, arousal and pathophysiology. *Progress in Neurobiology, 47*(2), 105–133.

Retson, T. A., & Van Bockstaele, E. J. (2013). Coordinate regulation of noradrenergic and serotonergic brain regions by amygdalar neurons. *Journal of Chemical Neuroanatomy, 52*, 9–19. doi:10.1016/j.jchemneu.2013.04.003

Sakai, K., & Crochet, S. (2001). Differentiation of presumed serotonergic dorsal raphe neurons in relation to behavior and wake-sleep states. *Neuroscience, 104*(4), 1141–1155.

Sari, Y. (2004). Serotonin1B receptors: from protein to physiological function and behavior. *Neuroscience and Biobehavior Reviews, 28*(6), 565–582. doi:10.1016/j.neubiorev.2004.08.008

Satake, S., Yamada, K., Melo, L. L., & Barbosa Silva, R. (2012). Effects of microinjections of apomorphine and haloperidol into the inferior colliculus on prepulse inhibition of the acoustic startle reflex in rat. *Neuroscience Letters, 509*(1), 60–63. doi:10.1016/j.neulet.2011.12.052

Schofield, B. R. (2010). Projections from auditory cortex to midbrain cholinergic neurons that project to the inferior colliculus. *Neuroscience, 166*(1), 231–240. doi:10.1016/j.neuroscience.2009.12.008

Schofield, B. R., & Cant, N. B. (1999). Descending auditory pathways: projections from the inferior colliculus contact superior olivary cells that project bilaterally to the cochlear nuclei. *Journal of Comparative Neurology, 409*(2), 210–223.

Schofield, B. R., & Hurley, L. M. (2018). Circuits for modulation of auditory function. In D. O. Oliver, N. B. Cant, A. N. Popper, & R. R. Fay (Eds.), *The mammalian auditory pathways: Synaptic organization and microcircuits* (Vol. 65). New York, NY: Springer-Verlag.

Schofield, B. R., & Motts, S. D. (2009). Projections from auditory cortex to cholinergic cells in the midbrain tegmentum of guinea pigs. *Brain Research Bulletin, 80*(3), 163–170. doi:10.1016/j.brainresbull.2009.06.015

Schofield, B. R., Motts, S. D., & Mellott, J. G. (2011). Cholinergic cells of the pontomesencephalic tegmentum: Connections with auditory structures from cochlear nucleus to cortex. *Hearing Research, 279*(1–2), 85–95. doi:10.1016/j.heares.2010.12.019

Sherriff, F. E., & Henderson, Z. (1994). Cholinergic neurons in the ventral trapezoid nucleus project to the cochlear nuclei in the rat. *Neuroscience, 58*(3), 627–633.

Shima, K., Nakahama, H., & Yamamoto, M. (1986). Firing properties of two types of nucleus raphe dorsalis neurons during the sleep-waking cycle and their responses to sensory stimuli. *Brain Research, 399*(2), 317–326.

Smith, A. R., Kwon, J. H., Navarro, M., & Hurley, L. M. (2014). Acoustic trauma triggers upregulation of serotonin receptor genes. *Hearing Research, 315*, 40–48. doi:10.1016/j.heares.2014.06.004

Stark, H., & Scheich, H. (1997). Dopaminergic and serotonergic neurotransmission systems are differentially involved in auditory cortex learning: a long-term microdialysis study of metabolites. *Journal of Neurochemistry, 68*(2), 691–697.

Stornetta, R. L., Macon, C. J., Nguyen, T. M., Coates, M. B., & Guyenet, P. G. (2013). Cholinergic neurons in the mouse rostral ventrolateral medulla target sensory afferent areas. *Brain Structure and Function, 218*(2), 455–475. doi:10.1007/s00429-012-0408-3

Tadros, S. F., D'Souza, M., Zettel, M. L., Zhu, X., Lynch-Erhardt, M., & Frisina, R. D. (2007). Serotonin 2B receptor: upregulated with age and hearing loss in mouse auditory system. *Neurobiology of Aging*, *28*(7), 1112–1123. doi:10.1016/j.neurobiolaging.2006.05.021

Tang, Z. Q., & Trussell, L. O. (2015). Serotonergic regulation of excitability of principal cells of the dorsal cochlear nucleus. *Journal of Neuroscience*, *35*(11), 4540–4551. doi:10.1523/JNEUROSCI.4825-14.2015

Tang, Z. Q., & Trussell, L. O. (2017). Serotonergic modulation of sensory representation in a central multisensory circuit is pathway specific. *Cell Reports*, *20*(8), 1844–1854. doi:10.1016/j.celrep.2017.07.079

Thompson, A. M., & Hurley, L. M. (2004). Dense serotonergic innervation of principal nuclei of the superior olivary complex in mouse. *Neuroscience Letters*, *356*(3), 179–182. doi:10.1016/j.neulet.2003.11.052

Thompson, A. M., & Schofield, B. R. (2000). Afferent projections of the superior olivary complex. *Microscopy Research Techniques*, *51*(4), 330–354. doi:10.1002/1097-0029(20001115)51:4<330::AID-JEMT4>3.0.CO;2-X

Thompson, A. M., & Thompson, G. C. (2001). Serotonin projection patterns to the cochlear nucleus. *Brain Research*, *907*(1–2), 195–207.

Thompson, G. C., Thompson, A. M., Garrett, K. M., & Britton, B. H. (1994). Serotonin and serotonin receptors in the central auditory system. *Otolaryngology—Head and Neck Surgery*, *110*(1), 93–102. doi:10.1177/019459989411000111

Tong, L., Altschuler, R. A., & Holt, A. G. (2005). Tyrosine hydroxylase in rat auditory midbrain: distribution and changes following deafness. *Hearing Research*, *206*(1–2), 28–41. doi:10.1016/j.heares.2005.03.006

Van Bockstaele, E. J., Biswas, A., & Pickel, V. M. (1993). Topography of serotonin neurons in the dorsal raphe nucleus that send axon collaterals to the rat prefrontal cortex and nucleus accumbens. *Brain Research*, *624*(1–2), 188–198.

Vasudeva, R. K., Lin, R. C., Simpson, K. L., & Waterhouse, B. D. (2011). Functional organization of the dorsal raphe efferent system with special consideration of nitrergic cell groups. *Journal of Chemical Neuroanatomy*, *41*(4), 281–293. doi:10.1016/j.jchemneu.2011.05.008

Villar, M. J., Vitale, M. L., Hokfelt, T., & Verhofstad, A. A. (1988). Dorsal raphe serotoninergic branching neurons projecting both to the lateral geniculate body and superior colliculus: a combined retrograde tracing-immunohistochemical study in the rat. *Journal of Comparative Neurology*, *277*(1), 126–140. doi:10.1002/cne.902770109

Wang, H. T., Luo, B., Huang, Y. N., Zhou, K. Q., & Chen, L. (2008). Sodium salicylate suppresses serotonin-induced enhancement of GABAergic spontaneous inhibitory postsynaptic currents in rat inferior colliculus in vitro. *Hearing Research*, *236*(1–2), 42–51. doi:10.1016/j.heares.2007.11.015

Wang, J., Palkovits, M., Usdin, T. B., & Dobolyi, A. (2006). Afferent connections of the subparafascicular area in rat. *Neuroscience*, *138*(1), 197–220. doi:10.1016/j.neuroscience.2005.11.010

Wang, X., & Robertson, D. (1997). Effects of bioamines and peptides on neurones in the ventral nucleus of trapezoid body and rostral periolivary regions of the rat superior olivary complex: An in vitro investigation. *Hearing Research*, *106*(1–2), 20–28.

Waterhouse, B. D., Border, B., Wahl, L., & Mihailoff, G. A. (1993). Topographic organization of rat locus coeruleus and dorsal raphe nuclei: distribution of cells projecting to visual system structures. *Journal of Comparative Neurology*, *336*(3), 345–361. doi:10.1002/cne.903360304

Waterhouse, B. D., Mihailoff, G. A., Baack, J. C., & Woodward, D. J. (1986). Topographical distribution of dorsal and median raphe neurons projecting to motor, sensorimotor, and visual cortical areas in the rat. *Journal of Comparative Neurology, 249*(4), 460–476, 478–481.

Weinberger, N. M. (2015). New perspectives on the auditory cortex: Learning and memory. *Handbook of Clinical Neurology, 129*, 117–147. doi:10.1016/B978-0-444-62630-1.00007-X

Woods, C. I., & Azeredo, W. J. (1999). Noradrenergic and serotonergic projections to the superior olive: Potential for modulation of olivocochlear neurons. *Brain Research, 836*(1–2), 9–18.

Wynne, B., & Robertson, D. (1996). Localization of dopamine-beta-hydroxylase-like immunoreactivity in the superior olivary complex of the rat. *Audiology and Neurotology, 1*(1), 54–64.

Yamada, R., Kuba, H., Ishii, T. M., & Ohmori, H. (2005). Hyperpolarization-activated cyclic nucleotide-gated cation channels regulate auditory coincidence detection in nucleus laminaris of the chick. *Journal of Neuroscience, 25*, 8867–8877.

Yasui, Y., Kayahara, T., Nakano, K., & Mizuno, N. (1990). The subparafascicular thalamic nucleus of the rat receives projection fibers from the inferior colliculus and auditory cortex. *Brain Research, 537*(1–2), 323–327.

Yasui, Y., Nakano, K., & Mizuno, N. (1992). Descending projections from the subparafascicular thalamic nucleus to the lower brain stem in the rat. *Experimental Brain Research, 90*(3), 508-518.

Yeomans, J. S., Lee, J., Yeomans, M. H., Steidl, S., & Li, L. (2006). Midbrain pathways for prepulse inhibition and startle activation in rat. *Neuroscience, 142*(4), 921–929. doi:10.1016/j.neuroscience.2006.06.025

Yigit, M., Keipert, C., & Backus, K. H. (2003). Muscarinic acetylcholine receptors potentiate the GABAergic transmission in the developing rat inferior colliculus. *Neuropharmacology, 45*(4), 504–513.

Zhou, J., & Shore, S. (2006). Convergence of spinal trigeminal and cochlear nucleus projections in the inferior colliculus of the guinea pig. *Journal of Comparative Neurology, 495*(1), 100–112. doi:10.1002/cne.20863

CHAPTER 22

DESCENDING AUDITORY PATHWAYS AND PLASTICITY

BRETT R. SCHOFIELD AND NICHOLE L. BEEBE

Abstract

Descending auditory pathways originate from multiple levels of the auditory system and use a variety of neurotransmitters, including glutamate, GABA, glycine, acetylcholine, and dopamine. Targets of descending projections include cells that project to higher or lower centers, setting up circuit loops and chains that provide top-down modulation of many ascending and descending circuits in the auditory system. Descending pathways from the auditory cortex can evoke plasticity in subcortical centers. Such plasticity relies, at least in part, on brainstem cholinergic systems that are closely tied to descending cortical projections. Finally, the ventral nucleus of the trapezoid body, a component of the superior olivary complex, is a major target of descending projections from the cortex and midbrain. Through its complement of different neurotransmitter phenotypes, and its wide array of projections, the ventral nucleus of the trapezoid body is positioned to serve as a hub in the descending auditory system.

Keywords: plasticity, modulation, top-down, feedback, acetylcholine, dopamine, GABA, glycine, glutamate, brainstem

How can organisms attend to salient sounds, while ignoring unimportant ones? How can a sound that was previously unimportant to an organism, such as a harmless tone, become salient when paired with another stimulus? How can a reflexive response, such as a startle resulting from a loud sound, be inhibited by preceding auditory cues? Questions like these have led to discoveries of plasticity at many levels of the auditory system, from the cochlear nucleus to the cortex (e.g., Irvine, 2010; Zhao & Tzounopoulos, 2011; Miranda et al., 2014). A particularly exciting development over the past few decades has been the recognition of a role for descending pathways in modulating, or even driving, such plasticity (e.g., Bajo & King, 2013). Descending pathways are important in many listening conditions and are currently being investigated as a contributor to clinical deficits associated with aging or damage to the system (e.g., Boyen et al., 2014; Markovitz et al., 2015). In this chapter, we will attempt to summarize the literature surrounding the descending auditory pathways and consider some specific areas of recent progress.

Our review focuses on three areas that have advanced significantly in recent years. First, continued physiological studies have extended our understanding of corticofugal effects in the inferior colliculus (IC; where the majority of early studies were conducted) and have expanded our view to corticofugal effects in other areas, both within and outside the traditional ascending auditory pathway. A second area of work involves the modulatory systems and their close relationships with descending auditory pathways. Recent work has begun to examine the interactions between descending auditory pathways and neuromodulatory systems, which will lead to advances in the understanding of plasticity in the normal auditory brainstem. Finally, there has been a resurgence of interest in neurotransmitter phenotypes associated with the descending pathways. This results in part from the general interest in neuromodulators and also from the advent of techniques that allow selective manipulation of neurotransmitter-specific circuits. While neurotransmitter phenotypes have long been a focus of studies in the ascending pathways, their roles in descending systems have been comparatively understudied. We begin with an update on the anatomy of the descending pathways to incorporate recent data and to review the associated neurotransmitters.

Descending Pathways

Previous reviews describe descending pathways within the auditory brainstem (Schofield, 2010, 2011; Malmierca & Ryugo, 2011). Here, we highlight new information, emphasizing neurotransmitter phenotype. Information about neurotransmitters is incomplete; confirmation with appropriate physiological approaches is limited to a small subset of pathways, but selective immunostains allow us to make tentative statements about the most likely neurotransmitters in many pathways. In some cases, the nucleus of origin may be largely homogenous in terms of neurotransmitter content, so the neurotransmitter present in the pathway can be inferred. Our discussion focuses on five neurotransmitters: glutamate, GABA, glycine, dopamine, and acetylcholine (ACh).

Subcortical Descending Projections to Auditory Brainstem Nuclei

Descending projections originate from a variety of subcortical auditory regions and, in contrast to projections from the auditory cortex, exhibit a variety of neurotransmitter phenotypes.

Glutamatergic descending projections

Glutamate is the dominant excitatory neurotransmitter in both ascending and descending auditory pathways. Glutamate has been implicated in descending projections from the medial geniculate body (MG), the nucleus of the brachium of the IC (NBIC), the ventral tectal longitudinal column (TLCv), and the IC (Figure 22.1A).

Descending projections from the thalamus (MG and surrounding regions) terminate in numerous areas, including the IC, superior olivary complex (SOC) and cochlear nucleus (CN). Projections to the ipsilateral IC have been demonstrated in numerous species, including cats, rats, squirrel monkeys, gerbils, and mice (Adams, 1980; Frisina et al., 1998; Kuwabara & Zook, 2000; Patel et al., 2017; Senatorov & Hu, 2002; Winer et al., 2002). They originate from the medial and suprageniculate subdivisions of the medial geniculate body (included in the multisensory "paralaminar thalamus" in Figure 22.1A) and, in some species, also from the dorsal or ventral subdivisions (MGd, MGv). In rodents, the MG contains almost exclusively glutamatergic neurons, so the MG-IC pathway must be largely glutamatergic (Patel et al., 2017; Winer & Larue, 1996). Projections from the auditory thalamus target the lateral cortex of the IC (IClc), and, to a lesser extent, the central nucleus of the IC (ICc) and the dorsal cortex of the IC (ICd) (Frisina et al., 1998; Kuwabara & Zook, 2000; Patel et al., 2017).

The NBIC, situated along the brachial pathway between the IC and the MG, also sends a descending projection to the IC (Senatorov & Hu, 2002; Patel et al., 2017). Glutamatergic cells are likely to contribute to this projection, although more direct experiments are needed to confirm this point (Patel et al., 2017).

The TLCv is an auditory-responsive nucleus located near the dorsal midline of the superior colliculi and rostral part of the inferior colliculi (Saldaña et al., 2007). A defining feature of the TLCv is a large descending projection to the SOC, which targets, at least in part, the superior paraolivary nucleus (SPN; Viñuela et al., 2011). A majority of TLCv neurons express vesicular glutamate transporters (a marker of glutamatergic cells), so the descending projection is likely to be at least partly glutamatergic, although this has not been demonstrated directly (Aparicio & Saldaña, 2014).

The IC is the origin of descending projections to the CN, the SOC, and regions in or around the nuclei of the lateral lemniscus (NLL; reviewed by Malmierca & Ryugo, 2011). Most, perhaps all, of the descending projections from the IC are glutamatergic (Milinkeviciute et al., 2017; Saint Marie, 1996).

Projections from the IC to the dorsal nucleus of the lateral lemniscus (DNLL) originate primarily from the ipsilateral ICc and are topographically organized (Caicedo & Herbert, 1993). Projections to the ipsilateral sagulum originate primarily from the IClc and ICd, and are not topographic.

Descending pathways from the IC to the SOC originate from the ICc and IClc (Faye-Lund, 1986; Hashikawa & Kawamura, 1983; Hashikawa, 1983; Okoyama et al., 2006) and primarily target the ventral nucleus of the trapezoid body (VNTB) and its rostral extension, the rostral periolivary area (Caicedo & Herbert, 1993; Faye-Lund, 1986; Malmierca et al., 1996; Schofield & Cant, 1999; Thompson & Thompson, 1993; Vetter

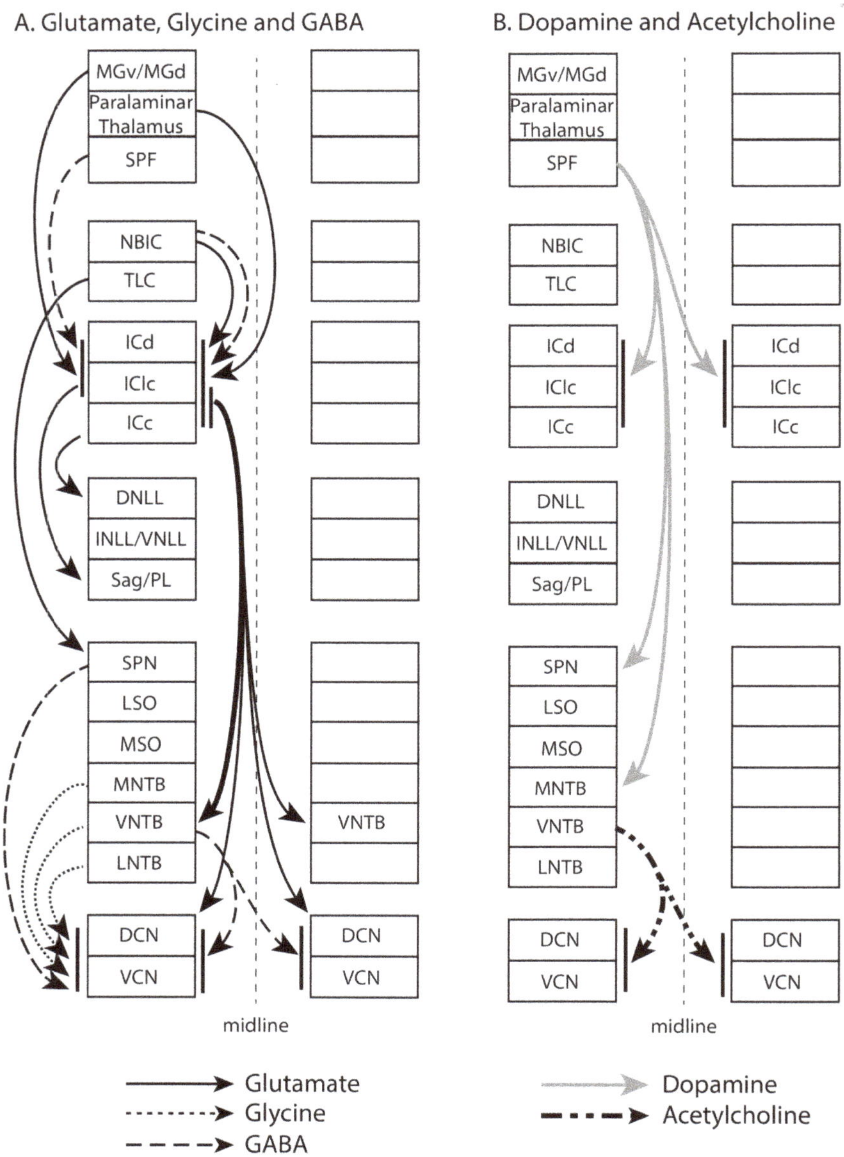

FIGURE 22.1. Descending auditory pathways use a variety of neurotransmitters. The major auditory nuclei are arranged hierarchically and grouped according to brain region (thalamus, midbrain, etc.). Nuclei are represented for both sides of the brain, separated by a midline. Arrows indicate the neurotransmitter attributed to specific pathways. (A) Descending pathways that use glutamate, glycine or GABA. (B) Descending pathways that use dopamine or acetylcholine. Note that some pathways are omitted if there is no evidence concerning their neurotransmitter phenotype.

et al., 1993). The projection terminates tonotopically and bilaterally with an ipsilateral dominance. Targets of IC projections include medial olivocochlear neurons (Suthakar & Ryugo, 2017; Vetter et al., 1993) and olivary cells that project to the CN ipsilaterally, contralaterally, or bilaterally (Gómez-Nieto et al., 2008; Schofield & Cant, 1999). Many olivary cells have projections to other nuclei within the SOC (reviewed in Thompson & Schofield, 2000), and it seems very likely that descending pathways contact some of these cells; however, there are very few data published on this issue.

Projections from the IC to the CN originate mostly in the IClc and the ICc (Caicedo & Herbert, 1993; Milinkeviciute et al., 2017; Schofield, 2001; Shore et al., 1991) and largely target the dorsal CN (DCN) bilaterally and tonotopically (Caicedo & Herbert, 1993; Malmierca et al., 1996; Milinkeviciute et al., 2017). Cellular targets within the DCN include fusiform and giant cells in the fusiform cell layer and the inner molecular layer, at least some of which make projections to the IC (Alibardi, 1999; Milinkeviciute et al., 2017). The IC–DCN projection is glutamatergic (Saint Marie, 1996; Ostapoff et al., 1997; Milinkeviciute et al., 2017).

GABAergic and glycinergic descending projections

Three areas of the auditory pathways give rise to substantial GABAergic or glycinergic descending projections (Figure 22.1A). These arise from the subparafascicular nucleus of the thalamus (SPF), the NBIC, and the SOC. The NLL contain large numbers of GABAergic and glycinergic neurons, but there is scant evidence for descending projections from these cells.

The SPF is a thalamic nucleus located medial to the MG. It has extensive connections with auditory nuclei, including reciprocal connections with auditory cortex (AC) and inputs from the IC (reviewed in Schofield, 2011). It also gives rise to descending projections to several auditory regions, including the IC, SOC, and CN. Projections to the IC terminate bilaterally, with an ipsilateral dominance, primarily in the IClc and ICd (Yasui et al., 1992). GABAergic cells in the SPF contribute to these projections, although their precise termination patterns are unknown (Moriizumi & Hattori, 1992).

As described earlier, the NBIC sends a descending projection to the IC. About half of the cells participating in this projection are GABAergic (Patel et al., 2017). The NBIC projections terminate primarily in the IClc and the ICd, but the characteristics of the target cells are otherwise unknown.

The SOC can be divided into principal nuclei (the medial and lateral superior olivary nuclei, MSO and LSO) and periolivary nuclei (the remaining nuclei, including the medial nucleus of the trapezoid body [MNTB], which others have sometimes called a principal SOC nucleus). The MSO has exclusively ascending projections. The LSO has ascending projections that arise from glutamatergic and glycinergic cells and descending projections to the cochlea (lateral olivocochlear cells) that are cholinergic. The periolivary nuclei vary across species in size, location and nomenclature (see discussions in Schwartz, 1992; Thompson & Schofield, 2000); nonetheless, there are generalizations that apply broadly to the periolivary projections to the CN.

The periolivary nuclei are the main source of extrinsic GABAergic and glycinergic inputs to CN cells. While periolivary cells can use a variety of neurotransmitter phenotypes (GABA, glycine, glutamate, acetylcholine as well as several neuropeptides), cells that use GABA or glycine constitute a majority (74–92%) of olivary cells that project to the CN (Ostapoff et al., 1997). Glycinergic projections arise from each of the ipsilateral periolivary nuclei; there are few glycinergic inputs from the contralateral SOC. Periolivary projections terminate throughout the CN, and a majority of CN cell types receive glycinergic inputs (Kolston et al., 1992; Altschuler et al., 1993; Oertel & Young, 2004), but rarely have the inputs been related to a specific source outside the CN. One exception is a glycinergic projection from principal cells of the MNTB, which project to the ipsilateral CN where their targets appear to include multipolar (stellate) cells and globular bushy cells (Schofield, 1994).

GABAergic inputs to the CN, in contrast, originate mainly from the VNTB and the SPN. Moreover, GABAergic inputs originate bilaterally from the VNTB. Some VNTB cells have axons that branch to innervate both left and right CN (Schofield & Cant, 1999); while the neurotransmitter phenotype was not identified in that study, the available evidence suggests that this bilateral projection is GABAergic. Although GABAergic boutons are found widely in the CN, there are few data relating extrinsic sources of GABA to specific CN cell types.

Dopaminergic descending projections

Figure 22.1B illustrates dopaminergic descending projections within the auditory brainstem. The paralaminar thalamus was mentioned earlier as a source of descending glutamatergic and GABAergic projections. The SPF, one of the paralaminar nuclei, also sends dopaminergic projections to lower centers, including the IC, where the projections terminate bilaterally with an ipsilateral dominance in the IClc and the ICd (Nevue et al., 2016a). Additional dopaminergic projections from the SPF terminate in the SOC (Nevue et al., 2016b). These projections are also bilateral with an ipsilateral dominance, and target primarily the SPN and MNTB. Individual dopaminergic cells in the SPF can send collateral projections to both the ipsilateral IC and SOC, suggesting that dopamine can be released nearly simultaneously in these two targets (Nevue et al., 2016b). The projections of the cells that are targeted by the dopaminergic axons are not known.

There are also projections from the SPF to the CN (Yasui et al., 1992). There is evidence for dopaminergic innervation of the CN, but it has yet to be determined whether the SPF is the source of the dopamine (reviewed in Altschuler & Shore, 2010; note that dopaminergic cells have been identified in several auditory regions and some in the SOC are known to project to the cochlea, but the projections of others are unknown).

Cholinergic descending projections

The SOC is the only auditory structure that contains a substantial number of cholinergic neurons. These cells have been associated exclusively with descending pathways. The best-known cholinergic projections are those of the olivocochlear system, which consists of medial and lateral subsystems (see Elgoyhen et al, Chapter 3). The SOC is also a source of cholinergic projections to the CN (Figure 22.1B). Some of these projections arise as collaterals of olivocochlear axons. The medial olivocochlear cells can project to the ipsilateral or contralateral cochlea, and most of these cells have axon collaterals that terminate in the CN on same side as the targeted cochlea. The medial olivocochlear axons contact large dendrites in the granule cell area (Benson & Brown, 1990; Brown et al., 1988). At least some of these dendrites belong to ventral CN multipolar cells; however, other ventral CN cell types with dendrites present in the granule cell area may be contacted as well (Benson & Brown, 1990). Reports differ on whether lateral olivocochlear cells, most of which are cholinergic, also send collaterals into the CN (Brown et al., 1988; Horváth et al., 2000; Ryan et al., 1990).

A second group of cholinergic cells in the SOC projects to the CN but does not project to the cochlea (Sherriff & Henderson, 1994). This group of small cells, located in the VNTB, projects into the CN bilaterally with a contralateral dominance. Some of these cholinergic projections contact cells of the auditory nerve nucleus (Gómez-Nieto et al., 2008); whether there are other targets within the CN is unknown.

Cortical Descending Projections to Auditory Brainstem Nuclei

It has been known for decades that higher functions can affect early auditory processing, including effects in the cochlea (reviewed in Delano & Elgoyhen, 2016). For much of that time, the underlying circuitry was assumed to be a three-neuron descending chain: (1) AC projects to the IC; (2) the IC projects to the SOC; (3) the SOC projects to the cochlea. The seminal discovery in 1995 of extensive projections from AC to subcollicular regions, including the CN, the SOC, and regions near the NLL, ushered in a renewed interest in corticofugal systems and top-down modulation of the auditory brainstem (Feliciano et al., 1995). Cortically driven plasticity has now been observed in several brainstem auditory nuclei; understanding the advantages (and possible disadvantages) of such plasticity requires a clear picture of the underlying circuitry.

AC projections to subcollicular targets appear to arise exclusively from layer V pyramidal cells and could be expected to be glutamatergic and to excite their targets. A major step toward characterizing the circuits is to identify the brainstem cells targeted by AC axons. In some areas, such as the cochlear nucleus, the targeted cell types have been identified. However, in many areas, most aspects of the target cells' phenotype, including the neurotransmitters used by target cells, are just beginning to be identified.

The AC projects directly to many of the brainstem auditory nuclei (Figure 22.2, gray shading). These projections are usually bilateral with an ipsilateral dominance. Additional details, particularly regarding the distribution of cortical terminals within a target area, are omitted from the figure but carry important implications about the circuits that are targeted (Malmierca & Ryugo, 2011; see Schofield, 2010). For example,

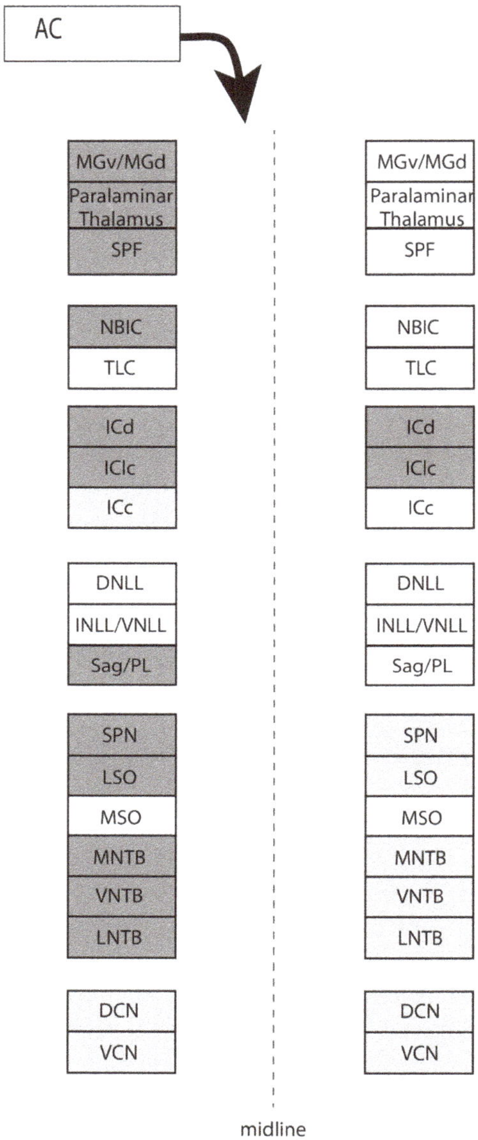

FIGURE 22.2. Descending projections from auditory cortex (AC) terminate in many subcortical nuclei that form the ascending auditory pathways. Projections arise from AC on both sides but are shown from a single side for clarity. The relative density of cortical terminations in each nucleus is indicated by shading: heavy—dark gray; moderate—light gray; minimal or none—white.

projections to the CN terminate heavily in the granule cell areas and, at least in guinea pigs, less densely in other regions of the CN. As its name implies, the SOC is particularly complex in this regard, with many distinguishable nuclei that vary from no cortical input (e.g., the medial superior olivary nucleus) to especially dense cortical inputs (e.g., the VNTB). The SOC as a whole gives rise to numerous ascending and descending auditory projections, and also contains substantial intra-olivary circuits, providing a rich array of targets for cortical axons. Work is continuing to dissect these circuits and their functions. Cortical projections to the IC terminate very densely in the outer shell areas, and less densely in the central nucleus (ICc). As we shall discuss, cortical effects can be observed in numerous IC subdivisions, where they are likely to play different functional roles. Finally, a number of cortical projections have been identified but not addressed in terms of target cell/circuit or function; many of these, such as projections to areas near the lateral lemniscus, are omitted from Figure 22.2.

Given the large number of pathways that are directly targeted by cortical axons, Figure 22.3 separates them into those pathways that project to higher centers (ascending pathways, Figure 22.3A) and those that project to lower centers (descending pathways, Figure 22.3B). A commissural pathway connecting the two ICs is also a target of AC projections (Figure 22.3A). Although the ascending and descending pathways are depicted separately, a simple examination shows that AC axons in a given target area (e.g., the IC) can contact ascending or descending pathways (e.g., IC–MG cells or IC–CN cells). An interesting question that has yet to be examined is whether single cortical axons contact both ascending and descending pathways, implying co-activation of the pathways. Perhaps the most striking aspect of Figure 22.3 is the large number of ascending and descending pathways, originating from almost all levels of the system, that are targeted directly by AC axons. Most of the pathways identified here were reviewed previously (Malmierca & Ryugo, 2011; Schofield, 2010, 2011); newer findings are described next.

AC projections to the NBIC

The NBIC has long been known as a target of AC projections, but the output pathways of the NBIC that are targeted have been unknown (Andersen et al., 1980; Budinger et al., 2006, 2013; Saldaña et al., 1996; Winer et al., 1998). The NBIC receives auditory input from the IC and is probably best known as the primary source of auditory projections to the superior colliculus, where it presumably contributes to orienting or avoidance responses to sounds (Mellott et al., 2018). The NBIC also projects directly to the MG, and is thus a component of ascending pathways to the AC. The projections to the MG originate from both GABAergic and non-GABAergic NBIC cells, suggesting inhibitory and excitatory effects on MG cells. Axons from the AC have now been identified as contacting both GABAergic and non-GABAergic NBIC cells that project to the thalamus (Mellott et al., 2014a). Whether AC axons contact NBIC cells that make descending projections to the IC is unknown.

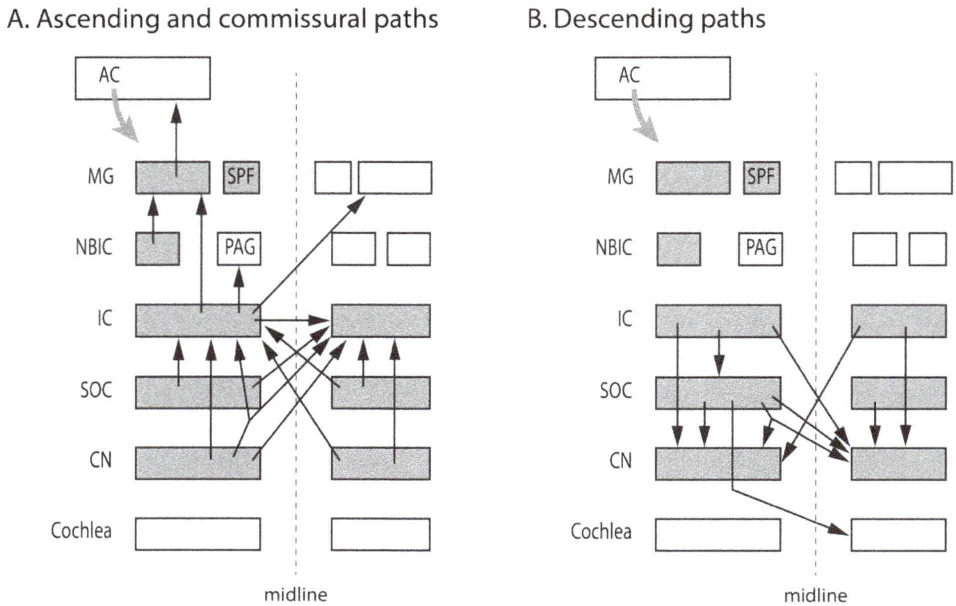

FIGURE 22.3. Axons from auditory cortex (AC) project to many brainstem nuclei, where they contact cells that give rise to ascending (A) or descending (B) pathways. (A) Arrows depict ascending or commissural pathways that appear to be contacted directly by AC axons. Gray shading—regions that receive direct AC projections. Note that arrows indicate *only* those pathways known to be targeted by the AC; many additional pathways (ascending as well as some commissural) have not been identified as AC targets. (B) Arrows depict descending pathways contacted directly by AC axons (conventions same as in A)

AC projections to the IC.

Bajo & King (2013) reviewed the corticocollicular pathway recently, and this topic continues to be a popular focus of research. The AC sends a dense projection to the ipsilateral IC and a sparse projection to the contralateral IC. The ipsilateral projections terminate densely in the IC shell areas and sparsely in the ICc; projections to the contralateral IC terminate only in the shell areas. Most physiological studies of the corticocollicular pathway have focused on the ICc, presumably because of its key role in the lemniscal pathway. Anatomical studies indicate that ascending and descending pathways from the IC originate from different, but intermingled, populations of IC cells (Coomes & Schofield, 2004; Okoyama et al., 2006; Schofield, 2001). Furthermore, AC axons appear to make direct contact with both ascending and descending IC output pathways (Coomes Peterson & Schofield, 2007; Schofield & Coomes, 2006). Unfortunately, very few physiological studies include information on the projections of the IC cells that are modulated by AC inputs, so it is unknown whether the effects observed in the study apply to ascending or descending pathways from the IC.

The IC commissural pathway is a recently discovered target of AC projections. Such a pathway could allow the AC on one side to affect the contralateral IC. While there is a direct projection from the AC to the contralateral IC, the large size of the ipsilateral AC-IC projection (roughly 10 times the size of the contralateral projection) along with the large size of the IC commissural pathway (Moore, 1988), suggests that a commissural route could play a significant role in corticofugal effects. Physiological studies indicate that the AC can affect activity in the *contralateral* IC (Torterolo et al., 1998; Ma & Suga, 2001). Nakamoto et al. (2013b) showed that AC axons that terminate in the ipsilateral IC appear to contact many IC commissural cells. Moreover, the commissural pathway originates from both excitatory glutamatergic neurons and inhibitory GABAergic IC neurons, both of which appear to be contacted directly by the AC axons (Nakamoto et al. 2013b). Thus, the large IC commissural pathway could provide a route for AC-evoked excitation and inhibition in the contralateral IC. Overall, the AC has multiple pathways by which it could potentially modulate ascending, descending and commissural pathways from the IC.

Corticocollicular cells form synapses in all IC subdivisions, where they release glutamate and excite their collicular targets (Feliciano & Potashner, 1995; Saldaña et al. 1996; Xiong et al., 2015). Corticocofugal projections activate both excitatory and inhibitory circuits in the IC (Gao et al., 2015; Mitani et al., 1983; Popelár et al., 2016; Peng et al., 2017). Cortical activation of inhibitory circuits has been assumed to result from cortical boutons contacting GABAergic cells in the IC. Nakamoto et al., (2013a) combined electron microscopy with immunochemistry to provide the first anatomical evidence for cortical inputs to IC GABAergic cells. The synaptic contacts were observed in the cortical regions of the IC (dorsal cortex and lateral cortex), where AC axons terminate densely. GABAergic cells in these regions project to the ICc, to the contralateral IC, or to the MG, and thus could distribute cortically driven inhibition to numerous target areas (González-Hernández et al., 1996; Jen et al., 2001; Mellott et al., 2014b).

Despite the fact that the AC projections terminate most heavily in the IC shell regions, the majority of physiologic data on corticocollicular effects has been collected from cells in the ICc. In a series of studies, Suga and colleagues demonstrated that AC activation can modulate the response of an IC cell to an acoustic stimulus (reviewed in Suga, 2012). The nature of the modulation depends on the similarity of tuning for the cortical and collicular sites. In brief, a cortical site can enhance the responses of collicular cells that have response properties similar to the cortical site and can shift the responses of nearby cells so that they respond more similarly to the cortical site. The responses of a collicular cell with more distant tuning properties are unaffected by the cortical stimulation. Suga referred to this as "egocentric" selection, whereby a cortical site can shift subcortical responses toward the inputs that would activate that cortical region. A remarkable level of specificity can be maintained in these effects; retuning can affect a neuron's response to stimulus duration, intensity, or location, in addition to the frequency effects described earlier. A particularly interesting aspect to these effects is that they can outlast, by minutes to hours, the period of cortical stimulation (Suga, 2012). If atropine was applied to block muscarinic receptors in the IC, a collicular cell's responses were retuned during cortical stimulation, but this retuning ceased once cortical stimulation ended. Thus, the cortically driven plasticity was dependent on cholinergic muscarinic receptors in the IC. This interplay between cortical projections and cholinergic systems will be discussed.

Recent work has also shown top-down effects on collicular cell responses to binaural cues. Nakamoto et al., (2010) showed that corticocollicular projections modulate IC responses to binaural cues. Such modulation may contribute to stream segregation, allowing a listener to distinguish sounds from different locations. The descending pathways may further contribute to filtering of different sounds by selectively enhancing or suppressing a sound based on its salience. Gao et al., (2015) suggested that corticocollicular projections enhance responses to biologically relevant vocalizations. Top-down modulation of binaural processing in the brainstem, with a role in stream segregation and the ability to hear one sound source in the presence of others, may be particularly relevant in the context of human hearing and age-related deficits.

Evidence for corticocollicular effects on IC responses to binaural cues led King and colleagues to investigate the ability of ferrets to localize sounds after selectively lesioning corticocollicular cells (Bajo et al., 2010). An adult ferret can normally be trained to localize sounds quite accurately and, with additional training, can recover that ability after localization cues are altered by placing an earplug in one ear. If the corticocollicular pathway is lesioned selectively, the ferret can localize sounds but is unable to adapt to an earplug. Thus, the corticocollicular pathway is critical for adaptation to the altered sensory input. The site, or more likely sites, of cellular plasticity that underlie these changes have not yet been determined; while the study manipulated corticocollicular projections, the targeted IC cells could project to higher centers (e.g., MG or superior colliculus) or lower centers (e.g., olivocochlear cells; see discussion in Bajo & King, 2013).

Many of the effects we have discussed demonstrate, or at least imply, frequency-specific effects of the corticocollicular pathway. To what extent are these pathways tonotopically organized? Corticocollicular projections arise from a wide array of auditory cortical fields, only some of which are tonotopically organized (reviewed by Malmierca & Ryugo, 2011; Bajo & King, 2013). Anatomical studies suggest that the projection from primary AC (A1) to the ICc is tonotopically organized (Saldaña et al., 1996; Budinger et al., 2013). Physiological studies now confirm such an arrangement (Markovitz et al., 2013). Another tonotopically organized projection to the ICc has been identified from a cortical area known in guinea pigs as the ventrorostral belt (Straka et al., 2015). The tonotopic organization of ventrorostral belt terminations in the ICc appears less precise than the organization of projections from A1. The two cortical areas also have different termination patterns: A1 projections terminate throughout the ICc iso-frequency laminae, whereas the ventrorostral belt projections terminate preferentially in the caudo-medial part of the laminae. Thus, different parts of a lamina receive input from different combinations of AC areas. The authors note that the ventrorostral belt may be specialized for processing vocalizations (Grimsley et al., 2012), but otherwise little is known about the functions of these two different projections.

Additional studies support the idea that corticofugal projections can have different effects on different parts of the IC. Anderson and Malmierca (2013) showed that inactivation of the AC affects stimulus specific adaptation of many cells located in the IC shell areas (see also Malmierca et al., Chapter 25). In a different study, bilateral ablation of the AC increased the response (fMRI BOLD signal) to noise and decreased response selectivity to vocalizations in the IC (Gao et al., 2015). Interestingly, the effect on noise responses was seen primarily in the ICc whereas the effect on vocalization selectivity was seen primarily in the IC shell. These data provide further support for differential effects of AC projections on different IC regions. The same study also showed that ablation of visual cortex had smaller but still differential effects on the IC regions.

Zhang and colleagues have added the pathway from the IC to the dorsolateral periaqueductal gray to the list of brainstem auditory pathways directly affected by AC projections (Xiong et al., 2015). Activation of this IC projection leads to flight behavior, and the authors speculate that the AC input to this pathway enhances the likelihood of an animal taking flight when the forebrain (i.e., AC and amygdala) detects a threatening stimulus. Of additional significance is that the authors attribute the main effects to the IC shell areas and conclude that the ICc plays, at most, a minor role in these defensive responses. This is one of the few studies that address the contributions of IC shell areas to corticofugal functions.

AC projections to the SOC (and effects on the cochlea)

AC axons terminate throughout most of the ipsilateral SOC, with the densest terminations in the VNTB and moderate terminations in all remaining nuclei except the MSO (Figure 22.2; reviewed by Malmierca and Ryugo, 2011). A sparser termination exists in the contralateral SOC, with the VNTB again receiving the strongest projection. The ascending and descending pathways from the SOC appear to arise largely from different populations of cells, although these cells can be intermingled within individual nuclei (Schofield, 2002). Many of the SOC cells that give rise to the ascending projections to the IC or descending projections to the CN or cochlea can receive direct inputs from AC axons (reviewed by Malmierca & Ryugo, 2011; Schofield, 2010). There has not yet been any direct study of the cortical effects on olivary cells. However, AC projections to olivocochlear cells were reported years ago (Mulders & Robertson, 2000), and many studies have described modulation of cochlear function via top-down mechanisms (see chapter by Elgoyhen et al. in this volume for an update on cochlear innervation, and several recent reviews for descending influences on the cochlea, e.g., Terreros & Delano, 2015; Delano & Elgoyhen, 2016). These descending effects are likely mediated via multiple descending inputs to olivocochlear cells, including inputs from the AC, IC, and various modulatory systems.

The anatomical studies suggest that a large proportion of the cortico-olivary axons terminate on olivary cells that are not olivocochlear. As mentioned previously, some of these cells probably project to the cochlear nucleus or to the inferior colliculus. In addition, there are extensive intra-olivary circuits, connecting nearby nuclei as well as nuclei across the midline (Thompson & Schofield, 2000). Cortical inputs to these circuits could affect both monaural and binaural processing in the SOC, but new studies are needed to characterize such cortical effects.

AC projections to the CN

AC projections terminate bilaterally in the CN in rats, mice, gerbils, and guinea pigs (Budinger et al., 2013; Malmierca & Ryugo, 2011). The majority of boutons are in the granule cell area and the DCN; in guinea pigs and gerbils, additional terminals have been observed in ventral CN. Physiological studies in mice have documented effects of A1 stimulation on CN responses bilaterally in the anteroventral CN and contralaterally in the DCN (e.g., Kong et al., 2014; Liu et al., 2010). The "egocentric" model described for corticofugal effects in the IC also applies in the CN. In other words, cortical stimulation tends to enhance responses of physiologically matched CN neurons and suppress responses in unmatched neurons. The study by Kong et al. (2014) also revealed that AC stimulation led to effects in the DCN that lasted for over an hour after cortical stimulation ended, showing cortically driven plasticity. While the direct projections from the AC to the CN likely play a key role in the observed effects, it is worth noting that there are several disynaptic pathways whereby the AC could affect the CN via relays in the IC or the SOC (reviewed in Schofield & Coomes, 2006). The extent to which these pathways interact is unknown.

Descending Pathways and Brainstem Modulatory Systems

Modulatory systems are increasingly recognized for their roles in subcortical auditory processing (Schofield and Hurley, 2018; see also Hurley, Chaprer 21). As mentioned earlier, recent discoveries have highlighted relationships between descending auditory pathways and neuromodulatory systems that use acetylcholine or dopamine. These connections probably serve a variety of important functions, including a role in top-down plasticity.

Circuits that Could Underlie AC-Driven Plasticity: Interactions between Descending and Cholinergic Systems

Auditory cortical projections to subcortical auditory nuclei likely control some details of how subcortical neurons are retuned for salient stimulus properties. At the same time, cortical projections to cholinergic centers in the midbrain tegmentum could determine whether ACh is also released in the auditory nuclei, and thus determine whether the retuning effects are sustained via long term plastic changes. Physiological evidence for a role of ACh in cortically driven plasticity predated the discovery of the underlying circuitry. The earliest studies focused on the IC, but evidence is accumulating for similar plasticity in other subcortical auditory centers.

Cortical and cholinergic inputs to the IC

A hallmark of cortically driven plasticity in the IC has been the high degree of specificity in the effects on cellular responses; that is, a collicular cell can be finely re-tuned in its selectivity for a specific stimulus parameter (e.g., frequency, location, duration, or intensity; see reviews by Suga, 2012; Bajo & King, 2013). Re-tuning typically includes increased firing to some stimuli and decreased firing to other stimuli, with the result that the tuning of the IC neuron shifts toward the tuning of the cortical site that was stimulated. At a circuit level, both excitatory and inhibitory components are involved; the AC projections are glutamatergic and excite IC cells, presumably including direct synaptic activation of glutamatergic and GABAergic IC cells (Nakamoto et al., 2013a). Plasticity is exhibited in that the retuning can outlast the period of cortical stimulation. Moreover, this plasticity is blocked by application of atropine to the IC, demonstrating that the plasticity is dependent on muscarinic cholinergic receptors in the IC. Acetylcholine in the IC originates primarily from the pontomesencephalic tegmentum (PMT, consisting of the pedunculopontine tegmental nucleus and the laterodorsal tegmental nucleus; Motts & Schofield, 2009). This cholinergic group extends through the tegmentum of the pons and midbrain from a caudal point just medial to the dorsal nucleus of the lateral lemniscus to a rostral and ventral location nearing the substantia nigra. The AC, including primary auditory cortex, projects directly to the PMT, where the cortical axons contact cholinergic cells, including some that project to the IC (reviewed in Schofield et al., 2011). Thus, stimulation of the AC, as done to activate the corticocollicular pathway, could also activate PMT cholinergic cells and lead to release of ACh in the IC (Figure 22.4A). We suggest that the highly detailed re-tuning is accomplished by the corticocollicular projections in conjunction with intra-collicular circuitry. The role of PMT-derived ACh is to provide a permissive signal for plasticity. If the cholinergic system is not active, then the cortical effects on IC cells would be short-lived; if the cholinergic system is activated concurrently with the corticocollicular system, then plasticity could enhance and prolong the cortical effects.

Cortical projections and cholinergic inputs to other auditory nuclei

Two main cholinergic groups innervate the subcortical auditory system: the PMT and the cholinergic groups of the SOC. The SOC groups are focused, perhaps exclusively, on the auditory system, whereas the PMT has connections with many systems across the brainstem and thalamus. Cholinergic cells in both areas have branching axons, allowing individual cells to innervate multiple auditory targets. Many olivocochlear cells have collateral branches that terminate in the CN. As a group, the PMT cholinergic cells have more widespread projections than do the olivary cells (reviewed in Schofield et al., 2011). Moreover, individual PMT cholinergic cells have branching axons that can

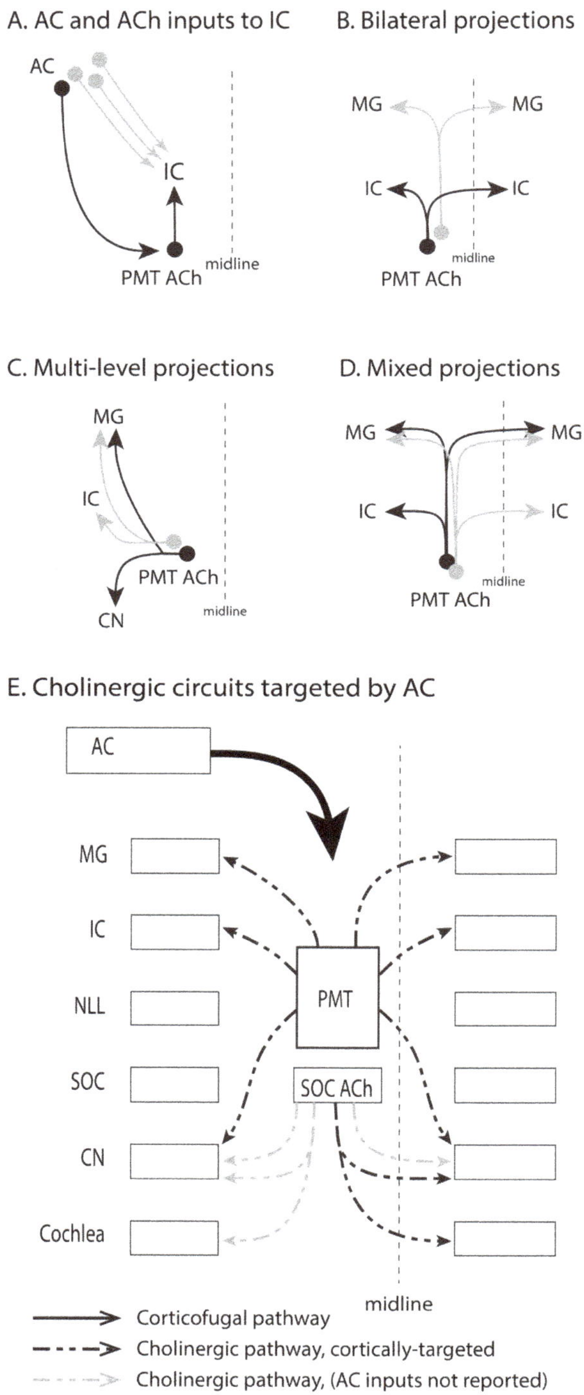

FIGURE 22.4. Brainstem cholinergic systems innervate many auditory nuclei and are closely tied to corticofugal projections. **A.** Auditory cortex (AC) projects directly to the inferior colliculus (IC, gray arrows) and also to the pontomesencephalic tegmentum (PMT), the cell group

innervate targets on both sides of the brain, that innervate different hierarchical levels of the auditory system, or combinations of such (Figure 22.4B–D; Motts & Schofield, 2011; Schofield & Beebe, 2018). At the population level, this allows the relatively small PMT (it contains ~7000 cholinergic cells in guinea pigs; ~6000 in rats; ~40,000 in humans) to innervate much of the brainstem and thalamus (Jones, 1990; Leonard et al., 1995; Manaye et al., 1999). It also means that activation of a small number of cells could lead to widespread release of acetylcholine.

The auditory corticofugal system is in a position to trigger acetylcholine release in auditory targets extending from the cochlea to the thalamus (Figure 22.4E). AC axons contact olivocochlear cells (Mulders & Robertson, 2000). AC axons can also contact PMT cholinergic cells, including those that project to the CN, to the MG, and to various combinations (Schofield, 2011; Schofield & Beebe, 2018). Such top-down control of acetylcholine release could play a key role in plasticity of the sort described earlier (Luo et al., 2011). Acetylcholine has also been implicated in other functions, such as gain control, and the descending inputs to cholinergic cells may allow for top-down influences on these functions as well.

Descending Pathways and Other Neuromodulatory Systems

The past decade has seen increasing interest in the role of neuromodulators in auditory processing and plasticity (see Hurley, Chapter 21). Significantly, these roles are being investigated at all levels of the auditory system, from cochlea to cortex. As discussed previously, dopamine appears to be a neurotransmitter in descending projections from

---

that provides the majority of cholinergic inputs to the IC. The AC axons make direct contact with PMT cholinergic cells that project to the ipsilateral IC (black arrows) and to the contralateral IC (not shown). The AC also projects to the contralateral PMT (not shown), where the axons contact cholinergic cells that innervate the IC. (B–D) PMT cholinergic cells commonly have branched axonal projections that innervate two or more auditory nuclei. Black versus gray arrows are used to show different branching patterns. Branching patterns allow individual cholinergic cells to innervate auditory nuclei bilaterally (B), or nuclei at multiple hierarchical levels of the auditory pathway (C), or both bilateral and multi-level (i.e., mixed; D). (E) Descending axons from the AC make direct contact with cholinergic cells that as a group project to many auditory structures, extending from the cochlea to the thalamus. The cholinergic projections arise from two regions: the PMT and the SOC. Cholinergic projections are shown with dashed arrows; those identified as direct targets of AC projections are shown in dashed black arrows; others are in gray. Note that AC axons also project to the contralateral PMT (not shown); this pathway is less dense than the ipsilateral one, but it also contacts cholinergic cells that project to multiple auditory nuclei. Of course, the unillustrated PMT would also receive corticofugal inputs from the AC on its own side. Together, the projections from left and right AC to the brainstem cholinergic groups are likely to elicit release of acetylcholine in many auditory structures.

the thalamus to the IC and to the SOC. These dopaminergic cells are located in the SPF, a region of the thalamus that receives ascending auditory input from the IC as well as descending input from the AC (reviewed in Schofield, 2010). It has not yet been determined whether the cortical axons directly contact SPF dopaminergic cells and, if so, where those cells project. Such a circuit could allow for auditory cortical projections to elicit dopamine release in the inferior colliculus and/or the superior olivary complex; new experiments will be needed to assess such a possibility.

Some Current Conceptual Issues

In this section, we touch briefly on the concepts of circuit loops and chains for understanding the descending auditory system. We then consider the ventral nucleus of the trapezoid body, a nucleus of the superior olivary complex and major component of the descending auditory system. We propose that this understudied nucleus serves as an inhibitory hub in the descending auditory pathways.

Loops and Chains

The concepts of feedback loops and multi-synaptic chains of neurons continue to be dominant themes for understanding the descending auditory pathways (Bajo & King, 2013; Malmierca & Ryugo, 2011; Schofield, 2010; Spangler & Warr, 1991;). Much of the early work was based on anatomical findings, and work has continued to more fully characterize descending chains (e.g., Brown et al., 2013). Loops can be technically more challenging to study, but physiological studies have reinforced views of extended loops that cross multiple levels of the auditory system. One early example is the AC–IC–MG–AC loop discussed by Yan and colleagues (Xiong et al., 2009; Luo & Yan, 2013). This work focuses on the multilevel components that interact to support cortically driven plasticity. Specifically, activation of the AC (by acoustic or artificial means) can lead to changes in the way cortical and subcortical cells respond to sounds. The largest changes are typically seen in the cortex. A key advance has been the recognition that the large changes seen in cortical responses reflect cellular changes, that is, plasticity, in both cortical and subcortical cells.

More recent work has promoted the idea of multiple interacting loops that allow top-down mechanisms to influence an even greater expanse of the central nervous system. Marsh and Campbell (2016) propose a brainstem-centered filter that controls the processing of complex sounds prior to that information being sent to higher (i.e., thalamic and cortical) levels. This brainstem filter relies on top-down influences from the AC and prefrontal cortex as well as the forebrain cholinergic system (which acts on the cortical areas). The filter, centered in the brainstem and controlled by the forebrain, exerts effects throughout the auditory system, extending even to the cochlea.

One intriguing aspect of this filter is that it allows higher functions—such as attention and expectancy—to play a key role in the perception of speech in a noisy or reverberant environment. Declining function of forebrain systems, as commonly occurs during aging, could affect processing the auditory brainstem through their effects on the brainstem filter.

The VNTB as an Inhibitory Hub in the Descending Auditory System

The VNTB stands out as a target of descending projections from both the AC and the IC. These latter regions project to numerous auditory regions below the IC, but their axons terminate most densely in the VNTB. The VNTB projects in turn to many auditory regions, including the cochlea, cochlear nucleus, other olivary nuclei, nuclei of the lateral lemniscus, inferior colliculus and auditory thalamus (Schofield et al., 2014; Warr & Beck, 1996). To date, there is direct evidence that descending pathways to the VNTB contact cells that project to the cochlea, cochlear nucleus or inferior colliculus. Specifically, projections from the IC contact VNTB cells that project contralaterally to the cochlea or contralaterally, ipsilaterally or bilaterally to the CN (Schofield & Cant, 1999). Projections from the AC contact VNTB cells that project to the cochlea or CN, and also VNTB cells that project to the IC (Coomes Peterson, & Schofield, 2007; Mulders & Robertson, 2000; Schofield & Coomes, 2006). Together, these facts suggest that the VNTB serves as a hub in the descending auditory system, distributing top-down influences from the AC and the IC to many parts of the subcortical auditory system (Figure 22.5).

What are the likely physiological effects in the descending system? The descending projections from the IC and the AC are glutamatergic and are expected to excite VNTB cells. The VNTB contains a multitude of neurotransmitter phenotypes, including cells that use GABA, glycine or acetylcholine. GABA and glycine are generally inhibitory whereas acetylcholine can be excitatory or inhibitory depending on the postsynaptic receptor. In guinea pigs, about 80% of the VNTB cells that project to the CN use GABA, glycine or both (Ostapoff et al., 1997). Accordingly, the VNTB is the primary source of inhibitory projections to the cochlear nucleus. As mentioned above, both AC and IC axons contact VNTB cells that project to the CN; if these cells use GABA or glycine, they could provide top-down inhibition to the CN. Assuming that the cortical and collicular projections excite their targets, the VNTB could serve as an inhibitory hub for higher order effects on the CN. Given the diverse projections from the VNTB (it projects to other olivary nuclei, to nuclei of the lateral lemniscus, to the IC and directly to the thalamus), the VNTB could possibly provide a route for AC and IC projections to exert effects throughout much of the subcortical auditory pathway. Future experiments will need to clarify the neurotransmitter phenotypes of VNTB cells targeted by descending axons and the projections of those VNTB cells.

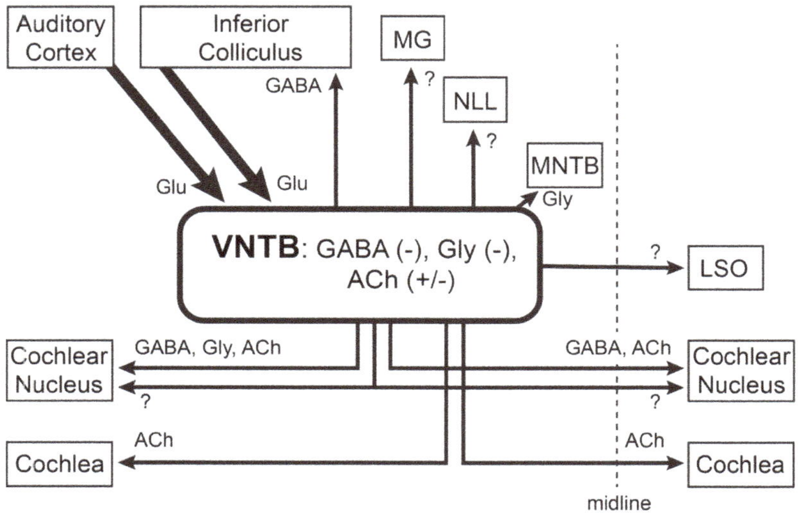

FIGURE 22.5. The ventral nucleus of the trapezoid body (VNTB) may serve as a hub in the descending auditory pathways. It is a primary target in two of the largest descending pathways, which originate from the auditory cortex (AC) and inferior colliculus (IC). The VNTB also is a source of projections to many auditory structures, from the cochlea to the thalamus. The VNTB contains multiple neurotransmitter phenotypes, including GABA, glycine, and acetylcholine. Among these, the inhibitory transmitters GABA and glycine are predominant in VNTB projections.

How does a "hub" fit into the loops and chains organization? The VNTB is likely to contribute to multiple loops and chains. The "hub" characteristic emphasizes the spatial overlap of the dense descending inputs and the multitude of VNTB outputs, raising the possibility of interactions or even shared components between loops and chains. Future experiments should be directed at characterizing the VNTB cells, their response properties, inputs, outputs, intrinsic properties, neurotransmitter phenotypes, and so on, so that the circuits can be related to their functions.

Remaining Questions

Many questions remain to be addressed to understand the contributions of descending auditory pathways to hearing. We list here a few that appear particularly relevant to the current discussion.

1. *What cell types give rise to descending pathways from a given area?* The characterization of these cells must include their neurotransmitters, the inputs they receive, their intrinsic properties, the receptors they express, and their projection

targets (again, at a resolution of cell type, not just brain area). The concept of different cell types implies different functions; correlating cell types with projection patterns will help in defining those functions and also contribute to distinguishing cell types (supporting existing schemes and/or suggesting their revision or refinement).

2. *Do cells with descending projections have branched axonal projections to multiple targets?* This is important for understanding function and also for designing and interpreting experiments. From a functional standpoint, do cells with descending projections send information (or commands) to multiple targets, or do those targets receive input from different populations of cells, allowing for independent effects on the targets? From the experimental perspective, it is critical for interpreting optogenetic experiments to know whether the axons making up a given pathway have collaterals that could lead to stimulation of additional (perhaps unintended) sites.
3. *What are the roles of tonotopic vs. non-tonotopic descending projections?* The IC gives rise to both types of projections. Moreover, the massive descending projections from the AC also includes both types. Much of the existing work on corticofugal physiology has involved stimulation or silencing of primary AC. What about projections from other cortical fields, including belt and parabelt areas, many of which are not tonotopically organized?
4. *To what extent do descending systems interact with the classic neuromodulatory systems?* There is growing evidence for close ties between corticofugal projections and the brainstem cholinergic systems. Do corticofugal projections activate, directly or indirectly, cells that use modulators like serotonin, dopamine, or noradrenaline (all of which are known to modulate brainstem auditory centers)? What functions are associated with such interactions?
5. *What roles do the descending pathways play during aging or after damage to the nervous system?* Marsh and Campbell (2016) suggest that top-down effects are critical for selecting signal from noise and represent a major site of failure in aging. Do descending pathways help compensate for diminishing input from an aging cochlea? Perhaps clinical symptoms arise *after* the descending systems have reached their limit of compensation. Or do some problems reflect dysfunction of the descending systems themselves?

CONCLUSION

This brief review has focused on the brainstem and descending inputs to it. Ongoing work is leading to better characterization of descending circuits. There remains a critical need for characterizing cell types/phenotypes of both the cells that give rise to descending projections and the cells and circuits they contact. This characterization must include neurotransmitters, the associated post-synaptic receptors and many other cellular properties that help to define function and distinguish cell types. Key advances are likely to include new insights into the relationships of descending auditory pathways with the various neuromodulatory systems. New experimental approaches, spurred by recent developments in chemogenetic and optogenetic methods, are expanding the range of functions associated with descending pathways. It will be of particular interest to learn the roles of descending pathways in contributing to the various forms of brainstem plasticity that play a role in hearing throughout the lifespan and in response to damage or degeneration in the auditory system.

Acknowledgments

The work described here that was completed in the authors' laboratory was supported by grants from the National Institutes of Health (R01 DC004391, F31 DC08463, F32 DC012450, F32 DC010958, and F31 DC014228). Space limitations prevent citation of many original studies. The authors acknowledge those researchers here with gratitude for their understanding. Special thanks to Will Noftz, Dr. Matthew Smith, and Dr. Michael Roberts for comments on an earlier draft.

References

Adams, J. C. (1980). Crossed and descending projections to the inferior colliculus. *Neuroscience Letters, 19*(1), 1–5.

Alibardi, L. (1999). Fine structure, synaptology and immunocytochemistry of large neurons in the rat dorsal cochlear nucleus connected to the inferior colliculus. *Journal für Hirnforschung, 39*(4), 429–439.

Altschuler, R. A., Juiz, J. M., Shore, S. E., Bledsoe, S. C., Helfert, R. H., Wenthold, R. J. (1993). Inhibitory amino acid synapses and pathways in the ventral cochlear nucleus. In M. A. Merchan (Ed.), *The Mammalian Cochlear Nuclei* (pp. 211–224). New York and London: Plenum Press.

Altschuler, R. A., & Shore, S. E. (2010). Central auditory neurotransmitters. In A. Rees & A. R. Palmer (Eds.), *Oxford Handbook of Auditory Neuroscience. Vol. 2: The Auditory Brain* (pp. 65–89). Oxford, England: Oxford University Press.

Andersen, R. A., Knight, P. L., & Merzenich, M. M. (1980). The thalamocortical and corticothalamic connections of AI, AII, and the anterior auditory field (AAF) in the cat: Evidence for two largely segregated systems of connections. *Journal of Comparative Neurology, 194*(3), 663–701.

Anderson, L.A., & Malmierca, M. S. (2013). The effect of auditory cortex deactivation on stimulus-specific adaptation in the inferior colliculus of the rat. *European Journal of Neuroscience, 37*(1), 52–62. doi:10.1111/ejn.12018

Aparicio, M. A., & Saldana, E. (2014). The dorsal tectal longitudinal column (TLCd): A second longitudinal column in the paramedian region of the midbrain tectum. *Brain Structure and Function, 219*(2), 607–630. doi:10.1007/s00429-013-0522-x

Bajo, V. M., & King, A. J. (2013). Cortical modulation of auditory processing in the midbrain. *Frontiers in Neural Circuits, 6*, 114. doi:10.3389/fncir.2012.00114

Bajo, V. M., Nodal, F. R., Moore, D. R., & King, A. J. (2010). The descending corticocollicular pathway mediates learning-induced auditory plasticity. *Nature Neuroscience, 13*(2), 253–260. doi:10.1038/nn.2466

Benson, T. E., & Brown, M. C. (1990). Synapses formed by olivocochlear axon branches in the mouse cochlear nucleus. *Journal of Comparative Neurology, 295*, 52–70.

Boyen, K., de Kleine, E., van Dijk, P., & Langers, D. R. (2014). Tinnitus-related dissociation between cortical and subcortical neural activity in humans with mild to moderate sensorineural hearing loss. *Hearing Research, 312*, 48–59. doi:10.1016/j.heares.2014.03.001

Brown, M. C., Liberman, M. C., Benson, T. E., & Ryugo, D. K. (1988). Brainstem branches from olivocochlear axons in cats and rodents. *Journal of Comparative Neurology, 278*, 591–603.

Brown, M. C., Mukerji, S., Drottar, M., Windsor, A. M., & Lee, D. J. (2013). Identification of inputs to olivocochlear neurons using transneuronal labeling with pseudorabies virus (PRV). *Journal of the Association for Research in Otolaryngology, 14*, 703–717.

Budinger, E., Heil, P., Hess, A., & Scheich, H. (2006). Multisensory processing via early cortical stages: Connections of the primary auditory cortical field with other sensory systems. *Neuroscience, 143*(4), 1065–1083.

Budinger, E., Brosch, M., Scheich, H., & Mylius, J. (2013). The subcortical auditory structures in the Mongolian gerbil: II. Frequency-related topography of the connections with cortical field AI. *Journal of Comparative Neurology, 521*(12), 2772–2797. doi:10.1002/cne.23314

Caicedo, A., Herbert, H. (1993). Topography of descending projections from the inferior colliculus to auditory brainstem nuclei in the rat. *Journal of Comparative Neurology, 328*, 377–392.

Coomes, D. L., Schofield, B. R. (2004). Separate projections from the inferior colliculus to the cochlear nucleus and thalamus in guinea pigs. *Hearing Research, 191*(1–2), 67–78.

Coomes Peterson, D., Schofield, B. R. (2007). Projections from auditory cortex contact ascending pathways that originate in the superior olive and inferior colliculus. *Hearing Research, 232*(1–2), 67–77. doi:10.1016/j.heares.2007.06.009

Delano, P. H., Elgoyhen, A. B. (2016). Editorial: Auditory efferent system: New insights from cortex to cochlea. *Frontiers in Systems Neuroscience, 10*, 50. doi:10.3389/fnsys.2016.00050

Faye-Lund, H. (1986). Projection from the inferior colliculus to the superior olivary complex in the albino rat. *Anatomy and Embryology, 175*, 35–52.

Feliciano, M., & Potashner, S. J. (1995). Evidence for a glutamatergic pathway from the guinea pig auditory cortex to the inferior colliculus. *Journal of Neurochemistry, 65*(3), 1348–1357.

Feliciano, M., Saldaña, E., & Mugnaini, E. (1995). Direct projections from the rat primary auditory neocortex to nucleus sagulum, paralemniscal regions, superior olivary complex and cochlear nuclei. *Auditory Neuroscience, 1*, 287–308.

Frisina, R. D., Walton, J. P., Lynch-Armour, M. A., & Byrd, J. D. (1998). Inputs to a physiologically characterized region of the inferior colliculus of the young adult CBA mouse. *Hearing Research, 115*(1–2), 61–81.

Gao, P. P., Zhang, J. W., Fan, S. J., Sanes, D. H., & Wu, E. X. (2015). Auditory midbrain processing is differentially modulated by auditory and visual cortices: An auditory fMRI study. *Neuroimage, 123*, 22–32. doi:10.1016/j.neuroimage.2015.08.040

Gómez-Nieto, R., Rubio, M. E., & Lopez, D. E. (2008). Cholinergic input from the ventral nucleus of the trapezoid body to cochlear root neurons in rats. *Journal of Comparative Neurology, 506*(3), 452–468. doi:10.1002/cne.21554

González-Hernández, T., Mantolán-Sarmiento, B., González-González, B., & Pérez-González, H. (1996). Sources of GABAergic input to the inferior colliculus of the rat. *Journal of Comparative Neurology*, *372*(2), 309–326.

Grimsley, J. M., Shanbhag, S. J., Palmer, A. R., & Wallace, M. N. (2012). Processing of communication calls in guinea pig auditory cortex. *PLoS One*, *7*(12), e51646. doi:10.1371/journal.pone.0051646

Hashikawa, T. (1983). The inferior colliculopontine neurons of the cat in relation to other collicular descending neurons. *Journal of Comparative Neurology 219*, 241–249.

Hashikawa, T., & Kawamura, K. (1983). Retrograde labeling of ascending and descending neurons in the inferior colliculus. A fluorescent double labeling study in the cat. *Experimental Brain Research*, *49*, 457–461.

Horváth, M., Kraus, K. S., & Illing, R. B. (2000). Olivocochlear neurons sending axon collaterals into the ventral cochlear nucleus of the rat. *Journal of Comparative Neurology*, *422*(1), 95–105.

Irvine, D. R. (2010). Plasticity in the auditory pathway. In A. Rees & A. R. Palmer (Eds.), *The Oxford Handbook of Auditory Neuroscience Vol. 2: The Auditory Brain* (pp. 387–415). Oxford, England: Oxford University Press.

Jen, P. H., Sun, X., & Chen, Q.C. (2001). An electrophysiological study of neural pathways for corticofugally inhibited neurons in the central nucleus of the inferior colliculus of the big brown bat, *Eptesicus fuscus*. *Experimental Brain Research*, *137*(3–4), 292–302.

Jones, B. E. (1990). Immunohistochemical study of choline acetyltransferase-immunoreactive processes and cells innervating the pontomedullary reticular formation in the rat. *Journal of Comparative Neurology*, *295*(3), 485–514. doi:10.1002/cne.902950311

Kolston, J., Osen, K. K., Hackney, C. M., Ottersen, O. P, & Storm-Mathisen, J. (1992). An atlas of glycine- and GABA-like immunoreactivity and colocalization in the cochlear nuclear complex of the guinea pig. *Anatomy and Embryology*, *186*, 443–465.

Kong, L., Xiong, C., Li, L., & Yan, J. (2014). Frequency-specific corticofugal modulation of the dorsal cochlear nucleus in mice. *Frontiers in Systems Neuroscience*, *8*, 125. doi:10.3389/fnsys.2014.00125

Kuwabara, N., & Zook, J. M. (2000). Geniculo-collicular descending projections in the gerbil. *Brain Research*, *878*(1–2), 79–87.

Leonard, C. S., Kerman, I., Blaha, G., Taveras, E., & Taylor, B. (1995). Interdigitation of nitric oxide synthase-, tyrosine hydroxylase-, and serotonin-containing neurons in and around the laterodorsal and pedunculopontine tegmental nuclei of the guinea pig. *Journal of Comparative Neurology*, *362*(3), 411–432.

Liu, X., Yan, Y., Wang, Y., & Yan, J. (2010). Corticofugal modulation of initial neural processing of sound information from the ipsilateral ear in the mouse. *PLoS One*, *5*(11), e14038. doi:10.1371/journal.pone.0014038

Luo, F., Liu, X., Wang, C., & Yan, J. (2011). The pedunculopontine tegmental nucleus: A second cholinergic source for frequency-specific auditory plasticity. *Journal of Neurophysiology*, *105*(1), 107–116. doi:10.1152/jn.00546.2010

Luo, F., & Yan, J. (2013). Sound-specific plasticity in the primary auditory cortex as induced by the cholinergic pedunculopontine tegmental nucleus. *European Journal of Neuroscience*, *37*(3), 393–399. doi:10.1111/ejn.12046

Ma, X., & Suga, N. (2001). Plasticity of bat's central auditory system evoked by focal electric stimulation of auditory and/or somatosensory cortices. *Journal of Neurophysiology*, *85*(3), 1078–1087.

Malmierca, M. S., Le Beau, F. E., & Rees, A. (1996). The topographical organization of descending projections from the central nucleus of the inferior colliculus in guinea pig. *Hearing Research*, *93*(1–2), 167–180.

Malmierca, M. S., & Ryugo, D. K. (2011). Descending connections of auditory cortex to the midbrain and brain stem. In J. A. Winer & C. E. Schreiner (Eds.), *The Auditory Cortex* (pp. 189–208). Berlin, Germany: Springer Science+Business Media.

Manaye, K. F., Zweig, R., Wu, D., Hersh, L. B., De Lacalle, S., Saper, C. B., & German, D. C. (1999). Quantification of cholinergic and select non-cholinergic mesopontine neuronal populations in the human brain. *Neuroscience*, *89*(3), 759–770.

Markovitz, C. D., Hogan, P. S., Wesen, K. A., & Lim, H. H. (2015). Pairing broadband noise with cortical stimulation induces extensive suppression of ascending sensory activity. *Journal of Neural Engineering*, *12*(2), 026006. doi:10.1088/1741-2560/12/2/026006

Markovitz, C. D., Tang, T. T., & Lim, H. H. (2013). Tonotopic and localized pathways from primary auditory cortex to the central nucleus of the inferior colliculus. *Front Neural Circuits*, *7*, 77. doi:10.3389/fncir.2013.00077

Marsh, J. E., & Campbell, T. A. (2016). Processing complex sounds passing through the rostral brainstem: The new early filter model. *Frontiers in Neuroscience*, *10*, 136. doi:10.3389/fnins.2016.00136

Mellott, J. G., Beebe, N. L., & Schofield, B. R. (2018). GABAergic and non-GABAergic projections to the superior colliculus from the auditory brainstem. *Brain Structure and Function*. doi:10.1007/s00429-017-1599-4

Mellott, J. G., Bickford, M. E., & Schofield, B. R. (2014a). Descending projections from auditory cortex to excitatory and inhibitory cells in the nucleus of the brachium of the inferior colliculus. *Frontiers in Systems Neuroscience*, *8*, 188. doi:10.3389/fnsys.2014.00188

Mellott, J. G., Foster, N. L., Nakamoto, K. T., Motts, S. D., & Schofield, B. R. (2014b). Distribution of GABAergic cells in the inferior colliculus that project to the thalamus. *Frontiers in Neuroanatomy*, *8*, 17. doi:10.3389/fnana.2014.00017

Milinkeviciute, G., Muniak, M.A., & Ryugo, D.K. (2017). Descending projections from the inferior colliculus to the dorsal cochlear nucleus are excitatory. *Journal of Comparative Neurology*, *525*(4), 773–793. doi:10.1002/cne.24095

Miranda, J. A., Shepard, K. N., McClintock, S. K., & Liu, R. C. (2014). Adult plasticity in the subcortical auditory pathway of the maternal mouse. *PLoS One*, *9*(7), e101630. doi:10.1371/journal.pone.0101630

Mitani, A., Shimokouchi, M., & Nomura, S. (1983). Effects of stimulation of the primary auditory cortex upon colliculogeniculate neurons in the inferior colliculus of the cat. *Neuroscience Letters*, *42*, 185–189.

Moore, D. R. (1988). Auditory brainstem of the ferret: Sources of projections to the inferior colliculus. *Journal of Comparative Neurology*, *269*, 342–354.

Moriizumi, T., & Hattori, T. (1992). Anatomical and functional compartmentalization of the subparafascicular thalamic nucleus in the rat. *Experimental Brain Research*, *90*, 175–179.

Motts, S. D., & Schofield, B. R. (2009). Sources of cholinergic input to the inferior colliculus. *Neuroscience* *160*, 103–114.

Motts, S. D., & Schofield, B. R. (2011). Cholinergic cells in the tegmentum send branching projections to the inferior colliculus and the medial geniculate body. *Neuroscience*, *179*, 120–130. doi:10.1016/j.neuroscience.2011.01.044

Mulders, W. H., & Robertson, D. (2000). Evidence for direct cortical innervation of medial olivocochlear neurones in rats. *Hearing Research*, *144*(1–2), 65–72.

Nakamoto, K. T., Mellott, J. G., Killius. J., Storey-Workley, M.E., Sowick, C. S., & Schofield, B. R. (2013a). Ultrastructural examination of the corticocollicular pathway in the guinea pig: A study using electron microscopy, neural tracers, and GABA immunocytochemistry. *Frontiers Neuroanatomy*, *7*, 13. doi:10.3389/fnana.2013.00013

Nakamoto, K. T., Shackleton, T. M., Palmer, A. R. (2010). Responses in the inferior colliculus of the guinea pig to concurrent harmonic series and the effect of inactivation of descending controls. *Journal of Neurophysiology*, *103*(4), 2050–2061. doi:10.1152/jn.00451.2009

Nakamoto, K. T., Sowick, C. S., Schofield, B. R. (2013b). Auditory cortical axons contact commissural cells throughout the guinea pig inferior colliculus. *Hearing Research*, *306*, 131–144.

Nevue, A. A., Elde, C.J., Perkel, D. J., & Portfors, C. V. (2016a). Dopaminergic input to the inferior colliculus in mice. *Frontiers in Neuroanatomy*, *9*, 168. doi:10.3389/fnana.2015.00168

Nevue A. A., Felix, R. A., & Portfors, C. V. (2016b) Dopaminergic projections of the subparafascicular thalamic nucleus to the auditory brainstem. *Hearing Research*, *341*, 202–209. doi:10.1016/j.heares.2016.09.001

Oertel, D., & Young, E. D. (2004). What's a cerebellar circuit doing in the auditory system? *Trends in Neuroscience*, *27*(2), 104–110. doi:10.1016/j.tins.2003.12.001 S0166223603003862 [pii]

Okoyama, S., Ohbayashi, M., Ito, M., & Harada, S. (2006). Neuronal organization of the rat inferior colliculus participating in four major auditory pathways. *Hearing Research*, *218*(1–2), 72–80.

Ostapoff, E.-M., Benson, C. G., & Saint Marie, R. L. (1997). GABA-and glycine-immunoreactive projections from the superior olivary complex to the cochlear nucleus in guinea pig. *Journal of Comparative Neurology*, *381*, 500–512.

Patel, M. B., Sons, S., Yudintsev, G., Lesicko, A. M., Yang, L, Taha, G. A., . . . Llano, D. A. (2017). Anatomical characterization of subcortical descending projections to the inferior colliculus in mouse. *Journal of Comparative Neurology*, *525*(4), 885–900. doi:10.1002/cne.24106

Peng, K., Peng, Y. J., Wang, J., Yang, M. J., Fu, Z. Y., Tang, J., & Chen, Q. C. (2017). Latency modulation of collicular neurons induced by electric stimulation of the auditory cortex in *Hipposideros pratti*: In vivo intracellular recording. *PLoS One*, *12*(9), e0184097. doi:10.1371/journal.pone.0184097

Popelár, J., Suta, D., Lindovsky, J., Bures, Z., Pysanenko, K., Chumak, T., & Syka, J. (2016). Cooling of the auditory cortex modifies neuronal activity in the inferior colliculus in rats. *Hearing Research*, *332*, 7–16. doi:10.1016/j.heares.2015.10.021

Ryan, A. F., Keithley, E. M., Wang, Z.-X., & Schwartz, I. R. (1990). Collaterals from lateral and medial olivocochlear efferent neurons innervate different regions of the cochlear nucleus and adjacent brainstem. *Journal of Comparative Neurology*, *300*, 572–582.

Saint Marie, R. L. (1996). Glutamatergic connections of the auditory midbrain: selective uptake and axonal transport of D-[3H]Aspartate. *Journal of Comparative Neurology*, *373*, 255–270.

Saldaña, E., Feliciano, M., & Mugnaini, E. (1996). Distribution of descending projections from primary auditory neocortex to inferior colliculus mimics the topography of intracollicular projections. *Journal of Comparative Neurology*, *371*(1), 15–40.

Saldaña, E., Viñuela, A., Marshall, A. F., Fitzpatrick, D. C., & Aparicio, M. A. (2007). The TLC: A novel auditory nucleus of the mammalian brain. *Journal of Neuroscience*, *27*(48), 13108–13116. doi:10.1523/JNEUROSCI.1892-07.2007

Schofield, B. R. (1994). Projections to the cochlear nuclei from principal cells in the medial nucleus of the trapezoid body in guinea pigs. *Journal of Comparative Neurology, 344*(1), 83–100.

Schofield, B. R. (2001). Origins of projections from the inferior colliculus to the cochlear nucleus in guinea pigs. *Journal of Comparative Neurology, 429*(2), 206–220.

Schofield, B. R. (2002). Ascending and descending projections from the superior olivary complex in guinea pigs: Different cells project to the cochlear nucleus and the inferior colliculus. *Journal of Comparative Neurology, 453*(3), 217–225.

Schofield, B. R. (2010). Structural organization of the descending auditory pathway. In A. Rees & A. R. Palmer (Eds.), *The Oxford Handbook of Auditory Neuroscience. Vol. 2: The Auditory Brain* (pp. 43–64). Oxford, England: Oxford University Press.

Schofield, B. R. (2011). Central descending auditory pathways. In D. K. Ryugo, A. N. Popper, & R. R. Fay (Eds.), *Springer Handbook of Auditory Research, Vol. 15, Auditory and Vestibular Efferents* (pp. 261–290). New York, NY: Springer-Verlag.

Schofield, B. R., & Beebe, N. L. (2018). Auditory cortex projects to brainstem cholinergic cells that innervate the thalamus and the cochlear nucleus. *Association for Research in Otolaryngology Abstracts, 41*, 27.

Schofield, B. R., & Cant, N. B. (1999). Descending auditory pathways: Projections from the inferior colliculus contact superior olivary cells that project bilaterally to the cochlear nuclei. *Journal of Comparative Neurology, 409*, 210–223.

Schofield, B. R., & Coomes, D. L. (2006). Pathways from auditory cortex to the cochlear nucleus in guinea pigs. *Hearing Research, 216–217*, 81–89.

Schofield, B. R., & Hurley, L. (2018). Circuits for modulation of auditory function. In: D. O. Oliver, N. B. Cant, A. N. Popper, R. R. Fay (Eds.). *Springer Handbook of Auditory Research, The Mammalian Auditory Pathways: Synaptic Organization and Microcircuits* (pp. 235–267). New York: Springer-Verlag.

Schofield, B. R., Mellott, J. G., & Motts, S. D. (2014). Subcollicular projections to the auditory thalamus and collateral projections to the inferior colliculus. *Frontiers in Neuroanatomy 8*, 70.

Schofield, B. R., Motts, S. D., & Mellott, J. G. (2011). Cholinergic cells of the pontomesencephalic tegmentum: Connections with auditory structures from cochlear nucleus to cortex. *Hearing Research, 279*(1–2), 85–95. doi:10.1016/j.heares.2010.12.019

Schwartz, I. R. (1992). The superior olivary complex and lateral lemniscal nuclei. In D. B. Webster, A. N. Popper, & R. R. Fay (Eds.), *The mammalian auditory pathway: Neuroanatomy* (pp. 117–167). New York, NY: Springer-Verlag.

Senatorov, V. V., & Hu, B. (2002). Extracortical descending projections to the rat inferior colliculus. *Neuroscience, 115*(1), 243–250.

Sherriff, F. E., & Henderson, Z. (1994). Cholinergic neurons in the ventral trapezoid nucleus project to the cochlear nuclei in the rat. *Neuroscience, 58*(3), 627–633.

Shore, S. E., Helfert, R. H., & Bledsoe, S. C. Jr., Altschuler, R. A., & Godfrey, D. A. (1991). Descending projections to the dorsal and ventral divisions of the cochlear nucleus in guinea pig. *Hearing Research, 52*, 255–268.

Spangler, K. M., & Warr, W. B. (1991). The descending auditory system. In R. A. Altschuler, R. P. Bobbin, B. M. Clopton, & D. W. Hoffman (Eds.), *Neurobiology of Hearing: the Central Auditory System* (pp. 27–45). New York, NY: Raven Press.

Straka, M. M., Hughes, R., Lee, P., & Lim, H. H. (2015). Descending and tonotopic projection patterns from the auditory cortex to the inferior colliculus. *Neuroscience, 300*, 325–337. doi:10.1016/j.neuroscience.2015.05.032

Suga, N. (2012). Tuning shifts of the auditory system by corticocortical and corticofugal projections and conditioning. *Neuroscience and Biobehavioral Reviews*, *36*(2), 969–988. doi:10.1016/j.neubiorev.2011.11.006

Suthakar, K., & Ryugo, D. K. (2017). Descending projections from the inferior colliculus to medial olivocochlear efferents: Mice with normal hearing, early onset hearing loss, and congenital deafness. *Hearing Research*, *343*, 34–49. doi:10.1016/j.heares.2016.06.014

Terreros, G., & Delano, P. H. (2015). Corticofugal modulation of peripheral auditory responses. *Frontiers in Systems Neuroscience* *9*, 134.

Thompson, A. M., Schofield, B. R. (2000). Afferent projections of the superior olivary complex. *Microscopy Research and Technique*, *51*(4), 330–354.

Thompson, A. M., & Thompson, G. C. (1993). Relationship of descending inferior colliculus projections to olivocochlear neurons. *Journal of Comparative Neurology*, *335*, 402–412.

Torterolo, P., Zurita, P., Pedemonte, M., & Velluti, R. A. (1998). Auditory cortical efferent actions upon inferior colliculus unitary activity in the guinea pig. *Neuroscience Letters*, *249*(2–3), 172–176.

Vetter, D. E., Saldaña, E., & Mugnaini, E. (1993). Input from the inferior colliculus to medial olivocochlear neurons in the rat: A double label study with PHA-L and cholera toxin. *Hearing Research*, *70*(2), 173–186.

Viñuela, A., Aparicio, M. A., Berrebi, A. S., & Saldaña, E. (2011). Connections of the superior paraolivary nucleus of the rat: II. Reciprocal connections with the tectal longitudinal column. *Frontiers in Neuroanatomy*, *5*, 1. doi:10.3389/fnana.2011.00001

Warr, W. B., & Beck, J. E. (1996). Multiple projections from the ventral nucleus of the trapezoid body in the rat. *Hearing Research*, *93*(1–2), 83–101.

Winer, J. A., & Larue, D. T. (1996). Evolution of GABAergic circuitry in the mammalian medial geniculate body. *Proceedings of the National Academy of Sciences USA*, *93*(7), 3083–3087.

Winer, J. A., Larue, D. T., Diehl, J. J., & Hefti, B. J. (1998). Auditory cortical projections to the cat inferior colliculus. *Journal of Comparative Neurology*, *400*(2), 147–174.

Winer, J. A., Chernock, M. L., Larue, D. T., & Cheung, S. W. (2002). Descending projections to the inferior colliculus from the posterior thalamus and the auditory cortex in rat, cat, and monkey. *Hearing Research*, *168*(1–2), 181–195.

Xiong, Y., Zhang, Y., & Yan, J. (2009). The neurobiology of sound-specific auditory plasticity: A core neural circuit. *Neuroscience Biobehavior Review*, *33*(8), 1178–1184. doi:10.1016/j.neubiorev.2008.10.006

Xiong, X. R., Liang, F., Zingg, B., Ji, X. Y., Ibrahim, L. A., Tao, H. W., & Zhang, L. I. (2015). Auditory cortex controls sound-driven innate defense behaviour through corticofugal projections to inferior colliculus. *Nature Communications*, *6*, 7224. doi:10.1038/ncomms8224

Yasui, Y., Nakano, K., & Mizuno, N. (1992). Descending projections from the subparafascicular thalamic nucleus to the lower brain stem in the rat. *Experimental Brain Research*, *90*(3), 508–518.

Zhao, Y., & Tzounopoulos, T. (2011). Physiological activation of cholinergic inputs controls associative synaptic plasticity via modulation of endocannabinoid signaling. *Journal of Neuroscience*, *31*(9), 3158–3168. doi:10.1523/JNEUROSCI.5303-10.2011

CHAPTER 23

AGING PROCESSES IN THE SUBCORTICAL AUDITORY SYSTEM

DONALD M. CASPARY AND DANIEL A. LLANO

Abstract

As arguably the third most common malady of industrialized populations, age-related hearing loss is associated with social isolation and depression in a subset of the population that will approach 25% by 2050. Development of behavioral or pharmacotherapeutic approaches to prevent or delay the onset of age-related hearing loss and mitigate the impact of hearing loss of speech understanding requires a better understanding of age-related changes that occur in the central auditory processor. This chapter critically reviews and discusses changes that occur in the auditory brainstem and thalamus with increased age. It briefly discusses age-related cellular changes that occur de novo within the central auditory system versus deafferentation plasticity and animal models of aging. Subsections discuss the cochlear nucleus, superior olivary complex, inferior colliculus, and the medial geniculate body with an emphasis on age-related changes in neurotransmission and how these changes could underpin the observed loss of precise temporal processing with increased age.

Keywords: age-related hearing loss, presbycusis, brainstem aging, central auditory system, dorsal cochlear nucleus, superior olivary complex, inferior colliculus, medial geniculate body

The Importance of Age-Related Hearing Loss

United States epidemiological studies suggest that the prevalence of age-related hearing loss and its significant companion, loss of speech understanding, doubles with every decade of life, affecting 30% of the US population aged 65 to 74 years, and 50% of the population over 75 years of age (F. R. Lin, Thorpe, Gordon-Salant, & Ferrucci, 2011). US census data predict that the over age 65 population will increase from 14% in 2014 to near 21% by 2040 (https://aoa.acl.gov/), substantially increasing the number of individuals with age-related declines in speech understanding. Age-related hearing loss is socially debilitating, decreasing quality of life and leading to social isolation and depression in a substantial number of older adults (Dalton et al., 2003). Even older adults with mild-to-moderate age-related hearing loss can show substantially impaired processing of speech, especially in complex listening environments (Dalton et al., 2003; Gordon-Salant, 2014; Humes et al., 2012). Human and animal models of presbycusis show large variations in the age-related loss of cochlear hair cells and auditory nerve fibers. Peripheral changes only partially correlate with the observed age-related loss of temporal discrimination/speech processing and with the ability to attend to acoustic stimuli. This lack of correlation suggests a significant contribution of central auditory changes to presbycusis (Alain & Woods, 1999; S. Anderson, Parbery-Clark, White-Schwoch, & Kraus, 2012; Caspary, Ling, Turner, & Hughes, 2008; de Villers-Sidani et al., 2010; Gordon-Salant & Fitzgibbons, 1993; Humes, Kewley-Port, Fogerty, & Kinney, 2010; Juarez-Salinas, Engle, Navarro, & Recanzone, 2010; Lister, Besing, & Koehnke, 2002; Pichora-Fuller, Alain, & Schneider, 2017; Snell, 1997; Takahashi & Bacon, 1992; Tremblay, Piskosz, & Souza, 2003). Here we review subcortical age-related changes, which likely reflects degraded up-stream/ascending temporal processing attributed, in part, to increased temporal jitter at successive nuclei along the ascending auditory neuraxis. Age-related auditory brainstem changes in the timing of coded environmental acoustic information also impact the ability of older adults to accurately localize sound, which further degrades their ability to extract speech signals in cluttered acoustic environments (Dubno, Ahlstrom, & Horwitz, 2008; Eddins & Hall, 2010; King, Hopkins, & Plack, 2014; Pichora-Fuller et al., 2017; Pichora-Fuller, Schneider, Macdonald, Pass, & Brown, 2007).

The ability to code rapidly time-varying signals such as speech is facilitated by time-locked and tonic inhibition at multiple levels of the auditory brainstem. Age-related loss of speech understanding, in part, likely reflects maladaptive age-related plastic changes in inhibitory neurotransmission in response to a loss of ascending glutamatergic excitatory drive (Caspary et al., 2008; Godfrey, Chen, O'Toole, & Mustapha, 2017; Gold & Bajo, 2014).

Each section of this chapter will focus on age-related changes in (1) anatomical and structural features, (2) excitatory (glutamate) and inhibitory (GABA and glycine) amino acid neurotransmitters and their ionotropic and metabotropic receptors. (3) neuromodulators and calcium homeostasis, and (4) functional/physiological properties, and how these changes may be reflected in the behavior of the whole organism.

Successive chapter sections will detail observed age-related changes in dorsal cochlear nucleus (DCN), superior olivary complex (SOC), inferior colliculus (IC), and auditory thalamus/medial geniculate body (MGB). Layered upon the age-related changes in primary auditory neurotransmission affecting temporal processing are age-related changes in auditory vigilance, which are performed less well by older adults, especially those individuals with cognitive and attentional declines (Harris, Wilson, Eckert, & Dubno, 2012; Humes et al., 2012).

Cellular Mechanisms of Aging and Age-Related Hearing Loss

At the tissue level, aging is generally characterized by an accumulation of cellular damage over time. Cellular aging was once thought to be caused by a stochastic decline in function (i.e., "wearing out") of cellular components (Abernethy, 1979). However, we now know that aging is driven by specific sets of genetically or epigenetically programmed sequences of events which cause both adaptive and non-adaptive changes in cellular function (reviewed in López-Otín, Blasco, Partridge, Serrano, & Kroemer, 2013). Here, we briefly review the major cellular changes thought to occur with aging, and how they relate to the auditory system.

DNA damage, both nuclear and mitochondrial, is one hallmark of aging. In the nucleus, DNA damage often leads to an adaptive cellular or replicative senescence response, which diminishes the replication of damaged cells or induces apoptosis (Grimes & Chandra, 2009; Rodriguez-Brenes, Wodarz, & Komarova, 2015). Concomitant with the age-related DNA changes is the shortening of telomeres, which are short strands of DNA that help protect chromosomes from damage or fusion with nearby chromosomes. Mitochondrial DNA contains diminished endogenous repair mechanisms relative to nuclear DNA and therefore is more vulnerable to age-related insults than nuclear DNA (López-Otín et al., 2013). Further, mitochondria are the source of oxygen-based free radical production, further exposing cells to threats over time. This age-related increase in free radicals has led to hypotheses suggesting that mitochondrial dysfunction underpins the aging process. In addition, aging is associated with the diminished ability of mitochondria to both produce ATP and to control the production of free radical molecules. Aging mitochondria also produce superoxide anion and hydrogen peroxide at increased rates compared to younger mitochondria (Lass, Sohal, Weindruch, Forster, & Sohal, 1998; Sohal, Agarwal, Candas, Forster, & Lal, 1994). Compounding this problem, the levels of endogenous anti-oxidant molecules diminish with aging (Rebrin, Forster, & Sohal, 2007; Rebrin, Kamzalov, & Sohal, 2003).

Efforts to extend the lifespans of experimental animals have led to the discovery of molecules that function, in part, to detect ambient cellular nutrient levels, and diminished function of these molecules may also lead to an aging phenotype. For example, sirtuins, which detect levels of NAD^+, function as deacetylase inhibitors, thereby altering age-related epigenetic modifications of nuclear DNA (Longo & Kennedy, 2006). Other molecules that are sensitive to nutrient levels are mTOR (mammalian target of rapamycin; Kapahi et al., 2010) and AMP-activated protein kinase (Salminen & Kaarniranta, 2012). These proteins have been implicated in the beneficial effects of caloric restriction on aging, which has been shown to protect against age-related hearing loss in experimental animals (Someya, Yamasoba, Weindruch, Prolla, & Tanokura, 2007).

Aging Mechanisms in the Auditory System

Although these mechanisms have been extensively studied in organisms ranging from yeast to humans, few studies have systematically examined their role in age-related hearing loss outside of the cochlea. Within the cochlea, multiple studies have revealed evidence for roles of mitochondrial dysfunction and oxidative stress (Fischel-Ghodsian et al., 1997; D. W. Hoffman, Whitworth, Jones-King, & Rybak, 1988; Someya & Prolla, 2010; Yamasoba et al., 2007), proteostatic dysfunction (W. Wang et al., 2015), and diminished sirtuin levels (Xiong et al., 2014; Zeng et al., 2014) with aging. However, very little work, to our knowledge, has been done to examine the relevance of these mechanisms in the central auditory system. At the level of the IC, and as reviewed in the next section, homogenates from aged Fischer 344 rats showed diminished levels of antioxidant enzymes superoxide dismutase and catalase and increased levels of lipid peroxidation (Mei, Gawai, Nie, Ramkumar, & Helfert, 1999). Electron microscopy also revealed a decrease in mitochondrial number with aging that was more pronounced in GABAergic neurons (Mei et al., 1999). The investigators also documented an increase in mitochondrial morphological abnormalities in the aged group (Mei et al., 1999). Supporting a potential age-related loss of proteostasis at the level of the IC is the finding that levels of heat-shock protein (Hsp) 72 are decreased by more than 50% in the aged Fischer 344 rat (Helfert, Glatz, Wilson, Ramkumar, & Hughes, 2002). At the level of the auditory cortex, aging in rodent models has been associated with a drop in sirtuin levels, as well as drops in superoxide dismutase and increases in mitochondrial DNA mutation rates (Xiong et al., 2014; Zeng et al., 2014). Further work is clearly needed to explore the potential contribution of cellular aging mechanisms to central auditory processing deficits in aging, described next.

The Auditory Periphery, Peripheral Deafferentation, and Age-Related Hearing Loss

A number of chapters in the present volume examine plastic compensatory changes in central auditory structures following loss of normal adult peripheral input due to damage/dysfunctional changes in the middle ear, cochlea, and/or acoustic nerve (see chapters by Trussell, Manis, Rubio, Kaltenbach, and Shore, in this volume). Age-related peripheral changes have been a focus of a considerable number of recent studies providing for an update of the elegant historic work described in Schuknecht and Gacek (1993). These recent studies find that age-related hearing loss or presbycusis likely consists of some combination of sensory, neural, strial, and conductive elements resulting in a net loss in the quality and intensity of environmental and communication sounds reaching the central auditory processor (Altschuler et al., 2015; Kujawa & Liberman, 2015; Liberman, 2017; Ohlemiller, 2004). Recently a series of studies suggest that even profound acoustic nerve fiber losses may not substantially alter pure tone thresholds (Cai, Montgomery, Graves, Caspary, & Cox, 2017; Kujawa & Liberman, 2009; H. W. Lin, Furman, Kujawa, & Liberman, 2011; Sergeyenko, Lall, Liberman, & Kujawa, 2013). However, it has long been understood that elderly individuals with near-normal pure-tone thresholds may show significant deficits in speech understanding especially in complex acoustic environments (Harris et al., 2012; Humes et al., 2012; Pichora-Fuller et al., 2017). As extensively reviewed by Gold and Bajo as well as Syka (Gold & Bajo, 2014; Syka, 2002), when comparing aging to hearing loss with sound exposure (Godfrey et al., 2017; Godfrey et al., 2012), there are similarities in the central neurotransmitter and functional changes irrespective of the source/cause of the peripheral deafferentation (also see Bauer, Turner, Caspary, Myers, & Brozoski, 2008). A series of studies by Wang and colleagues found that aging and mild acoustic trauma result in similar losses in glycine receptors and functional inhibition in the rat DCN (Brozoski, Bauer, & Caspary, 2002; Caspary, Schatteman, & Hughes, 2005; H. Wang, Brozoski, & Caspary, 2011; H. Wang, Brozoski, et al., 2009; H. Wang, Turner, et al., 2009). Superb early studies by Suneja and Potashner (Suneja, Benson, & Potashner, 1998; Suneja, Potashner, & Benson, 1998) examined neurochemical markers of neurotransmission at different levels of the brainstem auditory pathway and at different times following disarticulation or cochlear ablation. They found compensatory changes similar to aging and sound exposure with the milder disarticulation and less similar with complete ablation of the cochlea. A study that examined three different cochlear insults found similar levels of single unit hyperactivity in the chinchilla IC with all three insult types and concluded that cochlear trauma in general, rather than its specific features, leads to multiple changes in central activity (Bauer et al., 2008). Many other examples of the similarity of brainstem neurotransmission changes following partial peripheral deafferentation due to aging or other peripheral insults are described in the reviews just noted. It appears that over a wide range of degraded peripheral acoustic input, conceptually ranging between 10% and 80%, a remarkably similar set of compensatory changes in the balance between excitatory and inhibitory neurotransmission develops in the auditory brainstem over time.

Beyond the plastic downregulation of GABA neurotransmission following partial deafferentation, GABAergic neurons may also be selectively vulnerable to metabolic changes associated with aging. For example, clinical data involving syndromes presumably related to deafferentation-related maladaptive plasticity (e.g., tinnitus, phantom pain syndromes, Charles-Bonnet syndrome) suggest that many of these plastic changes are exacerbated in the aged brain (H. J. Hoffman & Reed, 2004; Rozycka & Liguz-Lecznar, 2017; Teunisse, Cruysberg, Verbeek, & Zitman, 1995; Werhagen, Budh, Hultling, & Molander, 2004). In addition, GABAergic neurons are particularly susceptible to metabolic insults such as ischemia (Francis & Pulsinelli, 1982; Ross & Duhaime, 1989; Smith, Auer, & Siesjö, 1984), hypoxia (Sloper, Johnson, & Powell, 1980), traumatic brain injury (Erb & Povlishock, 1991), induced seizures (Houser & Esclapez, 1996), and application of amyloid beta (Pakaski et al., 1998), which may be related to the high metabolic demands of inhibitory neurons relative to their excitatory counterparts (Kann, Papageorgiou, & Draguhn, 2014). These findings suggest that a *combination* of deafferentation-related plastic changes and age-related cellular factors conspire to produce changes in central auditory function with aging.

Rodent and Non-human Primate Models of Aging

Several species have been used in studies of the aging auditory system, though rats and mice have been the most commonly used. Aging studies have examined two mouse strains in particular: C57BL/6J and CBA/CaJ. The C57BL/6J strain shows early onset presbycusis and 50% survival over 27 months. Hair cell loss occurs as soon as 3–6 months of age in C57BL/6J mice due to a mutation in cadherin 23 (Johnson, Erway, Cook, Willott, & Zheng, 1997), a protein expressed in the tip links of hair cells. Studies of age-related hearing loss in this model are complicated by the expression of cadherin 23 in the brain (Di Palma et al., 2001; Diez-Roux et al., 2011). However, the majority of genetically modified mouse lines are made on a C57BL/6J background, making this strain important for study. The CBA strain shows mild progressive age-related hearing loss across the life span (Hunter & Willott, 1987; Parham, Sun, & Kim, 1999; Willott, Parham, & Hunter, 1991). Rat strains utilized in auditory aging studies include the Fischer 344 (F344) rat, developed for cancer research at Colombia University in the early 1960s and then adopted as a model of aging by the National Institute on Aging (NIA) with 50% survival at 22 months. Eventually the NIA Rodent Resource Group began providing a back-crossed Fischer-Brown Norway (F344xBN F1 or FBN) strain which was a Brown Norway male crossed with a F344 female. The FBN strain shows 50% mortality at 34 months of age (Lipman, Chrisp, Hazzard, & Bronson, 1996). Other common rat strains, including Sprague Dawley (SD), Wistar, and Long-Evans have also been used in numerous aging studies. Gerbils are an excellent rodent model of aging and have been used in peripheral and in central studies, as we will describe (Boettcher, Mills, Swerdloff, & Holley, 1996; Gratton, Schmiedt, & Schulte, 1996; Gratton, Smyth, Schulte, & Vincent, 1995). Finally, recent detailed series of non-human primate studies, using the macaque, have added to the aging animal literature, which we will also review.

Aging and the Cochlear Nucleus

The cochlear nucleus is the first nucleus of the central auditory neuroaxis. Glutamatergic acoustic nerve fibers enter the internal acoustic meatus and bifurcate into an ascending branch which innervates the anteroventral cochlear nucleus (AVCN), and a descending branch, which innervates the posteroventral (PVCN) and dorsal (DCN) cochlear nucleus. The anatomical circuitry and physiology of the cochlear nuclei are richly reviewed in the chapters by Oertel et al., Trussell, Manis, Rubio, Kaltenbach, and Shore, in this volume. This section will focus on age-related change in the anatomy, neurochemistry and physiology of the DCN with some references to aging in ventral cochlear nucleus (VCN) reviewed (see also Manis, this volume).

Impact of Aging on the Structure of the DCN

Willott and colleagues (Willott, Bross, & McFadden, 1992) working in CBA mouse, found no age-related changes in the number or volume of DCN neurons, while a second study in CBA mice described small, but significant losses in the number of DCN neurons with age (Idrizbegovic, Canlon, Bross, Willott, & Bogdanovic, 2001). In CBA mouse DCN a significant age-related decrease in the number of labeled projection neurons was observed following injection of a retrograde tracer into the contralateral IC (Frisina & Walton, 2001, 2006).

The FBN rat shows a parallel 20–30 dB age-related threshold shift across life span (Cai & Caspary, 2015; Cai et al., 2017; Caspary et al., 2005; H. Wang, Turner et al., 2009). Godfrey and colleagues (2017) found modest, but significant changes in DCN volume in the FBN rat across the life span with increases in the middle age group (22 months), but returns toward the young (6 months) volumes at the oldest age (33 months) examined. These authors found no significant reduction/change in dry weight for any layer of the DCN across lifespan. In addition, no age-related changes in the number of DCN neurons were observed across layers when comparing 3 and 24 month-old SD rats (Jalenques, Albuisson, Despres, & Romand, 1995). While mice show age-related decreases in DCN cell number, rats show a more complex set of age-related DCN changes, which include volume changes across life span with little or no changes in neuron number or DCN dry-weight.

Impact of Aging on Neurotransmitters in the DCN

Whether the association between age-related pre- and postsynaptic changes at inhibitory, glycinergic synapses in cochlear nuclei are due solely to deafferentation or in part to de novo aging, as discussed earlier, has not been conclusively established. It is reasonable to suggest that an age-related loss of ascending excitatory drive due to the loss of acoustic nerve fibers, loss of inner and outer hair cells, decreased metabolic/endocochlear potential, and/or loss of mechanical efficiency collectively result in activity-dependent changes at acoustic nerve synapses within cochlear nuclei (Cai et al., 2017; Sergeyenko et al., 2013). Age-related reductions in acoustic nerve input may be reflected in the profound age-related decline in ambient glutamate levels in cochlear nucleus (Banay-Schwartz, Lajtha, & Palkovits, 1989; Godfrey et al., 2017). Studies, in FBN and SD rats, report a greater than 20% age-related decrease in glutamate levels throughout the cochlear nucleus, where glutamate functions as the neurotransmitter released at acoustic nerve synapses and as the transmitter released at parallel fibers synapses in the DCN (Caspary, Havey, & Faingold, 1981; Martin & Adams, 1979; Petralia, Rubio, Wang, & Wenthold, 2000; Raman & Trussell, 1995). Glutamate is the most prevalent amino acid in the brain and has multiple roles in cellular metabolism as well as neurotransmission (Cooper, Bloom, & Roth, 2003). Although it has been established that both AMPA and NMDA type glutamate receptors are negatively impacted by aging (Wenk & Barnes, 2000), few, if any studies have examined the effects of aging on postsynaptic AMPA or NMDA receptors in the aging DCN. Additional studies by Manis (this volume), have shown age-related dysfunction at the endbulb/acoustic nerve synapses in AVCN (Y. Wang & Manis, 2005; Xie & Manis, 2017).

The primary inhibitory neurotransmitter in the cochlear nucleus is glycine (Caspary, Backoff, Finlayson, & Palombi, 1994; Caspary, Havey, & Faingold, 1979; Kolston, Osen, Hackney, Ottersen, & Storm-Mathisen, 1992). GABA may be a neurotransmitter at a minority of VCN synapses, primarily in PVCN, and there are likely GABAergic neurons in the superficial layers of the DCN which may project onto the apical dendrites of fusiform cells (Rubio & Juiz, 2004). It appears that at many glycinergic terminals/synapses, GABA is co-released along with glycine, where glycine functions as the primary postsynaptic inhibitory transmitter acting at ionotropic chloride fluxing glycine receptors (GlyRs) to inhibit the target neuron, while co-released GABA acts presynaptically at $GABA_B$ autoreceptors and possibly as a weak agonist at GlyRs to shorten postsynaptic glycinergic currents (Caspary, Rybak, & Faingold, 1984; Kolston et al., 1992; Lim, Alvarez, & Walmsley, 2000; T. Lu, Rubio, & Trussell, 2008). Presynaptic $GABA_B$ receptors also modulate excitatory neurotransmitter release in the cochlear nucleus (Caspary et al., 1984; Irie & Ohmori, 2008; Lujan, Shigemoto, Kulik, & Juiz, 2004). In DCN, glycinergic projections from neighboring vertical cells profoundly depress near-characteristic frequency (CF) tone-evoked responses by acting at GlyRs on the basal dendrites and somata of fusiform DCN projection neurons (Caspary, Pazara, Ko, & Faingold, 1987; Davis & Young, 2000; Rhode, 1999; Rhode, Smith, & Oertel, 1983; Voigt & Young, 1990). This micro-circuit controls near-CF discharge rate/dynamic range and gain while having only minor effects on the sharpness of tuning (Caspary et al., 1987). Glycine receptor radioligand binding studies have been carried out in mice and rats using the high affinity α_1 GlyR subunit ligand, strychnine (Frostholm & Rotter, 1985; Milbrandt & Caspary, 1995; H. Wang, Turner, et al., 2009; Willott, Milbrandt, Bross, & Caspary, 1997). These rodent studies show significant age-related losses of strychnine binding throughout the fusiform cell layer with the largest age-related losses in the medial or high frequency limb of DCN (Milbrandt & Caspary, 1995; H. Wang, Turner, et al., 2009; Willott et al., 1997). Age-related changes in GlyR subunit message and protein suggest an age-related change in the makeup of aged GlyRs in the DCN (Krenning, Hughes, Caspary, & Helfert, 1998; H. Wang, Turner, et al., 2009; Willott et al., 1997). Specifically, the wild-type α_1 GlyR subunit shows significant age-related declines in the fusiform cell layer with a paradoxical increase in the GlyR anchoring protein, gephrin (H. Wang, Turner et al., 2009). These age-related changes in near-CF inhibition significantly alter the temporal processing ability of DCN output neurons, as discussed next.

Impact of Aging on Calcium Binding Proteins, Glia, and Trophic Factors in DCN

Many theories of generalized aging have focused on dysfunctional calcium signaling because normal adult brain function, including synaptic transmission, transmitter and endocrine secretion, excitability, learning, and memory, relies on calcium homeostasis. A number of mouse DCN studies have shown age-related increases in levels of the major calcium binding proteins: calbindin, calretinin, and parvalbumin (Idrizbegovic, Bogdanovic, Viberg, & Canlon, 2003; Idrizbegovic, Bogdanovic, Willott, & Canlon, 2004; Idrizbegovic, Salman, Niu, & Canlon, 2006; Zettel, O'Neill, Trang, & Frisina, 2003). Contrary to these findings, a non-human primate aging study found no age-related change in parvalbumin in macaque DCN (Gray, Engle, & Recanzone, 2014). A postmortem human DCN study examined calcium-binding proteins across nine decades of life and found no age-related changes in calbindin and calretinin, but significant reductions in parvalbumin-positive neurons in the 6th and 8th decade with a nonsignificant trend in the 9th decade, likely due to the small number of subjects (Sharma, Nag, Thakar, Bhardwaj, & Roy, 2014). These investigators also examined age-related changes in glial fibrillary acidic protein (GFAP), considered a marker of gliosis and possibly for impaired synaptic plasticity (Finch, 2003). Few changes in GFAP across life span were found in human DCN (Sharma et al., 2014) unlike an earlier rat study which found significant increases in GFAP-positive cell numbers and density with aging (Jalenques et al., 1995). Wang and colleagues (2011) described no significant age-related changes in brain-derived neurotrophic factor (BDNF) or its receptor in rat DCN.

Impact of Aging on the Physiology of the DCN

DCN fusiform or pyramidal neurons represent the primary output to the contralateral IC (Cant & Benson, 2003; Oertel & Young, 2004; Rhode et al., 1983). These neurons show unique temporal response properties and areas of profound inhibition, which focused near the CF within their excitatory response areas (Young & Brownell, 1976). Thus, fusiform cell CF rate-level functions display a profound non-monotonicity reflecting the glycinergic input from neighboring vertical cells onto their basal dendrites and somata (Caspary et al., 1987; Caspary et al., 2005). Iontophoretic application of the GlyR antagonist strychnine transforms the non-monotonic rate-level function into more monotonic functions (Caspary et al., 1987; Davis & Young, 2000). One would predict that if aging negatively impacted glycinergic circuits within the DCN, rate-level functions from aged fusiform cells would show more monotonic functions. That is exactly what was found when comparing recordings from aged fusiform cells with fusiform cells from young adult DCN in FBN rat (Caspary et al., 2005). Likely reflecting age-related peripheral changes, aged fusiform cells showed significantly elevated CF thresholds, increased spontaneous activity, and higher driven rates at supra-threshold intensities. As might be predicted by the age-related loss of inhibition, this same population of fusiform cells showed a significant reduced ability to accurately code rapidly time varying modulated signals similar to speech sounds (Figure 23.1). Human studies show that loss of temporal processing is a hallmark of age-related hearing loss (Pichora-Fuller et al., 2007; Pichora-Fuller & Souza, 2003; Schatteman, Hughes, & Caspary, 2008). Thus when sinusoidally amplitude modulated (SAM) stimuli were used as a surrogate for speech, group data showed an age-related decrease in the peak vector-strength at the best modulation frequency (BMF) at different depths of modulation for aged fusiform cells relative to the young fusiform cells examined (Schatteman et al., 2008); Figure 23.1).

Cartwheel cells located in the superficial, molecular layer of the DCN, are excited by parallel fibers and likely project glycinergic/GABAergic inhibition onto the apical dendrites of fusiform cells and neighboring cartwheel cells (He, Wang, Petralia, & Brenowitz, 2014; Mancilla & Manis, 2009; Portfors & Roberts, 2007; Rubio & Juiz, 2004). Single unit recordings from aged cartwheel cells in FBN rat showed significantly higher thresholds, modestly increased spontaneous activity, and significantly altered rate-level functions characterized by hyperexcitability at higher intensities (Caspary, Hughes, Schatteman, & Turner, 2006). Aged cartwheel cells also showed reduced off-set suppression, suggesting a loss of tonic and perhaps sound-evoked inhibition.

In AVCN, markers for excitatory and inhibitory neurotransmission show age-related decreases in the mouse VCN and are reviewed in the chapter by Manis in this volume (Y. Wang & Manis, 2005; Xie & Manis, 2013, 2017).

Aging and the SOC

Cluttered acoustic environments such as restaurants and social settings represent a challenge to speech understanding for elderly adults, even those with relatively normal hearing (Gordon-Salant, 2014; Harris & Dubno, 2017; Pichora-Fuller et al., 2017; Pichora-Fuller & Souza, 2003). The ability to utilize binaural cues enables separation of relevant communication signals from irrelevant background distractors (Eddins & Hall, 2010; Ozmeral, Eddins, & Eddins, 2016). A key set of brainstem nuclei receiving time locked information primarily from VCN projection neurons comprise the SOC. Important nuclei for processing interaural time differences (ITDs) and interaural intensity differences (IIDs) include the medial superior olive (MSO) for low frequency ITD detection and the lateral superior olive (LSO)/medial nucleus of the trapezoid body (MNTB) for processing IIDs but also ITDs (see Grothe; Friauf; Kaczmarek; this volume). Human psychoacoustic studies have shown age-related binaural deficits

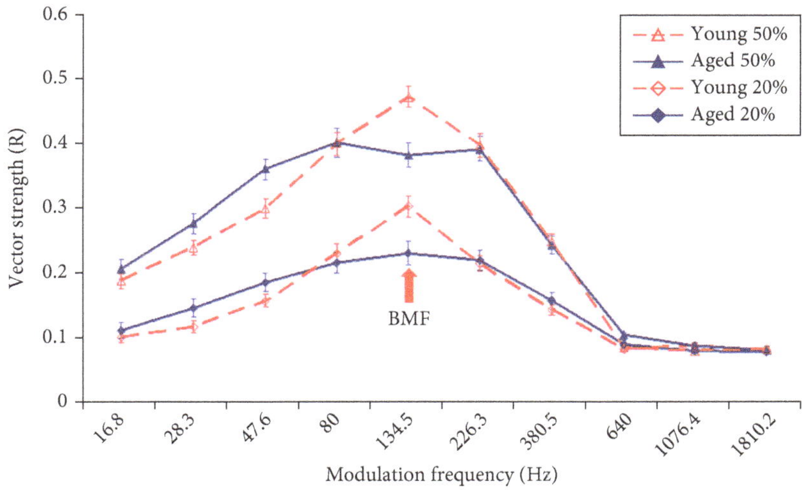

FIGURE 23.1. Age-related loss of temporal processing in dorsal cochlear nucleus. Temporal modulation transfer functions (tMTFs: vector strength) from young (n = 93; 4–6 mos) and aged (n = 88; 28–30 mos) fusiform cells at 50% and 20% depth of modulation. Note the clear band-pass nature of the young tMTFs at 50% and 20% modulation depth. With aging, fusiform cell tMTFs are flatter and broader likely reflecting an age-related loss of glycinergic inhibition. Error bars represent the S.E.M.

Reproduced from Schatteman, Hughes, & Caspary (2008), with permission from Elsevier.

negatively impact signal detection under a number of different listening conditions (Eddins & Hall, 2010; Pichora-Fuller et al., 2017).

Impact of Aging on the Structure of the SOC

Godfrey and colleagues (2017) found no significant differences in regional volume or dry weight for LSO, MSO, or MNTB between 6 month and 33 month-old FBN rat SOC. A series of anatomical aging studies in the 1980s focused on cellular changes in the MNTB of young and aged Sprague Dawley (SD) rats (Casey, 1990; Casey & Feldman, 1982, 1988). The MNTB provides contralateral inhibitory glycinergic input primarily to the LSO, but also to MSO and other nuclei within the SOC (Grothe & Pecka, 2014; Moore & Caspary, 1983). These studies initially used SD rats and showed a 34% loss of MNTB neurons between 2–3 months and 24 months of age (Casey & Feldman, 1982). Casey (1990) also counted the number of MNTB neuron in the F344 rat model of aging and found a significantly smaller 8% loss of principal neurons in this strain relative to the 34% loss in SD rats. A companion study in SD rats found that the volume density ratio of capillaries significantly decreased between 6 and 33 months of age (Casey & Feldman, 1985b). Aged SD rats showed degeneration of nerve endings including alterations in the endbulb input terminals from AVCN onto the principal neurons of the MNTB. The effect of aging on axosomatic MNTB synaptic terminals was measured using quantitative electron microscopy and revealed that the mean percentage of the principal cell surface areas contacted by synaptic terminals showed an age-related decrease from ~61% in young 3 month-old to ~43% in 27–33 month-old SD rats (Casey & Feldman, 1985a, 1988). Likewise, between 3 and 27–33 months of age, the average number of synaptic terminals present along a 100 micron length of principal cell surface decreases significantly, from 28.3 to 18.9. Only terminals derived from calyces of Held were lost in the aged animals described above (Casey & Feldman, 1988). These data support a partial age-related deafferentation of MNTB principal cells, potentially reducing both accurate IID and ITD coding in aged animals (discussed next).

Impact of Aging on Neurotransmitters in the SOC

Glutamate serves as the primary excitatory neurotransmitter providing well-timed drive from the VCN to endbulbs on MNTB neurons and onto the dendrites of ipsilateral LSO neurons and ipsi- and contralateral MSO neurons. The MNTB represents a large group of glycinergic neurons providing binaural/contralateral inhibition onto the medial dendrites of LSO neurons for IID detection and refining ITD coding in the MSO (see Grothe; Friauf, this volume; Grothe & Pecka, 2014; Myoga, Lehnert, Leibold, Felmy, & Grothe, 2014). Age-related changes in the magnitude or the timing of excitation or inhibition would certainly alter one's ability to accurately localize signals in the azimuthal plane. Age-related reductions in glutamate levels in areas of AVCN which project to SOC as well as all SOC subnuclei examined show significant age-related losses of ambient glutamate (Banay-Schwartz et al., 1989; Godfrey et al., 2017). Early SOC aging studies described above found a 34% loss of putative glycinergic principal cells in MNTB of SD rats but only an 8% loss in F344 rat MNTB (Casey, 1990; Casey & Feldman, 1982). Godfrey and colleagues (2017) show significant age-related decreases in glycine levels throughout the SOC with losses in the LSO and MNTB likely to directly impact azimuthal coding in the elderly. Functional studies described next tested the possible loss of IID coding due to the loss of glycinergic input onto LSO neurons in F344 and SD rats.

Impact of Aging on Calcium Binding Proteins and Neuromodulators in the SOC

A number of studies have examined age-related changes in calcium binding proteins, calbindin, calretinin, parvalbumin, and nitric oxide synthase NADPH-diaphorase (NADPHd) in rodent, non-human primates, and humans. Gray et al (Gray, Engle, & Recanzone, 2013; Gray, Engle, Rudolph, & Recanzone, 2014) observed an increase in parvalbumin-positive and calbindin-positive cells with age in macaque MSO, LSO, and nonsignificant changes in the MNTB. Calbindin-positive cells that co-localized with glutamic acid decarboxylase (GAD)-67 increased with age. NADPH showed a similar pattern of increase in MSO and LSO with aging (Gray, Engle, et al., 2013). Non-human primate results differed from results in certain mouse strains where calcium-binding proteins were seen to decrease in the SOC (O'Neill, Zettel, Whittemore, & Frisina, 1997).

Impact of Aging on the Physiology of the SOC

Few studies have examined age-related changes in the physiology of the SOC. Two studies evolved from the anatomical SOC studies described earlier and tested whether the age-related loss of putative glycinergic principal neurons of the MNTB would result in a shift in the interaural intensity functions derived from LSO neurons (Finlayson & Caspary, 1993). However, as might be predicted from the minor 8% age-related loss of MNTB neurons in the F344 rat, no significant aging changes were observed, although a trend toward loss of contralateral inhibition was noted (Finlayson & Caspary, 1993). When the SD rat LSO was similarly examined, the 34% age-related decrease in the numbers of MNTB neurons observed anatomically was not reflected in any age-related change in LSO IID coding. Despite these electrophysiological findings, age-related loss of azimuthal coding is well supported by psychoacoustic studies.

Aging and the IC

As reviewed in the chapters by Cant, Oliver et al., and Rees & Orton, in this volume, major inputs to the IC include ascending glutamatergic excitatory inputs from the cochlear nucleus, SOC, and descending from cortex, thalamus, and brachium of the IC. The IC comprises three subdivisions: the central nucleus, generally considered to be the lemniscal division, and two non-lemniscal divisions: the lateral nucleus (sometimes referred to as the lateral cortex or external cortex) and the dorsal cortex. Each division has a distinct synaptic and biochemical profile, which is potentially important since many studies have grouped segments of the IC together, potentially obscuring age-related differences between IC subdivisions.

Impact of Aging on the Structure of the IC

An early study by Willott et al. (1994) employed light microscopy to measure the volume of the IC, packing density and cellular volumes in mice ranging from 1.5 to 30 months of age. No differences in the IC were seen across ages in either CBA or C57BL/6J mice despite brainstem spongiform changes being observed in aged C57BL/6J mice (Willott et al., 1994). Similarly, Kazee et al. (1995) used a combination of light and electron microscopy to show preserved cellular volumes and synaptic numbers and types in aging

CBA mice (Kazee & West, 1999), but dramatic drops in synaptic number and somatic size in the central nucleus of IC neurons in C57BL/6 mice (Kazee et al., 1995). Consistent with these findings, using electron microscopy in the F344 rat, Helfert et al. (1999) observed no changes in cellular density across 3 to 28 months of age, but did report age-related decreases in excitatory and inhibitory synaptic number and proceeded to model how these changes might correlate with aging dendritic structure of IC disc shaped neurons. Specifically, they speculated that there is loss of GABAergic and non-GABAergic terminals on distal dendrites of both GABAergic and non-GABAergic neurons, but that there is a shift of these terminals to the proximal regions of GABAergic cells (Figure 23.2; Helfert et al., 1999). To our knowledge, only two studies examined age-related changes in connectivity between the IC and other brain regions (Frisina & Walton, 2001; Willott, Pankow, Hunter, & Kordyban, 1985). Willott et al. (1985) placed a retrograde tracer into the central nucleus of the IC of young and aged C57BL/6 mice and found no differences in the projection of the AVCN to the IC across the lifespan. A second study used a similar approach and found significant declines of inputs to the dorsomedial IC from all three divisions of the contralateral CN in aged CBA mice relative to young animals (Frisina & Walton, 2001). Taken together, these data suggest that gross morphological features of the IC (cell size and packing density) are relatively unchanged with aging, but neuropil features (synaptic number and density) decline with aging, and, given the accentuated synaptic loss in C57BL/J mice compared to CBA/CaJ mice, loss of peripheral hearing likely contributes to this loss of synaptic density. This loss in synaptic density is consistent with the many age-related changes in markers for both excitatory glutamate and inhibitory GABA neurotransmission in IC (Caspary et al., 1999; Caspary et al., 2008; Godfrey et al., 2017; Gold & Bajo, 2014; Ouda, Profant, & Syka, 2015) reviewed next.

Impact of Aging on Metabolism in the IC

The IC is one of the most metabolically active structures in the brain (Gross, Sposito, Pettersen, Panton, & Fenstermacher, 1987; Hevner, Liu, & Wong-Riley, 1995; Sokoloff et al., 1977). Given its high metabolic demand, one would predict that the IC may be particularly vulnerable to age-related metabolic stressors. This prediction is supported by data showing age-related decreases in the levels of antioxidant enzymes superoxide dismutase and catalase, as well as increases in lipid peroxidation in the aging rat IC (Mei et al., 1999). In addition, electron microscopic studies in the aging rat IC show decreases in mitochondrial density across both inhibitory and excitatory neurons when compared to younger animals (Mei et al., 1999), suggesting that metabolic energy failure may play a role in age-related IC dysfunction. Further, the aging F344 rat IC shows diminished levels of Hsp-72 (Helfert et al., 2002), which is an inducible heat-shock protein whose levels normally increase under conditions of environmental stress and function to chaperone misfolded proteins. Finally, expression of the BDNF receptor (tyrosine-kinase B or TrkB), is diminished in the aging F344 rat IC. Given the role of BDNF in supporting

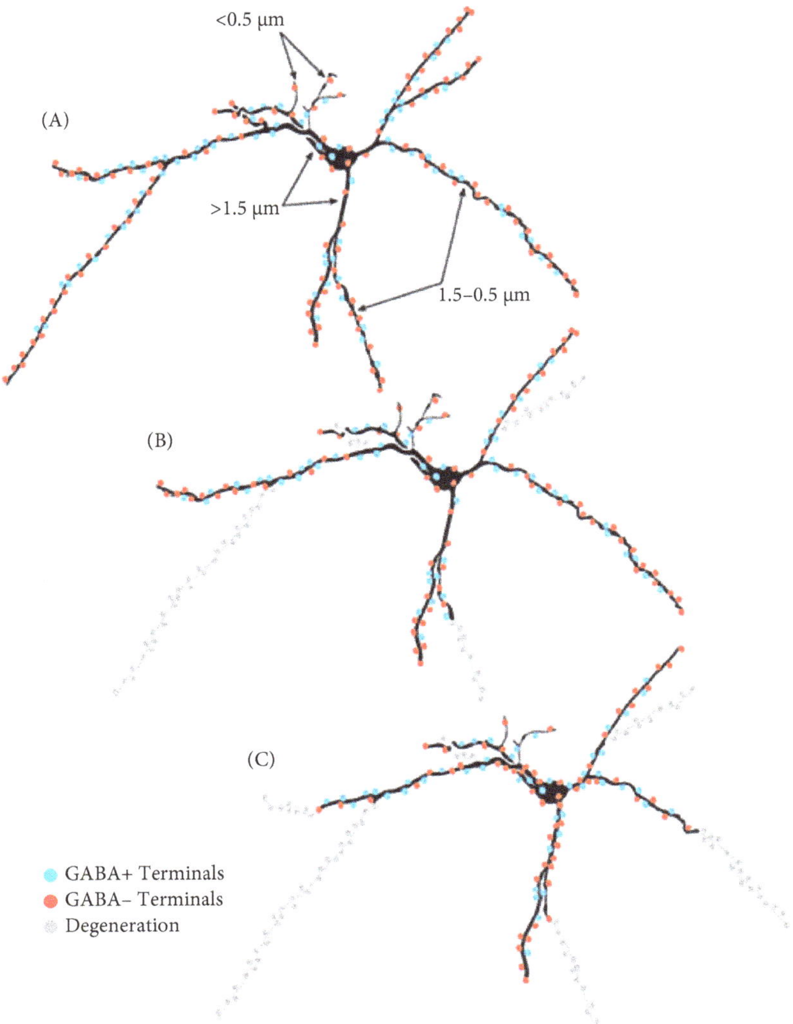

FIGURE 23.2. Model of age-related synaptic changes in the inferior colliculus
Impact of aging on the synaptic contacts of disc-shaped IC neurons. (A) Cartoon of a young IC neuron shows GABA– (excitatory) and GABA+ (inhibitory) terminals ending on secondary and tertiary dendrites. Both types of terminals are also located on the small numbers of dendritic spines and very thin dendrites throughout the dendritic arbor. (B) Cartoon of aged GABA– IC neuron shows GABA– and GABA+ synaptic terminals on remaining distal dendrites. (C) Cartoon of an aged GABA+ IC neuron showing loss of inhibitory and excitatory synaptic contacts on distal dendrites, with a shift of terminals onto more proximal portions of the dendritic tree.

Reproduced from Helfert, Sommer, Meeks, Hofstetter, & Hughes (1999), with permission from John Wiley & Sons.

synaptic health and its antioxidant function (Sato et al., 2001), the authors speculated that this diminishment in TrkB receptor activity may tie together the age-related synaptic losses and loss of antioxidant function already described.

In contrast, more direct measurements of neuronal metabolism using 2-deoxyglucose autoradiography have not revealed significant age-related changes in IC metabolic rate. Resting 2-deoxyglucose uptake in the aging rat and mouse IC appears to be unchanged relative to young controls (Clerici & Coleman, 1987; Willott, Hunter, & Coleman, 1988). In response to pure-tone stimulation, the sharpness of frequency tuning, as determined by the spatial spread of 2-deoxyglucose uptake, is diminished with aging in an SD rat model (Clerici & Coleman, 1987; Keithley, Lo, & Ryan, 1994). This finding is consistent with the in vivo single unit frequency tuning recordings that we shall review . The lack of overall metabolic changes at rest suggests that either compensatory mechanisms have permitted overall metabolic stability to occur despite the biochemical change noted previously, or that differences can only be seen with more sensitive techniques or under conditions of environmental stress. Further work is needed to elucidate these possibilities.

Impact of Aging on Neurotransmitters in the IC

The impact of aging on inhibitory neurotransmission in the IC has been extensively studied (Caspary et al., 2008; Godfrey et al., 2017; Gold & Bajo, 2014; Ouda et al., 2015). Resting GABA levels are significantly reduced in rodent models and in human aging studies (Banay-Schwartz et al., 1989; Banay-Schwartz, Palkovits, & Lajtha, 1993; Caspary, Raza, Armour, Pippin, & Arneric, 1990). Consistent with these findings are studies showing significant age-related loss in IC of both forms of GAD, the rate-limiting metabolic enzyme required for the production of both metabolic and neurotransmitter GABA in rodents and humans (Burianova, Ouda, Profant, & Syka, 2009; Caspary et al., 1990; Gutierrez, Khan, & De Blas, 1994; McGeer & McGeer, 1975; Milbrandt, Albin, & Caspary, 1994; Milbrandt, Holder, Wilson, Salvi, & Caspary, 2000; Raza, Milbrandt, Arneric, & Caspary, 1994). These age-related changes are observed in both the somata and terminals throughout the central nucleus of the IC (Caspary et al., 1990; Helfert et al., 1999). As one would predict, there is a commensurate reduction in potassium-evoked calcium mediated release of GABA from IC punches from the aged F344 rat IC (Caspary et al., 1990). $GABA_B$ receptors acting as presynaptic autoreceptors are known to control release of GABA from presynaptic terminals in the IC (C. L. Ma, Kelly, & Wu, 2002). Milbrandt and colleagues found a significant age-related loss of $GABA_B$ receptors in the IC of F344 rats (Milbrandt et al., 1994). Whether presynaptic age-related changes in production and release of GABA reflect a compensatory down-regulation of inhibition due to a loss of glutamatergic excitatory drive or age-related intrinsic changes has not been established, but as delineated later in the chapter, glutamate levels and excitatory terminals are also significantly reduced in aged rodent IC (Banay-Schwartz et al., 1989; Godfrey et al., 2017; Helfert et al., 1999).

The function and pharmacology of the heteromeric, pentameric chloride-fluxing $GABA_A$ receptor are determined by its subunit composition with different combinations of the 19 available subunits determining the magnitude/amplitude, and duration of evoked inhibitory post-synaptic potentials and ligand affinity (Rudolph & Möhler, 2006; Whiting, 2003). Thus, age-related changes in the subunit makeup of the primary excitatory and inhibitory neurotransmitters can have a profound effect on normal young adult physiology and the ability to accurately code acoustic information. Young-adult, wild-type $GABA_ARs$ are made up of $2\alpha_1 2\beta_2 \gamma_2$ subunits. Significant age-related changes in the message and protein of the $GABA_AR$ subunits have been reported in the IC and its subregions in two rat models (Caspary et al., 1999; Milbrandt, Hunter, & Caspary, 1997). The trend across all regions of the IC was for a decrease in wild-type $GABA_AR$ constructs which are replaced by constructs containing more developmental subunits, γ_1 and α_3, which have slower temporal kinetics (Caspary et al., 1999; Whiting, 2003). In addition to age-related changes in the subunit makeup of $GABA_ARs$, there is a significant loss in the number of metabotropic $GABA_BRs$ within the F344 rat IC (Milbrandt et al., 1994).

Glutamatergic signaling has been found to change in the aging IC. Glutamate levels were measured across multiple regions of the IC of young and aged rats, using quantitative microchemical analysis and high-performance liquid chromatography (HPLC; Godfrey et al., 2017). Working with FBN rats, Godfrey and colleagues found a roughly 20% decrease in glutamate levels throughout the IC, and that this drop was most prominent in the central nucleus of the IC (Figure 23.3), the most metabolically active part of the IC (Godfrey et al., 2017). This work in FBN rat is consistent with an early study which used HPLC to measure amino acid levels across whole structures in F344 rats (Banay-Schwartz et al., 1989). Perhaps in response to an age-related decrease in glutamate levels, Osumi et al. (2012) found diminished expression of the NMDA zeta1 subunit throughout the IC of middle-aged (12–15 months) compared to juvenile (1 month) C57BL/6J mice. Since "aged" animals in this study were relatively young, but had significant hearing loss, the authors speculated that such declines in NMDA receptor subunits may be related to loss of synaptic input from afferent fibers. It is possible that NMDA receptor subunit downregulation functions to diminish potential glutamate toxicity, given the metabolic vulnerability of this structure with aging (reviewed earlier). Consistent with this idea, Tadros et al. (2007) observed upregulation of the high-affinity glutamate transporter in the IC of aging CBA mice with advanced hearing loss, possibly functioning to clear excess glutamate. Thus, both the biochemical and structural data point to age-related decreases in both glutamatergic and GABAergic function in the IC with aging, but that GABAergic maybe dominant, tilting the balance in favor of excitation.

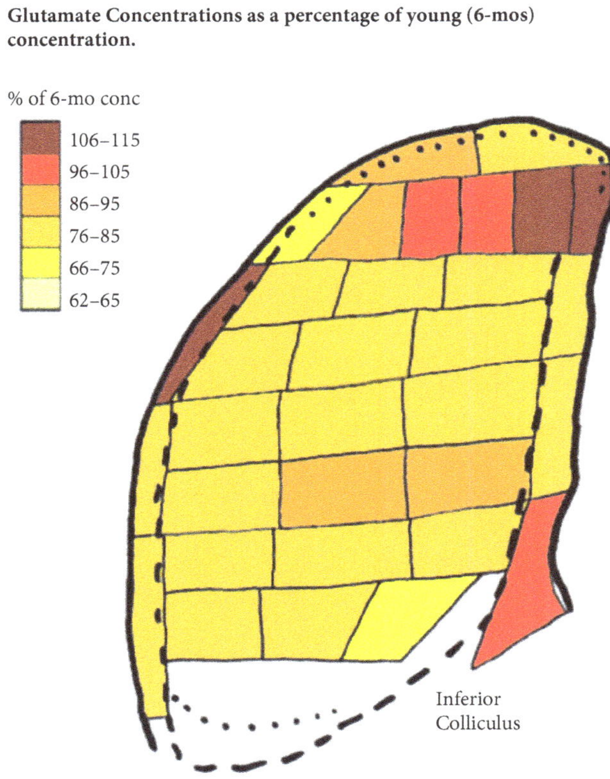

FIGURE 23.3. Age-related loss of glutamate in inferior colliculus
Map of the left inferior colliculus of 33-month-old rat with color coded percentages of glutamate levels in similarly located samples of 6-month-old rat. Young and old samples were microdissected on the same day and included in the same HPLC assay. Percentage values are coded as shown in the key.

Modified from Godfrey, Chen, O'Toole, & Mustapha (2017), with permission from Elsevier.

Impact of Aging on Calcium Binding Proteins and Neuromodulators in the IC

Expression of calcium-binding proteins is altered in the aging IC and aging effects appear to be species- and strain-specific. Normally, parvalbumin is strongly expressed in the central nucleus, as well as in discrete GABA-rich regions (containing both GABAergic somata and terminals) in the external cortex (Chernock, Larue, & Winer, 2004; Lesicko, Hristova, Maigler, & Llano, 2016). Calretinin, on the other hand, is present outside the GABA-rich regions of the external cortex (Dillingham, Gay, Behrooz, & Gabriele, 2017) while calbindin is only expressed in the nucleus of the commissure (Zettel, Frisina, Haider, & O'Neill, 1997). Zettel et al. (1997) observed substantial age-related increases in calretinin staining in the non-leminscal portions of the CBA/CaJ

IC, but not the C57BL/6J mice. Given the complementary staining for GABA and calretinin in the external cortex, the age-related increase in IC calretinin signal may reflect a relative decrease in GABA staining. Subsequent work on the CBA/CaJ mouse demonstrated that this calretinin increase is dependent on ongoing acoustic information processing and suggests that the difference between two strains maybe related to the poor hearing in C57BL/6 mice (Zettel, O'Neill, Trang, & Frisina, 2001). Data from rat have shown both increases (Hong et al., 2009) and decreases (Ouda, Burianova, & Syka, 2012) in calretinin staining in the IC with aging. Differences here may be related to strain as Wistar rats (24 months) were used in the Hong et al. (2009) study while Long-Evans and F344 rats (18-33 months) were used in the Ouda et al. (2012) study. Age-related upregulation was also seen in parvalbumin-positive neurons in the non-human primate IC with aging, and this increase correlated with peripheral hearing loss (Engle, Gray, Turner, Udell, & Recanzone, 2014). In the rat, the number of parvalbumin-positive neurons increases in the IC of aging Long-Evans rats, while the mean size of parvalbumin-positive neurons decreases in the IC of F344 rats (Ouda, Druga, & Syka, 2008). Given the disparate species and approaches used to examine the pattern of calcium binding proteins in the IC with aging, a unified picture of these proteins has yet to emerge.

In contrast to GABA and glutamate, where a number of studies provide a relatively coherent picture of age-related loss of both neurotransmitters in the IC, most studies of other neuroactive species have yet to provide consistent results. For example, the synthetic enzyme for nitric oxide, a gaseous neurotransmitter which has been implicated in toxicity associated with brain aging (Indo et al., 2015; McCann, 1997), is strongly expressed in the non-lemniscal portions of the IC (Coote & Rees, 2008). Two studies have measured changes in NADPH diaphorase staining (a marker for nitric oxide synthase-containing neurons) across young and aged Wistar rats, and found different results. Huh et al. (2008) observed a doubling of NADPH diaphorase-positive neurons in the IC in 24-month-old rats relative to 4-month-old rats. In contrast, Sánchez-Zuriaga and colleagues observed a significant drop (at least 50% in all IC subdivisions) in 28–30-month-old rats relative to 6–9-month-old rats (Sánchez-Zuriaga, Martí-Gutiérrez, La Cruz, Pérez, & Peris-Sanchis, 2007). Given the age differences between the control and the aged rats in these two studies, these results may point to a transient middle age increase in nitric oxide production, followed by a late-life decrease. Complicating the interpretation of these rodent findings is the finding of no age-related changes in the number of NADPH-positive cells in the non-human primate IC (Engle et al., 2014). More work is needed to add clarity in this area.

A single study probed changes in IC serotonergic function with aging. Expression of the $5HT_{2B}$ receptor was found to be upregulated in the external cortex of the IC of the aging CBA/J mouse (Tadros, D'Souza, Zettel, Zhu, Lynch-Erhardt, et al., 2007). This increased expression of $5HT_{2B}$ receptors has been correlated with hearing loss, and given the role of these receptors in inflammation, local blood flow, mitochondrial function, and calcium regulation, the authors speculated that the increase in $5HT_{2B}$ receptors may be a compensatory response to damage at the auditory periphery.

Impact of Aging on the Physiology of the IC

One of the most notable differences between young and aged IC neurons is the increase in average response threshold observed in aged animals (Leong, Barsz, Allen, & Walton, 2011; Palombi & Caspary, 1996b; Willott, 1986; Willott, Parham, & Hunter, 1988a, 1988b), likely reflecting peripheral hearing loss. Several studies also noted increases in spontaneous activity and/or reduction of the proportion of sound-responsive neurons in the aged IC (Chiu, Poon, Chan, & Yew, 2003; Palombi & Caspary, 1996b; Willott, Parham, et al., 1988a, 1988b). Increases in spontaneous firing rate have also been noted after acute hearing loss, and may reflect decreases in inhibitory tone (Bauer et al., 2008; Jastreboff, 1995; W. D. Ma, Hidaka, & May, 2006), as reviewed earlier. A majority of IC neurons across species are characterized by strongly non-monotonic CF input-output/rate-level functions likely reflecting GABAergic inhibition with their receptive fields (Palombi & Caspary, 1996a). The significant loss of markers for normal adult GABAergic inhibition in IC predicts the observed age-related loss of rate-level function non-monotonicity for IC neurons (Palombi & Caspary, 1996b). The combination of the increase in spontaneous firing, relative decrease of sound-responsive units and loss of damping at higher stimulus intensities would likely introduce temporal jitter and serve to diminish the overall signal-to-noise ratio of coded acoustic information in the IC of aged animals. Frequency representations in the aging IC tend to reflect changes in peripheral hearing, such that aged animals with high-frequency hearing loss have a lowered proportion of neurons representing this frequency range in the IC (Palombi & Caspary, 1996b; Willott, 1984, 1986). Sharpness of tuning functions also tends to be diminished with aging (Leong et al., 2011; Palombi & Caspary, 1996b; Willott, 1986). However, despite the age-related changes noted above, most investigators commented that, besides threshold shifts, increased spontaneous activity, and loss of non-monotonicity for rate-level functions, many basic response properties between young and aged IC were more similar than expected.

In contrast to the relatively subtle changes in the responses of IC neurons to simple stimuli, more robust age-related changes have been observed when temporally patterned stimuli are used. A number of studies have employed amplitude-modulated stimuli to probe the temporal processing characteristics of neurons in the young and aged IC. For example, Palombi et al. observed a significant shift in the proportion of band-pass neurons towards more low-pass neurons (i.e., a shift in toward neurons responding maximally to lower amplitude modulation rates) in aged F344 rats (Palombi, Backoff, & Caspary, 2001). A similar shift to lower rates of amplitude modulation was also seen in IC neurons of CBA mice (Walton, Simon, & Frisina, 2002). An age-related shift to more low-pass functions would also be seen with a drop in peak modulation frequency essentially turning a bandpass modulation transfer function into a more low-pass function. A study of young and aged Mongolian gerbils, Khouri et al. (2011) computed the selectivity to combinations of temporal parameters ("pulse matrix receptive field") when neurons were presented trains of pulses at varying rates and pulse durations. They found that aging was associated with a decline in temporal selectivity, and this drop in selectivity diminished the population encoding human speech sounds (Khouri et al., 2011).

Another commonly used paradigm to investigate temporal processing is gap detection, which is significantly compromised in behavioral studies of aged humans and rodents (Dubno, Horwitz, & Ahlstrom, 2003; Gordon-Salant & Fitzgibbons, 1993; Schneider, 1997; Snell, 1997; Strouse, Ashmead, Ohde, & Grantham, 1998; Walton, Frisina, Ison, & O'Neill, 1997; H. Wang, Brozoski, et al., 2009). Two studies in aging mice demonstrated impaired gap detection in aged IC neurons. In 24–28-month-old CBA/CaJ mice, Walton et al. observed both a shift in the minimal gap detection thresholds and a pronounced shift in the gap duration required to recover neuronal onset responses. More dramatically, in young mice, nearly all neurons recovered to 75% of their baseline responsiveness with gaps less than 10 msec, whereas very few aged IC neurons returned to 75% of baseline, even at gap widths of 50 msec (Walton, Frisina, & O'Neill, 1998). In addition, in 20 month-old Long Evans rats, Finlayson used paired tone stimuli to probe the effects of aging on forward masking recovery (Finlayson, 2002). It was found that the median time constant for suppression increased from 71.6 msec in young to 101.1 msec in aged IC neurons. This increase was not dependent on hearing loss, suggesting that the change was of central origin. Finally, a recent computational modeling study explored potential mechanisms by which the age-related temporal processing deficits described above may occur (Rabang et al., 2012). The authors constructed biologically realistic models of IC neurons based on anatomical and physiological data. They found that the shift from band-pass to low-pass neurons in response to SAM stimuli occurred as GABAergic inhibition was downregulated.

Humans show age-related loss in the ability to localize sound, which may well correlate to a loss in the ability to understand speech in complex acoustic environments (for review see (Eddins & Hall, 2010; Freigang, Richter, Rübsamen, & Ludwig, 2015)). Two studies measured binaural or free-field properties of IC neurons in aging rodent models. McFadden and Willott (1994) examined azimuthal tuning functions in C57BL/6J mice, which showed behavioral evidence of age-related declines in sound localization performance (Heffner & Donnal, 1993). In most respects, IC neurons showed similar azimuthal functions in young and aged mice. However, with aging, there was a shift in bias toward more neurons being ipsilaterally tuned, and this shift was not restricted to high-frequency sounds (where most hearing is lost), suggesting that the changes were due to central aging effects- and not purely hearing-loss related (McFadden & Willott, 1994). Similarly, in the F344 rat, only subtle differences (not reaching statistical significance) were seen in the binaural responses properties of aged IC neurons (Palombi & Caspary, 1996c). These data suggest that overall, sound localization properties of IC neurons are not substantially altered in aging rodents, but may reflect some minor loss of binaural inhibitory coding.

Taken together, the data suggest that the aged IC provides a lower fidelity representation of the external acoustic world, and that this representation is particularly vulnerable when temporally patterned stimuli are required. The computational work by Rabang et al. (2012) suggests that the biochemical and anatomical data demonstrating decreases in GABAergic tone in the aging IC described earlier may be, at least in part, responsible for age-related changes in temporal resolving power of IC neurons. Given that most real-life acoustic stimuli, such as speech and species-specific sounds, contain strong modulations in amplitude and frequency over time, the aging IC is likely to provide its target, the auditory thalamus, with a temporally smeared representation of the real-life acoustic world, relative to the young IC.

Aging and the Auditory Thalamus

The auditory thalamus, also known as the MGB, receives its main excitatory glutamatergic input from the IC and sends excitatory glutamatergic projections to the auditory cortex and the thalamic reticular nucleus (TRN). The MGB can be subdivided into a lemniscal ventral division (MGBv), and two non-lemniscal divisions: the dorsal division (MGBd), medial division (MGBm), as well as several paralaminar structures (suprageniculate, posterior intralaminar, and peripeduncular). The MGBv is the only tonotopically organized region and gets its main input from the central nucleus of the IC and projects to primary auditory cortical fields, whereas the other regions get their main input from the non-lemniscal portions of the IC and auditory cortex and project to non-primary auditory cortical fields as well as to the upper layers of the primary auditory cortex (reviewed in Lee, 2013).

GABAergic inhibitory input to the MGB stems from several sources. In non-rodent species, approximately 20% of MGB neurons are GABAergic, while in rodents as few as 1% of MGB neurons are GABAergic (Winer & Larue, 1988). In rodents, there is a major ascending GABAergic input from the IC (Peruzzi, Bartlett, Smith, & Oliver, 1997; Winer, Saint Marie, Larue, & Oliver, 1996). In addition, there is GABAergic input from the TRN, which partially surrounds the thalamus. Finally, there is a small GABAergic component from the zona incerta (Barthó, Freund, & Acsády, 2002). There is no known glycinergic input to the MGB.

Impact of Aging on Neurotransmitters in the MGB

Two carefully done rodent studies show significant reductions in ambient glutamate levels but unlike the IC, where GABA levels show significant age-related reductions, these same studies show nonsignificant reduction of endogenous GABA levels (Banay-Schwartz et al., 1989; Godfrey et al., 2017). Richardson et al. (2013) found small, but significant changes in GAD_{67} protein in Western blots from FBN rat MGB. This study also assessed whole-cell chloride currents in young (3-8 month) and aged (28-32 month) rat MGB neurons in a brain slice preparation. While age-related changes in synaptic chloride GABA currents were small, the authors observed a pronounced drop (~50%) in tonic chloride, extrasynaptic, currents from neurons in both the MGBv and MGBd with aging (see Figure 23.4). Given the multiple sources of GABAergic inhibition in the MGB, it is not clear if age-related changes in GABA release from one or more of these sources serve as the trigger for the compensatory decrease in extrasynaptic $GABA_ARs$. Down-regulation of extrasynaptic $GABA_ARs$ could be due to a loss of ambient GABA in response to an age-related decrease in GABA release, age-related changes in neuroactive steroids, or de novo aging.

Impact of Aging on Calcium Binding Proteins and Neuromodulators in the MGB

Three main calcium binding proteins (parvalbumin, calbindin, and calretinin) have different distributions within the MGB such that parvalbumin is primarily found in the MGBv, whereas calbindin and calretinin are found throughout the non-leminscal divisions (Cruikshank, Killackey, & Metherate, 2001; E. Lu, Llano, & Sherman, 2009; Molinari et al., 1995). To date, three studies have examined age-related changes of these proteins in rat MGB and one in monkey MGB, and have yielded conflicting results. Ouda and colleagues found drops in calbindin-positive cell density and cell volume in the rat MGBv (a structure with very little calbindin staining) and no changes in parvalbumin and calretinin (Ouda et al., 2012; Ouda et al., 2008). In contrast to the calbindin findings from Ouda et al., (2008; 2012) in F344 and Long-Evans rats, Hong et al. (2009) found no change in the numbers of calbindin-positive neurons in the aging MGB in Wistar rat. They also found no changes in calretinin neurons. Also in contrast to the Ouda parvalbumin study in rats, Gray et al. (2013) observed an increase in parvalbumin-positive cell density in the monkey MGBv with aging. The differences here likely relate to species differences since the rat MGBv has very few parvalbumin-positive cell bodies (most staining is in neuropil), whereas strong parvalbumin cellular staining was seen in the Gray et al. study in monkeys (see their figures 23.2A and B). The origin of the differences in calbindin changes with aging between the Ouda et al. (2008, 2012) and Hong et al. (2009) studies is not known, though it should be noted that the Hong et al. study did not parse MGB by subdivision. Clearly, more work is needed to resolve these differences across studies and to derive a coherent view of thalamic calcium homeostasis with aging.

Two recent studies examined the impact of aging on cholinergic function in the MGB. Using a combination of radioligand binding studies and whole-cell patch recordings from brain slices in FBN rats, findings from Sottile et al. (2017) are consistent with a reduction in β2-subunit containing post-synaptic neuronal nicotinic acetylcholine receptors on MGB neurons in the aging rat MGB (Figure 23.4 Sottile, Ling, et al., 2017). Sottile et al. (2017) also observed that pre-synaptic neuronal nicotinic acetylcholine

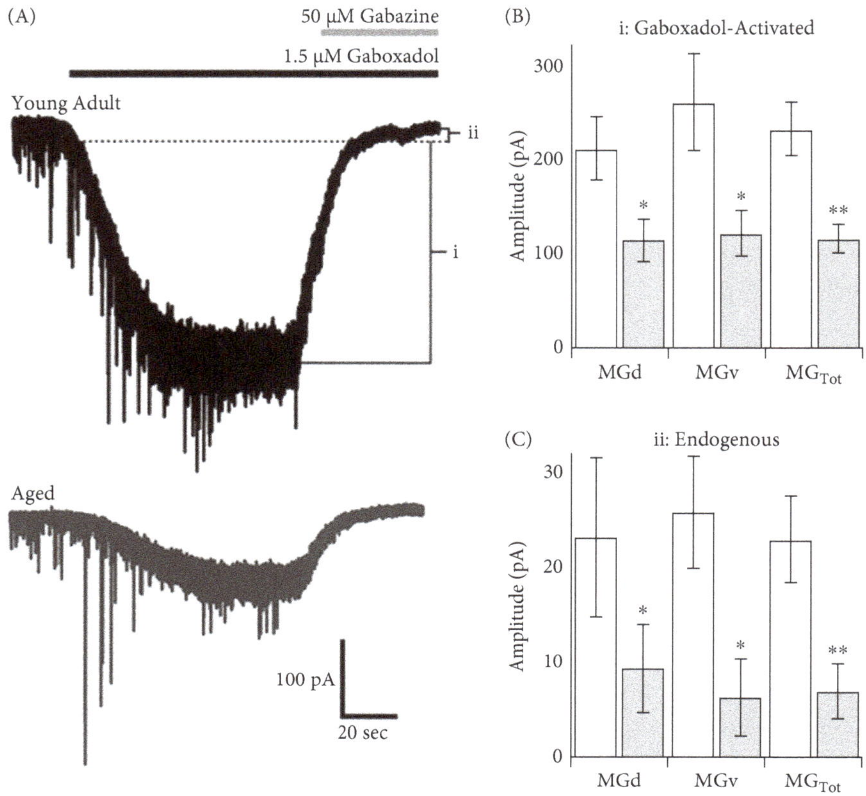

FIGURE 23.4. Age-related loss of extrasynaptic $GABA_ARs$ in rat MGB. $GABA_AR$-mediated tonic inhibitory currents are reduced with age. (A) Raw sample trace from a young adult MGB neuron (top, black) and an aged MGB neuron (bottom, gray) in response to application of gaboxadal (an agonist with high affinity for $\alpha_4\delta$ containing $GABA_ARs$). Addition of gabazine blocked all $GABA_A$ currents. Calibration applies to both traces. (B and C) Histogram (open bars, young adult; gray bars, aged rats) shows age-related differences between gaboxadol-activated (B) and endogenous (C) high-affinity $GABA_AR$-mediated tonic current amplitudes from MGd, MGv, and all MGB (MG_{Tot}) neurons. (B) Shows age-related tonic current amplitude difference in 1.5μM gaboxadol-evoked current $GABA_AR$ blockade. (C) Shows age-related tonic current amplitude difference between the baseline/endogenous current after blockade of $GABA_ARs$. $^*p < 0.05$; $^{**}p < 0.01$ (independent-sample t tests).

From Richardson, Hancock, & Caspary (2013), with permission from *Journal of Neuroscience*.

receptors on corticothalamic fibers and inhibitory tectothalamic fibers showed diminished effectiveness to applied acetylcholine and decreased epibatidine binding in the aged rat MGB. Given the evidence of cholinergic influences on attention (Klinkenberg, Sambeth, & Blokland, 2011), these data suggest that age-related changes in auditory attention may be mediated by pre- and post-synaptic changes in cholinergic function at the level of the MGB.

Impact of Aging on the Physiology of the MGB

To date, no studies have been published that examine basic response properties of MGB neurons with aging, though a recent abstract suggests that no differences exist in basic tuning properties between young (3 month) and aged (18 month) anesthetized CBA mice (L. A. Anderson, Quraishe, & Newman, 2017). A small number of studies examined changes in single MGB neurons in young and aged rodents and focused on selectivity for frequency modulation (Mendelson & Lui, 2004), amplitude modulation (Cai, Richardson, & Caspary, 2016), and novelty detection (Richardson, Hancock, & Caspary, 2013). In terms of responses to time-varying signals, Mendelson and Lui (2004) recorded from the MGBv of young (3-4 month) and aged (23-30 month) anesthetized Long Evans rats and found no differences in tuning for speed or directionality of frequency-modulated signals. The absence of a difference between groups contrasted with their previous work showing age-related changes in the auditory cortex using a similar experimental paradigm (Mendelson & Ricketts, 2001), suggesting that the negative result was not a result of lack of sensitivity of their approach, and that an age-related shift to preference for slow frequency modulation rates in the cortex was not inherited from the MGB.

Stimulus-specific adaptation (SSA) is a phenomenon reported in single units of the IC, MGB, and auditory cortex whereby units respond preferentially to novel stimuli (Malmierca, Cristaudo, Pérez-González, & Covey, 2009; Ulanovsky, Las, & Nelken, 2003). Although SSA is diminished in the auditory cortex of aged FBN rats (de Villers-Sidani et al., 2010), no age-related changes in SSA recorded from MGB neurons in awake FBN rats were found (Richardson, Hancock, et al., 2013). In a subsequent study, a more demanding, temporally complex novelty stimulus set was used in single unit recordings from young (4-6 month) and aged (28-30 month) awake FBN rat MGB neurons (Cai et al., 2016). SAM stimuli were modulated between 2 and 1024 Hz with the modulation frequency changing randomly across trials or presented in a predictable sequence. Units were found to be random-preferring, predictable-preferring, or non-selective based on total firing rate. When random versus predictable differences were examined across different modulation frequencies, the largest age-related differences were found at higher modulation frequencies, with aged MGB units preferring predictably presented SAM stimuli (see Figure 23.5, Cai et al., 2016). Figure 23.5, here, looks at the entire population of young and aged MGB neurons from Cai et al., (2016), in response to predictable presentation of a 512 Hz modulated carrier. While MGB neurons from young FBN rats are seen to adapt to repetitions of the SAM stimulus, neurons from the aged MGB increase their discharge rate across successive presentations (Figure 23.5). These findings suggest that aged MGB units/animals may employ increased top-down resources to enhance processing of "expected" temporally rich stimuli, especially at more challenging higher modulation rates These results suggest a neuronal substrate for an age-related increase in experience/attentional-based influences in processing temporally complex auditory information in the MGB. These findings are consistent with the body of psychophysical

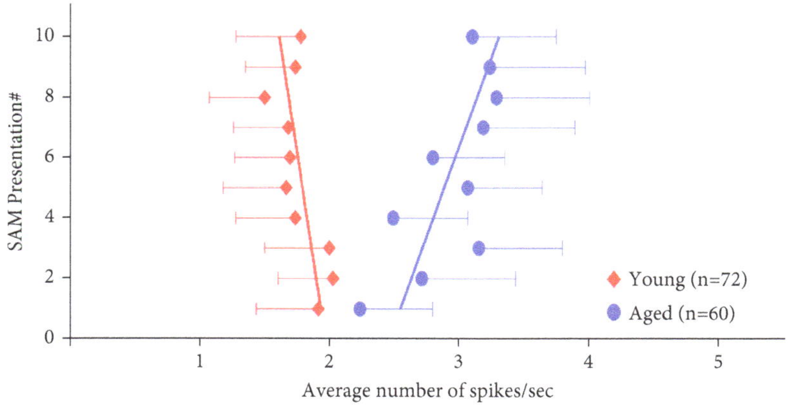

FIGURE 23.5. Aged MGB neurons show increasing responses to predictable stimuli. Trial-by-trial responses to a repeating SAM stimulus modulated at 512 Hz. Group data (mean ± SE) show statistically different trend lines slopes, when plotting average spikes against each successive presentation of the SAM stimulus, recorded from 60 old MGB neurons and 72 young MGB neurons (ANCOVA, 2-tailed, $p < 0.01$).

Modified from Cai, Richardson, & Caspary (2016), with permission from *Journal of Neuroscience*.

literature showing increasing dependence on top-down cues with aging, given the degradation in the processing of bottom-up signals (reviewed in Lesicko & Llano, 2017).

Conclusion

Age-related hearing loss is arguably the third major malady of industrialized populations causing social isolation and depression among a significant subset of this demographic. With the proportion of the elderly population approaching 25% by 2050, it is imperative that efforts be made to ameliorate this socially debilitating condition. It is accepted from human studies that presbycusis is multifactorial and that amplification of the input alone (i.e., hearing aids) frequently does not resolve issues of speech understanding especially in challenging acoustic environments.

It is our hope that this review has presented some of the many changes which occur in response to age-related peripheral deafferentation, as well as de novo central cellular aging. Many of issues highlighted in this review illustrate the disproportional downregulation of inhibitory processes and loss of temporal precision with aging. Development of non-sedating subunit selective GABA-related compounds to upregulate inhibition and training strategies shown to improve temporal processing in older individuals are indicative of future pharmacological and behavioral approaches toward ameliorating loss of speech understanding in the elderly.

ACKNOWLEDGMENTS

This work was supported by the National Institute on Deafness and Other Communication Disorders: DC000151-DMC; DC012125 & DC013073-DAL.

REFERENCES

Abernethy, J. D. (1979). The exponential increase in mortality rate with age attributed to wearing-out of biological components. *Journal of Theoretical Biology*, *80*(3), 333–354.

Alain, C., & Woods, D. L. (1999). Age-related changes in processing auditory stimuli during visual attention: Evidence for deficits in inhibitory control and sensory memory. *Psychology and Aging*, *14*(3), 507–519.

Altschuler, R. A., Dolan, D. F., Halsey, K., Kanicki, A., Deng, N., Martin, C., . . . Schacht, J. (2015). Age-related changes in auditory nerve-inner hair cell connections, hair cell numbers, auditory brain stem response and gap detection in UM-HET4 mice. *Neuroscience*, *292*, 22–33. doi:10.1016/j.neuroscience.2015.01.068

Anderson, L. A., Quraishe, S., & Newman, T. A. (2017). Age-related changes in neural gap-detection thresholds in the auditory thalamus. *Association for Research in Otolaryngology Meeting, PS 434*.

Anderson, S., Parbery-Clark, A., White-Schwoch, T., & Kraus, N. (2012). Aging affects neural precision of speech encoding. *Journal of Neuroscience*, *32*(41), 14156–14164. doi:10.1523/JNEUROSCI.2176-12.2012

Banay-Schwartz, M., Lajtha, A., & Palkovits, M. (1989). Changes with aging in the levels of amino acids in rat CNS structural elements. I. Glutamate and related amino acids. *Neurochemical Research*, *14*(6), 555–562.

Banay-Schwartz, M., Palkovits, M., & Lajtha, A. (1993). Heterogeneous distribution of functionally important amino acids in brain areas of adult and aging humans. *Neurochemical Research*, *18*(4), 417–423.

Barthó, P., Freund, T. F., & Acsády, L. (2002). Selective GABAergic innervation of thalamic nuclei from zona incerta. *European Journal of Neuroscience*, *16*(6), 999–1014. doi:10.1046/j.1460-9568.2002.02157.x

Bauer, C. A., Turner, J. G., Caspary, D. M., Myers, K. S., & Brozoski, T. J. (2008). Tinnitus and inferior colliculus activity in chinchillas related to three distinct patterns of cochlear trauma. *Journal of Neuroscience Research*, *86*(11), 2564–2578.

Boettcher, F. A., Mills, J. H., Swerdloff, J. L., & Holley, B. L. (1996). Auditory evoked potentials in aged gerbils: Responses elicited by noises separated by a silent gap. *Hearing Research*, *102*(1–2), 167–178.

Brozoski, T. J., Bauer, C. A., & Caspary, D. M. (2002). Elevated fusiform cell activity in the dorsal cochlear nucleus of chinchillas with psychophysical evidence of tinnitus. *Journal of Neuroscience*, *22*(6), 2383–2390.

Burianova, J., Ouda, L., Profant, O., & Syka, J. (2009). Age-related changes in GAD levels in the central auditory system of the rat. *Experimental Gerontology*, *44*(3), 161–169. doi:10.1016/j.exger.2008.09.012

Cai, R., & Caspary, D. M. (2015). GABAergic inhibition shapes SAM responses in rat auditory thalamus. *Neuroscience*, *299*, 146–155. doi:10.1016/j.neuroscience.2015.04.062

Cai, R., Montgomery, S. C., Graves, K. A., Caspary, D. M., & Cox, B. C. (2017). The FBN rat model of aging: Investigation of ABR waveforms and ribbon synapse changes. *Neurobiology of Aging*, *62*, 53–63. doi:10.1016/j.neurobiolaging.2017.09.034

Cai, R., Richardson, B. D., & Caspary, D. M. (2016). Responses to predictable versus random temporally complex stimuli from single units in auditory thalamus: Impact of aging and anesthesia. *Journal of Neuroscience*, *36*(41), 10696–10706.

Cant, N. B., & Benson, C. G. (2003). Parallel auditory pathways: projection patterns of the different neuronal populations in the dorsal and ventral cochlear nuclei. *Brain Research Bulletin*, *60*(5–6), 457–474.

Casey, M. A. (1990). The effects of aging on neuron number in the rat superior olivary complex. *Neurobiology of Aging*, *11*(4), 391–394.

Casey, M. A., & Feldman, M. L. (1982). Aging in the rat medial nucleus of the trapezoid body. I. Light microscopy. *Neurobiology of Aging*, *3*(3), 187–195.

Casey, M. A., & Feldman, M. L. (1985a). Aging in the rat medial nucleus of the trapezoid body. II. Electron microscopy. *Journal of Comparative Neurology*, *232*(3), 401–413. doi:10.1002/cne.902320311

Casey, M. A., & Feldman, M. L. (1985b). Aging in the rat medial nucleus of the trapezoid body. III. Alterations in capillaries. *Neurobiology of Aging*, *6*(1), 39–46.

Casey, M. A., & Feldman, M. L. (1988). Age-related loss of synaptic terminals in the rat medial nucleus of the trapezoid body. *Neuroscience*, *24*(1), 189–194.

Caspary, D. M., Backoff, P. M., Finlayson, P. G., & Palombi, P. S. (1994). Inhibitory inputs modulate discharge rate within frequency receptive fields of anteroventral cochlear nucleus neurons. *Journal of Neurophysiology*, *72*(5), 2124–2133. doi:10.1152/jn.1994.72.5.2124

Caspary, D. M., Havey, D. C., & Faingold, C. L. (1979). Effects of microiontophoretically applied glycine and GABA on neuronal response patterns in the cochlear nuclei. *Brain Research*, *172*(1), 179–185.

Caspary, D. M., Havey, D. C., & Faingold, C. L. (1981). Glutamate and aspartate: Alteration of thresholds and response patterns of auditory neurons. *Hearing Research*, *4*(3), 325–333.

Caspary, D. M., Holder, T. M., Hughes, L. F., Milbrandt, J. C., McKernan, R. M., & Naritoku, D. K. (1999). Age-related changes in GABA A receptor subunit composition and function in rat auditory system. *Neuroscience*, *93*(1), 307–312.

Caspary, D. M., Hughes, L. F., Schatteman, T. A., & Turner, J. G. (2006). Age-related changes in the response properties of cartwheel cells in rat dorsal cochlear nucleus. *Hearing Research*, *216–217*, 207–215. doi:S0378-5955(06)00075-X [pii] 10.1016/j.heares.2006.03.005

Caspary, D. M., Ling, L., Turner, J. G., & Hughes, L. F. (2008). Inhibitory neurotransmission, plasticity and aging in the mammalian central auditory system. *Journal of Experimental Biology*, *211*(11), 1781–1791.

Caspary, D. M., Pazara, K. E., Ko, M., & Faingold, C. L. (1987). Strychnine alters the fusiform cell output from the dorsal cochlear nucleus. *Brain Research*, *417*(2), 273–282.

Caspary, D. M., Raza, A., Armour, B. A., Pippin, J., & Arneric, S. P. (1990). Immunocytochemical and neurochemical evidence for age-related loss of GABA in the inferior colliculus: Implications for neural presbycusis. *Journal of Neuroscience*, *10*(7), 2363–2372.

Caspary, D. M., Rybak, L. P., & Faingold, C. L. (1984). Baclofen reduces tone-evoked activity of cochlear nucleus neurons. *Hearing Research*, *13*(2), 113–122.

Caspary, D. M., Schatteman, T. A., & Hughes, L. F. (2005). Age-related changes in the inhibitory response properties of dorsal cochlear nucleus output neurons: Role of inhibitory inputs. *Journal of Neuroscience*, *25*(47), 10952–10959.

Chernock, M. L., Larue, D. T., & Winer, J. A. (2004). A periodic network of neurochemical modules in the inferior colliculus. *Hearing Research, 188*(1), 12–20.

Chiu, T. W., Poon, P. W. F., Chan, W. Y., & Yew, D. T. W. (2003). Long-term changes of response in the inferior colliculus of senescence accelerated mice after early sound exposure. *Journal of the Neurological Sciences, 216*(1), 143–151.

Clerici, W. J., & Coleman, J. R. (1987). Resting and pure tone evoked metabolic responses in the inferior colliculus of young adult and senescent rats. *Neurobiology of Aging, 8*(2), 171–178.

Cooper, J. R., Bloom, F. E., & Roth, R. H. (2003). *The biochemical basis of neuropharmacology*: New York, NY: Oxford University Press.

Coote, E. J., & Rees, A. (2008). The distribution of nitric oxide synthase in the inferior colliculus of guinea pig. *Neuroscience, 154*(1), 218–225.

Cruikshank, S. J., Killackey, H. P., & Metherate, R. (2001). Parvalbumin and calbindin are differentially distributed within primary and secondary subregions of the mouse auditory forebrain. *Neuroscience, 105*(3), 553–569.

Dalton, D. S., Cruickshanks, K. J., Klein, B. E., Klein, R., Wiley, T. L., & Nondahl, D. M. (2003). The impact of hearing loss on quality of life in older adults. *Gerontologist, 43*(5), 661–668.

Davis, K. A., & Young, E. D. (2000). Pharmacological evidence of inhibitory and disinhibitory neuronal circuits in dorsal cochlear nucleus. *Journal of Neurophysiology, 83*(2), 926–940.

de Villers-Sidani, E., Alzghoul, L., Zhou, X., Simpson, K. L., Lin, R. C. S., & Merzenich, M. M. (2010). Recovery of functional and structural age-related changes in the rat primary auditory cortex with operant training. *Proceedings of the National Academy of Sciences, 107*(31), 13900–13905.

Di Palma, F., Holme, R. H., Bryda, E. C., Belyantseva, I. A., Pellegrino, R., Kachar, B., . . . Noben-Trauth, K. (2001). Mutations in Cdh23, encoding a new type of cadherin, cause stereocilia disorganization in waltzer, the mouse model for Usher syndrome type 1D. *Nature Genetics, 27*(1), 103–107. doi:10.1038/83660

Diez-Roux, G., Banfi, S., Sultan, M., Geffers, L., Anand, S., Rozado, D., . . . Ballabio, A. (2011). A high-resolution anatomical atlas of the transcriptome in the mouse embryo. *PLoS Biol, 9*(1), e1000582. doi:10.1371/journal.pbio.1000582

Dillingham, C. H., Gay, S. M., Behrooz, R., & Gabriele, M. L. (2017). Modular-extramodular organization in developing multisensory shell regions of the mouse inferior colliculus. *Journal of Comparative Neurology, 525*(17), 3742–3756. doi:10.1002/cne.24300

Dubno, J. R., Ahlstrom, J. B., & Horwitz, A. R. (2008). Binaural advantage for younger and older adults with normal hearing. *Journal of Speech, Language, and Hearing Research, 51*(2), 539–556. doi:10.1044/1092-4388(2008/039)

Dubno, J. R., Horwitz, A. R., & Ahlstrom, J. B. (2003). Recovery from prior stimulation: Masking of speech by interrupted noise for younger and older adults with normal hearing. *Journal of the Acoustical Society of America, 113*(4), 2084–2094.

Eddins, D. A., & Hall, J. W. (2010). Binaural processing and auditory asymmetries. In S. Gordon-Salant, R. D. Frisina, A. N. Popper, & R. R. Fay (Eds.), *The aging auditory system* (pp. 135–165). New York, NY: Springer New York.

Engle, J. R., Gray, D. T., Turner, H., Udell, J. B., & Recanzone, G. H. (2014). Age-related neurochemical changes in the rhesus macaque inferior colliculus. *Frontiers in Aging Neuroscience, 6*, 73. doi:10.3389/fnagi.2014.00073

Erb, D. E., & Povlishock, J. T. (1991). Neuroplasticity following traumatic brain injury: A study of GABAergic terminal loss and recovery in the cat dorsal lateral vestibular nucleus. *Experimental Brain Research, 83*(2), 253–267.

Finch, C. E. (2003). Neurons, glia, and plasticity in normal brain aging. *Neurobiology of Aging, 24*(Supplement 1), S123–S127. doi:https://doi.org/10.1016/S0197-4580(03)00051-4

Finlayson, P. G. (2002). Paired-tone stimuli reveal reductions and alterations in temporal processing in inferior colliculus neurons of aged animals. *Journal of the Association for Research in Otolaryngology, 3*(3), 321–331.

Finlayson, P. G., & Caspary, D. M. (1993). Response properties in young and old Fischer-344 rat lateral superior olive neurons: A quantitative approach. *Neurobiology of Aging, 14*(2), 127–139.

Fischel-Ghodsian, N., Bykhovskaya, Y., Taylor, K., Kahen, T., Cantor, R., Ehrenman, K., . . . Keithley, E. (1997). Temporal bone analysis of patients with presbycusis reveals high frequency of mitochondrial mutations. *Hearing Research, 110*(1), 147–154.

Francis, A., & Pulsinelli, W. (1982). The response of GABAergic and cholinergic neurons to transient cerebral ischemia. *Brain Research, 243*(2), 271–278.

Freigang, C., Richter, N., Rübsamen, R., & Ludwig, A. A. (2015). Age-related changes in sound localisation ability. *Cell and Tissue Research, 361*(1), 371–386.

Frisina, R. D., & Walton, J. P. (2001). Aging of the mouse central auditory system. In J. P. Willott (Ed.), *Handbook of mouse auditory research: From behavior to molecular biology* (chap. 24, pp. 339–379). New York, NY: CRC Press.

Frisina, R. D., & Walton, J. P. (2006). Age-related structural and functional changes in the cochlear nucleus. *Hearing Research, 216–217*, 216–223. doi:10.1016/j.heares.2006.02.003

Frostholm, A., & Rotter, A. (1985). Glycine receptor distribution in mouse CNS: Autoradiographic localization of [3H]strychnine binding sites. *Brain Research Bulletin, 15*(5), 473–486. doi:https://doi.org/10.1016/0361-9230(85)90038-3

Godfrey, D. A., Chen, K., O'Toole, T. R., & Mustapha, A. I. (2017). Amino acid and acetylcholine chemistry in the central auditory system of young, middle-aged and old rats. *Hearing Research, 350*, 173–188.

Godfrey, D. A., Kaltenbach, J. A., Chen, K., Ilyas, O., Liu, X., Licari, F., . . . McKnight, D. (2012). Amino acid concentrations in the hamster central auditory system and long-term effects of intense tone exposure. *Journal of Neuroscience Research, 90*(11), 2214–2224. doi:10.1002/jnr.23095

Gold, J. R., & Bajo, V. M. (2014). Insult-induced adaptive plasticity of the auditory system. *Frontiers in Neuroscience, 8*, 110. doi: 10.3389/fnins.2014.00110.

Gordon-Salant, S. (2014). Aging, hearing loss, and speech recognition: Stop shouting, I can't understand you. In A. N. Popper & R. R. Fay (Eds.), *Perspectives on auditory research* (pp. 211–228). New York, NY: Springer.

Gordon-Salant, S., & Fitzgibbons, P. J. (1993). Temporal factors and speech recognition performance in young and elderly listeners. *Journal of Speech, Language, and Hearing Research, 36*(6), 1276–1285.

Gratton, M. A., Schmiedt, R. A., & Schulte, B. A. (1996). Age-related decreases in endocochlear potential are associated with vascular abnormalities in the stria vascularis. *Hearing Research, 102*(1–2), 181–190.

Gratton, M. A., Smyth, B. J., Schulte, B. A., & Vincent, D. A., Jr. (1995). Na,K-ATPase activity decreases in the cochlear lateral wall of quiet-aged gerbils. *Hearing Research, 83*(1–2), 43–50.

Gray, D. T., Engle, J. R., & Recanzone, G. H. (2013). Age-related neurochemical changes in the rhesus macaque superior olivary complex. *Journal of Comparative Neurology, 522*(3), 573–591. doi:10.1002/cne.23427

Gray, D. T., Engle, J. R., & Recanzone, G. H. (2014). Age-related neurochemical changes in the rhesus macaque cochlear nucleus. *Journal of Comparative Neurology*, *522*(7), 1527–1541. doi:10.1002/cne.23479

Gray, D. T., Engle, J. R., Rudolph, M. L., & Recanzone, G. H. (2014). Regional and age-related differences in GAD67 expression of parvalbumin- and calbindin-expressing neurons in the rhesus macaque auditory midbrain and brainstem. *Journal of Comparative Neurology*, *522*(18), 4074–4084. doi:10.1002/cne.23659

Gray, D. T., Rudolph, M. L., Engle, J. R., & Recanzone, G. H. (2013). Parvalbumin increases in the medial and lateral geniculate nuclei of aged rhesus macaques. *Frontiers in Aging Neuroscience*, *5*, 69. doi:10.3389/fnagi.2013.00069

Grimes, A., & Chandra, S. B. C. (2009). Significance of cellular senescence in aging and cancer. *Cancer Research and Treatment: Official Journal of Korean Cancer Association*, *41*(4), 187.

Gross, P. M., Sposito, N. M., Pettersen, S. E., Panton, D. G., & Fenstermacher, J. D. (1987). Topography of capillary density, glucose metabolism, and microvascular function within the rat inferior colliculus. *Journal of Cerebral Blood Flow & Metabolism*, *7*(2), 154–160.

Grothe, B., & Pecka, M. (2014). The natural history of sound localization in mammals: A story of neuronal inhibition. *Frontiers in Neural Circuits*, *8*, 116. doi:10.3389/fncir.2014.00116

Gutierrez, A., Khan, Z. U., & De Blas, A. L. (1994). Immunocytochemical localization of gamma 2 short and gamma 2 long subunits of the GABAA receptor in the rat brain. *Journal of Neuroscience*, *14*(11), 7168–7179.

Harris, K. C., & Dubno, J. R. (2017). Age-related deficits in auditory temporal processing: Unique contributions of neural dyssynchrony and slowed neuronal processing. *Neurobiology of Aging*, *53*, 150–158. doi:10.1016/j.neurobiolaging.2017.01.008

Harris, K. C., Wilson, S., Eckert, M. A., & Dubno, J. R. (2012). Human evoked cortical activity to silent gaps in noise: Effects of age, attention, and cortical processing speed. *Ear and Hearing*, *33*(3), 330–339. doi:10.1097/AUD.0b013e31823fb585

He, S., Wang, Y. X., Petralia, R. S., & Brenowitz, S. D. (2014). Cholinergic modulation of large-conductance calcium-activated potassium channels regulates synaptic strength and spine calcium in cartwheel cells of the dorsal cochlear nucleus. *Journal of Neuroscience*, *34*(15), 5261–5272. doi:10.1523/jneurosci.3728-13.2014

Heffner, R. S., & Donnal, T. (1993). *Effect of high-frequency hearing loss on sound localization in mice (C57BL6J)*. Paper presented at the ARO Abstr.

Helfert, R. H., Glatz, F. R., Wilson, T. S., Ramkumar, V., & Hughes, L. F. (2002). Hsp70 in the inferior colliculus of Fischer-344 rats: Effects of age and acoustic stress. *Hearing Research*, *170*(1), 155–165.

Helfert, R. H., Sommer, T. J., Meeks, J., Hofstetter, P., & Hughes, L. F. (1999). Age-related synaptic changes in the central nucleus of the inferior colliculus of Fischer-344 rats. *Journal of Comparative Neurology*, *406*(3), 285–298.

Hevner, R. F., Liu, S., & Wong-Riley, M. T. T. (1995). A metabolic map of cytochrome oxidase in the rat brain: Histochemical, densitometric and biochemical studies. *Neuroscience*, *65*(2), 313–342.

Hoffman, D. W., Whitworth, C. A., Jones-King, K. L., & Rybak, L. P. (1988). Potentiation of ototoxicity by glutathione depletion. *Annals of Otology, Rhinology, & Laryngology*, *97*(1), 36–41. doi:10.1177/000348948809700107

Hoffman, H. J., & Reed, G. W. (2004). Epidemiology of tinnitus. In J. B. Snow (Ed.), *Tinnitus: Theory and Management* (pp. 16–41). Lewiston, NY: BC Decker Inc.

Hong, S. M., Chung, S. Y., Park, M. S., Huh, Y. B., Park, M. S., & Yeo, S. G. (2009). Immunoreactivity of calcium-binding proteins in the central auditory nervous system of aged rats. *Journal of Korean Neurosurgical Society, 45*(4), 231–235.

Houser, C. R., & Esclapez, M. (1996). Vulnerability and plasticity of the GABA system in the pilocarpine model of spontaneous recurrent seizures. *Epilepsy Research, 26*(1), 207–218.

Huh, Y. B., Choon Park, D., Geun Yeo, S., & Cha Il, C. (2008). Evidence for increased NADPH-diaphorase-positive neurons in the central auditory system of the aged rat. *Acta Oto-Laryngologica, 128*(6), 648–653.

Humes, L. E., Dubno, J. R., Gordon-Salant, S., Lister, J. J., Cacace, A. T., Cruickshanks, K. J., . . . Wingfield, A. (2012). Central presbycusis: A review and evaluation of the evidence. *Journal of the American Academy of Audiology, 23*(8), 635–666. doi:10.3766/jaaa.23.8.5

Humes, L. E., Kewley-Port, D., Fogerty, D., & Kinney, D. (2010). Measures of hearing threshold and temporal processing across the adult lifespan. *Hearing Research, 264*(1–2), 30–40.

Hunter, K. P., & Willott, J. F. (1987). Aging and the auditory brainstem response in mice with severe or minimal presbycusis. *Hearing Research, 30*(2–3), 207–218.

Idrizbegovic, E., Bogdanovic, N., Viberg, A., & Canlon, B. (2003). Auditory peripheral influences on calcium binding protein immunoreactivity in the cochlear nucleus during aging in the C57BL/6J mouse. *Hearing Research, 179*(1–2), 33–42.

Idrizbegovic, E., Bogdanovic, N., Willott, J. F., & Canlon, B. (2004). Age-related increases in calcium-binding protein immunoreactivity in the cochlear nucleus of hearing impaired C57BL/6J mice. *Neurobiology of Aging, 25*(8), 1085–1093. doi:10.1016/j.neurobiolaging.2003.11.004

Idrizbegovic, E., Canlon, B., Bross, L. S., Willott, J. F., & Bogdanovic, N. (2001). The total number of neurons and calcium binding protein positive neurons during aging in the cochlear nucleus of CBA/CaJ mice: a quantitative study. *Hearing Research, 158*(1–2), 102–115.

Idrizbegovic, E., Salman, H., Niu, X., & Canlon, B. (2006). Presbyacusis and calcium-binding protein immunoreactivity in the cochlear nucleus of BALB/c mice. *Hearing Research, 216–217*, 198–206.

Indo, H. P., Yen, H., Nakanishi, I., Matsumoto, K., Tamura, M., Nagano, Y., . . . Okuda, T. (2015). A mitochondrial superoxide theory for oxidative stress diseases and aging. *Journal of Clinical Biochemistry and Nutrition, 56*(1), 1–7.

Irie, T., & Ohmori, H. (2008). Presynaptic GABA(B) receptors modulate synaptic facilitation and depression at distinct synapses in fusiform cells of mouse dorsal cochlear nucleus. *Biochemical and Biophysical Research Communications, 367*(2), 503–508. doi:10.1016/j.bbrc.2008.01.001

Jalenques, I., Albuisson, E., Despres, G., & Romand, R. (1995). Distribution of glial fibrillary acidic protein (GFAP) in the cochlear nucleus of adult and aged rats. *Brain Research, 686*(2), 223–232. doi:https://doi.org/10.1016/0006-8993(95)00463-Z

Jastreboff, P. J. (1995). Salicylate-induced abnormal activity in the inferior colliculus of rats. *Hearing Research, 82*(2), 158–178.

Johnson, K. R., Erway, L. C., Cook, S. A., Willott, J. F., & Zheng, Q. Y. (1997). A major gene affecting age-related hearing loss in C57BL/6J mice. *Hearing Research, 114*(1–2), 83–92.

Juarez-Salinas, D. L., Engle, J. R., Navarro, X. O., & Recanzone, G. H. (2010). Hierarchical and serial processing in the spatial auditory cortical pathway is degraded by natural aging. *Journal of Neuroscience, 30*(44), 14795–14804. doi:10.1523/jneurosci.3393-10.2010

Kann, O., Papageorgiou, I. E., & Draguhn, A. (2014). Highly energized inhibitory interneurons are a central element for information processing in cortical networks. *Journal of Cerebral Blood Flow & Metabolism*, *34*(8), 1270–1282.

Kapahi, P., Chen, D., Rogers, A. N., Katewa, S. D., Li, P. W., Thomas, E. L., & Kockel, L. (2010). With TOR, less is more: A key role for the conserved nutrient-sensing TOR pathway in aging. *Cell Metabolism*, *11*(6), 453–465.

Kazee, A. M., Han, L. Y., Spongr, V. P., Walton, J. P., Salvi, R. J., & Flood, D. G. (1995). Synaptic loss in the central nucleus of the inferior colliculus correlates with sensorineural hearing loss in the C57BL/6 mouse model of presbycusis. *Hearing Research*, *89*(1), 109–120.

Kazee, A. M., & West, N. R. (1999). Preservation of synapses on principal cells of the central nucleus of the inferior colliculus with aging in the CBA mouse. *Hearing Research*, *133*(1), 98–106.

Keithley, E. M., Lo, J., & Ryan, A. F. (1994). 2-Deoxyglucose uptake patterns in response to pure tone stimuli in the aged rat inferior colliculus. *Hearing Research*, *80*(1), 79–85.

Khouri, L., Lesica, N. A., & Grothe, B. (2011). Impaired auditory temporal selectivity in the inferior colliculus of aged Mongolian gerbils. *Journal of Neuroscience*, *31*(27), 9958–9970.

King, A., Hopkins, K., & Plack, C. J. (2014). The effects of age and hearing loss on interaural phase difference discrimination. *Journal of the Acoustical Society of America*, *135*(1), 342–351. doi:10.1121/1.4838995

Klinkenberg, I., Sambeth, A., & Blokland, A. (2011). Acetylcholine and attention. *Behavioural Brain Research*, *221*(2), 430–442.

Kolston, J., Osen, K. K., Hackney, C. M., Ottersen, O. P., & Storm-Mathisen, J. (1992). An atlas of glycine- and GABA-like immunoreactivity and colocalization in the cochlear nuclear complex of the guinea pig. *Anatomy and Embryology (Berlin)*, *186*(5), 443–465.

Krenning, J., Hughes, L. F., Caspary, D. M., & Helfert, R. H. (1998). Age-related glycine receptor subunit changes in the cochlear nucleus of Fischer-344 rats. *Laryngoscope*, *108*(1 Pt 1), 26–31.

Kujawa, S. G., & Liberman, M. C. (2009). Adding insult to injury: cochlear nerve degeneration after "temporary" noise-induced hearing loss. *Journal of Neuroscience*, *29*(45), 14077–14085. doi:10.1523/JNEUROSCI.2845-09.2009

Kujawa, S. G., & Liberman, M. C. (2015). Synaptopathy in the noise-exposed and aging cochlea: Primary neural degeneration in acquired sensorineural hearing loss. *Hearing Research*, *330*(Pt B), 191–199. doi:10.1016/j.heares.2015.02.009

Lass, A., Sohal, B. H., Weindruch, R., Forster, M. J., & Sohal, R. S. (1998). Caloric restriction prevents age-associated accrual of oxidative damage to mouse skeletal muscle mitochondria. *Free Radical Biology and Medicine*, *25*(9), 1089–1097.

Lee, C. C. (2013). Thalamic and cortical pathways supporting auditory processing. *Brain and Language*, *126*(1), 22–28.

Leong, U., Barsz, K., Allen, P. D., & Walton, J. P. (2011). Neural correlates of age-related declines in frequency selectivity in the auditory midbrain. *Neurobiology of Aging*, *32*(1), 168–178.

Lesicko, A. M., Hristova, T., Maigler, K., & Llano, D. A. (2016). Connectional modularity of top-down and bottom-up multimodal inputs to the lateral cortex of the inferior colliculus. *Journal of Neuroscience*, *36*(43), 11037–11050.

Lesicko, A. M., & Llano, D. A. (2017). Impact of peripheral hearing loss on top-down auditory processing. *Hearing Research*, *343*, 4–13.

Liberman, M. C. (2017). Noise-induced and age-related hearing loss: New perspectives and potential therapies. *F1000Res*, *6*, 927. doi:10.12688/f1000research.11310.1

Lim, R., Alvarez, F. J., & Walmsley, B. (2000). GABA mediates presynaptic inhibition at glycinergic synapses in a rat auditory brainstem nucleus. *Journal of Physiology, 525 Pt 2*, 447–459.

Lin, F. R., Thorpe, R., Gordon-Salant, S., & Ferrucci, L. (2011). Hearing loss prevalence and risk factors among older adults in the United States. *Journal of Gerontology Series A, 66*(5), 582–590. doi:10.1093/gerona/glr002

Lin, H. W., Furman, A. C., Kujawa, S. G., & Liberman, M. C. (2011). Primary neural degeneration in the guinea pig cochlea after reversible noise-induced threshold shift. *Journal of the Association of Research Otolaryngology, 12*(5), 605–616. doi:10.1007/s10162-011-0277-0

Lipman, R. D., Chrisp, C. E., Hazzard, D. G., & Bronson, R. T. (1996). Pathologic characterization of brown Norway, brown Norway x Fischer 344, and Fischer 344 x brown Norway rats with relation to age. *Journal of Gerontology Series A, 51*(1), B54–B59.

Lister, J., Besing, J., & Koehnke, J. (2002). Effects of age and frequency disparity on gap discrimination. *Journal of the Acoustical Society of America, 111*(6), 2793–2800.

Longo, V. D., & Kennedy, B. K. (2006). Sirtuins in aging and age-related disease. *Cell, 126*(2), 257–268.

López-Otín, C., Blasco, M. A., Partridge, L., Serrano, M., & Kroemer, G. (2013). The hallmarks of aging. *Cell, 153*(6), 1194–1217.

Lu, E., Llano, D. A., & Sherman, S. M. (2009). Different distributions of calbindin and calretinin immunostaining across the medial and dorsal divisions of the mouse medial geniculate body. *Hearing Research, 257*(1–2), 16–23. doi:10.1016/j.heares.2009.07.009

Lu, T., Rubio, M. E., & Trussell, L. O. (2008). Glycinergic transmission shaped by the corelease of GABA in a mammalian auditory synapse. *Neuron, 57*(4), 524–535. doi:10.1016/j.neuron.2007.12.010

Lujan, R., Shigemoto, R., Kulik, A., & Juiz, J. M. (2004). Localization of the GABAB receptor 1a/b subunit relative to glutamatergic synapses in the dorsal cochlear nucleus of the rat. *Journal of Comparative Neurology, 475*(1), 36–46. doi:10.1002/cne.20160

Ma, C. L., Kelly, J. B., & Wu, S. H. (2002). Presynaptic modulation of GABAergic inhibition by GABA B receptors in the rat's inferior colliculus. *Neuroscience, 114*(1), 207–215.

Ma, W. D., Hidaka, H., & May, B. J. (2006). Spontaneous activity in the inferior colliculus of CBA/J mice after manipulations that induce tinnitus. *Hearing Research, 212*(1), 9–21.

Malmierca, M. S., Cristaudo, S., Pérez-González, D., & Covey, E. (2009). Stimulus-specific adaptation in the inferior colliculus of the anesthetized rat. *Journal of Neuroscience, 29*(17), 5483–5493.

Mancilla, J. G., & Manis, P. B. (2009). Two distinct types of inhibition mediated by cartwheel cells in the dorsal cochlear nucleus. *Journal of Neurophysiology, 102*(2), 1287–1295.

Martin, M. R., & Adams, J. C. (1979). Effects of DL-alpha-aminoadipate on synaptically and chemically evoked excitation of anteroventral cochlear nucleus neurons of the cat. *Neuroscience, 4*(8), 1097–1105.

McCann, S. M. (1997). The nitric oxide hypothesis of brain aging. *Experimental Gerontology, 32*(4), 431–440.

McFadden, S. L., & Willott, J. F. (1994). Responses of inferior colliculus neurons in C57BL/6J mice with and without sensorineural hearing loss: Effects of changing the azimuthal location of an unmasked pure-tone stimulus. *Hearing Research, 78*(2), 115–131.

McGeer, P. L., & McGeer, E. G. (1975). Evidence for glutamic acid decarboxylase-containing interneurons in the neostriatum. *Brain Research, 91*(2), 331–335.

Mei, Y., Gawai, K. R., Nie, Z., Ramkumar, V., & Helfert, R. H. (1999). Age-related reductions in the activities of antioxidant enzymes in the rat inferior colliculus. *Hearing Research, 135*(1), 169–180.

Mendelson, J. R., & Lui, B. (2004). The effects of aging in the medial geniculate nucleus: a comparison with the inferior colliculus and auditory cortex. *Hearing Research, 191*(1), 21–33.

Mendelson, J. R., & Ricketts, C. (2001). Age-related temporal processing speed deterioration in auditory cortex. *Hearing Research, 158*(1), 84–94.

Milbrandt, J. C., Albin, R. L., & Caspary, D. M. (1994). Age-related decrease in GABA B receptor binding in the Fischer 344 rat inferior colliculus. *Neurobiology of aging, 15*(6), 699–703.

Milbrandt, J. C., & Caspary, D. M. (1995). Age-related reduction of [3H]strychnine binding sites in the cochlear nucleus of the Fischer 344 rat. *Neuroscience, 67*(3), 713–719.

Milbrandt, J. C., Holder, T. M., Wilson, M. C., Salvi, R. J., & Caspary, D. M. (2000). GAD levels and muscimol binding in rat inferior colliculus following acoustic trauma. *Hearing Research, 147*(1), 251–260.

Milbrandt, J. C., Hunter, C., & Caspary, D. M. (1997). Alterations of GABAA receptor subunit mRNA levels in the aging Fischer 344 rat inferior colliculus. *Journal of Comparative Neurology, 379*(3), 455–465.

Molinari, M., Dell'Anna, M. E., Rausell, E., Leggio, M. G., Hashikawa, T., & Jones, E. G. (1995). Auditory thalamocortical pathways defined in monkeys by calcium-binding protein immunoreactivity. *Journal of Comparative Neurology, 362*(2), 171–194.

Moore, M. J., & Caspary, D. M. (1983). Strychnine blocks binaural inhibition in lateral superior olivary neurons. *Journal of Neuroscience, 3*(1), 237–242.

Myoga, M. H., Lehnert, S., Leibold, C., Felmy, F., & Grothe, B. (2014). Glycinergic inhibition tunes coincidence detection in the auditory brainstem. *Nature Communications, 5*, 3790. doi:10.1038/ncomms4790

O'Neill, W. E., Zettel, M. L., Whittemore, K. R., & Frisina, R. D. (1997). Calbindin D-28k immunoreactivity in the medial nucleus of the trapezoid body declines with age in C57BL/6, but not CBA/CaJ, mice. *Hearing Research, 112*(1–2), 158–166.

Oertel, D., & Young, E. D. (2004). What's a cerebellar circuit doing in the auditory system? *Trends in Neuroscience, 27*(2), 104–110. doi:10.1016/j.tins.2003.12.001

Ohlemiller, K. K. (2004). Age-related hearing loss: The status of Schuknecht's typology. *Current Opinion in Otolaryngology &Head and Neck Surgery, 12*(5), 439–443.

Osumi, Y., Shibata, S. B., Kanda, S., Yagi, M., Ooka, H., Shimano, T., . . . Inoue, T. (2012). Downregulation of N-methyl-d-aspartate receptor ζ1 subunit (GluN1) gene in inferior colliculus with aging. *Brain Research, 1454*, 23–32.

Ouda, L., Burianova, J., & Syka, J. (2012). Age-related changes in calbindin and calretinin immunoreactivity in the central auditory system of the rat. *Experimental Gerontology, 47*(7), 497–506.

Ouda, L., Druga, R., & Syka, J. (2008). Changes in parvalbumin immunoreactivity with aging in the central auditory system of the rat. *Experimental Gerontology, 43*(8), 782–789.

Ouda, L., Profant, O., & Syka, J. (2015). Age-related changes in the central auditory system. *Cell and Tissue Research, 361*(1), 337–358.

Ozmeral, E. J., Eddins, D. A., & Eddins, A. C. (2016). Reduced temporal processing in older, normal-hearing listeners evident from electrophysiological responses to shifts in interaural time difference. *Journal of Neurophysiology, 116*(6), 2720–2729. doi:10.1152/jn.00560.2016

Pakaski, M., Farkas, Z., Kasa, P., Forgon, M., Papp, H., Zarandi, M., & Penke, B. (1998). Vulnerability of small GABAergic neurons to human β-amyloid pentapeptide. *Brain Research*, *796*(1), 239–246.

Palombi, P. S., Backoff, P. M., & Caspary, D. M. (2001). Responses of young and aged rat inferior colliculus neurons to sinusoidally amplitude modulated stimuli. *Hearing Research*, *153*(1), 174–180.

Palombi, P. S., & Caspary, D. M. (1996a). GABA inputs control discharge rate primarily within frequency receptive fields of inferior colliculus neurons. *Journal of Neurophysiology*, *75*(6), 2211–2219.

Palombi, P. S., & Caspary, D. M. (1996b). Physiology of the aged Fischer 344 rat inferior colliculus: Responses to contralateral monaural stimuli. *Journal of Neurophysiology*, *76*(5), 3114–3125.

Palombi, P. S., & Caspary, D. M. (1996c). Responses of young and aged Fischer 344 rat inferior colliculus neurons to binaural tonal stimuli. *Hearing Research*, *100*(1), 59–67.

Parham, K., Sun, X. M., & Kim, D. O. (1999). Distortion product otoacoustic emissions in the CBA/J mouse model of presbycusis. *Hearing Research*, *134*(1–2), 29–38.

Peruzzi, D., Bartlett, E., Smith, P. H., & Oliver, D. L. (1997). A monosynaptic GABAergic input from the inferior colliculus to the medial geniculate body in rat. *The Journal of Neuroscience*, *17*(10), 3766–3777.

Petralia, R. S., Rubio, M. E., Wang, Y. X., & Wenthold, R. J. (2000). Differential distribution of glutamate receptors in the cochlear nuclei. *Hearing Research*, *147*(1–2), 59–69.

Pichora-Fuller, M. K., Alain, C., & Schneider, B. A. (2017). Older adults at the cocktail party. In J. C. Middlebrooks, J. Z. Simon, A. N. Popper, & R. R. Fay (Eds.), *The Auditory System at the Cocktail Party* (pp. 227–259). Cham, Switzerland: Springer International Publishing.

Pichora-Fuller, M. K., Schneider, B. A., Macdonald, E., Pass, H. E., & Brown, S. (2007). Temporal jitter disrupts speech intelligibility: A simulation of auditory aging. *Hearing Research*, *223*(1–2), 114–121. doi:S0378-5955(06)00305-4 [pii] 10.1016/j.heares.2006.10.009

Pichora-Fuller, M. K., & Souza, P. E. (2003). Effects of aging on auditory processing of speech. *International Journal of Audiology*, *42 Suppl 2*, 2S11–12S16.

Portfors, C. V., & Roberts, P. D. (2007). Temporal and frequency characteristics of cartwheel cells in the dorsal cochlear nucleus of the awake mouse. *Journal of Neurophysiology*, *98*(2), 744–756.

Rabang, C. F., Parthasarathy, A., Venkataraman, Y., Fisher, Z. L., Gardner, S. M., & Bartlett, E. L. (2012). A computational model of inferior colliculus responses to amplitude modulated sounds in young and aged rats. *Frontiers in Neural Circuits*, *6*, 77. doi:10.3389/fncir.2012.00077

Raman, I. M., & Trussell, L. O. (1995). The mechanism of alpha-amino-3-hydroxy-5-methyl-4-isoxazolepropionate receptor desensitization after removal of glutamate. *Biophysical Journal*, *68*(1), 137–146. doi:10.1016/s0006-3495(95)80168-2

Raza, A., Milbrandt, J. C., Arneric, S. P., & Caspary, D. M. (1994). Age-related changes in brainstem auditory neurotransmitters: Measures of GABA and acetylcholine function. *Hearing Research*, *77*(1), 221–230.

Rebrin, I., Forster, M. J., & Sohal, R. S. (2007). Effects of age and caloric intake on glutathione redox state in different brain regions of C57BL/6 and DBA/2 mice. *Brain Research*, *1127*, 10–18.

Rebrin, I., Kamzalov, S., & Sohal, R. S. (2003). Effects of age and caloric restriction on glutathione redox state in mice. *Free Radical Biology and Medicine*, *35*(6), 626–635.

Rhode, W. S. (1999). Vertical cell responses to sound in cat dorsal cochlear nucleus. *Journal of Neurophysiology, 82*(2), 1019–1032.

Rhode, W. S., Smith, P. H., & Oertel, D. (1983). Physiological response properties of cells labeled intracellularly with horseradish peroxidase in cat dorsal cochlear nucleus. *Journal of Comparative Neurology, 213*(4), 426–447. doi:10.1002/cne.902130407

Richardson, B. D., Hancock, K. E., & Caspary, D. M. (2013). Stimulus-specific adaptation in auditory thalamus of young and aged awake rats. *Journal of Neurophysiology, 110*(8), 1892–1902.

Richardson, B. D., Ling, L. L., Uteshev, V. V., & Caspary, D. M. (2013). Reduced GABA(A) receptor-mediated tonic inhibition in aged rat auditory thalamus. *Journal of Neuroscience, 33*(3), 1218–1227a. doi:10.1523/JNEUROSCI.3277-12.2013

Rodriguez-Brenes, I. A., Wodarz, D., & Komarova, N. L. (2015). Quantifying replicative senescence as a tumor suppressor pathway and a target for cancer therapy. *Scientific Reports, 5*. doi:10.1038/srep17660

Ross, D. T., & Duhaime, A. (1989). Degeneration of neurons in the thalamic reticular nucleus following transient ischemia due to raised intracranial pressure: Excitotoxic degeneration mediated via non-NMDA receptors? *Brain Research, 501*(1), 129–143.

Rozycka, A., & Liguz-Lecznar, M. (2017). The space where aging acts: Focus on the GABAergic synapse. *Aging Cell, 16*(4), 634–643. doi:10.1111/acel.12605

Rubio, M. E., & Juiz, J. M. (2004). Differential distribution of synaptic endings containing glutamate, glycine, and GABA in the rat dorsal cochlear nucleus. *Journal of Comparative Neurology, 477*(3), 253–272. doi:10.1002/cne.20248

Rudolph, U., & Möhler, H. (2006). GABA-based therapeutic approaches: GABA A receptor subtype functions. *Current Opinion in Pharmacology, 6*(1), 18–23.

Salminen, A., & Kaarniranta, K. (2012). AMP-activated protein kinase (AMPK) controls the aging process via an integrated signaling network. *Ageing Research Reviews, 11*(2), 230–241.

Sánchez-Zuriaga, D., Martí-Gutiérrez, N., La Cruz, D., Pérez, M. Á., & Peris-Sanchis, M. R. (2007). Age-related changes of NADPH-diaphorase-positive neurons in the rat inferior colliculus and auditory cortex. *Microscopy Research and Technique, 70*(12), 1051–1059.

Sato, T., Wilson, T. S., Hughes, L. F., Konrad, H. R., Nakayama, M., & Helfert, R. H. (2001). Age-related changes in levels of tyrosine kinase B receptor and fibroblast growth factor receptor 2 in the rat inferior colliculus: implications for neural senescence. *Neuroscience, 103*(3), 695–702.

Schatteman, T. A., Hughes, L. F., & Caspary, D. M. (2008). Aged-related loss of temporal processing: Altered responses to amplitude modulated tones in rat dorsal cochlear nucleus. *Neuroscience, 154*(1), 329–337.

Schneider, B. A. (1997). Psychoacoustics and aging: Implications for everyday listening. *Journal of Speech-Language Pathology and Audiology, 21*(2), 111–124.

Schuknecht, H. F., & Gacek, M. R. (1993). Cochlear pathology in presbycusis. *Annals of Otology, Rhinology, & Laryngology, 102*(1 Pt 2), 1–16. doi:10.1177/00034894931020S101

Sergeyenko, Y., Lall, K., Liberman, M. C., & Kujawa, S. G. (2013). Age-related cochlear synaptopathy: An early-onset contributor to auditory functional decline. *Journal of Neuroscience, 33*(34), 13686–13694. doi:10.1523/JNEUROSCI.1783-13.2013

Sharma, S., Nag, T. C., Thakar, A., Bhardwaj, D. N., & Roy, T. S. (2014). The aging human cochlear nucleus: Changes in the glial fibrillary acidic protein, intracellular calcium regulatory proteins, GABA neurotransmitter and cholinergic receptor. *Journal of Chemical Neuroanatomy, 56*, 1–12. doi:10.1016/j.jchemneu.2013.12.001

Sloper, J. J., Johnson, P., & Powell, T. P. S. (1980). Selective degeneration of interneurons in the motor cortex of infant monkeys following controlled hypoxia: A possible cause of epilepsy. *Brain Research, 198*(1), 204–209.

Smith, M. L., Auer, R. N., & Siesjö, B. K. (1984). The density and distribution of ischemic brain injury in the rat following 2–10 min of forebrain ischemia. *Acta Neuropathologica, 64*(4), 319–332.

Snell, K. B. (1997). Age-related changes in temporal gap detection. *Journal of the Acoustical Society of America, 101*(4), 2214–2220.

Sohal, R. S., Agarwal, S., Candas, M., Forster, M. J., & Lal, H. (1994). Effect of age and caloric restriction on DNA oxidative damage in different tissues of C57BL/6 mice. *Mechanisms of Ageing and Development, 76*(2), 215–224.

Sokoloff, L., Reivich, M., Kennedy, C., Des Rosiers, M. H., Patlak, C. S., & Pettigrew, K. D. (1977). Tomographic measurement of local cerebral glucose utilization: theory, procedure, and normal values in the conscious and anesthetized albino rat. *Journal of Neurochemistry, 28*, 897–916.

Someya, S., & Prolla, T. A. (2010). Mitochondrial oxidative damage and apoptosis in age-related hearing loss. *Mechanisms of Ageing and Development, 131*(7), 480–486.

Someya, S., Yamasoba, T., Weindruch, R., Prolla, T. A., & Tanokura, M. (2007). Caloric restriction suppresses apoptotic cell death in the mammalian cochlea and leads to prevention of presbycusis. *Neurobiology of Aging, 28*(10), 1613–1622.

Sottile, S. Y., Hackett, T. A., Cai, R., Ling, L., Llano, D. A., & Caspary, D. M. (2017). Presynaptic neuronal nicotinic receptors differentially shape select inputs to auditory thalamus and are negatively impacted by aging. *Journal of Neuroscience, 37*(47), 11377–11389. doi:10.1523/jneurosci.1795-17.2017

Sottile, S. Y., Ling, L., Cox, B. C., & Caspary, D. M. (2017). Impact of aging on postsynaptic neuronal nicotinic neurotransmission in auditory Thalamus. *Journal of Physiology, 595*(15), 5375–5385.

Strouse, A., Ashmead, D. H., Ohde, R. N., & Grantham, D. W. (1998). Temporal processing in the aging auditory system. *The Journal of the Acoustical Society of America, 104*(4), 2385–2399.

Suneja, S. K., Benson, C. G., & Potashner, S. J. (1998). Glycine receptors in adult guinea pig brain stem auditory nuclei: Regulation after unilateral cochlear ablation. *Experimental Neurology, 154*(2), 473–488. doi:10.1006/exnr.1998.6946

Suneja, S. K., Potashner, S. J., & Benson, C. G. (1998). Plastic changes in glycine and GABA release and uptake in adult brain stem auditory nuclei after unilateral middle ear ossicle removal and cochlear ablation. *Experimental Neurology, 151*(2), 273–288. doi:10.1006/exnr.1998.6812

Syka, J. (2002). Plastic changes in the central auditory system after hearing loss, restoration of function, and during learning. *Physiological Review, 82*(3), 601–636.

Tadros, S. F., D'Souza, M., Zettel, M. L., Zhu, X., Lynch-Erhardt, M., & Frisina, R. D. (2007). Serotonin 2B receptor: Upregulated with age and hearing loss in mouse auditory system. *Neurobiology of Aging, 28*(7), 1112–1123.

Tadros, S. F., D'Souza, M., Zettel, M. L., Zhu, X., Waxmonsky, N. C., & Frisina, R. D. (2007). Glutamate-related gene expression changes with age in the mouse auditory midbrain. *Brain Research, 1127*, 1–9.

Takahashi, G. A., & Bacon, S. P. (1992). Modulation detection, modulation masking, and speech understanding in noise in the elderly. *Journal of Speech Hearing Research, 35*(6), 1410–1421.

Teunisse, R. J., Cruysberg, J. R., Verbeek, A., & Zitman, F. G. (1995). The Charles Bonnet syndrome: A large prospective study in The Netherlands. A study of the prevalence of the Charles Bonnet syndrome and associated factors in 500 patients attending the University Department of Ophthalmology at Nijmegen. *The British Journal of Psychiatry*, *166*(2), 254–257.

Tremblay, K. L., Piskosz, M., & Souza, P. (2003). Effects of age and age-related hearing loss on the neural representation of speech cues. *Clinical Neurophysiology*, *114*(7), 1332–1343.

Ulanovsky, N., Las, L., & Nelken, I. (2003). Processing of low-probability sounds by cortical neurons. *Nature Neuroscience*, *6*(4), 391.

Voigt, H. F., & Young, E. D. (1990). Cross-correlation analysis of inhibitory interactions in dorsal cochlear nucleus. *Journal of Neurophysiology*, *64*(5), 1590–1610.

Walton, J. P., Frisina, R. D., Ison, J. R., & O'Neill, W. E. (1997). Neural correlates of behavioral gap detection in the inferior colliculus of the young CBA mouse. *Journal of Comparative Physiology A: Neuroethology, Sensory, Neural, and Behavioral Physiology*, *181*(2), 161–176.

Walton, J. P., Frisina, R. D., & O'Neill, W. E. (1998). Age-related alteration in processing of temporal sound features in the auditory midbrain of the CBA mouse. *Journal of Neuroscience*, *18*(7), 2764–2776.

Walton, J. P., Simon, H., & Frisina, R. D. (2002). Age-related alterations in the neural coding of envelope periodicities. *Journal of Neurophysiology*, *88*(2), 565–578.

Wang, H., Brozoski, T. J., & Caspary, D. M. (2011). Inhibitory neurotransmission in animal models of tinnitus: maladaptive plasticity. *Hearing Research*, *279*(1), 111–117.

Wang, H., Brozoski, T. J., Ling, L., Hughes, L. F., & Caspary, D. M. (2011). Impact of sound exposure and aging on brain-derived neurotrophic factor and tyrosine kinase B receptors levels in dorsal cochlear nucleus 80 days following sound exposure. *Neuroscience*, *172*, 453–459.

Wang, H., Brozoski, T. J., Turner, J. G., Ling, L., Parrish, J. L., Hughes, L. F., & Caspary, D. M. (2009). Plasticity at glycinergic synapses in dorsal cochlear nucleus of rats with behavioral evidence of tinnitus. *Neuroscience*, *164*(2), 747–759.

Wang, H., Turner, J. G., Ling, L., Parrish, J. L., Hughes, L. F., & Caspary, D. M. (2009). Age-related changes in glycine receptor subunit composition and binding in dorsal cochlear nucleus. *Neuroscience*, *160*(1), 227–239.

Wang, W., Sun, Y., Chen, S., Zhou, X., Wu, X., Kong, W., & Kong, W. (2015). Impaired unfolded protein response in the degeneration of cochlea cells in a mouse model of age-related hearing loss. *Experimental Gerontology*, *70*, 61–70.

Wang, Y., & Manis, P. B. (2005). Synaptic transmission at the cochlear nucleus endbulb synapse during age-related hearing loss in mice. *Journal of Neurophysiology*, *94*(3), 1814–1824. doi:10.1152/jn.00374.2005

Wenk, G. L., & Barnes, C. A. (2000). Regional changes in the hippocampal density of AMPA and NMDA receptors across the lifespan of the rat. *Brain Research*, *885*(1), 1–5. doi:https://doi.org/10.1016/S0006-8993(00)02792-X

Werhagen, L., Budh, C. N., Hultling, C., & Molander, C. (2004). Neuropathic pain after traumatic spinal cord injury–relations to gender, spinal level, completeness, and age at the time of injury. *Spinal Cord*, *42*(12), 665–673.

Whiting, P. J. (2003). GABA-A receptor subtypes in the brain: A paradigm for CNS drug discovery? *Drug Discovery Today*, *8*(10), 445–450.

Willott, J. F. (1984). Changes in frequency representation in the auditory system of mice with age-related hearing impairment. *Brain Research*, *309*(1), 159–162.

Willott, J. F. (1986). Effects of aging, hearing loss, and anatomical location on thresholds of inferior colliculus neurons in C57BL/6 and CBA mice. *Journal of Neurophysiology*, *56*(2), 391–408.

Willott, J. F., Bross, L. S., & McFadden, S. L. (1992). Morphology of the dorsal cochlear nucleus in C57BL/6J and CBA/J mice across the life span. *Journal of Comparative Neurology*, *321*(4), 666–678. doi:10.1002/cne.903210412

Willott, J. F., Bross, L. S., & McFadden, S. L. (1994). Morphology of the inferior colliculus in C57BL/6J and CBA/J mice across the life span. *Neurobiology of Aging*, *15*(2), 175–183.

Willott, J. F., Hunter, K. P., & Coleman, J. R. (1988). Aging and presbycusis: Effects on 2-deoxy-D-glucose uptake in the mouse auditory brain stem in quiet. *Experimental Neurology*, *99*(3), 615–621.

Willott, J. F., Milbrandt, J. C., Bross, L. S., & Caspary, D. M. (1997). Glycine immunoreactivity and receptor binding in the cochlear nucleus of C57BL/6J and CBA/CaJ mice: Effects of cochlear impairment and aging. *Journal of Comparative Neurology*, *385*(3), 405–414.

Willott, J. F., Pankow, D., Hunter, K. P., & Kordyban, M. (1985). Projections from the anterior ventral cochlear nucleus to the central nucleus of the inferior colliculus in young and aging C57BL/6 mice. *Journal of Comparative Neurology*, *237*(4), 545–551.

Willott, J. F., Parham, K., & Hunter, K. P. (1988a). Response properties of inferior colliculus neurons in middle-aged C57BL/6J mice with presbycusis. *Hearing Research*, *37*(1), 15–27.

Willott, J. F., Parham, K., & Hunter, K. P. (1988b). Response properties of inferior colliculus neurons in young and very old CBA/J mice. *Hearing Research*, *37*(1), 1–14.

Willott, J. F., Parham, K., & Hunter, K. P. (1991). Comparison of the auditory sensitivity of neurons in the cochlear nucleus and inferior colliculus of young and aging C57BL/6J and CBA/J mice. *Hearing Research*, *53*(1), 78–94.

Winer, J. A., & Larue, D. T. (1988). Anatomy of glutamic acid decarboxylase immunoreactive neurons and axons in the rat medial geniculate body. *Journal of Comparative Neurology*, *278*(1), 47–68. doi:10.1002/cne.902780104

Winer, J. A., Saint Marie, R. L., Larue, D. T., & Oliver, D. L. (1996). GABAergic feedforward projections from the inferior colliculus to the medial geniculate body. *Proceedings of the National Academy of Sciences USA*, *93*(15), 8005–8010.

Xie, R., & Manis, P. B. (2013). Glycinergic synaptic transmission in the cochlear nucleus of mice with normal hearing and age-related hearing loss. *Journal of Neurophysiology*, *110*(8), 1848–1859. doi:10.1152/jn.00151.2013

Xie, R., & Manis, P. B. (2017). Synaptic transmission at the endbulb of Held deteriorates during age-related hearing loss. *Journal of Physiology*, *595*(3), 919–934. doi:10.1113/jp272683

Xiong, H., Dai, M., Ou, Y., Pang, J., Yang, H., Huang, Q., . . . Cai, Y. (2014). SIRT1 expression in the cochlea and auditory cortex of a mouse model of age-related hearing loss. *Experimental Gerontology*, *51*, 8–14.

Yamasoba, T., Someya, S., Yamada, C., Weindruch, R., Prolla, T. A., & Tanokura, M. (2007). Role of mitochondrial dysfunction and mitochondrial DNA mutations in age-related hearing loss. *Hearing Research*, *226*(1), 185–193.

Young, E. D., & Brownell, W. E. (1976). Responses to tones and noise of single cells in dorsal cochlear nucleus of unanesthetized cats. *Journal Neurophysiology*, *39*(2), 282–300.

Zeng, L., Yang, Y., Hu, Y., Sun, Y., Du, Z., Xie, Z., . . . Kong, W. (2014). Age-related decrease in the mitochondrial sirtuin deacetylase Sirt3 expression associated with ROS accumulation in the auditory cortex of the mimetic aging rat model. *PloS One*, *9*(2), e88019.

Zettel, M. L., Frisina, R. D., Haider, S., & O'Neill, W. E. (1997). Age-related changes in calbindin D-28k and calretinin immunoreactivity in the inferior colliculus of CBA/CaJ and C57Bl/6 mice. *Journal of Comparative Neurology*, *386*(1), 92–110.

Zettel, M. L., O'Neill, W. E., Trang, T. T., & Frisina, R. D. (2001). Early bilateral deafening prevents calretinin up-regulation in the dorsal cortex of the inferior colliculus of aged CBA/CaJ mice. *Hearing Research*, *158*(1), 131–138.

Zettel, M. L., O'Neill, W. E., Trang, T. T., & Frisina, R. D. (2003). The effects of early bilateral deafening on calretinin expression in the dorsal cochlear nucleus of aged CBA/CaJ mice. *Hearing Research*, *183*(1), 57–66. doi:https://doi.org/10.1016/S0378-5955(03)00216-8

CHAPTER 24

GLIAL CELLS IN THE AUDITORY BRAINSTEM

GIEDRE MILINKEVICIUTE AND KARINA S. CRAMER

Abstract

The auditory brainstem carries out sound localization functions that require an extraordinary degree of precision. While many of the specializations needed for these functions reside in auditory neurons, additional adaptations are made possible by the functions of glial cells. Astrocytes, once thought to have mainly a supporting role in nervous system function, are now known to participate in synaptic function. In the auditory brainstem, they contribute to development of specialized synapses and to mature synaptic function. Oligodendrocytes play critical roles in regulating timing in sound localization circuitry. Microglia enter the central nervous system early in development, and also have important functions in the auditory system's response to injury. This chapter highlights the unique functions of these non-neuronal cells in the auditory system.

Keywords: astrocyte, oligodendrocyte, myelination, conduction velocity, calyx of Held, microglia, nucleus magnocellularis, nucleus laminaris

AUDITORY brainstem function emerges from precise and highly specialized neural circuits. Recent studies have demonstrated the remarkable extent to which the development and function of neuronal circuitry rely on multiple functions of glial cells. Notably, astrocytes (Allen & Eroglu, 2017; Chung et al., 2015), oligodendrocytes (Micu et al., 2017), and microglia (Mosser et al., 2017) are known to communicate closely with neurons during development, plasticity, and in response to brain injury. Astrocytes and oligodendrocytes are derived from neural lineages and, like neurons, display diversity appropriate for their specialized functions (Dimou & Simons, 2017; Farmer & Murai, 2017). In addition, they share some unexpected properties with neurons, including the ability to release and respond to neurotransmitters and, in some cases, excitability (Berret et al., 2017; Micu et al., 2017; Perea et al., 2014). Microglia, the immune cells of the brain, are derived from the myeloid lineage and migrate into the central nervous system early in development (Mosser et al., 2017). The highly motile branches of these cells interact dynamically with their environment (Gomez-Nicola & Perry, 2015). However, their gene expression profiles vary with brain region (Grabert et al., 2016), suggesting region-specific functions for subpopulations of microglia.

In this chapter, these aspects of glial cell function are explored in the context of the unique circuits of the auditory brainstem. We consider glial contributions to the formation of auditory brainstem circuits, to the function of synapses and circuits, and to the response of auditory nuclei to injury.

Sound Localization Pathways in Birds and Mammals

Both avian and mammalian animal models have led to insights on auditory brainstem function and on the roles of glial cells. The avian auditory brainstem (Figure 24.1) displays a well-characterized neuronal pathway from nucleus magnocellularis (NM) to nucleus laminaris (NL). NM, which is homologous to the anteroventral cochlear nucleus (AVCN), receives input from central projections of cochlear ganglion cells (Rubel & Fritzsch, 2002). NM axons branch and project bilaterally and tonotopically to NL, a laminated nucleus with bitufted dendrites oriented dorsally and ventrally (Figure 24.1A). The ipsilateral branch makes contacts with dorsal NL dendrites, while the contralateral branch contacts ventral NL dendrites (Hackett et al., 1982; Parks & Rubel, 1975; ; Young & Rubel, 1983). Coincidence detection by NL neurons together with axonal delay lines in the contralateral NM axon are used to reveal interaural time differences (ITDs), which are used to estimate the location of sound sources (Hyson, 2005; Koppl & Carr, 2008; Overholt et al., 1992). Coincidence detection in NL is improved with inhibitory input, which arises from the superior olivary nucleus (Burger et al., 2011; Lachica et al., 1994; Ohmori, 2014; Yang et al., 1999). In the developing chick embryo, NL is a single cell thick, and the cell body layer is surrounded by a region of neuropil free of cell bodies (Figure 24.1B). At the outer margins of the neuropil, the nucleus is surrounded by a tightly packed layer of glial cells (Figure 24.1B–E).

In mammals, ITDs are computed in the medial superior olive (MSO), which is analogous to NL (Grothe, 2003). Lateral MSO dendrites receive ipsilateral input from the AVCN and medial MSO dendrites receive contralateral AVCN input. Unlike the chick NL, MSO neurons rely on precisely timed inhibitory input in order to compute ITDs (Brand et al., 2002; Myoga et al., 2014; Pecka et al., 2008). In addition to ITDs, auditory brainstem nuclei are used to compute interaural level differences (ILDs). AVCN neurons project contralaterally to the medial nucleus of the trapezoid body (MNTB). The axon terminates in the large calyx of Held, encapsulating

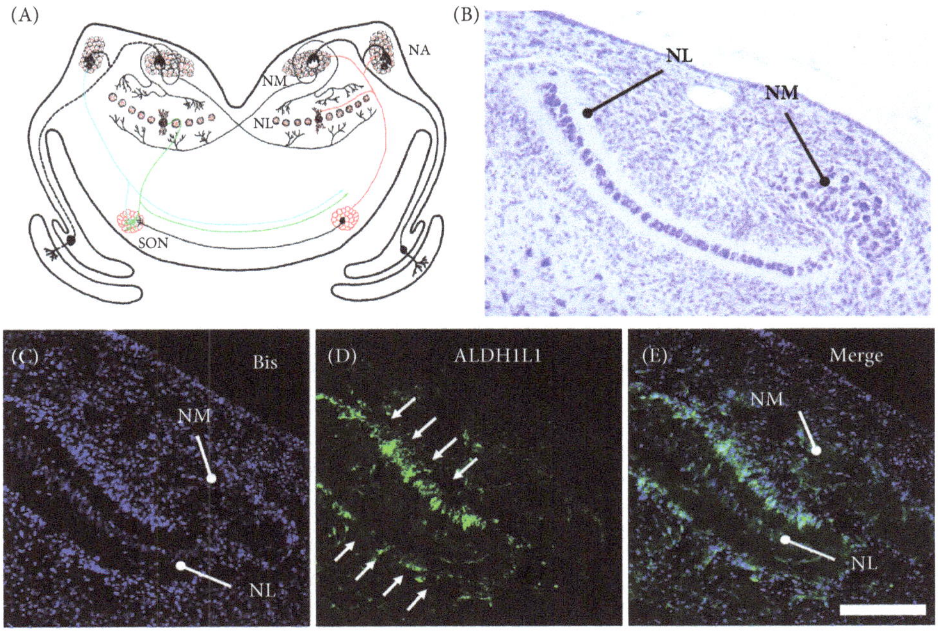

FIGURE 24.1. A: Auditory pathways in the chick. Nucleus magnocellularis (NM) receives VIIIth nerve input. NM axons branch and innervate nucleus laminaris (NL) bilaterally, with ipsilateral inputs on dorsal dendrites and contralateral inputs on ventral dendrites. Inhibitory input to NL arises from the superior olivary nucleus (SON). B: Glial cell bodies can be seen in Nissl stained sections in a margin (arrowheads) surrounding the cell-free zone around the NL cell body layer (arrow). C–E: Glial margin around NL is evident at E10 with bisbenzimide staining (bis) and ALDH1L1. Scale bar, 100 μm.

the MNTB neuron (Held, 1893; Kuwabara & Zook, 1992; Nakamura & Cramer 2011). MNTB provides inhibitory input to the lateral superior olive (LSO), which receives tonotopically matched excitatory input from AVCN. The balance of excitation and inhibition in LSO neurons is used to compute ILDs, which are used to determine the locations of sound sources (Glendenning et al., 1992; Kandler & Gillespie, 2005; Sanes, 1990; Tollin, 2003).

Glial Cells in Auditory Brainstem Development

Astrocytes, microglia, and oligodendrocytes arise in the auditory brainstem with a characteristic time course and morphological features. In some cases, their functions have been critically tested.

Astrocytes and Development of the Chick Auditory Brainstem Pathways

The emergence of glial cells in the developing chick auditory brainstem is evident at the time when NM-NL synapses are forming, at about embryonic day (E)10. Small cells expressing aldehyde dehydrogenase 1, family L1 (ALDH1L1), an astrocyte marker, are seen in the glial margin around NL (Cahoy et al., 2008; Rotschafer et al., 2016; Figure 24.1 C–E). At this age distinct populations of glial cells are present in the dorsal versus ventral regions of NL during the time of synaptic maturation. Astrocytes expressing glial fibrillary acidic protein (GFAP) emerge after the formation of excitatory connections and just prior to the maturation of inhibitory synapses in NL (Korn & Cramer, 2008) and at the beginning of a period of extensive dendritic remodeling (Smith & Rubel, 1979).

Late appearing GFAP-positive astrocytes may play a role in the maturation of inhibitory inputs. Organotypic slice cultures of the auditory brainstem from an age prior to the maturation of astrocytes were exposed to astrocyte-conditioned medium (ACM) from older brainstems taken at an age when GFAP-positive astrocytes were present. This treatment accelerated the formation of inhibitory inputs, whereas control cultures showed very little change in inhibitory inputs (Korn et al., 2012). These results suggest that astrocytes secrete factors needed for inhibitory synaptogenesis.

A second major role for astrocytes in chick auditory brainstem development appears to be the regulation of dendritic arbor morphology. Dendritic arbor size varies with the tonotopic location of NL neurons, whereby high frequency neurons have numerous short dendrites and low frequency neurons have fewer primary dendrites with longer branches (Smith & Rubel, 1979). This arrangement is thought to optimize the ability of NL neurons to perform computation of ITDs (Agmon-Snir et al., 1998). This gradient of dendritic arbor size emerges from a fairly uniform distribution at a relatively late stage of embryonic development, after the formation of synaptic connections and just after the emergence of GFAP-positive astrocytes. ACM derived from late brainstem astrocytes promoted maturation of these dendritic arbors in organotypic slices (Korn et al., 2011). In this study, the effects varied along the tonotopic axis, suggesting that elements that respond to astrocyte-derived cues reside in the dendrites in tonotopic gradients.

During chick auditory brainstem development, there appears to be significant communication between NM axons, NL dendrites, and the glial cells surrounding NL. We recently showed that cleaved caspase-3 is expressed in axons of the auditory pathway (Rotschafer et al., 2016). When caspase-3 was pharmacologically inhibited in the brainstem in whole embryo cultures, contralateral NM axon branches were mistargeted to dorsal regions of NL. In addition, there was disruption of both the NL cell lamination and the glial cell margin, with numerous ALDH1L1-positive astrocytes found in the normally cell-free NL neuropil region. The mechanism through which axonal caspase-3 non-cell-autonomously influences NL glial cells is not known. Entry of these glial cells into the neuropil region is also seen when the crossed fibers are experimentally severed

(Rubel et al., 1981); in this case the disruption is accompanied by rapid atrophy of ventral dendrites. Together, these experiments highlight the importance of signaling between NM axons and glia surrounding NL. They further suggest that the integrity of both the NL cell lamina and the NL glial margin relies on cues from NM axons.

Glial Cells in the Developing Mammalian Auditory Brainstem

ALDH1L1-positive astrocytes are seen in VCN and MNTB at P0 (Dinh et al., 2014) and their populations increase over the next two weeks. Another marker for astrocytes, the calcium binding protein, S100ß, is evident in VCN and MNTB by P6 (Dinh et al., 2014; Saliu et al., 2014), and the expression of GFAP is seen in these nuclei at later postnatal ages. Several studies have demonstrated the presence of astrocytes in the developing calyx of Held. At late ages, when the calyx of Held has formed, ALDH1L1 immunolabeling is associated with the encapsulating calyx around MNTB neurons (Dinh et al., 2014), and ultrastructural studies have demonstrated the interposition of astrocytes between the developing calyx and MNTB neurons (Holcomb et al., 2013). During postnatal development, astrocytic processes invade the calyx, producing numerous fenestrations in a time course that varies with tonotopic position (Ford et al. 2009). Microglia are also evident in the auditory brainstem during early postnatal development. Within MNTB, their branches are seen in close apposition with developing calyces, and their numbers peak at about two postnatal weeks in mice (Dinh et al., 2014). During the first postnatal week in mice, oligodendrocytes are present in both VCN and MNTB (Dinh et al., 2014; Kolson et al., 2016). Myelin basic protein in AVCN fibers projecting to MNTB is first expressed at P9 in the rat (Saliu et al., 2014) and P8 in the mouse (Sinclair et al., 2017). Myelin thickness continues to increase until P35, and its maturation is dependent on auditory input (Sinclair et al., 2017). Together these studies highlight the development of glial cells alongside the developing neuronal circuitry in the postnatal auditory brainstem.

Synaptic Functions of Astrocytes in the Auditory Brainstem

Astrocytes have important roles in synaptogenesis and synaptic function. Interestingly, the timing of synaptogenesis has been shown to be related to the arrival of astrocytes in the developing brain (Miller & Gauthier, 2007; Ullian et al., 2001). The involvement of astrocytes in synaptic function is captured in the concept of the "tripartite synapse," which includes close communication and apposition of the pre- and postsynaptic neurons as well as the astrocyte (Araque et al., 1999; Bosworth & Allen, 2017). Astrocytes respond to neurotransmitter release by elevating the intracellular Ca^{2+} concentration (Cornell-Bell et al., 1990; Cornell-Bell & Finkbeiner, 1991) and releasing their own chemical transmitters (Bezzi et al., 1998; Guthrie et al., 1999). Calcium increase is a necessary step for gliotransmission (Stout & Charles 2003), which results in feedback modulation of neurons and synaptic activity. This tripartite communication system enables astrocytic signals to control the timing, location, and strength of developing synapses (Allen, 2013; Ullian et al., 2001). Astrocytic molecules including thrombospondins and hevin induce silent synapses (Eroglu et al., 2009; Singh et al., 2016), while glypicans 4 and 6 prompt the formation of active synapses (Allen et al., 2012). In addition to their role in development, astrocytes regulate synaptic maturation through selective strengthening and weakening as well as refinement of neural connections (Risher et al., 2014; van Deijk et al., 2017). Astrocytes can directly phagocytose or remove synapses that have been tagged by microglia, thus contributing to synaptic pruning (Hakim et al., 2014; Tasdemir-Yilmaz & Freeman, 2014).

The involvement of astrocytes in synaptogenesis is facilitated by their location adjacent to synapses in various parts of the brain including the cerebellum, cortex, hippocampus, and brainstem (Satzler et al., 2002; Spacek, 1985; Ventura & Harris, 1999). This strategic positioning allows astrocytes to react rapidly to changes in synaptic activity. Increased synaptic activity leads to expansion of astrocytic volume, growth of astrocytic processes, followed by augmented ensheathment of synapses (Anderson et al., 1994; Genoud et al., 2006; Hawrylak et al., 1993; Jones & Greenough, 1996; Wenzel et al., 1991; Witcher et al., 2007). Astrocytic apposition to pre- and postsynaptic regions facilitates sequestering, releasing, and recycling of neurotransmitters and neuromodulators (Bardoni et al., 2010; Henneberger et al., 2010; Perea & Araque, 2007).

Like principal neurons in the MNTB, glial cells express both ionotropic and metabotropic glutamate receptors (Meguro et al., 1999; Reyes-Haro et al., 2010; Steinhauser & Gallo, 1996). These glial receptors mediate neuron-glia signaling in developing and mature animals (Steinhauser & Gallo, 1996; Vernadakis, 1996), in turn regulating neuronal maturation and synaptic plasticity as well as glial proliferation, differentiation, and gene expression (Condorelli et al., 1993; Gallo et al., 1996). Expression of different types of glutamate receptors can change throughout development and maturation, with occasional overlap. Studies in rats showed that metabotropic glutamate receptor mGluR4a is expressed in calyces of Held prior to hearing onset and expression declines thereafter (Elezgarai et al., 1999; Kandler & Friauf, 1993). The onset of hearing also appears to regulate mGluR3 localization, which shifts from the neuropil toward the cell bodies, in parallel with GFAP immunolabeling (Elezgarai et al., 2001). Taken together, these studies showed that mGluR3 expression in astrocytic processes parallels that of the mGluR4a in calyx of Held synapses and follows the same rise, peak, and decline timeline (Elezgarai et al., 1999). It is possible that astrocytic mGluR3 activates several intracellular mechanisms relevant for the development and maturation of both the neurons and the astrocytes. Additionally, it has been proposed that activation of mGluR3 could function as a way of maintaining glycogen stores for the high-energy levels required for developing and maturing CNS and, in particular, the calyx of Held (Elezgarai et al., 2001; Magistretti et al., 1993; Sorg & Magistretti, 1991).

Some literature suggests that glial transporters are left out of synaptic clefts in the calyx of Held and thus are not necessary for the control of the postsynaptic response (Renden et al., 2005). These data are further supported by the lack of glutamate-mediated uptake currents observed in astrocytes after the stimulation of presynaptic afferents. The slow inward currents in MNTB astrocytes may be due to increased extracellular potassium levels that follow neuronal activity (Reyes-Haro et al., 2010). Astrocytes in MNTB appear to signal to neurons through D-serine (Panatier et al., 2006), which acts as a co-agonist to evoke NMDA-mediated neuronal slow inward currents (Reyes-Haro et al., 2010). D-serine is only released by astrocytes (Panatier et al., 2006) and its content correlates with the distribution of NMDA receptors (Schell et al., 1995; Schell et al., 1997). These studies highlight the communication between astrocytes and the calyx of Held synapse.

In addition to neuron-glial communication via glutamate receptors, astrocytes are essential for glutamate recycling, which is imperative for the maintenance of neurotransmitter availability (Hertz et al., 1999; Laake et al., 1995; Pow & Robinson, 1994). Glutamate is released in the synaptic cleft and taken up by high-affinity excitatory amino acid transporters (Bak et al., 2006; Danbolt, 2001; Leke & Schousboe, 2016). Glutamate is then converted to glutamine by glutamine synthetase (Norenberg & Martinez-Hernandez, 1979), released from astrocytes and taken up by neurons (Chaudhry et al., 2002) that convert it back to glutamate (Kvamme et al., 2000). This glutamate-glutamine-glutamate cycle ensures a constant supply of glutamate, which is essential for fast and temporally precise high firing frequency (Hermann et al., 2007; Kopp-Scheinpflug et al., 2008) such as that which occurs between the calyx of Held and the MNTB principal neuron (Uwechue et al., 2012). The fenestrated morphology of the calyx of Held allows astroglial processes to closely appose the active sites where glutamate is released and subsequently taken up by astrocytic glutamate transporters terminating the synaptic events (Ford et al., 2009; Gegelashvili & Schousboe, 1997). Inhibition of astrocyte glutamate recycling cycle leads to altered synaptic transmission (Otis et al., 1996; Renden et al., 2005) and disrupts neuronal-glial communication pathway (Uwechue et al., 2012).

Oligodendrocytes and Control of Conduction Time

Auditory brainstem pathways are exquisitely sensitive to the timing of action potentials. In the chick auditory brainstem, coincident input in NL from ipsilateral and contralateral NM occurs for a range of interaural time delays and frequencies. However, NM and NL on each side reside in close proximity, after emerging from a common structure known as the auditory anlage (Book & Morest, 1990; Cramer et al., 2000; Harkmark, 1954). Consequently, the distance from NM to contralateral NL is much greater than the distance to ipsilateral NL. Early studies demonstrated the presence of a looped trajectory in the ipsilateral NM axon branch, and it was postulated that this circuitous pathway brought the conduction times into similar ranges (Young & Rubel, 1983). However, subsequent studies using careful reconstructions demonstrated that in fact, the contralateral axon branch is about twice the length of the ipsilateral axon branch (Seidl et al., 2014). Analysis of the internode distance (between nodes of Ranvier) and axon diameter, both of which are positively correlated with conduction velocity (Brill et al., 1977), revealed differences between the ipsilateral and contralateral NM axon branches that compensate for the disparities in length (Seidl, 2014; Seidl et al., 2014). Long projection segments of axon branches displayed longer internode distances and larger axon diameters than short projection regions. These differences suggest careful regulation of myelination at a subcellular, regional level, and further suggest close communication between axons and myelinating oligodendrocytes.

Adaptations to control conduction time are also evident in the excitatory ITD circuitry in the mammalian auditory brainstem. In gerbils, regulation of internode distance and axon diameter was similarly found to compensate for length disparities in the projection of spherical bushy cells (SBCs) in the AVCN to lateral and medial dendrites in ipsilateral and contralateral MSO, respectively (Seidl & Rubel, 2016). While the differences in axon diameter only became evident at about P20, the differences in internodal distance were already established at P10, prior to the time of hearing onset (Woolf & Ryan, 1984). Mechanisms that regulate timing in the inhibitory inputs are not known.

Auditory brainstem circuitry to detect ILDs also relies on precise timing of action potentials. LSO neurons compare excitatory input from the ipsilateral side and inhibitory input from the contralateral side. They receive excitatory input from SBCs in the ipsilateral AVCN and tonotopically matched inhibitory input from the ipsilateral MNTB, which is stimulated through the calyx of Held arising in globular bushy cells (GBCs) in contralateral AVCN. These inhibitory inputs arise in close temporal proximity, in spite of the longer distance and synaptic delay (Grothe et al., 2010). Morphometric analysis of axons and myelination in SBCs and GBCs in gerbils revealed some new insights into regulation of conduction time (Ford et al., 2015). GBCs showed larger diameter axons and greater internode distance than SBCs. However, GBCs varied according to whether they projected to low frequency, lateral regions of MNTB, or high frequency, medial regions of MNTB. Lateral GBCs had larger axon diameters and larger node of Ranvier diameters, but shorter internode length. Simulations of conduction time predict that lateral projecting GBCs conduct faster than medial GBCs, consistent with the longer path length of these axons. In addition, spatial aspects of nodes and axon diameter varied with distance from the axon termination; these were found to be optimized for fast, reliable propagation of action potentials to MTNB (Ford et al., 2015).

In the mouse trapezoid body, which includes axons projecting to MNTB, myelination, axon diameter, and conduction velocity mature after hearing onset (Sinclair et al.,

2017). While auditory input is needed for normal development of these fibers, reducing input with ear plugs in adult animals resulted in a reduction in large diameter axons and myelin thickness (Sinclair et al., 2017). This study suggests that axon and myelin specializations are regulated in an activity-dependent way throughout the lifespan.

There are several molecular pathways through which axons communicate with myelinating oligodendrocytes. They include neurotransmitters, such as glutamate, which is released from axons and taken up by glutamate receptors in oligodendrocytes (Bergles et al., 2000; Kukley et al., 2007). Additionally, the extracellular signal-regulated kinases 1 and 2 (ERK1/2) are crucial parts of the signal transduction pathway that initiates myelination during development, and sustained activation of ERK1/2 can reinstate myelination processes and increase auditory brainstem conduction velocity in adult mice (Jeffries et al., 2016). Oligodendrocyte precursor cells (OPCs) are excitable (De Biase et al., 2010) and later transition to immature pre-myelinating oligodendrocytes (pre-OLs), which attach to axons and retain excitable properties (Bakiri et al., 2011). Recent electrophysiological studies (Berret et al., 2017) demonstrated that pre-OLs in the developing rat MNTB displayed strong sodium currents, expressed $Na_v1.2$, and fired action potentials. This group further showed that a subpopulation of these cells remained through adulthood. Knockdown of $Na_v1.2$ using virally delivered RNA interference led to impaired morphological development of the pre-OLs and a reduction in myelination (Berret et al., 2017). These studies highlight the importance of ongoing neuron-oligodendrocyte communication throughout development.

Glial Cells in Auditory Brainstem Injury

Sensorineural hearing loss can result from a multitude of causes—genetics, exposure to ototoxic drugs, tumors, or other injuries—that compromise the function of hair cells in the cochlea and result in reduced neuronal input to spiral ganglion neurons (SGN). The most commonly used models of sensorineural hearing loss in animals are mechanical cochlear ablation, acoustic trauma or exposure to ototoxic drugs. All of these approaches allow for the study of degenerative and reparative mechanisms in the auditory system.

Loss of Afferent Input

Degeneration of SGNs starts with the loss of acoustic stimulation and initiates a cascade of activity-dependent changes along the auditory ascending pathway (Syka, 2002). Degenerating afferents are seen in the cochlear nucleus (CN) as early as 12–48 hours and disappear between ten days and one month after the lesion (Gentschev & Sotelo, 1973;

Morest et al., 1997). As a consequence of reduced or absent stimulation, cell atrophy has been observed in the CN (Moore, 1990; Tierney et al., 1997), as well as alterations to intracellular calcium signaling pathways (Caicedo et al., 1997; Fuentes-Santamaria et al., 2005; Lohmann & Friauf, 1996) and synaptic rearrangements (Du et al., 2012; Muly et al., 2002; Sie & Rubel, 1992). Following injury, synaptogenesis and initiation of axonal sprouting overlaps with degeneration. Recovery of synaptophysin (Benson et al., 1997) and upregulation of growth associated protein 43 (GAP-43), a marker of axonal sprouting, were observed one week after cochlear removal (Fredrich & Illing, 2010). Additionally, deafferentation caused glial proliferation and hypertrophy in the CN of a variety of animal species (Campos Torres et al., 1999; de Waele et al., 1996; Fuentes-Santamaria et al., 2012; Lurie & Durham, 2000; Lurie & Rubel, 1994; Insausti et al., 1999). It is still not entirely clear whether glial cells react to the injury as scavengers, removing the debris from degenerating axons, or whether they act to facilitate reorganization and formation of new synaptic connections and axonal sprouting, or both.

Microglia are activated early in the response to injury (Baizer et al., 2015; Colonna & Butovsky, 2017; Hanisch & Kettenmann, 2007). The microglial response leading to phagocytosis and plasticity has been studied in an experimental model of acoustic trauma. In this study, Baizer et al., (2015) exposed rats to prolonged loud sounds that resulted in the degeneration of the auditory nerve and the subsequent loss of synapses in the CN. The authors used antibodies that selectively identified resting versus activated microglia to characterize microglia in the CN and in the auditory nerve, labeled using silver stain to identify degenerating axons. While there were only minimal numbers of activated microglia in control animals, CN in experimental animals stained strongly for markers of activated microglia, and there was significant overlap between these markers and silver stained degenerating afferents at 30 days after acoustic trauma. This overlap is consistent with a phagocytic scavenging role for microglia, in which microglia act to remove dysfunctional inputs and clear the area for establishment of new synaptic connections (Kettenmann et al., 2013). Degenerating axons and activated microglia remained and showed overlapping regions at 60 days following acoustic trauma. At a six-month time point, evidence for degeneration remained, but the overlap with the activated microglial marker was reduced. At nine months after noise exposure, silver staining was still observed with an overlapping microglial region, but the microglia had shifted their marker profiles. Interestingly, many more activated microglia were observed in the adjacent brainstem (Baizer et al., 2015). These findings support the role of microglia as scavengers in response to injury. However, they do not rule out a role for microglia in plastic changes that occur during and after the time of nerve degeneration. Afferent degeneration and subsequent plasticity occur over a prolonged time course after acoustic trauma in comparison to the rapid responses after cochlear ablation, suggesting that these injury responses and recovery may be mediated by different mechanisms (Baizer et al., 2015; Morest et al., 1998).

Following bilateral cochlear ablation, a morphological transition in microglia from a quiescent surveying state to an activated amoeboid state was observed as early as 16 hours in the AVCN and PVCN (posterior VCN) in rats. The activation was characterized by an increase in cross-sectional area of microglial cells and in expression levels of the ionized calcium-binding molecule 1 (Iba-1). The activation peaked at 24 hours post-ablation, gradually declined thereafter, but remained statistically significant until 100 days later (Fuentes-Santamaria et al., 2012). In the unilateral cochlear ablation model, morphological changes in microglia, including compact cell bodies, thickened processes and decreased numbers of distal ramifications, were milder than in bilateral ablation (Janz & Illing, 2014). Microglial cells were observed in close apposition to the CN neurons after unilateral or bilateral cochlear ablations, (Fuentes-Santamaria et al., 2012). This juxtaposition may be related to a role for microglia in synaptic reorganization (Bruce-Keller, 1999; Hildebrandt et al., 2011; Muly et al., 2002) which includes synaptic stripping (Cullheim & Thams, 2007). Activated microglial processes contacted both excitatory and inhibitory synapses in deafferented ipsilateral AVCN and LSO but the cup-like structures partially surrounding the presynaptic endings favored glutamatergic synapses (Janz & Illing, 2014). This proximity is consistent with a role for microglia in a rapid response to neuronal signals following injury and possibly for facilitating axonal sprouting to reinstate synaptic homeostasis (Cullheim & Thams, 2007; Fuentes-Santamaria et al., 2012; Janz & Illing, 2014). It should be noted that microglia dynamically contact synapses in the normal course of surveying their microenvironment, and this contact lasts on the order of minutes (Wake et al., 2009). This contact enables microglia to rapidly detect and respond to any homeostatic deviations in the adult mammalian brain (Janz & Illing, 2014). The frequency and specificity of these ongoing contacts has yet to be compared in control versus experimentally lesioned animals. Such an analysis will be valuable in determining whether microglia-synapse interactions are features of the response to injury.

Microglial activation in response to auditory brainstem denervation is often accompanied by astrocytic activation (Canady & Rubel, 1992; Fuentes-Santamaria et al., 2012; Fuentes-Santamaria et al., 2013) and has been observed in rats (Campos-Torres et al., 2005; Fuentes-Santamaria et al., 2013), chickens (Lurie & Durham, 2000; Lurie & Rubel, 1994) and monkeys (Insausti et al., 1999). GFAP immunostaining peaks one week after bilateral cochlear ablation in rats (Fuentes-Santamaria et al., 2013). It appears that both glial cell types play a part in alteration and repair of auditory brainstem circuitry following cochlear damage, albeit with temporally distinct responses. Microglial transformation usually precedes astroglial changes (Fuentes-Santamaria et al., 2012; Fuentes-Santamaria et al., 2013; ; Fuentes-Santamaria et al., 2017; Janz & Illing, 2014), which may reflect their involvement in different parts of synaptic removal and reorganization. Work in other areas of the nervous system has shown that while microglial cells remove presynaptic boutons, astrocytes may facilitate the formation of new connections in areas denervated by the lesion (Cullheim & Thams, 2007; Jinno & Yamada, 2011; Reisert et al., 1984; Schiefer et al., 1999). Moreover, in cultured retinal ganglion cells, astrocyte-derived molecular signals were shown to be required for the formation of new functional synapses (Pfrieger & Barres, 1997; Ullian et al., 2001). This view is consistent with the close apposition of microglia and astrocytic processes in deafferented auditory neurons (Fuentes-Santamaria et al., 2012; Fuentes-Santamaria et al., 2013). Taken together, this evidence suggests the critical and coordinated roles of glial cells in synaptic degeneration and repair processes following the loss of afferent input.

Astrocytes have been shown to phagocytose cellular debris in the dentate gyrus and optic nerve as a response to degenerative processes (Bechmann & Nitsch, 1997; Vaughn & Pease, 1970). Numerous proteins become upregulated in response to injury, including some of the matrix metalloproteinases (MMPs). These molecules can cleave the extracellular matrix, altering the environment around neurons and allowing reinnervation to occur (Michaluk & Kaczmarek, 2007; Szklarczyk et al., 2002; Werb, 1997). MMP-9 was found to be upregulated in activated astrocytes following CN deafferentation in rats and occurred early in the degeneration phase (Fredrich et al., 2013). MMP-2 and polysialic acid, which is essential for activity-dependent plasticity (Dityatev et al., 2004; Muller et al., 1996), have been shown to be upregulated during reinnervation. Upregulation was similarly reported for ezrin, a protein that links the cell membrane with the actin cytoskeleton (Fredrich et al. 2013; Tsukita & Yonemura, 1997; Vaheri et al., 1997). Elevated expression of both MMP-9 and ezrin continued independently of the arrival of new GAP-43 positive axons in the denervated areas (Fredrich et al., 2013). GAP-43 has been known to be expressed by newly formed cholinergic collaterals that arrive from the ventral nucleus of the trapezoid body (VNTB) during the regenerative process (Fredrich et al,. 2013; Meidinger et al., 2006) and is thought of as a marker of synaptogenesis (Benowitz & Routtenberg, 1997; Grasselli et al., 2011). When VNTB was lesioned by injections of kainic acid, GAP-43 reactivity in AVCN in response to cochlear ablation was prevented, and reinnervation of the nucleus did not occur. Similarly, MMP-2 did not show its characteristic upregulation. In contrast, VNTB lesion did not affect MMP-9 and ezrin levels. It was concluded that these proteins take part in degenerative processes after injury. Astrocytes thus have multiple functions in injury and in regulation of axonal growth and synaptogenesis.

Cochlear ablation leads to effects along the auditory pathway in the CNS. The CN complex is the first auditory structure in the CNS and receives direct input from the auditory nerve. Accordingly, the CN is the first site where the pathological changes in response to the loss of auditory stimulus occur (Fuentes-Santamaria et al. 2012; Fuentes-Santamaria et al. 2013; Janz & Illing 2014). Downstream from the CN, morphological changes of microglia were present in the LSO, with a milder manifestation than that seen in the AVCN at 1 day after the cochlear ablation. By the 7th day, the changes were significant for microglial and astrocytic activation (Janz & Illing, 2014). The ripple of microglial response along the auditory pathway implies that trans-synaptic effects play a big part in response to the loss of auditory nerve input.

Activation of glial cells after an auditory insult induces the expression of various cellular mediators such as cytokines, consistent with restoration in synaptic homeostasis (Bruce-Keller, 1999; Cullheim & Thams, 2007; Hanisch & Kettenmann, 2007). However, some of these cytokines can have damaging roles and further contribute to inflammatory response (Fujioka et al., 2006; Touzani et al., 2002; Vezzani et al., 2002). It has been shown that blocking certain cytokines synthesized by microglia in the cochlea after noise exposure reduces subsequent hearing impairment in mice (Fujioka et al., 2006;

Wakabayashi et al., 2010). Interestingly, not all activity-dependent signaling molecules become upregulated and changes in expression depend on the location of the injury site. Proinflammatory cytokine IL-1β is produced and expressed by activated microglial cells in response to cellular damage (Vezzani et al., 1999; Hanisch, 2002) but does not get upregulated in the VCN after cochlear ablation. Instead, increased expression is observed in deafferented VCN neurons. The same effect is seen with insulin-growth factor 1 synthesis (Fuentes-Santamaria et al., 2013) in which expression increases after traumatic brain injury or ischemia (Hwang et al., 2004; Madathil et al., 2010; Touzani et al., 1999). Thus, not only glial cells but neurons themselves may augment the production of various activity-dependent signaling molecules in an attempt to re-establish functional connections (Fuentes-Santamaria et al., 2007).

Similar discoveries were made in a rat model of conductive hearing loss in which the tympanic membrane was punctured and the malleus and incus were removed unilaterally. This procedure disrupted the transmission of sound from the middle ear into the cochlea as evidenced by elevated auditory brainstem response (ABR) thresholds and reduction in auditory responses (Fuentes-Santamaria et al., 2014). Activation of microglia was evident one day after surgery, reached its peak by day 4 and microglia resumed their quiescent state by day 15. Surprisingly, activation of astrocytes was not detected. The neurotrophin NT-3, a neurotrophic survival factor expressed in developing and adult auditory system (Hafidi, 1999; Tierney et al., 2001), was found to be upregulated by day 4 in AVCN neurons rather than glial cells. The increased expression of NT-3 coincided with the peak of microglial activation suggesting but only few microglia and astrocytes co-localized NT-3 both in control and experimental groups (Fuentes-Santamaria et al., 2014). Several important conclusions are evident from this study. First, injury to middle ear resulting in reduced auditory input is enough to activate microglia. Second, an astrocytic response may require more severe auditory degeneration (as the one seen in cochlear ablation studies). Third, microglia may be functioning as broad responders, independent of the severity of the injury, e.g., conductive versus sensorineural hearing loss.

Demyelination

The auditory system relies on the precise and rapid neurotransmission that allows the comparison of the arrival of binaural signals on submillisecond scale (Carr et al., 2001). As noted previously, well-timed conduction is normally achieved through regulation of axon diameter and myelination and requires ongoing communication between axons and myelinating oligodendrocytes. However, in a number of neurodegenerative disorders the myelin sheath is disrupted, resulting in impaired nerve conduction and slowed conductance velocity (Kim et al., 2013b; Utzschneider et al., 1994).

Hearing loss is a common comorbid complaint in individuals with multiple sclerosis, which is associated with demyelination (Lewis et al., 2010; Noffsinger et al., 1972; Peyvandi et al., 2010). The Long Evans *shaker* (*LES*) rat is genetically predisposed to loss of myelin basic protein (MBP) and thus serves as an animal model for dysmyelination. In a study to investigate the effect of myelin loss on hearing status, ABRs were recorded in P15-P30 rats and showed increased threshold to high-frequency tone stimulation. These measurements demonstrated the loss of waves II and III in *LES* when compared to control rats and the latencies of waves I and IV were increased (Kim et al., 2013b). Waves I, II, III, and IV represent auditory response in the cochlea/AN, CN, SOC, and lateral lemniscus, respectively (Hall, 2007). Additionally, the action potential (AP) latency, measured as the time between the stimulation of the presynaptic afferent which terminates in the calyx of Held and the peak of postsynaptic AP in the MNTB neuron, was twofold longer and displayed often failures in *LES* rats (Kim et al., 2013b). The rate of failure was severely affected when firing at high frequencies (> 300 Hz) but could follow trains of APs up to 100 Hz without conduction problems (Kim et al. 2013a). The authors did not observe any difference in the pool of available neurotransmitter and no difference in the AP waveform in the stimulated MNTB neuron as well as the structure of the initial segments of MNTB neuron axons in control and *LES* rats. Taken together, these results indicate that the loss of myelin causes a defect in signal transduction in the auditory brainstem by increasing the conduction time and the rate of presynaptic failures (Kim et al., 2013b).

Myelin also contributes to ion channels clustering such as relocation of Na_v at the axon initial segment. A high density of Na_v channels at the AIS and sustained resurgent Na^+ current at axon heminodes is required for a reliable and precise AP propagation (Berret et al., 2016; Hamada & Kole, 2015). Due to the fact that dysmyelination reduces the reliability and precision of signal transduction (Kim et al., 2013a; Kim et al., 2013b), this group tested the hypothesis that myelin is essential for the final tuning of the AP at the last heminode (Berret et al., 2016). In the calyx of Held, Na_v channels form clusters at the nodes of Ranvier as well as at the last heminode, which separates the myelinated portion of the axon from the non-myelinated calyceal terminal (Leao et al., 2005). In control rats, following the AP Na^+ currents entered at the heminode first and then diffused to the terminal. In contrast, Na^+ currents in *LES* rats entered at the heminode and the terminal at the same time. The general increase of $[Na^+]_i$ was significantly higher at axon heminodes in control than in *LES* rats. However, the decay of Na^+ transient was much slower at heminodes and terminals of *LES* rats. Normally, Na_v channels are clustered in the heminode (10-20 μm away from the terminal) but in *LES* rats this cluster was much longer and invaded the calyx nerve terminal. The authors showed that it is the loss of $Na_v\beta4$ subunit at the last heminode that actually underlies the disruption of Na_v (Berret et al. 2016). Both $K_v1.2$ and $K_v3.1$ are essential for a consistent AP firing at the calyx of Held (Ishikawa et al., 2003; Johnston et al., 2010) and are located at nodes and perinodes, and at juxtaparanodes, respectively, in wild type rats. $K_v3.1$ expression was increased and dispersed at the heminode and the presynaptic calyceal terminal and $K_{v1}1.2$ expression at juxtaparanodes was completely disrupted in *LES* rats (Berret et al., 2016). The disruption of myelin thus affects not only conduction velocity, but also axonal excitability and reliability, factors that are critical for AP propagation in the auditory system.

Concluding Remarks

The auditory brainstem is a unique and specialized region of the nervous system with exceptionally high demands for synaptic precision and accurate timing. Its development is carefully orchestrated and its circuits are maintained for stable and reliable transmission of nerve impulses. We are now beginning to understand how astrocytes, microglia, and oligodendrocytes contribute to the specificity and specialized features needed for auditory brainstem function. Glial cells have been shown to guide multiple aspects of development. In the auditory brainstem astrocytes assist in the formation of appropriate synapses and in the regulation of dendritic arbors. Both astrocytes and microglia accompany the developing calyx of Held. Astrocytes contribute to auditory synaptic function, and oligodendrocytes communicate with neurons to adjust conduction times to obtain synchrony in sound localization circuits. Glial cells provide support for neural circuits and protect them from injury. In the auditory brainstem, they respond to denervation and acoustic trauma, likely contributing both to elimination of harmful elements and to adaptive generation of novel synapses.

References

Agmon-Snir, H., Carr, C. E., & Rinzel, J. (1998). The role of dendrites in auditory coincidence detection. *Nature*, *393*(6682), 268–272.

Allen, N. J. (2013). Role of glia in developmental synapse formation. *Current Opinion in Neurobiology*, *23*(6), 1027–1033.

Allen, N. J., & Eroglu, C. (2017). Cell biology of astrocyte-synapse interactions. *Neuron*, *96*(3), 697–708.

Allen, N. J., Bennett, M. L., Foo, L. C., Wang, G. X., Chakraborty, C., Smith, S. J., & Barres, B. A. (2012). Astrocyte glypicans 4 and 6 promote formation of excitatory synapses via GluA1 AMPA receptors. *Nature*, *486*(7403), 410–414.

Anderson, B. J., Li, X., Alcantara, A. A., Isaacs, K. R., Black, J. E., & Greenough, W. T. (1994). Glial hypertrophy is associated with synaptogenesis following motor-skill learning, but not with angiogenesis following exercise. *Glia*, *11*(1), 73–80.

Araque, A., Parpura, V., Sanzgiri, R. P., & Haydon, P. G. (1999). Tripartite synapses: Glia, the unacknowledged partner. *Trends in Neuroscience*, *22*(5), 208–215.

Baizer, J. S., Wong, K. M., Manohar, S., Hayes, S. H., Ding, D., Dingman, R., & Salvi, R. J. (2015). Effects of acoustic trauma on the auditory system of the rat: The role of microglia. *Neuroscience*, *303*, 299–311.

Bak, L. K., Schousboe, A., & Waagepetersen, H. S. (2006). The glutamate/GABA-glutamine cycle: Aspects of transport, neurotransmitter homeostasis and ammonia transfer. *Journal of Neurochemistry*, *98*(3), 641–653.

Bakiri, Y., Karadottir, R., Cossell, L., & Attwell, D. (2011). Morphological and electrical properties of oligodendrocytes in the white matter of the corpus callosum and cerebellum. *Journal of Physiology*, *589*(Pt 3), 559–573.

Bardoni, R., Ghirri, A., Zonta, M., Betelli, C., Vitale, G., Ruggieri, V., Sandrini, M., & Carmignoto, G. (2010). Glutamate-mediated astrocyte-to-neuron signalling in the rat dorsal horn. *Journal of Physiology*, *588*(Pt 5), 831–846.

Bechmann, I., & Nitsch, R. (1997). Astrocytes and microglial cells incorporate degenerating fibers following entorhinal lesion: A light, confocal, and electron microscopical study using a phagocytosis-dependent labeling technique. *Glia*, *20*(2), 145–154.

Benowitz, L. I., & Routtenberg, A. (1997). GAP-43: An intrinsic determinant of neuronal development and plasticity. *Trends in Neuroscience*, *20*(2), 84–91.

Benson, C. G., Gross, J. S., Suneja, S. K., & Potashner, S. J. (1997). Synaptophysin immunoreactivity in the cochlear nucleus after unilateral cochlear or ossicular removal. *Synapse*, *25*(3), 243–257.

Bergles, D. E., Roberts, J. D., Somogyi, P., & Jahr, C. E. (2000). Glutamatergic synapses on oligodendrocyte precursor cells in the hippocampus. *Nature*, *405*(6783), 187–191.

Berret, E., Kim, S. E., Lee, S. Y., Kushmerick, C., & Kim, J. H. (2016). Functional and structural properties of ion channels at the nerve terminal depends on compact myelin. *Journal of Physiology*, *594*(19), 5593–5609.

Berret, E., Barron, T., Xu, J., Debner, E., Kim, E. J., & Kim, J. H. (2017). Oligodendroglial excitability mediated by glutamatergic inputs and Nav1.2 activation. *Nature Communications*, *8*(1), 557.

Bezzi, P., Carmignoto, G., Pasti, L., Vesce, S., Rossi, D., Rizzini, B. L., Pozzan, T., & Volterra, A. (1998). Prostaglandins stimulate calcium-dependent glutamate release in astrocytes. *Nature*, *391*(6664), 281–285.

Book, K. J., & Morest, D. K. (1990). Migration of neuroblasts by perikaryal translocation: Role of cellular elongation and axonal outgrowth in the acoustic nuclei of the chick embryo medulla. *Journal of Comparative Neurology*, *297*(1), 55–76.

Bosworth, A. P., & Allen, N. J. (2017). The diverse actions of astrocytes during synaptic development. *Current Opinion in Neurobiology*, *47*, 38–43.

Brand, A., Behrend, O., Marquardt, T., McAlpine, D., & Grothe, B. (2002). Precise inhibition is essential for microsecond interaural time difference coding. *Nature*, *417*(6888), 543–547.

Brill, M. H., Waxman, S. G., Moore, J. W., & Joyner, R. W. (1977). Conduction velocity and spike configuration in myelinated fibres: Computed dependence on internode distance. *Journal of Neurology, Neurosurgery, and Psychiatry*, *40*(8), 769–774.

Bruce-Keller, A. J. (1999). Microglial-neuronal interactions in synaptic damage and recovery. *Journal of Neuroscience Research*, *58*(1), 191–201.

Burger, R. M., Fukui, I., Ohmori, H., & Rubel, E. W. (2011). Inhibition in the balance: Binaurally coupled inhibitory feedback in sound localization circuitry. *Journal of Neurophysiology*, *106*(1), 4–14.

Cahoy, J. D., Emery, B., Kaushal, A., Foo, L. C., Zamanian, J. L., Christopherson, K. S., . . . Barres, B. A. (2008). A transcriptome database for astrocytes, neurons, and oligodendrocytes: A new resource for understanding brain development and function. [Research Support, N.I.H., Extramural Research Support, Non-U.S. Gov't]. *The Journal of Neuroscience: The Official Journal of the Society for Neuroscience*, *28*(1), 264–278.

Caicedo, A., d'Aldin, C., Eybalin, M., & Puel, J. L. (1997). Temporary sensory deprivation changes calcium-binding proteins levels in the auditory brainstem. *Journal of Comparative Neurology*, *378*(1), 1–15.

Campos Torres, A., Vidal, P. P., & de Waele, C. (1999). Evidence for a microglial reaction within the vestibular and cochlear nuclei following inner ear lesion in the rat. *Neuroscience, 92*(4), 1475–1490.

Campos-Torres, A., Touret, M., Vidal, P. P., Barnum, S., & de Waele, C. (2005). The differential response of astrocytes within the vestibular and cochlear nuclei following unilateral labyrinthectomy or vestibular afferent activity blockade by transtympanic tetrodotoxin injection in the rat. *Neuroscience, 130*(4), 853–865.

Canady, K. S., & Rubel, E. W. (1992). Rapid and reversible astrocytic reaction to afferent activity blockade in chick cochlear nucleus. *Journal of Neuroscience, 12*(3), 1001–1009.

Carr, C. E., Soares, D., Parameshwaran, S., & Perney, T. (2001). Evolution and development of time coding systems. *Current Opinion in Neurobiology, 11*(6), 727–733.

Chaudhry, F. A., Reimer, R. J., & Edwards, R. H. (2002). The glutamine commute: Take the N line and transfer to the A. *Journal of Cell Biology, 157*(3), 349–355.

Chung, W. S., Allen, N. J., & Eroglu, C. (2015). Astrocytes control synapse formation, function, and elimination. *Cold Spring Harbor Perspectives in Biology, 7*(9), a020370.

Colonna, M., & Butovsky, O. (2017). Microglia function in the central nervous system during health and neurodegeneration. *Annual Review of Immunology,*35, 441–468.

Condorelli, D. F., Dell'Albani, P., Amico, C., Kaczmarek, L., Nicoletti, F., Lukasiuk, K., & Stella, A. M. (1993). Induction of primary response genes by excitatory amino acid receptor agonists in primary astroglial cultures. *Journal of Neurochemistry, 60*(3), 877–885.

Cornell-Bell, A. H., & Finkbeiner, S. M. (1991). Ca^{2+} waves in astrocytes. *Cell Calcium, 12*(2–3), 185–204.

Cornell-Bell, A. H., Finkbeiner, S. M., Cooper, M. S., & Smith, S. J. (1990). Glutamate induces calcium waves in cultured astrocytes: Long-range glial signaling. *Science, 247*(4941), 470–473.

Cramer, K. S., Fraser, S. E., & Rubel, E. W. (2000). Embryonic origins of auditory brain-stem nuclei in the chick hindbrain. *Developmental Biology, 224*(2), 138–151.

Cullheim, S., & Thams, S. (2007). The microglial networks of the brain and their role in neuronal network plasticity after lesion. *Brain Research Review, 55*(1), 89–96.

Danbolt, N. C. (2001). Glutamate uptake. *Progress in Neurobiology, 65*(1), 1–105.

De Biase, L. M., Nishiyama, A., & Bergles, D. E. (2010). Excitability and synaptic communication within the oligodendrocyte lineage. *Journal of Neuroscience, 30*(10), 3600–3611.

de Waele, C., Campos Torres, A., Josset, P., & Vidal, P. P. (1996). Evidence for reactive astrocytes in rat vestibular and cochlear nuclei following unilateral inner ear lesion. *European Journal of Neuroscience, 8*(9), 2006–2018.

Dimou, L., & Simons, M. (2017). Diversity of oligodendrocytes and their progenitors. *Current Opinion in Neurobiology, 47*, 73–79.

Dinh, M. L., Koppel, S. J., Korn, M. J., & Cramer, K. S. (2014). Distribution of glial cells in the auditory brainstem: Normal development and effects of unilateral lesion. [Research Support, N.I.H., Extramural]. *Neuroscience, 278*, 237–252.

Dityatev, A., Dityateva, G., Sytnyk, V., Delling, M., Toni, N., Nikonenko, I., Muller, D., & Schachner, M. (2004). Polysialylated neural cell adhesion molecule promotes remodeling and formation of hippocampal synapses. *Journal of Neuroscience, 24*(42), 9372–9382.

Du, X., Chen, K., Choi, C. H., Li, W., Cheng, W., Stewart, C., . . . Kopke, R. D. (2012). Selective degeneration of synapses in the dorsal cochlear nucleus of chinchilla following acoustic trauma and effects of antioxidant treatment. *Hearing Research, 283*(1–2), 1–13.

Elezgarai, I., Bilbao, A., Mateos, J. M., Azkue, J. J., Benitez, R., Osorio, A., . . . Grandes, P. (2001). Group II metabotropic glutamate receptors are differentially expressed in the medial nucleus of the trapezoid body in the developing and adult rat. *Neuroscience, 104*(2), 487–498.

Elezgarai, I., Benitez, R., Mateos, J. M., Lazaro, E., Osorio, A., Azkue, J. J., . . . Grandes, P. (1999). Developmental expression of the group III metabotropic glutamate receptor mGluR4a in the medial nucleus of the trapezoid body of the rat. *Journal of Comparative Neurology, 411*(3), 431–440.

Eroglu, C., Allen, N. J., Susman, M. W., O'Rourke, N. A., Park, C. Y., Ozkan, E., . . . Barres, B. A. (2009). Gabapentin receptor alpha2delta-1 is a neuronal thrombospondin receptor responsible for excitatory CNS synaptogenesis. *Cell, 139*(2), 380–392.

Farmer, W. T., & Murai, K. (2017). Resolving astrocyte heterogeneity in the CNS. *Frontiers in Cellular Neuroscience, 11*, 300.

Ford, M. C., Grothe, B., & Klug, A. (2009). Fenestration of the calyx of Held occurs sequentially along the tonotopic axis, is influenced by afferent activity, and facilitates glutamate clearance. *Journal of Comparative Neurology, 514*(1), 92–106.

Ford, M. C., Alexandrova, O., Cossell, L., Stange-Marten, A., Sinclair, J., Kopp-Scheinpflug, C., . . . Grothe, B. (2015). Tuning of Ranvier node and internode properties in myelinated axons to adjust action potential timing. *Nature Communications, 6*, 8073.

Fredrich, M., & Illing, R. B. (2010). MMP-2 is involved in synaptic remodeling after cochlear lesion. *Neuroreport, 21*(5), 324–327.

Fredrich, M., Zeber, A. C., Hildebrandt, H., & Illing, R. B. (2013). Differential molecular profiles of astrocytes in degeneration and re-innervation after sensory deafferentation of the adult rat cochlear nucleus. *European Journal of Neuroscience, 38*(1), 2041–2056.

Fuentes-Santamaria, V., Alvarado, J. C., & Juiz, J. M. (2012). Long-term interaction between microglial cells and cochlear nucleus neurons after bilateral cochlear ablation. *Journal of Comparative Neurology, 520*(13), 2974–2990.

Fuentes-Santamaria, V., Alvarado, J. C., Henkel, C. K., & Brunso-Bechtold, J. K. (2007). Cochlear ablation in adult ferrets results in changes in insulin-like growth factor-1 and synaptophysin immunostaining in the cochlear nucleus. *Neuroscience, 148*(4), 1033–1047.

Fuentes-Santamaria, V., Alvarado, J. C., Gabaldon-Ull, M. C., & Manuel Juiz, J. (2013). Upregulation of insulin-like growth factor and interleukin 1beta occurs in neurons but not in glial cells in the cochlear nucleus following cochlear ablation. *Journal of Comparative Neurology, 521*(15), 3478–3499.

Fuentes-Santamaria, V., Alvarado, J. C., Taylor, A. R., Brunso-Bechtold, J. K., & Henkel, C. K. (2005). Quantitative changes in calretinin immunostaining in the cochlear nuclei after unilateral cochlear removal in young ferrets. *Journal of Comparative Neurology, 483*(4), 458–475.

Fuentes-Santamaria, V., Alvarado, J. C., Lopez-Munoz, D. F., Melgar-Rojas, P., Gabaldon-Ull, M. C., & Juiz, J. M. (2014). Glia-related mechanisms in the anteroventral cochlear nucleus of the adult rat in response to unilateral conductive hearing loss. *Frontiers in Neuroscience, 8*, 319.

Fuentes-Santamaria, V., Alvarado, J. C., Melgar-Rojas, P., Gabaldon-Ull, M. C., Miller, J. M., & Juiz, J. M. (2017). The role of glia in the peripheral and central auditory system following noise overexposure: Contribution of TNF-alpha and IL-1beta to the pathogenesis of hearing loss. *Frontiers in Neuroanatomy, 11*, 9.

Fujioka, M., Kanzaki, S., Okano, H. J., Masuda, M., Ogawa, K., & Okano, H. (2006). Proinflammatory cytokines expression in noise-induced damaged cochlea. *Journal of Neuroscience Research, 83*(4), 575–583.

Gallo, V., Zhou, J. M., McBain, C. J., Wright, P., Knutson, P. L., & Armstrong, R. C. (1996). Oligodendrocyte progenitor cell proliferation and lineage progression are regulated by glutamate receptor-mediated K+ channel block. *Journal of Neuroscience, 16*(8), 2659–2670.

Gegelashvili, G., & Schousboe, A. (1997). High affinity glutamate transporters: Regulation of expression and activity. *Molecular Pharmacology, 52*(1), 6–15.

Genoud, C., Quairiaux, C., Steiner, P., Hirling, H., Welker, E., & Knott, G. W. (2006). Plasticity of astrocytic coverage and glutamate transporter expression in adult mouse cortex. *PLoS Biology, 4*(11), e343.

Gentschev, T., & Sotelo, C. (1973). Degenerative patterns in the ventral cochlear nucleus of the rat after primary deafferentation. An ultra-structural study. *Brain Research, 62*(1), 37–60.

Glendenning, K. K., Baker, B. N., Hutson, K. A., & Masterton, R. B. (1992). Acoustic chiasm V: inhibition and excitation in the ipsilateral and contralateral projections of LSO. *Journal of Comparative Neurology, 319*(1), 100–122.

Gomez-Nicola, D., & Perry, V. H. (2015). Microglial dynamics and role in the healthy and diseased brain: A paradigm of functional plasticity. *Neuroscientist, 21*(2), 169–184.

Grabert, K., Michoel, T., Karavolos, M. H., Clohisey, S., Baillie, J. K., Stevens, . . . McColl, B. W. (2016). Microglial brain region-dependent diversity and selective regional sensitivities to aging. *Nature Neuroscience, 19*(3), 504–516.

Grasselli, G., Mandolesi, G., Strata, P., & Cesare, P. (2011). Impaired sprouting and axonal atrophy in cerebellar climbing fibres following in vivo silencing of the growth-associated protein GAP-43. *PLoS ONE, 6*(6), e20791.

Grothe, B. (2003). New roles for synaptic inhibition in sound localization. *Nature Review Neuroscience, 4*(7), 540–550.

Grothe, B., Pecka, M., & McAlpine, D. (2010). Mechanisms of sound localization in mammals. *Physiology Reviews, 90*(3), 983–1012.

Guthrie, P. B., Knappenberger, J., Segal, M., Bennett, M. V., Charles, A. C., & Kater, S. B. (1999). ATP released from astrocytes mediates glial calcium waves. *Journal of Neuroscience, 19*(2), 520–528.

Hackett, J. T., Jackson, H., & Rubel, E. W. (1982). Synaptic excitation of the second and third order auditory neurons in the avian brain stem. *Neuroscience, 7*(6), 1455–1469.

Hafidi, A. (1999). Distribution of BDNF, NT-3 and NT-4 in the developing auditory brainstem. *International Journal of Developmental Neuroscience, 17*(4), 285–294.

Hakim, Y., Yaniv, S. P., & Schuldiner, O. (2014). Astrocytes play a key role in Drosophila mushroom body axon pruning. *PLoS ONE, 9*(1), e86178.

Hall, J. W. (2007). *New Handbook of Auditory Evoked Responses*. Boston, MA: Pearson.

Hamada, M. S., & Kole, M. H. (2015). Myelin loss and axonal ion channel adaptations associated with gray matter neuronal hyperexcitability. *Journal of Neuroscience, 35*(18), 7272–7286.

Hanisch, U. K. (2002). Microglia as a source and target of cytokines. *Glia, 40*(2), 140–155.

Hanisch, U. K., & Kettenmann, H. (2007). Microglia: Active sensor and versatile effector cells in the normal and pathologic brain. *Nature Neuroscience, 10*(11), 1387–1394.

Harkmark, W. (1954). Cell migrations from the rhombic lip to the inferior olive, the nucleus raphe and the pons; a morphological and experimental investigation on chick embryos. *Journal of Comparative Neurology, 100*(1), 115–209.

Hawrylak, N., Chang, F. L., & Greenough, W. T. (1993). Astrocytic and synaptic response to kindling in hippocampal subfield CA1. II. Synaptogenesis and astrocytic process increases to in vivo kindling. *Brain Research, 603*(2), 309–316.

Held, H. (1893). Die zentrale Gehörleitung. *Archiv für Anatomie, Physiologie und Anatomie, 17*, 201–248.

Henneberger, C., Papouin, T., Oliet, S. H., & Rusakov, D. A. (2010). Long-term potentiation depends on release of D-serine from astrocytes. *Nature, 463*(7278), 232–236.

Hermann, J., Pecka, M., von Gersdorff, H., Grothe, B., & Klug, A. (2007). Synaptic transmission at the calyx of Held under in vivo like activity levels. *J Neurophysiology, 98*(2), 807–820.

Hertz, L., Dringen, R., Schousboe, A., & Robinson, S. R. (1999). Astrocytes: Glutamate producers for neurons. *Journal of Neuroscience Research, 57*(4), 417–428.

Hildebrandt, H., Hoffmann, N. A., & Illing, R. B. (2011). Synaptic reorganization in the adult rat's ventral cochlear nucleus following its total sensory deafferentation. *PLoS ONE, 6*(8), e23686.

Holcomb, P. S., Hoffpauir, B. K., Hoyson, M. C., Jackson, D. R., Deerinck, T. J., Marrs, G. S., . . . Spirou, G. A. (2013). Synaptic inputs compete during rapid formation of the calyx of Held: A new model system for neural development. [In Vitro Research Support, N.I.H., Extramural]. *Journal of Neuroscience, 33*(32), 12954–12969.

Hwang, I. K., Yoo, K. Y., Park, S. K., An, S. J., Lee, J. Y., Choi, S. Y., . . . Won, M. H. (2004). Expression and changes of endogenous insulin-like growth factor-1 in neurons and glia in the gerbil hippocampus and dentate gyrus after ischemic insult. *Neurochemistry International, 45*(1), 149–156.

Hyson, R. L. (2005). The analysis of interaural time differences in the chick brain stem. *Physiology Behavior, 86*(3), 297–305.

Insausti, A. M., Cruz-Orive, L. M., Jauregui, I., Manrique, M., & Insausti, R. (1999). Stereological assessment of the glial reaction to chronic deafferentation of the cochlear nuclei in the macaque monkey (Macaca fascicularis). *Journal of Comparative Neurology, 414*(4), 485–494.

Ishikawa, T., Nakamura, Y., Saitoh, N., Li, W. B., Iwasaki, S., & Takahashi, T. (2003). Distinct roles of Kv1 and Kv3 potassium channels at the calyx of Held presynaptic terminal. *Journal of Neuroscience, 23*(32), 10445–10453.

Janz, P., & Illing, R. B. (2014). A role for microglial cells in reshaping neuronal circuitry of the adult rat auditory brainstem after its sensory deafferentation. *Journal of Neuroscience Research, 92*(4), 432–445.

Jeffries, M. A., Urbanek, K., Torres, L., Wendell, S. G., Rubio, M. E., & Fyffe-Maricich, S. L. (2016). ERK1/2 Activation in preexisting oligodendrocytes of adult mice drives new myelin synthesis and enhanced CNS function. *Journal of Neuroscience, 36*(35), 9186–9200.

Jinno, S., & Yamada, J. (2011). Using comparative anatomy in the axotomy model to identify distinct roles for microglia and astrocytes in synaptic stripping. *Neuron Glia Biology, 7*(1), 55–66.

Johnston, J., Forsythe, I. D., & Kopp-Scheinpflug, C. (2010). Going native: Voltage-gated potassium channels controlling neuronal excitability. *Journal of Physiology, 588*(Pt 17), 3187–3200.

Jones, T. A., & Greenough, W. T. (1996). Ultrastructural evidence for increased contact between astrocytes and synapses in rats reared in a complex environment. *Neurobiology of Learning and Memory, 65*(1), 48–56.

Kandler, K., & Friauf, E. (1993). Pre- and postnatal development of efferent connections of the cochlear nucleus in the rat. *Journal of Comparative Neurology, 328*(2), 161–184.

Kandler, K., & Gillespie, D. C. (2005). Developmental refinement of inhibitory sound-localization circuits. *Trends in Neuroscience, 28*(6), 290–296.

Kettenmann, H., Kirchhoff, F., & Verkhratsky, A. (2013). Microglia: New roles for the synaptic stripper. *Neuron, 77*(1), 10–18.

Kim, J. H., Renden, R., & von Gersdorff, H. (2013a). Dysmyelination of auditory afferent axons increases the jitter of action potential timing during high-frequency firing. *Journal of Neuroscience, 33*(22), 9402–9407.

Kim, S. E., Turkington, K., Kushmerick, C., & Kim, J. H. (2013b). Central dysmyelination reduces the temporal fidelity of synaptic transmission and the reliability of postsynaptic firing during high-frequency stimulation. *Journal of Neurophysiology, 110*(7), 1621–1630.

Kolson, D. R., Wan, J., Wu, J., Dehoff, M., Brandebura, A. N., Qian, J., . . . Spirou, G. A. (2016). Temporal patterns of gene expression during calyx of Held development. *Developmental Neurobiology*, 76, 166–189.

Kopp-Scheinpflug, C., Tolnai, S., Malmierca, M. S., & Rubsamen, R. (2008). The medial nucleus of the trapezoid body: comparative physiology. *Neuroscience, 154*(1), 160–170.

Koppl, C., & Carr, C. E. (2008). Maps of interaural time difference in the chicken's brainstem nucleus laminaris. *Biological Cybernetics, 98*(6), 541–559.

Korn, M. J., & Cramer, K. S. (2008). Distribution of glial-associated proteins in the developing chick auditory brainstem. *Developmental Neurobiology, 68*(8), 1093–1106.

Korn, M. J., Koppel, S. J., & Cramer, K. S. (2011). Astrocyte-secreted factors modulate a gradient of primary dendritic arbors in nucleus laminaris of the avian auditory brainstem. [Research Support, N.I.H., Extramural Research Support, U.S. Gov't, Non-P.H.S.]. *PLoS ONE, 6*(11), e27383.

Korn, M. J., Koppel, S. J., Li, L. H., Mehta, D., Mehta, S. B., Seidl, A. H., & Cramer, K. S. (2012). Astrocyte-secreted factors modulate the developmental distribution of inhibitory synapses in nucleus laminaris of the avian auditory brainstem. [Research Support, N.I.H., Extramural Research Support, U.S. Gov't, Non-P.H.S.]. *Journal of Comparative Neurology, 520*(6), 1262–1277.

Kukley, M., Capetillo-Zarate, E., & Dietrich, D. (2007). Vesicular glutamate release from axons in white matter. *Nature Neuroscience, 10*(3), 311–320.

Kuwabara, N., & Zook, J. M. (1992). Projections to the medial superior olive from the medial and lateral nuclei of the trapezoid body in rodents and bats. *Journal of Comparative Neurology, 324*(4), 522–538.

Kvamme, E., Roberg, B., & Torgner, I. A. (2000). Phosphate-activated glutaminase and mitochondrial glutamine transport in the brain. *Neurochemistry Research, 25*(9–10), 1407–1419.

Laake, J. H., Slyngstad, T. A., Haug, F. M., & Ottersen, O. P. (1995). Glutamine from glial cells is essential for the maintenance of the nerve terminal pool of glutamate: Immunogold evidence from hippocampal slice cultures. *Journal of Neurochemistry, 65*(2), 871–881.

Lachica, E. A., Rubsamen, R., & Rubel, E. W. (1994). GABAergic terminals in nucleus magnocellularis and laminaris originate from the superior olivary nucleus. *Journal of Comparative Neurology, 348*(3), 403–418.

Leao, R. M., Kushmerick, C., Pinaud, R., Renden, R., Li, G. L., Taschenberger, H., . . . von Gersdorff, H. (2005). Presynaptic Na^+ channels: locus, development, and recovery from inactivation at a high-fidelity synapse. *Journal of Neuroscience, 25*(14), 3724–3738.

Leke, R., & Schousboe, A. (2016). The glutamine transporters and their role in the glutamate/GABA-glutamine cycle. *Advances in Neurobiology, 13*, 223–257.

Lewis, M. S., Lilly, D. J., Hutter, M. M., Bourdette, D. N., McMillan, G. P., Fitzpatrick, M. A., & Fausti, S. A. (2010). Audiometric hearing status of individuals with and without multiple sclerosis. *Journal of Rehabilitation Research and Development, 47*(7), 669–678.

Lohmann, C., & Friauf, E. (1996). Distribution of the calcium-binding proteins parvalbumin and calretinin in the auditory brainstem of adult and developing rats. *Journal of Comparative Neurology, 367*(1), 90–109.

Lurie, D. I., & Rubel, E. W. (1994). Astrocyte proliferation in the chick auditory brainstem following cochlea removal. *Journal of Comparative Neurology, 346*(2), 276–288.

Lurie, D. I., & Durham, D. (2000). Neuronal death, not axonal degeneration, results in significant gliosis within the cochlear nucleus of adult chickens. *Hearing Research, 149*(1–2), 178–188.

Madathil, S. K., Evans, H. N., & Saatman, K. E. (2010). Temporal and regional changes in IGF-1/IGF-1R signaling in the mouse brain after traumatic brain injury. *Journal of Neurotrauma, 27*(1), 95–107.

Magistretti, P. J., Sorg, O., Yu, N., Martin, J. L., & Pellerin, L. (1993). Neurotransmitters regulate energy metabolism in astrocytes: implications for the metabolic trafficking between neural cells. *Developmental Neuroscience, 15*(3–5), 306–312.

Meguro, R., Ohishi, H., Hoshino, K., Hicks, T. P., & Norita, M. (1999). Metabotropic glutamate receptor 2/3 immunoreactivity in the developing rat cerebellar cortex. *Journal of Comparative Neurology, 410*(2), 243–255.

Meidinger, M. A., Hildebrandt-Schoenfeld, H., & Illing, R. B. (2006). Cochlear damage induces GAP-43 expression in cholinergic synapses of the cochlear nucleus in the adult rat: a light and electron microscopic study. *European Journal of Neuroscience, 23*(12), 3187–3199.

Michaluk, P., & Kaczmarek, L. (2007). Matrix metalloproteinase-9 in glutamate-dependent adult brain function and dysfunction. *Cell Death and Differentiation, 14*(7), 1255–1258.

Micu, I., Plemel, J. R., Caprariello, A. V., Nave, K. A., & Stys, P. K. (2017). Axo-myelinic neurotransmission: A novel mode of cell signalling in the central nervous system. *Nature Review Neuroscience.*

Miller, F. D., & Gauthier, A. S. (2007). Timing is everything: Making neurons versus glia in the developing cortex. *Neuron, 54*(3), 357–369.

Moore, D. R. (1990). Auditory brainstem of the ferret: Early cessation of developmental sensitivity of neurons in the cochlear nucleus to removal of the cochlea. *Journal of Comparative Neurology, 302*(4), 810–823.

Morest, D. K., Kim, J., & Bohne, B. A. (1997). Neuronal and transneuronal degeneration of auditory axons in the brainstem after cochlear lesions in the chinchilla: Cochleotopic and non-cochleotopic patterns. *Hearing Research, 103*(1–2), 151–168.

Morest, D. K., Kim, J., Potashner, S. J., & Bohne, B. A. (1998). Long-term degeneration in the cochlear nerve and cochlear nucleus of the adult chinchilla following acoustic overstimulation. *Microscopy Research and Technique, 41*(3), 205–216.

Mosser, C. A., Baptista, S., Arnoux, I., & Audinat, E. (2017). Microglia in CNS development: Shaping the brain for the future. *Progress in Neurobiology, 149–150*, 1–20.

Muller, D., Wang, C., Skibo, G., Toni, N., Cremer, H., Calaora, V., . . . Kiss, J. Z. (1996). PSA-NCAM is required for activity-induced synaptic plasticity. *Neuron, 17*(3), 413–422.

Muly, S. M., Gross, J. S., Morest, D. K., & Potashner, S. J. (2002). Synaptophysin in the cochlear nucleus following acoustic trauma. *Experimental Neurology, 177*(1), 202–221.

Myoga, M. H., Lehnert, S., Leibold, C., Felmy, F., & Grothe, B. (2014). Glycinergic inhibition tunes coincidence detection in the auditory brainstem. *Nature Communications, 5*, 3790.

Nakamura, P. A., & Cramer, K. S. (2011). Formation and maturation of the calyx of Held. [Research Support, N.I.H., Extramural Research Support, U.S. Gov't, Non-P.H.S. Review]. *Hearing Research, 276*(1–2), 70–78.

Noffsinger, D., Olsen, W. O., Carhart, R., Hart, C. W., & Sahgal, V. (1972). Auditory and vestibular aberrations in multiple sclerosis. *Acta Otolaryngologica Supplement, 303*, 1–63.

Norenberg, M. D., & Martinez-Hernandez, A. (1979). Fine structural localization of glutamine synthetase in astrocytes of rat brain. *Brain Research, 161*(2), 303–310.

Ohmori, H. (2014). Neuronal specializations for the processing of interaural difference cues in the chick. *Frontiers in Neural Circuits, 8*, 47.

Otis, T. S., Wu, Y. C., & Trussell, L. O. (1996). Delayed clearance of transmitter and the role of glutamate transporters at synapses with multiple release sites. *Journal of Neuroscience, 16*(5), 1634–1644.

Overholt, E. M., Rubel, E. W., & Hyson, R. L. (1992). A circuit for coding interaural time differences in the chick brainstem. *Journal Neuroscience, 12*(5), 1698–1708.

Panatier, A., Theodosis, D. T., Mothet, J. P., Touquet, B., Pollegioni, L., Poulain, D. A., & Oliet, S. H. (2006). Glia-derived D-serine controls NMDA receptor activity and synaptic memory. *Cell, 125*(4), 775–784.

Parks, T. N., & Rubel, E. W. (1975). Organization and development of brain stem auditory nuclei of the chicken: Organization of projections from n. magnocellularis to n. laminaris. *Journal of Comparative Neurology, 164*(4), 435–448.

Pecka, M., Brand, A., Behrend, O., & Grothe, B. (2008). Interaural time difference processing in the mammalian medial superior olive: The role of glycinergic inhibition. *Journal Neuroscience, 28*(27), 6914–6925.

Perea, G., & Araque, A. (2007). Astrocytes potentiate transmitter release at single hippocampal synapses. *Science, 317*(5841), 1083–1086.

Perea, G., Sur, M., & Araque, A. (2014). Neuron-glia networks: Integral gear of brain function. *Frontiers in Cellular Neuroscience, 8*, 378.

Peyvandi, A., Naghibzadeh, B., & Ahmady Roozbahany, N. (2010). Neuro-otologic manifestations of multiple sclerosis. *Archives of Iranian Medicine, 13*(3), 188–192.

Pfrieger, F. W., & Barres, B. A. (1997). Synaptic efficacy enhanced by glial cells in vitro. *Science, 277*(5332), 1684–1687.

Pow, D. V., & Robinson, S. R. (1994). Glutamate in some retinal neurons is derived solely from glia. *Neuroscience, 60*(2), 355–366.

Reisert, I., Wildemann, G., Grab, D., & Pilgrim, C. (1984). The glial reaction in the course of axon regeneration: A stereological study of the rat hypoglossal nucleus. *Journal of Comparative Neurology, 229*(1), 121–128.

Renden, R., Taschenberger, H., Puente, N., Rusakov, D. A., Duvoisin, R., Wang, L. Y., . . . von Gersdorff, H. (2005). Glutamate transporter studies reveal the pruning of metabotropic glutamate receptors and absence of AMPA receptor desensitization at mature calyx of Held synapses. *Journal of Neuroscience, 25*(37), 8482–8497.

Reyes-Haro, D., Muller, J., Boresch, M., Pivneva, T., Benedetti, B., Scheller, A., . . . Kettenmann, H. (2010). Neuron-astrocyte interactions in the medial nucleus of the trapezoid body. *Journal of General Physiology, 135*(6), 583–594.

Risher, W. C., Patel, S., Kim, I. H., Uezu, A., Bhagat, S., Wilton, D. K., . . . Eroglu, C. (2014). Astrocytes refine cortical connectivity at dendritic spines. *eLife, 17*, 3.

Rotschafer, S. E., Allen-Sharpley, M. R., & Cramer, K. S. (2016). Axonal cleaved Caspase-3 regulates axon targeting and morphogenesis in the developing auditory brainstem. *Frontiers in Neural Circuits, 10*, 84.

Rubel, E. W., & Fritzsch, B. (2002). Auditory system development: primary auditory neurons and their targets. *Annual Review of Neuroscience, 25*, 51–101.

Rubel, E. W., Smith, Z. D., & Steward, O. (1981). Sprouting in the avian brainstem auditory pathway: Dependence on dendritic integrity. *Journal of Comparative Neurology, 202*(3), 397–414.

Saliu, A., Adise, S., Xian, S., Kudelska, K., & Rodriguez-Contreras, A. (2014). Natural and lesion-induced decrease in cell proliferation in the medial nucleus of the trapezoid body during hearing development. [Research Support, N.I.H., Extramural Research Support, Non-U.S. Gov't]. *Journal of Comparative Neurology, 522*(5), 971–985.

Sanes, D. H. (1990). An in vitro analysis of sound localization mechanisms in the gerbil lateral superior olive. *Journal of Neuroscience, 10*(11), 3494–3506.

Satzler, K., Sohl, L. F., Bollmann, J. H., Borst, J. G., Frotscher, M., Sakmann, B., & Lubke, J. H. (2002). Three-dimensional reconstruction of a calyx of Held and its postsynaptic principal neuron in the medial nucleus of the trapezoid body. *Journal of Neuroscience, 22*(24), 10567–10579.

Schell, M. J., Molliver, M. E., & Snyder, S. H. (1995). D-serine, an endogenous synaptic modulator: Localization to astrocytes and glutamate-stimulated release. *Proceedings of the National Academy of Sciences USA, 92*(9), 3948–3952.

Schell, M. J., Brady, R. O., Jr., Molliver, M. E., & Snyder, S. H. (1997). D-serine as a neuromodulator: Regional and developmental localizations in rat brain glia resemble NMDA receptors. *Journal of Neurosciences, 17*(5), 1604–1615.

Schiefer, J., Kampe, K., Dodt, H. U., Zieglgansberger, W., & Kreutzberg, G. W. (1999). Microglial motility in the rat facial nucleus following peripheral axotomy. *Journal of Neurocytology, 28*(6), 439–453.

Seidl, A. H. (2014). Regulation of conduction time along axons. *Neuroscience, 276*, 126–134.

Seidl, A. H., & Rubel, E. W. (2016). Systematic and differential myelination of axon collaterals in the mammalian auditory brainstem. *Glia, 64*(4), 487–494.

Seidl, A. H., Rubel, E. W., & Barria, A. (2014). Differential conduction velocity regulation in ipsilateral and contralateral collaterals innervating brainstem coincidence detector neurons. *Journal of Neuroscience, 34*(14), 4914–4919.

Sie, K. C., & Rubel, E. W. (1992). Rapid changes in protein synthesis and cell size in the cochlear nucleus following eighth nerve activity blockade or cochlea ablation. *Journal of Comparative Neurology, 320*(4), 501–508.

Sinclair, J. L., Fischl, M. J., Alexandrova, O., Hebeta, M., Grothe, B., Leibold, C., & Kopp-Scheinpflug, C. (2017). Sound-evoked activity influences myelination of brainstem axons in the trapezoid body. *Journal of Neuroscience, 37*(34), 8239–8255.

Singh, S. K., Stogsdill, J. A., Pulimood, N. S., Dingsdale, H., Kim, Y. H., Pilaz, L. J., . . . Eroglu, C. (2016). Astrocytes assemble thalamocortical synapses by bridging NRX1alpha and NL1 via Hevin. *Cell, 164*(1–2), 183–196.

Smith, D. J., & Rubel, E. W. (1979). Organization and development of brain stem auditory nuclei of the chicken: Dendritic gradients in nucleus laminaris. *Journal of Comparative Neurology, 186*(2), 213–239.

Sorg, O., & Magistretti, P. J. (1991). Characterization of the glycogenolysis elicited by vasoactive intestinal peptide, noradrenaline and adenosine in primary cultures of mouse cerebral cortical astrocytes. *Brain Res, 563*(1–2), 227–233.

Spacek, J. (1985). Three-dimensional analysis of dendritic spines. III. Glial sheath. *Anatomy and Embryology, 171*(2), 245–252.

Steinhauser, C., & Gallo, V. (1996). News on glutamate receptors in glial cells. *Trends Neuroscience, 19*(8), 339–345.

Stout, C., & Charles, A. (2003). Modulation of intercellular calcium signaling in astrocytes by extracellular calcium and magnesium. *Glia, 43*(3), 265–273.

Syka, J. (2002). Plastic changes in the central auditory system after hearing loss, restoration of function, and during learning. *Physiology Review, 82*(3), 601–636.

Szklarczyk, A., Lapinska, J., Rylski, M., McKay, R. D., & Kaczmarek, L. (2002). Matrix metalloproteinase-9 undergoes expression and activation during dendritic remodeling in adult hippocampus. *Journal of Neuroscience, 22*(3), 920–930.

Tasdemir-Yilmaz, O. E., & Freeman, M. R. (2014). Astrocytes engage unique molecular programs to engulf pruned neuronal debris from distinct subsets of neurons. *Genes & Development, 28*(1), 20–33.

Tierney, T. S., Russell, F. A., & Moore, D. R. (1997). Susceptibility of developing cochlear nucleus neurons to deafferentation-induced death abruptly ends just before the onset of hearing. *Journal of Comparative Neurology, 378*(2), 295–306.

Tierney, T. S., Doubel, T. P., Xia, G., & Moore, D. R. (2001). Development of brain-derived neurotrophic factor and neurotrophin-3 immunoreactivity in the lower auditory brainstem of the postnatal gerbil. *European Journal of Neuroscience, 14*(5), 785–793.

Tollin, D. J. (2003). The lateral superior olive: a functional role in sound source localization. *Neuroscientist, 9*(2), 127–143.

Touzani, O., Boutin, H., Chuquet, J., & Rothwell, N. (1999). Potential mechanisms of interleukin-1 involvement in cerebral ischaemia. *Journal of Neuroimmunology, 100*(1–2), 203–215.

Touzani, O., Boutin, H., LeFeuvre, R., Parker, L., Miller, A., Luheshi, G., & Rothwell, N. (2002). Interleukin-1 influences ischemic brain damage in the mouse independently of the interleukin-1 type I receptor. *Journal of Neuroscience, 22*(1), 38–43.

Tsukita, S., & Yonemura, S. (1997). ERM (ezrin/radixin/moesin) family: From cytoskeleton to signal transduction. *Current Opinion in Cell Biology, 9*(1), 70–75.

Ullian, E. M., Sapperstein, S. K., Christopherson, K. S., & Barres, B. A. (2001). Control of synapse number by glia. *Science, 291*(5504), 657–661.

Utzschneider, D. A., Archer, D. R., Kocsis, J. D., Waxman, S. G., & Duncan, I. D. (1994). Transplantation of glial cells enhances action potential conduction of amyelinated spinal cord axons in the myelin-deficient rat. *Proceedings of the National Academy of Sciences USA, 91*(1), 53–57.

Uwechue, N. M., Marx, M. C., Chevy, Q., & Billups, B. (2012). Activation of glutamate transport evokes rapid glutamine release from perisynaptic astrocytes. *Journal of Physiology, 590*(10), 2317–2331.

Vaheri, A., Carpen, O., Heiska, L., Helander, T. S., Jaaskelainen, J., Majander-Nordenswan, P., . . . Turunen, O. (1997). The ezrin protein family: Membrane-cytoskeleton interactions and disease associations. *Current Opinion in Cell Biology, 9*(5), 659–666.

van Deijk, A. F., Camargo, N., Timmerman, J., Heistek, T., Brouwers, J. F., Mogavero, F., . . . Verheijen, M. H. (2017). Astrocyte lipid metabolism is critical for synapse development and function in vivo. *Glia, 65*(4), 670–682.

Vaughn, J. E., & Pease, D. C. (1970). Electron microscopic studies of wallerian degeneration in rat optic nerves. II. Astrocytes, oligodendrocytes and adventitial cells. *Journal of Comparative Neurology, 140*(2), 207–226.

Ventura, R., & Harris, K. M. (1999). Three-dimensional relationships between hippocampal synapses and astrocytes. *Journal of Neuroscience, 19*(16), 6897–6906.

Vernadakis, A. (1996). Glia-neuron intercommunications and synaptic plasticity. *Progress in Neurobiology, 49*(3), 185–214.

Vezzani, A., Conti, M., De Luigi, A., Ravizza, T., Moneta, D., Marchesi, F., & De Simoni, M. G. (1999). Interleukin-1beta immunoreactivity and microglia are enhanced in the rat hippocampus by focal kainate application: Functional evidence for enhancement of electrographic seizures. *Journal of Neuroscience*, *19*(12), 5054–5065.

Vezzani, A., Moneta, D., Richichi, C., Aliprandi, M., Burrows, S. J., Ravizza, T., . . . De Simoni, M. G. (2002). Functional role of inflammatory cytokines and antiinflammatory molecules in seizures and epileptogenesis. *Epilepsia*, *43 Suppl*, 5, 30–35.

Wakabayashi, K., Fujioka, M., Kanzaki, S., Okano, H. J., Shibata, S., Yamashita, D., . . . Okano, H. (2010). Blockade of interleukin-6 signaling suppressed cochlear inflammatory response and improved hearing impairment in noise-damaged mice cochlea. *Neuroscience Research*, *66*(4), 345–352.

Wake, H., Moorhouse, A. J., Jinno, S., Kohsaka, S., & Nabekura, J. (2009). Resting microglia directly monitor the functional state of synapses in vivo and determine the fate of ischemic terminals. *Journal of Neuroscience*, *29*(13), 3974–3980.

Wenzel, J., Lammert, G., Meyer, U., & Krug, M. (1991). The influence of long-term potentiation on the spatial relationship between astrocyte processes and potentiated synapses in the dentate gyrus neuropil of rat brain. *Brain Research*, *560*(1–2), 122–131.

Werb, Z. (1997). ECM and cell surface proteolysis: regulating cellular ecology. *Cell*, *91*(4), 439–442.

Witcher, M. R., Kirov, S. A., & Harris, K. M. (2007). Plasticity of perisynaptic astroglia during synaptogenesis in the mature rat hippocampus. *Glia*, *55*(1), 13–23.

Woolf, N. K., & Ryan, A. F. (1984). The development of auditory function in the cochlea of the mongolian gerbil. *Hearing Research*, *13*(3), 277–283.

Yang, L., Monsivais, P., & Rubel, E. W. (1999). The superior olivary nucleus and its influence on nucleus laminaris: A source of inhibitory feedback for coincidence detection in the avian auditory brainstem. *Journal of Neuroscience*, *19*(6), 2313–2325.

Young, S. R., & Rubel, E. W. (1983). Frequency-specific projections of individual neurons in chick brainstem auditory nuclei. *Journal of Neuroscience*, *3*(7), 1373–1378.

CHAPTER 25

DEVIANCE DETECTION AND ENCODING ACOUSTIC REGULARITY IN THE AUDITORY MIDBRAIN

MANUEL S. MALMIERCA, GUILLERMO V. CARBAJAL, AND CARLES ESCERA

Abstract

In the past, there was a rather corticocentric conception of the processing of relationships between sounds that used to mostly relegate the midbrain function to a mere relay. However, increasing neurophysiological evidence demonstrates that the midbrain is, in fact, playing a crucial role in encoding some sorts of regularities present in the flow of acoustic stimulation, adapting the neuronal response for processing efficiency. Midbrain neurons are capable of responding more rapidly and strongly when a new stimulus is not matching to a previously encoded regularity; a phenomenon referred to as deviance detection. This chapter discusses deviance detection evidence in the midbrain, mainly describing the characteristics and mechanisms of stimulus-specific adaptation (SSA), and closing with an interpretation from the standpoint of the predictive coding theory.

Keywords: SSA/stimulus-specific adaptation, MMN/mismatch negativity, MLR/middle-latency responses, deviance detection, repetition suppression, prediction error, GABA, acetylcholine, endocannabinoids, predictive coding

Introduction: Processing an Auditory World in Constant Change

In the everyday life of humans and animals, there is a plethora of events occurring simultaneously. Most of those events are routine, recurrent, or meaningless; whereas others might be of great importance. But all of them generate a profuse amount of sounds, mixing in an acoustic jumble that eventually reaches the eardrum. The tympanic membrane is hit by an incessant flow of fine air-pressure oscillations at every fraction of a second, and each oscillation is mechanically transduced into electrochemical impulses that the central nervous system has to process and interpret. This gargantuan sum of inputs could easily overwhelm the capacities of the auditory brain, which must implement processing strategies to avoid the loss of relevant sensory information.

Thus, the auditory system is equipped with efficient filtering mechanisms that progressively prune the original acoustic signal into more manageable and useful inputs, starting at very early stages of the auditory processing. Already at the auditory nerve, fibers respond vigorously when a stimulus is switched on, but after few tens of milliseconds their firing rate slows down until reaching a steady-state rate that follows the sound to its end (Feng et al., 1991; Nomoto et al., 1964; Sumner & Palmer, 2012). This decline over time from the initially high firing rate to a lower, "adapted" rate is known as *spike-frequency adaptation*, and its presumed function is to spare processing resources without losing sensory information. It has also been reported in nuclei of the auditory brainstem, like the superior olivary complex (Finlayson & Adam, 1997) and the inferior colliculus (Ingham & McAlpine, 2004).

Nonetheless, if spike-frequency adaptation were the only filter at play, auditory neurons would still have to respond to every sound. Overabundant auditory representations would be conveyed, ceaselessly and with similar saliency, to superior levels of processing. Higher brain regions would have to strive for distinguishing amongst all those representations which ones are the relevant perceptions for the ongoing tasks. A discriminative endeavor that could easily flood attention and affect cognition, thereby hampering an adaptive behavior, and eventually imperiling the survival of the hearing being.

Fortunately, the auditory system relies on yet another, more refined filtering strategy that makes it possible to discern the informative value of a sound based on its probability of occurrence, without fully processing it. Imagine, for example, the sudden unexpected burst of a droplet hitting the bottom of the sink. The bursts of the next couple of droplets are enough to deduce that the faucet is leaking. However, the ensuing droplet bursts are just providing confirmatory evidence, adding no new meaning to the represented event. Hence, every new droplet is less informative than the preceding one, but the processing cost remains constant. Only a change in that sequence of sounds would provide new information. If the droplets bursts suddenly become a stream, the water pipe may have broken! Therefore, it would be more efficient to just process the changes in the auditory scene, instead of fully representing each and every single sound in it.

Nature complies with this heuristic logic, as some neurons in the auditory system diminish or even cease their firing to repetitive stimulation, while still responding to the occurrence of new stimuli (Bibikov, 1977; Malone & Semple, 2001). Such filtering is appropriately referred to as stimulus-specific adaptation (SSA). The most widely-used paradigm to study SSA is the oddball sequence (Figure 25.1A), which consists in the repetition of a tone (named standard) featuring the random irruption of a rare tone (named deviant). During the oddball paradigm, SSA neurons keep the auditory system from overloading with mostly irrelevant input by preventing the representation of standard stimuli, thereby automatically providing perceptual saliency to deviant stimuli, which are potentially more informative. It is not surprising to find such refined selective processing widespread in the auditory cortex (Nieto-Diego & Malmierca, 2016; Ulanovsky et al., 2003). What might be somewhat unexpected, however, is to find neurons displaying SSA as early in the ascending auditory pathway as to in the midbrain level (Malmierca et al., 2009; Pérez-González et al., 2005; Duque et al., 2018). More precisely, robust and consistent SSA is present in the cortices of the inferior colliculus (IC), which reveals that this subcortical brain region is involved in higher-order functions of auditory processing.

General Properties of SSA in the Midbrain

The magnitude of SSA displayed by a neuron can be measured as an index of the difference between its respective responses to a given stimulus when presented as deviant or as standard in the oddball paradigm (Figure 25.1B). By systematically varying the physical parameters of the oddball sequence, it has been determined that SSA in the auditory midbrain is very sensitive to (1) the probability of occurrence of the deviant stimulus, (2) the pitch and the intensity of the stimuli, (3) the frequency contrast between standard and deviant, and (4) the repetition rate of the stimuli.

First, one important factor modulating SSA is the magnitude of the probability unbalance between standard and deviant. The rarity of the deviant is positively correlated with the magnitude of the SSA index. The differences between standard and deviant responses progressively diminish as their probability of occurrence in an oddball sequence tends to equalize. This means that higher SSA indices can be elicited when, e.g., deviant tones appear just 10% of the times than when they do it in 30% of the trials (Ayala et al., 2013; Malmierca et al., 2009). In this regard, it is worth mentioning that most studies report an effect of probability, not only in the total firing of a neuron, but also in the latency of the first spike fired to the stimulus (Malmierca et al., 2009; Zhao et al., 2011). However, this adaptation of the first spike latency was only observed at relatively fast presentation rates (≥ 4 Hz). It could be speculated that, under demanding sensory conditions, the repetition of a stimulus provokes a decline and delay of some neuronal

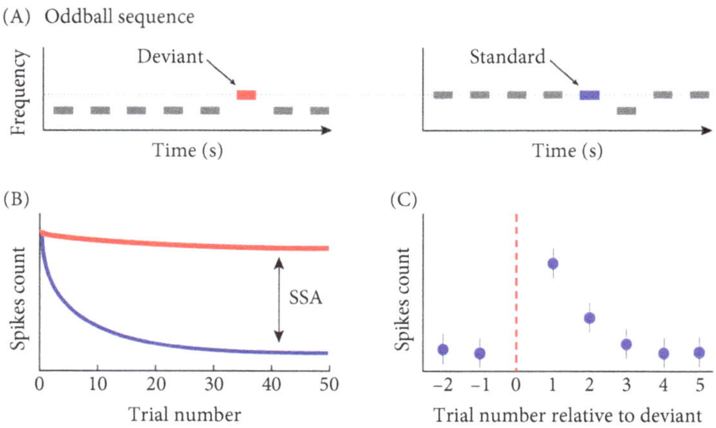

FIGURE 25.1. Oddball paradigm as a means of measuring SSA. **A.** Oddball sequence comprising two tones of different frequency. The unbalanced probability of appearance defines the deviant and standard conditions. Please note that the deviant and standard responses are always compared for a given tone (not between different tones), which requires the oddball sequence to be flipped in order to measure such tone in both conditions. **B.** Whereas the evolution in the response to deviant stimuli describes non-significant changes, the response to repetitive stimuli undergoes an initial sharp drop during the first presentations, which is followed by a slower exponential decay that reaches a maximum usually within 25 presentations. **C.** After every presentation of a deviant stimulus, the ensuing standard response partially remerges. This recovery is not complete, indicating that both short-term and long-term dynamics are at play in SSA.

responses, in order to prioritize a swift and favored processing of the rare events that might occur.

Second, SSA levels do not remain constant across the whole receptive field of a neuron. The strength of SSA is biased within the frequency response area (FRA) of IC neurons toward high-frequency and low-intensity regions (Duque et al., 2012). In other words, IC neurons adapt better to relatively softer and higher-pitched tones (Figure 25.2). The fact that SSA strength is not homogeneous within the receptive field indicates that SSA is not an intrinsic property of the neuron, but rather depends on its synaptic activity. Also regarding the neuronal receptive field, it is worth mentioning that there is a positive correlation between the width of the FRA of the neuron and the strength of its SSA (see Figure 25.4E, F for examples; Duque et al., 2012; Malmierca et al., 2009). This suggests that SSA is an integrative property of the network, conducted by neurons with extensive dendritic arbors and wide receptive fields that act as converges of auditory input.

Third, SSA strengthens as frequency contrast between standard and deviant increases (Ayala et al., 2013; Malmierca et al., 2009). Nevertheless, the excellent hyperacuity of the IC neurons enables SSA at frequency contrasts as small as 0.057 octaves

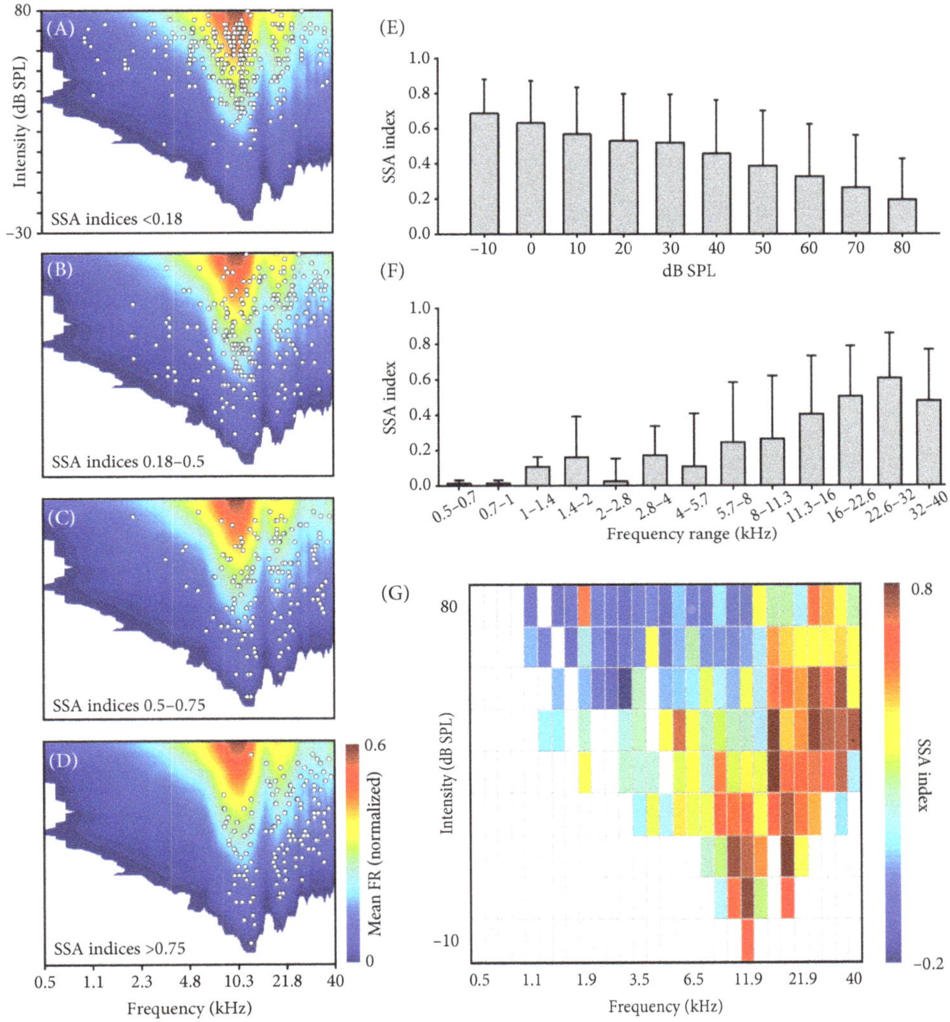

FIGURE 25.2. Distribution of SSA indices in a population of IC neurons, adapted form Duque et al. (2012). **A–D.** Cumulative receptive field of the population, generated by averaging the FRA of each neuron (normalized to its maximum firing rate) in the sample. Each white dot represents the center of a pair of frequencies tested in an oddball sequence. Note that the dot distribution progressively moves toward higher frequencies and low intensities as the indices of SSA increase. **A.** Topographic location of the lowest SSA indices. **B, C.** Topographic location for moderate SSA levels. **D.** Topographic location of the pairs of tones that evoked the highest SSA, visibly concentrated around the higher frequencies and low intensities of the receptive field. **E.** Distribution of SSA indices sorted by absolute intensities. **F.** Distribution of SSA indices sorted by frequency ranges. **G.** Distribution of SSA levels considering absolute intensity (10 dB steps) and frequency (grouped in 0.5 octave steps). Note the different distribution of high SSA indices (warm colors) and low SSA indices values (cold colors).

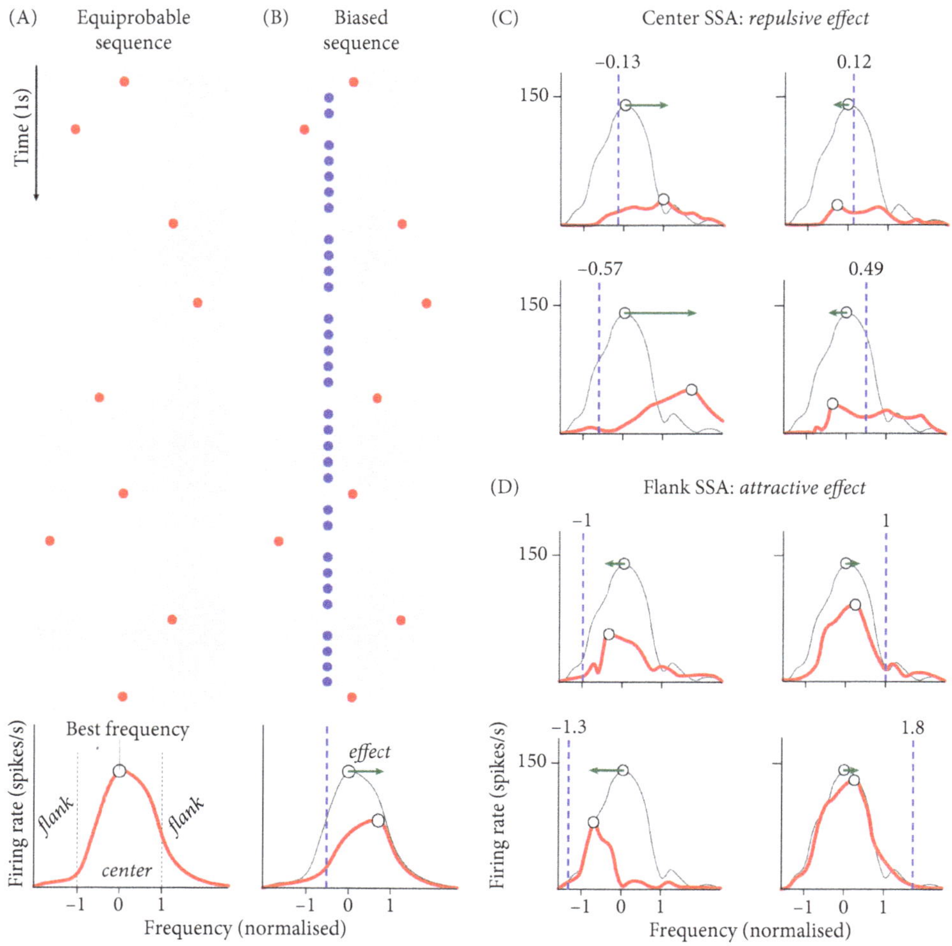

FIGURE 25.3. SSA may enhance neuronal stimulus discriminability, adapted from Shen et al. (2015). **A.** Equiprobable presentation of tones of the same intensity (red dots, only a segment of the sequence is represented) allows to define the tuning curve of the neuron (bottom chart, red line) and identify its best frequency (white dot), center, and flank areas. **B.** The introduction of a standard tone (blue) modifies the original tuning curve (thin grey line), resulting in a new adapted tuning curve (red line) where the best frequency has changed (green arrow). **C.** Example of an SSA neuron where 4 standard tones (blue dashed lines) close to the center of the tuning were tested. Standard tones falling in the central area elicit a SSA that exerts a repulsive effect on the best frequency, shifting it away from the adapted channel. **D.** Same example of SSA neuron, now testing 4 standard tones in the flanks of the tuning curve. In both flanks, SSA attracted the best frequency toward the adapted channel.

(Malmierca et al., 2009). Furthermore, SSA modulates the receptive field of auditory neurons in a way that could facilitate frequency discrimination (Ayala et al., 2013). Most neurons in the IC have an identifiable best frequency, which is the frequency that elicits the strongest firing in a tuning curve (Figure 25.3A). When the frequency of a standard tone is close to the best frequency of an SSA neuron, it shifts away that maximal response in the resulting adapted receptive field toward a contiguous frequency band (Figure 25.3B; Shen et al., 2015). Conversely, when the frequency of the standard tone is distant from the best frequency of an SSA neuron, the maximal response of the resulting receptive field is attracted closer to the adapted frequency band (Figure 25.3C; Shen et al., 2015).

Lastly, SSA also varies with the rate at which the stimuli are presented. SSA indices are positively correlated with presentation rate, up to a certain optimal point. Increasing the number of tones presented per second beyond that optimal point produces a reduction of SSA strength, due to temporal masking effects (Faure et al., 2003). The strongest SSA levels in the rat IC are reported at a rate of 4 Hz (inter-stimulus interval of 250 ms). Notwithstanding, notable SSA can be elicited presenting just one stimulus per second (Pérez-González et al., 2005; Zhao et al., 2011). In the case of the barn owl IC, SSA has been reported at inter-stimulus intervals as long as 10 seconds (Netser et al., 2011). This time scale of seconds allows to properly establish a connection between SSA and echoic memory already at the level of the midbrain. Furthermore, significant SSA could be appreciated at stimulation rates of 1 stimulus per minute in the barn owl optic tectum (OT, analogous to the mammalian superior colliculus, also in the midbrain), as well as in several nuclei of the avian forebrain compounded in the gaze control circuitry. The identification of long-lasting SSA in those kind of neural structures hints at a possible implication in behavioral habituation (Gutfreund, 2012; Netser et al., 2011).

SSA Dynamics: Sensitivity to Stimulus History

Stimulus history has an impact in SSA that can be decomposed in two components: short-term and long-term dynamics (Ulanovsky et al., 2004).

Only one repetition of a stimulus suffices to induct SSA. In consequence, SSA can emerge from a local effect prompted by the influence of the immediately preceding stimulus. Therefore, the response to a repeated stimulus A (r_{AA}) will always be weaker than if a different stimulus B would have come before A (r_{BA}), as it is the empirical case ($r_{BA} > r_{AA}$) in the auditory cortex (Ulanovsky et al., 2004) and the IC (Zhao et al., 2011). According to this one-trial effect, it does not matter if a stimulus is common (standard) or rare (deviant), just if it is repeated. This is known as the short-term dynamic of SSA (Ulanovsky et al., 2004; Zhao et al., 2011).

However, the short-term dynamic does not fully predict what can be observed in the context of an oddball paradigm. Even disregarding the global probabilities of the stimuli (e.g., 50% or 90% of the presentations in an oddball sequence), repetition creates a long-term accumulative effect. A stimulus will elicit a weaker response after several repetitions than after just one ($r_A > r_{AA} > r_{AAA} > r_{AAAA}$), implying an n-trial effect (Ulanovsky et al., 2004). Therefore, after enough presentations, the unbalanced probabilities of the oddball paradigm will have a great influence over the neuronal response. This global effect is referred to as the long-term dynamics of SSA (Ulanovsky et al., 2004; Zhao et al., 2011).

The long-term dynamic of SSA also explains why, during an oddball sequence, appearance of a deviant tone does not fully restore the response to the standard tone. SSA is taking into account several preceding trials, not just the last one. However, the standard response indeed recovers to some extent (Zhao et al., 2011), indicating that not only the global statistics of the stimuli are considered. If that were the case, after enough repetitions of the standard, a new standard coming after a deviant would display a similar level of SSA as the standard that came previously to that deviant tone. Inasmuch as the standard response partially remerges after a deviant tone, it implies that the one-trial effect is still at play throughout the whole oddball sequence (Figure 25.1C). The magnitude of the SSA that a neuronal response undergoes at each stimulus presentation is determined by the interplay of both local and global components, which represent two time scales of integration in the SSA dynamics (Ulanovsky et al., 2004).

SSA Time Course

As a rule of thumb for the rat IC, the response to the repetitive stimulus describes a rapid decay over the first 10 presentations, which is followed by a slower exponential decay that reached a maximum within 25 trials, and finally ensued by a late steady-state component (Figure 25.1B). During the oddball paradigm, interleaved deviant stimuli are not significantly affected by SSA (Figure 25.1B). However, its irruption partially restores the response to the subsequent standard stimulus (Figure 25.1C; Malmierca et al., 2009).

SSA Mechanics: The Model of Adaptation in Narrow Channels

The possible mechanisms underlying SSA are still under investigation and debate. Most types of adaptation can be understood as rather basic physiological mechanisms governed by the neuronal output. Thus, spike-frequency adaptation depends on the discharge history of the neuron, accounted for by activation of voltage-dependent conductance (Sánchez-Vives et al., 2000a, 2000b) or tonic hyperpolarization (Carandini & Ferster, 1997). However, since these mechanisms operate at the level of the somatic membrane potential, they cannot be stimulus specific (Ulanovsky et al., 2004), nor can they vary across the neuronal receptive field as SSA does (Duque et al., 2012). Considering that, SSA emergence must rely on physiological mechanisms operating at the input of the neuron, based on its synaptic history. Mechanisms such as synaptic depression and facilitation (Abbott et al., 1997; Tsodyks & Markram, 1997) or inhibition (Zhang et al., 2003) would affect differentially certain regions of the dendritic tree, thereby exerting stimulus-specific effects over the eventual response of the neuron.

The model of narrowly-tuned adaptation channels provides a functional explanation on how SSA may emerge from the differential adaptation of dendritic inputs (Taaseh et al., 2011). The repetition of a standard tone would adapt a particular frequency channel of the neuronal receptive field independently, leaving the rest mostly unaffected. Those channels have been estimated to stretch about ⅓ octaves on either side of the repeating frequency (Taaseh et al., 2011). Therefore, if the frequency contrast between the standard and the deviant tone is more than ⅓ octaves, the neuronal response to the deviant will not be adapted. Conversely, if the frequency contrast is less than ⅓ octaves, the deviant response will subdue some cross-frequency adaptation. This is why wider frequency separations between standard and deviant tones result in stronger SSA. Interestingly, the width of the adaptation channels in IC neurons seems even narrower at high frequencies and low intensities (Duque et al., 2016).

The model of adaptation channels, despite very comprehensive, suffers from some limitations to account for the empirical SSA data, revealing that complementary mechanisms may be at play (Hershenhoren et al., 2014; Taaseh et al., 2011). In this regard, recent efforts have attempted to reinterpret SSA from a more general framework based on the predictive coding theory (Carbajal & Malmierca, 2018a; Parras et al., 2017), as discussed in the last section of this chapter.

Neuroanatomical Features that Enable SSA Emergence in the Midbrain

Neuroanatomically speaking, the midbrain is the first structure in the ascending auditory pathway where SSA can be found (Ayala et al., 2013). The main auditory center in the midbrain is the IC, where nearly all ascending auditory pathways converge before passing the processed information to the auditory cortex via the thalamus. Besides, the IC receives rich descending auditory and non-auditory projections, and it possess a dense and complex microcircuitry of local and commissural connections. The integration of excitatory, inhibitory, and neuromodulatory input, coming from multiple sources, makes the IC a perfect gate for controlling the flow of relevant acoustic information before reaching the cortex. Neurons showing SSA have been found in the IC of frogs (Bibikov, 1977), gerbils (Malone & Semple, 2001), rats (Pérez-González et al., 2005), mice (Duque & Malmierca, 2015), bats (Thomas et al., 2012), and barn owls (Reches & Gutfreund, 2008), findings that reveal this filtering function is preserved across species. Additional evidence obtained from non-invasive approaches confirm that the IC may be the first gate of salient acoustic information also in humans (Cacciaglia et al., 2015; Shiga et al., 2015). The cytoarchitecture of the IC and its pattern of projections allows to differentiate at least two main structures: a central nucleus (Figure 25.4A) that is wrapped by a shell or cortices (Figure 25.4D).

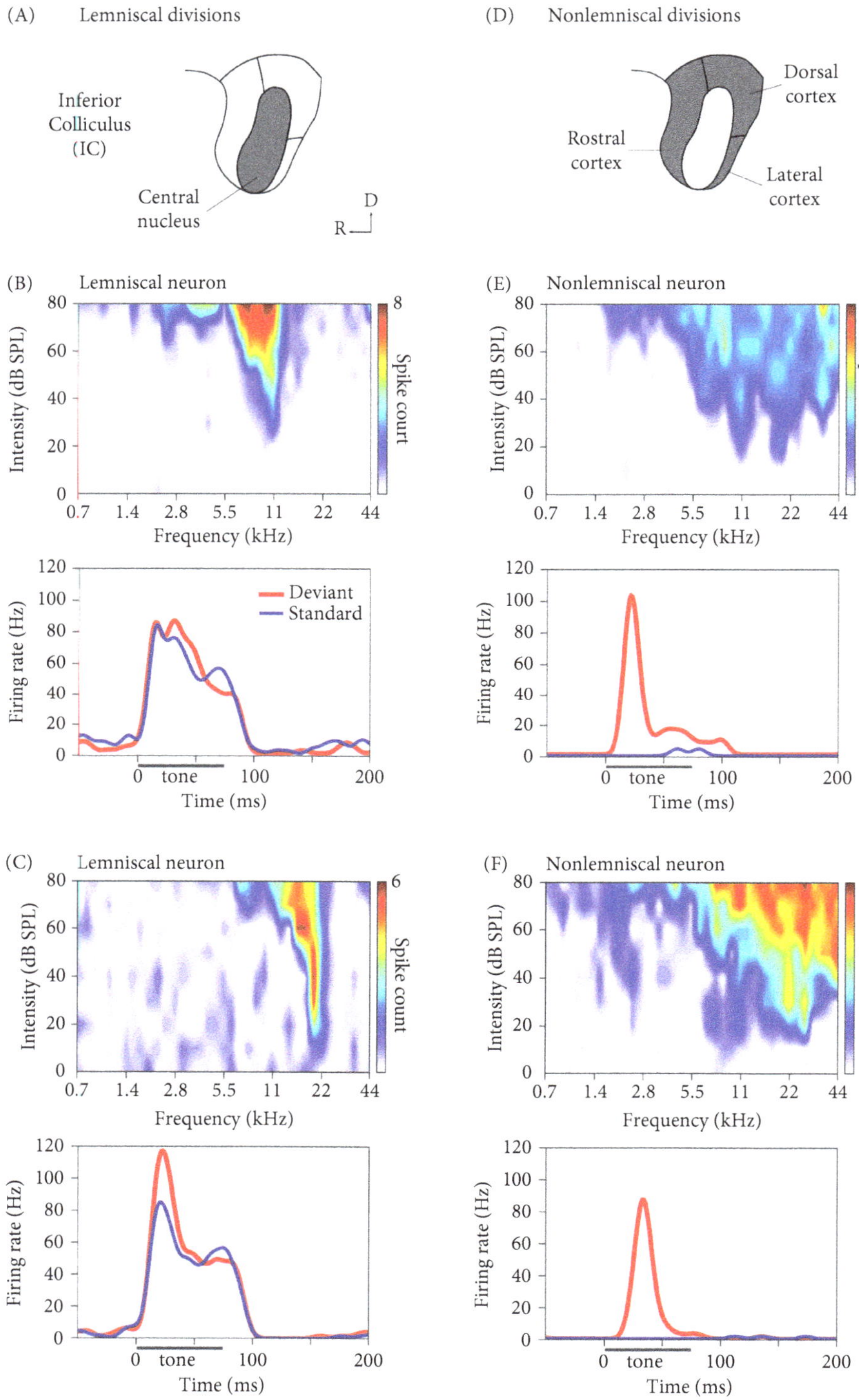

FIGURE 25.4. SSA in lemniscal and nonlemniscal IC neurons. **A.** The central nucleus of the IC highlighted in dark grey. **B, C.** Examples of typical lemniscal neurons from the IC. The upper frame displays their characteristically narrow FRAs of each neuron, indicating that their

The central nucleus of the IC receives most of its input from the lower auditory brainstem. It is organized in a tonotopic fashion, where sharply-tuned neurons (Figure 25.4B, C) are arranged in approximately 150 frequency laminae (Malmierca et al., 2008; Malmierca et al., 1993, 1995). They send tonotopically-arranged projections to the thalamus and cortex, forming the so-called *lemniscal pathway*. The response of lemniscal neurons is primarily determined by the physical features of the sound. Neurons located in the central nucleus of the IC tend to show only partial or rather poor SSA (Malmierca et al., 2009; Parras et al., 2017).

On the other hand, the neurons in the cortices of the IC are broadly-tuned (Figure 25.4E, F), with frequency-response areas so wide that any tonotopic arrangement is diffuse at best. As oppose to the central nucleus, the IC cortices receive less input from the main brainstem and more from a diversity of sources that include intrinsic connections from the central nucleus, the auditory cortex and other multimodal nuclei (Ito & Malmierca, 2018). Neurons in the IC cortices send ascending projections mainly to other non-lemniscal divisions of the auditory thalamus and cortex, constituting an adjunct ascending pathway known as the *nonlemniscal pathway*. Nonlemnical IC neurons possess large dendritic arbors (Malmierca et al., 2011), morphologically consistent with the wideness of their receptive fields. The capacity of the nonlemniscal neurons in the IC to converge inputs across many frequencies, along with the heavy cortical modulation these neurons are subjected to, denotes their integrative role in the auditory pathway (Carbajal & Malmierca, 2018b). In line with this, the neurons in the IC cortices show the highest and most robust levels of SSA in the midbrain, to the extent that many neurons cease firing completely after just few repetitions of a stimulus.

Three Classes of SSA Neurons in the Inferior Colliculus

The majority of IC neurons show at least some degree of SSA, varying in magnitude in a continuum from negligible to absolute. Three loosely defined functional groups of

receptive field is very sharply tuned. The lower frame shows the peristimulus time histogram of that neuron for the standard and deviant presentations of the same tone. Note that their responses tend to follow the sound (thick grey bar), and their vigorous firing rates are barely modulated by the experimental condition (although some weak SSA is visible in C). **D.** The cortices of the IC are highlighted in dark grey. **E, F.** Examples of typical nonlemniscal neurons from the IC. The upper frame displays their characteristically broad FRAs, indicating that their receptive field can process and integrate a wide range of frequencies. The lower frame shows the peristimulus time histogram of that neuron for the standard and deviant presentations of the same tone. Note that their responses tend to signal the onset of the deviant condition. The response to the standard condition is almost completely adapted, especially in the onset. No spontaneous activity can be appreciated (in time < 0 ms).

neurons can be distinguished in such continuum: non-adapting, partially-adapting and novelty neurons (Malmierca et al., 2009).

In one extreme of the continuum, *non-adapting neurons* are those lacking SSA in any configuration of the oddball paradigm. Non-adapting neurons will respond similarly to a tone when presented as standard as when presented as deviant (Figure 25.4B, C). As a rule of thumb, non-adapting neurons tend to have a narrow, V-shaped FRA, show more sustained responses during the whole presentation of the sound, and have shorter latencies than the adapting neurons. All of which suggests that the role of non-adapting neurons is to accurately represent the physical features of the stimulus, disregarding its context. Non-adapting neurons are commonly found in the central nucleus, i.e. the lemniscal IC (Figure 25.4A). In fact, these general trends seem particularly true in bats, whose central nucleus is greatly developed and resilient to SSA, probably due to the fundamental role of repetitive sounds in echolocation (Thomas et al., 2012).

On the other extreme, *novelty neurons* is the classic denomination given to those neurons that show great or even absolute levels of SSA consistently throughout their entire receptive field. Thus, while novelty neurons quickly cease to response to repeated stimuli they retain their full responses to deviant stimuli (Figure 25.4E, F). The FRAs of novelty neurons are always very broad, indicating they congregate a wide range of acoustic inputs. Most of novelty neurons are located in the cortices of the IC, i.e. in the nonlemniscal IC, where neurons have characteristically broadly-oriented dendritic arbors. Novelty neurons tend to be onset responders, or at least have a very pronounced onset component in their response, which is also the component most affected by SSA (Figure 25.4E, F). Furthermore, novelty neurons have virtually no spontaneous activity, so their firing reliably signals a change in the ongoing acoustic environment. In that regard, the term *novelty neurons* has lost popularity in recent years, in favor of other formulas like *deviance detectors*. The concept of deviance detection better emphasizes the sensitivity to a change in the stimulation, and it is better suited for interpretation from other more general theoretical frameworks about perception like the predictive coding theory (Carbajal & Malmierca, 2018a).

Between the extremes of non-adapting neurons and novelty neurons, there is a well-stocked and diverse group of neurons showing some degree of SSA. Those neurons are usually referred to as *partially-adapting neurons*, because they exhibit some levels of SSA, but not under all conditions. At certain oddball parameters (e.g., stimulation rate, rarity of the deviant, etc.) and at specific areas of the receptive field, these neurons may show SSA, whereas at other areas they may lose their deviance detection capacities completely. In general, *partially-adapting neurons* are not as finely tuned as the non-adapting neurons, but the broadness and shape of their FRAs are very variable. Partially-adapting neurons respond with a variety of discharge patterns. Nevertheless, the effects of SSA present in the partially-adapting neurons are most obvious in the onset portion of their response (the first 20-30 ms; Duque et al., 2012; Malmierca et al., 2009; Zhao et al., 2011). Indeed, this fact represents an interesting difference with the SSA observed in the auditory cortex, where SSA seems stronger in the sustained and late portions of the neuronal response (Nieto-Diego & Malmierca, 2016). The most characteristic feature of the partially-adapting neurons is their sensitivity to the internal context of the neuronal network. Whereas novelty neurons operate consistently filtering out redundant input, the function of partially-adapting neurons changes considerably depending on neuromodulation (Ayala & Malmierca, 2015), state of awareness (Duque & Malmierca, 2015), or cortical influences (Anderson & Malmierca, 2013). This suggests that, whereas novelty neurons behave as hard static filters against redundancy, partially-adapting neurons may act as finer dynamic filters that adjust their function dependent on other contextual aspects besides purely acoustic stimulus relationships. Partially-adapting neurons can be found in all subdivisions of the IC, but they tend to show stronger levels of SSA in the cortices.

The Origin of SSA in the Midbrain: Generated in Situ or Inherited from the Cortex?

The anatomical source of subcortical SSA has been a matter of discussion for the last 15 years. Selective adaptation had been described in the auditory midbrain of animal models long ago (Bibikov, 1977; Malone & Semple, 2001), implicitly assuming that such adaptation was being generated in situ. However, those pioneering studies were overlooked and their assumptions overwritten when a study using the oddball paradigm found SSA in primary auditory cortex of the cat (Ulanovsky et al., 2003). This seminal work was the first to propose that SSA could be the neuronal correlate of the mismatch negativity (MMN), a change-specific component of the auditory event-related potentials (ERP) recorded from the human scalp (Näätänen et al., 1978). The MMN is traditionally elicited using the oddball paradigm, although it can appear in response to any perceivable change in stimulation (Winkler & Schröger, 2015). The MMN has proven to be a central non-invasive tool for neurocognitive research (Näätänen et al., 2007), even showing promising potential diagnostic applications (Näätänen et al., 2012), as it appears altered in a great variety of clinical conditions. As a result, the suggested link between cortical SSA and MMN soon captured great scientific attention.

Unfortunately, this seminal study did not find significant traces of SSA in the auditory thalamus (Ulanovsky et al. 2003). Inasmuch as the anatomical sources of MMN had been firmly pinned down to the auditory cortex in humans (Alho, 1995), it was concluded that SSA was a purely cortical mechanism as well, leaving a profound and enduring impression in the literature. This conception had to be revised after the consistent confirmation of strong SSA using the oddball paradigm present in the nonlemniscal divisions of the IC (Ayala et al., 2015; Ayala & Malmierca, 2015, 2018; Duque et al., 2012, 2016; Duque & Malmierca, 2015; Gao et al., 2014; Herrmann et al., 2015; Lumani & Zhang, 2010; Malmierca et al., 2009; Netser et al., 2011; Parras et al., 2017; Patel et al., 2012; Pérez-González et al., 2005, 2012; Pérez-González & Malmierca, 2012; Reches & Gutfreund, 2008; Shen et al., 2015; Thomas et al., 2012; Valdés-Baizabal et al., 2017; Zhao et al., 2011) and thalamus (Anderson & Malmierca, 2013; Anderson et al., 2009; Antunes et al., 2010; Antunes & Malmierca, 2014; Duque et al. 2014; Parras et al., 2017; Yu et al., 2009). Notwithstanding, the corticocentric approach to understanding deviance detection was still not completely abandoned. It was suggested then that SSA had a cortical origin, to be passed down via corticofugal projections to the nonlemniscal divisions of the subcortical auditory nuclei (Nelken & Ulanovsky, 2007). Indeed, all SSA neurons located in the IC cortices receive descending cortical projections (Ayala et al., 2015). But it is not possible to determine the prime anatomical source of SSA just by investigating connectivity.

To properly address the question, studies of reversible deactivation of the auditory cortex using a cooling technique were conducted while recording from the nonlemniscal auditory thalamus (Antunes & Malmierca, 2011) and the IC cortices (Anderson & Malmierca, 2013). The general results demonstrated that, although the auditory cortex clearly modulated the firing rate of the nonlemniscal subcortical neurons in a gain-control manner (Malmierca et al., 2015), increasing the contrast between standard and deviant stimuli by affecting the response to both proportionally, the auditory cortex was not generating SSA by itself. Remarkable alterations were observed in many other response properties of the subcortical neurons during cortical deactivation, such as their FRA, spontaneous activity, and first spike latencies. However, the overall strength and dynamics of subcortical SSA were mostly unaffected by the deactivation of the auditory cortex. Only about half of the adapting neurons in the IC suffered changes in their SSA sensitivity. This confirms a prominent cortical modulation, but also demonstrates that SSA is emerging in the midbrain, independently from coticocollicular input. As a matter of fact, novelty neurons in the IC cortices remained mostly unaffected. Even the partially-adapting IC neurons that underwent reductions of their SSA sensitivity did not lose it completely. Furthermore, almost no changes in SSA sensitivity were detected in the non-lemniscal auditory thalamus after the cortical deactivation.

In light of these results, it is more plausible that the SSA present in the auditory cortex is inherited from subcortical structures than vice versa, albeit the possibility of SSA being generated de novo at the intrinsic microcircuitry of each station independently cannot be ruled out. Notwithstanding, since no other auditory nuclei lower than the midbrain seems to manifest SSA (Ayala et al., 2013), and given that cortical deactivation does not eliminate SSA from the midbrain, the IC cortices can be considered the most probable anatomical origin of SSA.

The Physiology of SSA: How Is Synaptic Adaptation Modulated?

Research in animal models has tried to disentangle the neurochemistry behind the emergence of SSA in IC neurons using microiontophoresis. During the extracellular recording of neuronal activity, the microiontophoresis technique is used to permeate the vicinity of the recorded neuron with neurotransmitter agonists or antagonists. By means of this local neuropharmacological manipulation, we have been able to characterize the contribution of some membrane receptors to the emergence of deviance detection in the auditory midbrain.

The Role of Inhibition: A Gain Control of Deviance Detection

Synaptic inhibition has been pointed at for long in the literature as one of the most probable mechanisms that could generate SSA (Figure 25.5B). The main inhibitory neurotransmitter in the IC is GABA, which binds to two main classes of receptors. $GABA_A$ receptors are ionotropic, part of a ligand-gated ion channel. $GABA_B$ receptors are metabotropic, regulating the opening or closing of ion channels via intermediate G proteins. In addition to GABA, in the mammalian IC inhibitory activity is also exerted by glycine through its ionotropic glycine receptors. Several studies have unraveled the role of inhibition in midbrain SSA emergence, using the oddball paradigm and the microiontophoresis technique.

The inhibition exerted through $GABA_A$ receptors, which regulate the postsynaptic membrane potential (Sivaramakrishnan et al. 2004), was analyzed using the antagonist gabazine in the rat IC (Pérez-González et al., 2012). Gabazine slowed down adaptation to the standard, having a profound effect on the magnitude and time course of SSA (Figure 25.5C). However, blocking $GABA_A$ receptors failed to abolish SSA, since the application of gabazine also increased the firing rate of the deviant response. Therefore, the response magnitude and latency still depended on the probability of the stimulus when $GABA_A$ receptors were blocked, maintaining the absolute difference between the responses to deviant and standard stimuli. What gabazine application actually achieved was the reduction of the proportional difference between the deviant and standard responses, whereby SSA indices dropped (Figure 25.5C). Thus, that general increase of neuronal responsiveness resulted in a reduction of SSA sensitivity. This reflects a gain control mechanism mediated by $GABA_A$ receptors in the IC. $GABA_A$-mediated inhibition facilitates the relative saliency of rare auditory events over the redundant ones by sharpening the contrast between their responses, as shown in the so-called *iceberg effect* (Ayala & Malmierca, 2018; Pérez-González et al., 2012). The iceberg effect describes the observation whereby the spike output of a neuron under inhibition is more sharply tuned than the underlying membrane potential, since only the strongest excitatory input sufficiently depolarizes the membrane to reach threshold for spike generation (Figure 25.5A; Isaacson & Scanziani, 2011). Such gain-control mechanism of SSA starting in the midbrain has been demonstrated to continue in the auditory thalamus (Duque et al., 2014), which suggests a progressive $GABA_A$-mediated filtering of redundant information before reaching the auditory cortex.

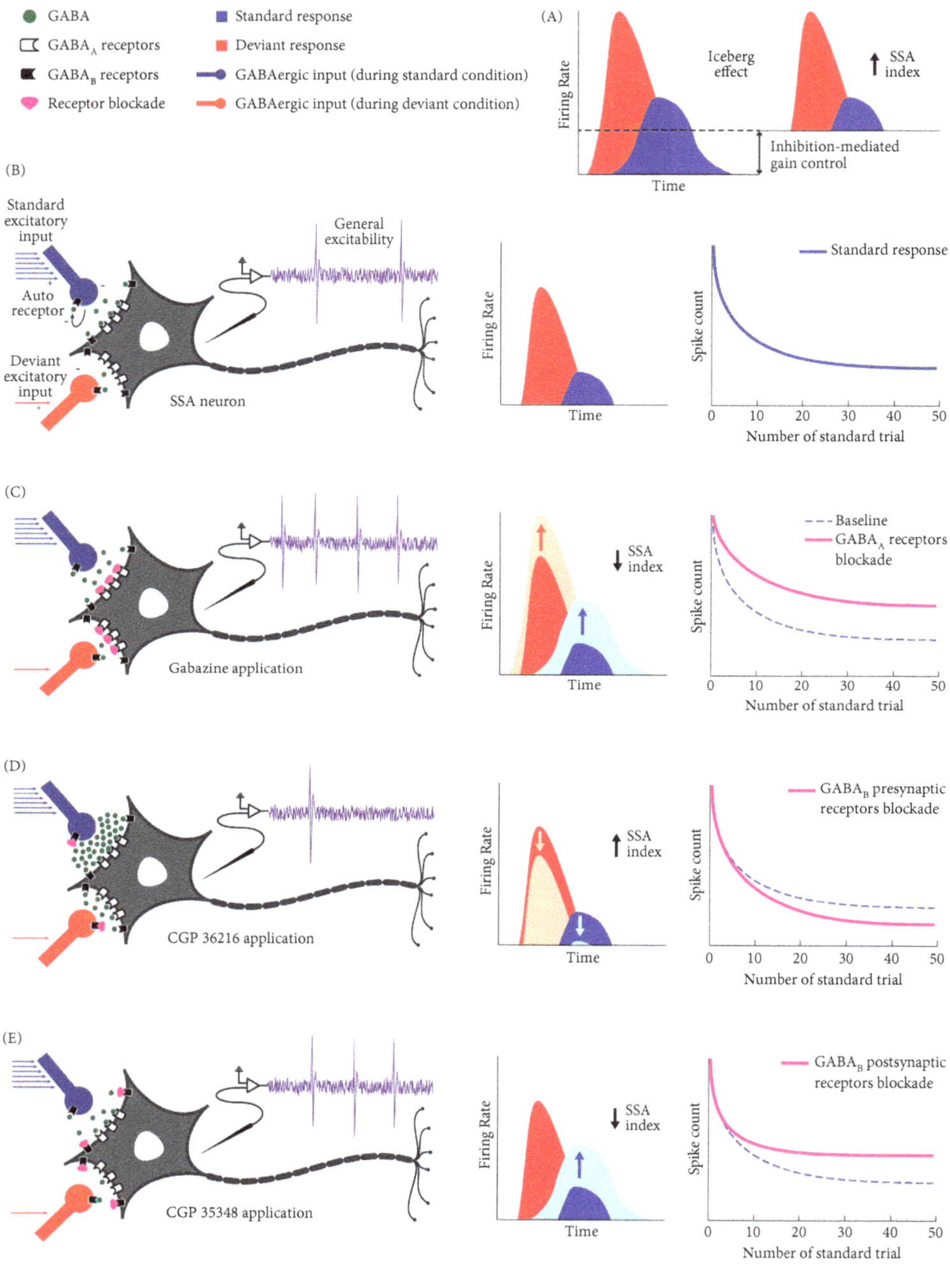

FIGURE 25.5. GABA-mediated inhibition modulates SSA. **A.** SSA enhancement resulting from the *iceberg effect*. **B.** In the left, a model of an SSA neuron (in gray) receiving GABAergic inhibition elicited by a given tone. The red GABAergic terminal represents the GABA release when such a tone is presented as a deviant, whereas the blue GABAergic terminal represents GABA release when the same tone is presented as a standard. Note that the repetitive and steady presentation of

More subtle gain control effects were found to be mediated by $GABA_B$ presynaptic receptors in the rat IC (Ayala & Malmierca, 2018), but in the opposite manner. Application of CGP 36216, a selective antagonist for presynaptic $GABA_B$ receptors (Ong et al., 2001), prompted a decrease of the neuron's overall excitability, producing an increase of SSA (Figure 25.5D). This is thought to occur because $GABA_B$ receptors act as autoreceptors at GABAergic terminals in the rat IC (Ma et al., 2002; Zhang & Wu, 2000). Activation of presynaptic $GABA_B$ receptors suppresses GABAergic inhibition, augmenting the overall responsiveness of the neuron, leading to a decrease in the relative difference of standard and deviant responses. When $GABA_B$ presynaptic receptors are blocked by CGP 36216, the continuous release of GABA on SSA neurons decreases its firing rate, maximizing the relative contrast between standard and deviant responses, therefore augmenting SSA indices (Figure 25.5D; Ayala & Malmierca, 2018).

Another preparation used CGP 35348, an antagonist that blocks both pre- and post-synaptic $GABA_B$ receptors (Luo et al., 2011; Magnusson et al., 2008; Sun et al., 2006), but shows a much higher affinity for the post-synaptic ones (Stäubli et al., 1999). Interestingly, that kind of blockade of $GABA_B$-mediated inhibition prompted an

---

a tone (blue arrows) is expected to generate more GABA release than the rare and sparse appearance of that same tone (red arrows). In consequence, enough GABA (green circles) is released from the blue terminal as to deluge the synaptic cleft and spill over the extrasynaptic space, where postsynaptic $GABA_B$ receptors (in black) are allegedly allocated (Ayala & Malmierca, 2018). The chart in the middle presents the normal peristimulus time histogram of that SSA neuron. In the right, a blue curve describes the decay of the response to the standard stimulus along the oddball sequence. C. Microiontophoretic application of gabazine (magenta plectra) blocks $GABA_A$ receptors (in white), augmenting the excitability of the SSA neuron (purple line). This dampens the iceberg effect, thereby reducing the SSA index (middle chart). The adaptation of the response to the standard becomes slower almost immediately, and the maximum it can reach diminishes severely (magenta line in left chart). D. Microiontophoretic application of CGP 36216 (magenta plectra) blocks presynaptic $GABA_B$ autoreceptors (in black), impeding self-regulation of GABA release and thereby augmenting postsynaptic inhibition. As the excitability of the postsynaptic neuron diminishes, the iceberg effect is more pronounced, increasing the SSA index (middle chart). The accumulation of GABA in the synaptic cleft requires some time to yield effects on SSA emergence, as the initial decay of the standard response remains unaffected. However, the maximum adaptation level ameliorates in the late steady-state component (magenta line in left chart). E. Microiontophoretic application of CGP 35348 (magenta plectra) blocks $GABA_B$ postsynaptic receptors (in black). As only repetitive input elicited enough GABA release as to spill over the synaptic cleft and reach extrasynaptic receptors, the reduced amount of inhibition will differentially increase the response to the standard condition, reducing the overall SSA index (middle chart). Rare tones did not elicit enough GABA release as to reach extrasynaptic receptors in the first place, so the blockade of such receptors would not elicit significant effects over the deviant response. As $GABA_B$ receptors are metabotropic and extrasynaptic, they require some time to reach and activate. Therefore, the blockade does not affect the initial decay of the standard response, but it dampens the maximum adaptation level reached in the late steady-state component (magenta line in left chart).

increase in the response to the standard tones that did not affect the response to the deviant ones, therefore reducing the total amount of SSA (Figure 25.5E). This selective effect can be explained by assuming that $GABA_B$ postsynaptic receptors on SSA neurons are mainly allocated extrasynaptically. Repetitive stimulation would generate larger amounts of GABA release than rare tones, which end up saturating the synaptic cleft. The spillovers would get to reach the additional extrasynaptic $GABA_B$ receptors. Therefore, blocking those $GABA_B$ postsynaptic receptors only diminishes the adaptation to the repetitive sound, and not the rare one (Figure 25.5E; Ayala & Malmierca, 2018).

Glycine-mediated inhibition displayed subtle paradoxical effects depending on the strength of SSA to different sets of frequencies in each partially-adapting neuron. Injections of strychnine, an antagonist of ionotropic glycine receptors, caused particular areas within the receptive field that showed strong levels of SSA to decrease it, while provoking enhancements of the salience of deviant responses in other areas with partial levels of SSA. This dual effect could be due to the differential effect of glycine in different parts of the receptive field of the IC neurons (Williams & Fuzessery, 2011), or a co-expression with other kinds of inputs in a frequency-dependent manner (e.g., with GABA for low intensities). The spread of strychnine in the surroundings of the SSA neuron, affecting also its sources of inputs, could be another possibility accounting for these paradoxical effects (Ayala & Malmierca, 2018). In any case, glycinergic receptors are expressed mainly in the ventral part of the central nucleus of the IC (Choy Buentello et al., 2015; Merchán et al., 2005), where SSA levels are weaker. Therefore, the implication of glycinergic inhibition in the generation of SSA must be secondary, if any.

Finally, this study tried all mixed inhibitory effects by co-applying different combinations of $GABA_A$, $GABA_B$ and glycinergic antagonists to block multiple receptors types at the same time. The augmented effects observed showed that the relative increase in neuronal responsiveness mostly affected the response to repetitive stimuli, and not all the sound-evoked responses. $GABA_A$-mediated inhibition proved to exert the most evident and profound modulatory effect on the SSA. Since $GABA_A$ receptor are ionotropic, their blockade rapidly affected the SSA time course from the beginning (Figure 25.5C). On the other hand, $GABA_B$ receptors are metabotropic, necessarily slower since they are coupled to ion channels through second messengers (Mott, 2015). Thus, $GABA_B$-mediated inhibition antagonists subtly affected the late steady-state component of the SSA time course only (Figure 25.5D, E), leaving the initial fast decay of the standard response untouched (Ayala & Malmierca, 2018).

In conclusion, local inhibition could account for about half of the relative difference between standard and deviant responses, therefore acting as an important modulator of SSA in the IC. Notwithstanding, inhibition alone could not fully account for SSA emergence, so other mechanisms must be contributing to its generation (Ayala & Malmierca, 2018; Pérez-González & Malmierca, 2012).

The Role of Acetylcholine: Enhancing Repetition Sensitivity

Cholinergic projections are known to play and important role in arousal, attention, and memory. MMN literature suggests that cholinergic modulation favors the encoding of ongoing stimulation (Hasselmo & McGaughy, 2004; Jääskeläinen et al., 2007; Moran et al., 2013; Sarter et al., 2005) and that it enhances responses to afferent sensory input in the auditory cortex (Hsieh et al. 2000; Metherate & Ashe 1993). In consequence, there is a possibility that acetylcholine (ACh) could be playing an important role in SSA.

This hypothesis was tested in the rat IC (Ayala & Malmierca, 2015) using microiontophoretic applications of Ach chloride to activate the two main kinds of cholinergic receptors: Nicotinic (ionotropic) and muscarinic (metabotropic) receptors. The infusion of the cholinergic agonist provoked a decrease in SSA levels on partially adapting neurons, whereas leaving the excitability of non-adapting neurons and novelty neurons mostly unaffected. SSA reduction affected the late steady-state component of its time course, and it was caused by a differential increase in the response to repetitive stimulation that did not generalized to the deviant responses (as in Figure 25.5E, middle and right charts). A decrease in SSA prompted by cholinergic input is coherent with the lower levels of SSA observed in awake animals (von der Behrens et al., 2009; Duque et al., 2014) in which ACh concentrations are higher (Kametani & Kawamura, 1990; Marrosu et al., 1995). Therefore, it is apparent that cholinergic modulation in the IC contributes to persistence of the encoding of repetitive acoustic stimulation by decreasing adaptation to high probability sounds.

In addition, preparations with antagonists for the two types of cholinergic receptors were also injected. Scopolamine was used for blocking muscarinic receptors, and mecamylamine for the nicotinic receptors. As expected, affected neurons tended to augment their SSA levels for both cholinergic antagonists. Notwithstanding, only scopolamine exhibited a significant increase of SSA at population level, implying a prominent role in cholinergic modulation of muscarinic receptors, most likely via M1-receptor subtype (Ayala & Malmierca, 2015). The activation of the M1-type receptor induces changes in potassium conductance that could act as an activity-dependent adaptation mechanism (Abolafia et al., 2011; Sánchez-Vives et al., 2000a, 2000b), making K^+-mediated adaptation a potential mechanism underlying SSA (Abolafia et al., 2011; Ayala & Malmierca, 2015; Malmierca et al., 2014).

The Role of Endocannabinoids: Modulating the Modulators

Unlike most neurotransmitters, endocannabinoids action is mostly presynaptic, and they are not stored in vesicles but rather synthesized "on demand," when and where they are needed (Mechoulam & Parker, 2013). The release of endocannabinoids can be stimulated by activity-dependent mechanisms (Di et al., 2005) and they play a role in short-term neural plasticity (Castillo et al., 2012), so their retrograde signaling could be also involved in the modulation of SSA (Figure 25.6A).

This was demonstrated by the application of two different agonists of CB1 cannabinoid receptors, anandamide (intravenously) and O-2545 (microiontophoretically), during the oddball paradigm (Valdés-Baizabal et al., 2017). Both systemic and local injections prompted a decrease of SSA in a subset of neurons in the rat IC, exerting its effects in the late steady-state component of the adaptation. This reduction was caused by the increased response to the standard condition, while the spike count of the deviant response remained unaffected (Figure 25.6B). The blockade of CB1 receptors, via microiontophoretic application of the antagonist AM251, leads to non-significant population effects. Nevertheless, there was a coherent tendency of some neurons to decrease their firing rate in response to the standard stimulus, increasing SSA levels in those neurons (Valdés-Baizabal et al., 2017).

Retrograde regulation of inhibitory and excitatory inputs by cannabinoids is found along the auditory pathway for both glutamatergic and GABAergic synapses (Zhao et al., 2009), describing a protective mechanism that could modulate SSA. Neurons in the IC displaying cannabinoid-mediated modulation of SSA probably receive inhibitory input from GABAergic neurons expressing CB1 receptors in their presynaptic terminals (Figure 25.6A; Merchán et al., 2005). The injection of CB1 agonists would decrease GABA release of presynaptic inhibitory neurons, exerting especially significant effects in the postsynaptic response to the standard condition, insofar as the repetitive stimulation is expected to elicit much more GABA release than rare tones (Figure 25.6B).

Mixed and complex interactions of the endocannabinoid system with other neuromodulators could be also at play. In any case, the capacity of the endocannabinoid system to exert modulation on SSA would depend on the strength and nature of the inputs that each adapting neuron receives (Valdés-Baizabal et al., 2017).

The Effects of Anesthesia: SSA During Deep Sleep

Most experiments on SSA are performed under anesthesia. The most common preparation uses urethane, for its stability and minimal disruptive impact on neuronal functioning (Hara & Harris, 2002; Maggi & Meli, 1986; Sceniak & MacIver, 2006). Some studies even show that the effects of moderate urethane doses on neurotransmission mimic those of natural sleep (Clement et al., 2008; Pagliardini et al., 2012, 2013). When compared, SSA levels in the IC of anaesthetized and awake rodents seem rather similar (Duque & Malmierca, 2015; Parras et al., 2017), confirming the automatic nature of SSA as a hardwired redundancy-filter.

Notwithstanding, both preparations are not identical, being the most obvious difference the drastic reduction of spontaneous neuronal activity caused by anesthesia (Duque & Malmierca, 2015; Parras et al., 2017). Such quietening of spontaneous activity

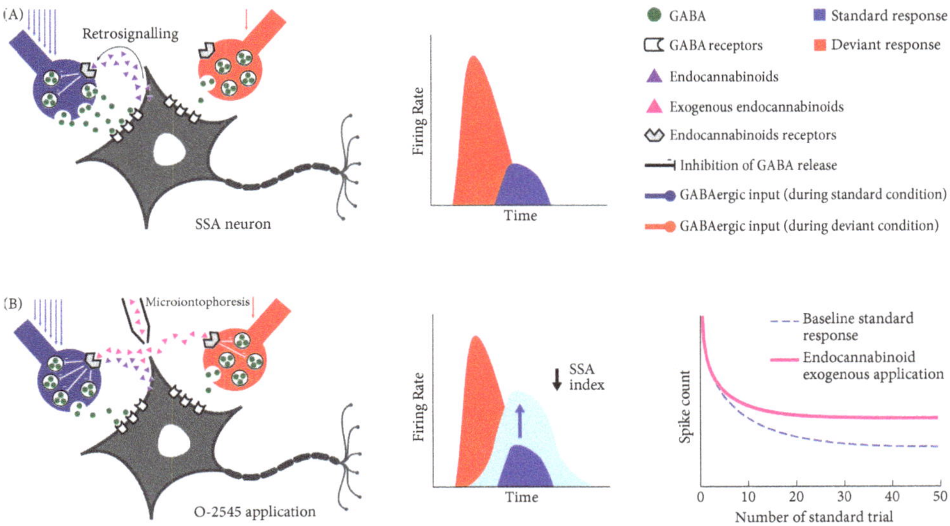

FIGURE 25.6. Endocannabinoid regulation of GABA release modulates SSA. **A.** A model of an SSA neuron (in gray) receiving GABAergic inhibition elicited by a given tone. The red GABAergic terminal represents the GABA release when such a tone is presented as a deviant, whereas the blue GABAergic terminal represents the GABA release when the same tone is presented as a standard. The repetitive input is expected to release much more GABA than rare tones. In consequence, the presynaptic neuron will synthesize "on demand" endocannabinoids (purple triangles) to regulate the excessive release of GABA elicited by the standard condition. **B.** The injection of exogenous endocannabinoids (magenta triangles) will enhance the inhibition of GABA release. As the deviant condition was prompting less GABA release, the effects of exogenous endocannabinoids may pass unnoticed. In the standard condition, however, the inhibition of GABA release will significantly disinhibit the response to the repetitive input. Those differential effects will eventually lead to a decrease in the SSA index, as shown in the peristimulus time response (middle chart). The neuromodulatory effect over the metabotropic endocannabinoids would take some time to regulate GABA release and significantly reduce the strength of the adaptation to the standard tone, not altering the initial decay in the standard response but reducing the maximum reachable (magenta line in right chart).

may further provide perceptual salience to deviant events that might take place during sleep-like states. Therefore, SSA could have an essential role during sleep, which is further supported by the large body of evidence demonstrating the existence of human MMN during sleep (Atienza et al., 2001). One of the functional roles of the deviance detection system, associated to MMN and by SSA, is driving attention involuntarily to unexpected stimuli (Escera et al., 1998; Escera et al., 2000). So during sleep, SSA could preserve the ability to filter out potentially disturbing noises, and thereby improve resting. But likewise, in a background of minimal spontaneous activity, SSA can prompt arresting responses to deviant sounds that might reveal some danger, eventually triggering awakening.

Auditory Deviance Detection in the Human Midbrain

Once firmly demonstrated with the oddball paradigm that SSA has presence (Malmierca et al., 2009) and origin (Anderson & Malmierca, 2013) in the midbrain of animal models, the suggested connection between SSA and the MMN (Ulanovsky et al., 2003) indirectly implied that deviance detection activity in humans could have subcortical roots as well (Carbajal & Malmierca, 2018a; Escera & Malmierca, 2014; Malmierca et al., 2014). In spite of the great technical challenge of recording non-invasively and correctly locating the source of a signal originated in such profound regions of the brain, several studies have since tried to find traces of deviance detection activity coming from the human midbrain.

Initial attempts to observe deviance detection used simple tones to analyze the classic auditory brainstem response (ABR) of the human ERP. No differences between standard and deviant tones could be identified at wave V (Althen et al., 2011; Slabu et al., 2010), which is the portion of the ABR that is thought to be generated in the IC (Picton, 2010; Stockard et al., 1979). Since SSA is present in the IC of animal models, contextual differences in wave V could be expected. However, the very short latency of the wave V (5–10 ms) contrasts with the timing of the changes in the firing rate observed at neuronal level in the IC, which spans throughout the first 20–30 ms (Malmierca et al., 2009; Pérez-González et al., 2005). This short latency of wave V indicates that it may be generated in the lemniscal portion of the IC, the central nucleus, where SSA population levels are rather low, when significant.

Using consonant–vowel vocalizations (Figure 25.7A) to build the oddball sequence made possible to elicit a "complex" ABR (Slabu et al., 2012; Skoe & Kraus, 2010). Contextual differences were detectable at the frequency-following responses (FFR; Figure 25.7B) that come after wave V (Shiga et al., 2015; Skoe et al., 2014; Slabu et al., 2012), indicating that the human midbrain is indeed contributing to deviance detection (Figure 25.7C). Research based in FFR analysis had for long emphasized an active and critical involvement of the brainstem in auditory plasticity regarding complex forms of sound processing (for review see Chandrasekaran et al., 2014). However, these claims might have been overestimated, since recent studies have discovered varying but significant cortical contributions to FFR, at least for eliciting stimuli of low fundamental frequency (F0) circa 100 Hz (Bidelman, 2018; Coffey et al., 2016, 2017), and therefore FFR evidence cannot be solely imputed to brainstem activity. Notwithstanding, deviance detection in the human IC has been also confirmed using fMRI (Cacciaglia et al., 2015), which could dissipate any possible doubts about the contribution of the human midbrain to the perceptual saliency of rare stimuli (Figure 25.8).

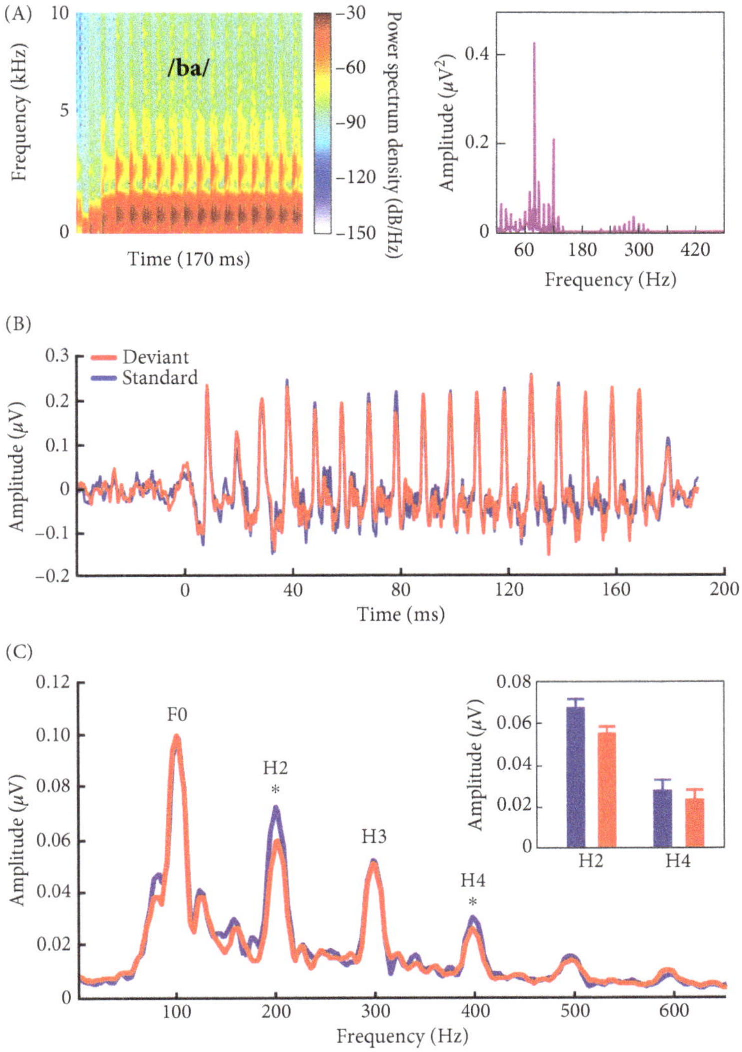

FIGURE 25.7. Deviance detection elicited in human auditory brainstem response by complex stimuli, adapted from Slabu et al. (2012). **A.** Spectrogram (left) and frequency spectrum (right) of the /ba/ syllable used in an oddball sequence together with different /wa/ vocalizations (not shown). **B.** Grand-average of the FFR elicited by the standard and deviant presentations of the /ba/ syllable. C. FFR spectrum of the /ba/ syllable, showing a significant difference between conditions in the amplitude of the second (H2) and fourth (H4) harmonics.

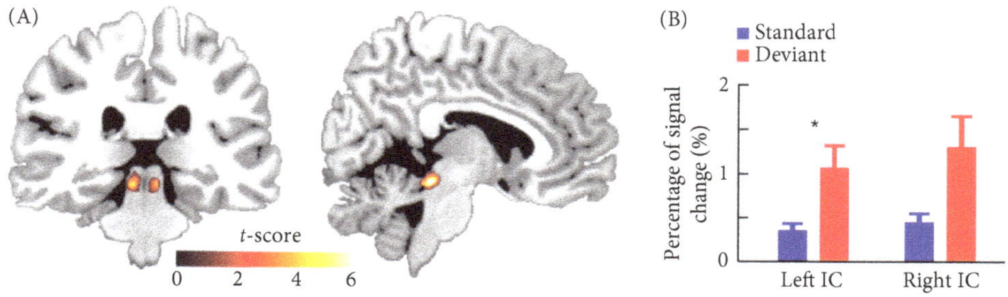

FIGURE 25.8. Deviance detection in the human IC shown in fMRI, adapted from Cacciaglia et al. (2015). **A.** For a contrast between standard and deviant conditions, the region of interest analysis revealed a significant activation of the left IC. **B.** Percentage of signal change.

Future Directions: Predictive Coding in the Auditory Midbrain

The proposal of cortical SSA as the neuronal correlate of the MMN (Ulanovsky et al., 2003) meant a great breakthrough in deviance detection research, boosting its exploration from a neurophysiological perspective, and improving our understanding of the early stages of perception emergence (Escera & Malmierca, 2014; Malmierca et al., 2014). However, the MMN clearly exceeds the explanatory potential of SSA as currently defined. The MMN can be elicited by any violation of an established regularity in the flow of stimulus (Winkler & Schröger, 2015). This includes even complex regularities that are well beyond the standard repetition featuring in the oddball paradigm. Even in sequences organized by abstract rules (e.g., tone pairs where the first tone can have any frequency but the second tone is always higher in pitch), the occurrence of deviant events (e.g., the second tone turns out to be lower in pitch) can prompt an MMN, something impossible to account for in terms of SSA. Whereas all SSA reflects a process of deviance detection at cellular level, deviance detection beyond sheer repetition cannot emerge from SSA as currently defined. Therefore, if MMN and SSA are indeed related, SSA must be just a specific manifestation of a more general mechanism of deviance detection. These limitations have encouraged a revision of SSA data from a more global approach, capable of accounting for MMN evidence as well. A new common framework arises based on the predictive coding theory (Carbajal & Malmierca, 2018a).

The predictive coding theory interprets the brain basically as a generative mechanism of Bayesian hierarchical inference (Friston, 2005; Friston, 2009). According to this general theory of neuronal function, higher-order processing stations send predictions (or expectations) to lower hierarchical levels based on a model extracted from the regularities in the flow of stimuli. The aim is to reduce or suppress any ascending input that can be anticipated by the perceptual model already represented in the system, in order to save processing resources. The suppressive effects on the firing rate of the neurons are resultant of short-term plasticity changes, exerted through mechanisms like synaptic adaptation. In turn, lower stations forward prediction errors to the higher hierarchical levels whenever their expectations fail, in order to favor the processing of those inputs that could not be anticipated, and mobilize resources to update the perceptual model. Hence, perception emerges from a dynamic multilevel interaction between top-down expectations and bottom-up prediction errors.

Based on the aforementioned, we can explain deviance detection resultant of the violation of both simple (repetition) and complex regularities (abstract rules). In the case of the oddball sequence, the representation of the repeating standard stimulus will quickly generate top-down predictions (i.e., "the upcoming stimulus will be similar to the previous one encoded"), efficiently explaining away the ascending sensory input and suppressing prediction error. But when the random deviant appears, its unpredictable occurrence will release the bottom-up input from suppression and forward a prediction error signal prompting an update of the predictive model. Hence, from a predictive coding standpoint, SSA would result from two processes: repetition suppression affecting the standard response, and prediction error emerging from deviances (Carbajal & Malmierca, 2018a). This has been empirically confirmed in a recent study, where it was possible to disentangle both components in the IC of anaesthetized rats and awake mice (Parras et al., 2017) using control conditions directly borrowed from MMN methodology for human research (Ruhnau et al., 2012). Prediction errors were only detected in the IC cortices, the parts which receive the strongest descending inputs from neocortex (Malmierca & Ryugo, 2011). Furthermore, a very recent study suggests that the IC could indeed have an important role in the early processing of complex regularities (Malmierca et al., 2018).

Hence, predictive coding provides a common framework to study both SSA and MMN as respectively the microscopic and macroscopic measurements of the same deviance detection mechanism, which generative roots can be trace down to the midbrain. The cortices of the IC are the first auditory nuclei to display such sophisticated predictive processing, as part of a larger multilevel modelling network. All of which highlights the pivotal role that the midbrain plays in the composition of meaningful perceptual representations of complex acoustic events. As a general conclusion, taking into account all the evidence discussed throughout this chapter, there is no doubt that the auditory midbrain is endowed with wondrous processing capacities, and its function is definitely more important in the attainment of complex and refined auditory perceptions than previous literature estimated.

Acknowledgments

Manuel S. Malmierca and Guillermo V. Carbajal have contributed equally. This work has been funded by Spanish MINECO (SAF2016-75803-P) and The European Union's Horizon 2020 research and innovation programme under the Marie Skłodowska-Curie grant agreement No 722098 (ITN-MCSA-LISTEN) to MSM and by MINECO/FEDER

(PSI2015-63664-P), the Generalitat de Catalunya (SGR2017-974), and the ICREA Acadèmia Distinguished Professorship award to CE. GVC held a fellowship from the Spanish MICINN (BES-2017-080030).

References

Abbott, L. F., Varela, J. A., Sen, K., & Nelson, S. B. (1997). Synaptic depression and cortical gain control. *Science*, 275(5297), 221–224. doi: 10.1126/science.275.5297.221

Abolafia, J. M., Vergara, R., Arnold, M. M., Reig, R., & Sánchez-Vives, M. V. (2011). Cortical auditory adaptation in the awake rat and the role of potassium currents. *Cerebral Cortex*, 21(5), 977–990. doi: 10.1093/cercor/bhq163

Alho, K. (1995). Cerebral generators of mismatch negativity (MMN) and its magnetic counterpart (MMNm) elicited by sound changes. *Ear and Hearing*, 16(1), 38–51.

Althen, H., Grimm, S., & Escera, C. (2011). Fast detection of unexpected sound intensity decrements as revealed by human evoked potentials. *PLoS ONE*, 6(12). doi: 10.1371/journal.pone.0028522

Anderson, L. A., Christianson, G. B., & Linden, J. F. (2009). Stimulus-specific adaptation occurs in the auditory thalamus. *Journal of Neuroscience*, 29(22), 7359–7363. doi: 10.1523/JNEUROSCI.0793-09.2009

Anderson, L. A., & Malmierca, M. S. (2013). The effect of auditory cortex deactivation on stimulus-specific adaptation in the inferior colliculus of the rat. *European Journal of Neuroscience*, 37(1), 52–62. doi: 10.1111/ejn.12018

Antunes, F. M., & Malmierca, M. S. (2011). Effect of auditory cortex deactivation on stimulus-specific adaptation in the medial geniculate body. *Journal of Neuroscience*, 31(47), 17306–17316. doi: 10.1523/JNEUROSCI.1915-11.2011

Antunes, F. M., & Malmierca, M. S. (2014). An overview of stimulus-specific adaptation in the auditory thalamus. *Brain Topography*, 27(4), 480–499. doi: 10.1007/s10548-013-0342-6

Antunes, F. M., Nelken, I., Covey, E., & Malmierca, M. S. (2010). Stimulus-specific adaptation in the auditory thalamus of the anesthetized rat. *PLoS ONE*, 5(11). e14071. doi: 10.1371/journal.pone.0014071

Atienza, M., Cantero, J. L., & Escera, C. (2001). Auditory information processing during human sleep as revealed by event-related brain potentials, *Clinical Neurophysiology*, 112/11: 2031–2045. doi: 10.1016/S1388-2457(01)00650-2

Ayala, Y. A., & Malmierca, M. S. (2015). Cholinergic modulation of stimulus-specific adaptation in the inferior colliculus. *Journal of Neuroscience*, 35(35), 12261–12272. doi: 10.1523/JNEUROSCI.0909-15.2015

Ayala, Y. A., & Malmierca, M. S. (2018). The effect of inhibition on stimulus-specific adaptation in the inferior colliculus. *Brain Structure and Function*, 223(3), 1391–1407. doi: 10.1007/s00429-017-1546-4

Ayala, Y. A., Pérez-González, D., Duque, D., Nelken, I., & Malmierca, M. S. (2013). Frequency discrimination and stimulus deviance in the inferior colliculus and cochlear nucleus. *Frontiers in Neural Circuits*, 6, 119. doi: 10.3389/fncir.2012.00119

Ayala, Y. A., Udeh, A., Dutta, K., Bishop, D., Malmierca, M. S., & Oliver, D. L. (2015). Differences in the strength of cortical and brainstem inputs to SSA and non-SSA neurons in the inferior colliculus. *Scientific Reports*, 5(April), 10383. DOI: 10.1038/srep10383 von der Behrens, W., Bauerle, P., Kossl, M., & Gaese, B. H. (2009). Correlating stimulus-specific adaptation of cortical neurons and local field potentials in the awake rat. *Journal of Neuroscience*, 29(44), 13837–13849. doi: 10.1523/JNEUROSCI.3475-09.2009

Bibikov, N. G. (1977). ['Novelty' neurons in the frog auditory system]. *Zh Vyssh Nerv Deiat Im I P Pavlova*, 27(5), 1075–1082.

Bidelman, G. M. (2018). Subcortical sources dominate the neuroelectric auditory frequency-following response to speech. *NeuroImage*, 175, 56–69. doi: 10.1016/j.neuroimage.2018.03.060

Cacciaglia, R., Escera, C., Slabu, L., Grimm, S., Sanjuán, A., Ventura-Campos, N., & Ávila, C. (2015). Involvement of the human midbrain and thalamus in auditory deviance detection. *Neuropsychologia*, 68, 51–58. doi: 10.1016/j.neuropsychologia.2015.01.001

Carandini, M., & Ferster, D. (1997). A tonic hyperpolarization underlying contrast adaptation in cat visual cortex. *Science*, 276(5314), 949–952. doi: 10.1126/science.276.5314.949

Carbajal, G. V., & Malmierca, M. S. (2018a). The neuronal basis of predictive coding along the auditory pathway: From the subcortical roots to cortical deviance detection. *Trends in Hearing*, 22, 233121651878482. https://doi.org/10.1177/2331216518784822

Carbajal, G. V., & Malmierca, M. S. (2018b). The unique role of the non-lemniscal pathway on stimulus-specific adaptation (SSA) in the auditory system. In Santurette S., Dau T., Dalsgaard J., Tranebjærg L., Andersen T., & Poulsen T. (eds.), *Proceedings of the International Symposium on Auditory and Audiological Research* (Vol. 6, pp. 95–106). Nyborg, Denmark: The Danavox Jubilee Foundation.

Castillo, P. E., Younts, T. J., Chávez, A. E., & Hashimotodani, Y. (2012). Endocannabinoid signaling and synaptic function. *Neuron*, 76(1), 70–81. doi: 10.1016/J.NEURON.2012.09.020

Chandrasekaran, B., Skoe, E., & Kraus, N. (2014). An integrative model of subcortical auditory plasticity. *Brain Topography*, 27(4), 539–552. doi: 10.1007/s10548-013-0323-9

Choy Buentello, D., Bishop, D. C., & Oliver, D. L. (2015). Differential distribution of GABA and glycine terminals in the inferior colliculus of rat and mouse. *Journal of Comparative Neurology*, 523(18), 2683–2697. doi: 10.1002/cne.23810

Clement, E. A., Richard, A., Thwaites, M., Ailon, J., Peters, S., & Dickson, C. T. (2008). Cyclic and sleep-like spontaneous alternations of brain state under urethane anaesthesia. *PLoS ONE*, 3(4): e2004. doi: 10.1371/journal.pone.0002004

Coffey, E. B. J., Herholz, S. C., Chepesiuk, A. M. P., Baillet, S., & Zatorre, R. J. (2016). Cortical contributions to the auditory frequency-following response revealed by MEG. *Nature Communications*, 7, 11070. doi: 10.1038/ncomms11070

Coffey, E. B. J., Musacchia, G., & Zatorre, R. J. (2017). Cortical correlates of the auditory frequency-following and onset responses: EEG and fMRI evidence. *Journal of Neuroscience*, 37(4). 830–838. doi: 10.1523/JNEUROSCI.1265-16.2017

Di, S., Boudaba, C., Popescu, I. R., Weng, F. J., Harris, C., Marcheselli, V. L., Bazan, N. G., et al. (2005). Activity-dependent release and actions of endocannabinoids in the rat hypothalamic supraoptic nucleus. *Journal of Physiology*, 569(3), 751–760. doi: 10.1113/jphysiol.2005.097477

Duque, D., & Malmierca, M. S. (2015). Stimulus-specific adaptation in the inferior colliculus of the mouse: Anesthesia and spontaneous activity effects. *Brain Structure and Function*, 220(6), 3385–3398. doi: 10.1007/s00429-014-0862-1

Duque, D., Malmierca, M. S., & Caspary, D. M. (2014). Modulation of stimulus-specific adaptation by GABAA receptor activation or blockade in the medial geniculate body of the anaesthetized rat. *Journal of Physiology*, 592(4), 729–743. doi: 10.1113/jphysiol.2013.261941

Duque, D., Perez-Gonzalez, D., Ayala, Y. A., Palmer, A. R., & Malmierca, M. S. (2012). Topographic distribution, frequency, and intensity dependence of stimulus-specific adaptation in the inferior colliculus of the rat. *Journal of Neuroscience*, 32(49), 17762–17774. doi: 10.1523/JNEUROSCI.3190-12.2012

Duque, D., Pais, R., & Malmierca M.S. (2018). Stimulus-specific adaptation in the anesthetized mouse revealed by brainstem auditory evoked potentials. *Hearing Research.* In press. doi: 10.1016/j.heares.2018.08.011.

Duque, D., Wang, X., Nieto-Diego, J., Krumbholz, K., & Malmierca, M. S. (2016). Neurons in the inferior colliculus of the rat show stimulus-specific adaptation for frequency, but not for intensity. *Scientific Reports*, 6(1), 24114. doi: 10.1038/srep24114

Escera, C., Alho, K., Winkler, I., & Näätänen, R. (1998). 'Neural mechanisms of involuntary attention to acoustic novelty and change', *Journal of Cognitive Neuroscience*, 10/5: 590–604. doi: 10.1162/089892998562997

Escera, C., Alho, K., Schröger, E., & Winkler, I. (2000). 'Involuntary attention and distractibility as evaluated with event-related brain potentials', *Audiology and Neuro-Otology*, 5/3–4: 151–166. doi: 10.1159/000013877

Escera, C., & Malmierca, M. S. (2014). The auditory novelty system: An attempt to integrate human and animal research. *Psychophysiology*, 51(2), 111–123. doi: 10.1111/psyp.12156

Faure, P. A., Fremouw, T., Casseday, J. H., & Covey, E. (2003). Temporal masking reveals properties of sound-evoked inhibition in duration-tuned neurons of the inferior colliculus. *Journal of Neuroscience*, 23(7): 3052–3065. doi: 23/7/3052 [pii]

Feng, A. S., Hall, J. C., & Siddique, S. (1991). Coding of temporal parameters of complex sounds by frog auditory nerve fibers. *Journal of Neurophysiology*, 65(3), 424–445. doi: 10.1152/jn.1991.65.3.424

Finlayson, P. G., & Adam, T. J. (1997). Excitatory and inhibitory response adaptation in the superior olive complex affects binaural acoustic processing. *Hearing Research*, 103(1–2), 1–18. doi: 10.1016/S0378-5955(96)00158-X

Friston, K. (2005). A theory of cortical responses. *Philosophical Transactions of the Royal Society B: Biological Sciences*, 360(1456), 815–836. doi: 10.1098/rstb.2005.1622

Friston, K. (2009). The free-energy principle: a rough guide to the brain? *Trends in Cognitive Sciences*, 13(7), 293–301. doi: 10.1016/j.tics.2009.04.005

Gao, P. P., Zhang, J. W., Cheng, J. S., Zhou, I. Y., & Wu, E. X. (2014). The inferior colliculus is involved in deviant sound detection as revealed by BOLD fMRI. *NeuroImage*, 91, 220–227. doi: 10.1016/j.neuroimage.2014.01.043

Gutfreund, Y. (2012). Stimulus-specific adaptation, habituation and change detection in the gaze control system. *Biological Cybernetics*, 106(11–12), 657–668. doi: 10.1007/s00422-012-0497-3

Hara, K., & Harris, R. A. (2002). The anesthetic mechanism of urethane: The effects on neurotransmitter-gated ion channels. *Anesthesia and Analgesia*, 94(2), 313–318. doi: 10.1213/00000539-200202000-00015

Hasselmo, M. E., & McGaughy, J. (2004). High acetylcholine levels set circuit dynamics for attention and encoding and low acetylcholine levels set dynamics for consolidation. *Progress in Brain Research*, 145, 207–231. doi: 10.1016/S0079-6123(03)45015-2

Herrmann, B., Parthasarathy, A., Han, E. X., Obleser, J., & Bartlett, E. L. (2015). Sensitivity of rat inferior colliculus neurons to frequency distributions. *Journal of Neurophysiology*, 114(5), 2941–2954. doi: 10.1152/jn.00555.2015

Hershenhoren, I., Taaseh, N., Antunes, F. M., & Nelken, I. (2014). Intracellular correlates of stimulus-specific adaptation. *Journal of Neuroscience*, 34(9), 3303–3319. doi: 10.1523/JNEUROSCI.2166-13.2014

Hsieh, C. Y., Cruikshank, S. J., & Metherate, R. (2000). Differential modulation of auditory thalamocortical and intracortical synaptic transmission by cholinergic agonist. *Brain Research*, 880(1–2), 51–64. doi: 10.1016/S0006-8993(00)02766-9

Ingham, N. J., & McAlpine, D. (2004). Spike-frequency adaptation in the inferior colliculus. *Journal of Neurophysiology*, 91(2), 632–645. doi: 10.1152/jn.00779.2003

Isaacson, J. S., & Scanziani, M. (2011). How inhibition shapes cortical activity. *Neuron*, 72(2), 231–243. doi: 10.1016/j.neuron.2011.09.027

Ito, T., & Malmierca, M. S. (2018). Neurons, connections, and microcircuits of the inferior colliculus. In D. Oliver, N. Cant, R. Fay, & A. Popper (eds.), *The Mammalian Auditory Pathways* (pp. 127–167). doi: 10.1007/978-3-319-71798-2_6

Jääskeläinen, I. P., Ahveninen, J., Belliveau, J. W., Raij, T., & Sams, M. (2007). Short-term plasticity in auditory cognition. *Trends in Neurosciences*, 30(12), 653–661 doi: 10.1016/j.tins.2007.09.003

Kametani, H., & Kawamura, H. (1990). Alterations in acetylcholine release in the rat hippocampus during sleep-wakefulness detected by intracerebral dialysis. *Life Sciences*, 47(5), 421–426. DOI: 10.1016/0024-3205(90)90300-G

Lumani, A., & Zhang, H. (2010). Responses of neurons in the rat's dorsal cortex of the inferior colliculus to monaural tone bursts. *Brain Research*, 1351, 115–129. Elsevier. DOI: 10.1016/j.brainres.2010.06.066

Luo, B., Wang, H. T., Su, Y. Y., Wu, S. H., & Chen, L. (2011). Activation of presynaptic GABAB receptors modulates GABAergic and glutamatergic inputs to the medial geniculate body. *Hearing Research*, 280(1–2), 157–165. DOI: 10.1016/j.heares.2011.05.018

Ma, C. L., Kelly, J. B., & Wu, S. H. (2002). Presynaptic modulation of GABAergic inhibition by GABAB receptors in the rat's inferior colliculus. *Neuroscience*, 114(1), 207–215. DOI: 10.1016/S0306-4522(02)00130-6

Maggi, C. A., & Meli, A. (1986). Suitability of urethane anesthesia for physiopharmacological investigations in various systems. Part 1: General considerations. *Experientia*, 42(2), 109–114. *DOI*: 10.1007/BF01952426

Magnusson, A. K., Park, T. J., Pecka, M., Grothe, B., & Koch, U. (2008). Retrograde GABA signaling adjusts sound localization by balancing excitation and inhibition in the brainstem. *Neuron*, 59(1), 125–137. doi: 10.1016/j.neuron.2008.05.011

Malmierca, M. S., Anderson, L. A., & Antunes, F. M. (2015). The cortical modulation of stimulus-specific adaptation in the auditory midbrain and thalamus: A potential neuronal correlate for predictive coding. *Frontiers in Systems Neuroscience*, 9(March: 19). doi: 10.3389/fnsys.2015.00019

Malmierca, M. S., Blackstad, T. W., & Osen, K. K. (2011). Computer-assisted 3-D reconstructions of Golgi-impregnated neurons in the cortical regions of the inferior colliculus of rat. *Hearing Research*, 274(1–2), 13–26. DOI: 10.1016/j.heares.2010.06.011

Malmierca, M. S., Blackstad, T. W., Osen, K. K., Karagülle, T., & Molowny, R. L. (1993). The central nucleus of the inferior colliculus in rat: A Golgi and computer reconstruction study of neuronal and laminar structure. *Journal of Comparative Neurology*, 333(1), 1–27. doi: 10.1002/cne.903330102

Malmierca, M. S., Cristaudo, S., Perez-Gonzalez, D., Covey, E., Pérez-González, D., & Covey, E. (2009). Stimulus-specific adaptation in the inferior colliculus of the anesthetized rat. *Journal of Neuroscience*, 29(17), 5483–5493. doi: 10.1523/JNEUROSCI.4153-08.2009

Malmierca, M. S., Izquierdo, M. A., Cristaudo, S., Hernandez, O., Perez-Gonzalez, D., Covey, E., & Oliver, D. L. (2008). A discontinuous tonotopic organization in the inferior colliculus of the rat. *Journal of Neuroscience*, 28(18). 4767–4776. doi: 10.1523/JNEUROSCI.0238-08.2008

Malmierca, M. S., Niño-Aguillón, B. E., Nieto-Diego, J., Porteros, Á., Pérez-González, D., & Escera, C. (2018). Pattern-sensitive neurons reveal encoding of complex auditory regularities in the rat inferior colliculus. *NeuroImage*. In press. doi: 10.1016/j.neuroimage.2018.10.012

Malmierca, M. S., Rees, A., Le Beau, F. E. N., & Bjaalie, J. G. (1995). Laminar organization of frequency-defined local axons within and between the inferior colliculi of the guinea pig. *Journal of Comparative Neurology*, 357(1), 124–144. Wiley-Blackwell. doi: 10.1002/cne.903570112

Malmierca, M. S., & Ryugo, D. K. (2011). 'Descending connections of auditory cortex to the midbrain and brain stem'. Winer J. A. & Schreiner C. E. (eds) *The Auditory Cortex*, 1st ed., pp. 189–208. Springer US: Boston, MA. doi: 10.1007/978-1-4419-0074-6

Malmierca, M. S., Sánchez-Vives, M. V, Escera, C., & Bendixen, A. (2014). Neuronal adaptation, novelty detection and regularity encoding in audition. *Frontiers in Systems Neuroscience*, 8(June), 111. doi: 10.3389/fnsys.2014.00111

Malone, B. J., & Semple, M. N. (2001). Effects of auditory stimulus context on the representation of frequency in the gerbil inferior colliculus. *Journal of Neurophysiology*, 86(3), 1113–1130.

Marrosu, F., Portas, C., Mascia, M. S., Casu, M. A., Fà, M., Giagheddu, M., Imperato, A., et al. (1995). Microdialysis measurement of cortical and hippocampal acetylcholine release during sleep-wake cycle in freely moving cats. *Brain Research*, 671(2), 329–332. doi: 10.1016/0006-8993(94)01399-3

Mechoulam, R., & Parker, L. A. (2013). The endocannabinoid system and the brain. *Annual Review of Psychology*, 64, 21–47. doi: 10.1146/annurev-psych-113011-143739

Merchán, M., Aguilar, L. A., Lopez-Poveda, E. A., & Malmierca, M. S. (2005). The inferior colliculus of the rat: Quantitative immunocytochemical study of GABA and glycine. *Neuroscience*, 136(3), 907–925. Pergamon. doi: 10.1016/j.neuroscience.2004.12.030

Metherate, R., & Ashe, J. H. (1993). Nucleus basalis stimulation facilitates thalamocortical synaptic transmission in the rat auditory cortex. *Synapse*, 14(2), 132–143. doi: 10.1002/syn.890140206

Moran, R. J., Campo, P., Symmonds, M., Stephan, K. E., Dolan, R. J., & Friston, K. J. (2013). Free energy, precision and learning: The role of cholinergic neuromodulation. *Journal of Neuroscience*, 33(19), 8227–8236. doi: 10.1523/JNEUROSCI.4255-12.2013

Mott, D. (2015). The metabotropic GABAB receptors. In C. Hammond (ed.), *Cellular and molecular neurophysiology* (4th ed., pp. 245–269). Cambridge, MA: Academic Press.

Näätänen, R., Gaillard, A. W. K., & Mäntysalo, S. (1978). Early selective-attention effect on evoked potential reinterpreted. *Acta Psychologica*, 42(4), 313–329. doi: 10.1016/0001-6918(78)90006-9

Näätänen, R., Kujala, T., Escera, C., Baldeweg, T., Kreegipuu, K., Carlson, S., & Ponton, C. (2012). The mismatch negativity (MMN): A unique window to disturbed central auditory processing in ageing and different clinical conditions. *Clinical Neurophysiology*, 123(3), 424–458. doi: 10.1016/j.clinph.2011.09.020

Näätänen, R., Paavilainen, P., Rinne, T., & Alho, K. (2007). The mismatch negativity (MMN) in basic research of central auditory processing: A review. *Clinical Neurophysiology*, 118(12), 2544–2590. doi: 10.1016/j.clinph.2007.04.026

Nelken, I., & Ulanovsky, N. (2007). Mismatch negativity and stimulus-specific adaptation in animal models. *Journal of Psychophysiology*, 21(3–4), 214–223. DOI: 10.1027/0269-8803.21.34.214

Netser, S., Zahar, Y., & Gutfreund, Y. (2011). Stimulus-specific adaptation: can it be a neural correlate of behavioral habituation? *Journal of Neuroscience*, 31(49), 17811–17820. doi: 10.1523/JNEUROSCI.4790-11.2011

Nieto-Diego, J., & Malmierca, M. S. (2016). Topographic distribution of stimulus-specific adaptation across auditory cortical fields in the anesthetized rat. *PLoS Biology*, 14(3): e1002397. doi: 10.1371/journal.pbio.1002397

Nomoto, M., Suga, N., & Katsuki, Y. (1964). Discharge pattern and inhibition of primary auditory nerve fibers in the monkey. *Journal of Neurophysiology*, 27, 768–787. doi: 10.1152/jn.1964.27.5.768

Ong, J., Bexis, S., Marino, V., Parker, D. A., & Froestl, W. (2001). CGP 36216 is a selective antagonist at GABAB presynaptic receptors in rat brain. *European Journal of Pharmacology*, 415(2–3), 191–195. doi: 10.1016/S0014-2999(01)00842-1

Pagliardini, S., Funk, G. D., & Dickson, C. T. (2013). Breathing and brain state: Urethane anesthesia as a model for natural sleep. *Respiratory Physiology and Neurobiology*, 188(3), 324–332. doi: 10.1016/j.resp.2013.05.035

Pagliardini, S., Greer, J. J., Funk, G. D., & Dickson, C. T. (2012). State-dependent modulation of breathing in urethane-anesthetized rats. *Journal of Neuroscience*, 32/33: 11259–11270. doi: 10.1523/JNEUROSCI.0948-12.2012

Parras, G. G., Nieto-Diego, J., Carbajal, G. V., Valdés-Baizabal, C., Escera, C., & Malmierca, M. S. (2017). Neurons along the auditory pathway exhibit a hierarchical organization of prediction error. *Nature Communications*, 8(1), 2148. doi: 10.1038/s41467-017-02038-6

Patel, C. R., Redhead, C., Cervi, A. L., & Zhang, H. (2012). Neural sensitivity to novel sounds in the rat's dorsal cortex of the inferior colliculus as revealed by evoked local field potentials. *Hearing Research*, 286(1–2), 41–54. doi: 10.1016/j.heares.2012.02.007

Pérez-González, D., Hernández, O., Covey, E., Malmierca, M. S., & Schulze, H. (2012). GABA A-mediated inhibition modulates stimulus-specific adaptation in the inferior colliculus. *PLoS ONE*, 7(3), e34297. doi: 10.1371/journal.pone.0034297

Pérez-González, D., & Malmierca, M. S. (2012). Variability of the time course of stimulus-specific adaptation in the inferior colliculus. *Frontiers in Neural Circuits*, 6, 107. doi: 10.3389/fncir.2012.00107

Pérez-González, D., Malmierca, M. S., & Covey, E. (2005). Novelty detector neurons in the mammalian auditory midbrain. *European Journal of Neuroscience*, 22(11), 2879–2885. doi: 10.1111/j.1460-9568.2005.04472.x

Picton, T. W. (2010). *Human auditory evoked potentials*. San Diego: Plural Publishing.

Reches, A., & Gutfreund, Y. (2008). Stimulus-specific adaptations in the gaze control system of the barn owl. *Journal of Neuroscience*, 28(6), 1523–1533. DOI: 10.1523/JNEUROSCI.3785-07.2008

Ruhnau, P., Herrmann, B., & Schröger, E. (2012). Finding the right control: The mismatch negativity under investigation. *Clinical Neurophysiology*, 123(3), 507–512. doi: 10.1016/j.clinph.2011.07.035

Sánchez-Vives, M. V., Nowak, L. G., & McCormick, D. A. (2000a). Membrane mechanisms underlying contrast adaptation in cat area 17 in vivo. *Journal of Neuroscience*, 20(11), 4267–4285. doi: 10.1523/JNEUROSCI.20-11-04267.2000

Sánchez-Vives, M. V., Nowak, L. G., & McCormick, D. A. (2000b). Cellular mechanisms of long-lasting adaptation in visual cortical neurons in vitro. *Journal of Neuroscience*, 20(11), 4286–4299. doi: 10.1523/JNEUROSCI.20-11-04286.2000

Sarter, M., Hasselmo, M. E., Bruno, J. P., & Givens, B. (2005). Unraveling the attentional functions of cortical cholinergic inputs: Interactions between signal-driven and cognitive modulation of signal detection. *Brain Research Reviews*, 48(1): 98–111. Elsevier. doi: 10.1016/j.brainresrev.2004.08.006

Sceniak, M. P., & MacIver, M. B. (2006). Cellular actions of urethane on rat visual cortical neurons in vitro. *Journal of Neurophysiology*, 95(6), 3865–3874. doi: 10.1152/jn.01196.2005

Shen, L., Zhao, L., & Hong, B. (2015). Frequency-specific adaptation and its underlying circuit model in the auditory midbrain. *Frontiers in Neural Circuits*, 9, 55. doi: 10.3389/fncir.2015.00055

Shiga, T., Althen, H., Cornella, M., Zarnowiec, K., Yabe, H., & Escera, C. (2015). Deviance-related responses along the auditory hierarchy: Combined FFR, MLR and MMN evidence. *PLoS ONE*, 10(9), 1–14. doi: 10.1371/journal.pone.0136794

Sivaramakrishnan, S., Sterbing-D'Angelo, S., Filipovic, B., D'Angelo, W., Oliver, D., & Kuwada, S. (2004). GABAA synapses shape neuronal responses to sound intensity in the inferior colliculus. *Journal of Neuroscience*, 24(21), 5031–5043. doi: 10.1523/JNEUROSCI.0357-04.2004

Skoe, E., Chandrasekaran, B., Spitzer, E. R., Wong, P. C. M., & Kraus, N. (2014). Human brainstem plasticity: The interaction of stimulus probability and auditory learning. *Neurobiology of Learning and Memory*, 109, 82–93. doi: 10.1016/j.nlm.2013.11.011

Skoe, E., & Kraus, N. (2010). Auditory brain stem response to complex sounds: A tutorial. *Ear and Hearing*, 31(3), 302–324. doi: 10.1097/AUD.0b013e3181cdb272

Slabu, L., Escera, C., Grimm, S., & Costa-Faidella, J. (2010). Early change detection in humans as revealed by auditory brainstem and middle-latency evoked potentials. *European Journal of Neuroscience*, 32(5), 859–865. doi: 10.1111/j.1460-9568.2010.07324.x

Slabu, L., Grimm, S., & Escera, C. (2012). Novelty detection in the human auditory brainstem. *Journal of Neuroscience*, 32(4), 1447–1452. doi: 32/4/1447 [pii]\r10.1523/JNEUROSCI.2557-11.2012

Stäubli, U., Scafidi, J., & Chun, D. (1999). GABAB receptor antagonism: Facilitatory effects on memory parallel those on LTP induced by TBS but not HFS. *Journal of Neuroscience*, 19(11) 4609–4615. doi: 10.1038/aps.2013.150

Stockard, J. J., Stockard, J. E., & Sharbrough, F. W. (1979). Brain-stem auditory-evoked responses. *Archives of Neurology*, 36(9), 597–598. doi: 10.1001/archneur.1979.00500450091025

Sumner, C. J., & Palmer, A. R. (2012). Auditory nerve fibre responses in the ferret. *European Journal of Neuroscience*, 36(4), 2428–2439.. doi: 10.1111/j.1460-9568.2012.08151.x

Sun, H., Ma, C. L., Kelly, J. B., & Wu, S. H. (2006). GABAB receptor-mediated presynaptic inhibition of glutamatergic transmission in the inferior colliculus. *Neuroscience Letters*, 399(1–2), 151–156. doi: 10.1016/j.neulet.2006.01.049

Taaseh, N., Yaron, A., & Nelken, I. (2011). Stimulus-Specific Adaptation and Deviance Detection in the Rat Auditory Cortex. (I. Sugihara, Ed.)*PLoS ONE*, 6/8: e23369. doi: 10.1371/journal.pone.0023369

Thomas, J. M., Morse, C., Kishline, L., O'Brien-Lambert, A., Simonton, A., Miller, K. E., & Covey, E. (2012). Stimulus-specific adaptation in specialized neurons in the inferior colliculus of the big brown bat, Eptesicus fuscus. *Hearing Research*, 291(1–2), 34–40. doi: 10.1016/j.heares.2012.06.004

Tsodyks, M. V., & Markram, H. (1997). The neural code between neocortical pyramidal neurons depends on neurotransmitter release probability. *Proceedings of the National Academy of Sciences of the United States of America*, 94(2), 719–723. doi: 10.1073/pnas.94.2.719

Ulanovsky, N., Las, L., Farkas, D., & Nelken, I. (2004). Multiple time scales of adaptation in auditory cortex neurons. *Journal of Neuroscience*, 24(46), 10440–10453. doi: 10.1523/JNEUROSCI.1905-04.2004

Ulanovsky, N., Las, L., & Nelken, I. (2003). Processing of low-probability sounds by cortical neurons. *Nature Neuroscience*, 6(4), 391–398. doi: 10.1038/nn1032

Valdés-Baizabal, C., Parras, G. G., Ayala, Y. A., & Malmierca, M. S. (2017). Endocannabinoid modulation of stimulus-specific adaptation in inferior colliculus neurons of the rat. *Scientific Reports*, 7(1): 6997. doi: 10.1038/s41598-017-07460-w

Williams, A. J., & Fuzessery, Z. M. (2011). Differential roles of GABAergic and glycinergic input on FM selectivity in the inferior colliculus of the pallid bat. *Journal of Neurophysiology*, 106(5), 2523–2535. doi: 10.1152/jn.00569.2011

Winkler, I., & Schröger, E. (2015). Auditory perceptual objects as generative models: Setting the stage for communication by sound. *Brain and Language*, 148, 1–22. doi: 10.1016/j.bandl.2015.05.003

Yu, X. J., Xu, X. X., He, S., & He, J. (2009). Change detection by thalamic reticular neurons. *Nature Neuroscience*, 12/9: 1165–1170. doi: 10.1038/nn.2373

Zhang, L. I., Tan, A. Y. Y., Schreiner, C. E., & Merzenich, M. M. (2003). Topography and synaptic shaping of direction selectivity in primary auditory cortex. *Nature*, 424(6945), 201–205. doi: 10.1038/nature01796

Zhang, Y., & Wu, S. H. (2000). Long-term potentiation in the inferior colliculus studied in rat brain slice. *Hearing Research*, 147(1–2: 92–103. doi: 10.1016/S0378-5955(00)00123-4

Zhao, L., Liu, Y., Shen, L., Feng, L., & Hong, B. (2011). Stimulus-specific adaptation and its dynamics in the inferior colliculus of rat. *Neuroscience*, 181, 163–174. doi: 10.1016/j.neuroscience.2011.01.060

Zhao, Y., Rubio, M. E., & Tzounopoulos, T. (2009). Distinct functional and anatomical architecture of the endocannabinoid system in the auditory brainstem. *Journal of Neurophysiology*, 101(5): 2434–2446. doi: 10.1152/jn.00047.2009

CHAPTER 26

BRAINSTEM ENCODING OF SPEECH AND MUSIC SOUNDS IN HUMANS

NINA KRAUS AND TRENT NICOL

Abstract

The encoding of speech and music in the auditory brainstem is available at the human scalp via the auditory-evoked frequency following response. The FFR, primarily reflecting activity in the inferior colliculus, may be evoked by speech or music stimulation and represents the combined activity of sensorimotor, cognitive, and reward centers in the brain. Its response properties, like the inferior colliculus itself, are influenced by long-term experience with sound. The transparency, individual-level reliability, and ability to gauge neural plasticity provide the researcher and clinician a powerful probe of auditory processing in the human brainstem. With it, we have learned a great deal about how mechanisms of decline, deprivation, and enrichment affect the processing of complex signals such as music and speech in the human brainstem.

Keywords: speech, music, auditory processing, inferior colliculus, frequency following response, encoding, neural plasticity

THE auditory brainstem, as detailed in earlier chapters of this book, comprises a number of structures that are specialized for certain sound-processing functions and, naturally, these structures are involved in the encoding of speech and music, as they are for any sound. In practice, however, when speaking of the brainstem encoding of speech and music in humans, we are largely limited in our investigation to the volume-conducted electrical potentials that can be picked up noninvasively from the scalp. This means that, for the most part, we are speaking of the rostral brainstem, including lateral lemniscus and inferior colliculus (Batra, Kuwada, & Maher, 1986; King, Hopkins, & Plack, 2016), the volume-conducted activity of which dominates the scalp-recorded sound-evoked response (Chandrasekaran & Kraus, 2010).

While this may seem limiting, it really is not, as the inferior colliculus is a major crossroads of afferent and efferent activity. If any single brainstem nucleus must stand as a representative of all, the IC is the worthiest to fulfill that role. In addition to receiving enervation from the lower brainstem nuclei, its response properties are profoundly impacted by learning via cortical, limbic and cerebellar feedback (Winer, 2006) and so likewise are the scalp-recorded responses (Kraus & White-Schwoch, 2015).

Speech, as anyone who has struggled to learn reading spectrograms in a speech-acoustics or phonetics class, comprises many components that overlap in time and frequency. Up to 72 phonemes are present in casually-spoken English alone (Mines, Hanson, & Shoup, 1978), and it goes without saying that for these phonemes to be accurately decoded by the listener, they must be accurately encoded by the auditory brain as discrete, unique, and discriminable auditory events. The subtleties present in music—the ever-changing timbres and textures—likewise are faithfully processed in the auditory brainstem.

A surprisingly faithful representation of both speech and music processing is available to the researcher or clinician at the human scalp. When considering volume-conducted voltage fluctuations emanating from a tiny structure deep below the scalp, we are extremely fortunate that the fidelity of complex sounds like speech or music is well maintained at the recording electrode. Although something of a parlor trick, it is nevertheless fascinating that a brain response that is sonified (played back) through a speaker is identifiable as the speech token that evoked it (Weiss & Bidelman, 2015). This maintenance of fidelity is not possible with blunt cortical evoked potentials, nor is it revealed in the brainstem response to a simple stimulus such as the click or tone pip that is familiar to the audiologist. In this chapter we will provide a very brief tutorial on the *frequency-following response* (FFR), the single best measurement of brainstem encoding of speech and music in humans, and then go on to harness its protean nature toward the description of the neural encoding of speech and music.

This is not to say that the IC in particular or the brainstem as a whole is the only neural structure where speech characteristics can be evaluated by human electrophysiology. There is a vast literature of cortical evoked responses to speech sounds, and the FFR itself is not entirely free of cortical input. However, the classic long-latency cortical evoked response is overwhelmingly blunt, signaling the detection of a speech sound or the detection of a change in a speech sound. However, there is a rather large chasm between *detection* and *encoding*. While the acoustic change complex (to name one cortical evoked-response) is able to *detect* very tiny changes in (for example) the pitch of a vowel (Martinez, Eisenberg, & Boothroyd, 2013), there is no way that the identity of the vowel or the pitch at which it was uttered could be ascertained from the ACC. In contrast, the *encoding* of speech or music by the brainstem permits one, via acoustic analysis of the FFR, to determine both the pitch and, within certain limitations, the identity of the evoking speech sound.

After a description of the FFR, we will unpack how selected classes of speech characteristics that combine to produce the 72 phonemes are encoded and subsequently recorded at the scalp as an FFR. (We will not cover music encoding to such a degree, but we will point out parallels as they arise.) Along the way, we will examine some pathologies that lead to poor brainstem encoding and some circumstances that lead to exceptional encoding.

The Frequency-Following Response

The best probe of speech and music encoding in the human brainstem is the frequency following response (FFR). First described in the 1960s via recordings in various auditory nuclei and species (Boudreau, 1965; Marsh, Worden, & Smith, 1970; Moushegian, Rupert, & Whitcomb, 1964; Worden & Marsh, 1968), it was mostly investigated with simple stimuli such as pure tones and found utility only as an adjunct to audiometry until the 1990s when Galbraith and colleagues (Galbraith, Arbagey, Branski, Comerci, & Rector, 1995; Galbraith, Bhuta, Choate, Kitahara, & Mullen, 1998; Galbraith, Jhaveri, & Kuo, 1997) began investigating the FFR to complex stimuli including speech. They and others discovered that the properties of an individual's brainstem encoding to complex sounds bears a relationship with more than peripheral hearing. Among these are attention, literacy, language, and musical experience.

Although not particularly more technically difficult to collect than a click-evoked auditory brainstem response (ABR), the analysis of the FFR is a bit more involved. Like the ABR, the timing of response peaks is an informative metric; but, because of the richness of the stimulus and, consequently, the response, the FFR lends itself to a variety of signal processing techniques that are beyond the scope of what most clinical ABR-focused evoked-response systems are able to provide. To a speech or music stimulus, the following FFR measures, among others, can be used to comprehensively investigate its encoding.

Timing. The latencies, referenced either to stimulus onset or to one another are measured. These can be either transient peaks in the response, such as those occurring to stimulus onset and offset, or tonic peaks representing the periodicity of the stimulus during a voiced period of speech, such as a vowel or a voiced formant transition, or during a musical note.

Magnitude. The size of the omnibus response is measured in the time domain by root-mean-square amplitude over a region of interest (e.g., the consonant-transition period of a response to a consonant-vowel syllable). Magnitude of individual peaks is usually not considered.

Frequency content and magnitude. Frequency content of the response is obtained by Fourier transform. Key frequencies in the spectrum, such as the fundamental frequency (fo) of the stimulus and its harmonics, are identified and the size is measured.

Frequency tracking. In the case of a response to a stimulus with a roving fo, the instantaneous frequency of both the stimulus and response are derived over the course of the waveforms by one of several techniques including autocorrelation, Fourier transform, cepstrum analysis, and more (Gerhard, 2003). Once pitches are established for both stimulus and response, the size of phase-locking at those frequencies can be determined, as well as the extent to which the response pitch hews to the stimulus pitch, e.g., by determining root-mean-square error between them.

Phase consistency. The strength of phaselocking at each time-frequency point is identified for each trial and normalized to a unit vector; the resultant vector length reflects the consistency of coding of time-frequency regions of interest such as the fo and its harmonics.

Intrinsic Factors. Two assessments of response "quality," contra its encoding fidelity or strength, can be derived independent of timing, size, or other acoustically-driven characteristics. 1) Stability of response morphology on a trial-by-trial basis, assessed by inter-response correlation. 2) Magnitude of background noise level, i.e., an averaged response to silence, usually the time between successive stimulus presentations.

Distinction between responses. Any of these FFR measures can be compared when evoked by the same stimulus under multiple conditions, such as a change in magnitude between monaural and binaural presentation or a change in timing between quiet and noise-masked presentation. Alternatively, the same measure may be assessed in contrasting speech or music sounds. In the latter case, the appropriate comparison is driven by the relevant acoustic contrasts of the stimuli, and may be in the time-, frequency- or time-frequency domains. For example, (1) a comparison of spectra might be made between responses elicited to the vowels /u/ and /e/. (2) Likewise, an investigation of consonant voicing-time between a /bo/ and a /po/ would rely on differences in the timing of transients in the response. (3) A cross-phase technique could be used to compare neural timing in response to contrasting consonant-vowel pairs in the time-frequency domain. The relative phase of the responses at frequencies corresponding to known acoustic differences between stop-consonant pairs is used to quantify the extent to which the nervous system discriminates them.

A quick word about techniques and terminology is in order before moving on. Briefly, the frequency following response to a pure tone is phase dependent. That is, the timing of the response is dependent on the phase of the stimulus. However, other components in the response, such as transient peaks, are phase independent. The FFR to more complex stimuli such as speech and music contains a mix of phase-dependent and phase-independent components. The phase-dependent and phase-independent components map onto fine-structure and envelope components of the stimulus, respectively. The latter also contains nonlinearities such as difference tones produced in the auditory system. The most widely used methodological technique to tease these two response components apart is to present the stimulus one-half of the time with inverted (i.e., pi, or 180 degrees out-of-phase) polarity. In this way, the envelope response, FFR_{env}, is constructed offline by adding the responses to the two stimulus types together; the temporal fine structure response, FFR_{tfs}, is a difference of the two response types. For a thorough treatment of the distinction in response properties of FFR_{env} and FFR_{tfs}, see (Aiken

& Picton, 2008). Some researchers who focus on the envelope component alone refer to the FFR_{env} as the envelope following response, or EFR. Others, ourselves included, in the past, termed it cABR (auditory brainstem response to complex stimulation). All are the frequency following response.

Encoding of Speech Features by the Auditory Brainstem

The inferior colliculus has an upper limit in its frequency coding ability that prevents the FFR from being a perfect representation of the evoking stimulus. This speed limit in the IC has been reported to be anywhere from 1 to 4 kHz (Liu, Palmer, & Wallace, 2006; Ping, Li, Galbraith, Wu, & Li, 2008; Warrier, Abrams, Nicol, & Kraus, 2011). Nevertheless, the gamut of acoustic-phonetic events—the flapping of the vocal folds, the plosive bursts, the stops, and so forth—results in corresponding, if imperfect, copies in the form of neural firing patterns in the IC. In this section, we will address particular classes of the speech sound, how they are reflected in the FFR, and what we have learned about this coding with respect to external manifestations, in other words real-life correlates, of auditory processing ability.

Vowels

The vowel sounds of speech are periodic in nature. Periodicity is imparted by vocal cord vibration, the rate of which is expressed perceptually as pitch in both global and local manifestations. A voice can be globally high or low on average, while roving higher or lower locally as emotion and intent vary over the course of running speech. Regardless of its pitch, this voicing sets up a harmonic series consisting of a fundamental frequency (fo) and integer harmonics, whereupon the shape and position of articulators (mouth, palate, tongue, nasal tract, etc.) cause selective filtering of the harmonic series. The resonances of the vocal tract, which appear as local peaks in the harmonic series, define the identity of the vowel. For example, if the first two energy concentrations (the first and second formants) are widely spaced at around 300 and 2500 Hz, the sound will typically be identifiable as an /i/ as in "beet." More closely spaced formants, perhaps at 800 and 1500 Hz, would produce an /ae/ as in "bat." These formant values hold for both high- and low-pitched voices; the approximate values given earlier will sound like /i/ and /ae/ whether spoken by a young child or a deep-voiced man. Both the identity of a vowel and the pitch at which it is spoken are coded in the FFR.

In music, there is a fairly direct parallel to the pitch and harmonic features in a vowel. Pitch has a one-to-one mapping in the two domains; the pitch of a vowel and the pitch of a note have an identical underpinning—the periodicity of the acoustic waveform. The shape of the harmonic series in music defines the identity of the instrument. Much like an /i/ and an /ae/ spoken by the same talker are readily distinguished, the same note played on an oboe and a flute are distinguishable—they have the same pitch with different emphases in the harmonic series.

Vowel pitch/fundamental frequency (fo)

The FFR to the fundamental frequency (or perhaps more accurately fundamental periodicity) of speech is an envelope component and, in fact, this aspect of the FFR is sometimes referred to as the "envelope following response." The fundamental frequency, by definition, is the lowest harmonic in a speech spectrum, but the fo is often very small or even missing. In this respect the speech signal is analogous to an amplitude modulated signal, with the modulator being the fo and the higher-frequency harmonics (and so, the formants) serving as the carrier. Modulation components are essentially phase invariant regardless of stimulus polarity and consequently, the fo response, along with other non-spectral components, is best viewed as a summation of responses evoked by stimuli of opposing polarities (FFR_{env}) as reviewed earlier. Figure 26.1 shows the spectrum of a speech utterance /a/ and its FFR_{env} and FFR_{tfs}. In this example, the fundamental frequency of the syllable, at 100 Hz, is rather small in the speech signal (left) and essentially absent from the FFR_{tfs} (right). In contrast, the fo dominates the FFR_{env} (center), along with some activity up to about 500 Hz that are distortion products of the first and second formants (i.e., 200 Hz = 2f1–f2; 500 Hz = f2–f1). The compass plots in the inset of the middle panel illustrate the relative phase *invariance* at 100 Hz in the FFR_{env}. In contrast, the phase *variance* of the harmonics of the fundamental is illustrated by the compass plot of 700 Hz activity in the FFR_{tfs} (inset, right).

Varieties of manipulated speech can be used in FFR research. For example, the encoding of a "missing fundamental" stimulus in the brainstem can be evaluated. A missing fundamental stimulus is one in which the spacing of the harmonics implies a particular fundamental frequency, but that frequency is absent from the stimulus. For example, a stimulus that contains spectral energy at 400, 500, 600, 700, . . . Hz has a percept of a 100 Hz pitch and the FFR will have a prominent 100 Hz peak—in fact it may be larger than the fo response to an fo-only stimulus. Although investigations of missing-fo with speech stimuli are relatively uncommon (Jeng, Costilow, Stangherlin, & Lin, 2011), tonal missing-fo FFR studies (Galbraith, 1994; Greenberg, Marsh, Brown, & Smith, 1987) remain relevant to speech encoding because these stimuli are analogous to the spectral characteristics of speech signals, wherein the fundamental is often much smaller than the peak amplitudes of the lower formants. Another speech manipulation is vocoded speech. Often studied in normal listeners to simulate cochlear implant processing strategies, vocoded speech is devoid of fine spectral content, consisting of

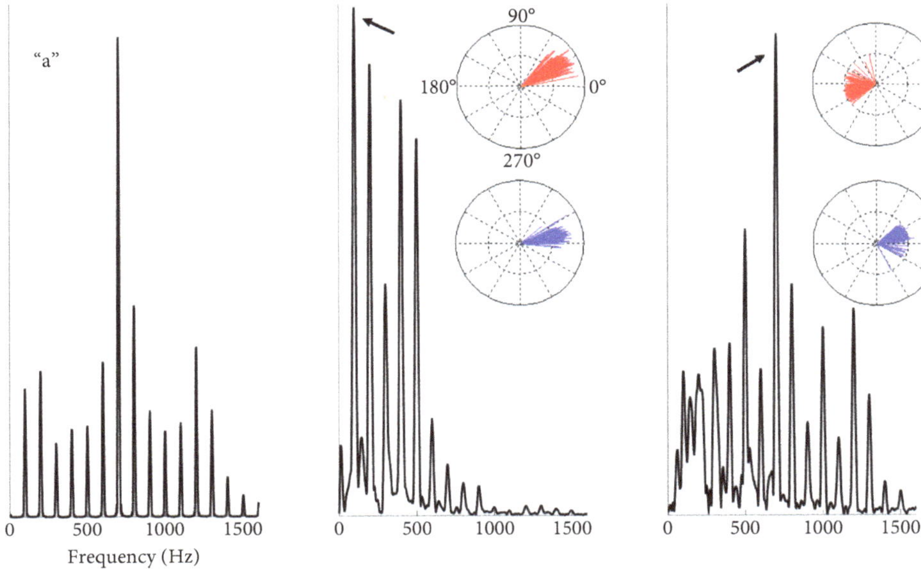

FIGURE 26.1. Left: spectrum to 1.5 kHz of speech syllable /a/ with a fundamental frequency of 100 Hz. The first and second formant frequencies, which define the vowel's identity, are visible as local spectral maxima at 700 and 1200 Hz. Center: the FFR_{env} response spectrum. The fo at 100 Hz (arrow) and some low harmonics dominate the spectrum. Inset: the neural responses at 100 Hz are approximately at the same phase regardless of polarity of stimulus presentation. Red and blue line segments represent the phase of individual response trials to the two stimulus presentation polarities. Regardless of stimulus phase, the 100 Hz brainstem response falls in the first quadrant of the phase compass within about a 0 to 45 degree range. Right: the FFR_{tfs} response. The fo is suppressed while local maxima at 700 (arrow) and 1200 Hz mirror the syllable's spectrum. Inset: the phase of the responses at 700 Hz are approximately 180 degrees out of phase to the two stimulus presentation polarities; consequently, a subtraction of the responses to stimuli of opposite polarity emphasizes this response feature.

modulated noise bands. The encoding of vocoded speech has been investigated with the FFR (Ananthakrishnan, Luo, & Krishnan, 2017) showing an agreement between its encoding and its perception.

A consistent finding in FFR literature is that the encoding of the speech fo is indicative of the ability to hear in noise. In normal hearing listeners of all ages, variability in the aptitude of understanding speech when masked by noise is mirrored in the amplitude of the fo components in speech (Anderson, Parbery-Clark, Yi, & Kraus, 2011; Anderson, Skoe, Chandrasekaran, Zecker, & Kraus, 2010; Coffey, Chepesiuk, Herholz, Baillet, & Zatorre, 2017; J. Song, Skoe, Banai, & Kraus, 2011). Relatedly, bilingual speakers have particularly strong fo encoding to speech (Krizman, Marian, Shook, Skoe, & Kraus, 2012), and the strength of phase-locking to the fo in the FFR to a speech sound of a foreign language relates to the ability to learn that language (Omote, Jasmin, & Tierney,

2017). This form of linguistic enrichment hones attention and memory—skills that improve the sort of auditory object formation that is essential for understanding speech in a noisy environment—so it follows that a bilingual speaker would have this characteristic enhancement in the brainstem response. Another fo finding has emerged wherein an increased FFR amplitude is seen in older adults with mild cognitive impairment, suggesting an overcompensation in sensory processing to offset cognitive processing inefficiencies (Bidelman, Lowther, Tak, & Alain, 2017).

Training explicitly designed to bolster listening in noise also has a positive influence on the fo response (Song, Skoe, Banai, & Kraus, 2012). These behavior-physiology relationships are maintained in the overall morphological similarity between evoking stimulus and FFR (Anderson et al., 2011; Cunningham, Nicol, Zecker, Bradlow, & Kraus, 2001; Kraus & White-Schwoch, 2016)—a metric that is influenced to a great extent by fo encoding.

The physiological-behavioral relationship between fo encoding and listening in noise is mirrored in individuals in clinical populations that are characterized by difficulty following speech in noise. An example is traumatic brain injury. People who have undergone sports-related concussions often complain of difficulty with sound processing (Gallun et al., 2012; Thompson et al., 2018) and their speech-evoked fo is indeed diminished, even after the concussion has been judged resolved (Kraus et al., 2017; Kraus et al., 2016).

Vowels with changing pitch

There are constant changes in the pitch of natural speech. These changes can signal intention, attitude, emphasis, or emotion in all languages and, in some, they have linguistic and grammatical meaning as well. These speech attributes are known as intention and tone, respectively, and both can be measured in the brainstem response to speech. Using standard signal-processing techniques for pitch extraction, the contour of the fundamental frequency in the response can be compared to its counterpart in the evoking speech utterance.

Experience with language has a bearing on the accuracy of neural pitch tracking. Speakers of tonal languages (in contrast to speakers of languages where varying pitch signals intention only) have more accurate responses in terms hewing to the pitch of the stimulus (Krishnan, Xu, Gandour, & Cariani, 2005; Wong, Skoe, Russo, Dees, & Kraus, 2007; Yu & Zhang, 2018). Another form of auditory expertise—musicianship—also produces stronger pitch-tracking responses (Wong et al., 2007). On the other hand, even within tone-language speakers, a decline in FFR pitch tracking is seen in older adults (Wang et al., 2016). Russo et al. (Russo et al., 2008) noted weaker pitch tracking in school-age children on the autism spectrum compared to typically developing peers, evocative of the characteristic flat affect in the speech of some autistic individuals and the diminished ability to perceive emotional valence (Matsumoto et al., 2016). Imperfect perception of the contours of speech pitch may have a bearing on aberrant speech production.

Vowel identity (harmonics)

Unlike the FFR to the fo of speech or music, the response to harmonic content of the stimulus is phase-dependent. So, as noted earlier, an appropriate manipulation must be made, the 180-degree inversion of the responses elicited by 180-degree out of phase stimuli, resulting in the FFR_{tfs}. An example spectrum of an FFR_{tfs} response to the vowel /a/ can be seen in the right panel of Figure 26.1. The spectrum matches well that of the evoking stimulus, especially past about 500 Hz, where clear local maxima at 700 and 1200 Hz, represent the first two formants of this particular /a/ vowel. Brainstem activity to contrasting vowels can be distinguished by spectral peaks in the FFRs (Aiken & Picton, 2008; Krishnan, 2002) and, when sonified (played audibly), responses to contrasting vowels can be distinguished (Weiss & Bidelman, 2015).

Of particular interest, from a clinical or diagnostic point of view, is not the ability to discern in the response the particular identity of the stimulus, but rather the strength of encoding of harmonics that are relevant to the identity of the syllable. There is a pattern that emerges in poor readers. Among other signs of response degradation, covered later in the chapter, individuals with dyslexia or who perform poorly in standardized measures of reading exhibit reduced harmonic encoding at frequencies corresponding to formant frequencies (Banai et al., 2009). Conversely, auditory enrichment via musical training boosts the harmonic representation of speech formants in the FFR (Strait & Kraus, 2014).

Consonants

Consonants are sometimes defined by what they are not—that is, they are the parts of speech that are not voiced like vowels, or at least not voiced with a stable spectrum. To be slightly more precise, they are partial or full obstructions of the breath that produces voicing in speech. Therefore, consonants are somewhat at odds with the nature of the frequency following response—the very name of which implies that there is a periodic component of the signal that is to be neurally followed. A response to a consonant in isolation (to the extent that such a thing exists) is a neural transient, in many respects like the brainstem response to a click that audiologists are familiar with. Nevertheless, it is possible to investigate consonant encoding in the brainstem using the FFR, even if in some cases we must loosen our definition of consonant to include its transition either to or from a conjoined fully voiced vowel.

Timing/transients.

Much speech FFR work, for better or worse, has focused on the consonant-vowel syllable "da." One in particular, a 40-ms variant, was chosen and created in our lab because it contains key acoustic elements important for speech perception, contains phonemes that are present in most world languages, and is short enough to be amenable to evoked response recording. This stimulus ships with many major clinical auditory evoked potential systems and has been widely used in research and, increasingly, in clinical settings. Norms are available for both the timing of well-characterized discrete peaks and for frequency-domain representation of features of the stimulus (Skoe, Krizman, Anderson, & Kraus, 2015). Although a very short utterance, during its 40-ms duration, the da progresses from a (relatively) broadband release burst, to a fully-voiced transition to a vowel. Figure 26.2 depicts a typical FFR_{env} to this short syllable. The response to the release burst (V and A), along with a response to the *offset* of the utterance (O), together can be viewed as qualitatively different than the intermediate peaks, D, E, and F, which arise from the periodicity of the stimulus fo and will be discussed further in the next section.

Some of the earliest findings equating the brainstem encoding of speech with language skills involved the timing of the onset transients of da. Cunningham et al. (Cunningham et al., 2001) noted that the timing of the V/A complex to a noise-masked da was delayed in children with a diagnosed reading disability. Later, a larger study relied on standardized tests of reading rather than external diagnoses. It found that discrete peaks elicited by the 40-ms da were consistently delayed in children (of any diagnosis) who scored poorly on reading assessments (Banai et al., 2009). Later investigations using the same stimulus confirmed this finding in children with reading impairment and extended it to auditory processing disorder (Rocha-Muniz, Befi-Lopes, & Schochat, 2012, 2014; White-Schwoch et al., 2015). In adults, on the other hand, the brainstem/

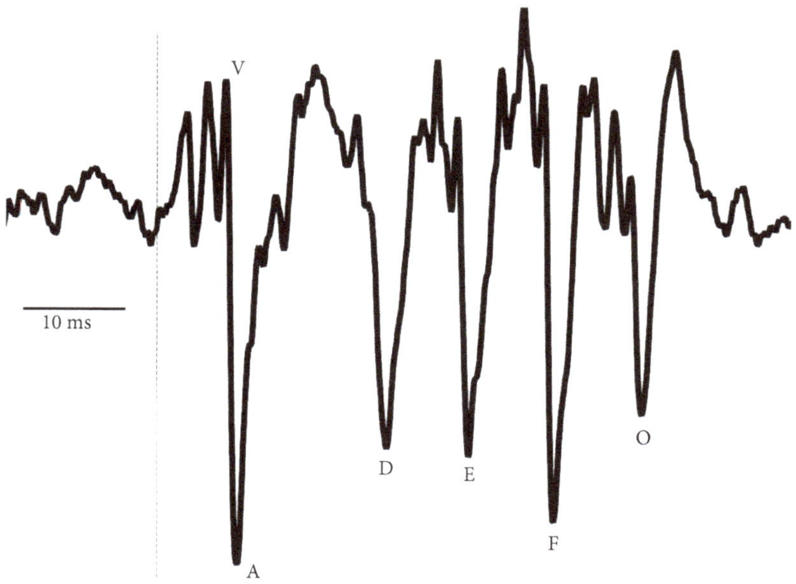

FIGURE 26.2. A response to a 40-ms da, with major peaks labeled. The vertical dashed line represents stimulus onset, time zero. Onset peak V (five) is analogous to wave V of the click-evoked auditory brainstem response. A is also considered an onset peak. D, E, and F are "following" the voicing of the syllable, at a period equivalent to the fo. O is an offset response.

reading relationship manifests itself differently, with earlier peak timing (Skoe, Brody, & Theodore, 2017). However, this is consistent with a more juvenile-like response, as response latencies prolong between childhood and adulthood (Skoe et al., 2015).

An intriguing corollary to the transient timing delays in poor readers is found in musicians. Listening experts, namely musicians whose precisely-driven auditory systems have been tuned by years of focused attention to the emotion-laden auditory input of their instruments (Patel, 2011), have enhancements in brainstem encoding that are evocative of the degraded response properties seen in poor readers. Among other response enhancements, transient timing to speech stimulation is, in fact, earlier in musicians (Kraus & White-Schwoch, 2016; Parbery-Clark, Anderson, & Hittner, 2012; Parbery-Clark, Anderson, Hittner, & Kraus, 2012).

Temporal-spectral (frequency sweeps)

As noted previously, a stop consonant is a near timeless event; a short-duration closure of the articulators (i.e., tongue, lips) that rapidly leads to or follows from a voiced segment of speech. However, this unvoiced-to-voiced transition (or voiced-to-unvoiced in the case of vowel-consonant syllables) is an important phonetic event that is rich in acoustic interest. In the case of consonant-vowel (CV) utterances, such as "go" or "bee," there is a distinct formant trajectory, visible in a spectrogram, that defines the identity of both the consonant and the vowel. Figure 26.3 illustrates spectrograms of three synthesized CV syllables, ba, da, and du. The first 2, ba and da conclude with the formants at the same frequencies, particularly well-depicted by dark F1 and F2 lines at about 700 and 1200 Hz, values typical for an "a" vowel. The difference between these two syllables is in the initial 50 ms—that is, the path the formants take to arrive at the shared steady-state vowel. F2 begins at about 900 Hz for ba and 1700 Hz for da, rising and falling, respectively, to 1200 Hz at 50 ms. In contrast, the origin frequency of F2 is 1700 Hz for both da and du, a frequency typical of the consonant "d," but the syllables end at very different places, with "u" attaining steady-state conclusions of 250 and 870 Hz for F1 and F2, respectively.

Different approaches are available to evaluate encoding of frequency-modulated formant glides. For one, there are transient peaks in the FFR during this period, such as D, E, and F, illustrated in Figure 26.2; these can be assessed for timing. Second, a spectrum over the formant transition can be produced and frequency encoding can be measured. Third, spectrograms, as those shown for the stimuli in Figure 26.3, offer a time-frequency approach. Finally, "cross-phase" approach can evaluate frequency-specific timing differences between the responses to stimulus pairs such as the da and ba in Figure 26.3.

Using one or more of these techniques, several investigations into reading (dis)ability, reading subskills such as phonological awareness, or the ability to understand speech in noise have revealed deficits in the encoding of consonant-vowel formant transitions in speech (Anderson, Skoe, Chandrasekaran, & Kraus, 2010; Hornickel, Anderson, Skoe, Yi, & Kraus, 2012; Hornickel, Skoe, Nicol, Zecker, & Kraus, 2009; Skoe, Nicol, & Kraus,

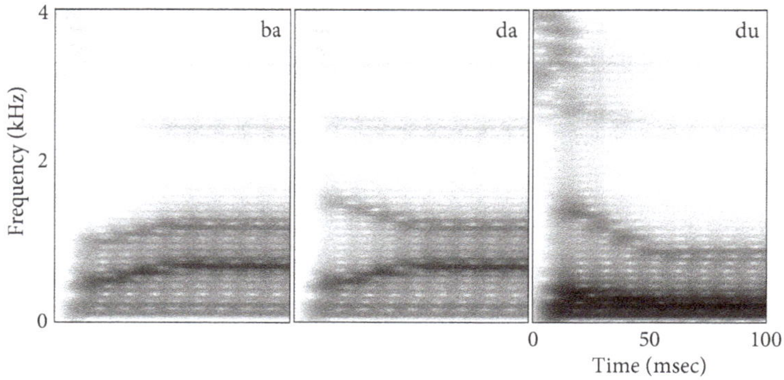

FIGURE 26.3. Spectrograms of three consonant-vowels syllables. The first two have a vowel in common, and so conclude with formants 1 and 2 at the same frequencies. The last two have a common consonant, so formants originate at the same frequencies, but conclude at frequencies prototypical of /a/ and /u/, respectively.

2011; White-Schwoch & Kraus, 2013). Musicians, a model for auditory expertise, on the other hand, excel in this aspect of speech encoding (Parbery-Clark, Tierney, Strait, & Kraus, 2012), even after a year-long music training program (Kraus et al., 2014).

Other Speech Features

A remaining feature of speech that to date remains largely unexplored is that of voicing timing. A major acoustical cue that identifies stop consonants is the extent to which they are fully voiced (g, b, d) or unvoiced (k, p, t). The brainstem encoding of voicing timing and its behavioral consequences are ripe for investigation. Also, only beginning to be explored is speech at a more macro level. Ongoing speech, such as full sentences, presents practical problems because of the large number of stimulus presentations typically required for satisfactory FFR collection. Recently, investigations have been undertaken that look at concatenated-word or full-sentence stimulation (Choi, Purcell, Coyne, & Aiken, 2013; Reichenbach, Braiman, Schiff, Hudspeth, & Reichenbach, 2016), demonstrating that even with a reduced presentation count, structural components of the stimulus are maintained in the response, and that an attentional effect can be discerned in the FFR (Forte, Etard, & Reichenbach, 2017).

Conclusion

Our life in sound has a cumulative impact on the biological response to sound in the inferior colliculus of the brainstem. Engagement with sound activates the cognitive, sensorimotor, and reward networks of the brain, and the auditory midbrain represents a crossroads where these networks converge and gel. In the past 20 years, research into the response properties of the auditory midbrain have provided us with insight into the biological legacy of experience, such as music engagement and bilingualism. Further, the brainstem's response to speech and other complex stimulation such as music has a connection to communication skills, such as literacy and listening in noise. This growing recognition of the valuable insights that can come from probing the auditory brainstem have moved the needle on interest in pursuing the measurement of the auditory brainstem. FFR is beginning to emerge as a clinical tool on the strength of its capacity for discerning impairment in auditory processing as well as expertise. As researchers who have been involved in FFR to speech for nearly two decades, we are gratified that the slow process of divorcing the FFR from its cousin the auditory brainstem response (ABR) is progressing. FFR is no longer met with a shrug, viewed only as a modestly valuable alternative to ABR for peripheral auditory screening.

Brainstem processing of speech and music, though still a comparatively new line of inquiry, is gaining traction. Much of the pioneering work has been done in terms of developing best practices for the collection and analysis of speech- and music-evoked frequency following responses. Norms are being established as the developmental time course of the FFR is becoming more understood (Skoe et al., 2015; Van Dyke, Lieberman, Presacco, & Anderson, 2017) and the evaluation of an individual's response component relative to a normative reference is increasing in validity. It is gaining prominence among auditory neuroscientists: its mindshare at conferences is rapidly growing for at least two reasons. One, from a basic science perspective, it is a direct and accessible metric of human communication. We can learn so much more by accessing the auditory circuit's systemic response to a complex sound than can be achieved by probing single neurons in experimental animals with a clicks, pure tones or pulse trains. FFR affords us the luxury of complex stimulation and the direct applicability of accessibility in humans. Second, from a clinical standpoint, is its value in *objectively assessing the encoding of the fast components of speech in individuals*. Fast components of speech elude cortical auditory evoked responses which also suffer from only moderate individual reliability. And imaging techniques, though reliable in individuals, are also severely limited in terms of their ability to probe the fast components of speech. As the best pure measure of objective auditory processing available, FFR is poised for immediate and near-future applications in the clinical realm.

References

Aiken, S. J., & Picton, T. W. (2008). Envelope and spectral frequency-following responses to vowel sounds. *Hearing Research*, 245(1–2), 35–47. doi:10.1016/j.heares.2008.08.004

Ananthakrishnan, S., Luo, X., & Krishnan, A. (2017). Human frequency following responses to vocoded speech. *Ear and Hearing*, 38(5), e256–e267. doi:10.1097/AUD.0000000000000432

Anderson, S., Parbery-Clark, A., Yi, H. G., & Kraus, N. (2011). A neural basis of speech-in-noise perception in older adults. *Ear and Hearing*, 32(6), 750–757. doi:10.1097/AUD.0b013e31822229d3

Anderson, S., Skoe, E., Chandrasekaran, B., & Kraus, N. (2010). Neural timing is linked to speech perception in noise. *Journal of Neuroscience*, *30*(14), 4922–4926. doi:10.1523/JNEUROSCI.0107-10.2010

Anderson, S., Skoe, E., Chandrasekaran, B., Zecker, S., & Kraus, N. (2010). Brainstem correlates of speech-in-noise perception in children. *Hearing Research*, *270*(1–2), 151–157. doi:10.1016/j.heares.2010.08.001

Banai, K., Hornickel, J. M., Skoe, E., Nicol, T., Zecker, S., & Kraus, N. (2009). Reading and subcortical auditory function. *Cerebral Cortex*, *19*(11), 2699–2707. doi:10.1093/cercor/bhp024

Batra, R., Kuwada, S., & Maher, V. L. (1986). The frequency-following response to continuous tones in humans. *Hearing Research*, *21*(2), 167–177.

Bidelman, G. M., Lowther, J. E., Tak, S. H., & Alain, C. (2017). Mild cognitive impairment is characterized by deficient brainstem and cortical representations of speech. *Journal of Neuroscience*, *37*(13), 3610–3620. doi:10.1523/JNEUROSCI.3700-16.2017

Boudreau, J. C. (1965). Neural volleying: Upper frequency limits detectable in the auditory system. *Nature*, *208*(5016), 1237–1238.

Chandrasekaran, B., & Kraus, N. (2010). The scalp-recorded brainstem response to speech: Neural origins and plasticity. *Psychophysiology*, *47*, 236–246. doi:10.1111/j.1469-8986.2009.00928.x

Choi, J. M., Purcell, D. W., Coyne, J. A., & Aiken, S. J. (2013). Envelope following responses elicited by English sentences. *Ear and Hearing*, *34*(5), 637–650. doi:10.1097/AUD.0b013e31828e4dad

Coffey, E. B. J., Chepesiuk, A. M. P., Herholz, S. C., Baillet, S., & Zatorre, R. J. (2017). Neural correlates of early sound encoding and their relationship to speech-in-noise perception. *Frontiers in Neuroscience*, *11*, 479. doi:10.3389/fnins.2017.00479

Cunningham, J., Nicol, T., Zecker, S. G., Bradlow, A., & Kraus, N. (2001). Neurobiologic responses to speech in noise in children with learning problems: Deficits and strategies for improvement. *Clinical Neurophysiology*, *112*, 758–767.

Forte, A. E., Etard, O., & Reichenbach, T. (2017). The human auditory brainstem response to running speech reveals a subcortical mechanism for selective attention. *Elife*, *6*. doi:10.7554/eLife.27203

Galbraith, G. C. (1994). Two-channel brain-stem frequency-following responses to pure tone and missing fundamental stimuli. *Electroencephalography & Clinical Neurophysiology*, *92*(4), 321–330.

Galbraith, G. C., Arbagey, P. W., Branski, R., Comerci, N., & Rector, P. M. (1995). Intelligible speech encoded in the human brain stem frequency-following response. *Neuroreport*, *6*(17), 2363–2367.

Galbraith, G. C., Bhuta, S. M., Choate, A. K., Kitahara, J. M., & Mullen, T. A. (1998). Brain stem frequency-following response to dichotic vowels during attention. *Neuroreport*, *9*(8), 1889–1893.

Galbraith, G. C., Jhaveri, S. P., & Kuo, J. (1997). Speech-evoked brainstem frequency-following responses during verbal transformations due to word repetition. *Electroencephalography & Clinical Neurophysiology*, *102*(1), 46–53.

Gallun, F. J., Diedesch, A. C., Kubli, L. R., Walden, T. C., Folmer, R. L., Lewis, M. S., . . . Leek, M. R. (2012). Performance on tests of central auditory processing by individuals exposed to high-intensity blasts. *Journal of Rehabilitation Research and Development*, *49*(7), 1005–1025.

Gerhard, D. (2003). *Pitch extraction and fundamental frequency: history and current techniques*. Retrieved from University of Regina Technical Report, Regina, Saskatchewan, Canada: http://citeseerx.ist.psu.edu/viewdoc/summary?doi=10.1.1.58.834

Greenberg, S., Marsh, J. T., Brown, W. S., & Smith, J. C. (1987). Neural temporal coding of low pitch. I. Human frequency-following responses to complex tones. *Hearing Research*, *25*(2–3), 91–114.

Hornickel, J., Anderson, S., Skoe, E., Yi, H. G., & Kraus, N. (2012). Subcortical representation of speech fine structure relates to reading ability. *Neuroreport*, *23*(1), 6–9. doi:10.1097/WNR.0b013e32834d2ffd

Hornickel, J., Skoe, E., Nicol, T., Zecker, S., & Kraus, N. (2009). Subcortical differentiation of stop consonants relates to reading and speech-in-noise perception. *Proceedings of the National Academy of Sciences USA*, *106*(31), 13022–13027. doi:10.1073/pnas.0901123106

Jeng, F. C., Costilow, C. E., Stangherlin, D. P., & Lin, C. D. (2011). Relative power of harmonics in human frequency-following responses associated with voice pitch in American and Chinese adults. *Perceptual and Motor Skills*, *113*(1), 67–86.

King, A., Hopkins, K., & Plack, C. J. (2016). Differential group delay of the frequency following response measured vertically and horizontally. *Journal of the Association for Research in Otolaryngology*, *17*(2), 133–143. doi:10.1007/s10162-016-0556-x

Kraus, N., Lindley, T., Colegrove, D., Krizman, J., Otto-Meyer, S., Thompson, E. C., & White-Schwoch, T. (2017). The neural legacy of a single concussion. *Neuroscience Letters*, *646*, 21–23. doi:10.1016/j.neulet.2017.03.008

Kraus, N., Slater, J., Thompson, E., Hornickel, J., Strait, D., Nicol, T., & White-Schwoch, T. (2014). Auditory learning through active engagement with sound: Biological impact of community music lessons in at-risk children. *Frontiers in Neuroscience*, *8*, 351. doi:10.3389/fnins.2014.00351

Kraus, N., Thompson, E. C., Krizman, J., Cook, K., White-Schwoch, T., & LaBella, C. R. (2016). Auditory biological marker of concussion in children. *Scientific Reports*, *6*, 39009. doi:10.1038/srep39009

Kraus, N., & White-Schwoch, T. (2015). Unraveling the biology of auditory learning: A cognitive-sensorimotor-reward framework. *Trends in Cognitive Sciences*, *19*(11), 642–654. doi:10.1016/j.tics.2015.08.017

Kraus, N., & White-Schwoch, T. (2016). Neurobiology of everyday communication: What have we learned from music? *Neuroscientist*, *23*(3), 287–298. doi:10.1177/1073858416653593

Krishnan, A. (2002). Human frequency-following responses: Representation of steady-state synthetic vowels. *Hearing Research*, *166*(1–2), 192–201. doi:10.1016/S0378-5955(02)00327-1

Krishnan, A., Xu, Y. S., Gandour, J., & Cariani, P. (2005). Encoding of pitch in the human brainstem is sensitive to language experience. *Cognitive Brain Research*, *25*(1), 161–168.

Krizman, J., Marian, V., Shook, A., Skoe, E., & Kraus, N. (2012). Subcortical encoding of sound is enhanced in bilinguals and relates to executive function advantages. *Proceedings of the National Academy of Sciences USA*, *109*(20), 7877–7881. doi:10.1073/pnas.1201575109

Liu, L. F., Palmer, A. R., & Wallace, M. N. (2006). Phase-locked responses to pure tones in the inferior colliculus. *Journal of Neurophysiology*, *95*(3), 1926–1935. doi:10.1152/jn.00497.2005

Marsh, J. T., Worden, F. G., & Smith, J. C. (1970). Auditory frequency-following response: Neural or artifact? *Science*, *169*(3951), 1222–1223.

Martinez, A. S., Eisenberg, L. S., & Boothroyd, A. (2013). The acoustic change complex in young children with hearing loss: A preliminary study. *Seminars in Hearing*, *34*(4), 278–287. doi:10.1055/s-0033-1356640

Matsumoto, K., Sugiyama, T., Saito, C., Kato, S., Kuriyama, K., Kanemoto, K., & Nakamura, A. (2016). Behavioral study on emotional voice perception in children with autism spectrum disorder. *Journal of Pediatric Neuropsychology*, *2*(3–4), 108–118. doi:10.1007/s40817-016-0021-0

Mines, M. A., Hanson, B. F., & Shoup, J. E. (1978). Frequency of occurrence of phonemes in conversational English. *Language and Speech*, *21*(3), 221–241. doi:10.1177/002383097802100302

Moushegian, G., Rupert, A., & Whitcomb, M. A. (1964). Brain-stem neuronal response patterns to monaural and binaural tones. *Journal of Neurophysiology*, *27*, 1174–1191.

Omote, A., Jasmin, K., & Tierney, A. (2017). Successful non-native speech perception is linked to frequency following response phase consistency. *Cortex*, *93*, 146–154. doi:10.1016/j.cortex.2017.05.005

Parbery-Clark, A., Anderson, S., & Hittner, E. (2012). Musical experience offsets age-related delays in neural timing. *Neurobiology of Aging*, *33*(7), 1483.e1–1483.e4. doi:10.1016/j.neurobiolaging.2011.12.015

Parbery-Clark, A., Anderson, S., Hittner, E., & Kraus, N. (2012). Musical experience strengthens the neural representation of sounds important for communication in middle-aged adults. *Frontiers in Aging Neuroscience*, *4*(30), 1–12. doi:10.3389/fnagi.2012.00030

Parbery-Clark, A., Tierney, A., Strait, D., & Kraus, N. (2012). Musicians have fine-tuned neural distinction of speech syllables. *Neuroscience*, *219*, 111–119. doi:10.1016/j.neuroscience.2012.05.042

Patel, A. D. (2011). Why would musical training benefit the neural encoding of speech? The OPERA hypothesis. *Frontiers in Psychology*, *2*, 142. doi:10.3389/fpsyg.2011.00142

Ping, J., Li, N., Galbraith, G. C., Wu, X., & Li, L. (2008). Auditory frequency-following responses in rat ipsilateral inferior colliculus. *Neuroreport*, *19*(14), 1377–1380. doi:10.1097/WNR.0b013e32830c1cfa

Reichenbach, C. S., Braiman, C., Schiff, N. D., Hudspeth, A. J., & Reichenbach, T. (2016). The auditory-brainstem response to continuous, non-repetitive speech is modulated by the speech envelope and reflects speech processing. *Frontiers in Computational Neuroscience*, *10*, 47. doi:10.3389/fncom.2016.00047

Rocha-Muniz, C. N., Befi-Lopes, D. M., & Schochat, E. (2012). Investigation of auditory processing disorder and language impairment using the speech-evoked auditory brainstem response. *Hearing Research*, *294*(1), 143–152. doi:10.1016/j.heares.2012.08.008

Rocha-Muniz, C. N., Befi-Lopes, D. M., & Schochat, E. (2014). Sensitivity, specificity and efficiency of speech-evoked ABR. *Hearing Research*, *317*, 15–22. doi:10.1016/j.heares.2014.09.004

Russo, N. M., Skoe, E., Trommer, B., Nicol, T., Zecker, S., Bradlow, A., & Kraus, N. (2008). Deficient brainstem encoding of pitch in children with autism spectrum disorders. *Clinical Neurophysiology*, *119*(8), 1720–1731. doi:10.1016/j.clinph.2008.01.108

Skoe, E., Brody, L., & Theodore, R. M. (2017). Reading ability reflects individual differences in auditory brainstem function, even into adulthood. *Brain and Language*, *164*, 25–31. doi:10.1016/j.bandl.2016.09.003

Skoe, E., Krizman, J., Anderson, S., & Kraus, N. (2015). Stability and plasticity of auditory brainstem function across the lifespan. *Cerebral Cortex*, *25*(6), 1415–1426. doi:10.1093/cercor/bht311

Skoe, E., Nicol, T., & Kraus, N. (2011). Cross-phaseogram: Objective neural index of speech sound differentiation. *Journal of Neuroscience Methods*, *196*(2), 308–317. doi:10.1016/j.jneumeth.2011.01.020

Song, J., Skoe, E., Banai, K., & Kraus, N. (2011). Perception of speech in noise: Neural correlates. *Journal of Cognitive Neuroscience, 23*(9), 2268–2279. doi:10.1162/jocn.2010.21556

Song, J. H., Skoe, E., Banai, K., & Kraus, N. (2012). Training to improve hearing speech in noise: Biological mechanisms. *Cerebral Cortex, 22*(5), 1180–1190. doi:10.1093/cercor/bhr196

Strait, D. L., & Kraus, N. (2014). Biological impact of auditory expertise across the life span: Musicians as a model of auditory learning. *Hearing Research, 308*, 109–121. doi:10.1016/j.heares.2013.08.004

Thompson, E. C., Krizman, J., White-Schwoch, T., Nicol, T., LaBella, C. R., & Kraus, N. (2018). Difficulty hearing in noise: A sequela of concussion in children. *Brain Injury, 32*(6), 763–769. doi:10.1080/02699052.2018.1447686

Van Dyke, K. B., Lieberman, R., Presacco, A., & Anderson, S. (2017). Development of phase locking and frequency representation in the infant frequency-following response. *Journal of Speech, Language, and Hearing Research, 60*, 2740–2751. doi:10.1044/2017_JSLHR-H-16-0263

Wang, S., Hu, J., Dong, R., Liu, D., Chen, J., Musacchia, G., & Liu, B. (2016). Voice pitch elicited frequency following response in Chinese elderlies. *Frontiers in Aging Neuroscience, 8*, 286. doi:10.3389/fnagi.2016.00286

Warrier, C. M., Abrams, D. A., Nicol, T. G., & Kraus, N. (2011). Inferior colliculus contributions to phase encoding of stop consonants in an animal model. *Hearing Research, 282*(1–2), 108–118. doi:10.1016/j.heares.2011.09.001

Weiss, M. W., & Bidelman, G. M. (2015). Listening to the brainstem: Musicianship enhances intelligibility of subcortical representations for speech. *Journal of Neuroscience, 35*(4), 1687–1691. doi:10.1523/jneurosci.3680-14.2015

White-Schwoch, T., & Kraus, N. (2013). Physiologic discrimination of stop consonants relates to phonological skills in pre-readers: A biomarker for subsequent reading ability? *Frontiers in Human Neuroscience, 7*, 899. doi:10.3389/fnhum.2013.00899

White-Schwoch, T., Woodruff Carr, K., Thompson, E. C., Anderson, S., Nicol, T., Bradlow, A. R., . . . Kraus, N. (2015). Auditory processing in noise: A preschool biomarker for literacy. *PLoS Biology, 13*(7), e1002196. doi:10.1371/journal.pbio.1002196

Winer, J. A. (2006). Decoding the auditory corticofugal systems. *Hearing Research, 212*(1–2), 1–8.

Wong, P. C. M., Skoe, E., Russo, N. M., Dees, T., & Kraus, N. (2007). Musical experience shapes human brainstem encoding of linguistic pitch patterns. *Nature Neuroscience, 10*(4), 420–422.

Worden, F. G., & Marsh, J. T. (1968). Frequency-following (microphonic-like) neural responses evoked by sound. *Electroencephalography & Clinical Neurophysiology, 25*(1), 42–52.

Yu, L., & Zhang, Y. (2018). Testing native language neural commitment at the brainstem level: A cross-linguistic investigation of the association between frequency-following response and speech perception. *Neuropsychologia, 109*, 140–148. doi:10.1016/j.neuropsychologia.2017.12.022

CHAPTER 27

THE AUDITORY BRAINSTEM IMPLANT

Restoration of Speech Understanding from Electric Stimulation of the Human Cochlear Nucleus

ROBERT V. SHANNON

Abstract

The auditory brainstem implant (ABI) is a surgically implanted device to electrically stimulate auditory neurons in the cochlear nucleus complex of the brainstem in humans to restore hearing sensations. The ABI is similar in function to a cochlear implant, but overall outcomes are poorer. However, recent applications of the ABI to new patient populations and improvements in surgical technique have led to significant improvements in outcomes. While the ABI provides hearing benefits to patients, the outcomes challenge our understanding of how the brain processes neural patterns of auditory information. The neural pattern of activation produced by an ABI is highly unnatural, yet some patients achieve high levels of speech understanding. Based on a meta-analysis of ABI surgeries and outcomes, a theory is proposed of a specialized sub-system of the cochlear nucleus that is critical for speech understanding.

Keywords: cochlear nucleus, auditory brainstem implant, auditory prosthesis, speech understanding, low spontaneous neurons, small cell cap

Introduction: Short History of the Auditory Brainstem Implant

Back in the late 1970s it was already becoming clear that cochlear implants (CIs), that is, electric stimulation of the cochlea, could produce functionally useful hearing and even some open set speech recognition without lipreading. There were clear cases of

CI patients conversing over the telephone using only the CI (Bilger & Hopkinson, 1977; Eddington, 1983; Spahr & Dorman, 2004). This result seemed impossible at the time and was met with much disbelief and skepticism. Auditory scientists were studying the complexities of basic cochlear biophysics and physiology. For example, phase locking in auditory nerve fibers was the rage, and researchers were trying to understand the role of phase-locking on auditory perception (Young & Sachs, 1979; Young, 2008). Basic auditory researchers thought that phase locking must be important for conveying fine timing information for speech, pitch and for localizing sounds in space. For more than 15 years, patients with cochlear implants have mostly been able to understand speech well enough to converse on the telephone. Children with cochlear implants at an early age are able to learn to speak and understand speech at high levels. The research community was skeptical and puzzled by the fact that some CI patients could understand speech with the crude pattern of nerve activation created by a cochlear implant because CIs provided neither fine time structure nor fine spectral structure.

One of the clinics that had pioneered cochlear implants, the House Ear Institute in Los Angeles, was also a large clinic that specialized in removal of vestibular schwannomas (VS) from patients with neurofibromatosis type 2 (NF2). Although NF2 is a rare genetic disorder, Drs. Bill House, a neurotologist, and Bill Hitselberger, a neurosurgeon, performed this tumor removal surgery in about 300 patients per year. It was traumatic to see NF2 patients lose all hearing in the tumor ear. The VIII nerve was removed along with the tumor, which had to be removed to save the patient's life. NF2 usually causes bilateral VS, so the patient will usually lose all hearing in both ears as both tumors required surgery.

House and Hitselberger decided to try something akin to a CI in these patients in an attempt to preserve some degree of hearing following VS removal. Since there was no remaining auditory nerve, a CI was not an option. They placed a ball electrode into the cochlear nucleus, near the root entry zone of the cochlear nerve (Hitselberger et al., 1984). This first auditory brainstem implant (ABI) was placed in a volunteer in 1979 and with a revision in 1981, and it has functioned stably until the present day, 2018 (House & Hitselberger, 2001). Although this innovation was met with skepticism and criticism, it did provide auditory perception at the level of a single-channel CI: sound awareness, an aid to lip reading, and identification of environmental sounds (Brackmann et al., 1993; Otto et al., 2002).

Later, around 2000, a significant proportion (about 30%) of ABI patients in some clinics were achieving high-level open-set speech recognition with only the ABI. The best ABI patients were performing at levels comparable to the best CI patients (Colletti & Shannon, 2005).

How is this possible? The ABI stimulates the rostral surface of the cochlear nucleus with multiple electrodes. But the surface of the cochlear nucleus (CN) does not have a simple tonotopic structure. There are many anatomically and physiologically different sub-structures within the CN, and each has its own tonotopic organization (Moore & Osen, 1979). They are not all near the CN surface, and the tonotopic axes don't all line up in the same orientation. While the ABI provides multiple points of stimulation, it is not clear how this stimulation maps onto the multiple tonotopic structures and multiple functional divisions within the CN. In spite of this, many ABI patients can understand speech well enough to have a relatively normal conversation by telephone. How can such a chaotic connection between the ABI electrode and the complex CN structure result in good speech recognition? In this chapter we discuss in more detail the factors that may have led to this good performance and propose a hypothesis to explain how it could happen.

The ABI Device

First, let us consider the design of a cochlear implant device. The design of a cochlear implant electrode is straightforward. The cochlea is organized tonotopically, so the CI electrode array consists of a linear array of 16–24 electrical contacts that are inserted into the scala tympani along the tonotopic axis. Electrodes near the round window activate neurons that would typically respond to high-frequency sound and those further in the cochlear would activate neurons that would typically respond to lower-frequency sound (Loizou, 1999).

However, it is not clear how to design an electrode to connect to the multiple tonotopic dimensions of the CN. Following removal of the VS, the surgeon cannot see any anatomical landmarks for the CN. If there is a remaining 8th cranial nerve (VIIIn) stump, the surgeon can follow that to the CN, but that is not often the case. Anatomical studies in human cadaver specimens has shown that the CN lies immediately along the dorsal side of the lateral recess of the IV ventricle. So an electrode array was designed as a mesh pad to be inserted into the lateral recess (LR) with the contacts facing dorsally and inferiorly. Over time additional electrodes were added, going from 1, to 3, to 8 and finally evolving to the 21-electrode system used in the Cochlear Corp ABI. The Cochlear Corp. ABI has electrodes arrayed along a 3 by 8 mm mesh substrate. An ABI is produced by Med-El that has 12 stimulating contact electrodes on a slightly smaller pad. The mesh substrate encourages fibrous in-growth to fix the array in position, which occurs within 1 to 2 weeks. At one time an ABI with penetrating microelectrodes was designed and used in 10 patients, but the results were no better than the surface electrode system (Otto et al., 2008).

In a CI there are very few non-auditory side effects from stimulation. Occasionally CI patients report a tingling or motor activation of the facial nerve. However, the CN is located in the brainstem, where there are many other neural structures that could be activated by the electrode. Anatomy and experience show that the primary points of non-auditory activation are the flocculus of the cerebellum (which is located on the opposite side of the LR from the CN) and the cerebellar peduncle, which is an uncrossed, ascending fiber tract in this location (Brackmann et al., 1993; Otto et al., 2002). Activation of the flocculus causes a sensation of the room jumping when stimulation occurs, presumably because it interferes with the fine ocular motor control. Activation of the peduncle produces a tickle or tingling sensation that occurs along the ipsilateral side of the body to the ABI. Activation of peduncle fibers can produce action potentials in both directions, causing sensations in the brain as well as motor activation at the peripheral terminus. Neither site of nonauditory activation is potentially harmful or unpleasant, and the sensations are eliminated if those electrodes are turned off. In a few instances more serious activation of the IXn was observed, causing and unpleasant coughing and tightness in the throat. In those few cases it was found that the entire electrode array had moved post-surgically and was located outside of the LR. The IXn passes near the mouth of the lateral recess of the IVth ventricle, so the IXn can be activated if the electrode array is extruded from the LR. Even in some of these cases, ABI use can still be useful by turning off electrodes that activate IXn and only using electrodes that remain inside the LR and produce auditory sensations.

ABI Outcomes

So what does an ABI sound like? Patients typically describe the sound of the ABI as bizarre and robotic. One patient said, "It's like you're trying to communicate with me by rattling a large sheet of plastic." At first, most patients are not able to make any use of the sound at all. It may take many months, or even years, to adapt to the sound patterns produced by the ABI, which are probably quite different from the normal tonotopic patterns of neural activation coming from the normal cochlea. Presumably the plasticity of the brain must map the strange new ABI pattern of information onto the stored patterns learned from a lifetime of sound experience. Most ABI patients eventually learn to use the device, but the individual differences in outcome are large. Some patients can only use the ABI at a level similar to single-channel CIs, that is, awareness of sound, aid to lip reading, and some identification of environmental sounds. A few patients achieve the ability to recognize speech without using lip reading. They can converse on the telephone without difficulty. One patient I know is a tradesman who relies on his cell phone for jobs. It is not clear what underlies the large differences in outcome across patients. Is it the electrode design and placement? Is it differences in the damage to the anatomy? Are there large individual differences in the ability to adapt to new patterns of information? Answers to some of these questions have developed over the last 20 years as ABI applications spread to more clinics and countries.

In the early 2000s Vittorio Colletti of Verona Italy reported CI-like speech recognition in ABI patients (Colletti & Shannon, 2005). These patients were not NF2 ABIs, but people who had lost their auditory nerves from non-tumor causes, such as trauma, infections, and so on. His initial reports were met with skepticism. However, further independent testing showed several non-tumor ABI patients who had outcomes comparable with good CI users. This observation suggested that the cause of poor ABI outcomes might be related to NF2. It was thought that the disease itself or damage from the tumor removal was the difference between good and bad performance with an ABI.

Soon, good outcomes were observed even in NF2 ABI patients. Two clinics in Germany, headed by Robert Behr and Cordula Matthies, both neurosurgeons, showed about 30% of their NF2 ABI patients able to recognize open-set speech at better than 30% correct (Behr et al., 2007, 2014; Matthies et al., 2013, 2014), a result similar to that obtained by Colletti on non-NF2 ABI patients. These result suggest that NF2 is not the limiting factor. This new pattern of results may help answer the question of how the ABI can work so well in some patients.

Colletti also pioneered the application of the ABI to children (Colletti et al., 2014). Sime children were born with no cochleas or auditory nerve and others lost the nerve due to disease process or trauma. He observed a wide range of outcomes, with the poorest performance in children with genetic syndromic disorders, such as CHARGE. However, he also observed speech development and speech understanding in some of the children, predominantly in children with damage only to the cochlea and auditory nerve and without other disabilities. This finding shows that the information provided by an ABI is even sufficient for children to learn auditory communication from the sound of the ABI and no prior auditory experience.

A meeting was held in Munich in 2012 to pool results across ABI clinics to see what factors might be related to ABI outcomes. Patient demographic information was collated as well as signal processing parameters and surgical procedure information. There was little correlation between demographics and signal processing with outcomes, but a strong relation between outcomes and surgical procedure. Patients with the best outcomes were from two clinics that used a semi-sitting neurosurgical position during surgery. There was consensus that it was not the patient position per se that made the difference, but something related to the position (Behr et al., 2014). The best guess is that the semi-sitting position produces lower vascular pressure in the surgical area so the surgeon needs little or no electrocautery because the intra-operative bleeding is minimal. Cautery can have two detrimental effects: excitotoxicity and direct tissue damage. If the VIIIn is interspersed in the tumor (which is common in NF2 tumors), then cautery applied to the tumor may cause high levels of activation in the neurons, possibly resulting in excitotoxicity in the VIIIn, as well as trans-synaptic injury in the CN regions receiving projections. It is also common that the anatomical landmarks are not clear in the case of large tumors, and application of cautery may impact the surface of the brainstem and CN directly. We will speculate in the next section as to how such excitotoxicity or surface damage to the CN may alter the outcome.

Hypothesis

At almost every step, performance of auditory prostheses has surpassed expectations. In the early single-channel cochlear implants, there was no frequency or tonotopically selective stimulation, yet most people found the stimulation useful and even indispensable in everyday life. A few patients even achieved some open set speech recognition (Berliner et al., 1989). In multichannel CIs, patients received separate channels of tonotopic information, and most were able to achieve open-set speech recognition (Spahr & Dorman, 2004). We now think we understand how such performance is possible (Shannon et al., 1995, 2004). Pattern recognition by the brain is a powerful system and speech patterns can be recognized using only temporal envelope fluctuations and four or more tonotopic channels (Shannon et al., 1995). The brain's powerful neural net must develop the ability to extract meaning from rapidly changing patterns in neurons across any listening situation and across different talkers, speaking styles, and accents. The ear and neural hearing system is capable of processing a wider range and complexity of information, like fine spectral resolution and fine temporal resolution, but not all of that complexity is necessary for speech. Musical melody recognition and localization of sounds in space require fine spectral resolution and fine time resolution (Smith et al., 2002; Shannon et al., 2004; Oxenham, 2012), but apparently speech recognition does not. Some aspects of speech also require fine spectral and temporal resolution, like voice pitch and prosody, and talker identification. While this information is not necessary to recognize the identity of the words, it is necessary to recognize the emotional content and emphasis of the spoken message. (Jiam et al., 2017)

Certainly, the brain's pattern recognition is part of the answer, but not the complete picture. No matter how impressive it is, even the brain cannot recognize sensory patterns based on no information—the key elements of the pattern must be transmitted to the brain. But what are the "key" elements? Are all portions of the auditory nerve involved or only a specialized subset? An important clue comes from the ABI results.

Most ABI patients hear sound from activation of the ABI. Most ABI patients hear temporal patterns of sound and some pitch changes, so even if they are not able to understand speech the ABI is activating auditory neurons and is connecting to the tonotopic dimension of the CN. But some ABI patients are able to understand speech well enough to converse on the telephone. This level of performance does not occur immediately but takes months to years of practice and adaptation. If the brain is slowly learning to use the new pattern of neural activity generated by an ABI, why don't all ABI patients learn to do it?

At that 2012 meeting in Munich it appeared that some aspect of the surgery was associated with the difference in outcomes across ABI patients. ABI patients who did the best were mostly ones who had surgery in the neurosurgical semi-sitting position. The participants thought that the differences in outcomes were due to the minimal use of cautery in these surgeries compared to other surgical approaches or patient positions. What might cautery be damaging that could cause such a significant difference in ABI performance?

VSs originate on the vestibular portion of the VIIIn near the myal/glial junction. As the tumor grows, it balloons out into the cerebellopontine angle and eventually fills the space between the medial opening of the internal auditory meatus and the surface of the brainstem. Large tumors contact the surface of the brainstem and draw a blood supply from there (angiogenesis). As the tumor is removed, the surface of the tumor must be teased away from the surface of the brainstem. Since the tumor draws its blood supply from the surface of the brainstem, there is often considerable bleeding from the shared vascularization. In most surgical positions, this bleeding is often halted using bipolar electrocautery. However, such cautery may damage the surface of the brainstem by excitotoxicity or direct electrical tissue damage. In the region of the tumor, the CN lies on the surface of the brainstem beneath a membrane. Thus, the surface of the CN may be in harm's way from the damaging effects of cautery. In the semi-sitting position there is less venous pressure and thus less need for cautery, so this damage may be less.

Let's review the anatomy of the human CN to see what portion might be affected by this potential cautery damage. Figure 27.1 shows schematic representation of the human CN adapted from Moore and Osen, 1979. The yellow shaded area, added by hand by Jean Moore, indicates the small cell cap (SCC). The SCC is a large structure in the human CN, significantly larger than almost all mammals except porpoises. The CN and SCC of the cat are shown for comparison. Little is known about the function of the cells in the SCC, but it is known that most of its innervation is received from the low-spontaneous rate (LSR) primary auditory afferents (Liberman, 1991). We know that the cells in the SCC are excellent at preserving modulation responses in firing rate (Goshal & Kim, 1996, 1997), probably because of the sloping saturation of the LSR fibers. We know that modulation sensitivity is one of the only psychophysical measures that correlates with speech perception (Fu, 2002; Colletti & Shannon, 2005). The low spontaneous rate fibers (LSR) arise from the non-pillar side of the inner hair calls (IHC) and have different synaptic connection to the IHC. Recent work by Kujawa and Liberman (2015) show that the LSR fibers are more susceptible to loud sounds and show significant mortality, even for sound levels that do not damage the IHCs. Such damage to LSR fibers seems to cause a loss of speech understanding even when there is no loss of threshold sensitivity and has been called "hidden hearing loss." IN CIs and ABIs as well, the variability in performance is not accompanied by an elevation in threshold or a degradation in any other psychophysical ability, except modulation detection. So if the LSR fibers play a special role in speech understanding, and primarily project to the SCC, and if the SCC region is damaged by cautery during tumor removal, then I suggest that the loss of this function may be a major factor in the individual differences in ABI speech understanding. Other regions can still carry general auditory information, including tonotopic information, but the LSR/SCC system may be essential for speech pattern perception.

This might seem like a dubious string of suppositions, but let us consider vision as an analogous system. The eye contains two receptor systems—rods and cones. Rods compose about 95% of the receptors and cones only 5%, similar to the relative proportion of HSR and LSR fibers in the ear. Rods and HSR fibers are highly sensitive to low energy levels but saturate at light and sound levels that occur in most daytime situations. The fovea, where most fine pattern recognition (like reading and facial recognition) takes place, contains mostly cones even though they are only 5% of the total receptor population. I suggest that the LSR fibers and SSC function similarly to the fovea of the eye—it is a separate and distinct subsystem that has an important function for pattern recognition. I suggest that both eye and ear have evolved separate subsystems for different sensory functions. HSR fibers in the ear and rods in the eye have extremely low thresholds, showing sensitivity that pushes the limits of physics. While such neurons/receptors have

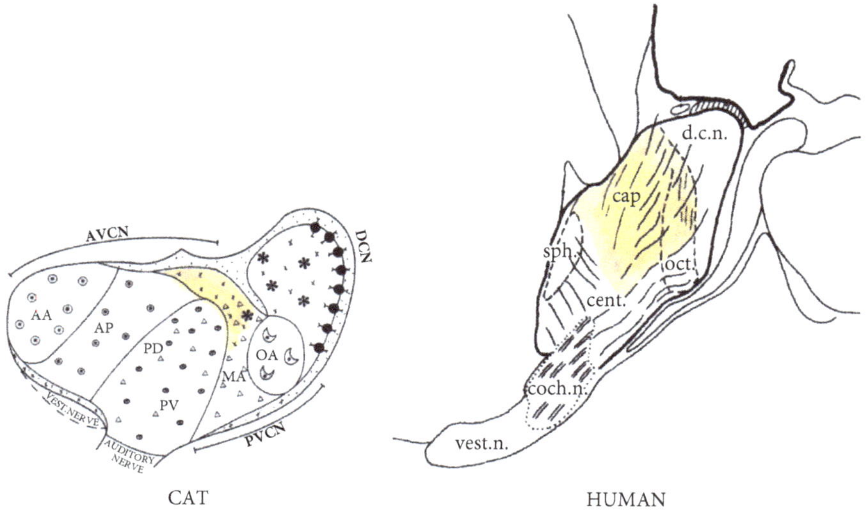

FIGURE 27.1. Comparative diagram of the cochlear nucleus from the cat (from Bahmer, 2007 based on Olsen, 1969) and human (after Moore & Olsen, 1976). Copyright © 1979 Wiley-Liss, Inc.).

The SCC is indicated in yellow as added by Jean Moore. Cap—dorsolateral cap area; AVCN—anteroventral cochlear nucleus; coch.n.—cochlear nerve; DCN—dorsal cochlear nucleus; PVCN—posteroventral cochlear nucleus; cent.—central region of ventral cochlear nucleus; oct.—octopus cell area; sph—spherical cell area; vest.n.—vestibular division of VIII nerve.

a clear evolutionary benefit, they have the disadvantage of saturating at low stimulus levels. The LSR neurons in the ear and cones in the eye have a larger dynamic range and may have preferential projection to higher neural regions that specialize in pattern recognition. In the eye there are distinct populations of primary receptors that feed the distinct subsystems. In the ear the segregation is accomplished by differences in the synaptic ribbons on the IHC membrane.

Summary

It is surprising that working with deaf people has helped us achieve new insights into auditory neuroscience. At first, it appears that the crude pattern of activation achieved by a CI or ABI won't be very helpful for hearing. As a field we were obsessed with the complexity and intricacies of the cochlea and auditory nerve firing patterns. Most people assumed that all of the detail was important—we were all acting like the proverbial shoemaker who sees the world through shoes. When phase-locking was discovered in the auditory nerve the zeitgeist turned to temporal coding, assuming that this temporal code was a critical part of pitch and vowel coding. Like the shoemaker, we all placed too much importance on what we were studying, and we forgot that there is a brain attached to the ear. The brain's pattern recognition is a powerful system that, once trained by millions of repetitions in childhood, can recognize speech patterns in our native language even in the presence of massive distortion and degradation. Vision scientists learned this lesson long ago in the study of face recognition (Harmon & Julesz, 1973). They visually degraded a famous picture of Abraham Lincoln by pixilizing it. To their surprise people could recognize the degraded picture with surprisingly few pixels. Interestingly, the surrealist artist Salvador Dali immediately recognized the perceptual significance of this finding and incorporated his own version of the pixilated Lincoln in many of his later paintings.

A second surprise from the work on auditory prosthesis is that it provides us with a hypothesis about the biological substrate of such pattern recognition. At present there is no hard evidence of the LSR/SCC system as an acoustic fovea, but it is at least broadly consistent with the outcomes of CI and ABI as well as a broad range of other auditory observations. How many times does science teach us that new insights can come from unexpected directions? Auditory research and auditory prostheses are intimately interconnected—as we discover more basic information about the normal auditory system we may be able to apply this new knowledge to the design of better prostheses devices. But I suggest that the arrow points both ways—insights from auditory prosthesis research may inform us about aspects of the normal system we could not have realized if not for the study of the disordered system. It is important to study both the forest and the trees.

References

Bahmer, A. (2007). Computer simulation of chopper neurons: intrinsic oscillations and temporal processing in the auditory system, PhD Dissertation, Technical University Darmstadt.

Behr, R., Colletti, V., Matthies, C., Morita, A., Nakatomi, H., Dominique, L., . . . Skarzynski, H. (2014). New outcomes with auditory brainstem implants in NF2 patients. *Otology & Neurotology* 35(10):1844–1851.

Behr, R., Müller, J., Shehata-Dieler, W., Schlake, H. P., Helms, J., Roosen, K. K., et al. (2007). The high rate CIS auditory brainstem implant for restoration of hearing in NF-2 patients. *Skull Base* 17:91–107.

Berliner, K. I., Tonokawa, L. L., Dye, L. M., & House, W. F. (1989). Open-set speech recognition in children with a single-channel cochlear implant. *Ear and Hearing* 10(4):237–242.

Bilger, R. C., & Hopkinson, N. T. (1977). Hearing performance with the auditory prosthesis. *Annals of Otology, Rhinology & Laryngology, Supplement* 86(3 Pt 3 Suppl 38):76–91.

Brackmann, D. E., Hitselberger, W. E., Nelson, R. A., Moore, J., Waring, M. D., Portillo, F., . . . Telischi, F. F. (1993). Auditory brainstem implant: I. Issues in surgical implantation. *Otolaryngology–Head and Neck Surgery* 108(6):624–633.

Colletti, V., & Shannon, R. V. (2005). Open set speech perception with auditory brainstem implant? *Laryngoscope* 115:1974–1978.

Colletti, L., Shannon, R. V., & Colletti, V. (2014). The development of auditory perception in children after auditory brainstem implantation. *Audiology & Neurotology* 19(6):386–394.

Eddington, D. K. (1983). Speech recognition in deaf subjects with multichannel intracochlear electrodes. *Annals of the New York Academy of Science* 405:241–258.

Fu, Q.-J. (2002). Temporal processing and speech recognition in cochlear implant users. *NeuroReport 13*:1635–1639.

Goshal, S., & Kim, D. O. (1996). Marginal shell of the anteroventral cochlear nucleus: Intensity coding in single units of the unanesthetized, decerebrate cat. *Neuroscience Letters, 205*: 71–74.

Ghoshal, S., & Kim, D.O. (1997). Marginal shell of the anteroventral cochlear nucleus: single-unit response properties in the unanesthetized decerebrate cat. *Journal of Neurophysiology 77*(4): 2083–2097.

Harmon, L. D., Julesz, B. (1973). Masking in visual recognition: effects of two-dimensional filtered noise. *Science 180*(4091):1194–1197.

Hitselberger, W. E., House, W. F., Edgerton, B. J., & Whitaker, S. (1984). Cochlear nucleus implants. *Otolaryngology–Head and Neck Surgery 92*(1):52–54.

House, W. F., Hitselberger, W. E.(2001). Twenty-year report of the first auditory brain stem nucleus implant. *Annals of Otology, Rhinology & Laryngology 110*(2):103–104.

Jiam, N. T., Caldwell, M., Deroche, M. L., Chatterjee, M., Limb, C. J. (2017). Voice emotion perception and production in cochlear implant users. *Hearing Research 352*:30–39.

Kujawa, S. G., Liberman, M. C. (2015). Synaptopathy in the noise-exposed and aging cochlea: Primary neural degeneration in acquired sensorineural hearing loss. *Hearing Research 330*(Pt B):191–199.

Liberman, M. C. (1991). Central projections of auditory nerve fibers of differing spontaneous rate: I. Anteroventral cochlear nucleus. *Journal of Comparative Neurology 313*:240–258.

Loizou, P. C. (1999). Introduction to cochlear implants. *IEEE Engineering in Medicine and Biology Magazine 18*(1): 32–42.

Matthies, C., Brill, S., Kaga, K., Morita, A., Kumakawa, K., Skarzynski, H., . . . Behr, R. (2013). Auditory brainstem implantation improves speech recognition in neurofibromatosis type II patients. *c ORL Journal of Otorhinolaryngology and Its Related Specialties 75*(5):282–295.

Matthies, C., Brill, S., Varallyay, C., Solymosi, L., Gelbrich, G., Roosen, K., . . . Müller, J. (2014). Auditory brainstem implants in neurofibromatosis Type 2: Is open speech perception feasible? *Journal of Neurosurgery 120*(2):546–558.

Moore, J. K., & Osen, K. K. (1979). The cochlear nuclei in man. *American Journal of Anatomy 154*(3):393–418.

Osen, K. K. (1969). Cytoarchitecture of the cochlear nuclei in the cat. *Journal of Comparative Neurology 136*(4):453–483.

Otto, S. R., Brackmann, D. E., Hitselberger, W. E., Shannon, R. V., & Kuchta, J. (2002). Multichannel auditory brainstem implant: Update on performance in 61 patients. *Journal of Neurosurgery 96*(6):1063–1071.

Otto, S. R., Shannon, R. V., Wilkinson, E. P., Hitselberger, W. E., McCreery, D. B., Moore, J. K., & Brackmann, D. E. (2008). Audiologic outcomes with the penetrating electrode auditory brainstem implant. *Otology & Neurotology 8*:1147–1154.

Oxenham A. J. (2012). Pitch perception. *Journal of Neuroscience 32*(39):13335–13338.

Shannon, R. V., Fu, Q-J., & Galvin, J. (2004). The number of spectral channels required for speech recognition depends on the difficulty of the listening situation. *Acta Oto-Laryngologica, Supplementum, 552*: 50–54.

Shannon, R. V., Zeng, F-G., Wygonski, J., Kamath, V., & Ekelid, M. (1995). Speech recognition with primarily temporal cues. *Science 270*:303–304.

Smith, Z. M., Delgutte, B., & Oxenham, A. J. (2002). Chimaeric sounds reveal dichotomies in auditory perception. *Nature 416*(6876):87–90.

Spahr, A. J., & Dorman, M. F. (2004). Performance of subjects fit with the Advanced Bionics CII and Nucleus 3G cochlear implant devices. *Archives of Otolaryngology—Head and Neck Surgery* 130(5):624–628.

Young, E. D. (2008). Neural representation of spectral and temporal information in speech. *Philosophical Transactions of the Royal Society of London Series B, Biological Sciences* 363(1493):923–945.

Young, E. D., & Sachs, M. B.(1979). Representation of steady-state vowels in the temporal aspects of the discharge patterns of populations of auditory-nerve fibers. *Journal of the Acoustical Society of America* 66(5):1381–1403.

Index

A

acetylcholine
  enhancing repetition sensitivity, 725
  in neuromodulation of DCN, 134–135
acetylcholine receptors, and STDP, 230*f*
acoustic and nonacoustic stimuli, neuromodulatory activity and, 586–587
acoustic regularity, encoding in auditory midbrain, 707
  acetylcholine, role of, 725
  anesthesia, effects of, 726–727
  classes of SSA neurons in inferior colliculus, 717–719
  deviance detection, in auditory midbrain, 728, 729*f*, 730*f*
  endocannabinoids, role of, 725–726, 727*f*
  inhibition, role of in deviance detection, 721, 722*f*, 723–724
  neuroanatomical features and SSA emergence, 715–720, 716*f*
  predictive coding, future research on, 730–731
  stimulus-specific adaptation (SSA), general properties, 709–715
  stimulus-specific adaptation (SSA), origin of, 719–720
  stimulus-specific adaptation (SSA), physiology of, 720–727
action potential generation, in MSO, 313
afferent input, brainstem injury and loss of, 689–693
age-related changes
  in auditory brainstem and thalamus, xxx
  cochlear nucleus and, 152–154
  descending auditory pathways and, 631
  in inferior colliculus, 533–536
  to neurotransmitter systems, 533–535
  physiological responses in inferior colliculus, 535–536
aging
  cellular mechanisms of, 641–642
  molecular changes during, 153
  morphological and structural changes during, 152–153
  rodent and non-human primate models of, 644
  ultrastructural synaptic changes during, 153–154
aging, processes in the subcortical system, 639, 664, 664*f*
  age-related hearing loss, significance of, 639–642
  aging mechanisms in the auditory system, 642
  auditory periphery, and age-related hearing loss, 642–644
  and auditory thalamus, 660–664, 662*f*
  cellular mechanisms of aging and related hearing loss, 641–642
  and cochlear nucleus, 644–648, 649*f*
  and inferior colliculus, 651–660
  and superior olivary complex, 648–651
anesthesia, effects of, 726–727
astrocytes
  and development of chick auditory brainstem pathways, 684–685
  synaptic functions in auditory brainstem, 685–687

auditory brainstem, glial cells in, 681–682, 683*f*, 695
  afferent input, brainstem injury and loss of, 689–693
  birds and mammals, sound localization pathways in, 682–683
  and brainstem development, 683–685
  and brainstem injury, 689–694
  chick auditory brainstem pathways, development of, 684–685
  demyelination, brainstem injury and, 693–694
  mammalian auditory brainstem, development of, 685
  oligodendrocytes, and control of conduction time, 687–689
  and synaptic functions of astrocytes, 685–687
auditory brainstem, introduction to, xxii*f*, xxx
  age-related changes in, xxx
  cochlear nucleus complex (CNC), xxiii–xxv
  descending auditory pathways, xxix–xxx
  glial cells in, xxx
  higher auditory functions in, xxix
  inferior colliculus, xxviii–xxix
  innervation of the cochlea, xxii–xxiii
  lateral lemniscus, nuclei of, xxviii
  superior olivary complex, nuclei of, xxv–xxvii
auditory brainstem implant (ABI), 759, 766–767
  cochlear nucleus, diagram of, 766*f*
  device design, 761–762
  history of development, 759–761
  hypothesis of effectiveness, 763–766
  outcomes of design and development, 762–767
auditory brainstem pathways, development of in chicks, 684–685
auditory function, MOC effect on, 75*f*
auditory information, filtering and processing, 707–709
auditory nerve (AN), changes after loss of activity, 166–167
auditory nerve fibers
  connections with bushy cells, 101–106, 104*f*
  D Stellate cells, connections with, 112
  histogram of responses, 98*f*
  octopus cells, connections with, 106–108, 107*f*
  T Stellate cells, connections with, 108–111, 111*f*
auditory pathways, plasticity and, 611–612, 630–632
  and brainstem modulatory systems, 624–628
  cortical descending projections to auditory brainstem nuclei, 617–624, 618*f*, 620*f*
  neuronal loops and chains, 628–629
  subcortical descending projections to auditory brainstem nuclei, 612–617, 614*f*
  VNTB as inhibitory hub in descending auditory system, 629–630, 630*f*
auditory periphery
  and age-related hearing loss, 642–644
  origin of tinnitus-related activity in, 198–199
auditory thalamus, aging and, 660–664, 662*f*, 664*f*
  impact on calcium-binding proteins and neuromodulators, 661–662
  impact on neurotransmitters, 660–661
  impact on physiology, 663–664
aversion, neuromodulatory regulation of, 593
axon trajectories, 473–475, 491–492, 492*f*
  ascending auditory axons, routes followed by, 475–486, 479*f*, 481*f*, 482*f*
  brainstem commissures, 489–491
  from cochlear nuclei to lateral lemniscus, 483–484
  descending auditory axons, routes followed by, 486–489
  descending pathways from auditory cortex, 486–487
  descending pathways from inferior colliculus to superior olivary complex, 487–488
  descending pathways from superior olivary complex to cochlear nucleus and cochlea, 488–489
  dorsal acoustic stria, 476
  intermediate acoustic stria, 476–477
  lateral lemniscus and paralemniscal fibers, 480–483

non-auditory inputs to auditory nuclei, routes followed by, 490–491
from superior olivary complex to lateral lemniscus, 485–486
ventral acoustic stria, 477–480

B

Beebe, Nichole L.
"Descending Auditory Pathways and Plasticity," 611–638
"benign" noise exposure, changes in cochlear nucleus after, 173
Berger, Joel I.
"Changes in the Inferior Colliculus Associated with Hearing Loss: Noise-Induced Hearing Loss, Age-Related Hearing Loss, Tinnitus and Hyperacusis," 527–547
binaural processing, MNTB and, 274–275, 275*f*
birds and mammals, sound localization pathways in, 682–683
brain development, critical periods of, 78–80
brainstem
brainstem injury, 689–694
higher auditory functions in, xxix
reciprocal interactions with cochlea, 17–19
brainstem modulatory systems, and descending auditory pathways, 624–628, 626*f*
Brandebura, Ashley
"Perinatal Development of the Medial Nucleus of the Trapezoid Body," 245–272
brevican
impact on hearing, 436
role in synaptic transmission and organization of subsynaptic space, 434, 435*f*, 436
bursting activity, and tinnitus, 192–193, 194*f*
bushy cells
connections with auditory nerve fibers, 101–106, 104*f*
subtypes of, 101

C

calcium-binding proteins, impacts of aging on
auditory thalamus, 661–662
dorsal cochlear nucleus, 647
inferior colliculus, 656–657
superior olivary complex, 650–651
calyx of Held, 245–246
formation of, 248–250, 249*f*
neuron maturation, 247*f*
postsynaptic excitability during growth, 256–257
regulation of calcium during growth, 257–258
specifying competition and growth, 261–262
spontaneous activity during growth, 253–256
Cant, Nell Beatty
"Axon Trajectories in the Auditory Brainstem," 473–502
Xiao-Jie Cao
"The Cochlear Nuclei: Synaptic Plasticity in Circuits and Synapses in the Ventral Cochlear Nuclei," 95–122
Carbajal, Guillermo V.
"Deviance Detection and Encoding Acoustic Regularity in the Auditory Midbrain," 707–739
Caspary, Donald M.
"Aging Processes in the Subcortical Auditory System," 639–679
cell types, and descending auditory pathways, 630–631
central axons, development of, 11–15
channelopathies, and tinnitus, 206–208
chick auditory brainstem pathways, development of, 684–685
cholinergic nicotinic hair cell receptor, 65–68
cholinergic systems, and descending auditory pathways, 624–627, 626*f*
chondroitin sulfate side chains, impact on neuronal excitability and synaptic plasticity, 433–434, 435*f*
cochlea
afferent and efferent innervation of, xxii–xxiii
cochlear innervation, 38*f*
cochlear trauma, changes following, 529–532
reciprocal interactions with brainstem, 17–19

cochlea, efferent innervation to, 59, 80
  cholinergic nicotinic hair cell receptor, 65–68
  critical periods of development, 78–80
  efferent responses, summation of, 74*f*
  efferent stimulation, hyperpolarization in response to, 73*f*
  medial olivocochlear (MOC) efferent synaptogenesis, 74–77
  molecular actors at MOC-hair cell synapse, 68–71, 69*f*
  olivocochlear innervation, 59–62, 60*f*
  physiology of MOC efferents, 62–63
  short-term synaptic plasticity, 71–74, 73*f*
  synaptic responses at the MOC-hair cell synapse, 63–65, 65*f*
cochlear afferents, form and function of, 37–58
  type I afferents, 38–42
  type I afferents, frequency selectivity, 39*f*
  type II afferents, 42–46, 44*f*
  type II afferents, functional role for, 48–49
  type II afferents, molecular specification of, 46–48, 47*f*
cochlear nuclei, 95–122
  auditory nerve fibers and bushy cells, connections between, 101–106, 104*f*
  auditory nerve fibers and D Stellate cells, connections between, 112
  auditory nerve fibers and octopus cells, connections between, 106–108, 107*f*
  auditory nerve fibers and T Stellate cells, connections between, 108–111, 111*f*
  synaptic plasticity in VCN circuits and synapses, 95–97, 113–114
  T and D Stellate cells, interconnections, 112–113
  and tonotopic organization of VCN, 97–101, 98*f*
cochlear nucleus
  age-related loss of temporal processing in DCN, 649*f*
  aging and, 644–648
  anatomy and function of, 143–145, 145*f*
  changes after "benign" noise exposure, 173
  comparative diagram of cat and human, 766*f*
  effect of synaptic activity on, 145–146
  multimodal integration in circuitry of, 225*f*
  noise-induced hearing loss and synaptic changes in, 171–172, 172*f*
  pathways innervating, 203*f*
cochlear nucleus, as generator of tinnitus-related signals, 189–190
  and agents causing tinnitus in humans, 190–195
  bursting activity, 192–193, 194*f*
  channelopathies, 206–208
  clinical implications, 210–211
  descending pathways, role of, 209
  dorsal *vs.* ventral cochlear nuclei, 209–210
  and higher-order nuclei, 198–200
  hyperactivity, 191–192, 192*f*
  imaging studies, 197
  issues, challenges, and controversies, 208–210
  mechanisms underlying, 200–297
  neural synchrony, 193–195, 195*f*
  synaptopathies, 200–206
  underlying activity changes, 195–197
cochlear nucleus, changes in response to hearing loss, 143, 154–155
  effect of synaptic activity, 145–146
  effects on contralateral side, 151–152
  protective mechanisms, 154
  structural and molecular age-related changes, 152–154
  structural and molecular postsynaptic effects, 149–152
  structural and molecular presynaptic effects, 146–149
cochlear nucleus, multimodal inputs to, 223, 237
  alterations to DCN circuit in tinnitus, 232–234
  CN neurons and tinnitus generation, 235
  and disinhibition-mediated synchrony, 234–235
  feed forward inhibition, role in STDP, 230–232
  function of inputs, 229
  fusiform cells, individual timing rules of, 227*f*
  fusiform cells, mechanisms underlying STDP in, 229–230, 230*f*

fusiform cells, neural signatures of tinnitus in, 233*f*
fusiform cells, STDP of, 226*f*
fusiform cells in animal models of tinnitus, 236
and long-term plasticity in the DCN, 224–229, 225*f*, 226*f*, 227*f*, 228*f*
multimodal innervation of CN, 223–224
multimodal integration of CN circuitry, 225*f*
retrograde signaling, role in STDP, 230–232
transdermal stimulation, 228*f*
and treating tinnitus, 236–237
cochlear nucleus complex (CNC), xxiii–xxv
projections of SGNs in, 12*f*
targeting and synaptogenesis in, 15–17
conduction time, oligodendrocytes and control of, 687–689
congenital deafness, and synaptic changes in cochlear nucleus, 176–178
consonants, and encoding of speech sounds, 749–752
spectrograms of three consonant-vowels syllables, 752*f*
timing, 749–751
cortical and cholinergic inputs to auditory nuclei, 625, 626*f*, 627
cortical descending projections to auditory brainstem nuclei, 617–624, 618*f*
AC projections to CN, 624
AC projections to IC, 620–623
AC projections to NBIC, 619, 620*f*
AC projections to SOC, 623–624
Cramer, Karina S.
"Glial Cells in the Auditory Brainstem, 681–706

D

deafferentation, peripheral, 642–644
demyelination, brainstem injury and, 693–694
descending auditory pathways, xxix–xxx
and neuromodulatory systems, 627–628
tinnitus, role in, 209
descending auditory pathways, plasticity and, 611–612, 630–632
and brainstem modulatory systems, 624–628
cortical descending projections to auditory brainstem nuclei, 617–624, 618*f*, 620*f*
neuronal loops and chains, 628–629
subcortical descending projections to auditory brainstem nuclei, 612–617, 614*f*
VNTB as inhibitory hub in descending auditory system, 629–630, 630*f*
desensitization, and short-term plasticity in DCN, 128
development, innervation of hair cells during, 61*f*
deviance detection, in auditory midbrain, 707, 728, 729*f*, 730*f*
acetylcholine, role of, 725
anesthesia, effects of, 726–727
classes of SSA neurons in inferior colliculus, 717–719
endocannabinoids, role of, 725–726, 727*f*
inhibition, role of, 721, 722*f*, 723–724
neuroanatomical features and SSA emergence, 715–720, 716*f*
predictive coding, future research on, 730–731
stimulus-specific adaptation (SSA), general properties, 709–715
stimulus-specific adaptation (SSA), origin of, 719–720
stimulus-specific adaptation (SSA), physiology of, 720–727
Di Guilmi, Mariano N.
"Efferent Innervation to the Cochlea," 59–93
disinhibition-mediated synchrony, 234–235
dopamine, in neuromodulation of DCN, 133
dorsal cochlear nucleus (DCN)
age-related loss of temporal processing, 649*f*
alterations to circuit in tinnitus, 232–234
function of multimodal inputs to, 229
fusiform cells, individual timing rules, 227*f*
fusiform cells, mechanisms underlying STDP in, 229–230, 230*f*
fusiform cells, STDP of, 226*f*
impact of aging on neurotransmitters, 645–647
impact of aging on physiology of, 647–648
impact of aging on structure of, 645
impacts of aging on calcium-binding proteins, glia, and trophic factors, 647
multimodal inputs and long-term plasticity, 224–229, 225*f*, 226*f*, 227*f*, 228*f*

dorsal cochlear nucleus (DCN), neuromodulation and plasticity in, 123–126, 136–137
  long-term plasticity, 129–130
  microcircuitry of DCN, 125*f*
  neuromodulation, 131–136
  short-term plasticity, 126–129
  spike timing dependent plasticity (STDP), 130–131
D Stellate cells
  auditory nerve fibers, connections with, 112
  interconnections with T Stellate cells, 112–113
  response to tones, 98*f*

E

efferent responses, summation of, 74*f*
efferent stimulation, hyperpolarization in response to, 73*f*
efferent transmitter release, facilitation of, 73*f*
electrophysiological maturation, of SGNs, 19–21
Elgoyhen, Ana Belén
  "Efferent Innervation to the Cochlea," 59–93
embryology, and origins of medial nucleus of trapezoid body, 246–248, 247*f*
endocannabinoids
  in neuromodulation of DCN, 134
  role in modulation, 725–726, 727*f*
Escera, Carles
  "Deviance Detection and Encoding Acoustic Regularity in the Auditory Midbrain," 707–739

F

Felmy, Felix
  "The Nuclei of the Lateral Lemniscus," 445–471
fiber patterns, and neuromodulatory inputs to inferior colliculus, 584–586
frequency-following response, and speech and music encoding, 743–745, 750*f*
frequency selectivity, 39*f*
Friauf, Eckhard
  "Lateral Superior Olive: Organization, Development, and Plasticity," 329–394
Fuchs, Paul Albert
  "The Diversified Form and Function of Cochlear Afferents," 37–58
fusiform cells
  and animal models of tinnitus, 236
  individual timing rules in vivo, 227*f*
  mechanisms underlying STDP in, 229–230
  neural signatures of tinnitus in, 233*f*
  spike-timing-dependent plasticity of, 226*f*

G

glial cells
  in auditory brainstem, xxx
  impact of aging on, 647
  neuron-glial cell interactions in MNTB, 293
  during perinatal development of MNTB, 258–260
glial cells, in auditory brainstem, 681–682, 683*f*, 695
  afferent input, brainstem injury and loss of, 689–693
  birds and mammals, sound localization pathways in, 682–683
  in brainstem development, 683–685
  and brainstem injury, 689–694
  chick auditory brainstem pathways, development of, 684–685
  demyelination, brainstem injury and, 693–694
  mammalian auditory brainstem, development of, 685
  oligodendrocytes, and control of conduction time, 687–689
  and synaptic functions of astrocytes, 685–687
globular bushy cell, responses to tones, 98*f*
glutamate, age-related loss in IC, 656*f*
Godfrey, D. A.
  "The Cochlear Nucleus as a Generator of Tinnitus-Related Signals, 189–221
Gómez-Álvarez, Marcelo
  "The Superior Paraolivary Nucleus," 395–420
Goodrich, Lisa V.
  "Wiring the Cochlea for Sound Perception," 1–35
Grothe, Benedikt
  "The Medial Superior Olivary Nucleus: Meeting the Need for Speed," 301–328

H

hair cells
  cholinergic nicotinic hair cell receptor, 65–68
  inner hair cells and formation of peripheral synapses, 8–11, 9*f*
  innervation by SGNs, 5*f*
  innervation during development, 61*f*
  outer hair cells and physiology of MOC efferents, 62–63
  synaptic responses at MOC-hair cell synapse, 63–65, 65*f*
harmonics, and encoding of speech sounds, 749
hearing loss
  auditory periphery and, 642–644
  changes in cochlear nucleus in response to, 143, 154–155
  effects on contralateral side, 151–152
  of genetic origin, 176–178
  physiological and anatomical changes after loss of AN activity, 166–167
  postsynaptic effects in the cochlear nucleus, 149–152
  presynaptic effects in the cochlear nucleus, 146–149
  protective mechanisms, 154
hearing loss, age-related, 163–164, 173–176, 179–180
  significance of, 639–642
  structural and molecular changes, 152–154
  synaptic changes, 174–176, 176*f*
  system-level functional studies, 174
hearing loss, noise-induced, 163–164, 167–173, 179–180
  "benign" noise exposure, changes in cochlear nucleus after, 173
  sequelae of, 529–532
  and synaptic changes in cochlear nucleus, 171–172, 172*f*
  system-level functional studies, 169–171
  and VCN neuroanatomy, 168–169
Heller, Daniel
  "Perinatal Development of the Medial Nucleus of the Trapezoid Body," 245–272
high-threshold potassium channels, in MNTB, 286–288, 288*f*
Holcomb, Paul
  "Perinatal Development of the Medial Nucleus of the Trapezoid Body," 245–272
Hurley, Laura
  "Neuromodulatory Feedback to the Inferior Colliculus," 577–609
hyperactivity, and tinnitus, 191–192, 192*f*

I

inferior colliculus, 503–504, xxviii–xxix
  classes of SSA neurons in, 717–719
  future research, 518–519
  innervation of, 583–586
  interactions with amygdala and modulatory systems, 595–596, 596*f*
  plasticity of, 516–518
inferior colliculus, aging and, 651–660
  impact on calcium-binding proteins and neuromodulators, 656–657
  impact on metabolism in, 652, 654
  impact on neurotransmitters, 654–655
  impact on physiology, 658–660
  impact on structure, 651–652
  loss of glutamate, 656*f*
  synaptic changes, 653*f*
inferior colliculus, changes associated with hearing loss, 527–528, 538–539
  age-related changes, 533–536
  cochlear trauma, changes following, 529–532
  future research directions, 539
  modulation of pathological activity, 536–538
  noise-induced hearing loss, 529–532,
inferior colliculus, commissure of, 549–550, 569–570
  anatomical organization of, 551–560, 552*f*, 561*f*
  commissural fibers outside the IC, 554–556
  commissural neurons, inputs and outputs of, 558–560
  commissural projections, functional properties of, 560–569
  connectivity of commissural fibers, 551–554, 555*f*
  functional properties of commissural projections, behavioral studies, 567–568

inferior colliculus, commissure of (*cont.*)
functional properties of commissural projections, in vitro studies of, 561–562
functional properties of commissural projections, in vivo studies of, 562–567, 564*f*, 566*f*
function of projections, 568–569, 569*f*
neurochemistry of commissural fibers, 556–557
neuronal morphologies contributing to connection, 557–558
inferior colliculus, intrinsic circuits, 514–516
future research into, 519
morphology of local circuits, 514–515
physiological properties of nearby neurons, 515–516
inferior colliculus, neuromodulatory activity in, 586–589
acoustic and nonacoustic stimuli, 586–587
internal state and experience, influence of, 587–589, 589*f*
measuring, 586
during social interaction, 587
inferior colliculus, neuromodulatory feedback to, 577–579
auditory and nonauditory integration, 596–597
auditory inputs to neuromodulatory neurons, 581–582, 582*f*
diverse inputs and integrative responses, 582–583
neuromodulation, behavioral functions of, 593–594
neuromodulators, functional reconfiguration of auditory circuitry, 589–592
neuromodulatory activity in IC and auditory brainstem, 586–589, 589*f*
neuromodulatory inputs, and diffuse projection, 583–584, 585*f*
neuromodulatory inputs, and fiber patterns, 584–586
neuromodulatory inputs and innervation of IC, 583–586
nonauditory inputs to neuromodulatory neurons, 582
sources of neuromodulatory input, 579–581
inferior colliculus, neuron types, 504–514
future research into, 519
intrinsic properties, 510–512
morphology, 504–507, 506*f*
neurotransmitter type, 507–508
response properties to sound, 512–514
synaptic organization, 508–510, 511*f*
inhibition, role in deviance detection, 721, 722*f*, 723–724
inner hair cells (IHCs)
and formation of peripheral synapses, 8–11, 9*f*
innervation by SGNs, 5*f*
innervation
cholinergic nicotinic hair cell receptor, 65–68
cochlear innervation, 38*f*
of hair cells during development, 61*f*
olivocochlear efferent innervation, anatomy of, 59–62, 60*f*
of VCN by spiral ganglion cells, 98*f*
interaural level differences (ILD)
center of detection in LSO, 329
fetal development of pathway, 353*f*
ILD coding of LSO neurons, 343*f*
and organization of LSO, 331*f*
prehearing and posthearing development of pathway, 358*f*
sensitivity of LSO principal neurons in vitro, 349*f*
interaural time difference (ITD)
coding of in MSO, 315*f*
computation of, 314–319
and medial superior olivary nucleus (MSO), 302–304
nature of internal delays, 316–319
sensitivity of LSO principal neurons in vitro, 349*f*
intermediate-threshold potassium channels, in MNTB, 286
ion channel expression, diversity of, 279–282, 280*f*, 281*f*

J

Jackson, Dakota
"Perinatal Development of the Medial Nucleus of the Trapezoid Body," 245–272

K

Kaczmarek, Leonard K.
  "Extraction of Auditory Information by Modulation of Neuronal Ion Channels," 273–300
Kaltenbach, J. A.
  "The Cochlear Nucleus as a Generator of Tinnitus-Related Signals, 189–221
Kandler, Karl
  "Introduction and Overview," xix
Kasten, Michael R.
  "Age-Related and Noise-Induced Hearing Loss," 163--188
Kolson, Douglas
  "Perinatal Development of the Medial Nucleus of the Trapezoid Body," 245–272
Krächan, Elisa G.
  "Lateral Superior Olive: Organization, Development, and Plasticity," 329–394
Kraus, Nina
  "Brainstem Encoding of Speech and Music Sounds in Humans," 741–757

L

lateral lemniscus, nuclei of, , xxviii, 445–446, 447*f*
  cellular features, 453–456
  cellular features, dorsal nucleus, 454–456
  cellular features, intermedial nucleus, 454
  cellular features, ventral nucleus, 453–454
  functional aspects, 456–463, 462*f*
  functional aspects, dorsal nucleus, 459–463, 462*f*
  functional aspects, intermedial nucleus, 458–459, 462*f*
  functional aspects, ventral nucleus, 456–458, 462*f*
  structure and connectivity, 446–452
  structure and connectivity, dorsal nucleus, 450–452
  structure and connectivity, intermedial nucleus, 450
  structure and connectivity, ventral nucleus, 446–450
lateral olivocochlea (LOC), firing behavior of neurons in vitro, 351*f*
lateral superior olive (LSO)
  afferent projections to, 339–341, 340*f*
  afferents to and efferents from, 340*f*
  anatomical organization of, 332, 333*f*
  biophysical adaptations, after onset of hearing, 365–366
  biophysical adaptations, before onset of hearing, 357–360
  circuit formation, 354–356
  circuit refinement, after onset of hearing, 367–369
  circuit refinement, before onset of hearing, 362–365
  cytology of, 332–338, 337
  development and plasticity after onset of hearing, 365–369
  development and plasticity before onset of hearing, 356–365
  efferent projects from, 340*f*, 341–342
  fetal development, 351–356, 353*f*
  firing behavior of neurons in vitro, 351*f*
  functional properties of neurons in vitro, 347–351
  functional properties of neurons in vivo, 342–347
  ILD and ITD sensitivity of principal neurons in vitro, 349*f*
  ILD coding of neurons, 343*f*
  inputs in vivo, 345*f*
  neurogenesis and differentiation of neurons, 352–354, 353*f*
  neurotransmitter phenotype of input, 360–362
  organization of, 329–351, 331*f*
  perineuronal nets in, 424–425
  postnatal development of synaptic parameters, 361*f*
  prehearing and posthearing development of ILD pathway, 358*f*
  short-term plasticity, before onset of hearing, 362
  size, contour, and audible frequency across species, 334*f*
leak K+ channels, in MNTB, 285
Leibold, Christian
  "The Medial Superior Olivary Nucleus: Meeting the Need for Speed," 301–328

Llano, Daniel A.
"Aging Processes in the Subcortical Auditory System," 639–679
low-threshold potassium channels, in MNTB, 284–285

M

Magnusson, Anna K.
"The Superior Paraolivary Nucleus," 395–420
Malmierca, Manuel S.
"Deviance Detection and Encoding Acoustic Regularity in the Auditory Midbrain," 707–739
mammalian auditory brainstem, glial cells in development of, 685
mammals and birds, sound localization pathways in, 682–683
Manis, Paul B.
"Age-Related and Noise-Induced Hearing Loss," 163–-188
Martel, David T.
"Multimodal Inputs to the Cochlear Nucleus and Their Role in the Generation of Tinnitus," 223–244
Mathers, Peter H.
"Perinatal Development of the Medial Nucleus of the Trapezoid Body," 245–272
medial nucleus of trapezoid body (MNTB)
binaural processing, 274–275, 275*f*
and distribution of perineuronal nets in superior olivary complex, 423–424
lateral interactions among neurons, 289–291, 290*f*
neuron-glial cell interactions in, 293
potassium channels, mechanisms for establishing K+ levels, 291–293, 292*f*
structure and composition of perineuronal nets in, 431–432
types of potassium channels in, 284–289
medial nucleus of trapezoid body (MNTB), perinatal development of, 245–246, 262
calyx of Held, formation of, 248–250, 249*f*
calyx of Held, postsynaptic excitability during growth, 256–257
calyx of Held, regulation of calcium during growth, 257–258
calyx of Held, specifying competition and growth, 261–262
calyx of Held, spontaneous activity during growth, 253–256
cell signaling, 250–253
embryonic origins of MNTB, 246–248, 247*f*
functional maturation of synaptic partners, 253–258
glial cells, 258–260
myelination, 260–261
neuron maturation, 247*f*
physiologic responses during embryonic and early postnatal ages, 254*f*
medial olivocochlear (MOC) efferent innervation, 62–63, 68–71, 69*f*
medial olivocochlear (MOC) efferent synaptogenesis, 74–77, 75*f*
medial olivocochlear (MOC) efferent system, 401–402
medial superior olivary nucleus (MSO), 301, 303*f*
biophysical properties, 308–314
circuit and anatomical adaptations for speed, 304–308, 305*f*
definition and computations, 302–304
interaural time differences, coding of, 315*f*
interaural time differences, computation of, 314–319, 317*f*
maturation of anatomy after hearing onset, 306*f*
spatial code and dynamics of spatial processing, 319–321
medial superior olivary nucleus (MSO), biophysical properties, 308–314
dendrite morphology and synaptic distributions, 308–309
modulatory influences, 313–314
subthreshold channels, 311–313
synaptic and membrane properties, 310*f*
synaptic kinetics and integration, 309–311
medial superior olive, perineuronal nets in, 425
metabolism, and impact of aging on IC, 652, 654
midbrain, stimulus-specific adaptation in, 709–715, 711*f*, 712*f*
dynamics and sensitivity to stimulus history, 713–714

means of measuring, *710*
mechanics and adaptation in narrow channels, 714–715
time course, 714
Milinkeviciute, Giedre
"Glial Cells in the Auditory Brainstem, 681–706
Morawski, Markus
"Perineuronal Nets in the Superior Olivary Complex," 421–444
Müller, Nicolas I. C.
"Lateral Superior Olive: Organization, Development, and Plasticity," 329–394
music sounds, brainstem encoding of, 741–743, 752–753
consonants, and encoding of speech sounds, 749–752
frequency-following response, 743–745, 750*f*
spectrograms of three consonant-vowels syllables, 752*f*
spectrum of speech sounds, 747*f*
voicing timing, 752
vowels, and encoding of speech sounds, 745–749
myelination, during perinatal development of MNTB, 260–261

N

neural phenotypes, influencing modulatory effects, 590
neural synchrony, and tinnitus, 193–195, 195*f*
neuromodulation, behavioral functions in inferior colliculus, 593–594
neuromodulation, in dorsal cochlear nucleus (DCN), 123–126, 125*f*, 131–136
acetylcholine, 134–135
dopamine, 133
endocannabinoids, 134
noradrenaline, 132
serotonin, 133–134
zinc, 135–136
neuromodulators, and functional reconfiguration of auditory circuitry, 589–592
functional outcomes of targeted effects, 591–592
neural phenotypes, influencing modulatory effects, 590
neuromodulator interactions, 592
receptors and modulatory effects, 589–590
subcellular targets, 591
neuromodulators, impact of aging on
auditory thalamus, 661–662
inferior colliculus, 656–657
superior olivary complex, 650–651
neuromodulatory activity, in inferior colliculus and auditory brainstem, 586–589
acoustic and nonacoustic stimuli, 586–587
internal state and experience, influence of, 587–589, 589*f*
measuring, 586
during social interaction, 587
neuromodulatory feedback, to inferior colliculus, 577–579
auditory and nonauditory integration, 596–597
auditory inputs to neuromodulatory neurons, 581–582, 582*f*
diverse inputs and integrative responses, 582–583
neuromodulation, behavioral functions of, 593–594
neuromodulators, functional reconfiguration of auditory circuitry, 589–592
neuromodulatory activity in IC and auditory brainstem, 586–589, 589*f*
neuromodulatory inputs, and diffuse projection, 583–584, 585*f*
neuromodulatory inputs, and fiber patterns, 584–586
neuromodulatory inputs and innervation of IC, 583–586
nonauditory inputs to neuromodulatory neurons, 582
sources of neuromodulatory input, 579–581
neuromodulatory systems
descending pathways and, 627–628, 631
feedback to auditory circuits, 594–596
interactions with inferior colliculus and amygdala, 595–596, 596*f*

neuronal death, and cochlear synaptic activity, 145–146
neuronal excitability, impact of chondroitin sulfate side chains on, 433–434
neuronal ion channels, modulation of, 273–274, 293–294
  binaural processing and the MNTB, 274–275, 275*f*
  high-threshold potassium channels, in MNTB, 286–288, 288*f*
  intermediate-threshold potassium channels, in MNTB, 286
  ion channel expression, diversity of, 279–282, 280*f*, 281*f*
  lateral interactions among MNTB neurons, 289–291, 290*f*
  leak K+ channels, in MNTB, 285
  low-threshold potassium channels, in MNTB, 284–285
  potassium channels, diversity of conductance, 281*f*, 282–284, 283*f*
  potassium channels, effects of alteration, 276–279, 278*f*
  potassium channels, mechanisms for establishing K+ levels, 291–293, 292*f*
  potassium channels, operation of, 275–276, 277*f*
  potassium channels, types in MNTB, 284–289
  transient A-type potassium channels, in MNTB, 289
neuronal loops and chains, and descending auditory pathways, 628–629
neurotransmitters, impact of aging on
  auditory thalamus, 660–661
  dorsal cochlear nucleus, 645–647
  inferior colliculus, 654–655
  superior olivary complex, 650
neurotransmitter systems, age-related changes to, 533–535
Nicol, Trent
  "Brainstem Encoding of Speech and Music Sounds in Humans," 741–757
N- methyl- D- aspartate acid (NMDA) receptors
  and STDP, 230*f*
noradrenaline, in neuromodulation of DCN, 132

O

octopus cells
  auditory nerve fibers, connections with, 106–108, 107*f*
  responses of, 98*f*
Oertel, Donata
  "The Cochlear Nuclei: Synaptic Plasticity in Circuits and Synapses in the Ventral Cochlear Nuclei," 95–122
oligodendrocytes, and control of conduction time, 687–689
olivocochlear efferent innervation
  anatomy of, 59–62
  olivocochlear reflex, 60*f*
  physiology of MOC efferents, 62–63
Orton, Llwyd D.
  "Unifying the Midbrain: The Commissure of the Inferior Colliculus," 549–576
outer hair cells (OHC), and physiology of MOC efferents, 62–63

P

Palmer, Alan R.
  "Changes in the Inferior Colliculus Associated with Hearing Loss: Noise-Induced Hearing Loss, Age-Related Hearing Loss, Tinnitus and Hyperacusis," 527–547
pathological activity, modulation of in inferior colliculus, 536–538
Pecka, Michael
  "The Medial Superior Olivary Nucleus: Meeting the Need for Speed," 301–328
perinatal development, of medial nucleus of trapezoid body (MNTB), 245–246, 262
  calyx of Held, formation of, 248–250, 249*f*
  calyx of Held, postsynaptic excitability during growth, 256–257
  calyx of Held, regulation of calcium during growth, 257–258
  calyx of Held, specifying competition and growth, 261–262
  calyx of Held, spontaneous activity during growth, 253–256
  cell signaling, 250–253
  embryonic origins of MNTB, 246–248, 247*f*

functional maturation of synaptic partners, 253–258
glial cells, 258–260
myelination, 260–261
neuron maturation, 247*f*
physiologic responses during embryonic and early postnatal ages, 254*f*
perineuronal nets, in superior olivary complex, 421–423, 437
brevican, role in synaptic transmission and organization of subsynaptic space, 434, 436
chondroitin sulfate side chains, impact on neuronal excitability and synaptic plasticity, 433–434, 435*f*
development of, 427, 429–431, 430*f*
distribution of, 423–426, 427*f*, 428*t*
function of, 432–433
and lateral superior olive, 424–425
and medial superior olive, 425
and MNTB, 423–424
structure and composition of nets in the MNTB, 431–432
peripheral deafferentation, 642–644
peripheral synapses, formation of, 8–11, 9*f*
physiology, impact of aging on
auditory thalamus, 663–664
dorsal cochlear nucleus, 647–648
inferior colliculus, 535–536, 658–660
superior olivary complex, 651
physiology, of stimulus-specific adaptation, 720–727
acetylcholine, role of, 725
endocannabinoids, role of, 725–726, 727*f*
inhibition, role in deviance detection, 721, 722*f*, 723–724
plasticity
circuits underlying AC-driven, 624–627
and development in LSO after onset of hearing, 365–369
and development in LSO before onset of hearing, 356–365
distinct types of, 96
in dorsal cochlear nucleus, 123–126, 125*f*, 126–129
of inferior colliculus, 516–518
short-term plasticity in LSO, after onset of hearing, 366–367
short-term plasticity in LSO, before onset of hearing, 362
short-term synaptic plasticity, 71–74, 73*f*, 74*f*
plasticity, and descending auditory pathways, 611–612, 630–632
and brainstem modulatory systems, 624–628
cortical descending projections to auditory brainstem nuclei, 617–624, 618*f*, 620*f*
neuronal loops and chains, 628–629
subcortical descending projections to auditory brainstem nuclei, 612–617, 614*f*
VNTB as inhibitory hub in descending auditory system, 629–630
plasticity, spike timing dependent (STDP)
in DCN, 130–131
feed forward inhibition, role of, 230–232
and fusiform cells, 226*f*
and NMDA and acetylcholine receptors, 230*f*
retrograde signaling, role of, 230–232
and transdermal stimulation, 228*f*
and treating tinnitus, 236–237
plasticity, synaptic
impact of chondroitin sulfate side chains on, 433–434
short-term synaptic plasticity, 71–74, 73*f*, 74*f*
in ventral cochlear nuclei, 95–97
potassium channels
diversity of conductance, 281*f*, 282–284, 283*f*
effects of alteration, 276–279, 278*f*
high-threshold channels, in MNTB, 286–288, 288*f*
intermediate-threshold channels, in MNTB, 286
leak K+ channels, in MNTB, 285
low-threshold channels, in MNTB, 284–285
mechanisms for establishing K+ levels, 291–293, 292*f*
operation of, 275–276, 277*f*
transient A-type channels, in MNTB, 289
types in MNTB, 284–289
predictive coding, in auditory midbrain, 730–731

prepulse inhibition, neuromodulatory regulation of, 594
prosodic information, early-level processing by SPON, 407–408

R

rebound spiking, 402–404
receptors, determining modulatory effects, 589–590
Recio-Spinoso, Alberto
  "The Cochlear Nuclei: Synaptic Plasticity in Circuits and Synapses in the Ventral Cochlear Nuclei," 95–122
Rees, Adrian
  "Unifying the Midbrain: The Commissure of the Inferior Colliculus," 549–576
repetition sensitivity, role of acetylcholine in enhancing, 725
Ropp, Tessa-Jonne F.
  "Age-Related and Noise-Induced Hearing Loss," 163––188
Rubio, Maria E.
  "Molecular and Structural Changes in the Cochlear Nucleus in Response to Hearing Loss," 143–162

S

Schofield, Brett R.
  "Descending Auditory Pathways and Plasticity," 611–638
sensory deprivation, resilience of SPON to, 406–407
serotonin, in neuromodulation of DCN, 133–134
Shannon, Robert V.
  "The Auditory Brainstem Implant: Restoration of Speech Understanding from Electric Stimulation of the Human Cochlear Nucleus," 759–769
Shore, Susan E.
  "Multimodal Inputs to the Cochlear Nucleus and Their Role in the Generation of Tinnitus," 223–244
Shrestha, Brikha R.
  "Wiring the Cochlea for Sound Perception," 1–35
Sivaramakrishnan, Shobhana
  "Perinatal Development of the Medial Nucleus of the Trapezoid Body," 245–272
social interaction, neuromodulatory activity during, 587
Sonntag, Mandy
  "Perineuronal Nets in the Superior Olivary Complex," 421–444
sound localization pathways, in birds and mammals, 682–683
spatial code and dynamics of spatial processing, of MSO, 319–321
speech sounds, brainstem encoding of, 741–743, 752–753
  consonants and, 749–752
  frequency-following response, 743–745, 750*f*
  spectrograms of three consonant-vowels syllables, 752*f*
  spectrum of speech sounds, 747*f*
  voicing timing, 752
  vowels and, 745–749
spike timing dependent plasticity (STDP)
  in DCN, 130–131
  feed forward inhibition, role of, 230–232
  and fusiform cells, 226*f*
  and NMDA and acetylcholine receptors, 230*f*
  retrograde signaling, role of, 230–232
  and transdermal stimulation, 228*f*
  and treating tinnitus, 236–237
spiking, rebound, 402–404
spiral ganglion cells
  innervation of VCN by, 98*f*
  and tonotopic organization of the VCN, 97–101, 98*f*
spiral ganglion neurons (SGNs), 1–2, 21
  and central axons, development of, 11–15
  development of, 2–3
  electrophysiological maturation of, 19–21
  and formation of peripheral synapses, 8–11, 9*f*
  innervation of hair cells by, 5*f*
  and interactions between cochlea and brainstem, 17–19
  peripheral processes, outgrowth and targeting of, 4–8
  production of, 3–4

projections in the cochlear nucleus complex, 12*f*
type II cochlear afferents, 47*f*
Spirou, George A.
"Perinatal Development of the Medial Nucleus of the Trapezoid Body," 245–272
spontaneous activity, and tinnitus, 191–192, 236–237
stimulation, hyperpolarization in response to, 73*f*
stimulus-driven activity, and tinnitus, 196
stimulus-specific adaptation (SSA), in inferior colliculus, 717–719
stimulus-specific adaptation (SSA), in midbrain, 709–715, 711*f*, 712*f*
acetylcholine, role of, 725
anesthesia, effects of, 726–727
dynamics and sensitivity to stimulus history, 713–714
endocannabinoids, role of, 725–726
means of measuring, *710*
mechanics and adaptation in narrow channels, 714–715
neuroanatomical features and, 715–720, 716*f*
origin of, 719–720
physiology of, 720–727
time course, 714
subcortical descending projections, to auditory brainstem nuclei, 614*f*
cholinergic descending projections, 616–617
dopaminergic descending projections, 616
GABAergic and glycinergic descending projections, 615–616
glutamatergic descending projections, 613–615
subsynaptic space, role of brevican in organization of, 434, 436
subthreshold channels, of MSO, 311–313
summation, of efferent responses, 74*f*
superior olivary complex, perineuronal nets in, 421–423, 437
brevican, role in synaptic transmission and organization of subsynaptic space, 434, 435*f*, 436
chondroitin sulfate side chains, impact on neuronal excitability and synaptic plasticity, 433–434, 435*f*
development of, 427, 429–431, 430*f*
distribution of, 423–426, 427*f*, 428*t*
function of, 432–433
and lateral superior olive, 424–425
and medial superior olive, 425
structure and composition of nets in the MNTB, 431–432
superior olivary complex (SOC), aging and, 648–651
impact on calcium-binding proteins and neuromodulators, 650–651
impact on neurotransmitters, 650
impact on physiology, 651
impact on structure, 649–650
superior olivary complex (SOC), nuclei of, xxv–xxvii
superior paraolivary nucleus (SPON), 395, 408
connectome, 398*f*
electrophysiological responses of neurons, 403*f*
medial olivocochlear efferent system, role in, 401–402
monaural temporal information, receipt of, 397–399
presence in mammals, 395–397
processing of prosodic information, 407–408
properties compatible with precise spiking, 405–406
rebound spiking, 402–404
resilience to sensory deprivation, 406–407
superior olivary complex, schematic representation of, 396*f*
temporally precise information, relay of, 399–400
synapses, formation of peripheral, 8–11, 9*f*
synaptic activity
age-related changes in IC, 653*f*
effect on cochlear nucleus, 145–146
synaptic adaptation, modulation of, 720–727
synaptic depression, 100*f*
bushy cells and, 103–104, 104*f*
and short-term plasticity in DCN, 126–128
synaptic facilitation, and short-term plasticity in DCN, 128–129
synaptic functions, of astrocytes in auditory brainstem, 685–687

synaptic inputs, responses of model neurons to, 278*f*
synaptic kinetics and integration, of MSO, 309–311
synaptic plasticity
  impact of chondroitin sulfate side chains on, 433–434
  in ventral cochlear nuclei, 95–97
synaptic responses
  at MOC-hair cell synapse, 63–65, 65*f*
synaptic transmission, role of brevican in, 434, 436
synaptogenesis
  MOC efferent, 74–77, 75*f*
  and targeting in CNC, 15–17
synaptopathies, and tinnitus, 200–206
  anatomical changes, 201
  chemical changes, 201–202
synchronous firing, and tinnitus, 195*f*
  disinhibition-mediated synchrony, 234–235
  and treating tinnitus, 236–237

T

temporal processing, age-related loss of, 649*f*
thalamus, age-related changes in, xxx
tinnitus, role of multimodal inputs in, 223, 237
  alterations to DCN circuit in tinnitus, 232–234
  and CN neurons, 235
  and disinhibition-mediated synchrony, 234–235
  and feed forward inhibition, role in STDP, 230–232
  function of inputs to DCN, 229
  fusiform cells, individual timing rules of, 227*f*
  fusiform cells, mechanisms underlying STDP in, 229–230, 230*f*
  fusiform cells, neural signatures of tinnitus in, 233*f*
  fusiform cells in animal models of tinnitus, 236
  and long-term plasticity in the DCN, 224–229, 225*f*, 226*f*, 227*f*, 228*f*
  multimodal innervation of cochlear nucleus, 223–224
  and multimodal integration of CN circuitry, 225*f*
  and retrograde signaling, role in STDP, 230–232
  and STDP of fusiform cells in DCN, 226*f*
  transdermal stimulation, 228*f*
  and treating tinnitus, 236–237
tinnitus-related signals, cochlear nucleus as generator of, 189–190
  and agents causing tinnitus in humans, 190–195
  bursting activity, 192–193, 194*f*
  changes in tonotopic map representation, 190–191
  channelopathies, 206–208
  clinical implications, 210–211
  descending pathways, role of, 209
  dorsal *vs.* ventral cochlear nuclei, 209–210
  and higher-order nuclei, 198–200
  hyperactivity, 191–192, 192*f*
  imaging studies, 197
  issues, challenges, and controversies, 208–210
  mechanisms underlying, 200–297
  neural synchrony, 193–195, 195*f*
  synaptopathies, 200–206
  underlying activity changes, 195–197
tonotopic organization, of VCN, 97–101, 98*f*
tonotopic *vs.* non-tonotopic descending projections, 631
transdermal stimulation, and STDP in DCN, 228*f*
transient A-type potassium channels, in MNTB, 289
transmitter release, facilitation of, 73*f*
trophic factors, impacts of aging on, 647
Trussell, Laurence O.
  "In Vitro Studies of Neuromodulation and Plasticity in the Dorsal Cochlear Nucleus," 123–141
T Stellate cells, 98*f*
  auditory nerve fibers, connections with, 108–111, 111*f*
  interconnections with D Stellate cells, 112–113

V

ventral cochlear nucleus (VCN), 95–122
  cells of, 165–166
  hearing loss, age-related and noise induced, 163–164, 179–180
  innervation by spiral ganglion cells, 98*f*
  neuroanatomy and noise-induced hearing loss, 168–169
  synaptic plasticity in, 95–97
  tonotopic organization of, 97–101, 98*f*
ventral nucleus of trapezoid body (VNTB), 629–630, 630*f*
voicing timing, and encoding of speech sounds, 752
vowels, and encoding of speech sounds, 745–749
  pitch and fundamental frequency, 746–748
  spectrograms of three consonant-vowels syllables, 752*f*
  vowel identity, 749
  vowels with changing pitch, 748–749

W

Wedemeyer, Carolina
  "Efferent Innervation to the Cochlea," 59–93

X

Ruili Xie
  "Age-Related and Noise-Induced Hearing Loss," 163––188

Z

zinc, in neuromodulation of DCN, 135–136

Printed in the USA
CPSIA information can be obtained
at www.ICGtesting.com
CBHW041622240924
14749CB00010B/55

9 780190 849061